KNEE SURGERY

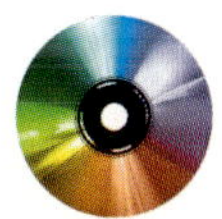

System requirement:

- Operating System—Windows XP or above
- Web Browser—Internet Explorer 8 or above, Google Chrome, Mozilla Firefox
- Essential plugins—Java and Flash Player
  - Facing problems in viewing content—it may be your system does not have Java enabled.
  - If videos do not show up—it may be the system requires Flash Player or need to manage Flash setting. To learn more about Flash setting click on the link in the help section.
  - You can test Java and Flash by using the links from the help section of the **CD/DVD**.

Accompanying DVD-ROM is playable only in Computer and not in DVD player.

CD/DVD has autorun function—it may take few seconds to load on your computer. If it does not work for you, then follow the steps below to access the contents manually:

- Click on my computer
- Select the **CD/DVD** drive and click open/explore—this will show list of files in the **CD/DVD**
- Find and double click file—"launch.html"

For more information about troubleshoot of autorun click on:
http://support.microsoft.com/kb/330135

DVD CONTENTS

KNEE SURGERY

Ashok Rajgopal MS MCh FRCS

Chairman
Medanta Bone and Joint Institute
Medanta—The Medicity
Gurgaon, Haryana, India

Forewords

Kim C Bertin
Chitranjan S Ranawat

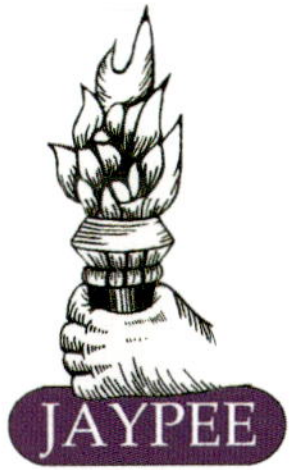

JAYPEE BROTHERS MEDICAL PUBLISHERS (P) LTD

New Delhi • London • Philadelphia • Panama

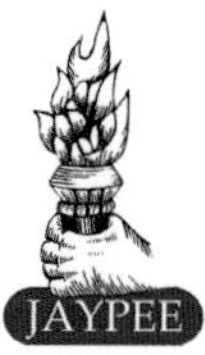

Jaypee Brothers Medical Publishers (P) Ltd

Headquarters
Jaypee Brothers Medical Publishers (P) Ltd.
4838/24, Ansari Road, Daryaganj
New Delhi 110 002, India
Phone: +91-11-43574357
Fax: +91-11-43574314
Email: jaypee@jaypeebrothers.com

Overseas Offices

J.P. Medical Ltd.
83, Victoria Street, London
SW1H 0HW (UK)
Phone: +44-2031708910
Fax: +02-03-0086180
Email: info@jpmedpub.com

Jaypee-Highlights Medical Publishers Inc.
City of Knowledge, Bld. 237, Clayton
Panama City, Panama
Phone: +1 507-301-0496
Fax: +1 507-301-0499
Email: cservice@jphmedical.com

Jaypee Medical Inc.
The Bourse
111, South Independence Mall East
Suite 835, Philadelphia, PA 19106, USA
Phone: +1 267-519-9789
Email: jpmed.us@gmail.com

Jaypee Brothers Medical Publishers (P) Ltd.
17/1-B, Babar Road, Block-B, Shaymali
Mohammadpur, Dhaka-1207
Bangladesh
Mobile: +08801912003485
Email: jaypeedhaka@gmail.com

Jaypee Brothers Medical Publishers (P) Ltd.
Bhotahity, Kathmandu, Nepal
Phone: +977-9741283608
Email: kathmandu@jaypeebrothers.com

Website: www.jaypeebrothers.com
Website: www.jaypeedigital.com

Inquiries for bulk sales may be solicited at: jaypee@jaypeebrothers.com

Knee Surgery

First Edition: 2014

ISBN : 978-93-5152-225-6

Printed at: Ajanta Offset & Packagings Ltd., New Delhi

Dedicated to

The Joy of Walking

CONTRIBUTORS

Aaron G Rosenberg
Professor of Surgery
Rush Medical College
1611 W Harrison
Chicago, Illinois, USA

Ajit J Deshmukh
Orthopedic Surgery Fellow
Insall Scott Kelly Institute
North Shore LIJ/Lenox Hill Hospital
New York, NY, USA

Alberto Combi
Clinica Ortopedica e Traumatologica
Università Degli Studi di Pavia
Fondazione IRCCS Policlinico
San Matteo Pavia
Pavia, Italy

Alfred J Tria Jr
Clinical Professor of Orthopedic Surgery
Director of Fellowship Training
Department of Orthopedic Surgery
Robert Wood Johnson Medical School
New Brunswick, New Jersey
Chief, Department of Orthopedic Surgery
St Peter's University Hospital
New Brunswick, New Jersey, USA

Alok Mohan
Domiciliary Physiotherapist
Medanta Bone and Joint Institute
Medanta—The Medicity
Gurgaon, Haryana, India

Amit Jawa
Consultant Radiologist
Dr Gulati Imaging Institute
New Delhi, India

Andrea Baldini
IFCA Clinic
Florence, Italy

Andrew A Freiberg
Arthroplasty Service Chief and
Vice Chairperson
Department of Orthopedic Surgery
Massachusetts General Hospital
Associate Professor
Harvard Medical School
Massachusetts, USA

Anoop Jhurani
Consultant Orthopedic Surgeon
Joint Replacement Service
Fortis Escorts Hospital
Jaipur, Rajasthan, India

Arun Mullaji
Director
The Arthritis Clinic, Cornelian
Kemp's Corner, Mumbai
Joint Replacement Surgeon
Breach Candy Hospital
Cumballa Hill Hospital and
Hinduja Healthcare
Mumbai, Maharashtra, India

Ashok Rajgopal
Chairman
Medanta Bone and Joint Institute
Medanta—The Medicity
Gurgaon, Haryana, India

Attique Vasdev
Associate Director, Knee Division
Medanta Bone and Joint Institute
Medanta—The Medicity
Gurgaon, Haryana, India

A Zahar
HELIOS ENDO-Klinik 22767
Hamburg, Germany

Azam Badar Khan
Specialist Orthopedic Surgery
PMC Dubai Health Authority (DHA)
Dubai, UAE

Bijaya Kumar Shadangi
Consultant Anesthesiologist
Medanta Institute of Critical Care
and Anesthesiology
Medanta—The Medicity
Gurgaon, Haryana, India

Brian Culp
Orthopedic Surgery Resident, PGY III
Department of Orthopedic Surgery
Robert Wood Johnson Medical School
New Brunswick
New Jersey, USA

Carlos A Higuera
Staff, Adult Reconstruction
Cleveland Clinic
Cleveland, Ohio, USA

Caterina Guarducci
IFCA Clinic
Florence, Italy

Charles H Brown
Abu Dhabi Knee and
Sports Medicine Center
Abu Dhabi, UAE

CJ Thakkar
Honorary Professor of Orthopedics
Maharashtra University of Health Science
Honorary Professor
Department of Orthopedics
Sion Hospital, Mumbai
Consultant Joint Specialist
Breach Candy and Lilavati Hospital
Mumbai, Maharashtra, India

David V Rajan
Orthopedic Speciality Center
Coimbatore
Tamil Nadu, India

Dinshaw Pardiwala
Director
Arthroscopy and Joint Preservation Service
Head
Center for Sports Medicine
Kokilaben Dhirubhai Ambani Hospital
Mumbai, Maharashtra, India

D Kendoff
HELIAS ENDO Klinik 22767
Hamburg, Germany

Douglas A Dennis
Adjunct Professor
Department of Biomedical Engineering
University of Tennessee
Adjunct Professor of Bioengineering
University of Denver
Assistant Clinical Professor
Department of Orthopedics
University of Colorado School of Medicine
Colorado, USA

Francesco Benazzo
Clinica Ortopedica e Traumatologica
Università Degli Studi di Pavia
Fondazione IRCCS Policlinico
San Matteo Pavia
Pavia, Italy

Francesco Traverso
Istituto Clinico Humanitas
Milan, Italy

Giles R Scuderi
210 East 64th Street 4th Floor
New York, USA

Hemant Wakankar
Specialist Joint Replacement Surgeon
Deenanath Mangeshkar Hospital
Pune, Maharashtra, India

Himanshu Gupta
Consultant, Knee Division
Medanta Bone and Joint Institute
Medanta—The Medicity
Gurgaon, Haryana, India

Jack W Shilling
Aria Health
Langhorne, Pennsylvania, USA

Jatinder Pal Singh
Senior Consultant
Department of Radiology
Medanta Bone and Joint Institute
Medanta—The Medicity
Gurgaon, Haryana, India

Javad Parvizi
Professor
Department of Orthopedic Surgery
Rothman Institute at Thomas
Jefferson University
Sheridan Building, 10th Floor
125 South 9th Street
Philadelphia, Pennsylvania, USA

J Clement Joseph
Senior Consultant
Head
Department of Arthroscopy and
Sports Medicine
Global Hospitals and Health City
Chennai, Tamil Nadu, India

Jean-Noel Argenson
Professor and Chairman
Department of Orthopedic Surgery
The Institute for Locomotion
Center for Arthritis Surgery
Aix-Marseille University
Sainte-Marguerite Hospital
Marseille, France

Jess H Lonner
Attending Orthopedic Surgeon
Rothman Institute
Associate Professor of Orthopedic Surgery
Thomas Jefferson University
Philadelphia, Pennsylvania, USA

Joel Kolmodin
Orthopedic Surgery Resident
Cleveland Clinic
Cleveland, Ohio, USA

Joseph W Greene
Norton Orthopedic Specialists-
Brownsboro
Norton Medical Plaza II
(Orthopedic and Hand Center)
9880 Angies Way, Suite 250
Louisville, Kentucky, USA

Justin Duke
Colorado Joint Replacement
Colorado, USA

Kalpana Aggarwal
Chief
Department of Physiotherapy
Medanta Bone and Joint Institute
Medanta—The Medicity
Gurgaon, Haryana, India

Karthikeyan Chinnakkannu
Research Fellow
Rothman Institute at Thomas
Jefferson University
Philadelphia, USA
Assistant Professor in Orthopedics
Melmaruvathur Adhiparasakthi
Institute of Medical
Sciences and Research
Melmaruvathur, Tamil Nadu, India

Kelly G Vince
Consultant Surgeon
Department of Orthopedic Surgery
Whangarei Medical Center
Northland District Health Board
Whangarei, New Zealand

K Santosh Sahanand
Orthopedic Speciality Center
Coimbatore, Tamil Nadu, India

Matteo Ghiara
Clinica Ortopedica e Traumatologica
Università Degli Studi di Pavia
Fondazione IRCCS Policlinico
San Matteo Pavia
Pavia, Italy

Matthew J Dietz
Assistant Professor
Department of Orthopedic Surgery
West Virginia University
West Virginia, USA

Matthieu Ollivier
Department of Orthopedic Surgery
The Institute for Locomotion
Center for Arthritis Surgery
Aix-Marseille University
Sainte-Marguerite Hospital
Marseille, France

Michael A Kelly
Chairman
Department of Orthopedic Surgery
Hackensack University Medical Center
New Jersey
Fellowship Director
Insall Scott Kelly Institute for
Orthopedic Surgery and Sports Medicine
New York, USA

Michel Malo
Assistant Professor
Department of Surgery
University of Montreal
Chief of Orthopedics
Sacré-Coeur Hospital
Montreal, Quebec, Canada

Mohamed Elfekky
Senior Specialist Orthopedic Surgery
Dubai Health Authority
Dubai, UAE

Mojieb Manzary
Consultant Orthopedic and
Reconstructive Surgeon
Dhahran Health Center
Dhahran, Saudi Arabia

Nicholas A Antao
Consultant Orthopedic
Arthroscopic, Sports Medicine,
Joint Reconstruction and
Replacement Surgeon
Head
Department of Orthopedics
Holy Family Hospital and
Holy Spirit Hospital
Mumbai, Maharashtra, India

Nirav N Antao
Molecular and Cellular Biology
University of Illinois Urbana-Champaign
Medical Student
Midwestern University
Illinois, USA

Nishith Shah
Fellow, Arthroscopy Association
of North America (AANA)
President, Indian Arthroscopy Society
Head
Arthroscopy, General Hospital, Ahmedabad
Aash Arthroscopy Center
Ahmedabad, Gujarat, India

Parveen Gulati
Director and Chief Radiologist
Dr Gulati Imaging Institute
New Delhi, India

Pierpaolo Summa
IFCA Clinic
Florence, Italy

Pranjal Kodkani
Fellowships in Arthroscopy
Shoulder and Knee Surgery
USA, Norway, Japan, Germany
Consultant Arthroscopy
Sports Injuries and Joint
Preservation Surgery
Bombay Hospital
Sports Medicine, Shushruta Hospital
Mumbai, Maharashtra, India

P Sripathi Rao
Medcare Orthopedics Spine Hospital
Dubai, UAE

Raju Easwaran
Senior Consultant
Shree Meenakshi Orthopedics and
Sports Medicine Clinic, New Delhi
Department of Orthopedics
Max Super Specialty Hospital
Saket and Shalimar Bagh
New Delhi, India

Robert E Booth
Aria Health
Langhorne, Pennsylvania, USA

Rohan K Vakta
Consultant Orthopedic Surgeon
Ahmedabad, Gujarat, India

Sachin Tapaswi
Director
Department of Orthopedics
Sports Injuries and Joint Replacement
The Orthopedic Specialty Clinic and
Oyster Pearl Hospital
Pune, Maharashtra, India

Samih Tarabichi
Director of Tarabichi Institute for
Joint Surgeries
Burjeel Hospital
Dubai, UAE

Sandeep Vijayan
Associate Professor
Department of Orthopedics
Kasturba Medical College and Hospital
Manipal, Karnataka, India

Saumitra Goyal
Senior Resident
Kasturba Medical College and Hospital
Manipal, Karnataka, India

Sebastien Parratte
Department of Orthopedic Surgery
The Institute for Locomotion
Center for Arthritis Surgery
Aix-Marseille University
Sainte-Marguerite Hospital
Marseille, France

Sharath K Rao
Professor and Head
Department of Orthopedics
Kasturba Medical College and Hospital
Manipal, Karnataka, India

Shivani Jain
Senior Physiotherapist
Medanta Bone and Joint Institute
Medanta—The Medicity,
Gurgaon, Haryana, India

Sinukumar Bhaskaran
Consultant
Orthopedics and Joint
Replacement Surgery
Columbia Asia Hospital
Pune, Maharashtra, India

Stefano Marco Paolo Rossi
Clinica Ortopedica e Traumatologica
Università Degli Studi di Pavia
Fondazione IRCCS Policlinico
San Matteo Pavia
Pavia, Italy

Sujit Kadrekar
Clinical Associate
Arthroscopy and Joint
Preservation Service
Kokilaben Dhirubhai Ambani Hospital
Mumbai, Maharashtra, India

Suryanarayan P
Senior Consultant
Department of Orthopedic Surgery
Apollo Hospitals
Chennai, Tamil Nadu, India

Vipin Tyagi
Consultant, Knee Division
Medanta Bone and Joint Institute
Medanta—The Medicity
Gurgaon, Haryana, India

Vivek Dahiya
Consultant, Knee Division
Medanta Bone and Joint Institute
Medanta—The Medicity
Gurgaon, Haryana, India

Vivek Pandey
Associate Professor
Sports Injury Division
Department of Orthopedics
Kasturba Medical College and Hospital
Manipal, Karnataka, India

Waseem Siddiqui
Clinical Associate
Arthroscopy and Joint
Preservation Service
Kokilaben Dhirubhai Ambani Hospital
Mumbai, Maharashtra, India

William Baione
Orthopedic Surgery Resident, PGY III
Department of Orthopedic Surgery
Robert Wood Johnson Medical School
New Brunswick, New Jersey, USA

W Klauser
HELIAS ENDO Klinik 22767
Hamburg, Germany

Xavier Flecher
Professor
Department of Orthopedic Surgery
The Institute for Locomotion
Center for Arthritis Surgery
Aix-Marseille University
Sainte-Marguerite Hospital
Marseille, France

Yair D Kissin
Attending Orthopedic Surgeon
Department of Orthopedic Surgery
Hackensack University Medical Center
New Jersey
Assistant Clinical Professor
University of Medicine and Dentistry of
New Jersey-Newark
New Jersey, USA

Yatin Mehta
Chairman
Medanta Institute of Critical Care and
Anesthesiology
Medanta—The Medicity
Gurgaon, Haryana, India

FOREWORD

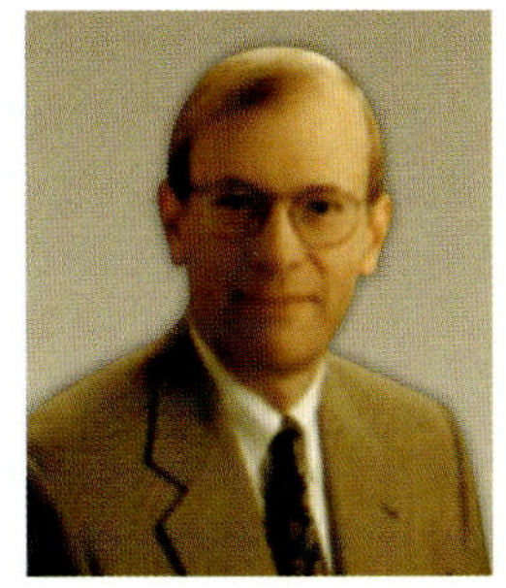

Treatment of disorders of the knee has become the most commonly performed group procedures for the practicing orthopedic surgeons. Presently, there are almost over one million knee replacements and more than two million knee arthroscopic procedures performed in the world every year. This book is a timeless resource for the practicing orthopedic surgeons to understand and master these two procedures.

This book of *Knee Surgery* comprehensively handles the state-of-the-art knee replacement. The readers will be exposed to every essential aspect of knee replacement surgery. Single compartment replacement, through total knee replacement, is thoughtfully addressed. In a unique way, the readers will understand the advantages and disadvantages of different techniques and current options in knee arthroplasty.

This book also addresses most common arthroscopic interventions. The chapters begin with anatomy and examination and proceed through more difficult and complex topics of posterior cruciate ligament (PCL) and posterolateral corner reconstruction. Each chapter is well-written and the illustrations help clearly convey the authors' intended message.

The assembled contributors are established experts in their respective fields and have written authoritative chapters sharing their expertise. The chapters are well-designed to build on each other and construct a solid foundation of knowledge for treating a wide variety of knee problems. The experienced surgeon and the novice alike will appreciate the book as each seeks to better his skill. The clinical utility of the book is made evident by the inclusive discussion on anesthesia, postoperative pain management and rehabilitation of the knee.

As a student of knee surgery for over three decades, I would compliment the contributors and strongly recommend the book to the residents and surgeons for increasing their understandings of knee pathology and treatment.

Kim C Bertin MD
Orthopedic Surgeon
Utah Bone and Joint Center
5323, Woodrow Street
Suite-202
Salt Lake City
Utah, USA

FOREWORD

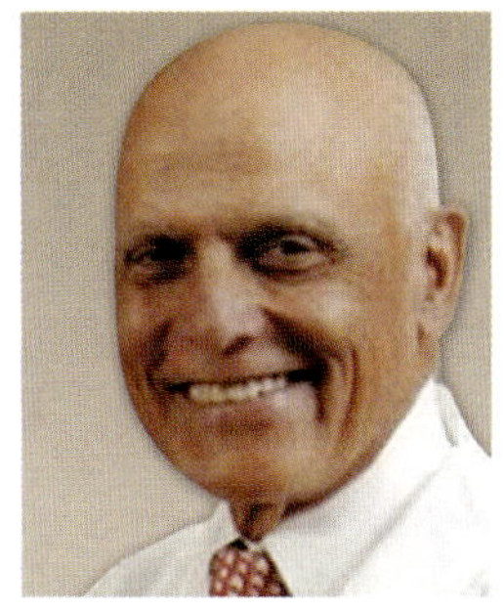

Ashok Rajgopal has invited various authors who are experts in the field of knee surgery. Many of these authors have extensive publication expertise in their respective specialties.

Knee Surgery covers topics on total knee surgery and sports medicine which are of current interest, some of which deal with controversial issues. These include management of major and minor cartilage defects, meniscal transplant, tibial osteotomy and isolated patellar femoral replacement.

Looking towards the future, the book offers many insightful points of view on custom-jig, robotic surgery, pain control, patient satisfaction, early diagnosis of infection and noncemented fixation.

It is with great pleasure and honor that I write the foreword for this multi-authored book on surgery of the knee, which I strongly recommend for postgraduates, practicing orthopedic surgeons and individuals interested in research.

CS Ranawat

Chitranjan S Ranawat MD
Orthopedic Surgeon
535, East 70th Street
6th Floor
Hospital for Special Surgery
New York, USA

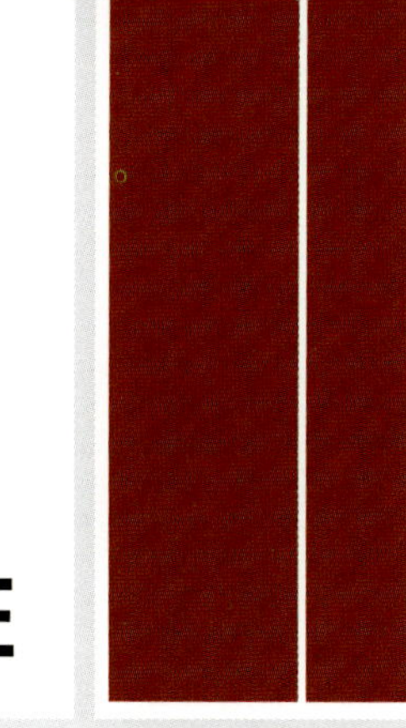

PREFACE

The field of orthopedics, especially that of the knee, has evolved over the years. Our understanding of the kinematics and biomechanics of the knee has evolved by leaps and bounds in recent years. Better understanding of the knee biomechanics is leading to design changes at a very fast pace. While certain concepts, which were thought to be flawed earlier, are the gold standards today, others are open to debate. To retain or sacrifice the posterior cruciate ligament, fixed or mobile-bearing surfaces, cemented or uncemented are all issues which have still not seen a conclusive end. Computer navigation, patient-specific instrumentation and robotics are all emerging concepts. Wear pattern analysis and newer technology have led to the introduction of highly crosslinked polyethylene and ceramics that were previously unknown.

Anatomic reconstruction of the anterior cruciate ligament (ACL) has, today, replaced the transtibial ACL reconstruction. Open ligament reconstructions are a thing of the past era.

Encouraged by my peers and friends, I undertook to put together in *Knee Surgery*. As I embarked on this endeavor, the enormity of this gratifying and enriching challenge dawned upon me.

The book focuses on total knee replacement and arthroscopy of the knee. It represents present-day concepts, on various aspects of knee surgery, sports medicine and biomechanics. It also represents current issues such as recent advances and evolving technology. The book is intended to be a reference guide for orthopedic surgeons with abundant pictorial contents and an atlas on MRI images and arthroscopic appearances of normal and pathological situations.

Contributors, renowned in the similar field, have unhesitatingly made the time and effort to write the chapters. Each of them is an expert in his respective field, with extensive personal contributions in peer-reviewed journals, enhancing the art and science of knee surgery. Each chapter in the book goes beyond the present available literature, incorporating new thoughts and ideas based on the knowledge and experience of years by the contributors to provide a clear thought process to the reader. I would like to express my gratitude for their contribution.

I would also like to acknowledge the tremendous help from my own group and friends for their constant encouragement during the innumerable hours spent in putting the book together. A special word of thanks to Drs Attique Vasdev, Vivek Dahiya and Puneet Puri for burning the midnight oil with me. I would also like to acknowledge my patients without whom my journey of knee surgery, over the years, would not have been possible. Finally, a grateful appreciation to my family, who put up with my long hours devoted to the compilation of the book.

Ashok Rajgopal

ACKNOWLEDGMENTS

An acknowledgment to the people who impacted my career:

- **John Charley**
- **John Insall**
- **Grahm Hayes**
- **Arjun Dev Sehgal**
- **Madan G Abbot**

CONTENTS

SECTION 1: KNEE ARTHROPLASTY

SECTION 2: ARTHROSCOPY AND SPORTS INJURIES OF THE KNEE

SECTION 1

Knee Arthroplasty

Chapter 1

History of Total Knee Arthroplasty

Michael A Kelly, Yair D Kissin

INTRODUCTION

It is remarkable to discuss the history of total knee arthroplasty (TKA) when one considers the current devices and modern techniques that are readily available and how in a short period of time, these incredible advancements balance on the foundation of the first-generation TKAs. The concepts from 30 to 40 years ago still resonate in today's modern designs. Ironically, even vestiges from the initial disastrous failures, such as early partial knee replacement, hinged prostheses, and uncemented implants, still remain in our armamentarium as knee surgeons.

Generally speaking, both the advancements and the failures that have taken place have allowed TKA to become a modern day routine procedure that is performed in well over half a million cases in the United States annually with a highly successful track record.

The purpose of this chapter is to discuss the origins of the development of what we identify today as contemporary TKA and how the ideas from years ago, before much of our modern technology was available, have advanced us to where we operate today.

TOTAL KNEE ARTHROPLASTY DEVELOPMENT

Advancement of TKA has taken several directions, and it does not involve only the implants themselves. Prosthesis design is only one aspect of development that has taken major leaps forward since early generation implants. Concepts such as fit, bearing surface design, patellar tracking, polyethylene characteristics, and fixation options are among the design features that have been improved in modern designs. Additionally, much attention has also been paid to improving the procedure itself and the outcomes that patients achieve. While this chapter focuses on the progress of the implants, it is important to remember that much effort has been devoted to improve the way we perform TKA, not just the device itself.

Preoperative medical optimization, improved surgical techniques, operating room efficiency, perioperative pain management and standardizing postoperative protocols have also evolved and play an important role in the success of modern day TKA.

EVOLUTION

The advancements available to us today originate from a true evolution that began over 150 years ago in attempts made to reconstruct the knee to treat degenerative joint disease. Artificial implants began as hemi-resurfacings on one or both sides of the joint, followed by linked and unlinked implants and other designs that did not survive in the short term in most cases. Initial early failures led to the first well-functioning TKAs in the early mid-1970s, which ultimately became the basis of today's designs.

However, some of the failures, which were actually quite impressive concepts considering the lack of knowledge and technology at that time, have now found a place in the algorithm of treating degenerative knees. Hemi-resurfacings evolved into unicondylar knee replacement that is applied today in selective cases. Early attempts on knee replacement involved hinged implants that will be discussed later in this chapter, and while they were not successful initially, they serve as salvage procedures today for some of the most complex primary and revision cases. Additionally, until the advent of polymethylmethacralate, uncemented implants were attempted, and while initially disappointing, they have recently seen resurgence as an option for the fixation of modern implants. It is, therefore, important to respect the historical attempts on knee reconstruction, whether successful or failed, as both have contributed to what we use today.

The first documented attempt at joint reconstruction to improve motion is thought to have been attempted by Verneuil in 1860, who interposed various soft tissues into the joint and Ferguson in 1861 who resected bone to gain motion while sacrificing stability. Both techniques were mainly used as salvage procedures for the most severely diseased joints, such as those suffering from sepsis, and were not very encouraging. Similar resection arthroplasty, along with arthrodesis, is, albeit rarely, used today as salvage procedures in the worst of cases.

Nearly 100 years later, after attempts were made to implant ivory, fascia lata, bursa, among others, metal was introduced as a viable implant in the knee. Perhaps the two most noted originators of effectual metal implants were MacIntosh from Canada and McKeever from the United States, around 1958. The two independently developed metallic interposition arthroplasties that covered the tibia to correct varus or valgus deformities by the insertion of the implant on the diseased side. These implants had no fixation and were prone to migration and subsidence and did not enjoy any long-term success.

On the heels of successful implantations of early cemented metal on plastic hip replacements, Gunston, a student of Sir John Charnley, developed the first cemented implant in 1971, called a polycentric prosthesis. This was a four-part system, consisting of two hemiarthroplasties, where thin femoral runners articulated on tibial polyethylene surfaces. The prosthesis enjoyed some limited success, but aligning the individual parts proved difficult, and these tended to fail by subsidence into the tibia. Essentially, these were isolated resurfacings and did not adequately address soft tissue causes of deformity.

Two years later, the Freeman-Swanson design (**Figure 1.1**) used a single metal femur and single polyethylene tibia to replace the medial and lateral joint

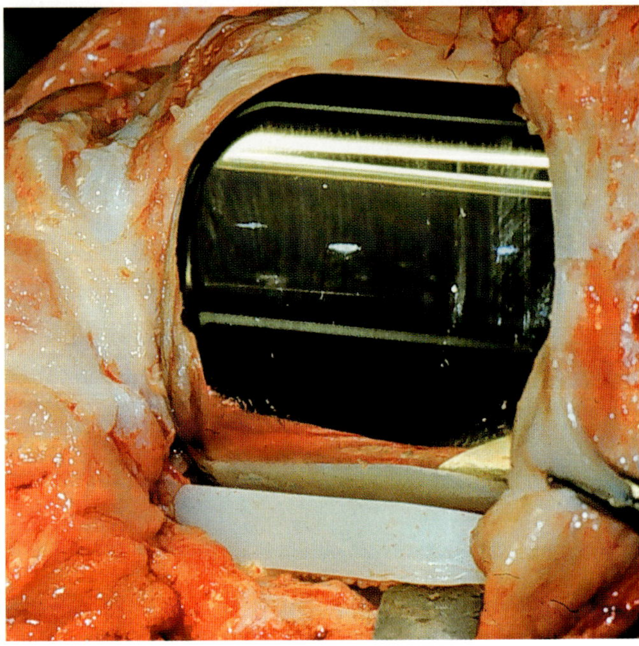

Figure 1.1 Freeman-Swanson

in a roller-on-trough design. Perhaps more important than the implant itself, Freeman's group outlined principles of performing a TKA that still holds true almost half a century later in the techniques we employ today. Their recommendations included enlarging the contact area between the femoral and tibial components, minimal bone resection, implantation onto a flat surface of cancellous bone, minimizing friction at the articulating surface, minimizing wear debris, allowing a physiologic range of motion without too much freedom and minimizing forces at the bone-implant interface by not over constraining the joint. The group also addressed two of today's biggest concerns, infection and bleeding, by urging the limitation of dead space and operative time and by obtaining adequate bone coverage and avoiding the intramedullary canals. They also stressed the importance of obtaining proper alignment through the use of standard instrumentation as well as balancing the knee with spacer blocks. Two unsolved aspects of the surgery at that time, the fate of the cruciate ligaments and the patella, remain hotly debated topics today.

Two other tibiofemoral replacements of note were developed shortly thereafter. The first was called geometric knee (**Figures 1.2A and B**), which was designed at the Mayo Clinic by Coventry and colleagues. This was a single femoral and single tibial implant. The second was called the Duocondylar (**Figure 1.3**) that had a single femur, two separate tibial polyethylene surfaces, and retained the anterior cruciate ligament (ACL) and posterior cruciate ligament (PCL). Up to this point, tibial subsidence was a frequent cause of failure and the patellofemoral was largely left unaddressed. It was becoming clear that the tibial component needed better fixation and that patellofemoral pain was a cause of patient complaints following these surgeries. Furthermore, the developers began to realize

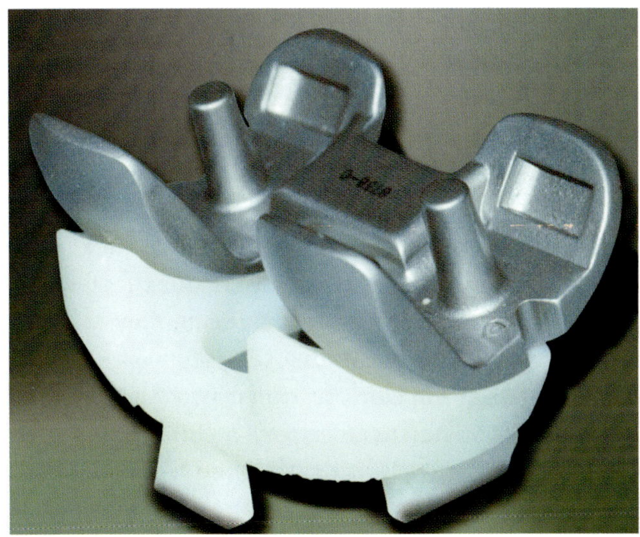

Figure 1.3 Duocondylar

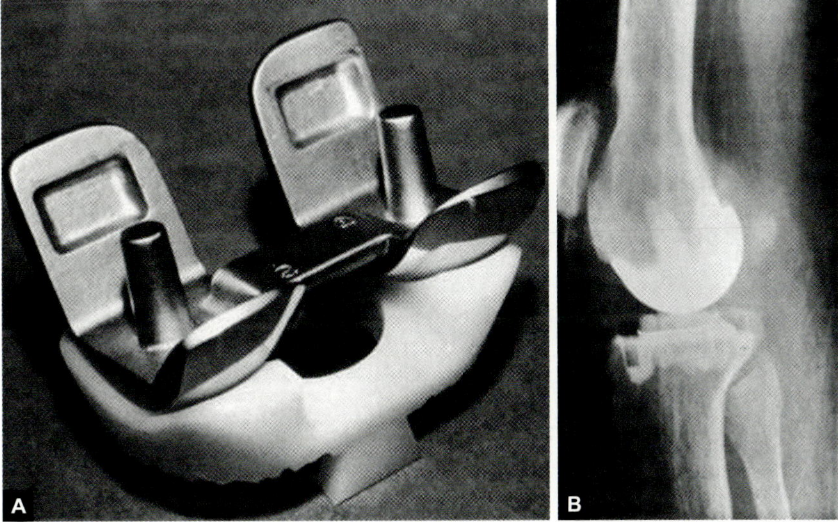

Figures 1.2A and B Geometric prosthesis

that the retention of both cruciate ligaments interfered with deformity correction.

The next critical and truly revolutionary stage in TKA advancement began at the Hospital for Special Surgery as Drs Ranawat and Insall further refined the principles introduced by Freeman's group. Consideration of the PCL, the need for deformity correction, obtaining better motion without sacrificing stability, and improving implant fixation were all emphasized as vital to success. Furthermore, options were developed for difficult cases with greater deformity and severe bone loss that had no viable options prior to this point.

A dichotomy developed in 1974, where one line of thought designed the Duopatellar implant, which sacrificed the ACL, preserved the PCL and included an anterior femoral flange and a patellar button, which became a basis for many current cruciate retaining (CR) designs. Simultaneously, a second group developed the total condylar prosthesis (TCP) (**Figure 1.4**), which sacrificed the ACL and PCL and also had an anterior flange and a patellar button. The latter employed a calculated degree of conformity between the femur and tibia to allow a balance between stability and laxity. Both implants finally addressed the as yet ignored patellofemoral joint and used a central keel on the tibial implant to remedy two major aforementioned problems recognized in prior implants.

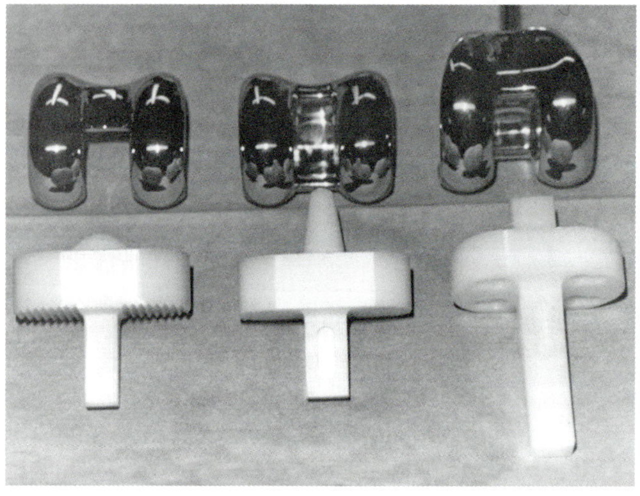

Figure 1.4 TCP, TCP-II, TCO-III

Both of these early designs were initially available only with all-polyethylene tibial components that have proved quite durable. Although largely replaced with the advent of metal backed tibial components, there has been a resurgence of these successful all-poly tibial components mainly as a partial solution to today's economic issues of joint replacement. The addition of metal backing of tibial components began in 1980 to enhance load transmission to the underlying bone, and will be discussed further in this chapter.

MOBILE-BEARING

The fixed bearing versus mobile bearing debate was fueled by the desire to lessen polyethylene wear as a failure mode for TKA. As conformity between the femoral component and tibial polyethylene increased in order to obtain a stable articulation, edgeloading increased as well due to increased contact stress. The theoretical advantage behind mobile bearing implants was to transfer some of the forces to the backside of the tibial polyethylene by allowing the physiological freedom of rotation, thereby lessening that contact stress and decreasing wear. It is not fully clear as yet what the correct balance between conformity and laxity is, and whether mobile bearing implants help lower wear. Actually, concern for backside wear at this added articulation has unfortunately been seen in the literature, and comparative studies have not shown the superiority of these implants as compared to the fixed bearing ones.

Credit for the first impactful design in mobile bearing TKA is probably attributable to the work of Pappas and Buechel in the late 1970s who introduced the New Jersey Knee System, which later became the basis for the low contact stress implant.

Currently, it is unclear whether the theoretical benefits of mobile bearing designs are the actual answer to obtaining more natural kinematics of the knee and thereby reducing wear.

MODULARITY

During this period, modularity was also introduced. Initially, this helped surgeons with enhanced

intraoperative versatility with tibial polyethylene sizes and knee stability. The advantages of modular tibial components came with a cost. The availability of such interchangeable parts seemed advantageous, but concerns quickly developed regarding another interface of poly and metal that may be susceptible to wear. Modularity introduced a new term 'backside wear' to describe polyethylene wear that occurred on the posterior aspect of the tibial component. This was seen in many designs, and inadequacies of the tibial-locking mechanism were largely responsible for this. Flat-on-flat articulations between femoral and tibial components especially CR designs and polyethylene issues further contributed to enhanced polyethylene wear. These wear particles contributed to a new family of TKA complications involving osteolysis of bone, loosening of components, and severe bone defects. Fortunately, more conforming designs, along with better tibial-locking mechanisms and improved quality of polyethylene, have markedly minimized these problems in today's implants.

It was in 1978, with the advent of the Insall-Burstein knee (**Figure 1.5**), that PCL sacrifice morphed into PCL substitution utilizing a spine-cam mechanism, as the designers noted some important limitations of the TCP. These included an inability to reliably achieve greater ranges of motion and satisfactory stair climbing as well as inadequate posterior stability needed in greater degrees of flexion, especially in postpatellectomy patients. While highly successful in long-term survivorship, the average flexion achieved with the TCP was only 90°. The term 'posterior-stabilized' (PS) was coined, representing PCL substitution, which has enjoyed abundant clinical success for many years, achieving an average flexion of 115° in this early design. Initial criticisms included issues related to increased prosthetic constraint possibly leading to early and increased loosening. However, this proved to be an unfounded concern as the PS knee has enjoyed great long-term success without significant loosening.

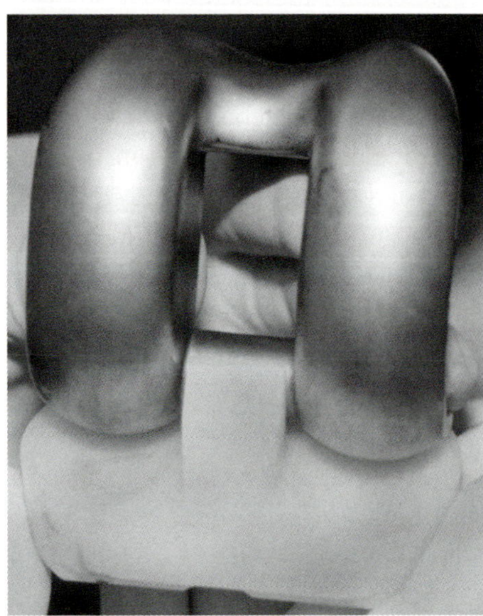

Figure 1.5 IB-I

Thus, the PCL debate began in the TKA implant design. The retention of the PCL in TKA included anterior-posterior flexion stability and more importantly supposed enhanced posterior condylar rollback as the knee flexed. Among other arguments, favoring PCL excision included the ease of the tibial cut, correction of angular deformity, and more conforming prosthetic design features. Virtually every orthopedic implant company had their own CR and PCL substituting designs during the ensuing decade.

Another idea, which coined the natural knee, was developed by Dr Aaron Hoffman as a CR design. This knee could be used either with or without cement fixation. The tibial component was asymmetric, mimicking the natural dimensions of the proximal tibia. As more CR surgeons recognized the occasional need for increased anterior-posterior stability, a unique design called the ultracongruent poly was developed in the 'Natural' family of TKAs. They designed a PCL substituting implant without the need for traditional PS-type cam and postmechanism. Only minor surgical alterations were needed such as minimizing the tibial slope, with no need for an additional femoral notch cut or different femoral components.

The essential concepts introduced in these last renditions of TKA development provided the templates for today's modern implants, and while there have been many modifications to these concepts, the fundamental principles remain valid today. Furthermore, as the long-term clinical results emerged from these early PS and CR TKAs, new supersystems were developed, capitalizing on successful design features and developing new features to correct observed deficiencies. These systems include Nexgen, Sigma, Natural Knee II, Vanguard, and others.

HINGED PROSTHESES

Around the same time as unlinked implants were undergoing early development, linked TKAs were being designed utilizing intramedullary stems and a hinge attaching the femoral and tibial components. The idea behind these implants was to simplify implantation, ligament balance, and alignment through complete constraint afforded by the prosthesis itself. Unfortunately, unlike a hip's relatively simple ball-in-socket arc of movement, the knee endures a much more complex freedom of motion that proved difficult to constrain with such an implant, which is why many early designs failed.

The first hinged implant was introduced by Judet et al. in 1947, followed by several other designs, including both cemented and uncemented options. These included designs by Wallidus in 1951, Shiers, and the Guepar cemented implant (**Figure 1.6**).

While initially appealing as a concept, these early implants suffered from a high infection rate and loosening, and they proved to be nonanatomic, as the knee is not a simple hinge joint. Ultimately, the concept did not restore function as too much force was transferred to the bone-implant interface, leading to loosening. It is important to remember that these implants were commonly used to treat the worst of knees at a time when both understanding of disease and treatment were very limited, so perhaps too much was being asked of these implants.

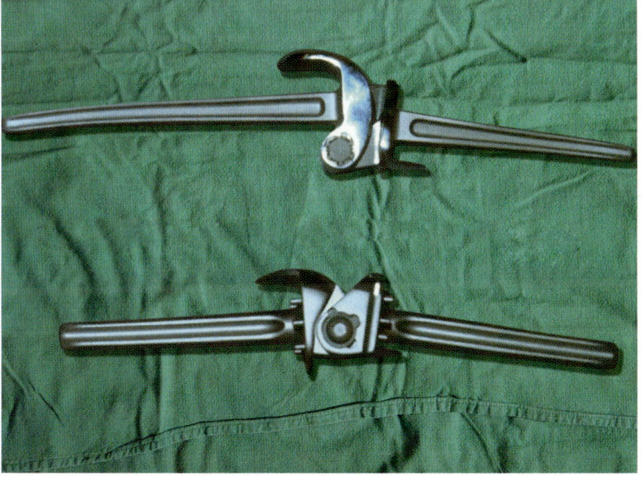

Figure 1.6 Guepar linked prosthesis

Evolution of these implants developed by allowing a degree of rotation while maintaining the hinge coupling. Presently, hinged prostheses are accepted as the last option along the algorithm of treating severely diseased knees such as those with significant bone loss and ligament insufficiency, usually in a complex revision setting. Besides giving today's surgeons a tool in treating the most difficult cases, hinged implants added to the understanding of controlling some of the movement of TKA.

TOTAL KNEE ARTHROPLASTY SYSTEMS

Early in the evolution of the TKA design, surgeons desired a graduated system of implants to manage especially complex cases, both primary and revision. With the early failures of hinged prostheses, an unlinked design providing increased constraint evolved with the total condylar III (TCP III) (**Figure 1.4**). This prosthesis provided markedly increased varus and valgus constraint by means of an enlarged central peg on the tibial component and deepened notch on the femur. Additionally, an uncemented femoral stem was added for improved fixation. This prosthesis proved quite successful and provides a blueprint for improved and more versatile designs to come. In the early 1980s, joint surgeons were faced with extremely complex revision procedures involving severe bone loss, ligament instability, and component fixation issues associated with failed early generation TKAs. In an effort to manage these cases, some surgeons began to utilize custom TKA designs with metal augments to better manage bone loss, with a variety of intramedullary stems for enhanced fixations and tibial polys to provide varied implant constraint as needed. While quite successful, disadvantages of these implants were that they were time consuming to be created, afforded limited intraoperative versatility, and were costly.

A modular knee system known as the constrained condylar knee (CCK) evolved, providing surgeons tremendous intraoperative versatility. This modular system essentially allowed one the flexibility to utilize a variety of intramedullary stems, femoral and tibial augments and tibial polys for both PCL substitution and significant varus-valgus constraint similar to the TCP III in a case-by-case basis. Custom designs were rarely needed after the CCK emerged. Many similar systems arose over

the ensuing decade. Clinical results of the CCK have proved excellent and durable both in complex primary and revision TKA.

These modular CCK-like knee systems have continued to expand in their offerings of intramedullary stems and metal augments. Both cemented and uncemented intramedullary stem fixation have indications in difficult cases and have been clinically successful. These indications are subject to surgeon discretion. Modular augments to manage bone loss on the femur and tibia have also evolved to manage greater degrees of bone loss that may be encountered. More recently, the emergence of cementless femoral and tibial cones utilizing tantalum metal has greatly enhanced surgeons' ability to manage these very large bone defects. Early clinical success with these cones has been reported by several authors but long-term results are not yet available.

CEMENTLESS FIXATION

Loosening was an early concern of TKA designs giving rise to concerns regarding cement fixation of these implants. Cementless fixation has received attention during the evolution of TKA design. Polymethylmethacralate cement was approved by the FDA for use in TKA in the early 1970s and is widely used today. Removing this interface would be an attractive prospect in eliminating a possible source of TKA failure by fixing the implant itself to the patient's bone.

While some modest successes have been reported with cementless fixation, cemented TKA has been the gold standard regarding fixation. Investigators such as Hungerford, Whiteside, Hoffman, Galante, and others continued to pioneer cementless fixation. Some recent advancements, such as porous trabecular metal (TM), have ignited some renewed interest in this prospect. Especially, in the young, more active patients are undergoing TKA today. Many systems today are available in cementless forms, but long-term results are lacking as yet. A recent five-year follow-up of TM monoblocktibial components using radiostereometric analysis showed stable implants in all cases reviewed.

PATELLAR RESURFACING

In the 1980s, in an otherwise increasingly successful surgery, roughly 30% of patients undergoing TKA suffered from complications related to the patellofemoral joint. While patellar resurfacing became a standard part of TKA with Insall's TCP implant in 1973, it was, and still is, not completely clear whether or not the patella should be resurfaced in all cases. Multiple studies have shown no difference in TKA outcome as far as anterior knee pain whether the patella is resurfaced or not. Consistently, there is roughly a 10% reoperation rate in knees with unresurfaced patellae. Perhaps a more important factor in reducing anterior knee pain related to the patellofemoral articulation is actually trochlear design. As femoral components evolved, they were designed to be more 'patellar-friendly' than prior implants. In one study, lateral release rates were significantly reduced as implant design was improved to accommodate the patella better, along with a better understanding of component rotation (**Flow chart 1.1**).

CONCLUSION

TKA is a very successful procedure that has undergone an evolution with many developments over a course of roughly half a century. While early designs failed, we must remember that they were used in the worst of knees, and our implants today are highly derivative of those failures. It is imperative that we respect the failures as much as the successes as both were essential to what we utilize today. Progress is ongoing as many patients are still unhappy after the surgery, and we are still charged with the task of improving the procedure and explaining why in so many cases, a 'perfect' looking X-ray can still be a painful TKA.

ACKNOWLEDGMENT

We wish to acknowledge that we have received the pictures from Dr Russel E Windsor, Hospital for Special Surgery and Zimmer.

Flow chart 1.1 Evolution of TKA

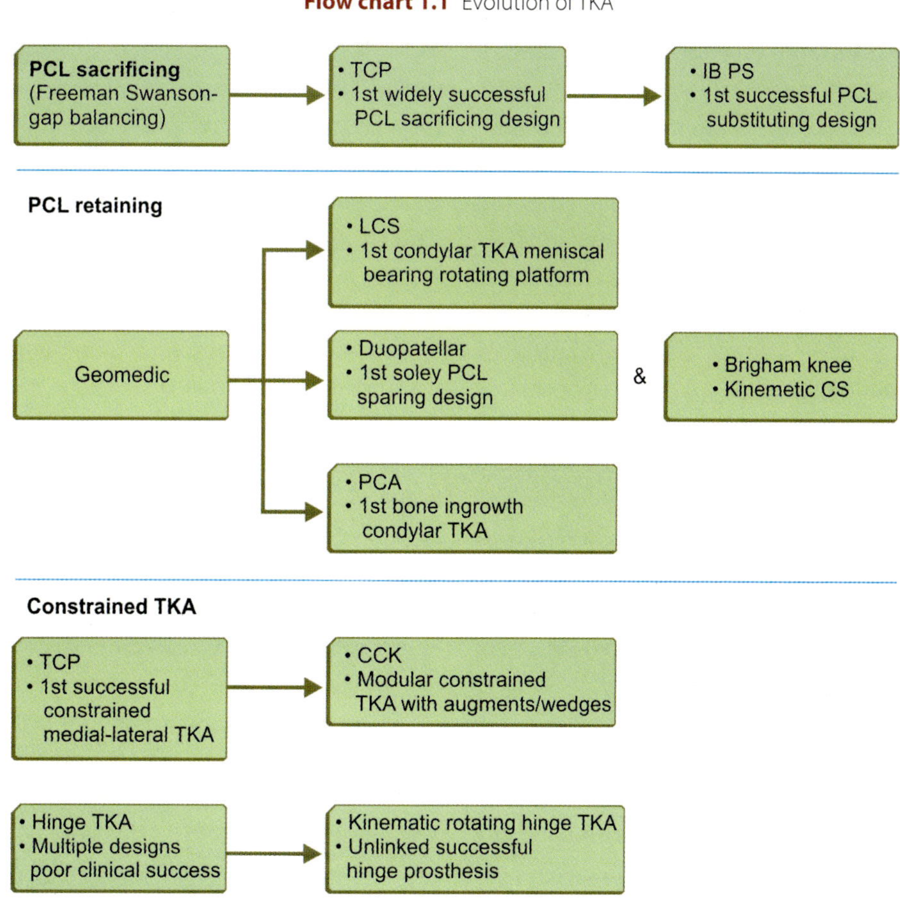

BIBLIOGRAPHY

1. Abdeen AR, Collen SB, Vince KG. 15 to 19-year follow-up of the Insall-Burstein-1 total knee arthroplasty. J Arthroplasty. 2010;25:173-8.
2. Abraham W, Buchanan JR, Daubert H, et al. Should the patella be resurfaced in total knee arthroplasty? Efficacy of patellar resurfacing. Clin Orthop Relat Res. 1988;236:128.
3. Aglietti P, Buzzi R, Gaudenzi A. Patellofemoral functional results and complications with the posterior stabilized total condylar knee prosthesis. J Arthroplasty. 1988;3:17.
4. Aglietti P, Buzzi R. Posteriorly stabilised total-condylar knee replacement: three to eight years' follow-up of 85 knees. J Bone Joint Surg Br. 1988;70:211.
5. Aglietti P, Rinonapoli E. Total condylar knee arthroplasty: a five-year follow-up study of 33 knees. Clin Orthop Relat Res. 1984;186:104.
6. Andriacchi TP, Galante JO. Retention of the posterior cruciate in total knee arthroplasty. J Arthroplasty. 1988;3:S13.
7. Bargar WL, Cracchiolo IIIA, Amstutz HC. Results with the constrained total knee prosthesis in treating severely disabled patients and patients with failed total knee replacements. J Bone Joint Surg Am. 1980;62:504.
8. Barrack RL. Evolution of the rotating hinge for complex total knee arthroplasty. Clin Orthop Relat Res. 2001;392:292.
9. Bertin KC, Freeman MAR, Samuelson KM, et al. Stemmed revision arthroplasty for aseptic loosening of total knee replacement. J Bone Joint Surg Br. 1985;67:242.
10. Bertin KC, Lloyd WW. Effect of total knee prosthesis design on patellar tracking and need for lateral retinacular release. J Arthroplasty. 2013;28:772-7.
11. Blaha JD, Insler HP, Freeman MAR, et al. The fixation of a proximal tibial polyethylene prosthesis without cement. J Bone Joint Surg Br. 1982;64:326.
12. Bourne RB, Burnett RSJ. The consequences of not resurfacing the patella. Clin Orthop Relat Res. 2004; 428:166.

13. Brooks PJ, Walker PS, Scott RD. Tibial component fixation in deficient tibial bone stock. Clin Orthop. 1984;184:302.
14. Bryce CD, Long WJ, Scott WN, et al. Long term outcomes of TKA in patients under 55 years of age with osteoarthritis. Knee society meeting, Garden City, NJ. 12 September 2012.
15. Buechel FF, Pappas MJ. Long-term survivorship analysis of cruciate-sparing versus cruciate-sacrificing knee prostheses using meniscal bearings. Clin Orthop Relat Res. 1990;260:162.
16. Burnett RS, Haydon CM, Rorabeck CH, Bourne RB. Patella resurfacing versus nonresurfacing in total knee arthroplasty. Results of a randomized controlled clinical trial at a minimum of 10 years' follow-up. Clin Orthop Relat Res. 2004;428:12.
17. Campbell WC. Arthroplasty of the knee-report of cases. J Orthop Surg. 1921;3:430-6.
18. Colizza WA, Insall JN, Scuderi GR. The posterior stabilized total knee prosthesis: assessment of polyethylene damage and osteolysis after a ten-year-minimum follow-up. J Bone Joint Surg Am. 1995;77:1713.
19. Conditt, MA, Ismaily SK, Noble PC. Modular tibial insert micromotion during the gait cycle: effects of cold flow and implantation time. Program and abstracts of the AAOS 68th Annual Meeting, San Francisco, CA. 29 February–4 March 2001; Paper No. 190.
20. Deburge A, Guepar. GUEPAR hinge prosthesis: complications and results with two years' follow-up. Clin Orthop Relat Res. 1976;120:47.
21. Diduch DR, Insall JN, Scott WN, et al. Total knee replacement in young active patients: long-term follow-up and functional outcome. J Bone Joint Surg Am. 1997;79:575.
22. Donaldson III WF, Sculco TP, Insall JN, et al. Total condylar III knee prosthesis: long-term follow-up study. Clin Orthop Relat Res. 1988;226:21.
23. Ferguson W. Excision of the knee joint-recovery with a false joint and useful limb. Med Times Gazette. 1861;1:601.
24. Freeman MAR, Samuelson KM, Bertin KC. Freeman-Samuelson total arthroplasty of the knee. Clin Orthop Relat Res. 1985;192:46.
25. Gluck T. Die invaginations methode der osteo-und arthroplastik. Berliner KlinischeWochenschrift. 1890;27:732-6.
26. Gunston FH. Polycentric knee arthroplasty: prosthetic simulation of normal knee movement. J Bone Joint Surg Br. 1971;53:272.
27. Haas SB, Insall JN, Montgomery III W, et al. Revision total knee arthroplasty with use of modular components with stems inserted without cement. J Bone Joint Surg Am. 1995;77:1700.
28. Hanssen AD, Rand JA. A comparison of primary and revision total knee arthroplasty using the kinematic stabilizer prosthesis. J Bone Joint Surg Am. 1988;70:491.
29. Hungerford DS, Kenna RV, Krackow KA. The porous-coated anatomic total knee. Orthop Clin North Am. 1982;13:103.
30. Hungerford DS, Krackow KA. Total joint arthroplasty of the knee. Clin Orthop Relat Res. 1985;192:23.
31. Insall JN, Freeman MAR, Matthews LS, et al. Present status of total knee replacement [symposium]. Contemp Orthop. 1980;2:592.
32. Insall JN, Kelly M. The total condylar prosthesis. Clin Orthop. 1986;205:43.
33. Insall JN, Lachiewicz PF, Burstein AH. The posterior stabilized condylar prosthesis: a modification of the total condylar design: two to four-year clinical experience. J Bone Joint Surg Am. 1982;64:1317.
34. Insall JN, Ranawat CS, Scott WN, et al. Total condylar knee replacement: preliminary report. Clin Orthop Relat Res. 1976;120:149.
35. Insall JN, Scott WN, Ranawat CS. The total condylar knee prosthesis: a report of two hundred and twenty cases. J Bone Joint Surg Am. 1979;61:173.
36. Jones EC, Insall JN, Inglis AE, et al. GUEPAR knee arthroplasty results and late complications. Clin Orthop Relat Res. 1979;140:145.
37. Judet J, Judet R, Crepin GT. Essais de prostheseosteso-articulaire. Presse Med. 1947;52:302.
38. Kavolus CH, Faris PM, Ritter MA, et al. The total condylar III knee prosthesis in elderly patients. J Arthroplasty. 1991;6:39.
39. Kim YH, Kim JS, Choe JW, Kim HJ, et al. Long term comparison of fixed-bearing and mobile bearing TKR in patients younger than 51 years of age with osteoarthritis. J Bone Joint Surg Am. 2012;94:866-73.
40. Kim Y-H. Salvage of failed hinge knee arthroplasty with a total condylar III type prosthesis. Clin Orthop Relat Res. 1987;221:272.
41. MacIntosh DL. Hemiarthroplasty of the knee using a space occupying prosthesis for painful varus and valgus deformities. J Bone Joint Surg Am. 1958;40:1431.

42. McKeever DC. Tibial plateau prosthesis. Clin Orthop Relat Res. 1960;18:86-95.
43. Murphy JB. Ankylosis, arthroplasty: clinical and experimental. JAMA. 1905;44:1573, 1671-94.
44. Pappas MJ, Mokris G, Bucchel FF. Wear in prosthetic knee joints. 72nd AAOS. 23–27 February 2005; Washington, DC.
45. Pappas MJ. Engineering design of the LCS knee replacement. In: Hamelynck KJ, Stiehl JB (Eds). LCS mobile bearing knee arthroplasty—a 25 years worldwide review. Heidelberg: Springer; 2002.pp.39-52.
46. Pilling, RWD, et al. Patellar resurfacing in primary total knee replacement: a meta-analysis. J Bone Joint Surg Am. 2012;94(24):2270-8.
47. Ranawat CS, Boachie-Adjei O. Survivorship analysis and results of total condylar knee arthroplasty. Eight- to 11-year follow-up period. Clin Orthop Relat Res. 1988;226:6.
48. Rhoads DD, Noble PC, Reuben JD, Mahoney OM, Tullos HS. The effect of femoral component position on patellar tracking after total knee arthroplasty. Clin Orthop Relat Res. 1990;260:43-51.
49. Robinson RP. The early innovators of today's resurfacing condylar knees. J Arthroplasty. 2005;20(Suppl. 1):2.
50. Samuelson K, Nelson L. An all-polyethylene cementless tibial component: a five- to nine-year follow-up study. Clin Orthop Relat Res. 1990;260:93.
51. Scott RD, Volatile TB. Twelve years' experience with posterior cruciate-retaining total knee arthroplasty. Clin Orthop Relat Res. 1986;205:100.
52. Scott WN, Rubinstein M, Scuderi G. Results after knee replacement with a posterior cruciate-substituting prosthesis. J Bone Joint Surg Am. 1988;70:1163.
53. Sledge CB, Stern P, Thomas WH, et al. Two-year follow-up of the duocondylar total knee replacement. Orthop Trans. 1978;2:193.
54. Springer BD, Hanssen AD, Sim FH, Lewallen DG. The kinematic rotating hinge prosthesis for complex knee arthroplasty. Clin Orthop Relat Res. 2001;392:283.
55. Townley CO. The anatomic total knee resurfacing arthroplasty. Clin Orthop Relat Res. 1985;192:82.
56. Vince KG, Insall JN, Kelly MA. The total condylar prosthesis: 10- to 12-year results of a cemented knee replacement. J Bone Joint Surg Br. 1989;71:793.
57. Wilson DAJ, Richardson G, Hennigor A, Dunbar MJ. Continued stabilization of trabecular Metzl tibial monoblock TKA components of 5 years-measured with radiostereometric analysis. Acta Orthop. 2012; 83(1)136-40.
58. Wilson FC, Fajgenbaum DM, Venters GC. Results of knee replacement with the Walldius and geometric prostheses: a comparative study. J Bone Joint Surg Am. 1980;62:497.

Chapter 2

Biomechanics of Normal and Replaced Knee

Sharath K Rao, Sandeep Vijayan

INTRODUCTION

Biomechanics of the knee describes the various functions of the knee in relation to mechanical components. Knee joint is the largest and most complex synovial joint of the body. Capsule, musculotendinous units, and ligaments of the knee have varied and overlapping functions. Knee can be considered as having three different types of joints, namely patellofemoral joint, medial, and lateral tibiofemoral joints. The knee has passive elastic structures in the form of ligaments, active elastic structures in the form of musculotendinous units and nonelastic structures in the form of bone.[1]

MECHANICAL AXIS

The mechanical axis refers to the line drawn from the center of the head of the femur to the center of the ankle. This is a straight line and corresponds to the weight-bearing axis of the lower limb. This line passes through the center or near center of the knee. The mechanical axis passes through the three-dimensional center of the knee. Because the hip is more widely separated compared to knee and ankle, the mechanical axis is 3 degrees valgus to the vertical axis (**Figure 2.1**). The weight-bearing is done by the tibiofemoral joint and passes from the femur to the tibia. The anatomical axis of the femur is at an angle of 5–7° valgus to the mechanical axis. The tibial articular surface is approximately 3 degrees of varus with respect to the mechanical axis. Joint reaction force in tibiofemoral joint is 3 times the body weight while walking and 4 times the body weight while climbing stairs.

PATELLOFEMORAL JOINT

This joint transmits the tensile forces generated by the quadriceps tendon to the patellar tendon. It increases the lever arm of quadriceps mechanism. Patellectomy decreases the extension force by 30%. Joint reaction force in patellofemoral joint is 7 times the body weight during squatting and 3 times the body weight during descending stairs.[2]

The articulation of the patellofemoral joint permits sliding movement. The patella moves 7 cm caudally during full knee flexion. Maximum contact between the femur and patella is at 45° of knee flexion. Primary

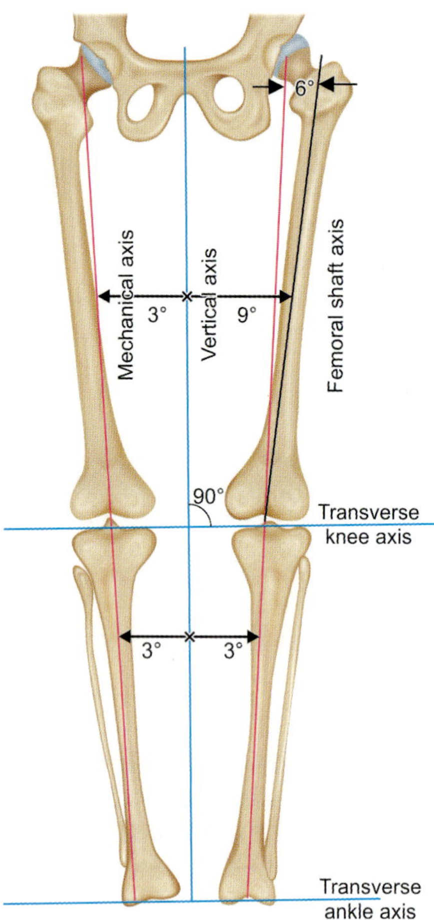

Figure 2.1 Diagram showing vertical axis, mechanical axis and femoral shaft axis

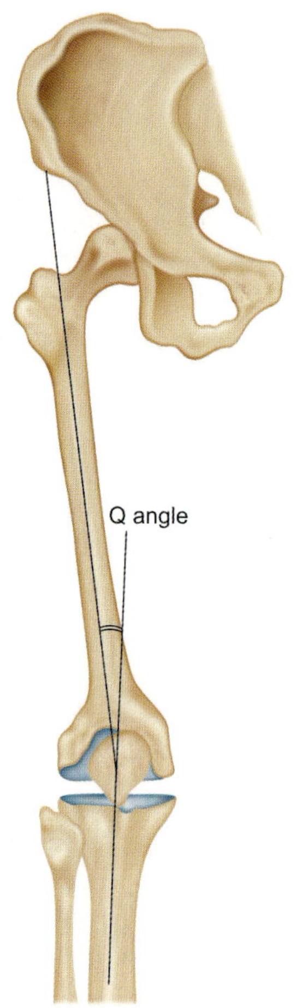

Figure 2.2 Q angle

passive restraint to lateral subluxation of the patella is the medial patellofemoral ligament, acting maximally at 20° of knee flexion. Sixty percent of the restraining force is from the medial patellofemoral ligament. The medial patellomeniscal ligament (13%) and the lateral retinaculum (10%) are the other contributors to the restraining force. Dynamic restraint of the patellofemoral joint is the quadriceps muscle.

Q Angle

The Q angle, also called the quadriceps angle, depicts the angle of pull of quadriceps muscle. A line is drawn from the anterior superior iliac spine to middle of the patella and from the middle of the patella to the tibial tuberosity. The angle subtended between these two lines is the Q angle (**Figure 2.2**). Normally, the Q angle is about 8°. In flexion, the Q angle increases and is 13° in males and 18° in females.

TIBIOFEMORAL ARTICULATION

Movement

In the sagittal plane, the knee moves from 3° of hyperextension to 155° of flexion. The thigh-calf contact while flexing limits the flexion. Normal gait requires a range of 0–70° of flexion in the knee. Due to the contour of femoral and tibial condyles, the flexion of the knee is not a simple hinge movement unlike what occurs in the elbow.

Flexion and extension do not occur about a fixed transverse axis of rotation, but they occur through an instant center of rotation, which is polycentric. When plotted, this instant center of rotation moves posteriorly in the femoral condyle in a J-shaped pattern. The point of contact between the tibial and femoral surfaces moves posteriorly as the knee flexes. With rolling alone the femoral condyle will roll off the tibial plateau before the full flexion is achieved. With gliding alone the femoral shaft would impinge on the tibia, thus the knee both glides and rolls. This allows an increased flexion of the knee without causing impingement. This movement is similar to the one that occurs in a rocking chair. This mechanism is brought about by the cross bar linkage of the anterior and posterior cruciates. Rolling and gliding are also helped by the posterior tibial slope.

The exact ratio between the rolling and gliding varies in different individuals. It is around 1:2 in early flexion and reaches to 1:4 in terminal flexion movement.

Screw Home Mechanism

Femur internally rotates about 5° in the last 15° of extension of the knee producing a screw home mechanism. As the knee is extended, the shorter and more highly curved lateral condyle exhausts its articular surface and is checked by the anterior cruciate ligament (ACL). The larger and less curved medial condyle continues its forward roll and skids backward assisted by the posterior cruciate ligament (PCL). This results in the medial rotation of the femur, which tightens the collaterals and accounts for the screw home movement. This locking of the knee helps to decrease the force generated by the quadriceps during standing. The same action is produced by the external rotation of the tibia when the knee is extended and not bearing weight. Similarly, flexion of knee during the stance phase unlocks the knee by externally rotating the femur. This is produced by the popliteus muscle. This relaxes the tension in collateral ligaments to produce the flexion of the knee. This is called the unlocking of the knee and in non-weight-bearing position, the tibia internally rotates to do it. This is due to the action of the popliteus muscle from both directions of origin and insertion.

Stability of Knee

The lateral collateral ligament is the stabilizer of the knee during varus stress. Superficial portion of the medial collateral ligament stabilizes the knee during valgus stress. Tibial spines provide the mediolateral stability to an extended knee.

The ACL provides stability for anterior translation. The ACL is attached to a semicircular area on the posteromedial aspect of the lateral femoral condyle and anterior to and between the intercondylar eminences of the tibia. The ACL has an anteromedial bundle that is tight in flexion and a posterolateral bundle, which is tight in extension. The ACL apart from being a primary static restrainer of anterior translation also plays a role in axial rotation (**Figures 2.3 to 2.5**).

The PCL provides stability for posterior translation. The PCL is attached proximally to the anterolateral aspect of the medial femoral condyle and distally to the tibial sulcus below the articular surface. The PCL has an anterolateral bundle that is tight in flexion and a posteromedial bundle, which is tight in extension. The PCL is a primary static restrainer of posterior translation. External tibial rotation is stabilized by the posterolateral corner.

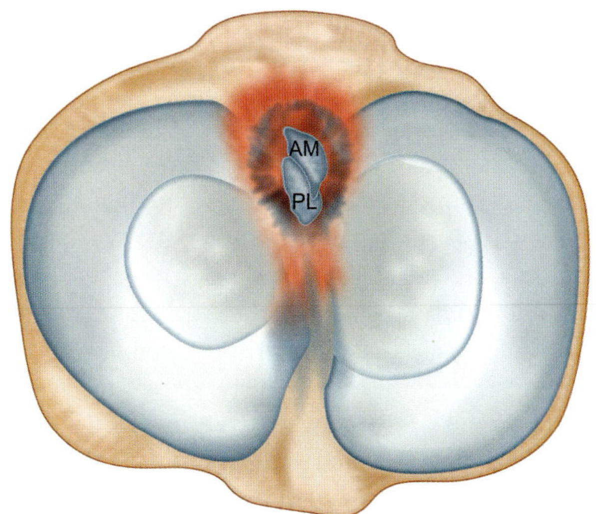

Figure 2.3 Tibial attachment of an anterior cruciate ligament (ACL). *Abbreviations:* AM, anteromedial bundle; PL, posterolateral bundle

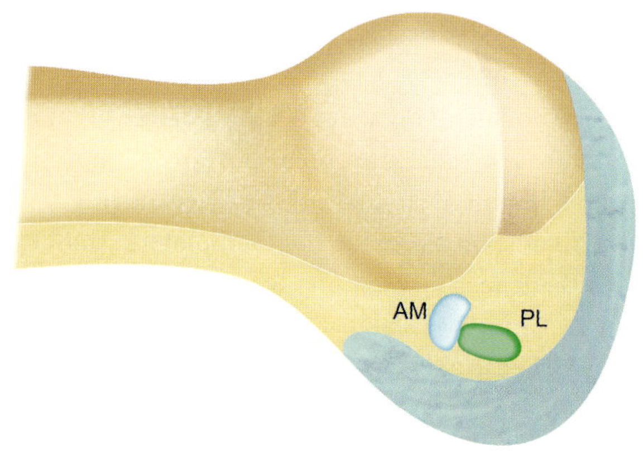

Figure 2.4 Femoral attachment of anterior cruciate ligament. *Abbreviations:* AM, anteromedial bundle; PL, posterolateral bundle

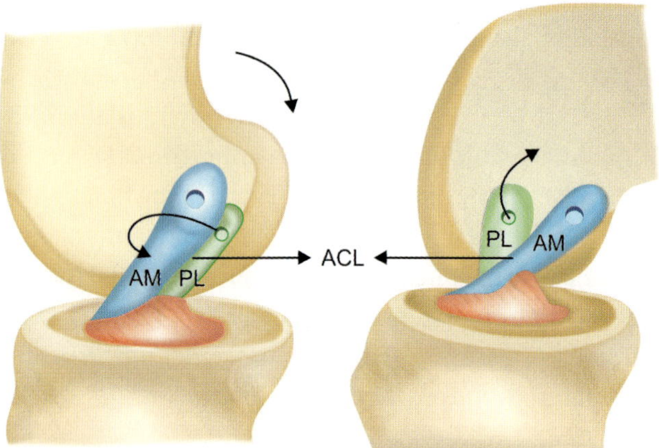

Figure 2.5 Anterior cruciate ligament (ACL) showing two bundles. *Abbreviations:* AM, anteromedial bundle; PL, posterolateral bundle

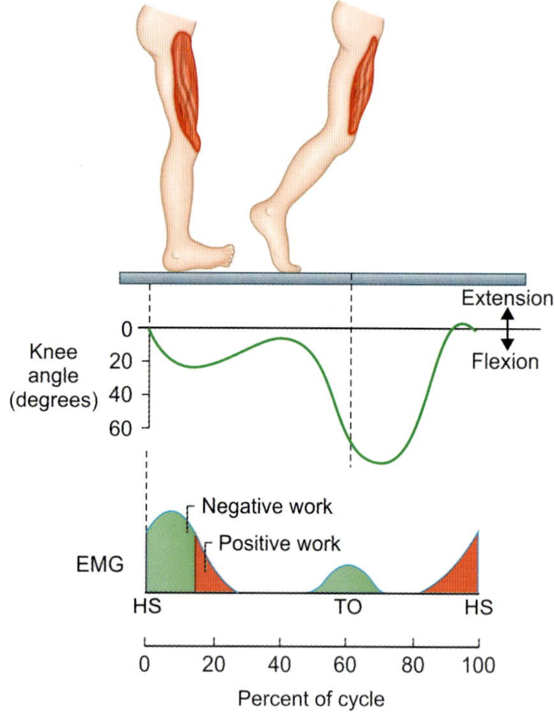

Figure 2.6 Quadriceps activity during gait cycle

KNEE IN NORMAL GAIT

In the normal gait, the center of the gravity is brought to the point of support in the single leg stance phase. This is not necessary if a crutch or a cane is used on the opposite side. A narrow-based gait is more energy efficient than a broad-based gait, because of the decrease in the side-to-side shift of the center of gravity.[3] The normal gait is divided into two phases: stance phase and swing phase. In walking at some phase of the gait cycle the feet are on the ground as double support unlike in running. The stance phase is divided into heel strike, foot flat, midstance, heel off and toe off. The length of the double support depends on the rate of the gait cycle. Normally, the double support constitutes 10–12% of the gait cycle.

Knee flexion starts occurring immediately after the heel strike and reaches to around 20°. This returns to full extension during foot flat and midstance. Knee starts flexing further during heel off and toe off, and reaches to a maximum of 60° immediately after the toe off.

Quadriceps starts contracting at the end of the swing phase to prepare for the heel strike and stabilizes the knee during the heel strike. From heel strike to foot flat knee flexes up to 20° and quadriceps lengthens showing negative activity in EMG. As the knee starts extending during the midstance, quadriceps again shows positive activity due to contraction. Small burst of activity before and after the toe off is to limit knee flexion in the swing phase (**Figure 2.6**).

Hamstring muscle shows contraction and positive EMG immediately after the heel strike. This is exactly opposite to the action of quadriceps, thus stabilizing the knee. During toe off, hamstring again contracts helping to flex the knee to produce the toe off. Hamstring shows electromyography activity throughout the swing phase, but the quadriceps is silent (**Figure 2.7**).

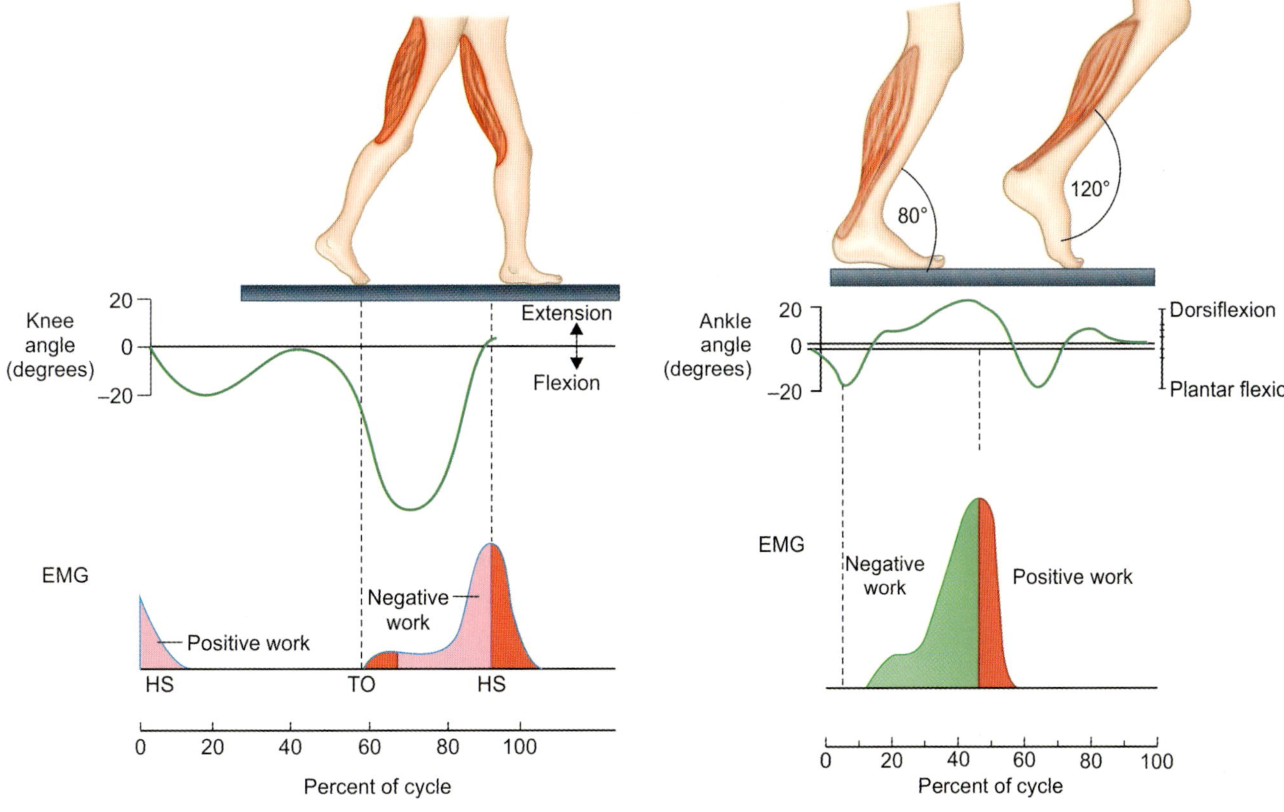

Figure 2.7 Hamstring activity during gait cycle

Figure 2.8 Triceps surae activity during gait cycle

Triceps surae shows maximum activity from foot flat to toe off since they are directly related to ankle plantar flexion. Gastrocnemius part of the triceps surae as it crosses the knee joint also stabilizes the knee during the stance phase of the gait cycle (**Figure 2.8**).

Stair Climbing and Descending

Ascending stairs is always easier than descending stairs. The amount of knee flexion needed to ascend the stair depends on height of the patient and the height of the stair. For a regular 7-inch stair, the amount of knee flexion needed is 65°. It appears that the amount of flexion needed in the knee is less than that required for normal walking. But the difference is that the knee is not loaded in walking at 70° of flexion, but in stair climbing the knee is loaded at 65° of flexion. The patellofemoral joint force is half that of the body weight during normal walking, but it reaches 3.8 times the body weight during stair climbing.[4] This is because the body weight acts from a long lever arm. This force can be reduced by decreasing the lever arm by bending the body forward during stair climbing. The tibia remains vertical during stair climbing, thereby preventing the anterior subluxation of the femur (**Figure 2.9**).

To descend a 7-inch step, the required flexion of the knee is 85°. While descending the stairs, the tibia is inclined forward, bringing the tibial plateaus to an oblique orientation. Here, the femur tends to subluxate forward under the body weight. This is prevented by the joint reaction forces of the patellofemoral joint and the tension created in the PCL. In the absence of the PCL, only the collaterals remain to assist the patellofemoral joint. The unreplaced patellofemoral joint, absent PCL and unbalanced collateral ligaments are detrimental to a replaced joint during descending the stairs (**Figure 2.10**).

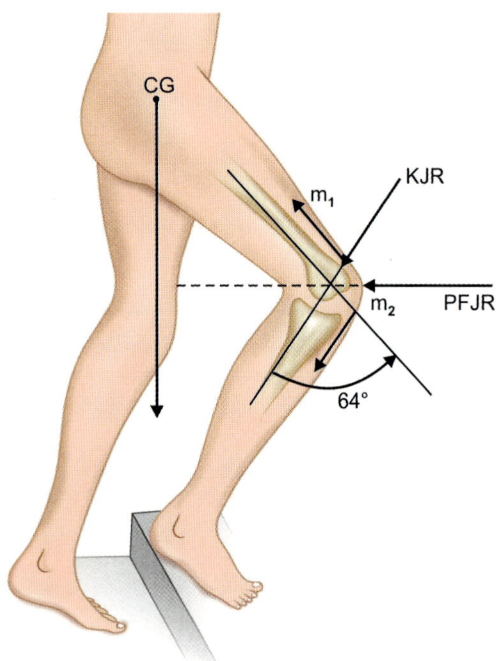

Figure 2.9 Mechanics of ascending stairs

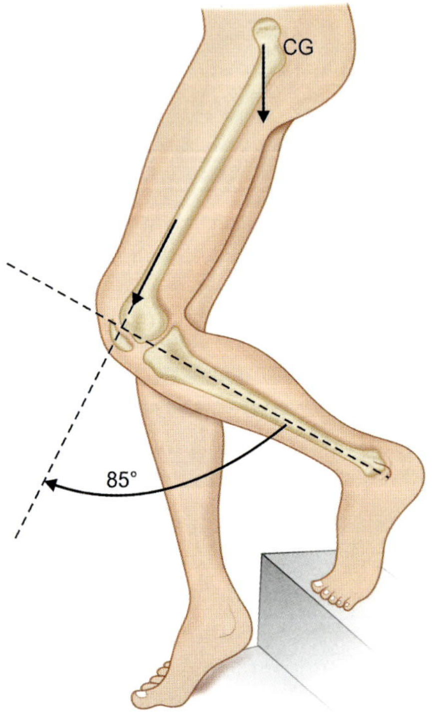

Figure 2.10 Descending stairs

Descending the stairs initially backward or sideways helps the patient to rehabilitate better for stair descending.

BIOMECHANICS OF AN ARTHRITIC KNEE

Introduction

Osteoarthritis of the knee is a common joint disease. This disease produces pain, deformity, muscle weakness and loss of function. Primary change in osteoarthritis occurs in the articular cartilage and later in the subchondral bone.[5] The etiology of osteoarthritis is multifactorial. Aging is one factor and overweight is the other. Excessive activity, damage to knee, posture and occupation, all contribute to the degeneration of the joint.

There is a significant contribution from biomechanical variations in the knee toward the development and progression of arthritis of the knee. Degenerative arthritis of the knee most commonly starts in the medial compartment of the knee. The external knee adduction moment usually distributes 60–80% of the compressive load of the knee to the medial compartment normally. An increase in the adduction moment occurs in medially degenerated knees, which further increases the compressive load on the medial compartment.[6,7] The knee adduction moment seems to be both the cause and the effect of degenerative arthritis of the knee.

Quadriceps weakness, which initially starts because of a response to arthritic pain in the knee, also contributes to the progression of the disease. Quadriceps weakness produces a myriad of biomechanical changes in the knee joint especially during the normal gait and stair climbing. This also may have a role in increasing the adductor moment of the knee.[8]

Cartilage

Structure and Function

Cartilage consists of mainly an extracellular matrix devoid of blood supply, lymphatics and nerves. There is very less metabolic activity in the cartilage even though the cartilage cells are capable of undergoing cell division.[9] The extracellular matrix consists of tissue fluid and a framework of type II collagen fibers and proteoglycans. The appropriate mixture of these makes the articular cartilage elastic and also highly tensile.[10]

Cartilage in Osteoarthritis

The cartilage cells fail to maintain the homeostasis between the production and destruction of the extracellular matrix.[11] This leads to an increase in the water content and a decrease in the proteoglycans in the extracellular matrix. Collagen fibers are also synthesized less and the existing collagens breakdown. This reduces the resiliency and tensile strength of the cartilage.

Cartilage Overloading

An excessive load on the joint can induce changes in the articular cartilage. In experimental settings, it has been shown that cartilage cannot withstand more than 25MPa of impulsive contact stress.[11] This leads to microfracture, cartilage fissure, chondrocyte death and proteoglycan release. Apart from the load, the rate of loading and generation of shear stresses also play an important role in cartilage damage.[12] This cartilage overloading in the knee occurs in obesity, high contact sports, postmeniscectomy, deformities and post-traumatic malalignment.

Cartilage Defects

Cartilage defects are described according to their thickness, partial and complete. Complete cartilage defects predispose to degenerative arthrosis. There is an increased load on the rim of the defect triggering overload changes in the cartilage. The pain in these situations is mainly due to the exposure of the subchondral bone. Partial defects have not been shown to cause arthritis.

Malalignment

In a normal knee in stance phase the forces pass through the medial side of the center of the knee by about 4–8 mm.[13] The forces can reach 3 times the body weight in walking and up to 6 times the body weight during stair climbing. The forces run much more medially in the flexion of the knee. Varus and valgus malalignments alter these biomechanics. A mild increase of 4° of varus increases the loading in the medial compartment by 20%.[14] Articular cartilage damage and subchondral bone changes following the increase in load may further increase the malalignment. Malalignment has been shown to increase incidence and progression of radiographic changes of osteoarthritis.

Meniscectomy

The loss of meniscal tissue either by trauma or by surgery alters the biologic and mechanical environment of the knee joint. The risk of developing arthritis is 14 folds in patients who have undergone meniscectomy.[15] Concomitant cartilage damage and ligament injury further increase the chances of developing the degeneration of the cartilage. Meniscus transmits 50% and 70% of the medial and lateral compartment load, respectively, with the knee in extension. This will increase to 85% when the knee is flexed to 90°.[16] Excision of the meniscus also decreases the contact area, further increasing the local contact stresses.

Joint Stability

Joint instability is one of the causes for developing degenerative arthrosis.[17] Joint instability usually shifts the load to a peripheral area rather than the central area resulting in the overloading of the peripheral area articular cartilage. However, there is no evidence-based support to conclude that restoring the stability in the way of ligament reconstruction may prevent the arthrosis. Isolated ligament injuries are also complex injuries, often with cartilage or meniscal damage, which might contribute to the development of arthritis.

Summary

Malalignment, meniscectomy and ligament injuries change the mechanical loading pattern of the knee joint. The contact stresses increase on the cartilage. Cartilage damage either due to trauma or disease predisposes to the changes in the cartilage. Load- and age-related changes in the cartilage make it less elastic prone to break down.

These combined with obesity and excessive activity trigger the degeneration.

ROLE OF POSTERIOR CRUCIATE LIGAMENT IN KNEE REPLACEMENT

Despite the excellent data published relating to total knee arthroplasty (TKA) using cruciate sacrificing, cruciate substituting and cruciate retaining knees, the debate on whether 'to preserve the PCL or not' still continues.[18-20] Even though the cruciate sacrificing total condylar knee's survivorship toward revision was 90.8% at the end of 21 years, there were problems related to the range of movement, stair climbing and descending and posterior subluxation. The concept of cruciate substituting designs came into existence. Cruciate substituting mechanism can either be due to spine and cam (posterior stabilized) or deep dish.

Wear

When the PCL is retained and the knee is flexed, the femur rolls back by the pull of the PCL. To produce an effective rollback of the femur, the tibial surface has to be nonconforming (flat). A conformed surface of the tibia produces posterior lip in the tibial surface and as the femur rolls up in this inclined plane it further tightens the PCL. This prevents the smooth rollback. Nonconformity of the tibial surface reduces the contact between the femur and the tibia. This increases the load per square cm and thus produces more wear. This was described as 'Kinematic Conflict.' When a flat-on-flat design is used with cruciate retaining, the chance of polyethylene wear is high. A moderate conformity is produced in the cruciate retaining implants that are in the market today. This when combined with cruciate recession when the PCL is tight reduces the polythene wear significantly. A moderate conformity design combined with cruciate substitution also reduces the poly wear.

Mechanics

Retaining the PCL in anatomical models has shown, posterior rollback of the femur, more efficient stair climbing and better patellofemoral kinematics (**Figure 2.11**). The shift of the weight-bearing point in the knee posteriorly by femoral rollback increases the quadriceps lever arm. But the more recent studies have shown that in cruciate retaining knees, the contact point moves anteriorly rather than posteriorly as the knee is flexed. This paradoxical anterior translation of the femur may produce more wear. Posterior-stabilized designs (those with spine and cam)did show the posterior rollback of the femur, but it was not similar to normal knees. In a biomechanical study by Mahoney et al.,[21] cruciate retaining designs showed 36% loss and cruciate substituting designs 12% loss in the posterior rollback of the femur compared to normal knees. Extensor mechanism efficiency is decreased by 15% and 11%, respectively, in both designs.

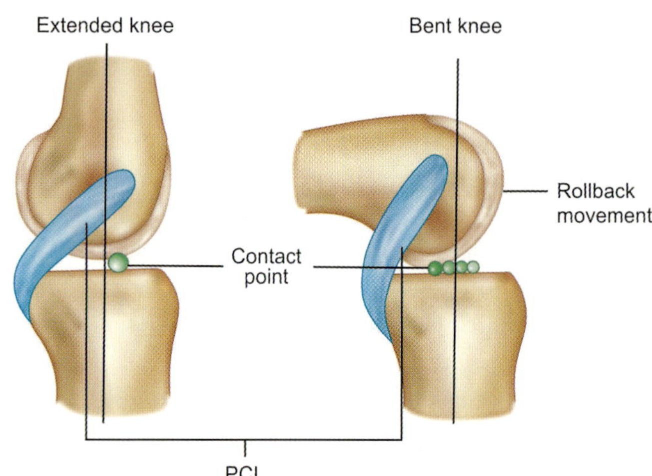

Figure 2.11 Rollback by the posterior cruciate ligament (PCL)

Range of Motion

The comparison of the range of motion between cruciate sacrificing knees, cruciate retaining knees and cruciate substituting knees showed that the cruciate substituting knees had a better range of motion (mean 112°) as compared to the other two (cruciate retaining 104° and cruciate sacrificing 103°). The increase in the usage of the cruciate recession technique in cruciate retaining knees has improved the flexion in these knees up to 110–115.[18,19]

Proprioception

It has been postulated earlier that proprioception is better with the cruciate retaining implants. In arthritic knees, age-related changes in the proprioception also occur in the PCL. Some studies have shown that cruciate retaining TKA showed better proprioception than the posterior-stabilized TKA. When the degree of preoperative arthritis is severe, posterior-stabilized knees performed better than cruciate retaining knees.

Gait Analysis

Initial studies revealed that stair climbing was better with cruciate retaining designs.[22] A forward-bending posture while climbing stairs was noted in patients who underwent cruciate sacrificing or substituting TKA, and it was suggested that this happens because of the lack of femoral rollback. Studies by Wilson et al.[23] showed no difference in the range of motion or isokinetic muscle strength between the normal and posterior-stabilized knees.

Correction of Deformities

In deformities amounting to more than 15° in any plane, correction is easier when the PCL is sacrificed and substituted. Soft tissue balancing may be more demanding if the PCL is retained in such situations. This may even lead to an increase in wear over a period of time.[18] In severe deformities, PCL recession combined with PCL retention has shown results similar to PCL substitution.[16]

PATELLOFEMORAL JOINT

In earlier posterior-stabilized designs, there were problems with the patella in the form of fracture and patellar clunk syndrome, and these complications amounted to 10–11% of all failures.[24] Improvement in designs has decreased these complications. The preservation of the joint line is important for cruciate retaining knees to exactly balance the PCL. A change of joint line up to 10 mm does not have an effect on the knee range of motion or patellofemoral function. At present, patellofemoral problems with TKA have been reduced to 3–5%, irrespective of cruciate retaining or substituting design.

BONE LOSS

To produce a cam mechanism, the intercondylar area of the femur has to loose bone in the form of a notch cut in posterior-stabilized knees. The amount of bone removed varies with the design of the prosthesis. There are prostheses with open or closed box accommodating the spine of the tibial insert. In cruciate retaining knees there is no box cut and hence there is bone preservation. Whether this bone preservation really makes difference in the outcome of revision surgery later has not been proved yet in the literature.

Summary

Earlier claims of a better range of motion, better joint stability, near normal gait, enhanced longevity of prosthesis in PCL retaining TKA, have not been substantiated in the recent literature. Both the designs match very well in terms of stability, gait, longevity and stair climbing. The range of motion seems to be better with cruciate substituting prosthesis. Deformity correction is better when the cruciate is sacrificed. Proprioception may still be better with cruciate retaining knees except in severely arthritic knees. Excessive bone loss in the form of box cut may be an issue of the future.

MOBILE-BEARING KNEES

Introduction

Mobile-bearing knees were introduced to serve two main purposes. The first was to increase the contact area and thus reduces the load and wear. The second was to improve the knee kinematics by adding rotational element to the biomechanics. It is important for the surgeon to understand the design kinematics, constraint-conformity conflict, wear progression and additional complications of spin-off and dislocation while using mobile-bearing knees.[25,26]

Designs

Basically there are four type of designs of mobile-bearing knee.[27]

1. **Internal-external rotation only:** Allows the knee to orient itself in varied rotation during flexion and extension. Forward movement of one condyle is associated with backward movement of the other.[28]
2. **Internal-external rotation about a medial axis:** This rotates through the longitudinal axis on the medial tibial plateau and simulates the anatomic motion better.[29,30]
3. **Internal-external rotation and anterior-posterior translation**: This relies on ligament balancing and has both PCL retaining and sacrificing types.[28]
4. **Guided motion type:** This allows rotation and anteroposterior translation and is guided by intercondylar cams. This has a posterior-stabilized design that allows posterior rollback in flexion. The other saddle cam design allows posterior rollback in flexion and anterior roll forward in the extension.[31]

Kinematics of Mobile-bearing Devices

With the progressive flexion, normal knee undergoes the rollback of the femur and internal rotation of the tibia. The aim of designing the mobile-bearing implants was to improve and reproduce the normal knee kinematics. The recent literature suggests that no mobile-bearing knee closely mimics the normal knee. Studies have shown that paradoxical femoral condyle anterior translation, reverse axial rotation and femoral condyle lift-off still occur similar to the fixed-bearing knees.[32,33] The range of movement achieved in the mobile bearing options is also not significantly greater when compared to posterior-stabilized implants.

Contact Stress and Wear

Wear in the poly occurs at the femur-poly surface (superior surface) and tibial-poly surface (backside wear) in both fixed-bearing and mobile-bearing knees. Two types of wear are common in the knee: abrasive wear and fatigue wear. The fatigue wear produces delamination and pitting of poly. An increase in the surface load produces the fatigue wear. This is commonly seen in the round on a flat surface where the contact stresses are more. Increasing the conformity decreases the contact stress and thus the fatigue wear. However, increasing the conformity also increases the constraint and thus more torque forces are distributed on the poly and on the cement-implant interface again producing wear and loosening. This is the constraint-conformity conflict. Mobile-bearing designs try to answer this conflict by providing low stress articulations and free rotations. There is a high rate of volumetric wear in the mobile bearing from two distinctive surfaces when compared to the fixed-bearing knees. It is important to understand that all these findings were noted in in vitro studies. Rotating platform devices also tolerate a moderate amount of tibial malrotation.

Reduction in Torque Forces

In the fixed-bearing knees, there is some amount of torque forces that is transmitted to the prosthesis bone interphase. These torque forces are less in flat designs. As the designs become more conforming, the amount of the torque force generated at the prosthesis bone interphase increases. Adding axial rotation in mobile-bearing knees is an attractive option to reduce these torque forces.

Breakage and Spin-off

Dislocation of the bearing and breakage are the two most commonly encountered problems with mobile bearings. Dislocation or subluxation produces soft tissue impingement. The rates have been described in the literature varying from 2.5 to 7.6%. A good surgical technique and proper flexion extension gap balancing are the keys to the prevention of these complications.

Summary

Mobile-bearing total knee replacements have theoretical advantage when compared to the fixed-bearing knees by providing better biomechanics. Better axial constraint and the increase in conformity reduce the wear rate. They also compensate for the tibial malrotation error to a certain extent. But long-term results clinically are yet to show the superiority compared to fixed bearing. The number of different designs available in the market makes a comparative study difficult. Mobile-bearing designs also need a better surgical technique and gap balancing for it to be successful.

KNEE BIOMECHANICS IN HIGH FLEXION

For a normal function, less than 120° of knee movement is required. In Eastern culture because of the habit of sitting cross-legged, squatting and kneeling, high flexion is needed.[34,35] Following TKA, the knee shows a reduced amount of posterior femoral translation and internal tibial rotation in flexion.[36,37] Another usual mechanism that occurs in high flexion in replaced knees is the lateral femoral condyle lift-off.[38] This femorotibial lift-off is a concern for wear and survival of the prosthesis.[39] Cam post-disengagement occurs at high knee flexion further assisted by posterior femoral translation. Although need for high flexion is well understood, instability and early loosening are still the concern in these high flexing knees.

GENDER DIFFERENCES IN KNEES

There are differences in bony anatomy of male and female knees.[40] Men have a higher anteroposterior height, transepicondylar width and lateral and medial condylar heights of the distal femur when compared to females.[41,42] For the same anteroposterior height of the distal femur, females have narrower transepicondylar width.[43] Trochlear groove is rotated internally in males and externally in females with respect to the transepicondylar axis.

Females have a larger Q angle.[44] Females have more patella alta (larger ratio between the patellar tendon and the greatest diagonal length of the patella in the lateral radiograph of the knee) and more negative congruence angle (lowest portion of the patella is more medial to the line bisecting the sulcus angle). At knee flexion angles of more than 30°, males have more patellofemoral contact area as compared to females.[45] Patellofemoral contact pressure is higher in females at 0°, 30° and 60° of knee flexion. But the literature has never proved the gender difference in the functional outcome when the same prosthesis is used for the knee replacement. The question of improvement in the survival in females after using a gender-specific knee is still to be proven.

REHABILITATION BIOMECHANICS

Narrow-based gait decreases the lateral shift of the center of gravity and conserves energy. Short steps and decreasing the rate of gait increase the double stance phase. Knowing the maximum quadriceps activity during gait cycle helps in rehabilitation. The quadriceps in an arthritic knee would have wasted and this will produce feeling of instability and giving way after TKA.

In patients who have walked with stiff knee gait preoperatively will have difficulty in relearning the controlled knee flexion between heel strike and toe off. Initially, they tend to stabilize their knees by hyperextending, producing capsular stretch posteriorly and posterior knee pain.

REFERENCES

1. Frankel VH, Burstein AH, Brooks DD. Biomechanics of internal derangement of the knee. J Bone Joint Surg Am. 1971;53:945-62.
2. Morrison JB. Bioengineering analysis of forces transmitted by the knee joint. Biomed J Eng. 1968;3:164.
3. Inman VT, Rolston HJ, Todd F. Human walking. Baltimore, MD: Williams & Wilkins; 1981.
4. Reilly DT, Martens Mt. Experimental analysis of quadriceps muscle force and patellofemoral joint reaction force for various activities. Acta Orthop Scand. 1972;43:126.
5. Buckwalter JA, Mankin HJ, Grodzinsky AJ. Articular cartilage and osteoarthritis. Instr Course Lect. 2005;54:465-80.
6. Felson DT, Naimark A, Anderson J, et al. The prevalence of knee osteoarthritis in the elderly. The Framingham Osteoarthritis Study. Arthritis Rheum. 1987;30:914-8.
7. Sharma L, Hurwitz DE, Thonar EJMA, et al. Knee adduction moment, serum hyaluronan level, and disease severity in medial tibiofemoral osteoarthritis. Arthritis Rheum. 1998;41:1223-40.
8. Sharma L, Dunlop DD, Cahue S, et al. Quadriceps strength and osteoarthritis progression in malaligned and lax knees. Ann Intern Med. 2003;138:613-9.
9. Aigner T, Rose J, Martin J, Buckwalter J. Aging theories of primary osteoarthritis: from epidemiology to molecular biology. Rejuvenation Res. 2004;7:134-45.

10. Buckwalter JA, Mankin HJ, Grodzinsky AJ. Articular cartilage and osteoarthritis. Instr Course Lect. 2005;54:465-80.
11. Buckwalter JA, Martin JA, Brown TD. Perspectives on chondrocyte mechanobiology and osteoarthritis. Biorheology. 2006;43:603-9.
12. Atkinson TS, Haut RC, Altiero NJ. An investigation of biphasic failure criteria for impact-induced fissuring of articular cartilage. J Biomech Eng. 1998;120:536-7.
13. Paley D, Pfeil J. Principles of deformity correction around the knee. Orthopade. 2000;29:18-38.
14. Tetsworth K, Paley D. Malalignment and degenerative arthropathy. Orthop Clin North Am. 1994;25:367-77.
15. McNicholas MJ, Rowley DI, McGurty D, et al. Total meniscectomy in adolescence. A thirty-year follow-up. J Bone Joint Surg Br. 2000;82:217-21.
16. Ahmed AM, Burke DL. *In vitro* measurement of static pressure distribution in synovial joints - part I: tibial surface of the knee. J Biomech Eng. 1983;105:216-25.
17. Lohmander LS, Englund PM, Dahl LL, Roos EM. The long-term consequence of anterior cruciate ligament and meniscus injuries: osteoarthritis. Am J Sports Med. 2007;35:1756-69.
18. Stern SH, Insall JN. Total knee arthroplasty with posterior cruciate ligament substitution designs. In: Insall JN, Windsor RE, Scott WN, Kelly MA, Aglietti P (Eds), Surgery of the knee, vol. 2, 2nd edn. New York: Churchill Livingstone; 1994. pp. 829-67.
19. Rand JA. Posterior cruciate retaining total knee arthroplasty. In: Morrey BF (Ed.), Reconstructive surgery of the joints, vol. 2, 2nd edn. New York: Churchill Livingstone; 1996. pp. 1401-8.
20. Barnes CL, Sledge CB. Total knee arthroplasty with posterior cruciate ligament retention designs. In: Insall JN, Windsor RE, Scott WN, Kelly MA, Aglietti P (Eds), Surgery of the knee, vol. 2, 2nd edn. New York: Churchill Livingstone; 1993. pp. 815-27.
21. Mahoney OM, Nobel PC, Rhoads DD, Alexander JW, Tullos HS. Posterior cruciate function following total knee arthroplasty: a biomechanical study. J Arthroplasty. 1994;9:569.
22. Andriacchi T. Gait analysis and total knee replacement. In: Insall J, Scott W, Scuderi GR (Eds), Current concepts in primary and revision total knee arthroplasty. Philadelphia, PA: Lippincott-Raven; 1996.
23. Wilson SA, McCann PD, Gotlin RS, et al. Comprehensive gait analysis in posterior-stabilized knee arthroplasty. J Arthroplasty. 1996;11:359.
24. Scuderi GR, Insall JN. Performance of posterior cruciate ligament substituting total knee arthroplasty. In: Insall JN, Scott WN, Scuderi GR (Eds), Current concepts in primary and revision total knee arthroplasty. Philadelphia, PA: Lippincott-Raven; 1996. pp. 41-5.
25. Connor JJ, Goodfellow JW. Theory and practice of meniscal knee replacement: designing against wear. ProcInst Mech Eng H. 1996;210:217-22.
26. Menchetti PPM, Walker PS. Mechanical evaluation of mobile bearing knees. Am J Knee Surg. 1997;10:73-82.
27. Walker PS, Sathasivam S. Design forms of total knee replacement. Proc Inst Mech Eng H. 2000;214:101-19.
28. Callaghan JJ, Insall JN, Greenwald AS, et al. Mobile-bearing knee replacement: concepts and results. J Bone Joint Surg Am. 2000;82:1020-41.
29. Hollister AM, Jatana S, Singh AK, Sullivan WW, Lupichuk AG. The axes of rotation of the knee. Clin Orthop. 1993;290:259-68.
30. Churchill DL, Incavo SJ, Johnson CC, Beynnon BD. The transepicondylar axis approximates the optimal flexion axis of the knee. Clin Orthop. 1998;356:111-8.
31. Walker PS, Sathasivam S. Controlling the motion of total knee replacements using intercondylar guide surfaces. J Orthop Res. 2000;18:48-55.
32. D'Lima DD, Trice M, Urquhart AG, Colwell CW Jr. Comparison between the kinematics of fixed and rotating bearing knee prostheses. Clin Orthop. 2000;380:151-7.
33. Insall JN, Aglietti P, Baldini A, Easley ME. Meniscal-bearing knee replacement. In: Insall JN, Scott WN (Eds), Surgery of the knee, 3rd edn. New York: Churchill Livingstone; 2001. pp. 1717-38.
34. Hemmerich A, Brown H, Smith S, Marthandam SS, Wyss UP. Hip, knee, and ankle kinematics of high range of motion activities of daily living. J Orthop Res. 2006;24:770-81.
35. Mulholland SJ, Wyss UP. Activities of daily living in non-Western cultures: range of motion requirements for hip and knee joint implants. Int J Rehabil Res. 2001;24:191-8.
36. Delport HP, Banks SA, De Schepper J, Bellemans J. A kinematic comparison of fixed- and mobile-bearing knee replacements. J Bone Joint Surg Br. 2006;88:1016-21.

37. Hanson GR, Suggs JF, Freiberg AA, Durbhakula S, Li G. Investigation of in vivo 6DOF total knee arthroplasty kinematics using a dual orthogonal fluoroscopic system. J Orthop Res. 2006;24:974-81.
38. Hanson GR, Park SE, Suggs JF, et al. *In vivo* kneeling biomechanics after posterior stabilized total knee arthroplasty. J Orthop Sci. 2007;12:476-83.
39. Jennings LM, Bell CJ, Ingham E, et al. The influence of femoral condylar lift-off on the wear of artificial knee joints. Proc Inst Mech Eng H. 2007;221:305-14.
40. Woodland LH, Francis RS. Parameters and comparisons of the quadriceps angle of college-aged men and women in the supine and standing positions. Am J Sports Med. 1992;20:208-11.
41. Poilvache PL, Insall JN, Scuderi GR, Font-Rodriguez DE. Rotational landmarks and sizing of the distal femur in total knee arthroplasty. Clin Orthop Relat Res. 1996;331:35-46.
42. Chin KR, Dalury DF, Zurakowski D, Scott RD. Intraoperative measurements of male and female distal femurs during primary total knee arthroplasty. J Knee Surg. 2002;15:213-7.
43. Hitt K, Shurman JR, Greene K, et al. Anthropometric measurements of the human knee: correlation to the sizing of current knee arthroplasty systems. J Bone Joint Surg Am. 2003;85:115-22.
44. Aglietti P, Insall JN, Cerulli G. Patellar pain and incongruence: I. Measurements of incongruence. Clin Orthop Relat Res. 1983;176:217-24.
45. Csintalan RP, Schulz MM, Woo J, McMahon PJ, Lee TQ. Gender differences in patellofemoral joint biomechanics. Clin Orthop Relat Res. 2002;402:260-9.

Chapter 3

Surgical Approaches to Total Knee Arthroplasty

Sharath K Rao, Sandeep Vijayan

INTRODUCTION

The surgical approach selected for total knee arthroplasty should be simple, surgeon-friendly and reproducible. For the surgeon, it is an important decision to choose the appropriate surgical approach. The approach selected should be flexible enough to adjust for intraoperative modifications and innovative enough for difficult primary cases.

ANATOMY

Thorough understanding of the local anatomy of the knee is essential for the surgeon to perform the various surgical approaches used in primary and revision total knee arthroplasty. Wound dehiscence and wound edge necrosis are the complications seen in the cases of revision and in primary knees with previous surgical scars. Because of this reason, it is essential to know the local blood supply to the skin and other different regions of the knee. Thorough knowledge of vascular anatomy also helps in preventing patellar osteonecrosis and postoperative hematomas.

Blood Supply to Skin

Blood supply to skin (**Figure 3.1**) around the knee is well documented. Microanatomical studies have demonstrated an anastomosis just superficial to the deep fascia. Perforators passing through the deep fascia feed this anastomosis.[1] Blood vessels penetrate the superficial fascia from this anastomosis to feed the skin (**Figure 3.1**). There is little or no communication between them in the superficial layer. Because of this reason superficial dissection above the deep fascia is likely to hamper the blood supply to the skin. For this reason, making an incision to 5–10 mm close to the old scar produces edge necrosis. Perforators to the skin usually come from the medial side from the saphenous artery.

Nerves are also similarly distributed traversing from medial to lateral. Infrapatellar branch of saphenous nerve is frequently transected in routine anterior and anteromedial incisions. This might leave a transient or permanent area of hypoesthesia on the anterolateral aspect of skin below the knee.

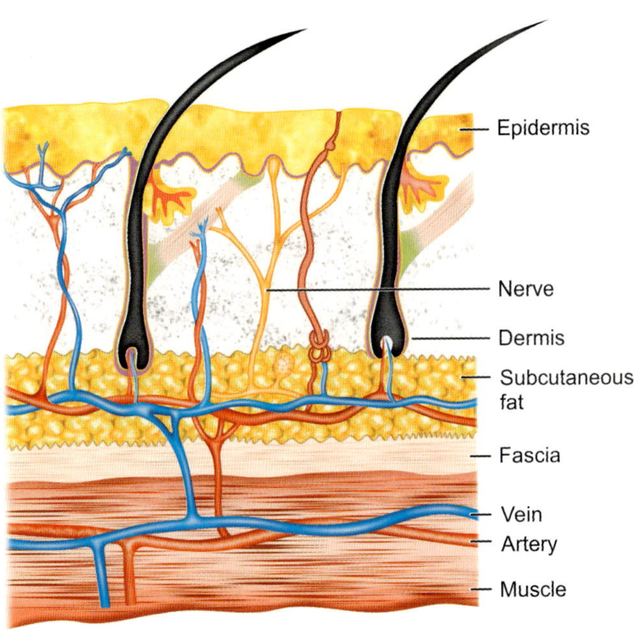

Figure 3.1 Blood supply to the skin over the knee

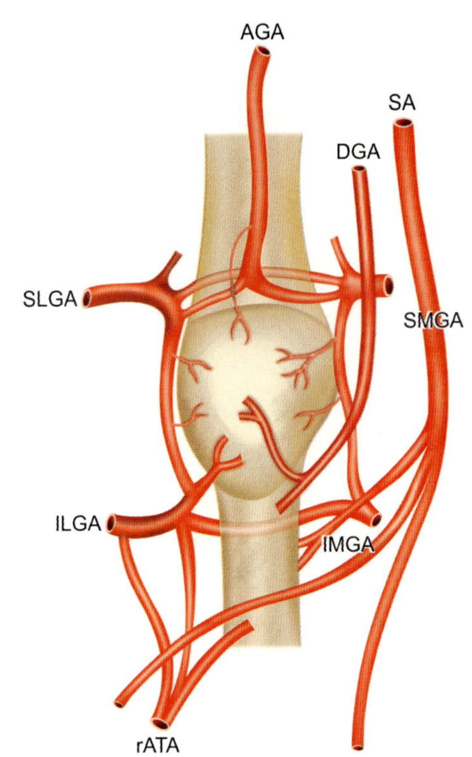

Figure 3.2 Blood supply to the patella and arterial anastomoses around the knee. *Abbreviations:* AGA, anterior genicular artery; DGA, descending genicular artery; SA, saphenous artery; SMGA, superior medial genicular artery; IMGA, inferior medial genicular artery, SLGA, superior lateral genicular artery; ILGA, inferior lateral genicular artery; rATA, recurrent branch of anterior tibial artery

Blood Supply to Patella

There is a rich plexus of arteries surrounding the patella (**Figure 3.2**). This plexus is contributed by four genicular arteries, namely superior medial genicular artery (SMGA), inferior medial genicular artery (IMGA), superior lateral genicular artery (SLGA) and inferior lateral genicular artery (ILGA). This plexus is also joined by descending genicular artery (DGA) and anterior tibial recurrent arteries (rATA).[2-4] Medial parapatellar incision will disrupt the three medial blood vessels feeding the plexus. If in addition lateral retinacular release is done, the lateral genicular vessel may also be disrupted. Excision of patellar fat pad disrupts the recurrent anterior tibial artery and excision of lateral meniscus disrupts the ILGA. Hence, the incidence of patellar vascular disruption and patellar fragmentation incidence are higher when medial parapatellar incision is combined with lateral release.[5,6]

Skin Incision

Vascularity of the skin on the anterior aspect of the knee is medially based; hence, lateral flaps are more hypoxic.[7,8] Basically, three skin incisions are described—anterior midline, medial parapatellar and curved medial (**Figure 3.3**). Medial parapatellar incision is oriented relative to Langer's lines.[9] During knee flexion, the medial parapatellar skin incision is under less tension as compared to anterior midline incision.[10] The curved medial approach is more likely to produce lateral flap hypoxia leading to wound dehiscence when compared to the anterior midline and medial parapatellar incisions. Based on its extensibility, and the authors need for further exposure and its potential for subsequent healing the anterior midline approach is prefered (**Figiure 3.4**). The incision is centered over the patella and extends proximally and distally to ~10 cm. Distally, it ends 1 cm medial to the tibial tubercle. The same skin incision can be readily used if there is the need of revision.

When there are previous scars, the longitudinal part of the scar is incorporated with the incision and the

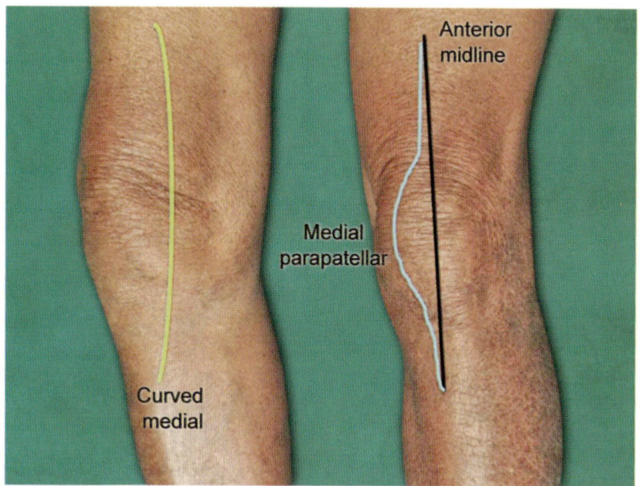

Figure 3.3 Basic skin incisions on the knee for total knee arthroplasty. Anterior midline (black), medial parapatellar (blue) and curved medial (yellow)

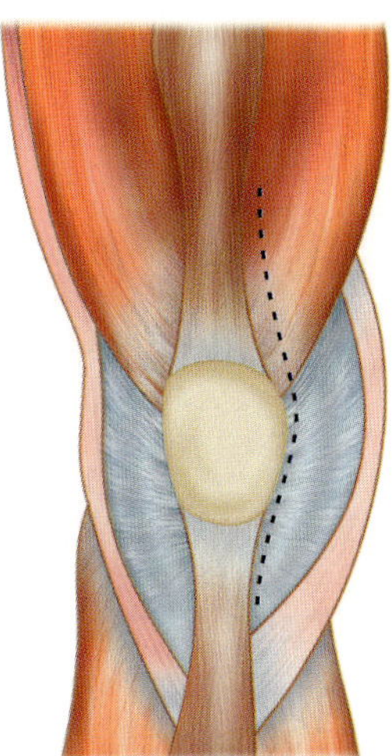

Figure 3.5 Langenbeck's medial parapatellar approach

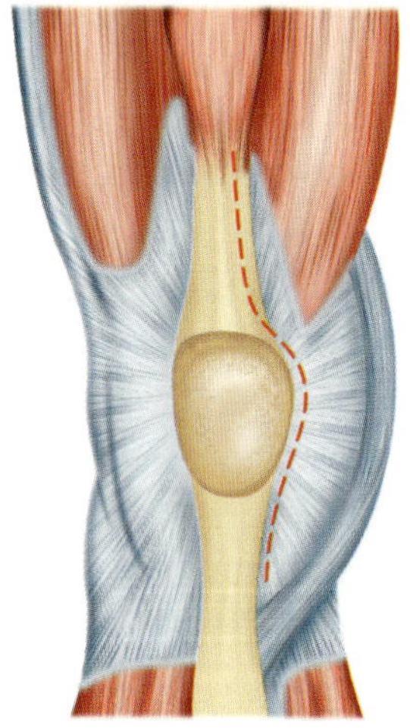

Figure 3.4 Authors preferred medial parapatellar approach

horizontal part of the scar is crossed vertically rather than at an acute angle to avoid necrosis. If there is more than one longitudinal scar, the lateral most scar is used for the incision.

Deep dissection after skin incision should be carried directly through the subcutaneous fat and deep fascia to the extensor mechanism. No flap should be elevated between the skin and fat especially on the lateral side to avoid hypoxia. This incision is made with the knee in flexion.

MEDIAL PARAPATELLAR APPROACH

Introduction

The medial parapatellar approach is the workhorse as far as any surgery on the knee joint is concerned. This is also the primary approach to total knee arthroplasty. Further modifications of this approach are described later to minimize the tissue damage, maximize the exposure and address specific problems.

Procedure

The original description of Langenbeck involved the superior dissection through the vastus medialis, which is no longer followed for the fear of knee stiffness (**Figure 3.5**). Insall's modification of incising the quadriceps tendon at the junction of medial one-third and lateral two-thirds is classically followed.[11] Insall described peeling of the quadriceps from the medial border of the patella (**Figure 3.6**). Langenbeck described leaving a cuff of tissue on the medial border of the patella for the future closure. Distally, incision is carried out 5 mm medial to the patellar tendon. The author's bias is to make the proximal incision 0.5–1 cm medial to the tendon. The incision leaves a 5 mm cuff of tissue attached to the medial border of the patella to facilitate closure. A 5 mm cuff of tissue is also

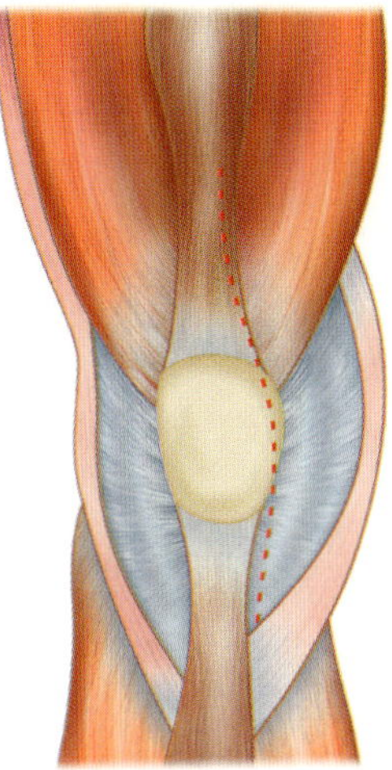

Figure 3.6 Insall's medial parapatellar approach

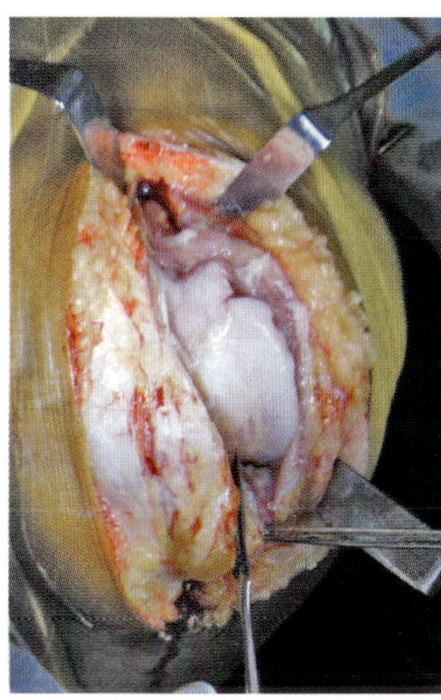

Figure 3.7 Cutting of the anterior horn of medial meniscus

left along the medial border of the patellar tendon. This entire deep dissection can easily be done with the knee in extension.

The anterior horn of medial meniscus is cut at this juncture (**Figure 3.7**). Further dissection can be done either in the extension or flexion of the knee depending on the surgeon's preference. The medial dissection is carried out at this juncture. The extent of medial dissection depends on the existing deformity. The external rotation of the tibia aids in this dissection.

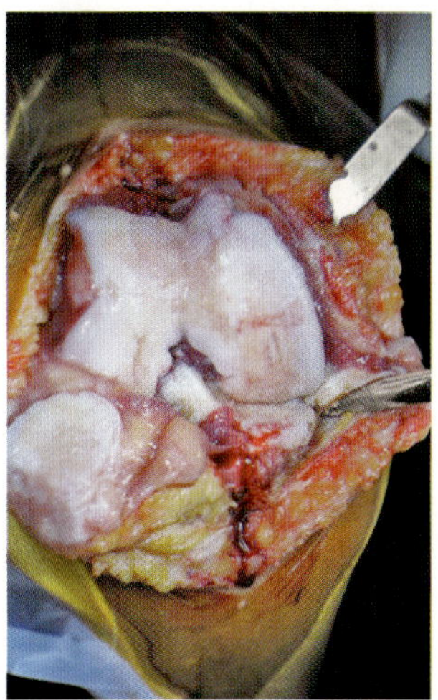

Figure 3.8 Medial dissection showing elevated periosteal sleeve with the medial meniscus

Initially, in the proximal tibia, medial release is done at least 1 cm distal from the joint line till the posteromedial aspect exposes the entire osteophytes. This is done either with cautery or the periosteal elevator. The author prefers to retain the entire medial meniscus with the sleeve at this juncture to protect the medial collateral ligament (**Figure 3.8**). Osteophytes from the medial side of tibia and femur are excised.

From here on, a systematic approach in a clockwise direction in the left knee and an anticlockwise direction in the right knee will greatly help.[12] The medial gutter is inspected, adhesions are released and excessive synovium is excised. Anterior synovium from the distal femur is reflected to expose the supracondylar region of the femur for anterior referencing. The lateral gutter is then inspected, adhesions are released and if needed synovectomy is performed. Osteophytes from the lateral femur are excised. The fat pad is detached from the meniscus and anterior horn of lateral meniscus is incised vertically. The excision of lateral meniscus at this stage helps in everting the patella. The patella is everted and the knee is slowly taken into flexion. When the knee is flexed and the patella is everted, the fat pad is assessed and some amount of fat pad may be excised, depending on the hypertrophy (**Figure 3.9**).

The anterior cruciate ligament is excised at this stage and the tibia can easily be subluxated forward.

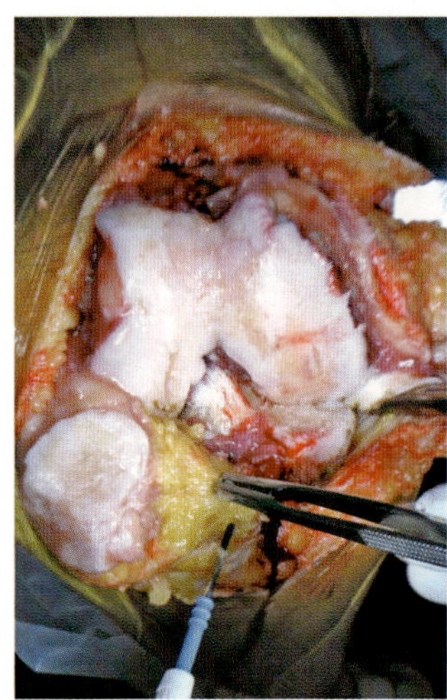

Figure 3.9 Partial removal of fat pad and patellar eversion

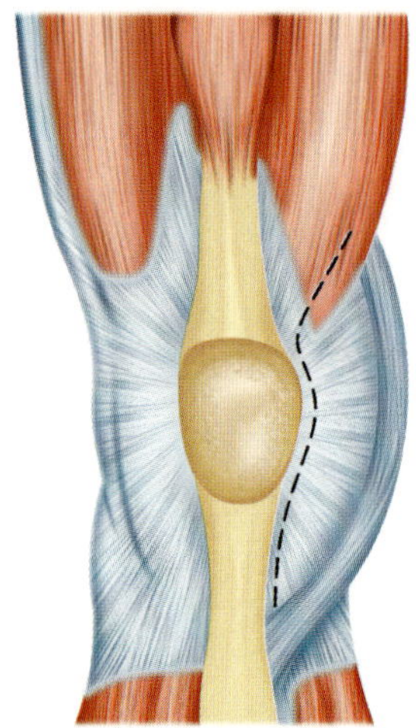

Figure 3.10 Midvastus approach

Surgical Tips

- Horizontal markings with the marking pen or electrocautery on the medial side of the patella on two cut edges of soft tissue helps in the proper approximation during later suturing.
- Release of lateral patellofemoral ligament and excision of the adequate fat pad help in the exposure of the lateral tibial plateau.
- If the patellar tendon is at risk of avulsion, fixation pins can be used at the tendon insertion.
- Retaining the medial meniscus till the end protects the medial sleeve of soft tissues, especially the medial collateral ligament.
- Resection of the lateral meniscus is done early for the better exposure of the lateral side.

MIDVASTUS APPROACH

Introduction

This approach was described and popularized by Engh and Parks.[13] Starting at the superomedial border of the patella, the vastus medialis muscle fibers are split (**Figure 3.10**). This approach maintains the intact extensor mechanism above the patella. The patellar blood supply is also less compromised. Parentis et al. observed electromyographic evidence of nerve injury while using this approach.[14] The relative contraindications to this approach are obesity, hypertrophic arthritis, flexion of less than 80° in the knee and previous high tibial osteotomy. If further exposure is needed, a quadriceps snip cannot be combined with this approach. For a further extensile approach, one has to combine tibial tubercle osteotomy with the midvastus approach.

Procedure

A standard anterior midline skin incision is made and dissection is continued through subcutaneous fat and superficial fascia. With the knee in flexion, vastus medialis muscle with its insertion to patella and quadriceps tendon is identified. The superomedial border of the patella is identified and the vastus medialis muscle is split 4 cm from the patella to its medial border. Underneath a capsule is incised leaving a cuff of tissue attached to the patella and the dissection is carried till the patellar tendon insertion to tibial tubercle. The joint is entered superiorly by incising the capsule deep to the split vastus medialis. Patella is everted and if necessary more of vastus medialis muscle can be split by blunt dissection. Closure of the capsule is done at 60° of knee flexion and the split muscle need not be sutured.

Surgical Tips

- The sharp dissection with a scalpel should be restricted only up to 4 cm from the patella into the vastus medialis muscle.
- Medial dissection on the proximal tibia is completed before trying to evert the patella. Further blunt dissection of the vastus medialis muscle while trying to evert the patella is facilitated by this medial dissection.

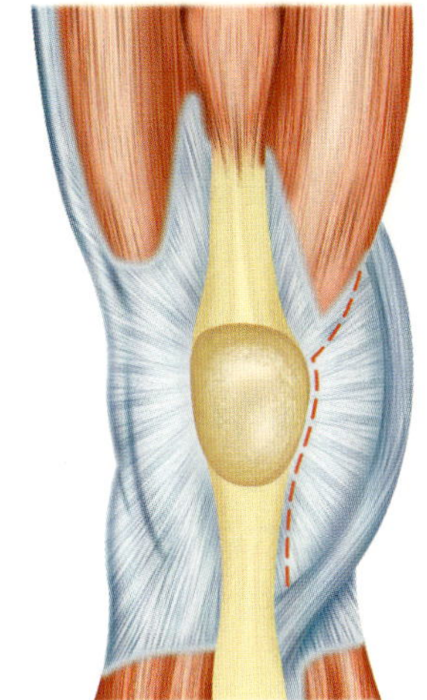

Figure 3.11 Subvastus approach

SUBVASTUS APPROACH

Introduction

This approach was popularized by Hoffmann et al.[15] This is a more anatomic nature of arthrotomy. The extensor mechanism is left intact (**Figure 3.11**). Patellar tracking is better with this approach and the incidence of lateral release is less. Medial vascularity of the patella is undisturbed and is an important issue when the lateral retinacular release is done for better patellar tracking. This approach is, however, difficult to use in obese patients' knees where previous arthrotomy was done, post-high-tibial osteotomy and in revision situations. The only way to convert this approach into an extensile approach is by doing a tibial tubercle osteotomy. Stiff knees and valgus knees that require a fair amount of dissection laterally may be contraindication for this approach.

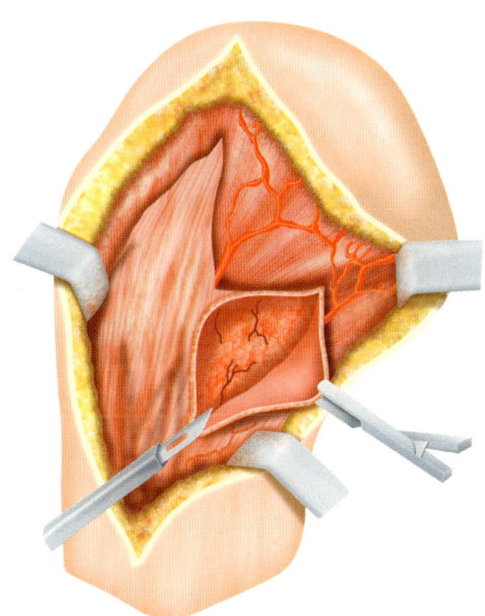

Figure 3.12 Subvastus—'L' incision on capsule

Procedure

A standard anterior midline skin incision is made and dissection is continued through subcutaneous fat and superficial fascia with knee in 90° of flexion. Blunt dissection is used to separate the epimuscular fascia from the vastus medialis down to its insertion. At this juncture, the knee can be extended and the inferior edge of the vastus medialis is identified. Vastus medialis muscle is lifted from the medial intermuscular septum and the periosteum using blunt finger dissection. At the midpatellar level, tendinous insertion of vastus medialis to the capsule is incised transversely (**Figure 3.12**). The entire extensor mechanism is retracted laterally and arthrotomy is done. The patella can be everted and the knee can be slowly flexed. Further dissection of the vastus medialis from the septum and periosteum can be done at this stage if needed. After arthroplasty, patellar tracking can be visualized through the inferomedial window. If lateral retinacular release is necessary it can be done from outside in, looking and palpating the tight structures. The capsular closure is done beginning at the apex of L-shaped incision.

Surgical Tips

- Extension of vastus medialis blunt dissection beyond 10 cm is avoided, because this dissection can injure the septal or articular branch of DGA artery.
- While using this approach, excessive dissection can be avoided if the entire arthroplasty procedure is done without everting the patella and by laterally displacing it.

LATERAL APPROACH

Introduction

Keblish is the originator of this approach for valgus knees.[16] In valgus knees, the lateral structures are tight and this approach directly deals with the contracted structures. With this approach, extensive lateral retinacular release is incorporated in the lateral arthrotomy. This approach naturally corrects the external rotation. The medial blood supply to patella is not hampered. With the medial approach and extensive lateral release, the blood supply to the patella may get jeopardized. The stability of the medial structures is not compromised with this approach. The posterolateral corner of the knee can be easily accessed with this approach.[17] Rehabilitation is easier since the medial tissues are intact. In stiff knees, the extensile approach can be used by adding either lateral to medial quadriceps snip or tibial tubercle osteotomy to this approach.

The disadvantages of this approach are relatively poor visualization of the medial side, difficult orientation to anatomy and difficulty in everting the patella medially. The large lateral defect may invariably be created but can be avoided by coronal Z plasty of soft tissues.

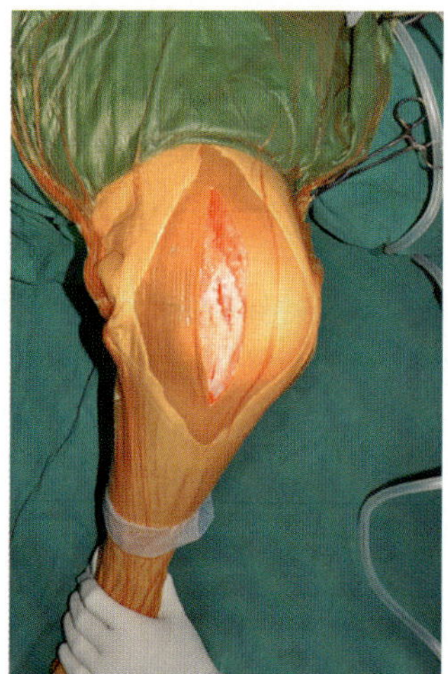

Figure 3.13 Skin incision for lateral approach

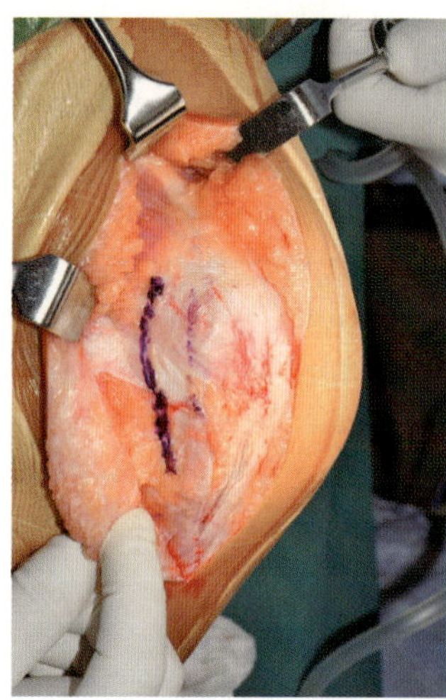

Figure 3.14 Coronal Z plasty—thick line represents the more lateral retinacular incision and thinner line the more medial capsulo-synovial incision

Procedure

Skin incision is on the lateral patellar border in line with the Q angle. The incision is taken lateral to the tibial tubercle by 1–2 cm (**Figure 3.13**).

The iliotibial (IT) band is exposed by separating the vastus lateralis muscle, and the IT band is fingerstriped from the femur till the posterolateral corner. Varus stress to knee in extension further tightens the IT band and 'pie crusting' and lengthening of the IT band is done under digital control. This release is performed 10 cm above the joint line.

The incision is extended superiorly to the center of the quadriceps tendon. The lateral retinaculum is divided laterally leaving 2–4 cm cuff of tissue attached to the patella. This is carried out till the middle of Gerdy's tubercle. Incision to the deeper capsule, synovium and fat pad is made medially almost at the rim of the patella (**Figures 3.14 and 3.15**). This ensures coronal soft tissue Z plasty (**Figures 3.16 and 3.17**). When the lateral edge of the retinaculum is sutured to the medial edge of

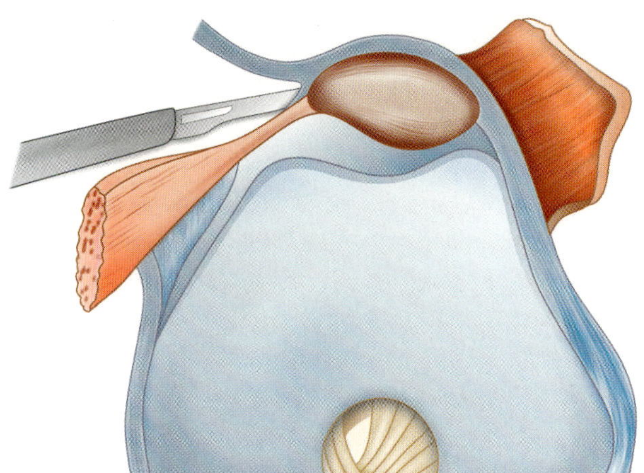

Figure 3.15 Cross-sectional diagram of coronal Z plasty incision

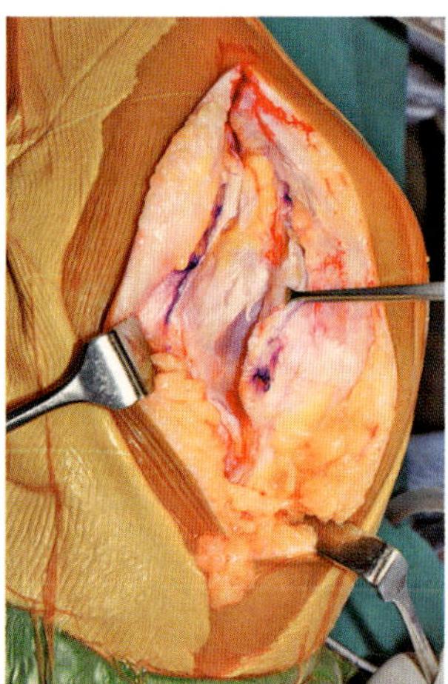

Figure 3.16 Coronal Z plasty showing the lateral incision of the retinaculum

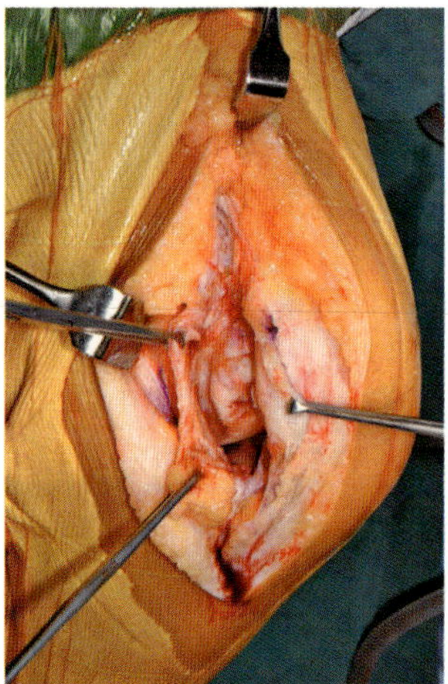

Figure 3.17 Coronal Z plasty showing the medial incision of the capsulo-synovial tissue and exposure of the joint

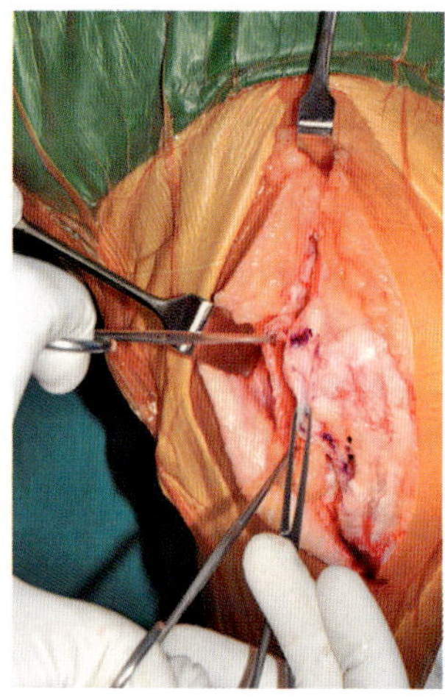

Figure 3.18 Coronal Z plasty showing the two layers to achieve closure

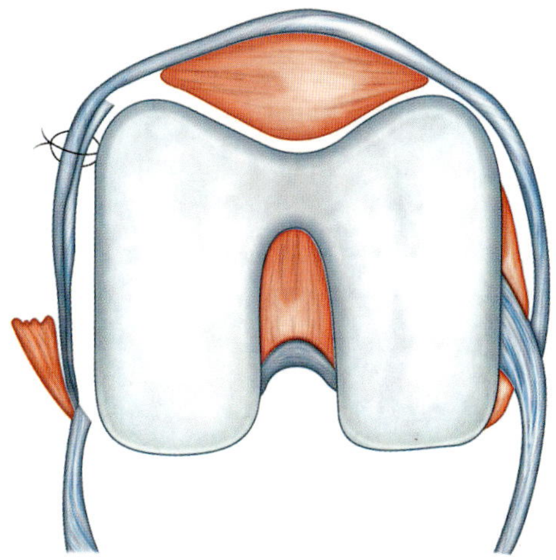

Figure 3.19 Coronal section diagram depicting the closure of the Z plasty

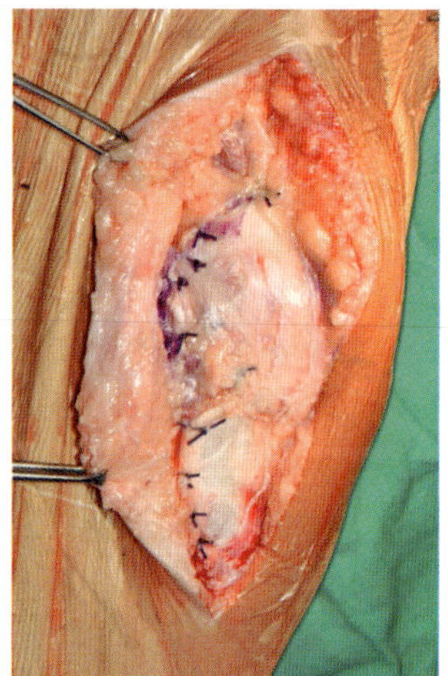

Figure 3.20 Final closure of the coronal Z plasty

capsule—synovial complex, the adequate soft tissue coverage of the prosthesis is achieved (**Figures 3.18 to 3.20**).

Keblish recommends elevating the fascial sleeve from the Gerdy's tubercle for valgus deformities of more than 40°. The patella can be dislocated or everted medially as the knee is flexed. This can be assisted by holding the patella with the Weber's forceps. Release of the soft tissue sleeve from the lateral tibia can be easily done. After completing the TKA, coronal Z plasty of the anterior soft tissue sleeve is closed as described earlier.

Surgical Tips

- Proximal quadriceps, middle vastus lateralis and inferior fat pad dissection need to be considered separately.
- The avulsion of the patellar tendon can be avoided by using fixation pins on the tibial tubercle.
- If the medial evertion or dislocation of the patella is problematic, the surgeon has two choices: either to do a tibial tubercle osteotomy or preferably a lateral to medial rectus (quadriceps) snip.

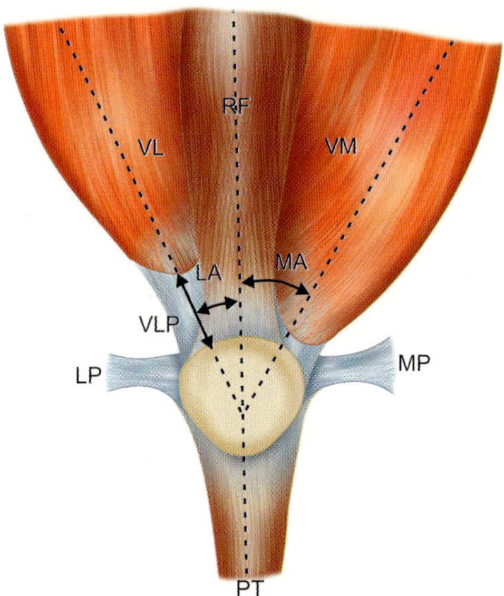

Figure 3.21 Principle of the trivector approach. *Abbreviations:* RF, rectus femoris; VM, vastus medialis; VL, vastus lateralis; MP, medial patellofemoral ligament; LP, lateral patellofemoral ligament; MA, angle between VM and RF (55–70°); LA, angle between VL and RF (22–45°); VLP, the distance between distal fibers of VL and superolateral corner of patella

TRIVECTOR APPROACH

Introduction

The trivector approach is based on the concept of the quadriceps pull of extension being directed in a trivector fashion and retaining the integrity of these three vectors (**Figure 3.21**). This is a good approach for optimal patellar tracking and to avoid patellar clunks.

Procedure

Standard midline skin incision is made. Quadriceps tendon and vastus medialis muscle junction is exposed. One to two cm cuff is retained medial to the patella and 1 cm medial to the patellar tendon. Superiorly, 1-2 cm medial to the quadriceps tendon and 6 cm superior to the patella, the vastus medialis is incised and continued inferiorly (**Figure 3.22**). Here the quadriceps tendon is not affected.

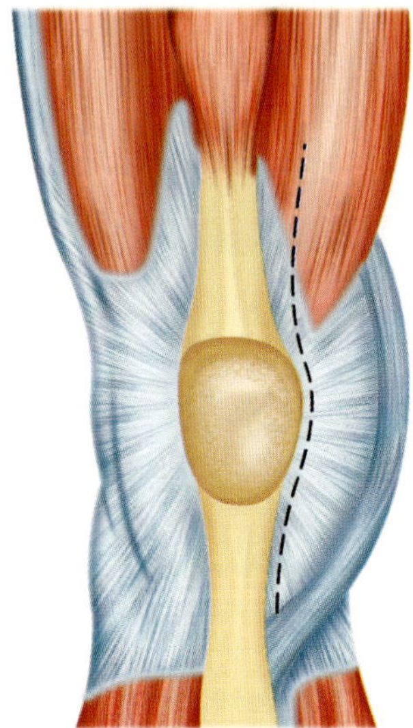

Figure 3.22 Trivector approach

Surgical Tips

At least 60% of the vastus medialis muscle fibers are kept intact on the medial side. Closure is preferably done in 100° of knee flexion.

QUADRICEPS (RECTUS) SNIP

Introduction

Quadriceps or rectus snip was described by Garvin.[18] This was further modified by Insall.[5] This is a technically simple procedure that can be easily combined with a medial parapatellar approach and is useful in stiff knees. It does not affect the recovery and the function of quadriceps muscle and invariably spares superior lateral genicular vessels.

Procedure

A standard medial parapatellar arthrotomy is performed. All the scar tissues from the lateral and medial gutters and osteophytes are removed. The guideline to do a lateral retinacular snip is when there is difficulty in everting the patella without placing the patellar tendon at risk. At this juncture, a decision on performing the quadriceps snip is taken. The proximal limit of the rectus incision is extended proximally and laterally at approximately 45° to transect the rectus femoris tendon at its musculotendinous junction. After this, the patella can be mobilized distally and laterally. If the exposure is inadequate, a lateral retinacular release can be added and if the exposure is still inadequate, quadriceps turndown is done.

Surgical Tips

- An attempt to preserve the SLGAs done to prevent the devascularization of the patella.
- Medial rectus snip can be done while using the lateral approach to the knee, to enhance the exposure.
- Active knee extension can be started immediately after surgery.

QUADRICEPS TURNDOWN

Introduction

This approach, initially described by Coonse and Adams, has undergone many modifications over the years.[19] This approach is preferred for stiff knee, ankylosed knee, severe varus, and revision knees. This approach should be used only if and after quadriceps snip is unable to expose the knee and evert the patella.[20]

Procedure

The anterior midline standard approach is applied. Medial and lateral parapatellar gutters are cleared off adhesions. Osteophytes from the femur and tibia are excised. The quadriceps snip is performed at an angle of 45° in the lateral oblique direction and extended proximally till the musculotendinous junction (**Figure 3.23**). If patellar eversion is still not possible, a lateral release is done (**Figure 3.24**). If the exposure is still limited, a quadriceps modified V-Y turndown is done by connecting the lateral release incision to the quadriceps snip incision (**Figure 3.25**). The patella along with the quadriceps tendon is turned down and kept moist with a wet gauze throughout the procedure (**Figure 3.26**). After the surgery, medial parapatellar and quadriceps snip are closed and the lateral release incision can be left open.

Surgical Tips

- The posterior aspect of the patellar tendon is released adequately before the procedure is undertaken.
- Vastus medialis and vastus lateralis bridges are kept intact for further suturing.

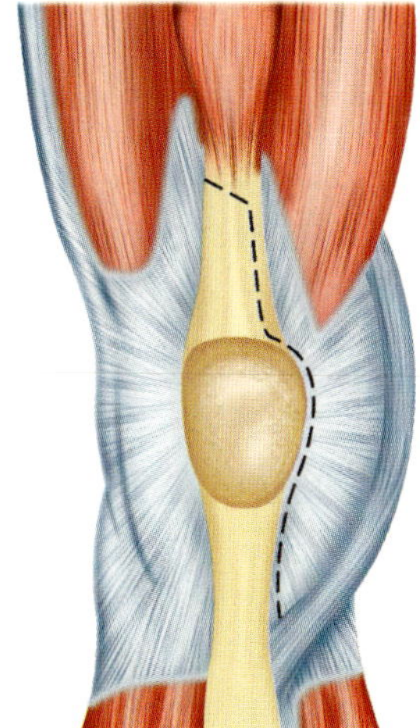

Figure 3.23 Quadriceps turndown—step 1 depicting a quadriceps snip

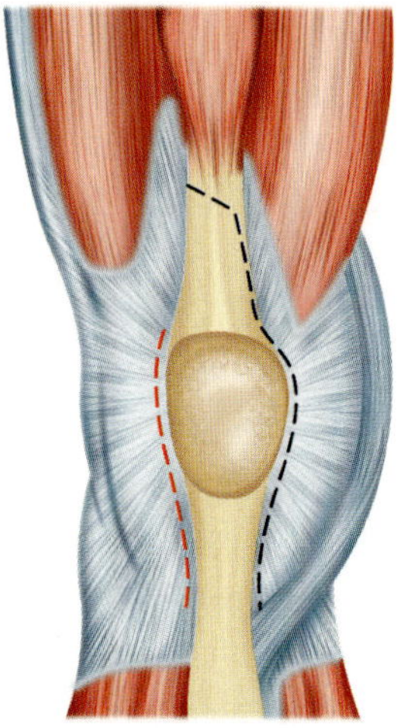

Figure 3.24 Quadriceps turndown—step 2 depicting lateral retinacular incision (red dotted lines) along with the quadriceps snip (black dotted lines)

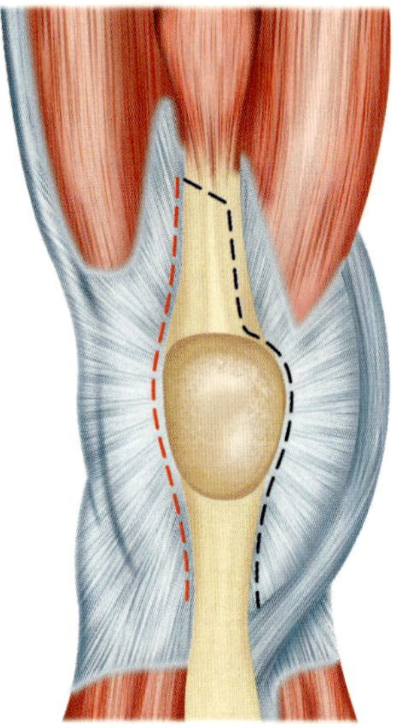

Figure 3.25 Quadriceps turndown—step 3 connecting the lateral retinacular incision to the rectus snip

- Usage of a fixation pin at the patellar tendon insertion is a useful technique to avoid the rupture of the patellar tendon.
- Knee bracing for two weeks is necessary after this procedure.
- While this approach affords excellent visibility, the persistent extensor lag is the major disadvantage that restricts its usage.

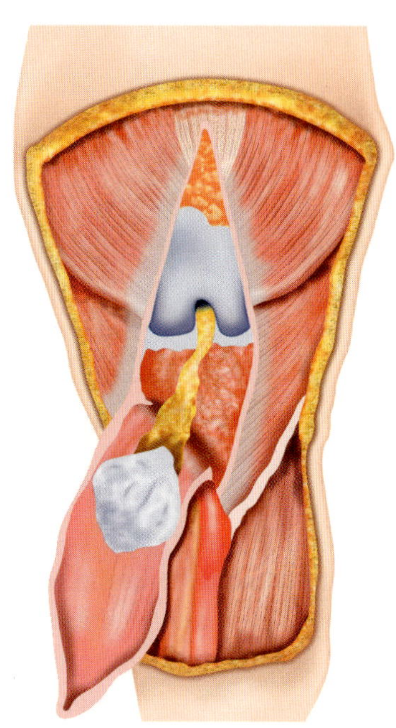

Figure 3.26 Quadriceps turned down

TIBIAL TUBERCLE OSTEOTOMY

Introduction

This is a technique adopted for stiff knees, when there is a patella baja, in revision situations and in previous severe varus deformities.[21,22]

Procedure

Anterior midline standard TKA incision that is extended distally medial to the tibial tubercle for 6–8 cm is made. An oscillating saw is used to do a transverse osteotomy of the tibial tubercle. The osteotomy extends at least 6–8 cm distally from the proximal edge of the tibial tubercle. A curved osteotome is used to complete the osteotomy laterally. The periosteal hinge and lateral muscular attachment are kept intact to the tubercle on the lateral side (**Figure 3.27**). The entire osteotomized fragment is osteoclased and the exposure completed. Three SS wires are necessary to repair the osteotomy and at least one of them should be through the medial cortex of the tibia (**Figure 3.28**).

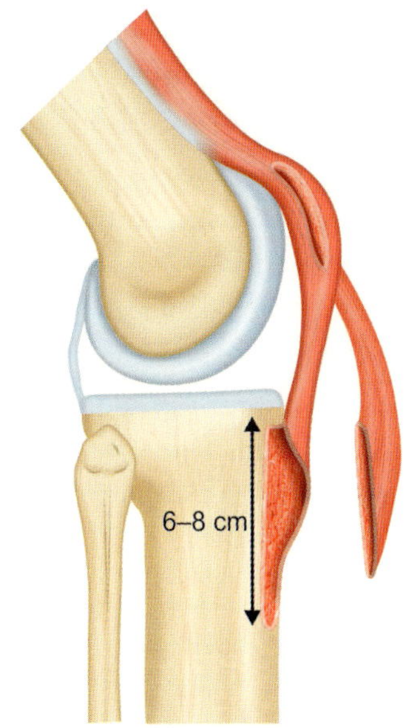

Figure 3.27 Tibial tubercle osteotomy

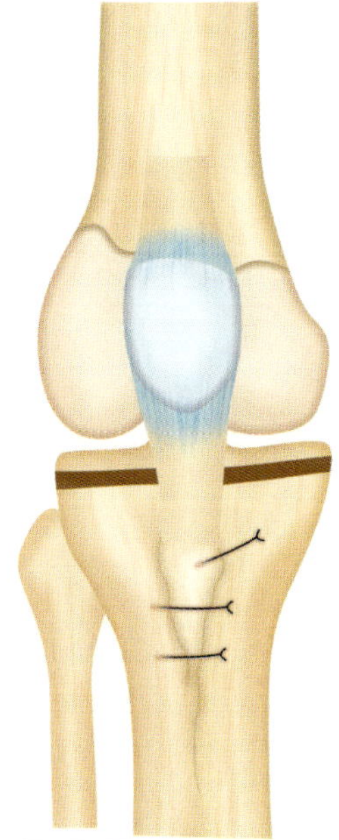

Figure 3.28 Tibial tubercle osteotomy fixation

Surgical Tips

- The skin incision is avoided on the tibial tubercle, but it is done medial to it.
- While using the tibial tray, using a stem to bypass the osteotomy safeguards the weak bone.
- Less than 3 cm of osteotomy length is avoided and fixing the osteotomy with screws is also avoided.
- In patients who kneel down, osteotomy is not a good choice because of skin irritation.

REFERENCES

1. Haertsch PA. The blood supply to the skin of the leg: a post-mortem investigation. Br J Plast Surg. 1981;34:470-77.
2. Scapinelli R. Blood supply of the human patella: its relation to ischaemic necrosis after fracture. J Bone Joint Surg Br. 1967;49:563-70.
3. Laskin RS. Soft tissue techniques in total knee replacement. In: Laskin RS (Ed.), Total knee replacement. London: Springer-Verlag; 1991. pp. 41-53.
4. Insall JN, Kelly MA. Anatomy. In: Insall JN, Windsor RE, Scott WN, Kelly MA, Aglietti P (Eds), Surgery of the knee, vol. 1, 2nd edn. New York: Churchill Livingstone; 1993. pp. 1-20.
5. Insall JN. Surgical approaches. In: Insall JN, Windsor RE, Scott WN, Kelly MA, Aglietti P (Eds), Surgery of the knee, vol. 1, 2nd edn. New York: Churchill Livingstone; 1993. pp. 135-48.
6. Ritter MA, Herbst SA, Keating EM, Faris PM, Meding JB. Patellofemoral complications following total knee arthroplasty: effect of a lateral release and sacrifice of the superior lateral genicular artery. J Arthroplasty. 1996;11:368-72.
7. Younger ASE, Duncan CP, Masri BA. Surgical approaches in revision total knee arthroplasty. J Am Acad Orthop Surg. 1998;6:55-64.
8. Johnson DP. Midline or parapatellar incision for knee arthroplasty. J Bone Joint Surg Br. 1988;70:656-8.
9. Langer K. On the anatomy and physiology of the skin. Br J Plast Surg. 1978;31:3-8.
10. Johnson DP, Houghton TA, Radford P. Anterior midline or medial parapatellar incision for arthroplasty of the knee. J Bone Joint Surg Br. 1986;68:812-4.
11. Insall J. A midline approach to the knee. J Bone Joint Surg Am. 1971;53:1584-6.
12. Douglas DR, Broune RB. In: Paul AL, Jess HL (Eds), Knee arthroplasty, vol. 1, 3rd edn. Philadelphia, PA: Lippincott Williams and Wilkins; 2009. pp. 1-18.
13. Engh GA, Parks NL. Surgical technique of the mid vastus arthrotomy. Clin Orthop. 1998;351:270-4.

14. Parentis MA, Rumi MN, Deol GS, et al. A comparison of the vastus splitting and median parapatellar approaches in total knee arthroplasty. Clin Orthop. 1999;367:107-16.
15. Hoffmann AA, Plaster RL, Murdock LE. Subvastus (southern) approach for primary total knee arthroplasty. Clin Orthop. 1991;269:70-7.
16. Keblish PA. The lateral approach to the valgus knee. Surgical technique and analysis of 53 cases with over two-year follow-up evaluation. Clin Orthop. 1991;271:52-62.
17. Munzinger V, Boldt J, Keblish P (Eds). Primary knee arthroplasty. Heidelberg: Springer-Verlag; 2005.
18. Garvin KL, Scuderi G, Insall JN. Evolution of the quadriceps snip. Clin Orthop. 1995;321:131-7.
19. Coonse K, Adams JD. A new operative approach to the knee joint. Surg Gynecol Obstet. 1943;77:344-7.
20. Scott RD, SIliski JM. The use of a modified V - Y quadricepsplasty during total knee replacement to gain exposure and improve flexion in the ankylosed knee. Orthopedics. 1985;8:45-8.
21. Whiteside LA. Exposure in difficult total knee arthroplasty using tibial tubercle osteotomy. Clin Orthop. 1995;321:32-5.
22. Whiteside LA, Ohl MD. Tibial tubercle osteotomy for exposure of the difficult total knee arthroplasty. Clin Orthop. 1990;260:6-9.

Chapter 4

Role of MRI in Evaluation of the Knee

Parveen Gulati, Amit Jawa

INTRODUCTION

The introduction of dedicated radiofrequency coils/digital radiofrequency technology, high magnetic field systems, and other technical advancements has made magnetic resonance imaging (MRI) the modality of choice for the evaluation of the knee. It has an established role in knee imaging for the evaluation of ligaments, articular cartilage, muscles, tendons, synovial structures or bursae, vessels, and subcutaneous tissue in addition to the evaluation of subchondral bone and bone marrow.

TECHNIQUE

The knee is ideally imaged using a dedicated knee coil in a 1.5 or 3.0 T MRI system for optimal quality. The patient lies supine, feet first with leg in full extension and mild external rotation. Imaging is performed in all three orthogonal planes—sagittal, axial, and coronal. The anatomy of the joint is complex, and it is essential to evaluate the joint in at least two planes, preferably in all three planes. Spin echo (SE), fast spin echo (FSE), various gradient echo (GRE) sequences, and 3D imaging sequences are used in various combinations depending upon the clinical indication. T1, T2, proton density (PD) and FATSAT images are obtained—T1/PD images being ideal to assess the normal anatomy and FATSAT/T2 images to assess the pathology. The sagittal plane is best for evaluating the cruciate ligaments and menisci with other views for confirming the pathology. Likewise, collateral ligaments are best viewed in the coronal plane. The tibiofemoral articular cartilage is best assessed in the sagittal and coronal planes, while the patellofemoral articular cartilage is seen best in the axial plane. Dedicated cartilage imaging is performed using special sequences with the calculation of T2* relaxation values of the cartilage at various points and creation of cartigrams.

MR arthrography combines the technique of arthrography with MRI to benefit from the added imaging information afforded by intra-articular distention. It is most commonly used for the evaluation of recurrent meniscal tears after partial meniscectomy or meniscal repair. In patients with partial meniscectomy, retears may demonstrate contrast tracking into the substance of the meniscus. Menisci that have not retorn should not depict the intrasubstance extension of contrast. MR arthrography can also be useful to further evaluate the articular hyaline cartilage and has been shown to provide an advantage over conventional MRI when evaluating the stability of chondral and osseous fragments. The presence of intra-articular contrast better demonstrates the size and depth of defects in the articular cartilage and can assist when grading chondromalacia. When contrast is seen tracking between cartilaginous flap tears and subchondral bone, it strongly suggests fragment instability. Loose bodies are also better delineated when surrounded by contrast and can be differentiated from synovial processes when the diagnosis is unclear on conventional images.

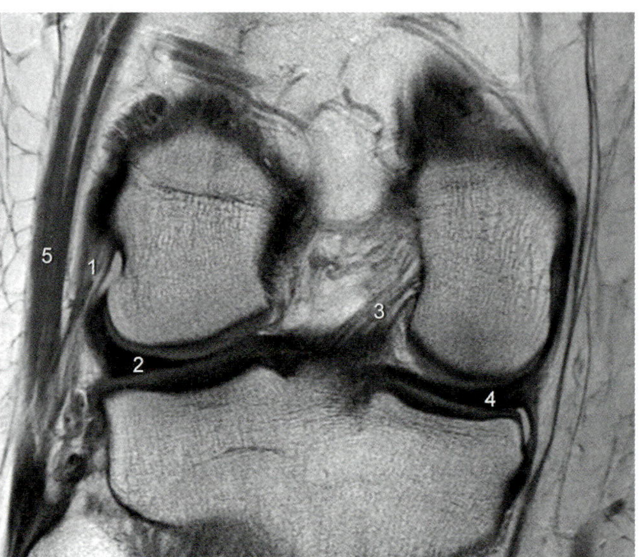

Figure 4.1 Coronal PD image showing lateral collateral ligament (1), posterior horn of lateral meniscus (2), posterior cruciate ligament (3), posterior horn of medial meniscus (4), biceps femoris (5). Note homogeneous low-intense signal of the meniscus

MENISCI

Normal menisci are triangular in shape in the sagittal plane and normally measure about 3–5 mm in height. The medial meniscus measures about 6 mm in width at the anterior horn to about 12 mm at the posterior horn. The lateral meniscus is about 10 mm in width uniformly (**Figures 4.1 to 4.3**). The normal menisci show a diffusely homogeneous low signal on all MRI sequences.

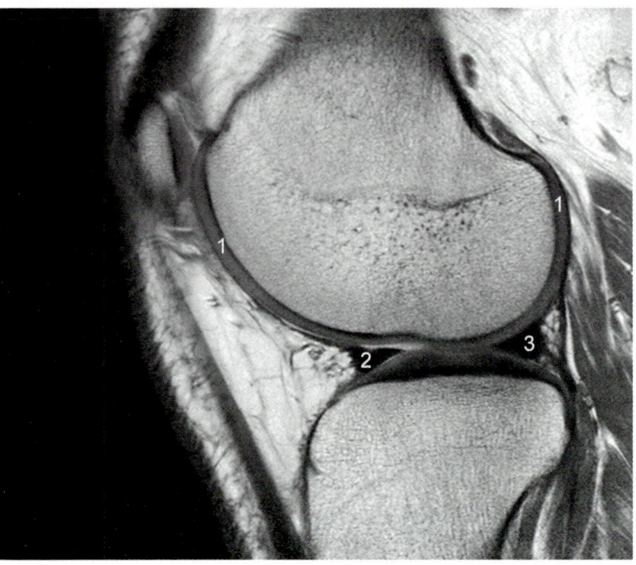

Figure 4.2 Sagittal PD image showing articular cartilage (1), anterior horn of medial meniscus (2), posterior horn of the medial meniscus (3). Note homogeneous low-intense signal of the meniscus

Meniscal Tear

Meniscal degeneration and meniscal tears exhibit increased signal intensity on T2-weighted and short-tau inversion recovery (STIR) images. Increased signal intensity within the menisci is categorized into three grades depending upon its configuration and its relation to the articular surface of meniscus.[1]

Grade 1 signal—a focal intrasubstance hyperintense signal on T2 or STIR images. It may represent early mucinous degeneration and is not clinically significant.

Grade 2 signal—is a linear, horizontal intrasubstance hyperintense signal not communicating with the meniscal articular surface.

Grade 1 and grade 2 signals in the menisci do not represent tears. These may or may not progress to tears.

Grade 3 signal—is actually a meniscal tear where the hyperintense intrameniscal signal is seen to communicate with at least one of the meniscal articular surfaces. Two findings on MRI that are diagnostic for tears are—the increased signal on T2 as well as PD images (**Figures 4.4A and B**) unequivocally reaching an articular surface and an abnormal shape of menisci with no prior history of surgery.

The treatment of meniscal tears depends upon the type, location, and extent of the tear. Most of the information required can be obtained with MRI.

A meniscal tear is either horizontal or vertical. Vertical tears can be longitudinal or radial depending on the axis of the meniscus. A complex tear is a combination of these tears.

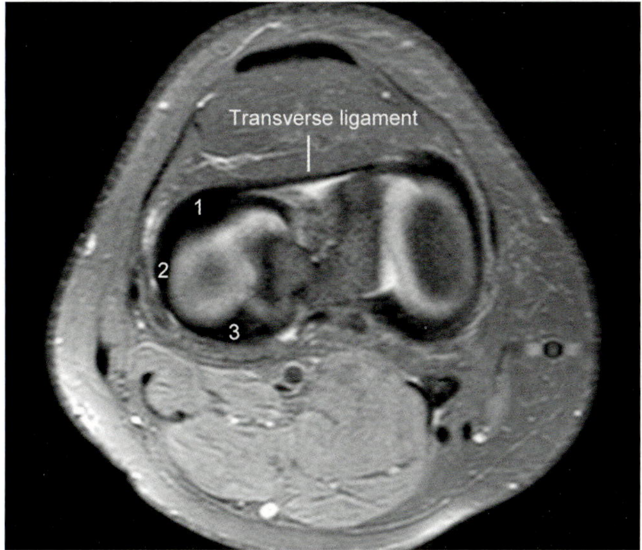

Figure 4.3 Axial FATSAT sequence showing transverse ligament, anterior horn (1), body (2) and posterior horn (3) of lateral meniscus. All three components of medial meniscus are also well seen

Horizontal meniscal tears or cleavage tears, also called the fishmouth tear or parrot tear, are parallel to the tibial plateau and divide the meniscus into the superior and inferior fragments.[2] These tears are usually secondary to meniscal degeneration and may be associated with an intrameniscal or parameniscal cyst.

The diagnostic feature suggestive of: a longitudinal tear parallel to the outer margin of the meniscus and the point where the tear contacts the articular surface remains at the same distance from the outer margin on the sequential images. They usually involve the posterior horn initially. A Bucket Handle tear is a displaced longitudinal tear. A displaced meniscal fragment may lodge in the intercondylar notch to give a 'double posterior cruciate ligament (PCL) sign'[3] (**Figures 4.5A to D**). The displaced meniscal fragment may flip over the anterior horn of the affected meniscus. A truncated inner margin of the meniscus on coronal images can indicate a meniscal tear.

Radial tears are perpendicular to the long axis of the meniscus. These tears usually begin at the inner margin and extend peripherally to a variable distance. These tears are frequently missed on MRI.

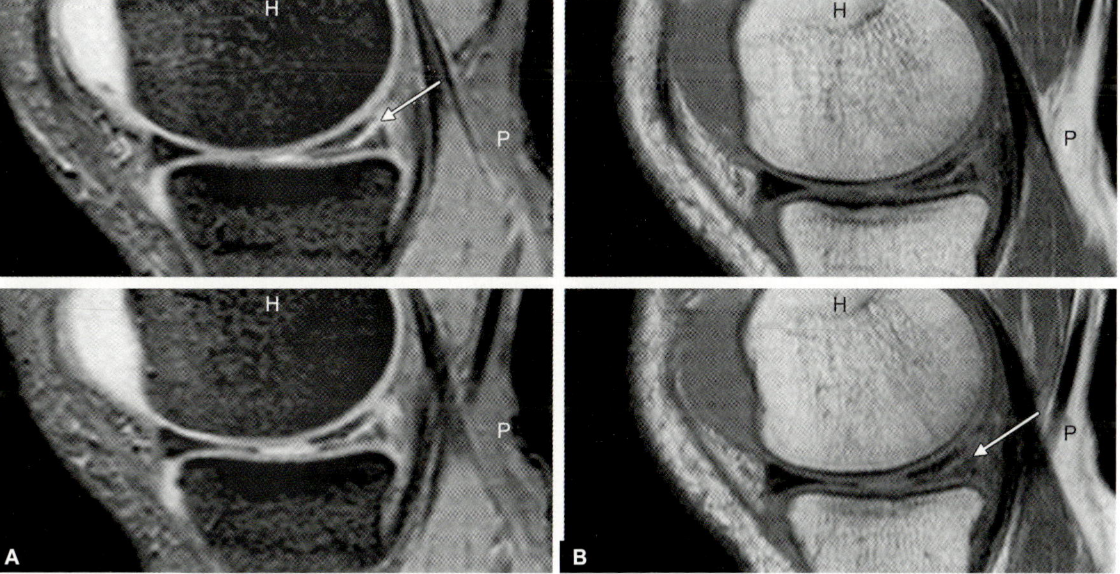

Figures 4.4A and B Sagittal STIR and PD weighted images showing horizontal-cleavage tear of posterior horn of medial meniscus seen as linear horizontal fluid signal (arrow)

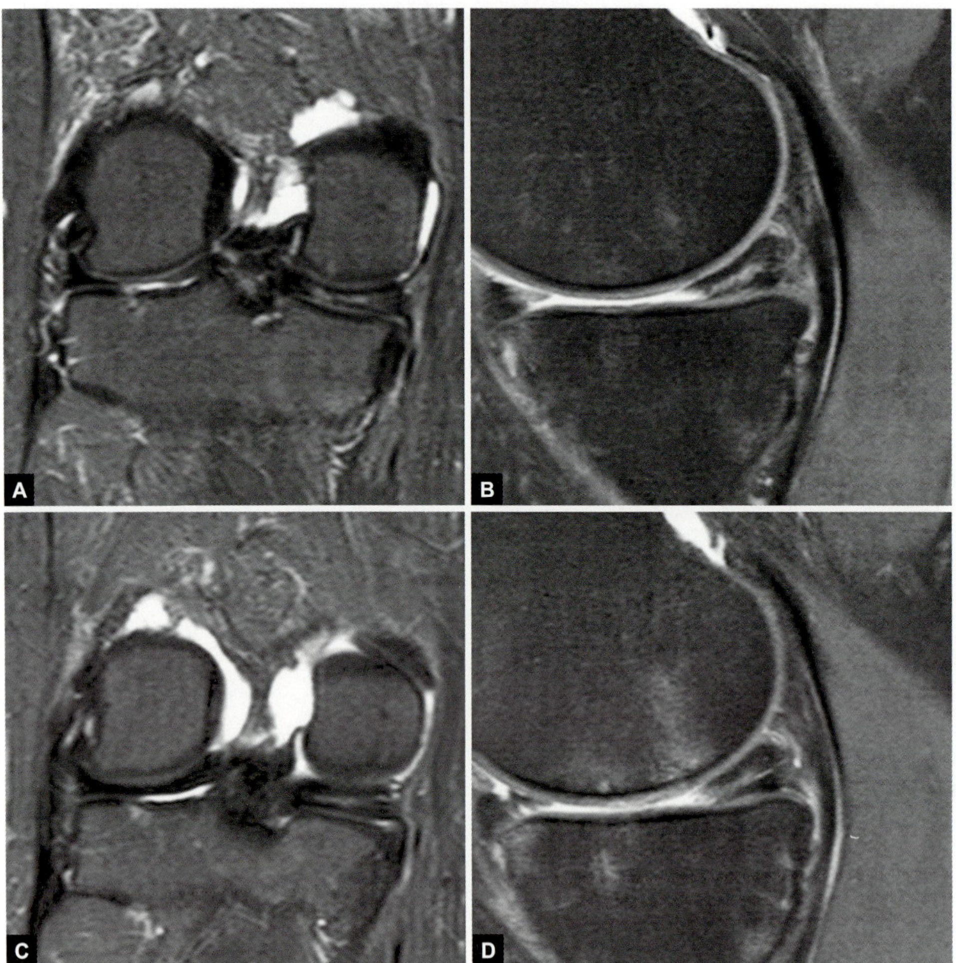

Figures 4.5A to D Coronal (A and C) and sagittal (B and D) STIR images showing a linear hyperintense signal in the posterior horn of the medial meniscus dividing it into upper and lower portion suggestive of horizontal tear

A meniscal root tear (**Figures 4.6A to D**) is a radial tear at the meniscal root or at its tibial attachment.[4] Root tears and complete radial tears are usually associated with meniscal extrusion.[5]

An oblique tear, also called the Parrot Beak tear, is a type of radial tear beginning radially at the inner meniscal edge and then taking a curve into a longitudinal orientation as it extends peripherally.

A peripheral tear is a tear involving the outer one-third of the meniscus. These tears are likely to heal with conservative therapy due to good blood supply in the peripheral zone.

A discoid meniscus (**Figures 4.7A and B**) is an anatomic variant in which the meniscus is abnormally large and is disk shaped (commonly lateral meniscus). On sagittal MR images, a discoid meniscus exhibits continuous or bow-tie appearance on 3 or more consecutive 4 mm slice thickness or a meniscal body on coronal images more than 15 mm in width or extending into the intercondylar notch.[6] These menisci are more prone to tears and degeneration.

Meniscal extrusion: Extrusion of the medial meniscus more than 3 mm and extrusion of the lateral meniscus more than 1 mm are abnormal. These are measured from the outer meniscal edge to the tibial margin.

Meniscal ossicles are small ossific foci found typically in the posterior horn of the medial meniscus. They are associated with meniscal tears and can be asymptomatic.

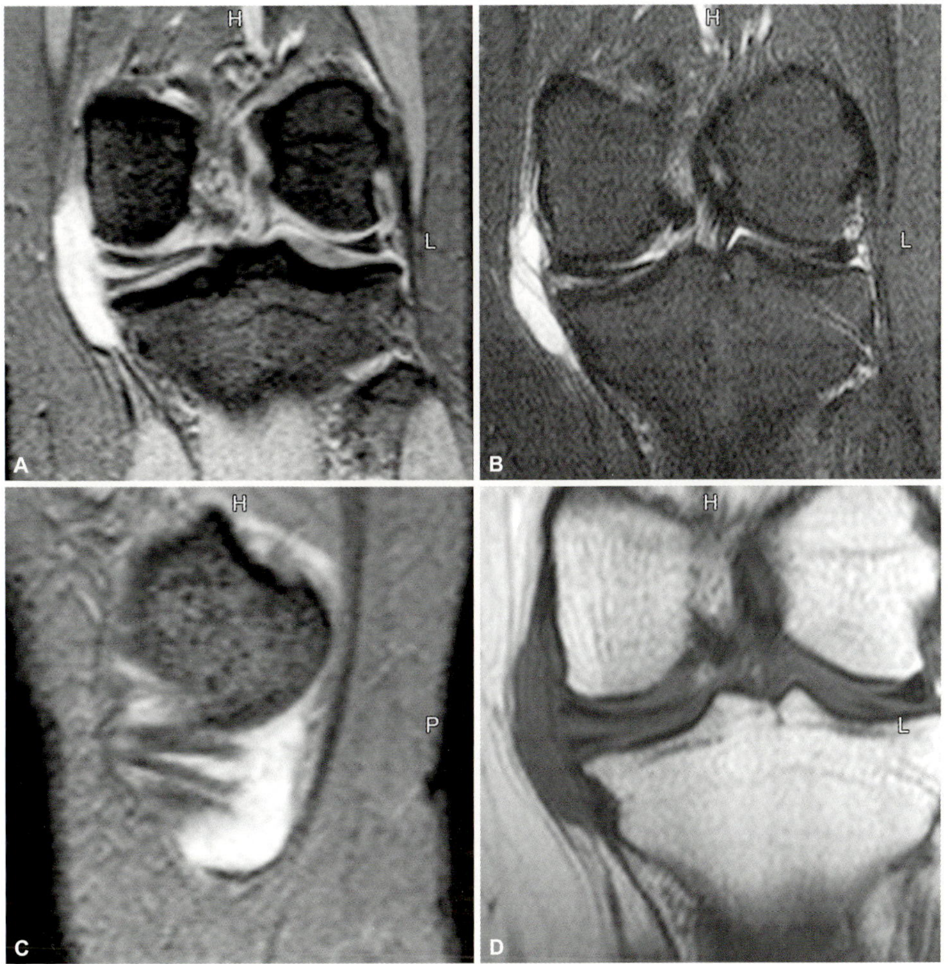

Figures 4.6A to D Coronal STIR (A and B); Sagittal STIR (C) and coronal PD (D) images show a horizontal cleavage tear of the posterior horn of medial meniscus with parameniscal cyst

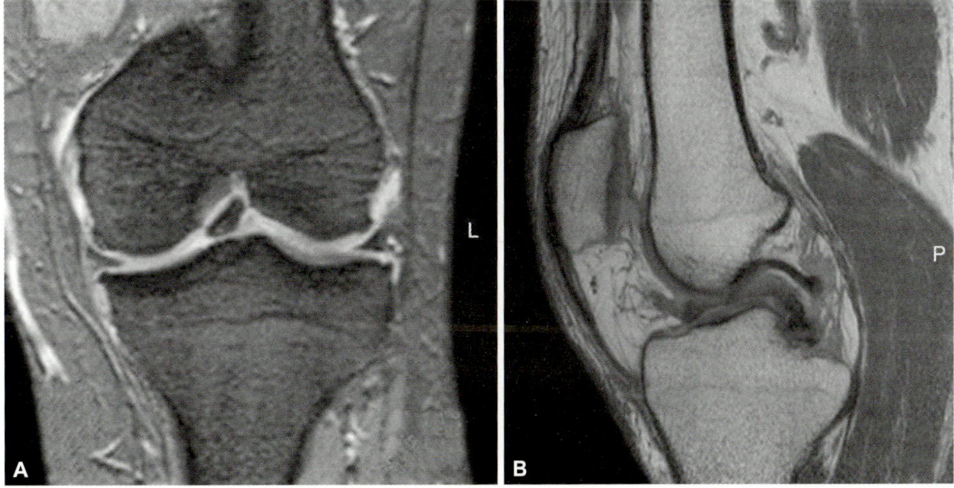

Figures 4.7A and B Coronal T2 (A) and sagittal PD (B) images showing a bucket handle tear of the medial meniscus with torn fragment flipped to intercondylar notch giving a double PCL sign on sagittal image

Postoperative Meniscus

Magnetic resonance imaging especially with standard protocols is relatively less reliable for the evaluation of postoperative menisci. Contour abnormalities and signal intensity abnormalities reaching the articular surface are less reliable signs of meniscal tears with an accuracy of 66–80% that is much less compared to the accuracy for primary tears. The specific but not sensitive signs for retears in an operated meniscus are high signal intensity fluid on T2 or STIR images extending into a cleft within the meniscal fragment or a displaced meniscal fragment.[7,8] The accuracy for diagnosing meniscal tears in postoperative cases can be improved by performing an MR arthrogram. A tear on the arthrogram will be seen as an area of an increased signal within the meniscal fragment.

All knee pains following meniscal surgery may not be due to retears, and it is also essential to assess osseous as well as chondral lesions.

CRUCIATE LIGAMENTS

Anterior Cruciate Ligament

Anterior cruciate ligament (ACL) is a fan-shaped ligament within the lateral aspect of the intercondylar notch coursing

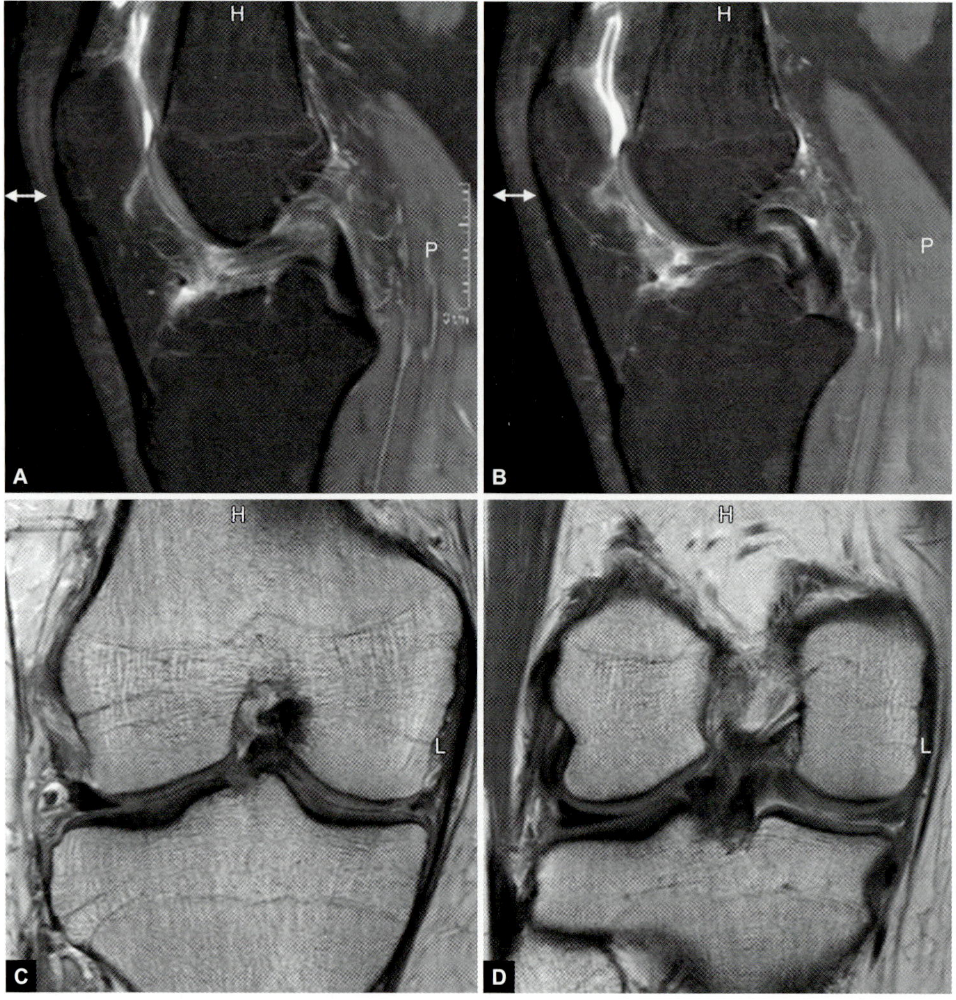

Figures 4.8A to D STIR sagittal (A and B) and coronal PD (C and D) show displaced bucket handle tear of medial meniscus with sagittal images demonstrating double PCL sign—displaced meniscal fragment anterior and parallel to PCL. There is associated tear of the anterior cruciate ligament

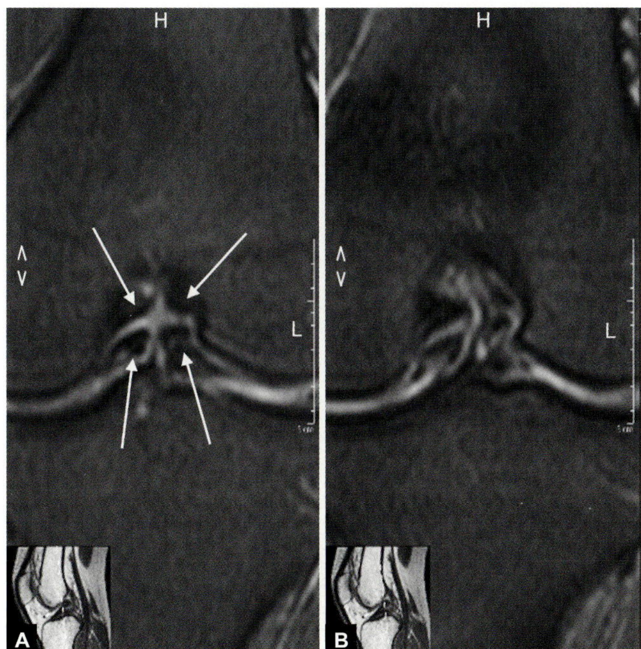

Figures 4.9A and B Coronal STIR images reveal two additional structures in the intercondylar notch apart from ACl and PCL consistent with displaced bucket handle tear of both medial and lateral meniscus—"Quadruple cruciate sign"

parallel to the roof of the intercondylar notch. It is an intra-articular extrasynovial structure. It has two components—the anteromedial bundle and the posterolateral bundle. The normal ACL is straightened and appears isointense to hypointense on all imaging sequences. The ACL is best evaluated on the sagittal PD and STIR images (**Figures 4.8A to D**).

On MRI, the primary signs of ACL tears are: abnormal course, abnormal signal intensity, and discontinuity (**Figures 4.9A and B**). The ACL course can be assessed by measuring the Blumensaat angle—the angle between the Blumensaat line (the line parallel to the roof of the intercondylar notch) and a line along the distal portion of the ACL. An angle of more than 10° is highly suggestive of ACL tear. The signal alteration may be focal or diffuse and is usually seen as a hyperintense signal on T2 and FATSAT (STIR) images.

An acute or subacute tear is seen as a hyperintense signal on T2W and PD images. The locations of the tear may be proximal, midsubstance, distal, or at the femoral/tibial attachment.

Injuries commonly associated with the ACL tear are[9,10] as follows.

- Bone bruises at the posterior lateral tibial plateau (most sensitive secondary sign) and midlateral femoral condyle. These are seen as areas of the heterogeneous hyperintense signal on T2 and STIR images and the iso- to low-intense signal on T1-weighted and PD images.
- Impaction fracture along the lateral femoral condyle.
- Avulsion fracture involving the lateral tibial rim—Segond fracture.
- Anterior tibial subluxation/translocation >5–7 mm with respect to the posterior aspect of the femoral condyle on sagittal images.
- Posterior cruciate ligament buckling—any reduction in the PCL angle from 115°.

Meniscal injuries are frequently associated with ACL tears, with the medial meniscus showing tears more frequently than the lateral.

Avulsion of the ACL from the tibial attachment site is more common in children/young adults[10] (**Figures 4.10A to D**).

An ACL ganglion is usually an incidental finding and should not be confused with a tear. The exact etiopathogenesis of a ganglion is not clear but is usually attributed to mucinous degeneration. On MRI, the ganglia may present as discrete fluid signal intensity cystic structures within the substance of the ligament or on the surface or it may give a celery stalk appearance—ligament showing diffuse thickening with intrasubstance hyperintensity on T2 or FATSAT PD images. It can be differentiated from an ACL tear by demonstrating fibers coursing through the ligament substance[11,12] (**Figures 4.11A and B**).

ACL Reconstruction

An ACL is the most commonly reconstructed ligament of the body. The clinical evaluation of the postoperative knee may be difficult. MRI is the imaging modality of choice for assessing the integrity of the ACL graft as well as in diagnosing any complication.

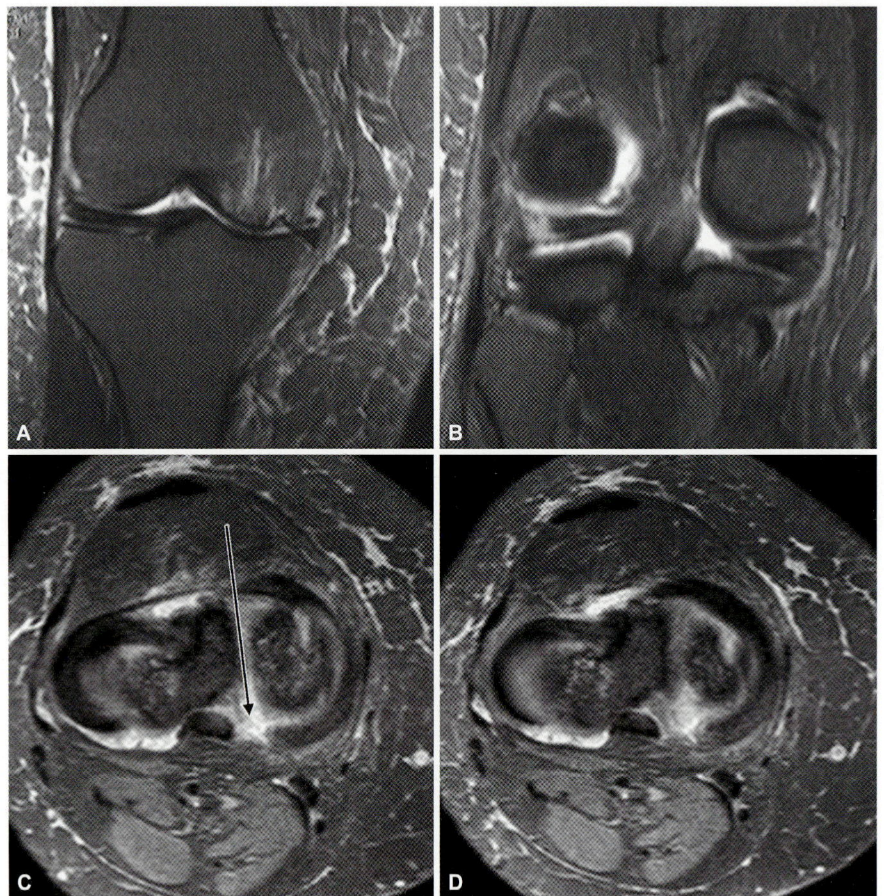

Figures 4.10A to D Coronal (A and B) and axial (C and D) STIR images showing posterior root tear of medial meniscus seen as fluid filled gap with medial extrusion of medial meniscus. Other findings are sprain of MCL and subchondral marrow edema in medial femoral condyle

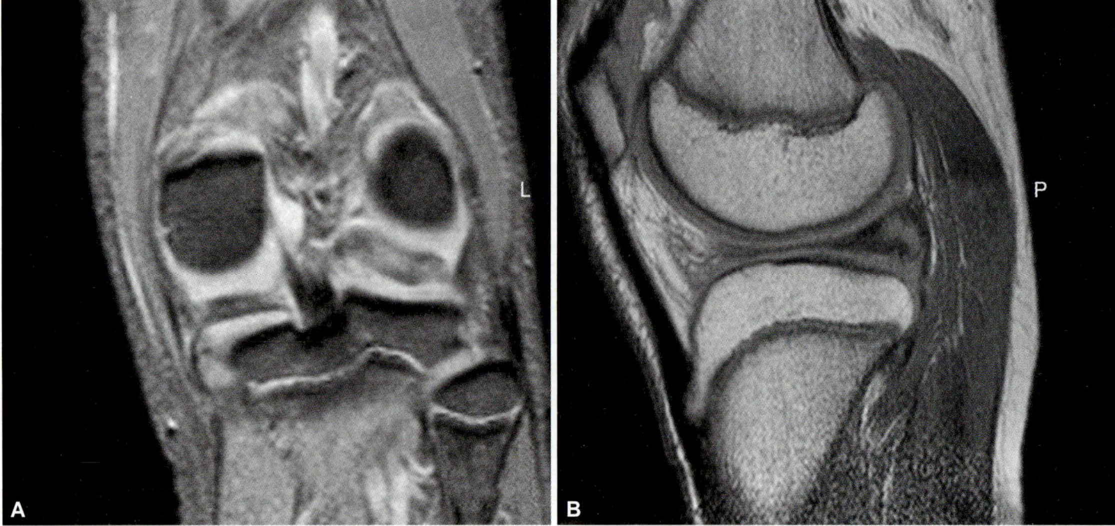

Figures 4.11A and B Coronal T2 (A) and sagittal PD (B) images showing bulky posterior horn of the medial meniscus suggestive of discoid meniscus. There is associated intrameniscal hyperintense signal suggestive of myxoid degeneration

Normal Postoperative Appearance

The femoral graft tunnel should normally be located at the junction of the intercondylar roof and posterior femoral cortex on sagittal images. The tibial tunnel should normally be located parallel and posterior to the Blumensaat line between the anterior tibial tubercle and the posterior border of the tibia near the midline. The normal femoral tunnel should be at 11 o'clock in the right and at 1 o'clock in the left knee on coronal images and should open on the intercondylar eminence.[7,13]

The MRI signal of the graft depends on its composition and postoperative period. By 5–8 months, the graft can be seen as a focal or diffusely increased T2 hyperintensity. After 1 year, the graft returns to its normal low signal.

Complications of an ACL graft[7,13-15] are as follows.

- *Graft tear:* T2-weighted/FATSAT PD imaging is essential to assess the graft tear/disruption. It is seen as a break in the intact graft fibers and a signal similar to that of fluid in the region of the graft. Partial tears are seen as focal areas of the increased signal within the graft with some intact fibers.
- Flexion contracture or extension loss/extension lag is another complication of ACL repair and can happen due to graft impingement or localized anterior arthrofibrosis. These two may be difficult to differentiate clinically but can easily be differentiated on MRI. The tibial tunnel placed too far anteriorly can result in graft impingement along the intercondylar notch roof. The tibial tunnel placed too far laterally can result in graft impingement along the medial aspect of the lateral femoral condyle.
- Localized arthrofibrosis in the anterior aspect of the knee is the other cause of extension loss. It appears as a low intense signal fibrous tissue in Hoffa's fat pad (**Figure 4.12**). Cyclops lesion is focal arthrofibrosis anterior to the distal aspect of the graft.
- A complication seen with patellar tendon autograft is patellar fracture.

Posterior Cruciate Ligament

The PCL is larger and stronger than the ACL, present along the medial side of the intercondylar notch. It extends from the lateral surface of the medial femoral condyle to the posterior aspect of the tibia. It has two components: anterolateral and posteromedial bundles. Meniscofemoral ligaments extend from the posterior horn of the lateral meniscus to the medial femoral condyle. The meniscofemoral ligament lying posterior to the PCL is known as the ligament of Wrisberg and the one lying anterior to it is called the ligament of Humphrey. The meniscofemoral ligaments of Wrisberg and Humphrey are taken as part of the PCL complex. On MRI, the PCL shows a smooth posterior convex curve with a homogeneously low-intense signal on T1- as well as T2-weighted images. The ligament of Humphrey is seen anterior and the ligament of Wrisberg posterior to the PCL as low-intense signal structures (**Figure 4.13**).

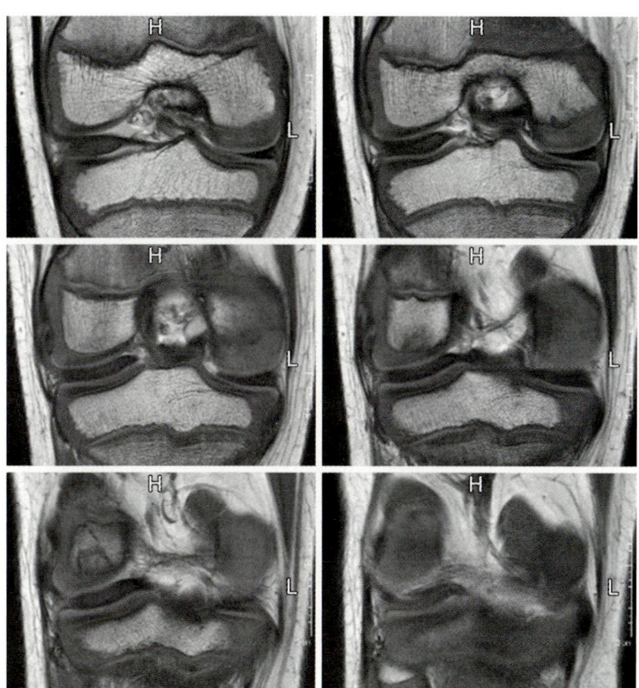

Figure 4.12 Coronal PD images showing bulky posterior horn of the lateral meniscus suggestive of discoid meniscus. There is associated focal area of signal alteration in the lateral femoral condyle suggestive of osteochondritis

The PCL is less commonly injured with most common tears at the midportion of the ligament. PCL tears are associated with posterolateral corner injuries. MRI delineates associated injuries of bone, other ligaments, menisci, and cartilage. A chronically injured PCL may be thickened or elongated.[16]

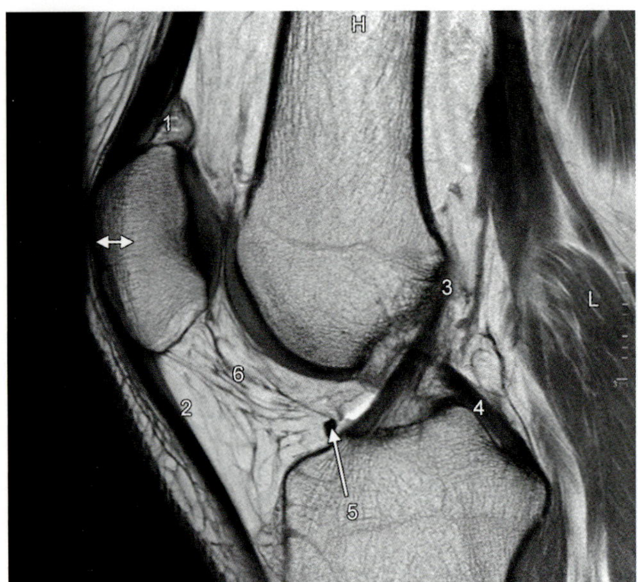

Figure 4.13 Almost mid-sagittal PD image showing quadriceps tendon (1), patellar ligament (2), anterior cruciate ligament (3), posterior cruciate ligament (4), transverse ligament (5) and Hoffa's pad of fat (6)

Full thickness PCL tears may be associated with the posterior translation of the tibia with respect to the femur.

Depending upon the extent of the ligamentous tear these are classified as follows:

Grade I—intraligamentous high signal consistent with edema with intact ligament margins.

Grade II—partial tear of the ligament.

Grade III—complete tear (**Figures 4.14A to D**).

As with the ACL there may be the avulsion of the PCL with a normal integrity of the ligament per se (**Figures 4.15A and B**). Avulsion is more common at the tibial insertion.

MEDIAL COLLATERAL LIGAMENT

It comprises of two layers—a superficial layer formed by the tibial collateral ligament with a deeper layer formed by meniscofemoral and meniscotibial ligaments. Best seen on T2-weighted coronal images, the medial collateral ligament (MCL) is seen as a smooth hypointense structure extending from medial femoral epicondyle to proximal tibial metaphysis. MCL injuries are classified as:

Grade I—(sprain) irregularity of contour/thickening of the ligament. No discontinuity of fibers. Periligamentous edema seen as a high signal on STIR images.

Grade II—(partial tear) shows an increased signal both within and surrounding the ligament.

Grade III—complete tear.

Chronic MCL tear results in thickening without associated fluid.

Posterolateral Knee

The key to posterolateral knee stabilization is the arcuate ligament complex that includes the lateral collateral ligament, biceps femoris tendon, popliteus muscle and tendon, popliteal meniscal and popliteal fibular ligaments, oblique popliteal, arcuate and fabellofibular ligaments and the lateral gastrocnemius muscle.

Lateral collateral ligament (LCL) arises from the tubercle of the lateral femoral condyle and inserts on the fibular head in conjugation with the biceps femoris tendon.

Acute ligamentous injury is evidenced by periligamentous soft tissue edema seen as a high STIR signal. Chronic injuries are evidenced by irregularity and thickening of the ligament.

The complete rupture of the LCL is usually associated with damage to the posterolateral knee structures such as capsular tears, detachment fracture of superior rim of the tibia, biceps femoris tendon tears, popliteus tendon lesions, etc.

Popliteus tendon: inserts at the lateral femoral condyle anteroinferior to the LCL. Popliteus insertion injury is common at its musculotendinous junction and is usually associated with damage to other knee structures such as the arcuate ligament complex, cruciate ligament, menisci, bones, etc. Isolated popliteus injuries are seen only in about 10% patients.[17] MRI findings vary depending upon the level and grade of injury. The avulsion of the tendon from the femoral attachment is seen as an irregular contour of the avulsed tendon at the popliteus hiatus with edema in/around the muscle. Interruption in continuity with possible retraction is suggestive of complete tear.

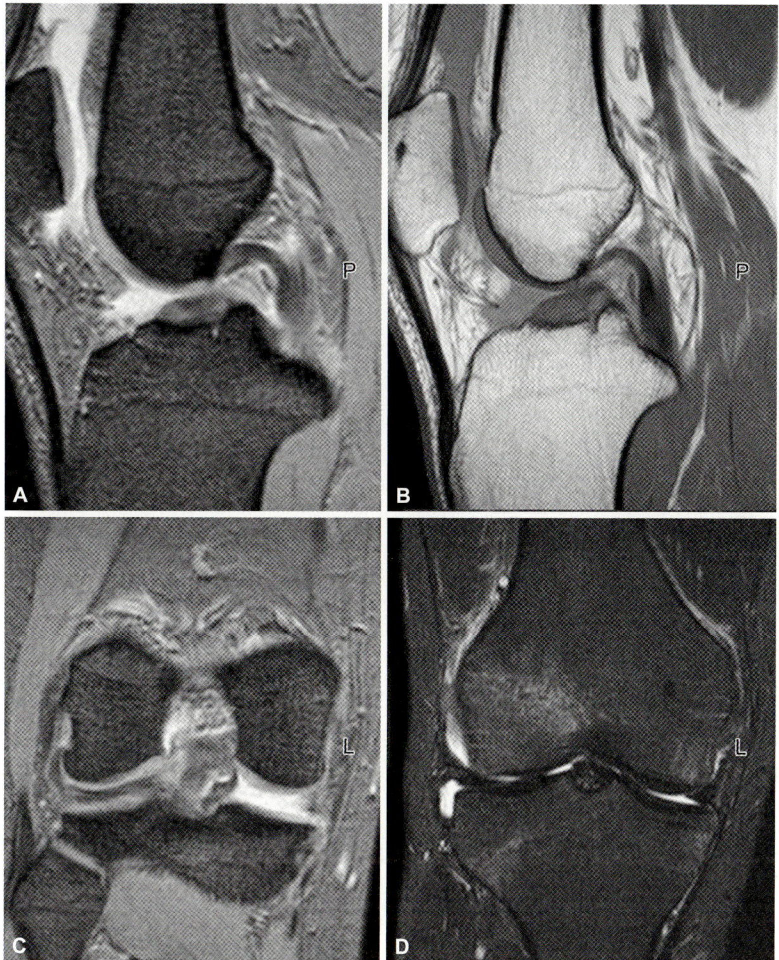

Figures 4.14A to D Sagittal T2 (A); PD (B); Coronal T2 (C) and STIR (D) images showing ACL tear evidenced by break in the continuity of ligament near femoral end with buckling of PCL (A and B) and associated bucket handle tear of the posterior horn of medial meniscus (C) with contusion of lateral femoral condyle and lateral tibial plateau seen as hyperintense signal on STIR images (D). There is moderate joint effusion

Anterior Knee Structures

These form the extensor mechanism of knee and are as follows.

- *Quadriceps tendon:* It is inserted at the superior pole of the patella and is best evaluated in sagittal sections showing hypointense bands with an intervening fat signal in keeping with its layered configuration. Partial tears or complete transection may be seen depending on the layers involved. Complete transection is associated with a low riding patella (patella baja).
- *Patellar tendon:* It extends from the inferior pole of the patella to tibial tuberosity.
- Medial and lateral patellar retinacula—medial patellar retinacular tears are usually associated with transient lateral patellar dislocation injury.

Rupture of patellar tendon: The patellar tendon can rupture due to acute trauma or secondary to repeated microtrauma. Underlying systemic disease like diabetes, systemic lupus erythematosus or chronic renal failure may result in tendon rupture with relatively minor trauma. T2-weighted or FATSAT PD images are the sequences of choice to assess the patellar tendon integrity.

Patellofemoral joint: The patellar facet configuration is described as per Wiberg classification:[18]

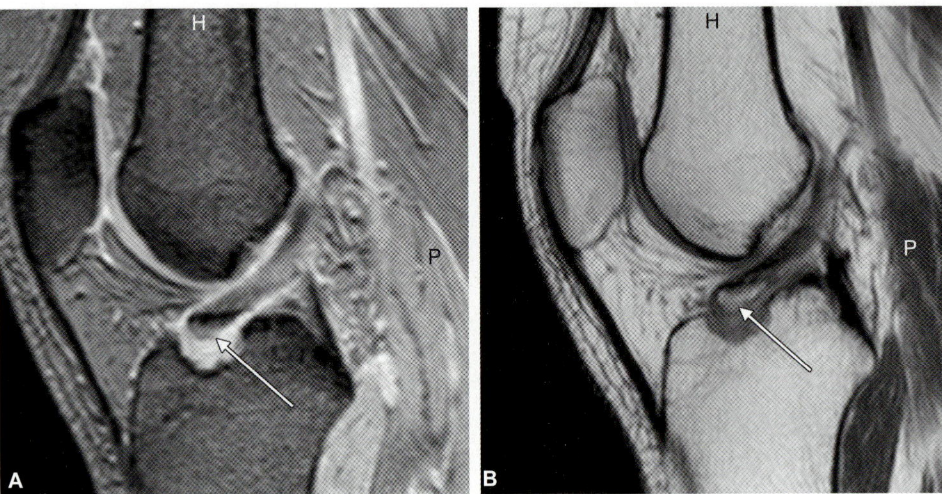

Figures 4.15A and B Sagittal STIR (A) and PD (B) images showing avulsion of the ACL (arrows) at the tibial insertion. The ACL in the rest of the course is normal

- *Type I:* The facets are concave, symmetrical and of equal size.
- *Type II:* The medial facet is rather smaller than the lateral facet. The lateral facet is concave.
- *Type III:* The medial facet is markedly smaller than the lateral facet.

FEMORAL TROCHLEAR GROOVE

The sulcus angle also called the trochlear angle is defined by the intersection of the lines connecting the highest point of the femoral condyle to the deepest point of the trochlear groove and measures about 138° (141–143°).[19] Shallow sulcus angle predisposes to patellar instability.

The position of the patella in the vertical plane is assessed using the Insall-Salvati ratio that is the ratio of the patella tendon length (TL) to the length of the patella (PL) measured on a lateral image with knee ideally in 30° flexion. The normal ratio is <1.2. Anything more than 1.2 indicates a patella alta or a high riding patella and less than 0.8 patella baja or a low-lying patella.[20]

TRANSIENT LATERAL PATELLAR DISLOCATION

This injury results in characteristic contusions of the anterolateral femoral condyle and the inferomedial aspect of the patella. Actual patellar malalignment may or may not be apparent on MRI as the patella almost always relocates spontaneously with the extension of the knee. Osteochondral injuries of the inferomedial patella may be seen. The medial patellofemoral ligament or medial patellar retinaculum can show disruption with a high T2 signal.

There are certain conditions that predispose to patellar dislocation and include patellar dysplasia (flattened articular surface of patella), shallow trochlear groove of the femur, dysplastic distal third of the vastus medialis and a large Q angle (the angle between the vertical axis of the femoral shaft and the vertical axis of the patella—normally 10–20°).[21,22]

EVALUATION OF ARTICULAR CARTILAGE

Advancements in cartilage imaging have made it the best available technique for diagnosing cartilage diseases at an early stage and monitoring the drug effects. Morphological imaging can be performed using standard SE and gradient recalled echo (GRE) sequences, FSE and 3D SE as well as GRE sequences. These sequences demonstrate fissuring, partial or full thickness defects and can provide an accurate assessment of the cartilage thickness, demonstrate morphological changes on the surface of the cartilage, changes in internal cartilage as well as in the underlying subchondral bone (**Figures 4.16 and 4.17**).

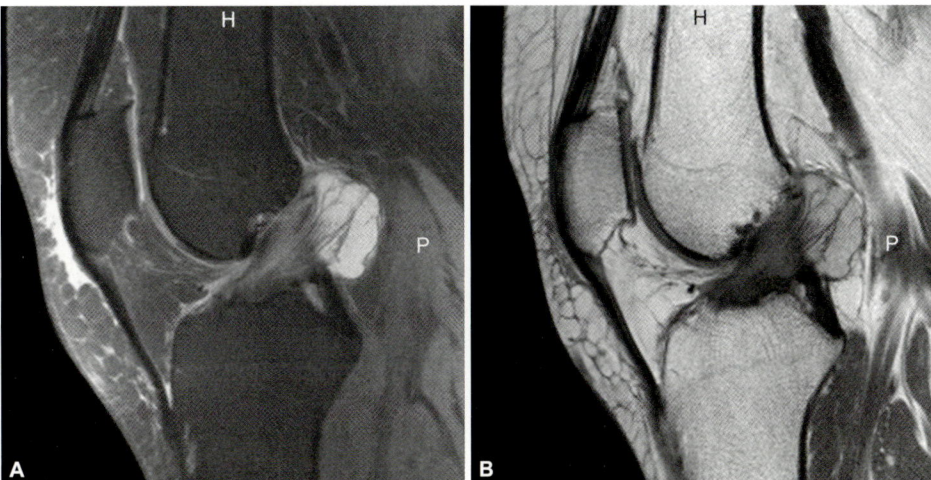

Figures 4.16A and B Sagittal STIR (A) and PD (B) images showing focal expansion of the ACL in the mid substance and near femoral end with a cystic lesion near femoral end. Linear strands of the ligament can be seen traversing the expanded portion of ACL and the cyst suggesting a ganglion at the femoral end of ACL with myxoid degeneration in the rest of the portion

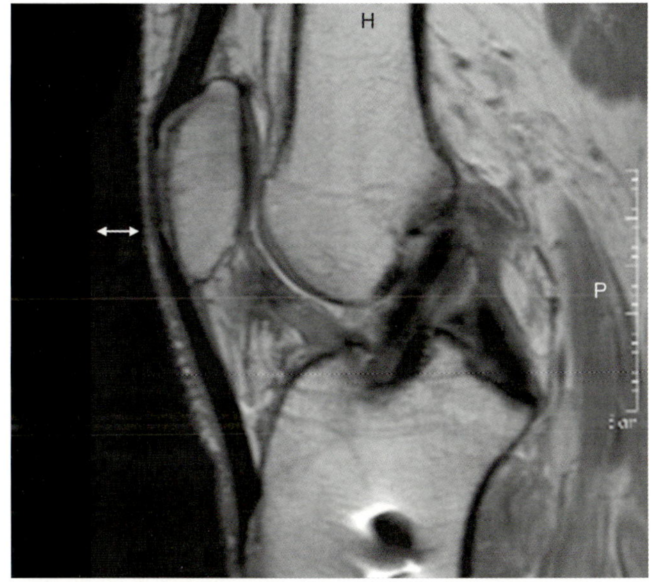

Figure 4.17 Sagittal PD image showing normal integrity of the reconstructed ACL, however there is low-intense signal (arrow) in the anterior pad of fat suggestive of anterior arthrofibrosis

The advanced MR techniques such as T2 mapping, delayed gadolinium enhanced cartilage imaging, T1p imaging, sodium imaging and diffusion-weighted imaging can provide information about the collagen network and proteoglycan content in the cartilage matrix. Of these, T2 mapping is gradually being used more often for early diagnosis and follow-up of cartilage degeneration. T2 relaxation time reflects the water content and an increase in T2 relaxation time indicates degeneration. T2 mapping holds good promise in the quantitative assessment of the cartilage, especially in patients with the cartilage repair procedure.[23-25]

Cartilage disease is broadly categorized into:

- Acute chondral/osteochondral injury
- Degenerative/osteoarthritis
- Inflammatory arthritis.

An acute chondral/osteochondral injury has sharp margins oriented perpendicular to the bone surface. It usually occurs on weight-bearing surfaces and is associated with subjacent bone marrow edema. The fractured cartilage/cartilage-bone can dislodge as a loose body.

Cartilage lesions in osteoarthritis typically occur in the weight-bearing portions and are shallower, showing wide, horizontal, or obtuse margins with respect to the bone surface. Subchondral cysts are common. It is possible to quantify the changes with dedicated special software packages by computing a number of parameters of the cartilage like size/area of the subchondral zone, area of cartilage surface, denuded and covered subchondral bone area, cartilage thickness over the total area of subchondral bone, cartilage volume, etc.

Cartilage loss is more diffuse and uniform in inflammatory arthritis due to cartilage breakdown by the enzymes produced by the pannus. Focal lesions are less common. Inflammatory changes of the subchondral bone and chondrocalcinosis can be seen.

Osteochondritis dissecans (OCD)—a disease of teenagers—usually involves the lateral aspect of the medial femoral condyle, but the lateral condyle, patella, and other areas of the knee may get involved. The MRI classification of the extent correlates with the surgical/arthroscopic classification. The role of MRI is to assess the stability of the defect. The instability of the lesion is evidenced by torn overlying articular cartilage, fluid signal under the osteochondral fragment, osteochondral defect with fluid-filled cavity and cystic change (>5 mm) deep to the lesion[26] (**Figures 4.18A and B**).

Synovial disease of knee: normal synovium is barely visible on conventional MRI. The visualization of the synovium indicates an underlying disease. The effusion in the joint is another indicator of synovial pathology. These are sensitive but not specific features. MRI cannot only detect joint effusion and synovitis but also quantify synovial and effusion volume that may help in assessing disease severity and response to therapy. It may be of immense help in directing synovial biopsy.

Figures 4.18A and B Coronal STIR images showing collection in the femoral tunnel of the ACL graft. The collection is extending up to the skin surface

Synovial disorders may be inflammatory or noninflammatory. Common inflammatory arthropathies include rheumatoid arthritis, psoriatic arthritis, septic arthritis, etc. The findings on MRI in most of these cases are nonspecific. The common noninflammatory arthropathies include osteoarthritis, post-traumatic synovitis, hemorrhagic arthropathies, synovial chondromatosis, pigmented villonodular synovitis (PVNS), lipoma arborescens, etc.

Synovial osteochondromatosis of knee: It is characterized by the metaplasia of the synovium resulting in the creation of lobulated cartilaginous masses of varying sizes that frequently involve the joint. These cartilaginous soft tissue masses may or may not ossify. MRI shows diffuse synovial proliferation with isointense to hypointense nodules in the tibiofemoral joint space, intercondylar notch and suprapatellar bursa (**Figure 4.19**). Postgadolinium T1-weighted scans reveal the intense enhancement of the synovium and the nodules with focal well-defined central areas of nonenhancement.

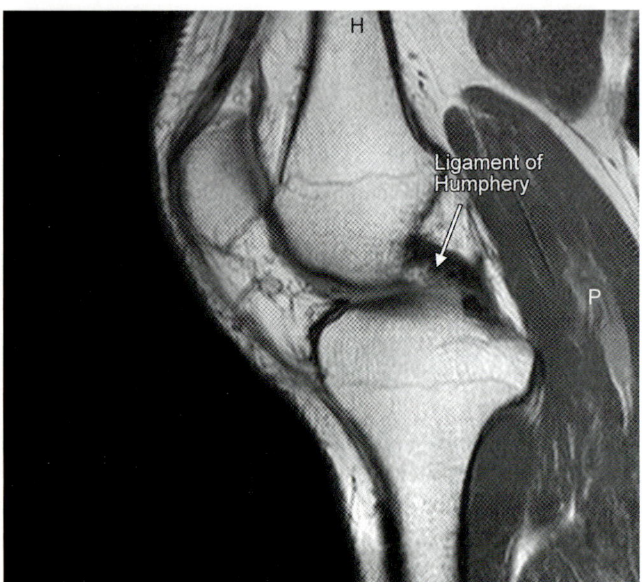

Figure 4.19 Sagittal PD image showing ligament of Humphrey (arrow) anterior to PCL

Pigmented villonodular synovitis (PVNS): It is an uncommon benign process characterized by hyperplastic synovial proliferation within the joint or along the tendon sheaths, periarticular fascial planes or within the bursae. If outside the joint, it is called the giant cell tumor of tendon sheath.

Magnetic resonance imaging is the preferred modality for diagnosing PVNS that is seen as a mass—like synovial proliferation with lobulated margins showing low-signal intensity on T1- and T2-weighted images and magnetic susceptibility artifact (blooming) within a gradient sequence. This artifact is related to the local magnetic field that is created by iron present in the hemosiderin-laden synovial tissue.[27] The suprapatellar bursa, infrapatellar fat pad, and posterior to the cruciate ligament are the common sites involved.

Magnetic resonance imaging findings in chronic hemophilic arthropathy can mimic those of PVNS. Differentiating factors in the favor of hemophilic arthropathy include the lack of prominent nodularity, more pronounced cartilage, and subchondral bone injury, and, in some instances, widening of the intercondylar notch.[28]

CYSTS, BURSAE, AND GANGLION

The most common cyst around the knee is the popliteal also known as Baker's cyst. It represents fluid extending through a communication between the gastrocnemius and semimembranosus bursa and is usually located in the posteromedial aspect of the knee (**Figures 4.20A and B**). Two diagnostic features for popliteal cyst are—anatomic communication between the gastrocnemius—semimembranosus bursa and joint effusion. These cysts are seen in association with the internal derangement of the knee especially a tear of the medial meniscus, joint effusion, and osteoarthritis. Popliteal cyst is the most common synovial cyst around the knee; however, synovial cysts may extend along the medial, lateral, and anterior plane as well. All the cysts on MRI are seen as well-defined lesions with thin low-intense wall and hyperintense contents on T2 as well as STIR images. These may be simple unioculated or multiple/septated and may contain debris or osseous loose bodies. Being synovial cysts, other associated synovial pathologies like synovial chondromatosis or pigmented villonodular sinusitis may be there.

Ganglions are other cystic lesions seen in the knee joint. These are structures filled with gelatinous fluid with dense connective tissue around. These may be juxta-articular, intra-articular, and periosteal. Intra-articular ganglia are usually associated with cruciate ligaments, the anterior cruciate being involved more frequently. Their exact cause is not certain but is presumed to be secondary to mucoid degeneration. On MRI, ACL ganglia are fusiform with a

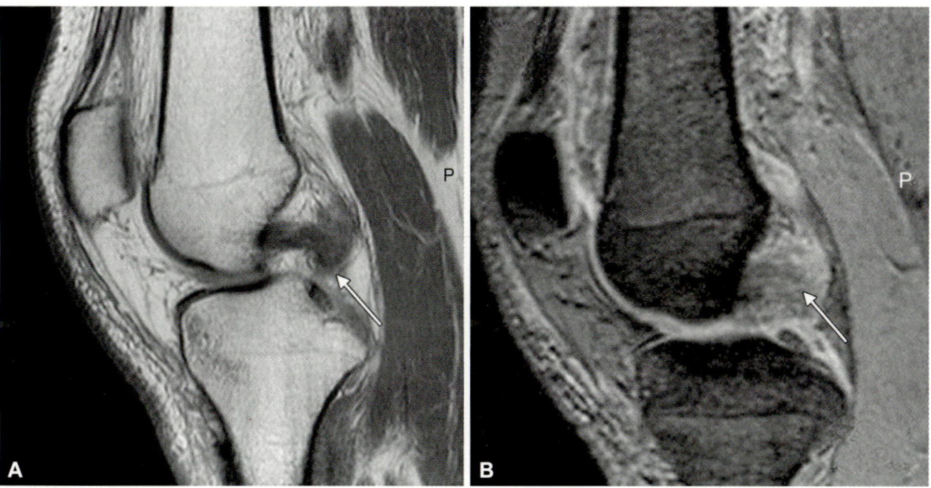

Figures 4.20A and B (A) Sagittal PD and (B) STIR image show complete PCL tear at tibial insertion (arrows)

bright signal on T2 and SPIR images with an isointense to a low-intense signal on T1 and PD images. The fibers of the ligament are seen interspersed within this signal. PCL ganglions are better defined and cystic.[11,12,29]

Bursae are synovial lined structures that act to reduce the friction between the moving structures. These are collapsed under normal circumstances and may contain a small amount of fluid. There are a number of bursae around the knee and these may get inflamed and fluid distended resulting in well-defined simple, lobulated or multifocal cyst like lesions around the tendons. There are a number of conditions that result in the bursae getting inflamed or distended—common being overuse from exercise or repetitive trauma, systemic inflammatory arthritis like rheumatoid arthritis, trauma, etc. Irrespective of the cause, MRI features remain the same—typically low intense on T1-weighted and hyperintense on T2-weighted images.

Bursae around the knee are many and based upon anatomic location these may be anterior, posterior, medial, and lateral. Sagittal scans are best to assess the anterior and posterior groups, while coronal and axial scans are ideal for medial and lateral groups. Anteriorly located bursae are suprapatellar bursa, prepatellar bursa (inflammation resulting in Housemaid's knee), and superficial and deep infrapatellar bursa. Gastrocnemius semimembranosus bursa is the main bursa in the posterior group presenting as Baker's cyst. The medial group includes pes anserine bursa (inflammation resulting in pes anserine bursitis), tibial collateral ligament bursa (vertically oriented bursa between the superficial and deep layers of the MCL) and semimembranosus—tibial collateral ligament bursa. The iliotibial band bursa and fibular collateral ligament and biceps femoris bursa are the main lateral group bursae.

INFECTIONS

Magnetic resonance imaging is helpful in evaluating cases of cellulitis, fasciitis, abscess, septic arthritis, and osteomyelitis about the knee. It is a useful tool for early detection in evaluating the extent of infection and in facilitating adequate debridement and drainage.

Magnetic resonance imaging demonstrates infection as increased signal intensity in the bone, muscle/soft tissue on fluid sensitive sequences –STIR with a corresponding low signal on T1-weighted images (**Figures 4.21A to D**). Infected areas are enhanced with intravenous gadolinium. On MRI, marrow signal abnormality is more sensitive than lytic changes on X-ray and findings become positive earlier in the disease process.

Magnetic resonance imaging findings in osteomyelitis usually are related to the replacement of marrow fat with water secondary to edema, exudate, hyperemia, and bone ischemia. There is decreased signal intensity in the involved bone on T1-weighted images with increased signal intensity on T2-weighted and STIR images.[30]

Sequestrum of cortical bone appears hypointense on all imaging sequences showing no gadolinium enhancement. Sequestrum of cancellous bone is hyperintense relative to cortical sequestrum on all sequences and shows no gadolinium enhancement. The involucrum is hypointense on all sequences and shows gadolinium enhancement.

Granulation tissue is hypointense on T1-weighted images, hyperintense on T2-weighted and STIR images, and shows gadolinium enhancement. Draining sinuses and soft tissue inflammation are hypointense on T1-weighted images and hyperintense on T2-weighted and STIR images.

TUBERCULAR KNEE

Magnetic resonance imaging features of the tuberculous infection of the knee are nonspecific and include fluid collections in the joint, synovial hypertrophy with abnormally increased enhancement, low intensity nonenhancing foci in the synovial fluid (representing debris and caseous material), intra-articular and periarticular abscesses, cortical erosions, marrow edema, and osteomyelitis.

SUMMARY

Multiplanar imaging capabilities with excellent soft tissue contrast coupled with noninvasive nature make MRI the

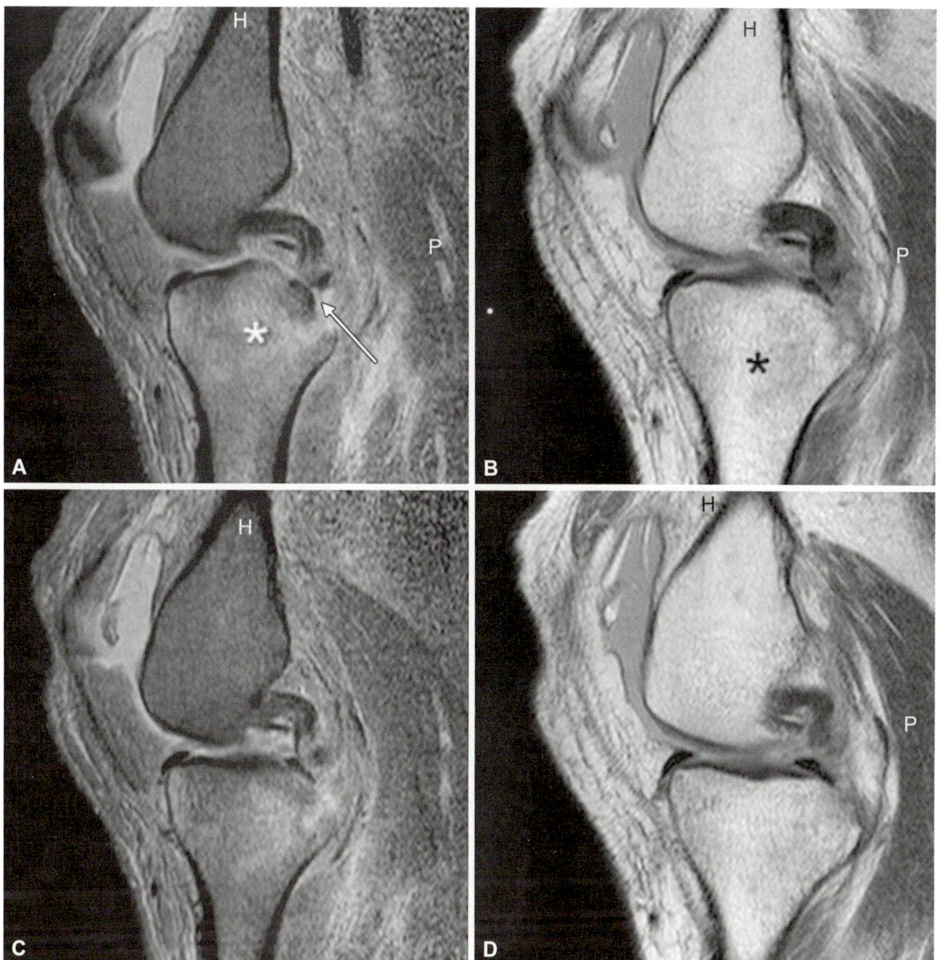

Figures 4.21A to D Sagittal STIR (A and C) and PD (B and D) images show PCL avulsion from tibial attachment (arrows) with subjacent bone marrow edema (*) seen as hyperintese signal on STIR images and hypointese signal on PD images

modality of choice for the evaluation of the knee. The ligaments, menisci, bones as well as soft tissues are well assessed. Recent advancement in technology with the development of new sequences has made it possible to assess the cartilage noninvasively. It has made it possible not only to assess the early damage to cartilage but also monitor the therapeutic response. Improvements in dynamic contrast imaging, T2 mapping, diffusion and diffusion tensor imaging, sodium imaging with the introduction of digital RF technology and newer sequences are expected to further improve diagnostic capabilities of MRI.

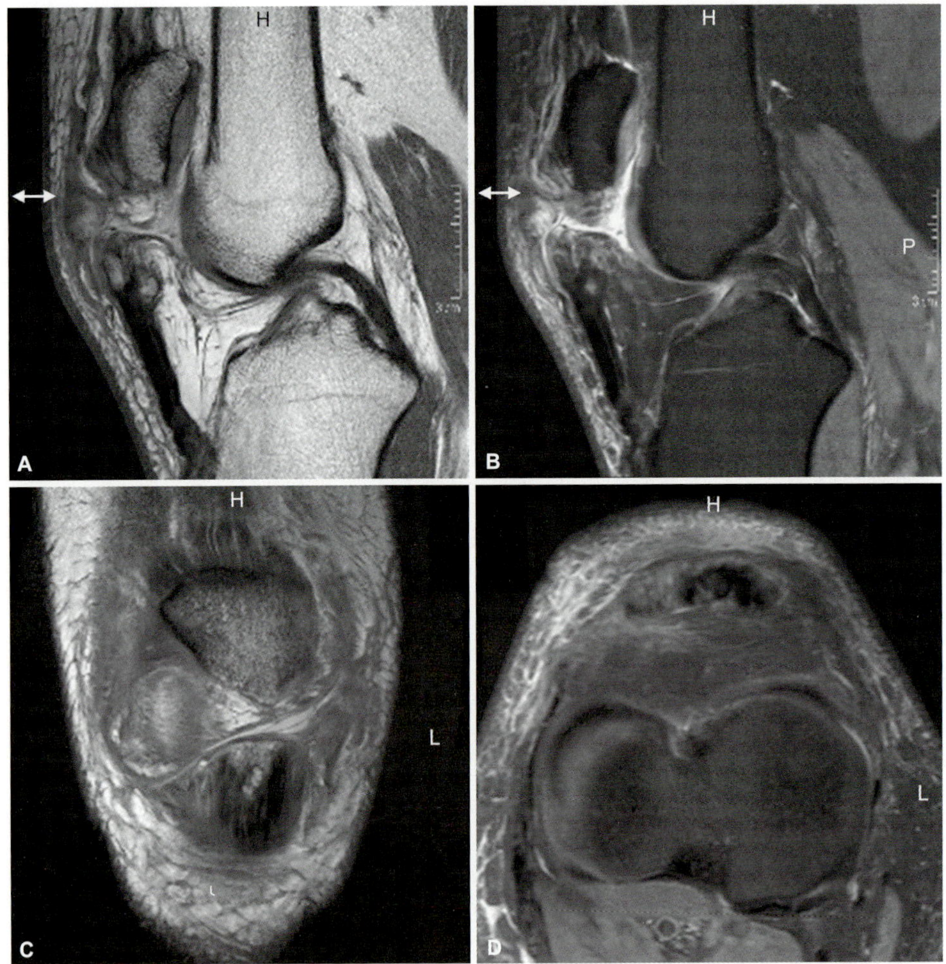

Figures 4.22A to D Sagittal PD (A); Sagittal STIR (B); Coronal and axial STIR (C and D) images show complete tear of the patellar ligament at its patellar attachment

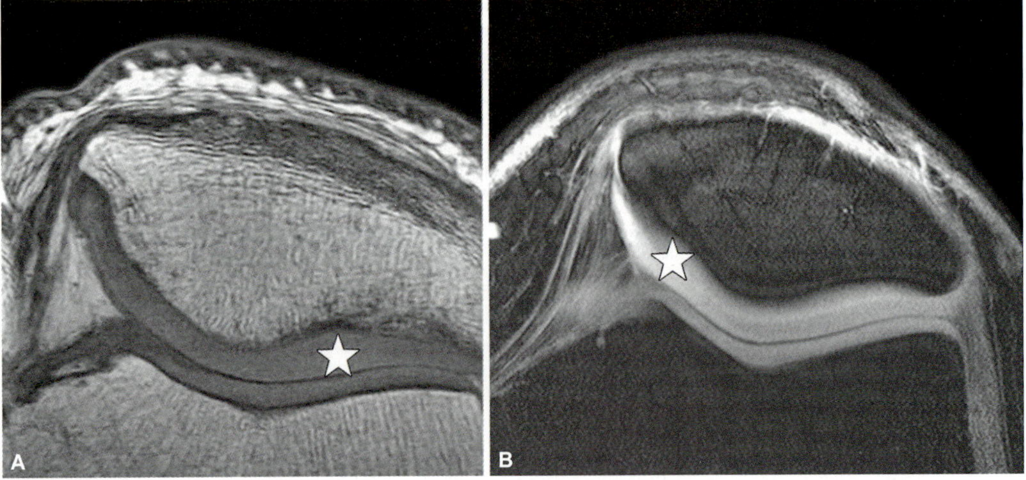

Figures 4.23A and B Normal patellar articular cartilage (*) as seen on high resolution PD axial images (A). Corresponding 3D FATSAT sequence (B)

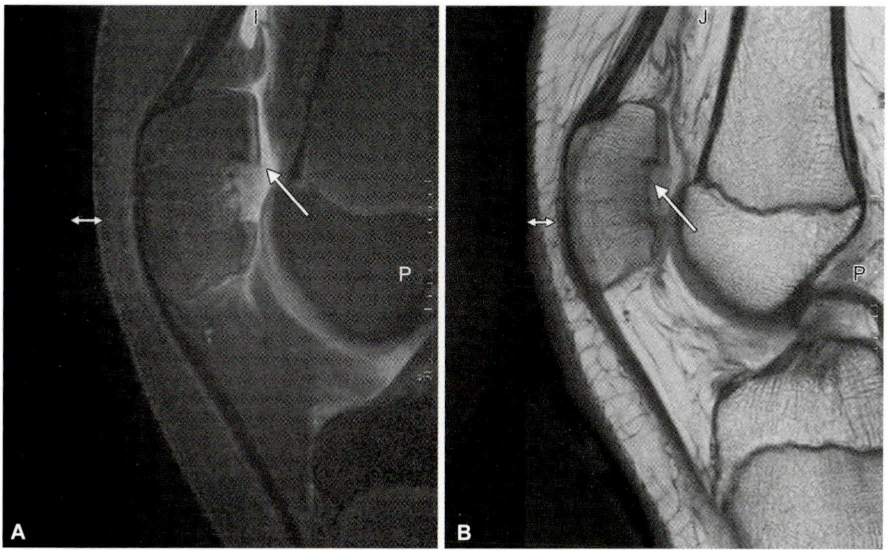

Figures 4.24A and B Sagittal STIR (A) and PD (B) images showing focal patellar full thickness articular cartilage and underlying bony defect (arrows)—osteochondral defect

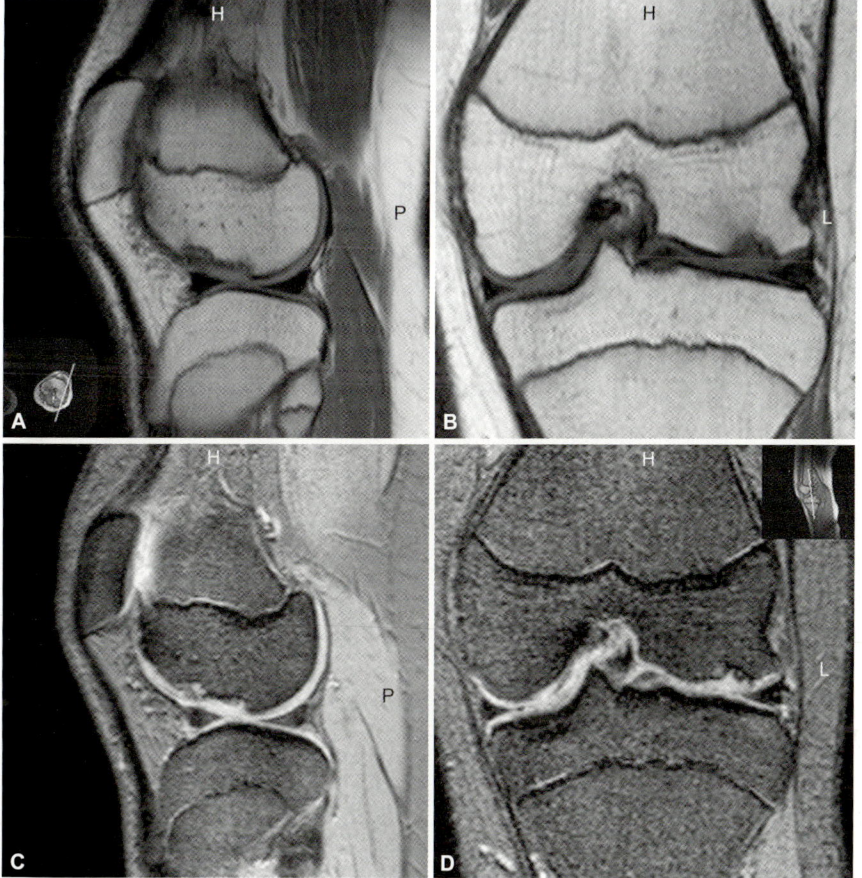

Figures 4.25A to D Sagittal: (A) Coronal; (B) PD and sagittal; (C) Coronal (D) T2 weighted images in a 15-year-old male showing focal osteochondral defect in the lateral femoral condyle—osteochondritis dissicans. There is no free fragment

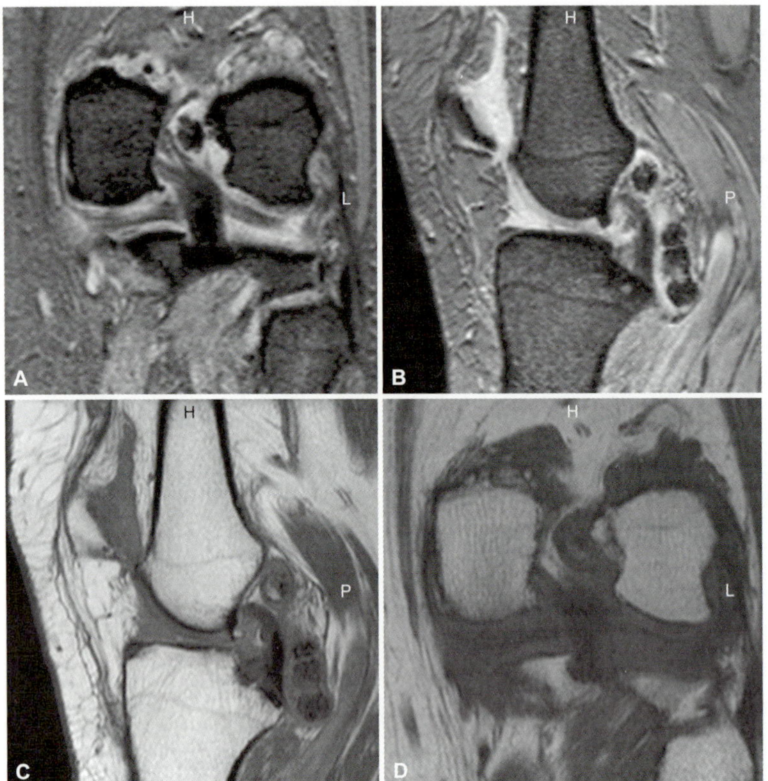

Figures 4.26A to D Coronal: (A) Sagittal; (B) T2 and Sagittal; (C) Coronal (D) PD weighted images showing multiple calcified osteochondral loose bodies in the knee joint seen as hypointense foci on all imaging sequences suggestive of osteochondromatosis

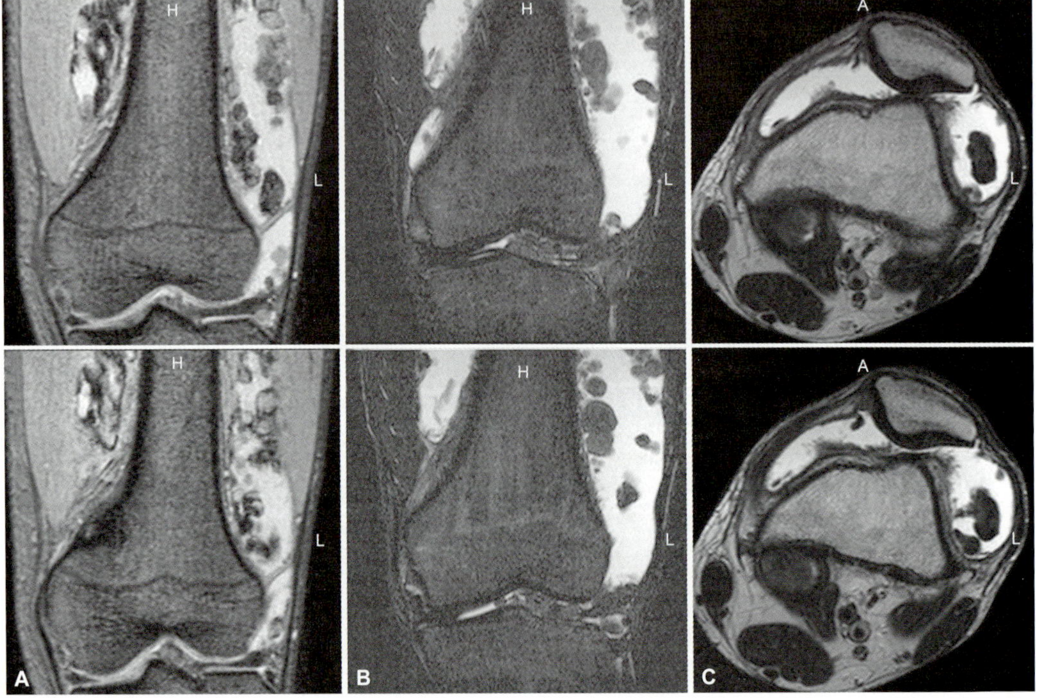

Figures 4.27A to C Coronal T2 (A); STIR (B) and axial PD (C) images show moderate knee joint effusion with diffuse synovial thickening with multiple hypointense nodules/loose bodies—synovial osteochondromatosis

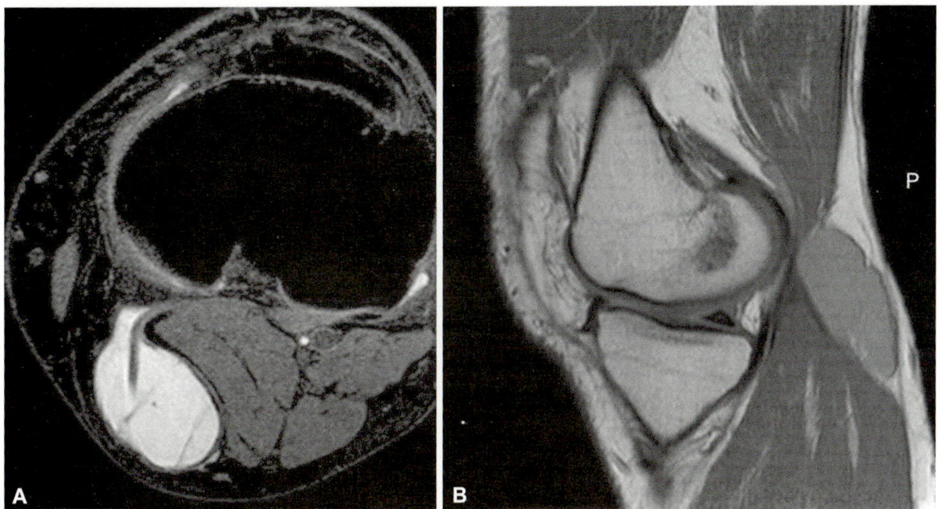

Figures 4.28A and B Axial T2 FATSAT (A) and sagittal PD (B) images showing distension of gastrocnemius—semimembranosus . A thin neck communicating with joint can be seen—popliteal/Bakers cyst

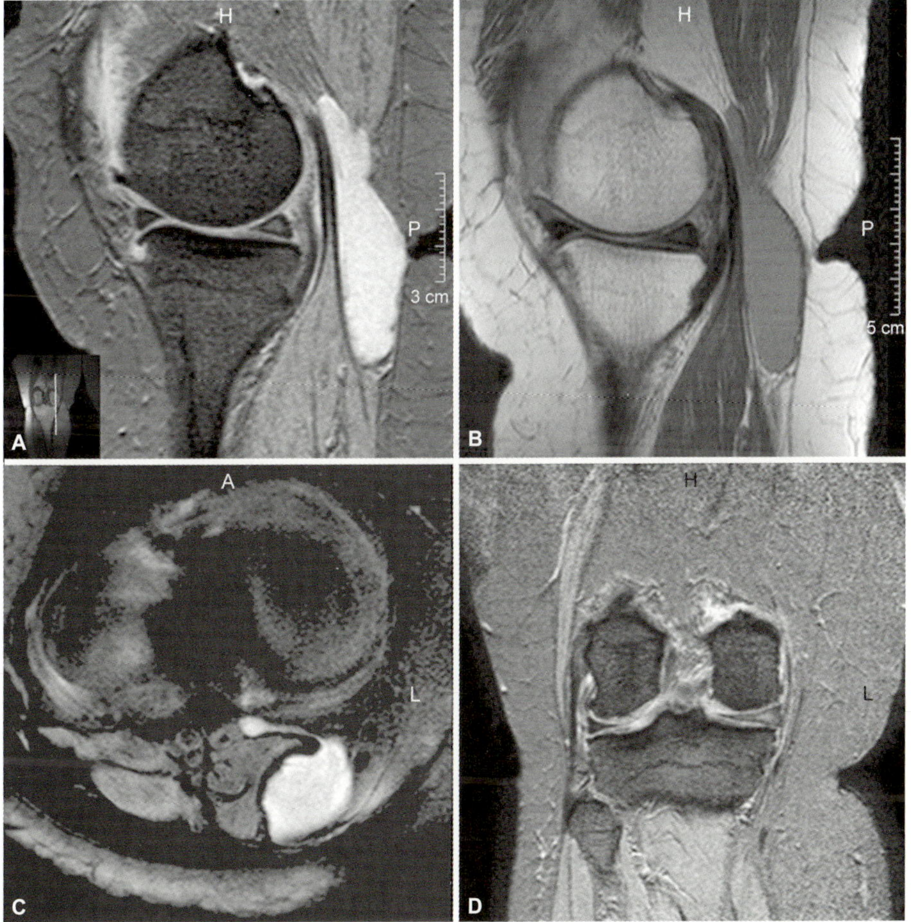

Figures 4.29A to D Sagittal STIR and PD, an axial STIR images show a loculated collection in the popliteal fossa between the tendon of semimembranosus muscle and medial head of gastrocnemius communicating with the knee joint—Baker's cyst. Grade II myxoid degenerative changes seen in the posterior horn of medial meniscus seen as intrameniscal hyperintensity not contacting the meniscal articular surface

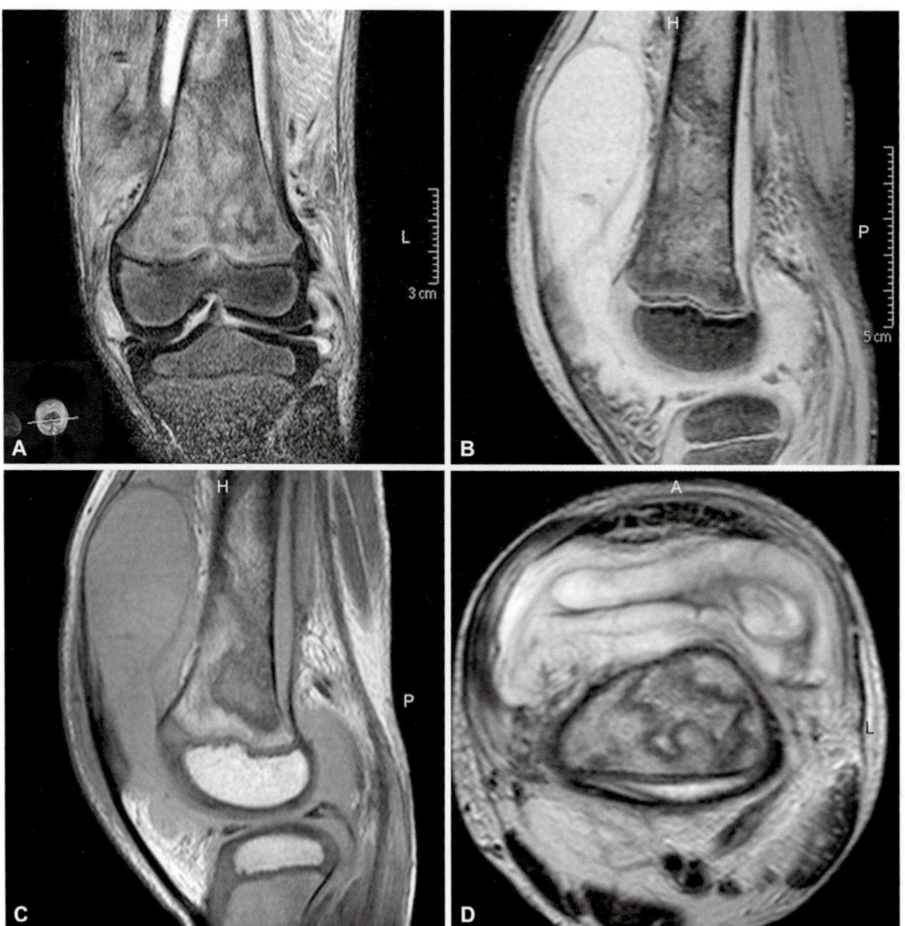

Figures 4.30A to D Coronal STIR (A); Sagittal STIR (B); Sagittal PD (C); Axial T2 (D); images showing large knee joint effusion with diffuse synovial thickening with heterogeneous signal alteration of the marrow with geographical lesions in the marrow suggestive of medullary bone infarcts in distal femur—pyogenic osteomyelitis

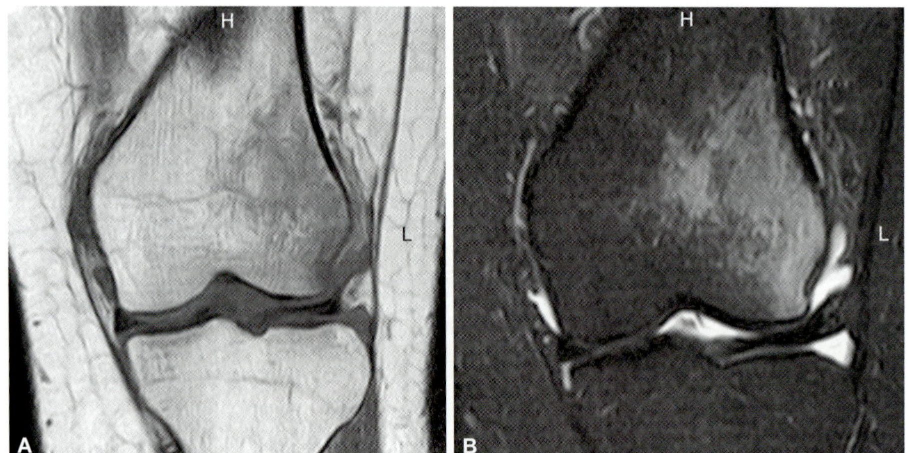

Figures 4.31A and B Coronal T1 (A) and STIR (B) images in a 23-year-old with no history of trauma showing heterogeneous low-intense signal on T1 and hyperintense signal on STIR images in the medial femoral condyle. Soft tissue edema seen in tissues overlying MFC with small amount of effusion—fluid aspiration revealed tubercular etiology

REFERENCES

1. De Smet AA, Norris MA, Yandow DR, et al. MR diagnosis of meniscal tears of the knee: importance of high signal in the meniscus that extends to the surface. Am J Roentgenol. 1993;161(1):101-7.
2. Jee WH, McCauley TR, Kim JM, et al. Meniscal tear configurations: categorization with MR imaging. Am J Roentgenol. 2003;180(1):93-7.
3. Ruff C, Weingardt JP, Russ PD, et al. MR imaging patterns of displaced meniscus injuries of the knee. Am J Roentgenol. 1998;170(1):63-7.
4. Tuckman GA, Miller WJ, Remo JW, et al. Radial tears of the menisci: MR findings. Am J Roentgenol. 1994;163(2):395-400.
5. Brody JM, Lin HM, Hulstyn MJ, et al. Lateral meniscus root tear and meniscus extrusion with anterior cruciate ligament tear. Radiology. 2006;239(3):805-10.
6. Singh K, Helms CA, Jacobs MT, et al. MRI appearance of Wrisberg variant of discoid lateral meniscus. Am J Roentgenol. 2006;187(2):384-7.
7. Recht MP, Kramer J. MR imaging if the postoperative knee: a pictorial essay. Radiographics. 2002;22:765-74.
8. Tomus AP, White LM, Marshall TJ, Donell ST. Imaging the postoperative meniscus. Eur J Radiol. 2005;54(2):189-98.
9. Gentili A, Seeger LL, Yao L, et al. Anterior cruciate ligament tear: indirect signs at MR imaging. Radiology 1994;193(3):835-40.
10. Lee K, Siegel MJ, Lau DM, et al. Anterior cruciate ligament tears: MR imaging-based diagnosis in a pediatric population. Radiology. 1999;213:697-704.
11. Do-Dai DD, Youngberg RA, Lanchbury FD, et al. Intraligamentous ganglion cysts of the anterior cruciate ligament: MR findings with clinical and arthroscopic correlations. J Comput Assist Tomogr. 1996;20(1):80-4.
12. McIntyre J, Moelleken S, Tirman P. Mucoid degeneration of the anterior cruciate ligament mistaken for ligamentous tears. Skeletal Radiol. 2001;30(6):312-5.
13. Sanders TG. MR imaging of postoperative ligaments of the knee. Semin Musculoskelet Radiol. 2002;6(1):19-33.
14. Cheung Y, Magee TH, Rosenberg ZS, et al. MRI of anterior cruciate ligament reconstruction. J Comput Assist Tomogr. 1992;16(1):134-7.
15. Papakonstantinou O, Chung CB, Chanchairujira K, et al. Complications of anterior cruciate ligament reconstruction: MR imaging. Eur Radiol. 2003; 13(5):1106-17.
16. Malone AA, Dowd GS, Saifuddin A. Injuries of the posterior cruciate ligament and posterolateral corner of the knee. Injury. 2006;37(6):485-501.
17. Mirkopulos N, Myer TJ. Isolated avulsion of the popliteus tendon: a case report. Am J Sports Med. 1991;19:417-9.
18. Wiberg G. Roentgenographic and anatomic studies of the femoropatellar joint with special reference to chondromalacia patella. Acta Orthop Scand. 1941; 121:319-40.
19. Pfirmann CWA, Zanetti M, Romero J, Hodler J. Femoral trochlear dysplasia: MR findings. Radiology. 2000;216:858-64.
20. Miller TT, Staron RB, Feldman F. Patellar height on sagittal MR imaging of the knee. Am J Roentgenol. 1996;167:339-41.
21. Dupuis CS, Westra SJ, Makris J, Wallace EC. Injuries and conditions of the extensor mechanism of the pediatric knee Radiographics. 2009;29:877-86.
22. Elias DA, White LM, Fithian DC. Acute lateral patellar dislocation at MR imaging: injury patterns of medial patellar soft-tissue restraints and osteochondral injuries of the inferomedial patella. Radiology. 2002;225(3):736-43.
23. Crema MD, Roemer FW, Marra MD, et al. Articular cartilage in the knee: current MR imaging techniques and applications in clinical practice and research. Radiographics. 2011;31:37-61.
24. Gold GE, McCauley TR, Gray ML, et al. Special focus session: what's new in cartilage. Radiographics. 2003;23:1227-42.
25. Jeffrey DR, Watt I. Imaging hyaline cartilage. Br J Radiol. 2003;76:777-87.
26. De Smet AA, Ilahi OA, Graf BK. Untreated osteochondritis dissecans of the femoral condyles: prediction of patient outcome using radiographic and MR findings. Skeletal Radiol. 1997;26:463-7.
27. Hughes TH, Sartoris DJ, Schweitzer ME, et al. Pigmented villonodular synovitis: MRI characteristics. Skeletal Radiol. 1995;24(1):7-12.
28. Dobon M, Lucia JF, Aguilar C, et al. Value of magnetic resonance imaging for the diagnosis and follow-up of haemophilic arthropathy. Haemophilia. 2003;9:76-85.
29. Bergin D, Morrison WB, Carrino JA, et al. Anterior cruciate ligament ganglia and mucoid degeneration: coexistence and clinical correlation. Am J Roentgenol. 2004;182:1283-7.
30. Karchevsky M, Schweitzer ME, Morrison WB, et al. MRI findings of septic arthritis and associated osteomyelitis in adults. Am J Roentgenol. 2004;182:119-22.

Chapter 5

Current Principles of High Tibial Osteotomy, and its Role in Management of Unicompartmental Degenerative Joint Disease

Suryanarayan P

INTRODUCTION

Osteotomy for limb malalignment and the consequent functional disturbances is a well-established treatment option for many decades. However, its precise role, scope, and the appropriate indications are being constantly debated and challenged. With the improved performance and long-term survival of unicompartmental and total knee replacements,[1-6] there is considerable debate generated on this issue. Data from the United States show a constant decline in the absolute number of osteotomies for monocompartmental arthrosis when compared with the number of replacements being performed for the same.[7-9] A better understanding of the indications, improvement in the designs, techniques, and better mid-term outcomes have led to a resurgence of interest in the unicompartment replacement, thus challenging the space and scope for high tibial osteotomies.

From a purely mechanical standpoint a good long-term function requires that the principle segments of the limb be under an appropriate alignment, so that the biological integrity of the articular cartilage is preserved and its potential for the normal function and repair is maintained. Malalignment induces abnormal biomechanics and eccentric overload, which over time predisposes the subject to arthritis. The damaging effects of excessive focal pressures on normal cartilage are well documented.[10,11] Osteotomy principally attempts to reverse this and improves the lifespan of the knee joint by force redistribution.[12] This preservation of the native joint surface supports pain-free high-impact functional demands, which otherwise is precluded with prosthetic options.

There is often a tendency to compare the outcomes of the alternative procedures with the historically reported outcomes of high tibial osteotomies. However, a better understanding of the pathological process, defined principles of correction, precise correction techniques, and stable fixation options have resulted in significantly improved outcomes.[13-19] Careful patient selection, precise preoperative planning, and execution of the surgical steps are fundamental to successful outcomes with tibial osteotomies.The correction of the axial malalignment today is increasingly used as an adjuvant to a variety of joint and cartilage preserving procedures such as cartilage transplants, meniscus allograft, etc.[20-23]

MALALIGNMENT AND OSTEOARTHRITIS

In practice, it is not uncommon to see a lack of correlation between the pain, symptoms, and the radiographic findings. In some instances, changes in the tibiofemoral compartments, in addition to rotational malalignment, fails to provoke any symptoms.[24] Only few published longitudinal study reports have addressed to the outcomes of pre-existing malalignment, and the onset and progress of osteoarthritis. Nilsson et al.[25] in their review (n = 94) found >50% cases showing deterioration of the affected compartment over a 17-year follow-up. This was aggravated by pre-existing axial deviation and instability, clearly establishing a correlation. Odenbring et al. [26] in their 14-year review of 189 cases with medial arthrosis concluded that untreated osteoarthritis has a poor prognosis and has a relentless progression.

VARUS DEFORMITY AND OSTEOARTHRITIS

Progression of symptomatic arthritis in the presence of varus deformity is clearly dictated by two elements:

1. The static limb malalignment which can be easily measured on long leg films, defined as MAD (mechanical axis deviation). In addition, the measurement of the joint orientation angles and the angles of convergence help us to identify the source of MAD, whether it is the femur, tibia, or the stretching of the lateral ligaments (**Figures 5.1A and B**).
2. However, during the normal gait, the joint reaction forces from the muscles and ligaments around the knee determine the actual load on the medial compartment. This is defined as the ground reaction force, and a medial displacement of this vector increases the medial compartmental load.

Hence, the overall increase in the medial compartment load is both due to the static malalignment and the dynamic responses of the surrounding musculoskeletal structures. This dynamic contribution of the muscles has a profound impact on the overall compartmental load. Weak muscles and stretched incompetent ligaments have a negative influence and consequently a faster progression of symptoms and deterioration.

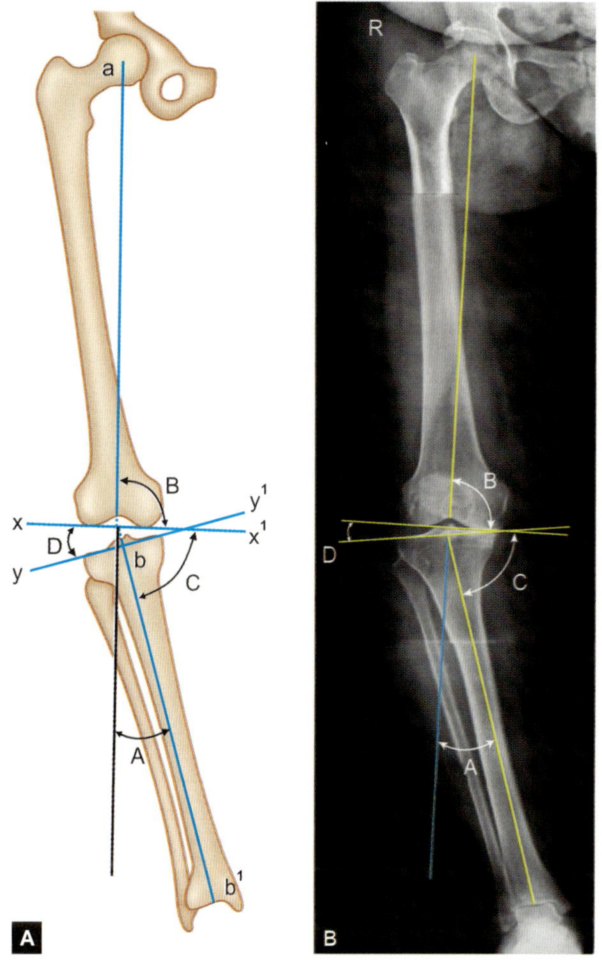

Figures 5.1A and B Radiological assessment; (A) xx', femoral transcondylar line; yy', tibial plateau line; (B) Transcondylar angle; B, tibial plateau shaft angle; C, angle of convergence; D, varus angle

In theory, MAD deviation to 6° varus results in the 100% load on the medial compartment. Neutral MAD results in a distribution of the 70% load on the medial side and 30% on the lateral side.[27] However, anatomy-based mathematical models that factor the muscle forces show a more equitable distribution of forces across the knee,[28,29] thus highlighting the importance of the muscles and ligaments in the overall pathogenesis and management of osteoarthritis. The clinical significance being that weak muscle mass or power can accelerate deterioration. Conversely, early symptoms can be addressed to, with muscle strengthening exercises, namely the gluteus maximus, tensor fascia lata, etc. It is also a clinical observation that is well built, and muscular individuals with the same degree of static deformity seem to present with less symptoms than those with weak tissues. Supporting this statement is the improved outcomes of osteotomy reported in the subset of physically active people.[30]

The predominant contribution to the overall varus alignment is the increase in the condylar plateau angle, depicting loss or erosion of the medial cartilage accentuated in more severe cases by the lateral opening of the joint due to stretching of the lateral ligaments. Cooke et al.[24] have reported the following observations in their studies and this deserves mention:

- Decreased valgus angulation of the distal femur in a certain proportion of symptomatic people (CH angle). This shows the pathological element on the femoral side in varus deformities.[31]
- Varus alignment with an oblique joint line showing a pronounced inward slope of the tibial articular surface. This is seen in approximately 5% of the subjects. The distal femur in this subset shows increased valgus angulation. There is an increased tendency for tibial subluxation, probably due to the shear forces generated by the joint line obliquity. The clinical relevance of this observation is that the correction by a valgus osteotomy alone may yield less than the optimal result and one will need to consider getting the joint line horizontal, if need be with a correction on the femoral side as well.

The model proposed by Maquet best describes the biomechanical implications of malalignment.[32-34] The eccentric force P imposed on the knee by the body above is neutralized by the muscle forces L and passive ligament stress. This results in force R that is the sum of all these forces, that acts perpendicular to the weight-bearing surface of the joint (**Figure 5.2**). In a normal homeostatic state, this is symmetric and in a state of equilibrium. This uniform distribution of the stresses on the joint surface is reflected on the X-rays by the even thickness of the subchondral bone. Bone mineral density studies have shown an increased density in the medial tibial and femoral condyles in subjects with varus osteoarthritis. This increase in density reverts back to normal after the correction of the deformity with an osteotomy. This response depicting increased bone stress and tissue response to the increased load has also been confirmed by bone scintigraphic studies.[35,36]

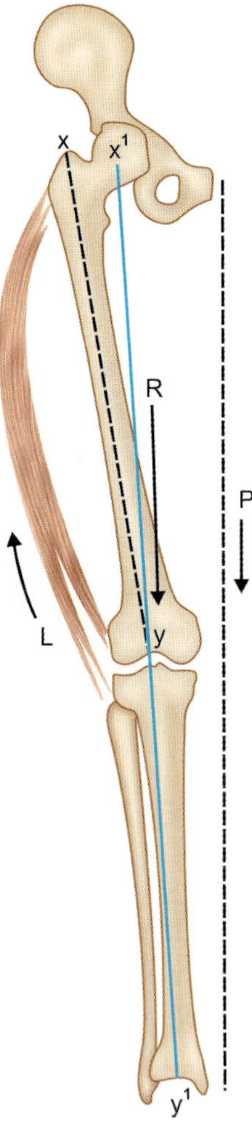

Figure 5.2 xy, femoral anatomical axis; x^{1}y, femoral mechanical axis; yy^1, tibial axis; P, the body force; L, muscular forces (Tensor fascia lata, biceps femoris); R, resultant load on the knee

In a well-aligned limb, the mechanical axis of the femur is defined by a line drawn from the center of the femoral head through the center of the knee. The anatomical axis of the femur is defined by a line from the piriformis fossa to the center of the knee. The angle between the anatomic axis of the femur and a line through the long axis of the tibia represents the normal 6° of valgus angle of the knee. In a neutrally aligned limb, the hip-knee-ankle (HKA) angle is about 180° (**Figure 5.2**). At this point, the femoral mechanical axis and the tibial mechanical axis are collinear and pass through the center of the knee. The forces across the tibiofemoral joint are a result of body weight, center of gravity, musculature (acting as a tension band), and joint alignment. The joint is stressed maximally during the single-limb stance phase of the gait cycle, when it sustains a force approximately 6 times the body weight. The medial compression loads increase to 70–75% of the load at the knee in the midstance phase of the gait secondary to varus thrust or adduction moment occurring in this phase. Electrophysiologic studies by Blaimont et al.[37,38] have shown that biceps femoris and TFL are the main stabilizers that laterally attempt to neutralize the adductor moment and maintain the balance (**Figure 5.2**). The forces of these muscles are weak in subjects with varus arthrosis, resulting in the inability to close the lateral opening of the joint. This insufficiency of the muscles (force L) results in the varus thrust. It is postulated that in the early stage of this pathology if the varus is minimal, the process can be reversed by strengthening of these muscles in addition to some alterations in the footwear and gait patterns that help minimize the varus thrust.

A better understanding of the concept of the adductor moment around the knee is important since it is becoming increasingly evident that it has significant bearing on the treatment decisions and outcomes. **Figures 5.3A and B** depicts schematically the forces around the normal knee. The lever arm of the gravity force P can be split into extrinsic and intrinsic. The extrinsic varus distance (EVD) is the distance between the mechanical axis (knee center) and the line of force of the gravity. The intrinsic varus distance (IVD) is the distance between the theoretical mechanical axis and the center of the knee (in subjects with a varus deformity). The sum total of EVD + IVD constitutes the total varus distance [global varus distance (GVD)].

The EVD is influenced by the patient morphology. Broad pelvis, coax vara, femoral bowing, short femur, and hip adduction increase the EVD. This plays a major role in the development of arthritis and explains the weak muscle force L and increased varus thrust in this situation. This is typically seen in short stocky women presenting with medial joint pain with significant opening of the lateral joint space and exaggerated adductor thrust on the gait. Hence, some overcorrection is necessary to re-establish the equilibrium in these cases.[37,38]

The adductor moment is the factor that is responsible for the increased joint reaction forces and thereby the medial compartmental load. Clinical outcomes of the corrective

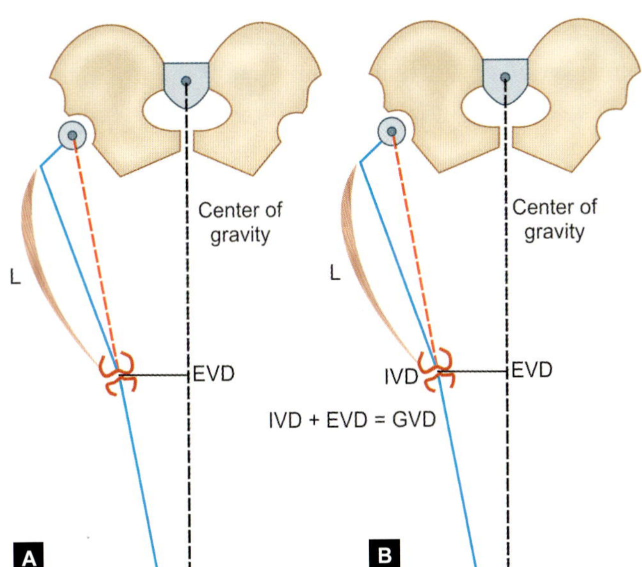

Figures 5.3A and B Adductor movement around the knee. (A) Normal; EVD, extrinsic varus distance; L, muscular forces; (B) Varus deformity; IVD, intrinsic varus distance; GVD, global varus distance

surgeries have been closely related to the magnitude of the adductor thrust seen preoperatively.[39-41] Low adductor moments preoperatively show better clinical results, and the correction is seen to be better maintained in 79% of the individuals compared to only 20% in the group with a high adductor moment.

Historically, most studies and publications on the subject of deformity and arthrosis emphasized on the issue of static deformity, malalignment, and its correction. However, recent studies,[42] have laid more stress on joint laxity as another important variable, since this can result in dynamic malalignment during gait with associated changes in the absolute load on the compartment. Lateral collateral laxity is commonly seen with varus deformity, and this has clinical implications in the evaluation, planning, and treatment.

PATIENT SELECTION

The criteria and desirable features of an ideal candidate for high tibial osteotomy (HTO) have been defined and reported in numerous studies. A middle-aged, physically active, and well-motivated individual with monocompartmental degenerative changes and pain with no fixed deformity and a range of motion greater than

120° typically describes most of the desirable features. However, in practice not more than 15% of the patients fall into this category. The following issues deserve careful consideration before a decision for an osteotomy is made:

- Malalignment with coexisting inflammatory arthritis will result in less than optimal outcome. Osteotomy in this situation is not recommended.[43]
- Ideal indications are primary osteoarthritis and secondary arthritis following trauma, osteochondritis dissecans, postmenisectomy arthritis or in conjunction with salvage procedures such as cartilage transplants, meniscal allograft, etc. However, arthritis following combined medial and lateral meniscectomies has shown poor outcomes.[44,45]
- Candidates with morphologic features imposing high adductor thrust and with significant instability need to be carefully assessed before an osteotomy is planned.
- For a long time, patellofemoral changes were considered a significant contraindication for HTO. However, a number of reports do not support this assumption and they have shown fewer failures attributable to the patellofemoral joint. In fact, it is observed that the patellofemoral symptoms can benefit with upper tibial osteotomy.[46,47] Mild-to-moderate degree of patellofemoral changes is today not considered a contraindication.[48-50]
- It is clear that a numerical age bar seems inappropriate. Rather, one needs to take into account the level of their physical activities, their needs, and the social background. A less active sedentary individual of similar age and disease level may have a better outcome with the alternate arthroplasty option. However, an upper age limit of 50–55 for osteotomy seems appropriate considering the diminishing capacity of the cartilage to heal spontaneously with age and the predictable good successful outcomes of total knees at 15–20 years.
- Obesity has been shown to influence the outcome, and it is not a good candidate for osteotomy.[51-53] This could be attributed to the high thrust and poor muscle tone in addition to the body weight.
- Patient motivation too is a very important element. Candidates should have a clear idea of the limitation, outcomes, the alternate options, and the prolonged rehabilitation. An active involvement of the candidate in the decision-making process helps in selecting a well-informed, motivated, and compliant patient, thus improving the possibility of a good outcome.

Radiographic Examination

It is ideal to perform the following X-rays for a complete evaluation of the knee joint and for the assessment and quantification of the deformity. This enables proper case selection and planning of the surgery:

- Anteroposterior and lateral radiographs in supine position and knee in extension.
- Varus and valgus stress views (anteroposterior). Enables the assessment of tibiofemoral compartments and the integrity of collateral ligaments. It is important to differentiate between the lax and contracted MCL on the stress views. This influences the choice of the procedure. If the MCL is contracted, to avoid further stretch on the ligament, planning an osteotomy distal to the ligament insertion is appropriate. On the other hand, if the MCL is lax and stretched, the deformity is better corrected with an intraligamentous procedure that will overcome the laxity.
- Standing posteroanterior radiographs with the knee in 30° flexion. This helps define the intercondylar notch and the presence of any osteophytes.
- HKA long-leg radiograph on a 51 × 14-inch film with the patient standing on both legs. This projection helps in the overall assessment of the extremity and the knee, and in the calculation of the degree of varus deformity and the adductor moment. This is best done with the patient standing on both legs, which gives a correct estimation of the axial alignment of the limb. This is easy to standardize and reproduce in all cases. It is not recommended to do this in a one-leg stance, since the pelvis tends to tilt to the side of the weight-bearing limb. This minimizes the varus distance and the calculation of the adductor moment. Also, it is difficult to position a painful varus limb in this position.
- Skyline view of the patella to evaluate and study this joint. Patella alignment and patella height could sometimes have an influence on the planning.[54,55]

Radiographic Assessment (*see* Figure 5.1)

- Mechanical axis of the femur—from the center of the hip to the center of the intercondylar notch
- Mechanical axis tibia—from the center of the proximal physis to the center of the ankle
- HKA angle—the angle between the mechanical axis of the femur and the mechanical axis of the tibia. Normal value 0–1.2°.[56,57]
- Transcondylar angle—the angle between the tangent line of the femoral condyles and the femoral mechanical axis. This is seen to be decreased in a certain percentage of cases contributing to the varus deformity. This may signify developmental abnormality, focal cartilage loss, or an adaptive remodeling response of osteoarthritis.
- Tibial plateau-tibial shaft angle—the angle between the tangent line of tibial plateau and the mechanical axis of the tibia.
- Varizing distances—extrinsic (EVD), intrinsic (IVD), global (EVD + IVD).

Principles in Planning the Steps of Osteotomy

Osteotomy at best is a time-buying procedure in most situations. Symptomatic deterioration over time may necessitate the need for arthroplasty. Reported outcomes of arthroplasty following HTO are inferior to those of primary osteoarthritis. Implants used for fixation, previous surgical scars, changes in the upper tibial morphology, patella baja are some of the issues that may impact the future arthroplasty. These need to be carefully considered during the planning.

Historical Overview

Jackson and Waugh[58] first published the concept of HTO. This was a report of eight cases with osteotomy performed distal to the tibial tuberosity. In response to the reported difficulties of healing with this osteotomy distal to the tibial tubercle, Coventry[59] published the closing wedge osteotomy proximal to the tibial tubercle. This osteotomy described by Coventry became synonymous with HTO.

The varus deformity results in the progressive shift of the weight-bearing point medially. The objective of the osteotomy is to bring the weight-bearing line to the center of the knee. Based on the static load distribution studies,[27] most studies recommend the restoration of the mechanical alignment to 2–6° of mechanical valgus.[59-62] This was validated in the long-term outcome of a large series reported by Hernigou et al.[63] who showed the best results with a correction band between 3° and 6°.

Taking the absolute point of load transfer within the knee, the recommendation is to correct the deformity for placing the mechanical axis to pass 30–40% lateral to the center of the tibial spine.[60] This is called the Fujisawa point, first described by the authors.

Based on the current understanding of the various issues and variables involved, namely the role of ligaments, adductor thrust, and the influence of the subject morphotype, Paley[64,65] and coworkers have suggested an ala carte approach based on the type of the deformity. They recommend that while planning the location of the osteotomy, it is necessary to consider the level of the center of rotation of angulation (CORA). Normally, it is at the level of the joint or just distal to it. If the osteotomy is made proximal to the tuberosity, only angulation is needed. However, if it is further away and distal, it will require both angulation and translation.

The four elements in the planning of correction are:

1. Type of osteotomy
2. Level of the osteotomy
3. Planning the degree of correction
4. Fixation options.

OPEN WEDGE OSTEOTOMY

This technique was first reported by Debeyre.[66-68] The availability of better fixation methods and encouraging results has generated a new wave of interest with this technique. There are several advantages of this technique which to date remains our personal preference:

- No violation of the proximal tibiofemoral joint.
- Correction can be precise and controlled.
- Biplane corrections can be achieved easily by adjusting the shape and thickness of the spacer wedges. Mild degrees of flexion contractures are correctable with the appropriate placement of the spacer wedges more posteriorly.

- Open wedge osteotomy does not result in any metadiaphyseal offset deformity. This is commonly seen in a closed wedge technique, especially larger corrections leading to difficulties in subsequent TKA (Need for offset stems, short keel base plates, etc.).
- The proximal tibial morphology is preserved.
- Intraligamentous osteotomy proximal to the tuberosity tightens the pseudolaxity of the MCL, often seen due to the cartilage loss. It has also been observed that small degrees of subluxation seen in some cases also tend to be corrected, secondary to the tightening of the MCL. This is subject to the ACL being intact and functional.
- Greater degrees of deformity are amenable to correction by the opening wedge technique.
- Dissection away from the peroneal nerve.
- The main disadvantage of this technique is the need for an additional graft, with the incidental donor site morbidity. Collapse and recurrence of the deformity and delayed bone healing are the other major concerns.

Variations of Open Wedge Osteotomy

- Open wedge osteotomy with acute correction
- Open wedge with callus distraction.

Open Wedge with Acute Correction

This procedure can be performed both proximal and distal to the tuberosity. Proximal to the tubercle has an influence on the tension of the MCL. This is an ideal technique in cases with moderate deformity associated with the pseudolaxity of the MCL. The advantage of performing at this level is, it is still cancellous bone and healing is more predictable.

Distal osteotomy is advocated when greater degrees of corrections are required. Also, if the MCL is tight, it is preferable to plan a distal osteotomy to avoid increasing the medial joint tension and load. The main disadvantage being, it is through the cortical bone with potential possibility of delay in healing. Also, it is necessary to bear on mind that being away from the joint line, the correction may need a combination of angulation and translation to be in line with CORA.

Planning the Osteotomy (Figures 5.4A and B)

- Divide the tibial plateau as shown in the figure from 0% to 100%. Identify the point ~62%, which often is over the medial aspect of the lateral condyle. This is the planned coordinate based on the measured MAD.
- Standing radiographs can at times overestimate the required degree of correction. This may be due to the stretched ligaments. Typically 1 mm wedge is equal to 1° of deformity (at a tibia width of 55–60 mm). If there is significant lateral opening, subtract the lateral joint space width of the opposite side to avoid overcorrection.
- Draw lines from the center of the femoral head and the ankle center to this coordinate.
- The angle formed defines the amount of angular correction required.
- Define the desired level of the osteotomy on a true A-P film. A point 3–3.5 cm from the joint line directed toward the fibular head is ideal. Advantages are as

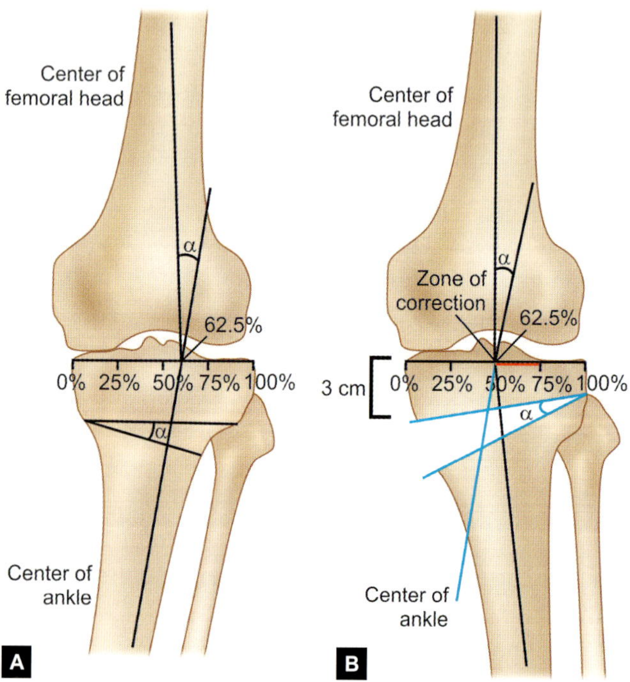

Figures 5.4A and B Preoperative planning. (A) Closed wedge osteotomy. α—angle of correction; (B) Open wedge osteotomy. Fujisawa point—center of the zone of correction

follows. It avoids intra-articular penetration of the osteotomy. Also, there is adequate bone for screw placement on the medial cortex.

- Draw the distal converging line to the osteotomy at the planned angle.
- Maintain the neutral slope in the sagittal plane to avoid tightening the ACL. Deliberate modification of the slope may be needed only under special circumstances like PCL deficiency or to decompress the patellofemoral joint.

Surgical Techniques—Medial Open Wedge Osteotomy (Figures 5.5A and B)

- The patient is positioned supine on the radiolucent table. A tricortical iliac graft, if planned, is harvested from the ipsilateral iliac crest. The extremity is draped free, and the tourniquet elevated straight incision is made midway between tibial tubercle and posteromedial border 2 cm proximal to joint line and 6–7 cm distally. The length may vary depending on the girth of the limb. It is desirable to have the length approximately 60% more than the width of the tibia at the level of the osteotomy. This helps in smooth the retraction of the composite osteoperiosteal sleeve without transverse tear. Incise the Sartorius fascia along the line of the skin incision
- Retract gracilis and semitendinosus posteriorly. Alternately, it may be incised transversely to be resutured later. Identify the superficial MCL. We propose a composite subperiosteal flap elevation both anteriorly and posterior, adequate to comfortably visualize the breadth of the tibia at the proposed site of osteotomy. Flex the knee 40° and continue the subperiosteal dissection posteriorly to retract the posterior structures. Place retractors anteriorly beneath the patellar tendon and subperiosteally posteriorly.
- Approximately 3.5 cm from joint line insert a guidewire directed toward the fibular head under fluoroscopy guidance if a sagittal slope is planned insert a second wire at the appropriate angle. Use a thin bladed saw to perform the osteotomy under fluoroscopic guide along the guidewire. Do not cut the lateral cortex. Stop short by 1 cm. Use a 2.5 mm drill to make 3–4 hole in the lateral cortex for controlled osteoclysis. Cut the remaining cancellous bone with a sharp osteotome.
- Under fluoroscopy, gradually open the osteotomy with a lamina spreader. Take care to avoid breaching the lateral cortex. Open the osteotomy to the desired amount as planned. Verify the correction. Insert the appropriate size wedge plate/synthetic wedge/bone graft as planned. Control the sagittal position according to the planned sagittal correction, if any. Secure the plate, if used. Alternately, correction can be adequately stabilized purely with a tricortical graft alone without the use of any fixation device. The prime requirement being the graft width should be equal to the desired degree of correction and of good quality. One important step in this method is ensuring cortex-to-cortex apposition of the graft and the medial tibial cortex. In this method, the limb is immobilized in a long leg cast for 4–6 weeks. Close the osteoperiosteal sleeve. And close the wound in layers.

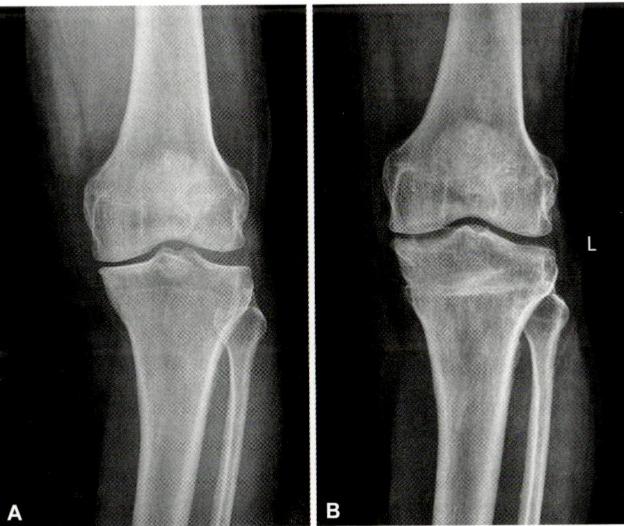

Figures 5.5A and B (A) Preoperative X-ray with varus deformity; (B) Correction with tricortical iliac graft-3 years postoperative

The newer implants developed especially for this osteotomy like the Puddu plate[69] and TomoFix, with dedicated instruments facilitate a precise correction and stable fixation (**Figures 5.6 and 5.7**). The plate with blocks of varying heights is fixed, such that the block buttresses

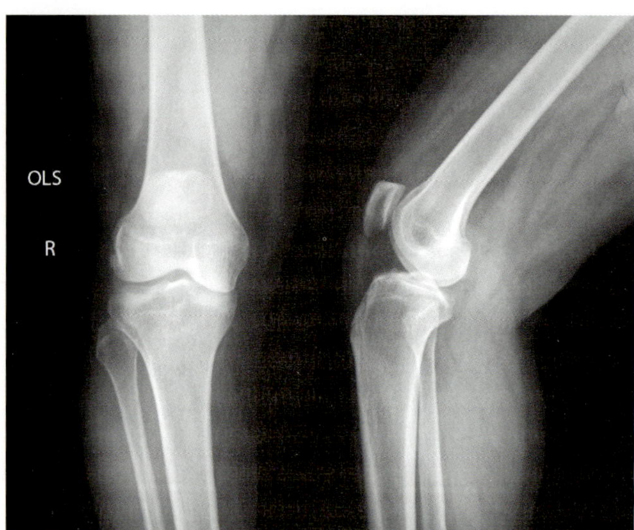

Figure 5.6 Preoperative X-rays with varus deformity

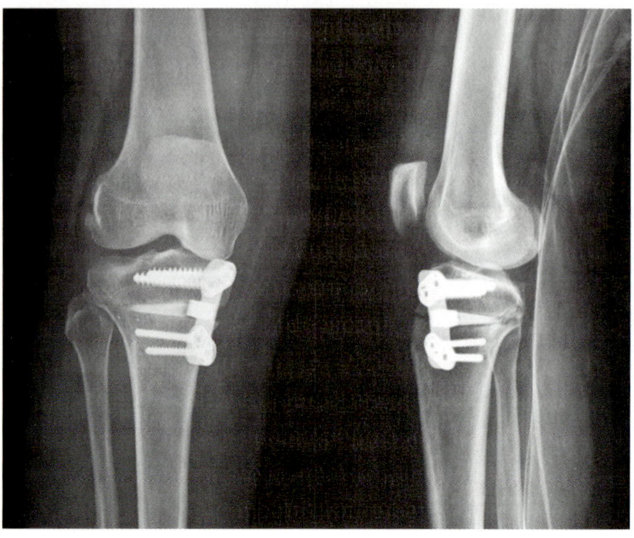

Figure 5.7 Postoperative correction with Puddu plate

precisely on the cortex of the osteotomy gap and prevents loss of correction. TomoFix is a plate-fixator adapted to the anatomy of the upper tibia, which works on the principle of the internal fixator. *In vitro* studies show a mechanical superiority of this device even in the presence of a breach of the lateral cortex.[70,71]

Open Wedge Osteotomy with Callus Distraction

Precise, controlled progressive opening wedge osteotomy has become increasingly popular in the recent years. Various types of external fixator devices are available like the T-Fixator, medial uniplanar fixator with a lockable ball joint; Illzarov frames are some of the popular constructs in use. One could perform the osteotomy proximal to the tubercle or distal to it. The advantages of this technique are as follows:

- It is less invasive.
- Fixators are relatively simple to apply.
- The distraction can be precisely controlled. The current fixator designs allow multiplanar adjustments during the process of distraction. With a precise preoperative plan, one could carry out simultaneous angulation and translation, if needed. The sagittal plane control is better.
- Partial weight-bearing is allowed immediately.
- There is no requirement of any graft or other filler devices.

The main disadvantage is the concern of pin tract infection.[72] Another potential risk is the loss of correction, if the fixator is removed prior to full maturation of the new bone. Overall this is a well-accepted popular technique these days. Patient personality too plays a part in the acceptance of this procedure since some people are wary of having the fixator for a prolonged period of time.

LATERAL CLOSING WEDGE OSTEOTOMY (*SEE* FIGURE 5.4A)

This technique is relatively more straightforward and since the time it was first described by Coventry,[53] it has remained a preferred method with many surgeons. The main advantages of this method are:

- It is performed proximal to the tubercle in the cancellous bone.
- No bone graft is required.
- The good bone to bone contact enables more aggressive rehabilitation.

- The healing is more predictable.
- The stabilization of the osteotomy is achieved with bone staples. The correction with the use of the angled swan-neck plate is preferred by the European surgeons.[73-75] On the other hand, a simple closure of the wedge with no fixation and only cast immobilization with early weight-bearing is a technique effectively adopted by many surgeons in India.

Surgical Technique

- The patient is positioned supine on the radiolucent table. The extremity is draped free, and the tourniquet is elevated. A short oblique incision is made from the fibular head toward the tibial tuberosity, 7–8 cm long. Various modifications to the incision have been proposed by various authors, ranging from transverse to curvilinear incisions. A relatively more straight incision is preferred, since this lends itself well to future revisions, minimizing the scar-related complications. This needs to be considered in the planning of the incision. Split the IT band anteriorly parallel to the incision. Confirm the location of the peroneal nerve by palpation. It is not always necessary to dissect and expose the nerve.
- For the effective closure of the wedge osteotomy, it is necessary that the tibiofibular articulation is dissociated in one of the three following ways: (1) percutaneous osteotomy at the lower third junction, (2) excision of the medial half of the fibular head and (3) complete capsulotomy of the superior tibiofibular joint. These maneuvers allow the dissociation of the tibiofemoral articulation, which helps in the complete closure of the osteotomy. Elevate the anterior tibial muscles subperiosteally. With the knee being in the flexion of 40°, continue the subperiosteal exposure posteriorly and insert a malleable retractor to guard the posterior structures. Place another retractor anteriorly between the patellar tendon and the tibia.
- Locate the joint line with a fine K-wire passed through the joint and confirmed with fluoroscopy. Pass a K-wire parallel to the joint line of the tibia 2.5 cm distally from the lateral to medial cortex. Pass a second wire obliquely at an angle based on the preoperative planning to intersect the first wire at the medial cortex. This determines the amount of wedge that needs to be resected. Osteotomy is made with a broad saw blade between the two wires (below the first and above the second). Care should be taken to remain parallel to the native tibia slope, unless any deliberate alteration has been planned preoperatively. Advance the osteotomy to 75% of the width and remove this partial wedge. It is extremely crucial to maintain the medial cortical continuity and avoid inadvertent osteotomy. Hence, it is preferable to perform the medial osteoclysis under vision. Proceed to complete the osteotomy gently with a fine sharp osteotome. Three to four drill holes with a 2.5 mm drill on the medial cortex is an effective way to perform a controlled osteoclysis. Ensure that the posterior cortex is cut completely and all the cortical bone is removed.
- Confirm with fluoroscopy and gently close the osteotomy with a valgus stress on the extremity in full extension. Confirm the alignment and correction. Proceed with the stabilization of osteotomy with the staples or the buttress plate as planned. Hemostasis is achieved and the wound is closed in layers under drains.

The potential limitations of this techniquc are:

- It is difficult to achieve large corrections.
- Injury to the peroneal nerve is a concern.
- Intraoperative adjustments are difficult. Also, this technique does not address the soft tissue laxity.
- Difficult to control the tibia slope.
- This alters the shape of the proximal tibia morphology impacting future conversions as discussed earlier.
- Violation of fibula or the syndesmosis is necessary.
- Alterations in the patella height, pseudopatella alta (patella riding proximal), retro patellar scarring and tethering of the retinaculum are the other undesirable consequences that affect future revisions.

Complications

- *Loss of correction:* Over and under correction are reflective of improper preoperative planning or the execution of the procedure. Late recurrence of the deformity has been reported in some long-term studies.[76] Hernigou[63] in a 20-year follow-up of 35 cases reported a recurrence in 50% of the cases despite a correction within the accepted range of 3–6° valgus. Deformity recurred within 10 years if the initial correction was less than 3°.

- *Patella baja:* This is a problem seen with the intraligamentous osteotomy; closing wedge osteotomy distal to the tubercle would potentially avoid this. This can be minimized by early mobilization following the surgery.
- *Intra-articular fractures:* Reported incidence is 2%.[77] Reported incidence is more with the opening wedge osteotomy.
- *Nonunion:* Delayed union or nonunion is rare. Most studies report a rate of 0.5–1%.
- Infection
- *Peroneal nerve dysfunction:* This could be related to the surgical dissection around the fibular head or during the closed wedge osteotomies. This has also been attributed to the application of the external fixator pins. Two areas seem prone to injury namely 30 mm and 153 mm from the fibular head.[78]
- Compartment syndrome.

CONCLUSION

A large number of studies performed on the pathogenesis and progression of osteoarthritis have led to a better understanding of the key issues involved. Contrary to the earlier understanding, it is clear today that besides the static malalignment, dynamic factors, such as the adductor thrust, the patient morphotype, alterations in the gait pattern, influence the outcome of these corrective surgeries. The modifications in the technique proposed by various authors address both the bone and the soft tissue deformities. Improved fixation options enable the early mobilization of the joint and maintenance of the correction.

Critical to the success of the procedure is the careful patient selection. This is a technique-sensitive procedure. Meticulous planning and restoration of the mechanical axis to 3–6° of mechanical valgus seem to give the best outcomes. Correction with the use of fixators and hemicallus distraction is becoming popular, given the fact that precise multiplane correction, infratubercle osteotomy, and early mobilization with a less invasive approach can be achieved. Despite the increasing popularity of the alternate options, tibial osteotomy still has a significant role in the active middle-aged with monocompartmental disease or in conjunction with other joint conserving procedures. A well-performed procedure does add 10–20 years to the life of the natural joint, allowing high-impact activities and burns no bridges for the future procedures.

REFERENCES

1. Descamps L, Jarsaillon B, Schuster P, et al. Angular synthesis in upper tibial valgus osteotomy in osteoarthritis: apropos of a series of 544 cases. Rev Chir Orthop Reparatrice Appar Mot. 1987;73:231-6.
2. Font-Rodriguez DE, Scuderi GR, Insall JN. Survivorship of cemented total knee arthroplasty. Clin Orthop. 1967;345:79-86.
3. Rand JA, Ilstrup DM. Survivorship analysis of total knee arthroplasty: cumulative rates of survival of 9200 total knee arthroplasties. J Bone Joint Surg Am. 1991;73:397-409.
4. Carr A, Keyes G, Miller R, et al. Medial unicompartmental arthroplasty: a survival study of the Oxford meniscal knee. Clin Orthop. 1993;295:205-13.
5. Tabor OB Jr, Tabor OB. Unicompartmental arthroplasty: a long-term follow-up study. J Arthroplasty. 1998;13:373-9.
6. Murray DW, Goodfellow JM, O'Connor J. The Oxford medial unicompartmental arthroplasty: a ten-year survival study. J Bone Joint Surg Br. 1998;80:983-9.
7. Berger RA, Meneghini RM, Sheinkop MB, et al. The progression of patellofemoral arthrosis after medial unicompartmental replacement: results at 11 to 15 years. Clin Orthop. 2004;428:92-9.
8. Mont MA, Stuchin SA, Paley D, et al. Different surgical options for monocompartmental osteoarthritis of the knee: high tibial osteotomy versus unicompartmental knee arthroplasty versus total knee arthroplasty: indications, techniques, results, and controversies Instr Course Lect. 2004;53:265-83.
9. Swienckowski JJ, Pennington DW. Unicompartmental knee arthroplasty in patients sixty years of age or younger. J Bone Joint Surg Am. 2004;86(Suppl 1):131-42.

10. Wu DD, Burr DB, Boyd RD, et al. Bone and cartilage changes following experimental varus or valgus tibial angulation. J Orthop Res. 1990;8:572-85.
11. McKellop HA, Sim FH, Redfern FC, et al. The effect of simulated fracture-angulations of the tibia on cartilage pressures in the knee joint. J Bone Joint Surg Am. 1991;73:1382-91.
12. Hanssen AD, Stuart MJ, Scott RD, Scuderi FR. Surgical options for the middle-aged patient with osteoarthritis of the knee joint. Instr Course Lect. 2001;50:499-511.
13. Amendola A, Fowler PJ, Litchfield R, et al. Opening wedge high tibial osteotomy using a novel technique: early results and complications. J Knee Surg. 2004;17:164-9.
14. Koshino T, Murase T, Saito T. Medial opening-wedge high tibial osteotomy with use of porous hydroxyapatite to treat medial compartment osteoarthritis of the knee. J Bone Joint Surg Am. 2003;85:78-85.
15. Lobenhoffer P, Agneskirchner JD. Improvements in surgical technique of valgus high tibial osteotomy. Knee Surg Sports Traumatol Arthrosc. 2003;11:132-8.
16. Staubli AE, De Simoni C, Babst R, Lobenhoffer P. TomoFix: a new LCP-concept for open wedge osteotomy of the medial proximal tibia-early results in 92 cases. Injury. 2003;34(Suppl 2):B55-B62.
17. Stoffel K, Stachowiak G, Kuster M. Open wedge high tibial osteotomy: biomechanical investigation of the modified Arthrex Osteotomy Plate (Puddu Plate) and the TomoFix Plate. Clin Biomech. 2004;19:944-50.
18. Sen C, Kocaoglu M, Eralp. The advantages of circular external fixation used in high tibial osteotomy (average 6 years follow-up). Knee Surg Sports Traumatol Arthrosc. 2003;11:139-44.
19. Weale AE, Lee AS, MacEachern AG. High tibial osteotomy using a dynamic axial external fixator. Clin Orthop. 2001;382:154-67.
20. Badhe NP, Forster IW. High tibial osteotomy in knee instability: the rationale of treatment and early results. Knee Surg Sports Traumatol Arthrosc. 2002;10:38-43.
21. Bonin N, Ait Si Selmi T, Donell ST, et al. Anterior cruciate reconstruction combined with valgus upper tibial osteotomy: 12 years follow-up. Knee. 2004;11:431-7.
22. McGuire DA, Carter TR, Shelton WR. Complex knee reconstruction: osteotomies, ligament reconstruction, transplants, and cartilage treatment options. Arthroscopy. 2002;18(9, Suppl 2):90-103.
23. Sterett WI, Steadman JR. Chondral resurfacing and high tibial osteotomy in the varus knee. Am J Sports Med. 2004;32:1243-9.
24. Cooke TDV, Pichora D, Siu D, Scudamore RA, Bryant JT. Surgical implications of varus deformity of the knee with obliquity of joint surfaces. J Bone Joint Surg. 1989;71B:560-5.
25. Hernborg JS, Nilsson BE. The natural course of untreated osteoarthritis of the knee. Clin Orthop. 1977;123:130-7.
26. Odenbring S, Lindstrand A, Egund N, et al. Prognosis for patients with medial gonarthrosis. A 16-year follow-up study of 189 knees. Clin Orthop. 1991;266:152-5.
27. Hsu RW, Himeno S, Coventry MB, Chao EY. Normal axial alignment of the lower extremity and load-bearing distribution at the knee. Clin Orthop Relat Res. 1990;255:215-27.
28. Huss RA, Holstein H, O'Connor JJ. A mathematical model of forces in the knee under isometric quadriceps contractions. Clin Biomech. 2000;15:112-22.
29. Lu TW, O'Connor JJ. Lines of action and moment arms of the major force-bearing crossing the human knee joint: comparison between theory and experiment. J Anat. 1996;189:575-85.
30. Korovessis P, Katsoudas G, Salonikides P, et al. Medium- and long-term results of high tibial osteotomy for varus gonarthrosis in an agricultural population. Orthopedics. 1999;22(8):729-36.
31. Lawrence JS, Bremner JM, Bier F. Osteoarthrosis: prevalence in the population and relationship between symptoms and X-ray changes. Ann Rheum Dis. 1996;25:1-24.
32. Maquet P. Osteotomy. In: Freeman MAR (Ed), Arthritis of the Knee Clinical Features and Surgical Management. Berlin: Springer-Verlag; 1980. pp. 148-83.
33. Maquet P. Surgical treatment of femoro-tibial arthrosis. Acta Orthop Belg. 1982;48:172-89.
34. Maquet P. The treatment of choice in osteoarthritis of the Knee. Clin Orthop. 1985;192:108-12.
35. Akamatsu Y, Koshino T, Saito T, et al. Changes in osteosclerosis of the osteoarthritic knee after high tibial osteotomy. Clin Orthop. 1997;334:207-14.
36. Koshino T, Ranawat NS. Healing process of osteoarthritis in the knee after high tibial osteotomy through observation of strontium-85 scintimetry. Clin Orthop. 1672;82:149-56.

37. Blaimont P, Burnotte J, Baillon JM, et al. Contribution biomecanique a l'etude des conditions d'equilibre dans le genou normal et pathologique: application au traitement de l'arthrose varisante. Acta Orthop Belg. 1971;37:573-91.
38. Blaimont P, Burnotte J, Halleux P. La prearthrose du genou: Pathogenie biomecanique et traitement prophylactique. Acta Orthop Belg. 1975;41:177-200.
39. Andriacchi TP. Dynamics of knee malalignment. Orthop Clin North Am. 1994;25:395-403.
40. Prodromos CC, Andriacchi TP, Galante JO. A relationship between gait and clinical changes following high tibial osteotomy. J Bone Joint Surg Am. 1985;67:1188-94.
41. Wang JW, Kuo KN, Andriacchi TP, Galante JO. The influence of walking mechanics and time on the results of proximal tibial osteotomy. J Bone Joint Surg Am. 1990;72:905-9.
42. Sharma L, Lou C, Felson DT, et al. Laxity in healthy and osteoarthritic knees. Arthritis Rheum. 1999;42:861-70.
43. Coventry MB. Upper tibial osteotomy. Clin Orthop. 1984;182-46-52.
44. Morrey BF. Upper tibial osteotomy for secondary osteoarthritis of the knee. J Bone Joint Surg Br. 1996;71:554-9.
45. Slawski DP. High tibial osteotomy in the treatment of adult osteochondritis dissecans. Clin Orthop. 1997;341:155-61.
46. Coventry MB, Ilstrup DM, Wallrichs SL. Proximal tibial osteotomy. A critical long-term study of eighty-seven cases. J Bone Joint Surg Am. 1993;75:196-201.
47. Grelsamer R. High tibial osteotomy (HTO) is an effective procedure for medial and patellofemoral disease. Clin Orthop. 1990;260:310,311.
48. Insall J, Shoji H, Mayer V. High tibial osteotomy: a five-year evaluation. J Bone Joint Surg Am. 1974;56:1397-1405.
49. Insall JN. Osteotomy. In: Insall JN, Windsor RE, Scott WN, et al. (Eds), Surgery of the knee, 2nd edn. New York: Churchill Livingstone; 1993. pp. 635-75.
50. Insall JN, Joseph DM, Msika C. High tibial osteotomy for varus gonarthrosis: a long-term follow-up study. J Bone Joint Surg Am. 1984;66:1040-8.
51. Matthews LS, Goldstein SA, Malvitz TA, et al. Proximal tibial osteotomy: factors that influence the duration of satisfactory function. Clin Orthop. 1988;229:193-200.
52. Levigne CH, Bonnin M. Ostetomie tibiale de valgisation pour arthrose femoro-tibiale interne: Resultats d' un echantillon de 217 osteotomies revues avec un recul de 1 a 21 ans. In: Dejour H, Neyret P (Eds), Journees Lyonnaises de Chirurgie du Genou. Lyon: Hopital Lyon Sud; 1991. pp. 142-68.
53. Coventry MB. Osteotomy about the knee for degenerative and rheumatoid arthritis. J Bone Joint Surg Am. 1973;55:23-48.
54. Scuderi GR, Windsor RE, Insall JN. Observations on patellar height after proximal tibial osteotomy. J Bone Joint Surg Am. 1989;71:245-8.
55. Tigani D, Ferari D, Trentani P, et al. Patellar height after high tibial osteotomy. Int Orthop. 2001;24:331-4.
56. Moreland JR, Basset LW, Hanker GJ. Radiographic analysis of the axial alignment of the lower extremity. J Bone Joint Surg Am. 1987;69:745-9.
57. Ramadier Jo, Buard Je, Lortat-Jacob A, et al. Mesure radiologique des deformations frontales du genou: Procede du profil vrai radiologique. Rev Chir Orthop. 1982;68:75-8.
58. Jackson JP, Waugh W. Tibial osteotomy for osteoarthritis of the knee. J Bone Joint Surg Br. 1961:43:746-51.
59. Coventry Mb. Osteotomy of the upper portion of the tibia for degenerative arthritis of the knee: a preliminary report. J Bone Joint Surg Am. 1965;47:984-90.
60. Fujisawa Y, Masuhara K, Shiomi S. The effect of the high tibial osteotomy on osteoarthritis of the knee: an arthroscopic study of 54 knee joints. Orthop Clin North Am. 1979;10:585-608.
61. Hernigou P, Medevielle D, Debeyre J, Goutallier D. Proximal tibial osteotomy for osteoarthritis with varus deformity: a ten to thirteen-year follow-up study. J Bone Joint Surg Am. 1987;69:332-54.
62. Jacobi M, Jakob RP. Open wedge osteotomy in the treatment medial osteoarthritis of the knee. Tech Knee Surg. 2005;4:70-78.
63. Hernigou P. A 20-year follow-up study of internal gonarthrosis after tibial valgus osteotomy: single versus repeated osteotomy. Rev Chir Orthop Reparatrice Appar Mot. 1996;82:241-50.
64. Paley D, Maar DC, Herzenberg JE. New concepts in high tibial osteotomy for medial compartment osteoarthritis. Orthop Clin North Am. 1994;24:483-98.
65. Paley D. Principles of Deformity Correction. 1st edn. Berlin: Springer-Verlag; 2005 (revised edn.).

66. Debeyre J, Artigou JM. Long-term results of 260 tibial osteotomies for frontal deviations of the knee. Rev Chir Orthop Reparatrice Appar Mot. 1972;58:335-9.
67. Debeyre J, Artigou JM. Indications and results of tibial osteotomy: influence of laxity. Rev Chir Orthop Reparatrice Appar Mot. 1973;59:641-56.
68. Debeyre J, Patte D. Place des osteotomies de correction dans le traitement de la gonarthrose. Acta Orthop Bleg. 1961;27:374-83.
69. Puddu G, Cerullo G, Cipolla M, et al. A plate for open wedge tibial osteotomy. Personal communication; 1997.
70. Staubli AE, De Simoni C, Babst R, et al. TomoFix: a new LCP-concept for open wedge osteotomy of the medial proximal tibia-early results in 92 cases. Injury. 2003;34(Suppl 2): B55-B62.
71. Stoffel K, Stachowiak G, Kuster M. Open wedge high tibial osteotomy: biomechanical investigation of the modified Arthrex Osteotomy Plate (Puddu Plate) and the TomoFix Plate. Clin Biomech. 2004;19:944-50.
72. Perusi M, Baietta B, Pizzoli A. Surgical correction of osteoarthritic genu varum by the hemicallotasis technique. Rev Chir Orthop Reparatrice Appar Mot. 1994;80:739-43.
73. Postel M, Langlais F. Osteotomies du genou pour gonarthrose. In: Encyclopèdie Medico-chirurgicale: Techniques Chirurgicales, Orthopedie. Paris, Editions Techniques; 1997. pp. 1-17.
74. Merle d'Aubigne R. Joint realignment in the management of osteoarthritis. In: Straub LR, Wilson PD Jr (Eds), Clinical Trends in Orthopedics. New York: Thieme-Stratton; 1982. p. 246.
75. Segal P, Burdin PH, Cartier PH, et al. Les echecs des osteotomies tibiales de valgisation pour gonarthrose et leurs reprises: symposium. Rev Chir Orthop. 1992;78:85-128.
76. Stuart MJ, Grace JN, Ilstrup DM, et al. Late recurrence of varus deformity after proximal tibial osteotomy. Clin Orthrop. 1990;260:61-5.
77. Healy WL, Wilk RM. Osteotomy in treatment of the arthritic knee. In: Scott WN (Ed.), The Knee. St. Louis: Mosby; 1994. pp. 1019-43.
78. Kirgis A, Albrecht S. Palsy of the deep peroneal nerve after proximal tibial osteotomy: an anatomical study. J Bone Joint Surg Am. 1992;74:1180-85.

Chapter 6

Choice of Knee Implant

CJ Thakkar, Anoop Jhurani

INTRODUCTION

The success of total knee replacement as a treatment for arthritis has led to an exponential rise in number of surgeries all over the world. With the growing number of surgeries, there has been a parallel growth in the number of knee implants as well. Some implants have been successfully used for last two decades while others have been recently introduced. The number and variety of knee implants pushed with a strong marketing force often confuse the surgeon regarding the choice of knee implant. Some of the potential advantages of these newer knee prosthesis are questionable and not based on evidence. The purpose of this chapter is to evaluate the long-term results of each device through best evidence and consider other important factors to form a guideline for the practicing orthopedic surgeon regarding the choice and use of total knee prosthesis. The following factors should be considered while choosing a knee implant:

- History and long-term results of the knee prosthesis
- Body mass index (BMI), type of arthritis, age of the patient
- Ligament laxity and condition of the ligaments (Posterior cruciate ligament, Medial collateral ligament, Lateral collateral ligament)
- Bone quality and bone defects
- Preoperative range of movement and deformity
- Training and surgical skills.

HISTORY AND LONG-TERM RESULTS OF KNEE PROSTHESIS

Cruciate-retaining and Cruciate-substituting Knees

The role of the posterior cruciate ligament (PCL) remains controversial in total knee arthroplasty (TKA), with some surgeons who believe in PCL sacrifice and substitution and others who believe in PCL preservation for stability. Manufacturers have developed both cruciate-substituting/posterior-stabilized (PS) implants typically used when the ligament is sacrificed and the cruciate-retaining (CR) implants designed for ligament preservation (**Figures 6.1 and 6.2**).

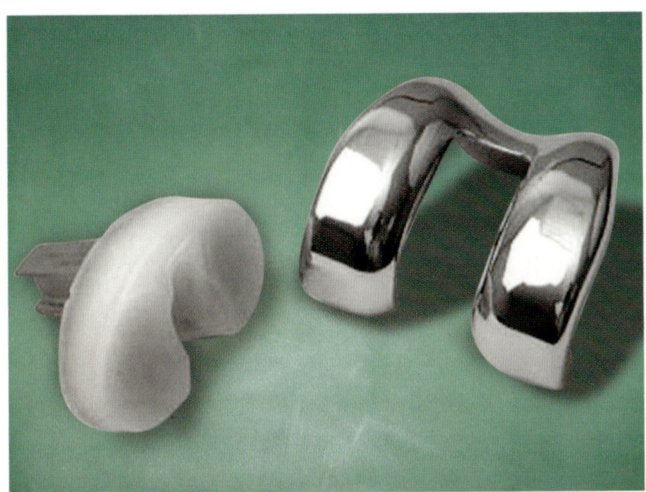

Figure 6.1 Cruciate-retaining knee

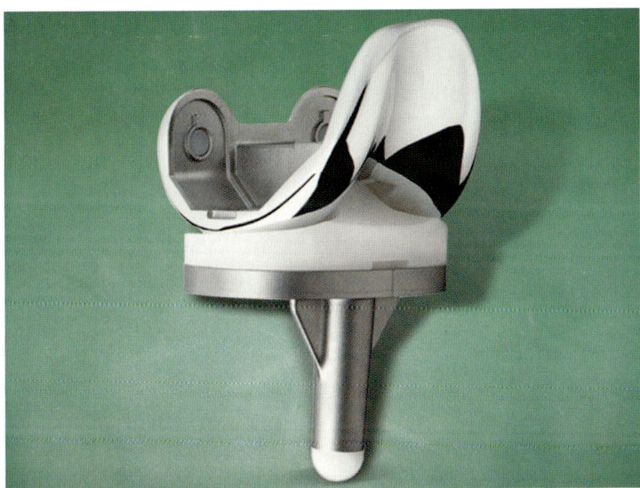

Figure 6.2 Cruciate-substituting knee

Advantages of PCL Retention

The potential advantages of preserving the PCL are many. As a natural ligament imparts stability, the prosthesis does not need a box-cam mechanism for stability and hence is less constrained; therefore, less force is imparted to the insert-tray interface and the prosthesis-to-bone interface.

With the PCL preservation, it is also possible to maintain the joint line at a near-normal location. When the PCL is cut, the flexion gap increases by 2–3 mm and there is a requirement for thicker polyethylene to fill the flexion space. This thicker polyethylene in turn requires greater distal femoral resection to allow full extension of the knee. Thus, the joint line is elevated in both flexion and extension by a few millimeters with cruciate-sacrificing designs leading to distortion of the collateral ligament kinematics. Finally, CR knees allow the preservation of the intercondylar bone stock for future revision, and it also prevents condylar fractures in small-sized Asian knees.

Disadvantages of PCL Retention

There are some potential disadvantages of PCL retention. There is the possibility of late anterior-posterior instability if the PCL stretches or ruptures over time. Another criticism is a higher incidence of late polyethylene wear. Since early designs of CR knees were mostly round on flat, the higher stresses led to a higher incidence of wear compared to cruciate-sacrificing designs with curved-on-curved articulations. This experience led to the evolution of PCL-preserving designs with curved tibial topography in the sagittal plane that has reduced the amount of the late polyethylene wear.

Indications for Posterior-stabilized Primary TKA

The advantages of the PCL substitution are that it is easier and more forgiving to balance deformity. The knee is more forgiving of slight flexion laxity. Modern designs of cruciate substitution provide controlled rollback for better potential range of motion, especially in preoperatively stiff knees. Finally, the partial rotational constraint between the post and the femoral housing allows the surgeon to have more control in selecting the Q-angle of the knee to facilitate patellar tracking in cases having patellar instability.

Following are the ideal candidates for PCL substitution: the ankylosed knee, the knee with severe deformities especially flexion contracture, the knee with chronic patellar dislocation, the postpatellectomy knee and knee with severe inflammatory arthritis in which PCL may be insufficient.

Disadvantages of PCL Substitution

Several possible disadvantages can be sighted for the PCL substitution technique. Because of the higher constraint in the articulation, greater stress is transferred to the modular insert-tray or bone-cement interface. These forces lead to increased motion between the insert and tray and initiate backside wear. These same forces could also increase the potential for loosening of the prosthesis at the fixation interface in both modular and nonmodular designs.

A second problem specific to PCL-substituting designs is the patellar clunk syndrome. This occurs when there is a build-up of the scar tissue above the superior pole of the patella on the quadriceps tendon. This scar gets entrapped in the intercondylar notch of the femoral component in flexion, causing painful crepitus as the knee is extended. A third disadvantage of the PCL substitution is the removal of the intercondylar bone stock for the housing of the femoral component.

Posterior CR and PS TKA have similar clinical outcomes with regard to the knee function, postoperative knee pain and other complications. Prosthesis survivorship for both posterior CR and PS TKA is satisfactory, and there are no differences between them at a middle-term follow-up. With regard to the longevity of implant, the CR knee appears to have an edge over the PS design in the Australian and Mayo registry with a lower risk of revision at 15 years.

The decision to use one design versus the other should rest with the surgeon's preference and comfort with a particular design.

FIXED COMPARED WITH MOBILE-BEARINGS FOR KNEE REPLACEMENT

The original low contact stress (LCS) mobile-bearing implant was developed to reduce wear and improve function after the TKA. This device originally had two principal designs: meniscal bearing and rotating platform. The rotating-platform design was the more widely used because of the greater frequency of dislocations associated with the meniscal-bearing design. Currently, many new mobile-bearing designs are available, and the safety and effectiveness of mobile bearings in general and of the individual designs have not been well studied. The dislocation of mobile-bearing total knee implants seems to be a unique phenomenon related to this bearing design, and this subtle instability may present as pain or stiffness.

BIOMECHANICS OF A MOBILE-BEARING KNEE

Fixed-bearing knees, whether CR or substituting, have a good track record at 10–15 years of the follow-up. The small incidence of the late tibial insert wear requiring revision is the problem that in theory might be addressed by mobile-bearing articulations. These were designed to allow high conformity between metal and plastic to minimize stresses and lower the incidence of the wear. This type of articulation can provide high conformity on the topside to minimize the surface wear without the adverse effects of constraint. Backside wear is addressed by allowing the undersurface of the insert to move freely as determined by the dynamic forces across the knee on a flat-on-flat surface that provides the least amount of stress to the polyethylene (**Figure 6.3**).

A second advantage of a rotating-platform mobile bearing is the ability of the prosthetic articulation to accommodate to malrotation between the femur and the tibia that either is created at operation by the surgeon or occurs postoperatively during functional activities.

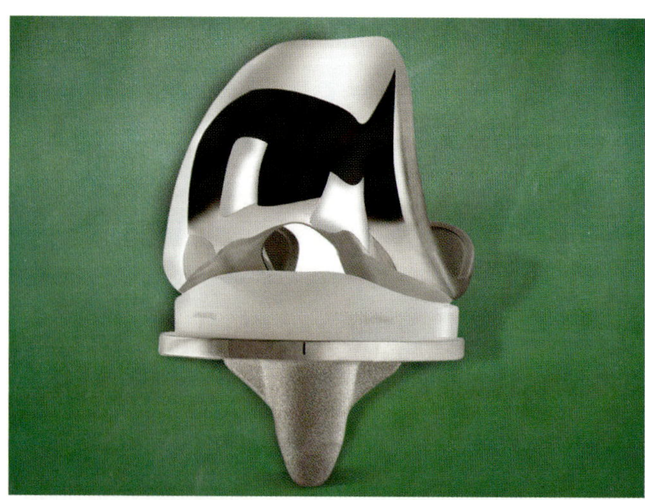

Figure 6.3 Rotating-platform knee

Disadvantages of Mobile-Bearings

Mobile bearings without stops can subluxate, impinging on soft tissues, and even possibly dislocate. Bearings with stops, however, might be subject to wear because of repetitive impingement on the stop. To prevent impingement, most mobile-bearing inserts are slightly smaller than equivalent fixed-bearing inserts. This allows a certain amount of rotation or translation to occur on top of the tray before soft tissue impingement can occur.

Mobile-bearing knees are also somewhat more sensitive to certain technical considerations, while they are forgiving to others, such as malrotation. For rotating-platform knees, the most significant technical complication is 'spinout' of the bearing (dislocation), usually a result of flexion gap asymmetry. As a consequence of flexion gap asymmetry with or without posterior cruciate tightness, a mobile bearing could fail early with spinout. Fixed-bearing knees, however, may be able to tolerate flexion gap asymmetry for a much longer period of time, failing late as a result of progressive instability problems or polyethylene wear.

The finding of most prospective randomized trials, registry reports, and meta-analyses shows no evidence of the superiority of mobile-bearing designs compared with fixed-bearing designs with respect to survival of implants, range of movement and overall function. The LCS and other rotating-platform implants have been associated with a greater revision rate compared with contemporary fixed-bearing implants in the Norwegian and Australian national registry.

ALL POLYETHYLENE VERSUS METAL-BACKED TIBIAL COMPONENTS IN TOTAL KNEE ARTHROPLASTY

The advantages of all polytibial component are the lack of backside wear and its cost effectiveness. The potential disadvantages are subsidence in cases with bone defects, lack of modularity and difficulty in changing the liner in cases of infection.

While the benefits have been well proven in the literature, the evidence for the potential pitfalls is scant. To circumvent the perceived disadvantages of the all polytibial component, 'highly polished' cobalt-chromium tibial trays have been introduced to reduce wear and osteolysis (**Figure 6.4**). Whether these expensive trays will provide improved longevity over the time tested all polytibial component remains to be seen.

The criticism of all polytibial components on its strength of fixation and unequal distribution of forces on the tibial plateau when compared to the metal-backed component is unfounded.

Several studies have described equivalent performance on radiostereometric analysis of all-polyethylene and metal-backed tibial components in the TKA. While metal-backed prosthesis was introduced to bring modularity in polysize and distribute joint reaction forces more evenly, they brought in a new problem of backside wear.

Numerous studies support the use of all polyethylene tibial design for primary knee arthroplasty in the majority of patients. The metal-backed tibial component offers intraoperative flexibility and the choice for using stems when required. The contribution of backside wear to overall volumetric wear and subsequent osteolysis is essentially nonexistent with use of all polyethylene tibial designs and is a problem seen with metal-backed devices. Finally, the issue of cost clearly favors the all polyethylene tibial component. In light of the current evidence, equal consideration should be given to the use of all polyethylene tibial implants in the primary TKA.

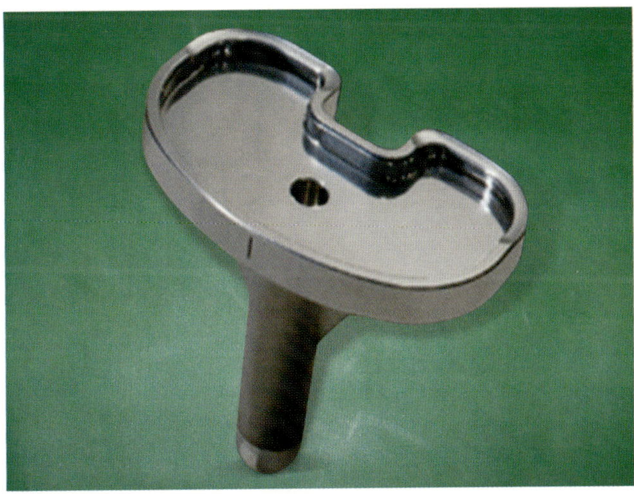

Figure 6.4 Highly polished Co–Cr tray

MONOBLOCK TIBIA WITH COMPRESSION-MOLDED POLYETHYLENE: A CASE FOR REDUCED WEAR

In an effort to reduce the backside wear in the metal-backed modular tibia and offset the disadvantages of the all poly tibia, the monoblock metal back tibia was introduced along with the compression-molded polyethylene (AGC, Biomet, USA), (**Figure 6.5**). The potential advantages were the elimination of the backside wear and the increased longevity of implant. This metal-backed monoblock tibia has been proven to have survivorship of more than 95% at 15-year follow-up in many studies. It has also given excellent long-term results in young active patients aged less than 55 years proving that minimizing poly and backside wear improves longevity of knee implants. The poly in this particular type of implant is compression molded poly wherein most other knee prosthesis have bar extruded poly. Direct compression molded polyethylene is a process of creating a net-shaped component with finished articular surfaces from ultrahigh molecular weight polyethylene by applying heat and pressure to the raw resin (usually Hi-fax 1900) with the use of fixed geometry metallic tools. The final product has no machining or finishing. This polyethylene has proven track record in both *in vivo* and *in vitro* settings. The Swedish registry considers AGC implant as the baseline to compare other prosthesis as AGC has 97.5% survivorship at 10 years in Swedish registry.

HIGH FLEXION KNEES

The demand of increased knee bending from patients all over the world, especially the Asian countries, is increasing. This has promoted many companies to launch and promote high flexion implants. Whether these implants truly give the patient the benefit of high flexion in weight-bearing positions is the contentious issue that remains unanswered.

Some designs also require the surgeon to remove up to 4 mm of bone from the posterior condyles (**Figure 6.6**). The potential long-term effect of this on femoral fixation and its efficacy to achieve few more degrees of flexion needs to be assessed. Initial reports of radiolucent lines along the posterior condyles of high flexion knees may well be the initial warning sign.

In an effort to give high flexion, manufacturers have brought in design changes in the femoral implant and the Polyliner without substantial investigation about its long-term effects on wear and damage to box-cam mechanism. Many of these 'new' high flexion knees have gone into disrepute because of increased incidence of patellar crepitus and loosening of the femur component. The ill-effects and the increased cost of high flexion devices along

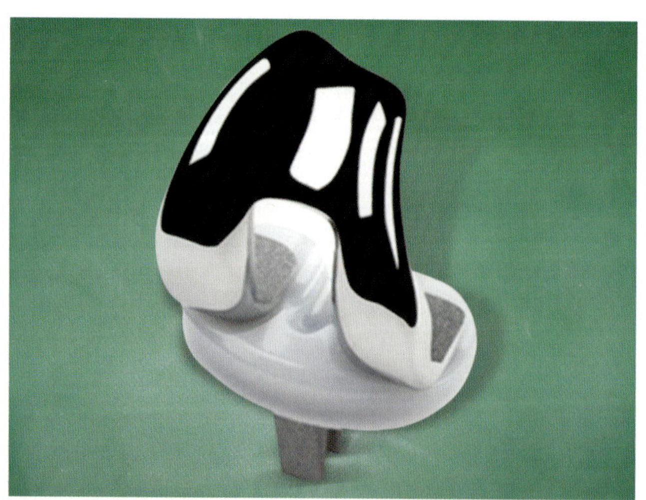

Figure 6.5 Metal-backed monoblock tibia

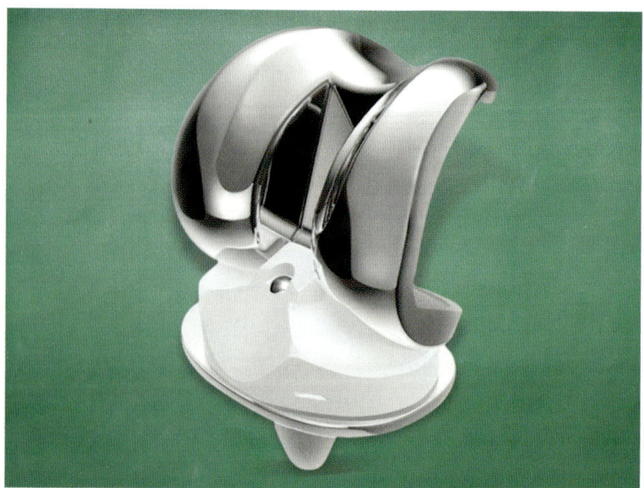

Figure 6.6 Rotating-platform high flexion knee

with the evidence of comparable results with the standard prosthesis certainly do not make a case for their use in everyday practice.

OXINIUM FEMORAL COMPONENT

Polyethylene wear is one of the most common causes for TKA failure after 5 years. The etiology of wear is multifactorial but usually occurs at the bearing surface. Recent advances in implant design have focused on reducing the number of biologically active wear particles. This can be achieved either by improving the polyethylene liner or by the use of alternative bearing surfaces to improve the wear characteristics of the femoral component.

Femoral components are usually manufactured with a standard cobalt-chromium alloy with a polished articular surface. A new bearing surface has been manufactured from wrought zirconium alloy (Zr–niobium [Nb] 2.5%) oxidized by thermal diffusion to create a 5 mm oxidized zirconium layer (oxinium; Smith and Nephew). The surface oxide is a transformation of the underlying metal surface into zirconium oxide ceramic, resulting in an implant that combines the strength of metal with the wear properties of ceramic in terms of its superior lubrication properties and resistance to abrasive scratching (**Figure 6.7**). Whether this surface will prove to be superior to conventional cobalt chrome and prove its worth in clinical practice needs critical assessment.

While the *in vitro* trials with oxinium suggest better lubrication properties and lesser wear as compared to the conventional cobalt-chromium femur, the clinical results with both these implants seem similar in most randomized prospective studies.

GENDER-SPECIFIC KNEE

The difference in male and female femoral anatomy is well known. While man's femur is shorter anteroposteriorly and wider mediolaterally, the female's femoral anatomy is reverse. A woman's femur is taller anteroposteriorly and narrower mediolaterally. Hence, it is common to find overhang of the femoral component on the lateral side in many women. Whether this overhang is clinically significant and causes any relevant symptoms is unclear.

To solve this problem, a special implant for the female gender was developed and marketed as the gender knee. This implant is narrower mediolaterally on the anterior flange and has a wider Q-angle to mimic the female anatomy (**Figure 6.8**).

Though the idea of having gender-specific knee prosthesis was attractive and gained popularity, the long-term advantages of this knee over others has not been proven. Patient subjective preferences for gender-specific knees in female total knee patients showed no advantages over standard unisex knees in terms of clinical or radiologic outcomes.

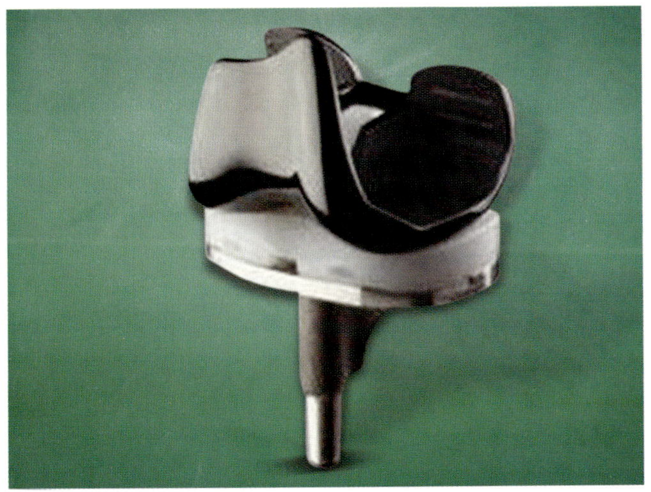

Figure 6.7 Oxinium knee

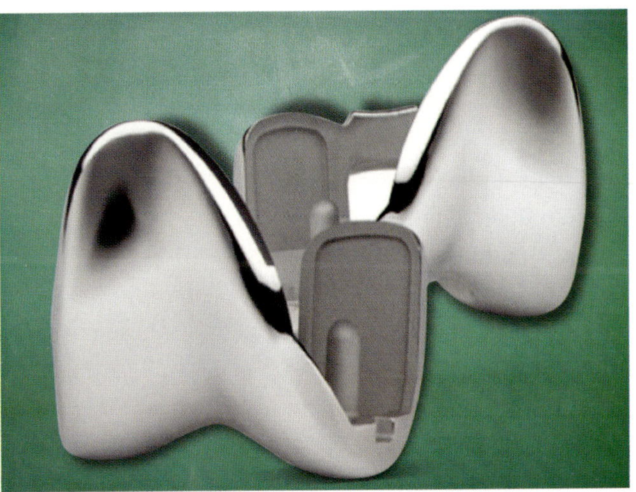

Figure 6.8 Gender knee

A careful analysis of all available evidence proves superior long-term results of fixed-bearing knees when compared to rotating-bearing prosthesis. The claim that rotating-platform or other high flexion knees gives more flexion in weight-bearing positions is unfounded. Improved outcomes have not been found with new surfaces like oxinium and newer designs like the gender knee. The old workhorse, all polytibial component, continues to give excellent long-term results.

Finally, orthopedic surgeons ought to be evidence based in their approach to choose a prosthesis. Restraint must be exercised before believing in advertisements and industrial claims. It would be wise to accept a new prosthesis only if there is sufficient evidence that it is likely to perform better than the implants with proven long-term results.

BODY MASS INDEX (BMI), AGE, AND TYPES OF ARTHRITIS

The spectrum of patients undergoing TKA has changed over the last decade. Younger patients with degenerative arthritis are presenting for total knee replacement and so are the elderly whose longevity and quality of life are improving. It is common to see patients from age of 50–85 years presenting for the treatment of knee arthritis.

The age of the patient has a bearing on the choice of prosthesis. Younger the patient, better be the implant with a proven track record of 20 years and lowest risk of revision. The young active high demand patients should be implanted with a CR knee, if the surgeon is trained and familiar with the technique as the longevity of CR knees surpasses that of PS knees in Mayo and Australian registry. If the surgeon is of the PS philosophy, then highly polished cobalt-chromium tibia or a monoblock metal-backed tibia is recommended to reduce wear and delay revision.

If the patient has inflammatory arthritis, then the PS metal-backed knee should be the implant of choice as the posterior cruciate is often incompetent in these patients. An elderly patient of over 70 years could well be offered a metal-backed device or an all polytibia.

The percentage of obese patients presenting for knee arthroplasty is increasing as well. These patients present with lax ligaments and associated osteopenia because of multiple metabolic disturbances associated with obesity. Most studies favor the use of PS metal-backed knees for these patients.

LIGAMENT LAXITY AND CONDITION OF LIGAMENTS

The clinical examination before and after anesthesia is of paramount importance in deciding on the nature of prosthesis to be used for that particular patient. A patient with lax ligaments will do well with a PS metal-backed knee, more so in a patient with hyperextension of knee. The patients with recurvatum deformity tend to develop recurrence of deformity because of lax collaterals and loose posterior capsule and are best treated with a cruciate-substituting knee.

A patient presenting with a severely deformed valgus knee with lax MCL may need a constrained knee to prevent instability after surgery.

Patient having deficient or incompetent MCL/LCL in a primary setting have to be implanted with a constrained or rarely a hinged knee.

BONE QUALITY AND BONE DEFECTS

Bone quality and bone defects play a significant role in determining the choice of implant for a patient undergoing TKA. The osteopenic bone will dictate a metal-backed tibia, while a tibia with large bone defect will necessitate a tibial component with provision for augments and a stem. A severely deformed valgus knee with a deficient lateral femoral condyle may need a primary implant with a provision for augment on the distal femoral condyle and a stem in a femur.

PREOPERATIVE RANGE OF MOVEMENT AND DEFORMITY

Severe deformities especially more than 20° in any given plane require soft tissue releases to correct the deformity during knee replacement, and may also require partial or complete release of the PCL to balance the knee and hence should be treated by using a PS knee, preferably with a metal-backed tibia to give modular options till the last trial. A CR knee may be difficult to balance, especially in severe fixed flexion deformities, where release of the PCL is required to balance the flexion and extension space.

Patients presenting with challenging problems like extrarticular femoral or tibial deformities, previous high tibial osteotomies or stress fractures are best treated by a PS knee with modular tibia as these cases are difficult to balance and may have some degree of ligament laxity in extension or flexion. It is best to keep the modular option till the last trial and have the choice for a stem, may it be necessary.

TRAINING AND SURGICAL SKILLS

The training of a surgeon plays a decisive role in his choice of prosthesis. A surgeon who is mentored by a CR surgeon and trained in the philosophy of retaining the PCL is likely to follow suit in his practice and may find it difficult to switch to a PS knee while a surgeon trained in a hospital, where PS usage is predominant will be comfortable using a PS knee for his patients. As the PS knee is more forgiving and less exacting in technique compared to a CR knee most budding surgeons choose a PS knee for their patients.

CONCLUSION

Multiple factors come into consideration when choosing an implant for a patient undergoing total knee replacement. While the training and surgical skill may tilt the surgeon's choice one way or the other, age and BMI of the patient form an important baseline factor for the choice of prosthesis. For patients with severe deformities, bone defects, obesity, and inflammatory arthritis, the PS knee with a metal-backed tibia is the optimum choice. A young, active patient will benefit from a CR knee or PS knee with a highly polished surface to reduce the wear and maximize longevity, while an old patient with limited activity could well be implanted with an all polytibia. The algorithm of choosing a knee implant is summarized in **Flow chart 6.1**.

Flow chart 6.1 Algorithm of choosing a knee implant

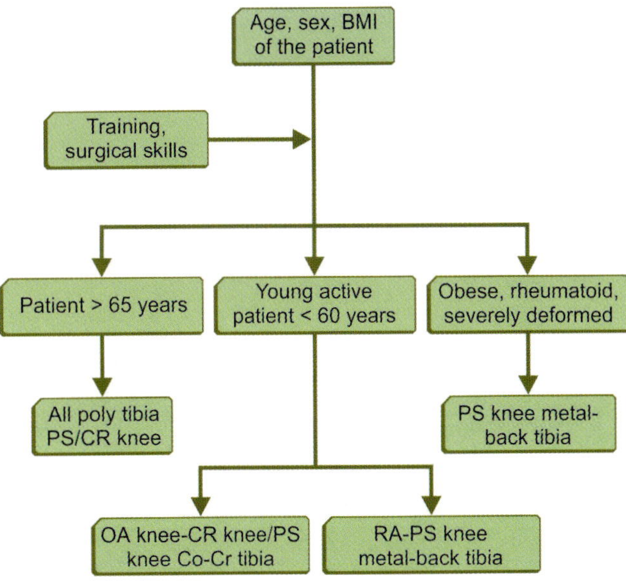

BIBLIOGRAPHY

1. 7th Annual Report of the National Joint Registry of England and Wales 2010. www.njrcentre.org.uk/NjrCentre/Portals/0/NJR%207th%20Annual%20Report%202010.pdf (Retrieved on 25 September 2012).
2. Abdel MP, Morrey ME, Jensen MR, Morrey BF. Increased long-term survival of posterior cruciate-retaining versus posterior cruciate-stabilizing total knee replacements. J Bone Joint Surg Am. 2011;93(22):2072-8.
3. Adalberth G, Nilsson KG, Byström S, Kolstad K, Milbrink J. All-polyethylene versus metal-backed and stemmed tibial components in cemented total knee arthroplasty: a prospective, randomized RSA study. J Bone Joint Surg Br. 2001;83:825-31.
4. American Academy of Orthopaedic Surgeons. Position statement. Value driven use of orthopaedic implants. http://www.aaos.org/about/papers/position/1104.asp (Retrieved on 25 September 2012).
5. Anand R, Graves SE, de Steiger RN, et al. What is the benefit of introducing new hip and knee prostheses? J Bone Joint Surg Am. 2011;93:51-4.

6. Australian Orthopaedic Association, National Joint Replacement Registry. 2011 www.dmac.adelaide.edu.au/aoanjrr/documents/AnnualReports2011/AnnualReport_2011_WebVersion.pdf.
7. Bankston AB, Keating EM, Ranawat C, Faris PM, Ritter MA. Comparison of polyethylene wear in machined versus molded polyethylene. Clin Orthop Rel Res. 1995;317:37-43.
8. Barrack RL. The results of TKA: what the registries do not tell us. Orthopedics. 2011;34(9):e485-7.
9. Bauman RD, Johnson DR, Menge TJ, Kim RH, Dennis DA. Can a high-flexion total knee arthroplasty relieve pain and restore function without premature failure? Clin Orthop Relat Res. 2012;470(1):150-8.
10. Bercik MJ, Joshi A, Parvizi J. Posterior cruciate-retaining versus posterior-stabilized total knee arthroplasty: a meta-analysis. J Arthroplasty. 2013;28(3):439-44.
11. Bettinson KA, Pinder IM, Moran CG, Weir DJ, Lingard EA. All-polyethylene compared with metal-backed tibial components in total knee arthroplasty at ten years: a prospective, randomized controlled trial. J Bone Joint Surg Am. 2009;91(7):1587-94.
12. Bistolfi A, Massazza G, Lee GC, et al. Comparison of fixed and mobile-bearing total knee arthroplasty at a mean follow-up of 116 Months. J Bone Joint Surg Am. 2013;95(12):e831-7.
13. Bollars P, Luyckx JP, Innocenti B, et al. Femoral component loosening in high-flexion total knee replacement: an in vitro comparison of high-flexion versus conventional designs. J Bone Joint Surg Br. 2011;93(10):1355-61.
14. Bourne R, et al. A gender-specific prosthesis was similar to a standard prosthesis in women having total knee replacement. J Bone Joint Surg Am. 2011;93(4):396.
15. Bozic KJ, Durbhakula S, Berry DJ, et al. Differences in patient and procedure characteristics and hospital resource use in primary and revision total joint arthroplasty: a multicenter study. J Arthroplasty. 2005;20:17-25.
16. Choi WC, Lee S, Seong SC, Jung JH, Lee MC. Comparison between standard and high-flexion posterior-stabilized rotating-platform mobile-bearing total knee arthroplasties: a randomized controlled study. J Bone Joint Surg Br. 2010;92(10):1429-34.
17. Clark CR. Cost containment: total joint implants. J Bone Joint Surg Am. 1994;76:799-800.
18. Conditt MA, Stein JA, Noble PC. Factors affecting the severity of backside wear of modular tibial inserts. J Bone Joint Surg Am. 2004;86:305-11.
19. Conditt MA, Thompson MT, Usrey MM, Ismaily SK, Noble PC. Backside wear of polyethylene tibial inserts: mechanism and magnitude of material loss. J Bone Joint Surg Am. 2005;87:326-31.
20. Dargel J, Michael JW, Feiser J, Ivo R, Koebke J. Human knee joint anatomy revisited: morphometry in the light of sex-specific total knee arthroplasty. J Arthroplasty. 2011;26(3):346-53.
21. Delanois R, Mont A, Mahone OM. Comparison between standard and high-flexion posterior-stabilized rotating-platform mobile-bearing total knee arthroplasties: a randomized controlled study. J Bone Joint Surg Am. 2010;92(16):e29.
22. Dennis DA, Heekin RD, Clark CR, et al. Effect of implant design on knee flexion. J Arthroplasty. 2012;pii: S0883-5403(12):00546.
23. Dixon MC, Brown RR, Parsch D, Scott RD. Modular fixed-bearing total knee arthroplasty with retention of the posterior cruciate ligament. A study of patients followed for a minimum of fifteen years. J Bone Joint Surg Am. 2005;87:598-603.
24. Engh GA, Lounici S, Rao AR, Collier MB. In vivo deterioration of tibial baseplate locking mechanisms in contemporary modular total knee components. J Bone Joint Surg Am. 2001;83:1660-5.
25. Gioe TJ, Glynn J, Sembrano J, et al. Mobile and fixed-bearing (all-polyethylene tibial component) total knee arthroplasty designs: a prospective randomized trial. J Bone Joint Surg Am. 2009;91:2104-12.
26. Gioe TJ, Sharma A, Tatman P, Mehle S. Do premium joint implants add value? Analysis of high cost joint implants in a community registry. Clin Orthop Relat Res. 2011;469(1):48-54.
27. Gioe TJ, Sinner P, Mehle S, Ma W, Killeen KK. Excellent survival of all-polyethylene tibial components in a community joint registry. Clin Orthop Relat Res. 2007;464:88-92.
28. Haider H, Garvin K. Rotating platform versus fixed-bearing total knees: an in vitro study of wear. Clin Orthop Relat Res. 2008;466(11):2677-85.
29. Hamilton WG, Sritulanondha S, Engh CA Jr. Prospective randomized comparison of high-flex and standard rotating platform total knee arthroplasty. J Arthroplasty. 2011;26:28-34.

30. Hamilton WG, Sritulanondha S, Engh CA Jr. Results of prospective, randomized clinical trials comparing standard and high-flexion posterior-stabilized TKA: a focused review. Orthopedics. 2011;34(9):e500-3.
31. Hanusch B, Lou TN, Warriner G, Hui A, Gregg P. Functional outcome of PFC sigma fixed and rotating-platform total knee arthroplasty: a prospective randomised controlled trial. Int Orthop. 2010;34(3):349-54.
32. Harrington MA, Hopkinson WJ, Hsu P, Manion L. Fixed- vs mobile-bearing total knee arthroplasty: does it make a difference? A prospective randomized study. J Arthroplasty. 2009;24:24-7.
33. Hino K, Ishimaru M, Iseki Y, et al. Mid-flexion laxity is greater after posterior-stabilised total knee replacement than with cruciate-retaining procedures: a computer navigation study. Bone Joint J. 2013;95-B(4):493-7.
34. Hui C, Salmon L, Maeno S, et al. Five-year comparison of oxidized zirconium and cobalt-chromium femoral components in total knee arthroplasty: a randomized controlled trial. J Bone Joint Surg Am. 2011;93(7):624-30.
35. Hyldahl H, Regnér L, Carlsson L, Kärrholm J, Weidenhielm L. All-polyethylene vs metal-backed tibial component in total knee arthroplasty: a randomized RSA study comparing early fixation of horizontally and completely cemented tibial components: part 1. Horizontally cemented components: AP better fixated than MB. Acta Orthop. 2005;76:769-77.
36. Joglekar S, Gioe TJ, Yoon P, Schwartz MH. Gait analysis comparison of cruciate retaining and substituting TKA following PCL sacrifice. Knee. 2012;19(4):279-85.
37. Johnson AJ, Costa CR, Mont MA. Do we need gender-specific total joint arthroplasty? Clin Orthop Relat Res. 2011;469(7):1852-8.
38. Jung WH, Jeong JH, Ha YC, Lee YK, Koo KH. High early failure rate of the Columbus posterior stabilized high-flexion knee prosthesis. Clin Orthop Relat Res. 2012;470(5):1472-81.
39. Kalisvaart MM, Pagnano MW, Trousdale RT, Stuart MJ, Hanssen AD. Randomized clinical trial of rotating-platform and fixed bearing total knee arthroplasty: no clinically detectable differences at five years. J Bone Joint Surg Am. 2012;94(6):481-9.
40. Kim YH, Choi Y, Kwon OR, Kim JS. Range of motion of standard and high-flexion posterior cruciate-retaining total knee prostheses: a prospective randomized study. J Bone Joint Surg Am. 2009;91:753-60.
41. Kim YH, Kim JS, Choe JW, Kim HJ. Long-term comparison of fixed-bearing and mobile-bearing total knee replacements in patients younger than fifty-one years of age with osteoarthritis. J Bone Joint Surg Am. 2012;94(10):866-73.
42. Kim YH, Kim JS, Huh W, Lee KH. Weight of polyethylene wear particles is similar in TKAs with oxidized zirconium and cobalt-chrome prostheses. Clin Orthop Relat Res. 2010;468:1296-304.
43. Kim YH, Sohn KS, Kim JS. Range of motion of standard and high-flexion posterior stabilized total knee prostheses: a prospective, randomized study. J Bone Joint Surg Am. 2005;87:1470-75.
44. Kim YH, Yoon SH, Kim JS. The long-term results of simultaneous fixed-bearing and mobile-bearing total knee replacements performed in the same patient. J Bone Joint Surg Br. 2007;89:1317-23.
45. Kim YH, Choi Y, Kim JS. Comparison of a standard and a gender-specific posterior cruciate-substituting high-flexion knee prosthesis: a prospective, randomized, short-term outcome study. J Bone Joint Surg Am. 2010;92(10):1911-20.
46. Lachiewicz PF, Soileau ES. Results of a second-generation constrained condylar prosthesis in primary total knee arthroplasty. J Arthroplasty. 2011;26(8):1228-31.
47. Li N, Tan Y, Deng Y, Chen L. Posterior cruciate-retaining versus posterior stabilized total knee arthroplasty: a meta-analysis of randomized controlled trials. Knee Surg Sports Traumatol Arthrosc. 2012. (Epub ahead of print)
48. Mehin R, Burnett RS, Brasher PM. Does the new generation of high-flex knee prostheses improve the postoperative range of movement?: a meta-analysis. J Bone Joint Surg Br. 2010;92:1429-34.
49. Mullaji AB, Padmanabhan V, Jindal G. Total knee arthroplasty for profound varus deformity: technique and radiological results in 173 knees with varus of more than 20 degrees. J Arthroplasty. 2005;20(5):550-61.
50. Namba RS, Inacio MC, Paxton EW, et al. Risk of revision for fixed versus mobile-bearing primary total knee replacements. J Bone Joint Surg Am. 2012;94(21):1929-35.
51. Namba RS, Inacio MC, Paxton EW, Robertsson O, Graves SE. The role of registry data in the evaluation of mobile bearing total knee arthroplasty. J Bone Joint Surg Am. 2011;93:48-50.
52. Norgren B. All polytibial component better than metal-backed: a randomized RSA study. Knee. 2004;11(3):189-96.

53. Parks NL, Engh GA, Topoleski LD, Emperado J. Modular tibial insert micro-motion: a concern with contemporary knee implants. Clin Orthop Relat Res. 1998;356:10-5.
54. Petrisor BA, Bhandari M. The hierarchy of evidence: levels and grades of recommendation. Indian J Orthop. 2007;41(1):11-5.
55. Rajgopal A, Dahiya V, Vasdev A, Kochhar H, Tyagi V. Long-term results of total knee arthroplasty for valgus knees: soft-tissue release technique and implant selection. J Orthop Surg Hong Kong. 2011;19(1):60-3.
56. Ranawat AS, Mohanty SS, Goldsmith SE, et al. Experience with an all-polyethylene total knee arthroplasty in younger, active patients with follow-up from 2 to 11 years. J Arthroplasty. 2005;20:7-11.
57. Rand JA, Trousdale RT, Ilstrup DM, Harmsen WS. Factors affecting the durability of primary total knee prostheses. J Bone Joint Surg Am. 2003;85A(2):259-65.
58. Ritter MA, Berend ME, Meding JB, et al. Long-term follow-up of anatomic graduated components posterior cruciate retaining total knee replacement. Clin Orthop Relat Res. 2001;388:51-7.
59. Ritter MA, Davis KE, Meding JB, Farris A. The role of the posterior cruciate ligament in total knee replacement. Bone Joint Res. 2012;1(4):64-70.
60. Ritter MA,Lutgring JD,Davis KE, Faris PM,Berend ME. Total knee arthroplasty effectiveness in patients 55 years old and younger: osteoarthritis versus rheumatoid arthritis. Knee. 2007;14(1):9-11.
61. Ritter MA. Direct compression molded polyethylene for total hip and knee replacements. Clin Orthop Relat Res. 2001;393:94-100.
62. Ritter MA. The Anatomical Graduated Component total knee replacement: a long term evaluation with 2-year survival analysis. J Bone Joint Surg Br. 2009;91:745-9.
63. Song EK, Jung WB, Yoon TR, et al. Comparison of outcomes after bilateral simultaneous total knee arthroplasty using gender-specific and unisex knees. J Arthroplasty. 2012;27(2):226-31.
64. Spicer DD, Pomeroy DL, Badenhausen WE, et al. Body mass index as a predictor of outcome in total knee replacement. Int Orthop. 2001;25(4):246-9.
65. Sumino T, Gadikota HR, Varadarajan KM, et al. Do high flexion posterior stabilised total knee arthroplasty designs increase knee flexion? A meta-analysis. Int Orthop. 2011;35(9):1309-19.
66. Swedish Knee Register, 2012 Annual Report.
67. Thomsen MG, Husted H, Bencke J, et al. Do we need a gender-specific total knee replacement? A randomized controlled trial comparing a high-flex and a gender-specific posterior design. J Bone Joint Surg Br. 2012;94(6):787-92.
68. Udomkiat P, Dorr LD, Long W. Matched-pair analysis of all-polyethylene versus metal-backed tibial components. J Arthroplasty. 2001;16:689-96.
69. Voigt J, Mosier M. Cemented all-polyethylene and metal-backed polyethylene tibial components used for primary total knee arthroplasty: a systematic review of the literature and meta-analysis of randomized controlled trials involving 1798 primary total knee implants. J Bone Joint Surg Am. 2011;93:1790-8.

Chapter 7

Role of Unicompartmental Arthroplasty in Arthritis of the Knee

Matthieu Ollivier, Sebastien Parratte, Xavier Flecher, Jean-Noel Argenson

ABSTRACT

Unicondylar knee replacement should not be considered as a temporary procedure, and the 10-year survival can be as good as with total knee arthroplasty (TKA) if patient selection and surgical principles are followed carefully. The advantages of unicompartmental knee arthroplasty (UKA) compared with TKA include bone-stock protection, physiologic kinematics, retention of main knee ligament, as well as better functional results. For young patients, a modern UKA is now a valid alternative to bridge the gap between high tibial osteotomy and TKA, although component loosening and progression of arthritis in the remaining compartments have become rare with appropriate patient selection and an adequate surgical technique. On the other hand, polyethylene wear, an associated metal-backed component, remains a problem, particularly in active and heavy patients. The last decade evolution in terms of the surgical technique, instrumentation and implant designs has made unicompartmental arthroplasty the standard of treatment for patients with severe osteoarthritis limited to one tibiofemoral compartment.

INTRODUCTION

Isolated unicompartmental knee arthritis in the young patient is a challenging problem.[1] Surgical management of unicompartmental knee arthritis includes nonprosthetic treatments such as arthroscopic debridement, meniscus transplantation, high tibial osteotomy (HTO), unicompartmental knee arthroplasty (UKA) or conventional total knee arthroplasty (TKA).[2] These procedures, however, have a finite lifespan in the young and active patients and some concerns, such as functional recovery, possibility of returning to sports activities, should be considered.[1,3-5] The risk of failure after HTO for patients whose osteoarthritis is rated,[6] Ahlback's grade 2 or higher had convinced surgeons to decrease the number of HTO performed to a higher number of nonconservative treatment even in a younger patient.[1] Thus, in 2006, medial-UKA was the preferred procedure for 11.4% of the American surgeons for a 45-year-old active male and for 29.5% of the surgeons for a 45-year-old active female to manage a medial compartment arthritis (assuming only little deformation of the knee).[7] Moreover, UKA in a patient in whom only one compartment of the knee is affected may provide a better physiological function and quicker recovery when compared to TKA, and it also preserves the bone stock.[1,7-12] An improper patient selection combined with the limited instrumentation and suboptimal designs may provide less than the satisfactory results originally published for UKA and the subsequent decreased interest especially in the United States.[11] A more precise selection and a more reliable surgical technique actually permitted the expect survivorship to be greater than 90% after 10 years of follow-up.[8]

The most important evolution in UKA during the last decade is the so-called minimally invasive surgery (MIS).[13] Concerning UKA, MIS is defined as the ability to implant the components without an incision in the quadriceps tendon or the vastus medialis or lateralis (depending on the compartment to be replaced) and without everting the patella.[13] With the evolution in instrumentation over the last 5 years, it is now possible to perform partial knee arthroplasty with cutting guides fixed only on the replaced compartment preserving the integrity of the unaffected tibiofemoral compartment.[9,14] New worldwide interest in UKA is due to the possibilities of fast recovery and minimal surgical morbidity permitted by MIS and improvement in the UKA design, allowing greater and safer motion capabilities, especially for active patients who are candidates for UKA.[3,10,14]

PATIENT SELECTION AND INDICATIONS

The indications for UKA are painful osteoarthritis (OA) or osteonecrosis limited to one compartment of the knee associated with a significant loss of joint space on the radiographs.[1,2,8,14] In fact, results after UKA for osteonecrosis limited to one compartment of the knee (i.e. idiopathic or post-traumatic osteonecrosis) were comparable to those observed for OA at a mean of 12 years.[2] Mild chondrocalcinosis may also be accepted as an indication to perform UKA; in contrast, any type of inflammatory arthritis, such as rheumatoid arthritis, is recognized as a formal contraindication for UKA because this can be a cause of a rapid degeneration of the unreplaced compartments. Preoperative physical exam should ensure: a range of knee flexion >100°; full knee extension and a stable knee in the anteroposterior (AP) and sagittal planes. The patellofemoral joint should be clinically asymptomatic.

RADIOLOGICAL EVALUATION

The radiological analysis should include full-length X-rays, AP and ML view of the knee, skyline views and stress radiographs.[15] The radiographic analysis should ensure that there is no patellofemoral loss of joint space on skyline views at 30°, 60°, and 90° of flexion, and confirm full-thickness articular cartilage in the uninvolved compartment.

The full correction of the deformity to neutral on stress radiographs performed with the patient supine using a dedicated knee stress system is also mandatory. The angle between the mechanical axis of the femur and the anatomical axis of the femur should be calculated on the full-length X-ray as well as the mechanical axis of the lower limb. A varus or valgus deformation of the lower limb greater than 15° degrees may represent a contraindication for UKA as the correction of such deformation may require soft tissue release which should not be performed when doing UKA.

If the anterior cruciate ligament (ACL) status is unclear during the clinical exam, magnetic resonance imaging may be useful to confirm that the ACL is intact.

AGE AND WEIGHT

Age and weight may still represent debatable issues for the indication of UKA as the procedure is often presented as an alternative to either osteotomy or TKA. As previously mentioned and according to the results of previously published series, we do consider the HTO as an attractive and efficient conservative procedure for patient below 50 with a low-grade unicompartmental osteoarthritis and a varus knee.[4] However, the HTO risk of failure increased dramatically for the patient with osteoarthritis rated Ahlback's grade 2 or more, and that is why in those cases we do consider UKA even in younger patients.[16,17] Thus, we recently reported very good survivorship of the patients younger than 50, despite greater polyethylene wear than that for the older patient, as observed also after TKA.[1,18] Nevertheless, early reports of UKA considered obesity as a relative contraindication for UKA, but recent studies found no correlation between weight and outcomes, and we do concur with the idea that wear is more related to activity than to weight.[19] Obesity itself is consequently not a contraindication.

SURGICAL TECHNIQUES

Approach

The procedure can be performed under general or epidural anesthesia on a routine operating table. The knee is flexed at 90° for skin incision, and the thigh tourniquet is inflated with the foot resting on the table. A minimally invasive parapatellar approach is performed either medial for the medial UKA or lateral for the lateral UKA. The approach extends proximally at the level of the proximal pole of the patella extending distally toward either medial for a medial UKA or the lateral one for a lateral UKA of the tibial tuberosity but ending 2 cm under the joint line previously located. The length of the skin incision varies from 8 to 10 cm depending on skin elasticity. It is important to maintain proper visualization throughout the procedure which in part depends on the variation in tissue elasticity. The proximal part of the incision is more essential for the procedure and two-thirds of the incision should be located above the joint line. Once the synovial cavity is opened, the part of the fat pad in the way of the condyle is excised to properly visualize the condyle, the ACL and the corresponding tibial side of the tibial plateau. Then it is important to note that the principles of ligament balancing existing in TKA cannot be applied to UKA because the collateral ligaments should not be released in UKA. Before proceeding to the bone cuts or anything else, the first step is to bring the knee to 60° of flexion to evaluate the joint by checking the resistance of the ACL with an appropriate hook and evaluating the state of both the opposite tibiofemoral and patellofemoral joints. The osteophytes are then removed in the intercondylar notch to avoid late impingement with the ACL on the notch.

Tibial Cut

Once the status of the patella, the ACL and the opposite compartment has been checked, the next step is to progress to the bone cuts. It is important to recall that in UKA the proper tension of the ligaments will be restored while filling the gap left by the worn cartilage with the unicompartmental components and therefore UKA is a so-called surfacing procedure.

In our practice, the tibial cut is always performed first. The entire procedure can be performed either using extramedullary or intramedullary instrumentation. The extramedullary technique is based on the correction of the deformity of the leg in extension using an extramedullary rod that references the ankle and the femoral head.

In our technique, the tibial cut is made using an extramedullary road. The guide is placed distally around the ankle with the axis of the guide lying slightly medial to the center of the ankle joint. The proximal part of the guide is resting on the anterior tibia pointing toward the axis of the tibial spines and with modern instrumentation. The diaphyseal part of the guide is parallel to the anterior tibial crest, and the AP position of the guide is adjusted distally to reproduce the natural upper tibial slope, usually between 5° and 7° of the posterior slope. The amount of resection is decided after using a 4 mm probe located on the deepest part of the affected plateau, and particular care should be taken to properly define the level of the cut. To complete the tibial cut, the sagittal tibial cut should be done. This could be done using one of the sagittal marks provided by the guide or made as a freehand cut. At this step, once again, particular care should be taken to protect the ACL.

Femoral Cut

The entrance hole of the distal femur for the intramedullary technique is centered above the roof of the intercondylar notch and prepares using an adaptated osteotomy to conserve the cartilage. We then bring the knee to 60° of flexion to drill the medullary canal. Once the guide has been properly introduced, the distal femoral cut can be made, reporting the angle between the anatomic and mechanical axis previously calculated on the full weight bearing view. This angle is usually 4°–6°. The amount of bone resected from the distal femur corresponds exactly millimeter for millimeter to the femoral prosthesis.

We then check the extension space using a dedicated spacer block. The next challenge concerns the remainder of the femoral cuts (posterior cut and chamfers), which will then be completed using the appropriate cutting block. The rotation setup of the cutting block is the crucial point of the procedure. The size of the cutting block is determined once this femoral finishing guide is positioned on the distal femoral cut, searching for the best compromise between an anatomically centered position on the femoral condyle and a long axis perpendicular to the resected tibial plateau. The top of this finishing guide should be localized 1–2 mm above the deepest layer of the cartilage to avoid a potential notch between the femoral implant and the patella. The control of the mediolateral position of the femoral cutting guide, which determines the position of the final implant, as previously mentioned, is crucial. Once the posterior cut and the chamfers have been made and the cutting guide removed, removal of any posterior osteophytes is necessary using a curved osteotome to increase the range of flexion and avoid any posterior impingement with the polyethylene in high flexion.

TIBIAL FINISHING AND TRIALS

The size of the tibial tray should now be determined, resulting in the best compromise between the maximal tibial coverage and overhang, which might induce pain. The AP size of the tibial plateau sometimes differs from the mediolateral one, especially for female knees; thus different sizing trials are necessary to find the best compromise. It is important to keep the depth of the tibial cut as conservative as possible to take advantage of the strength of the tibial cortex and the increased area of contact proximally. The knee is then brought into maximal flexion and internally rotated. The final preparation of the tibia is completed with the appropriate guide with the underlying keel impacted in the subchondral bone. The flexion-extension gaps should then be tested with the trial components in place and inserting a trial polyethylene liner. At that step, it is important to search for any impingement of the femur against the spine eminence in extension due to a lack of external rotation in flexion. Once this has been verified, it is important to look for a 2 mm protective laxity checked close to full extension to avoid any overcorrection of the deformity leading to the progression of osteoarthritis in the medial compartment. The polyethylene insert is often thicker than that for the medial side in the case of femoral dysplasia, even if the principle of under correction of the deformity for all cases of the lateral UKA remains the basis for successful long-term results. All components should be cemented for better fixation because the long-term results suggest that loosening is not a common mode of failure with modern cemented, metal-backed components. The tibial component is cemented first with the knee in full flexion and internally rotated to improve the exposure of the lateral compartment. Once the femoral implant has been cemented, bringing the knee close to the extension helps to remove any posterior cement. Finally, the polyethylene can be inserted in flexion after the cleaning and the drying of the tibial implant.

The ideal correction as measured on the postoperative full weight-bearing view will probably consist of a tibiofemoral axis crossing the knee between the tibial spines and the lateral third of the tibial plateau for a medial UKA.

We cement all components for better fixation because the long-term results suggest that loosening is not a common mode of failure with modern cemented, metal-backed components.

The tibial component is cemented first with the knee in full flexion and externally rotated for a medial UKA to improve the exposure of the medial compartment. When cementing the components, it is important to avoid leaving any cement at the posterior aspect of the knee, and the 90° curved probe is useful to remove any posterior cement when using a minimal incision. Once the femoral implant has been cemented, bringing the knee close to the extension helps remove any posterior cement with the polyethylene inserted last.

In our practice, one intra-articular drain is left for 36 h. Postoperatively, an immediate weight-bearing is recommended after the removal of the femoral nerve block catheter (left 24 h postoperatively). The painless, passive manual range of motion physiotherapy is carried out the day after surgery. The active range of motion training then continues.

RESULTS OF MODERN UNICOMPARTMENT KNEE ARTHROPLASTY

UKA through Minimally Invasive Surgery

Only a few reports are available at the midterm follow-up for the evaluation of UKA performed through a mini-incision.[8,12,13,20-25] Romanowski and Repicci[23] evaluated, at 8-year follow-up, a group of 136 knees implanted with UKA performed through a mini-incision. The revision rate was 7%, and they suggested that the procedure was only temporary to relieve pain and improve the function with minimal morbidity.[26] These results contrast with the long-term results reported for the UKA performed through a conventional incision with a survival rate greater than 94% at 10 or 13 years.[8,11] We believe that the results and technical errors reported by Romanowski[23] highlight the difficulty performing the procedure through a minimal incision if the visualization is not appropriate. Moreover, there is probably less tolerance in UKA compared to TKA in component malpositioning. Hamilton et al. reported about 221 UKAs performed through a mini-incision and an overall revision rate for aseptic loosening of 3.7% in the mini-incision group compared with 1% in the group with the open technique.[21]

When following the first group of 44 consecutive patients with 48 UKA knees implanted in our institution using a minimal incision, we found no difference, in terms of implant positioning, compared with a group previously operated on with the 'classic' approach; however, one case of femoral divergence up to 9° was noted with the mini-incision technique.[9] There is no doubt that limiting extensor mechanism disruption during the procedure provided more rapid recovery with less morbidity as mentioned in the original report by Price et al. using the Oxford knee.[18] This accelerated recovery is associated with a decreased hospital stay in all the recent reports of UKA performed through a mini-incision. We have found that patients can perform active exercises for one week compared with three weeks with the open technique.[9]

Mobile-bearing UKA

Mobile-bearing UKA, using a specific design (Oxford; Biomet, Warsaw, IN, USA) has shown a recent increase in use. The challenges with the mobile-bearing design include technical issues of ligament balancing with the potential risk of bearing dislocation. Murray et al.[27] reported 98% cumulative prosthetic survivorship at 10-year follow-up. Price et al.[28] using the same implant, found a 15-year survivorship of up to 92%. However, they noted a high frequency of complete radiolucent lines around the tibial component in half of the tibial components. Other studies, however, suggest contradictory results with similar mobile-bearing implants. Vorlat et al.[29] reported an 84% survival of 149 consecutive Oxford knees at 5.5 years. In the US Investigative Device Exemption study, 125 Oxford UKAs were followed at eight sites,[16] and the authors found at 7 years only 80.6% of survivorship, with a clinical success rate of only 74.2%. In the actual literature, we found three comparison studies evaluating fixed-bearing versus mobile-bearing designs. Confalonieri et al.[30] found no statistical difference in outcome. Gleeson et al.[17] found three bearing dislocations in the mobile-bearing group and four additional revisions (versus three revisions in the fixed bearing group). To sum these studies, the functional results of both implants are similar, and comparative studies show no consensus between the mobile- and fixed-bearing designs in regard to function, success or recovery. We do prefer to use the fixed-bearing implant because mobile-bearing designs still present the potential of bearing dislocation.

Fixed-bearing UKA

To comfort our feelings on mobile- versus fixed-bearing design, we presented, in 2011, our results in terms of the survivorship of the fixed- versus mobile-bearing UKA in young patients.[31] We retrospectively reviewed 75 patients (79 knees) with a fixed-bearing UKA and 72 patients (77 knees) with a mobile-bearing UKA operated on between 1989 and 1992. The mean age of the patients was 63 years; gender and body mass index (26 kg/m^2) were comparable in the two groups. We obtained the knee society function and radiographic scores and determined survival. The minimum follow-up was 15 years (mean, 17.2 ± 4.8 years; range, 15–21.2 years). Radiographically, the number of overcorrections and the number of radiolucencies were statistically higher in the mobile-bearing group (69% versus 24%) but at the final follow-up, considering the revision for any reason, 12 of 77 (15%) UKAs were revised (for aseptic loosening, dislocation and arthritis progression) in the mobile-bearing group and 10 of 79 (12%) in the fixed-bearing group (for wear and arthritis progression). This difference did not reach the significance level. Thus, biomechanical study demonstrated that running and jumping produce surface loads that exceed the limits of polyethylene resistance.[19]

The rate of polyethylene wear seems to be higher when using the mobile-bearing UKA to recommend specific activities after UKA. Factors such as wear, joint load and the type of prosthesis must be taken into account for each patient.[19,32-34] Based on our results and previous reports, decreasing wear seems to be the main factor in improving the long-term results of UKA.[19,35] Two major symptoms can be observed when polyethylene wear occurred: medial knee pain without signs of inflammation and progressive nontraumatic frontal instability. There was no clinical or biological sign of infection. Physical examination is important to confirm the development of frontal instability in these patients. When these symptoms occurred, we performed weight-bearing and varus and valgus stress radiographs to confirm wear and look for osteolysis. Usually, the exchange of the polyethylene insert is an affordable option when no evidence of infection, loosening or osteolysis has been found. In all the other cases, a revision of UKA should be discussed with the patient.

Lateral UKA

Mid- and long-term studies suggest reasonable outcome at 10 years with the survivorship greater than 95% of UKA performed for medial osteoarthritis or osteonecrosis,[2] but limited long-term follow-up data are available for lateral UKA in the literature.[36-38] The authors of one small series of UKA in the lateral compartment reported only one failure out of 19 patients at 89 months of follow-up.[38] As both of anatomic and biomechanical characteristics are different in each of the knee femorotibial compartments, similar surgical treatment may not provide reproducible results when applied to a different compartment.[36-38] UKA in the lateral compartment is technically more challenging and 10 times less performed than medial UKA (representing less than 1% of all knee arthroplasty procedures).[39] In 2008, we presented the result of a consecutive series of 39 lateral UKA.[40] Our data demonstrate that the lateral UKA can provide reasonable clinical and radiographic results, with the survivorship at 10 and 16 years comparable to the survivorship obtained for medial UKA (Sah and Scott),[38] who reported no revision at 5 years in a group of 49 knees implanted with the lateral UKA, and the rate of radiolucencies observed in those two series (10% of nonprogressive tibial radiolucencies) was comparable with those observed in previous series of the lateral UKA at the same follow-up. In the other hand, Gunther et al.[37] reported a 21% failure rate using the mobile-bearing Oxford unicompartmental prosthesis in the lateral compartment with a 10% rate of bearing dislocation. This difference with the commonly reported high functioning long-term outcomes using the same implant for the medial compartment may be explained by the amount of femoral translation of the lateral condyle while the medial one remains fairly stationary.[37] When studying the *in vivo* kinematics of patients implanted with either a medial or a lateral UKA, we showed an important posterior femoral translation of the lateral condyle during flexion compared with the medial one.[41,42]

To conclude, because anatomic and the biomechanical characteristics are different in each of the knee's compartments, some pitfalls must be outlined for the lateral UKA.

- The rule of undercorrection of the deformity should be strictly applied to the lateral UKA to avoid medial OA progression. Furthermore, the positioning of the femoral component should accommodate the femoral divergence of the lateral condyle when the knee is flexed to avoid impingement with the tibial spines when brought into extension.

- The mediolateral positioning of the femoral component should also avoid the excessive lateral placement in extension, which may lead to an overload of the lateral part of the tibial plateau when the knee is flexed to 30°.
- Additionally, the internal rotation of the tibial component when performing the lateral UKA accommodates the typical 'screw-home' mechanism occurring during knee flexion, and this should be included when performing the sagittal tibial cut.[43]

UKA after Osteonecrosis

Osteonecrosis of the knee classically includes two distinct entities: spontaneous or secondary osteonecrosis.[44-50] Spontaneous osteonecrosis occurs most often in patients older than 55, unilaterally, and in one compartment of the knee.[44,45,47,48] Secondary osteonecrosis could appear after corticosteroid therapy, renal and systemic disease, or barotrauma, and occurs most often in younger patients with bilateral multicompartmental disease.[44,48] For both types of osteonecrosis, the natural evolution without treatment is arthritis.[44,49,50] Four stages of the radiographic evolution of the lesion have been described according to Mont et al.[47] The final evolution of the necrosis is often associated with severe clinical symptoms, and TKA[51-53] or UKA[54-57] have been advocated. To date, there are limited data to analyze the clinical and radiological outcomes after modern UKA for spontaneous and secondary osteonecrosis of the knee and these outcomes should be clarified. The utility of UKA in secondary osteonecrosis should be clarified, as this entity typically involves the metaphyseal region and both compartments.[44] Furthermore, the place of UKA for secondary osteonecrosis that more often involves the metaphyseal regions and both compartments should be determined.[44] We presented in 2007,[2] a series of 31 UKA performed after osteonecrosis of the knee; according to the Ahlback classification, two patients (6%) were graded

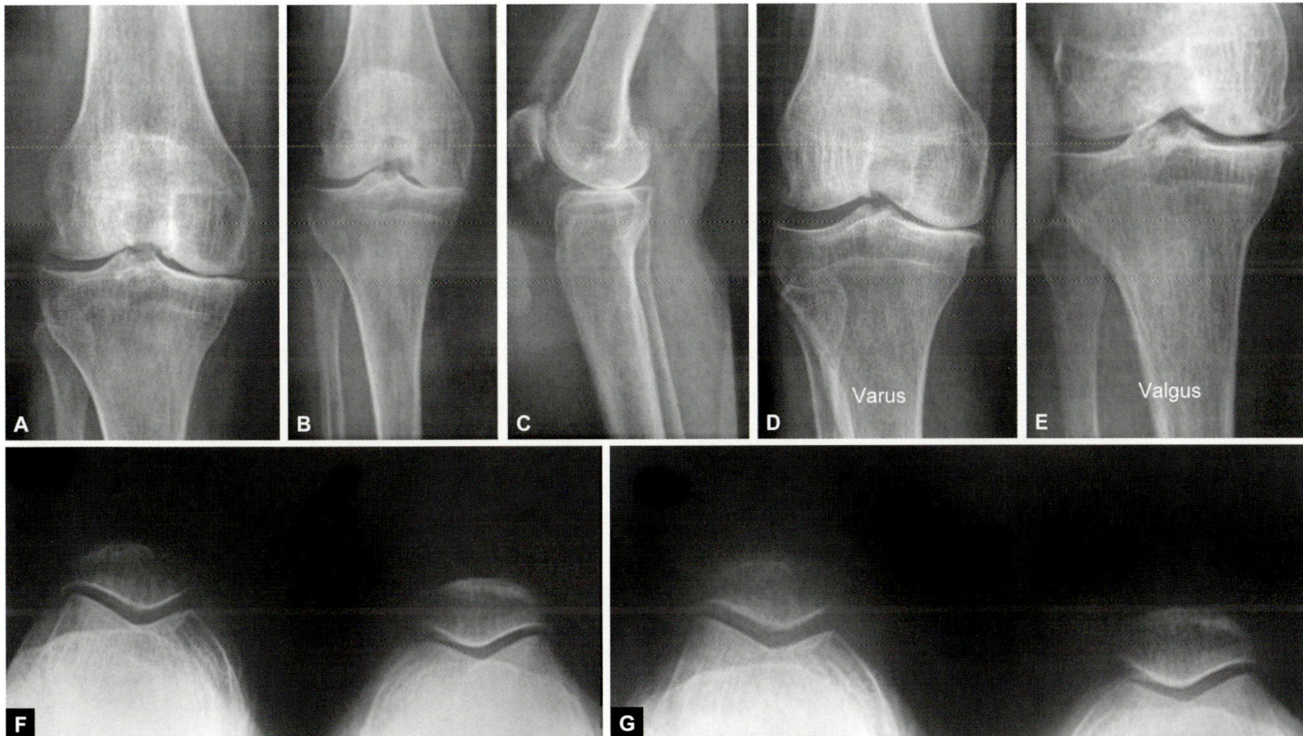

Figures 7.1A to G Preoperative radiological analysis. (A to C) The frontal view and sagittal view of the right knee: OA limited to one compartment of the knee (medial) associated with significant loss of joint space; (C and D) Stress radiograph with full correction of the deformity to neutral on valgus stress radiographs; (E to G) No patellofemoral loss of joint space on skyline views at 30°, 60°, and 90° of flexion

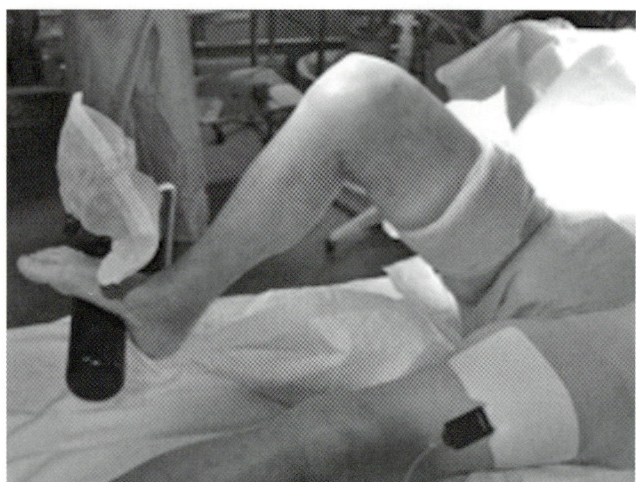

Figure 7.2 Patient's installation: the knee is flexed 90° for skin incision, the thigh tourniquet inflated and the foot resting on the table

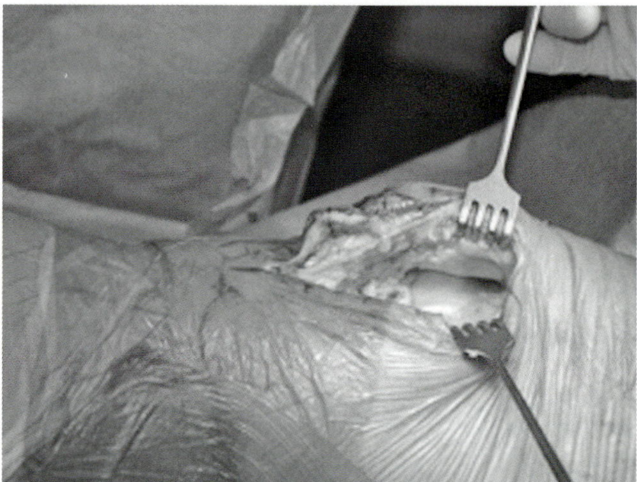

Figure 7.4 Once the synovial cavity is opened, the part of the fat pad in the way of the condyle is excised to properly visualize the condyle

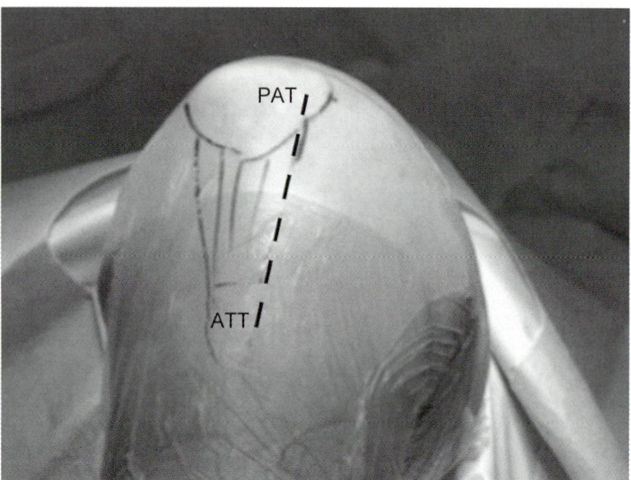

Figure 7.3 The upper limit of the incision is the superior pole of the patella (P) extending distally toward the lateral side of the anterior tibial tuberosity but ending 2 cm under the joint line previously located. The proximal part of the incision is more essential for the procedure and two-thirds of the incision should be located above the joint line

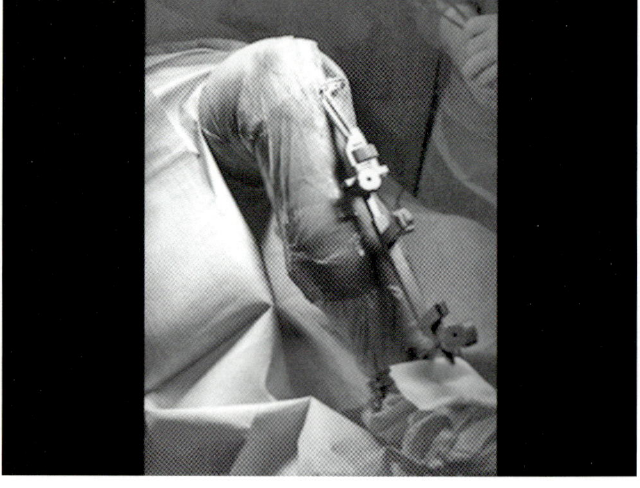

Figure 7.5 Tibial cut: the extramedullary guide is placed distally around the ankle with the axis of the guide lying slightly medial to the center of the ankle joint

1, 14 (45%) were graded 2 and 15 (49%) were graded 3. The etiologies of the osteonecrosis were spontaneous in 21 knees (67%) and secondary in 10 knees (33%), including steroid-induced osteonecrosis in seven patients and barotraumatic osteonecrosis in professional scuba divers in three patients. All cases of steroid-induced osteonecrosis have had a long-term steroid therapy, in four cases for a systematic lupus erythematous and in three cases after a renal transplantation.

In this retrospective study,[2] we analyzed the results of UKA for osteonecrosis using a modern implant and strict inclusion criteria, and the 12-year survival rate was 96.7% ± 3% with revision for any reason or radiographic loosening as the end point. Only one knee underwent revision with a

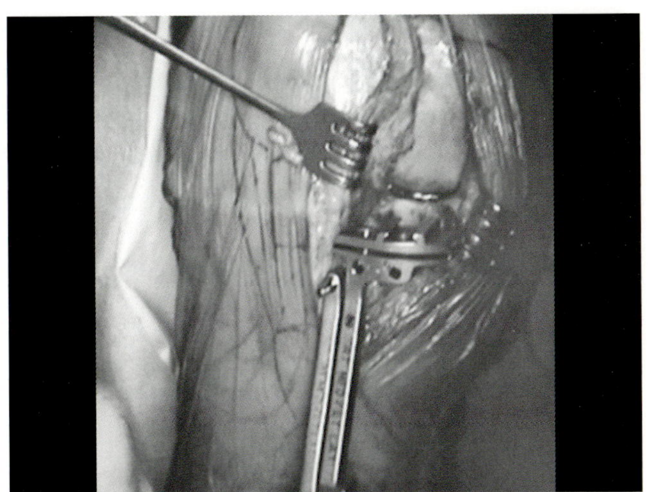

Figure 7.6 Tibial cut: the amount of resection is decided after using a 4 mm probe located on the deepest part of the affected plateau

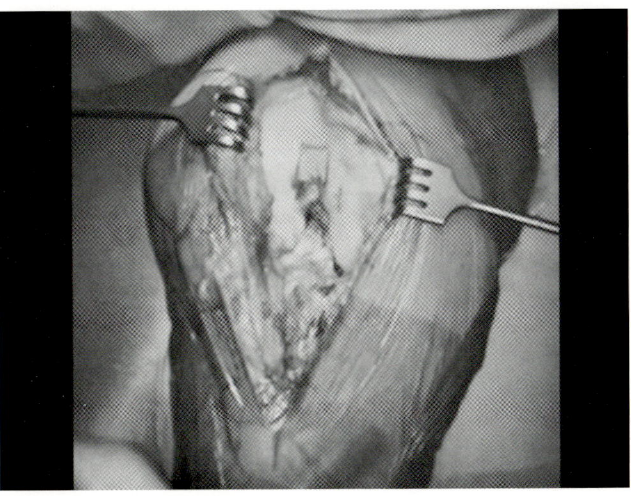

Figure 7.7 The entrance hole of the distal femur for the intra-medullary technique is centered above the roof of the intercondylar notch and prepares using an adapted osteotomy

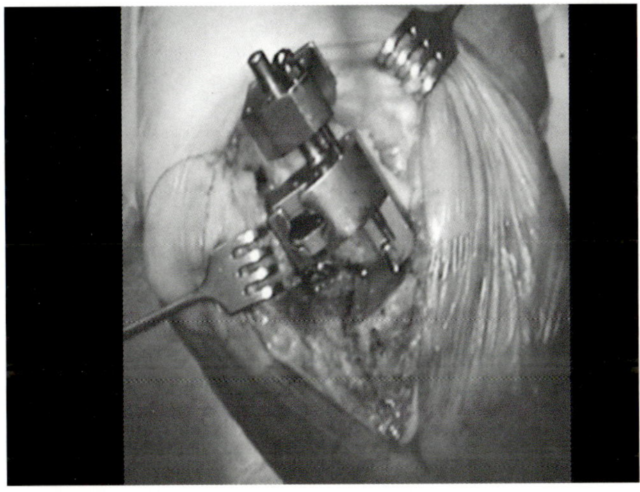

Figure 7.8 The distal femoral cut is made by reporting the angle between the anatomic and mechanical axis previously calculated on the full weight-bearing view (4°–6°)

cemented TKA for aseptic loosening at 30 months suggesting that the UKA is reliable in osteonecrosis for alleviating pain and improving function, restoring the proper lower-limb mechanical axis, and achieving a durable survivorship.

CONCLUSION

Unicompartmental arthroplasty has become the standard of treatment for patients with full loss of cartilage limited to one femorotibial compartment. When the indications are satisfied and the surgical principles respected, it is possible to restore full knee function after UKA. The recent evolution in surgical technique and instrumentation has allowed the surgeon to perform the procedure through a reliable mini-incision approach and to extend the indication to lateral compartment osteoarthritis, osteonecrosis or post-traumatic disorder.

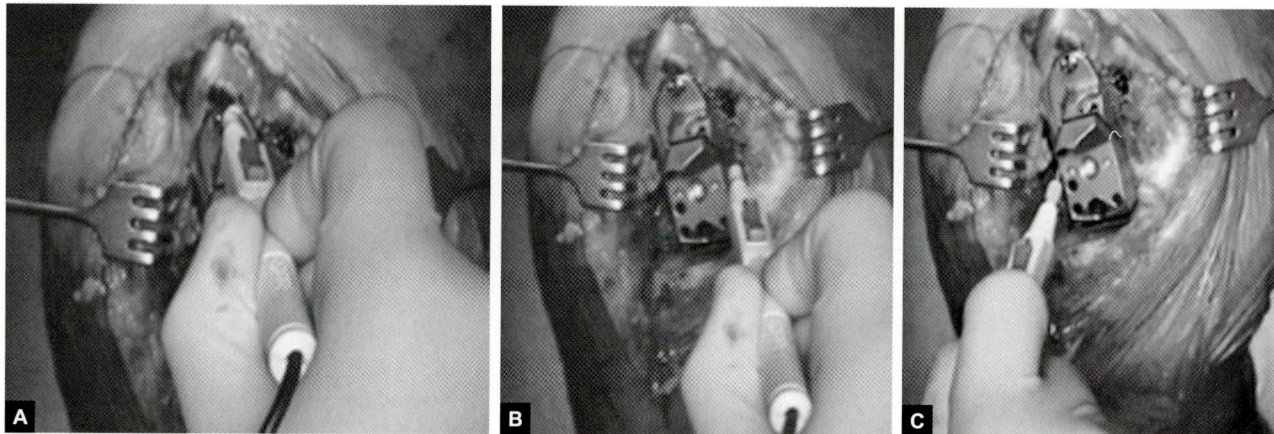

Figures 7.9A to C The femoral finishing guide is positioned on the distal femoral cut, searching for the best compromise between an anatomically centered position on the femoral condyle and a long-axis perpendicular to the resected tibial plateau. The top of this finishing guide should be localized 1–2 mm above the deepest layer of the cartilage to avoid a potential notch between the femoral implant and the patella

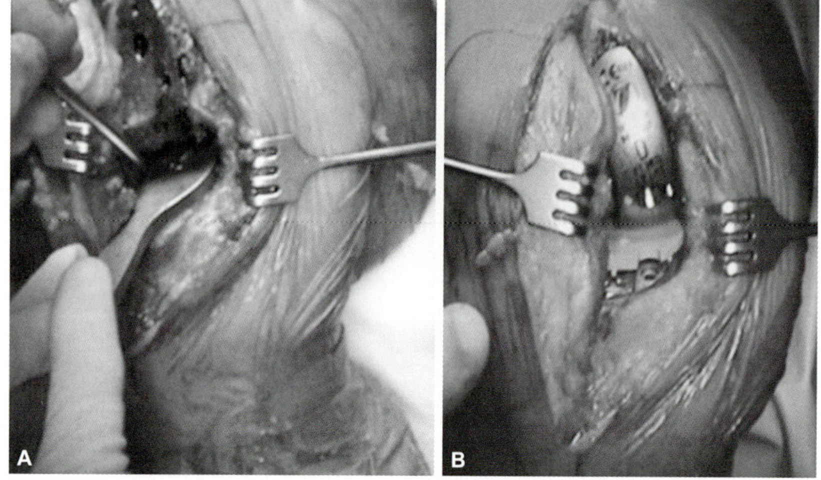

Figures 7.10A and B The tibial plateau is finishing, trying to find the best compromise between maximal tibial coverage and overhang

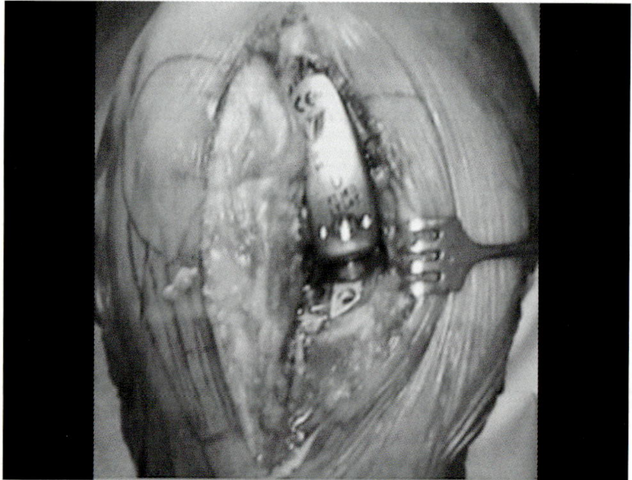

Figure 7.11 Tibial trials. The flexion-extension gaps are tested with the trial components in place and a trial polyethylene liner

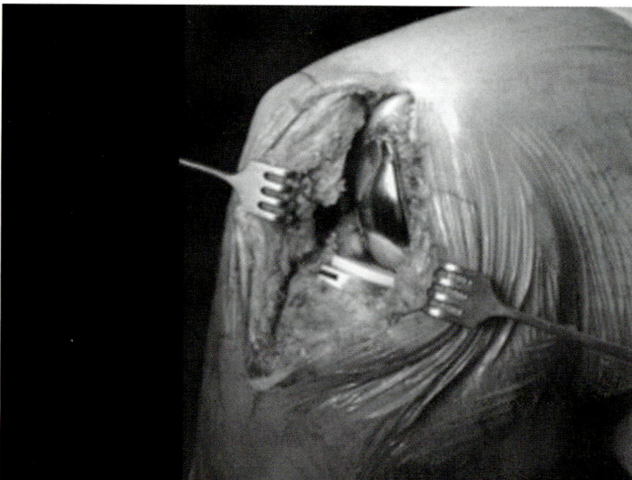

Figure 7.12 Final aspect with cemented implants

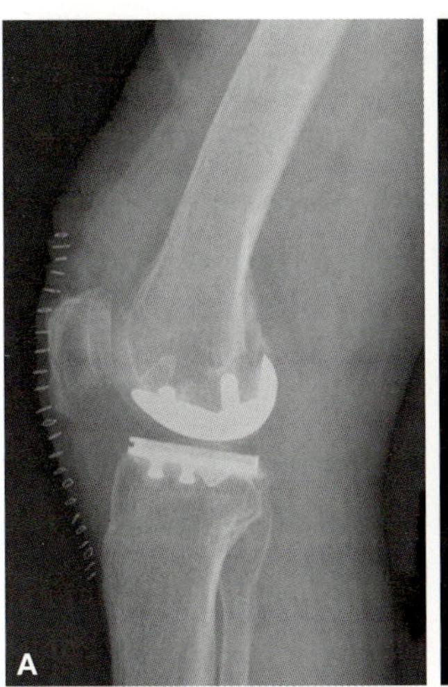

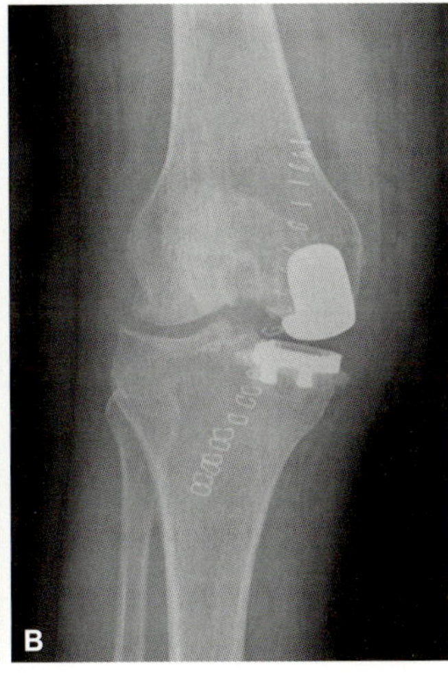

Figures 7.13A and B Postoperative X-rays (frontal and sagittal) analysis of the medial UKA

REFERENCES

1. Parratte S, Argenson JN, Pearce O, et al. Medial unicompartmental knee replacement in the under-50s. J Bone Joint Surg Br. 2009;91:351-6.
2. Parratte S, Argenson JN, Dumas J, Aubaniac JM. Unicompartmental knee arthroplasty for avascular osteonecrosis. Clin Orthop Relat Res. 2007;464:37-42.
3. Argenson JN, Parratte S, Bertani S, et al. The new arthritic patient and arthroplasty treatment options. J Bone Joint Surg Am. 2009;(Suppl. 5):43-8.
4. Flecher X, Parratte S, Aubaniac JM, Argenson JN. A 12-28-year follow-up study of closing wedge high tibial osteotomy. Clin Orthop Relat Res. 2006;452:91-6.
5. Pagnano MW, Clarke HD, Jacofsky DJ, Amendola A, Repicci JA. Surgical treatment of the middle-aged patient with arthritic knees. Instr Course Lect. 2005;54:251-9.
6. Ahlback S. Osteoarthrosis of the knee. A radiographic investigation. Acta Radiol Diagn. 1968; 277:7-72.
7. Barnes CL, Mesko JW, Teeny SM, York SC. Treatment of medial compartment arthritis of the knee: a survey of the American Association of Hip and Knee Surgeons. J Arthroplasty. 2006;21:950-6.
8. Argenson JN, Chevrol-Benkeddache Y, Aubaniac JM. Modern unicompartmental knee arthroplasty with cement: a three to ten-year follow-up study. J Bone Joint Surg Am. 2002;84-A:2235-9.
9. Argenson JN, Flecher X. Minimally invasive unicompartmental knee arthroplasty. Knee. 2004;11:341-7.
10. Argenson JN, Flecher X, Parratte S. [Mini-invasive implantation of an uni-compartmental medial knee prosthesis]. Rev Chir Orthop Reparatrice Appar Mot. 2006;92:193-9.
11. Berger RA, Meneghini RM, Jacobs JJ, et al. Results of unicompartmental knee arthroplasty at a minimum of ten years of follow-up. J Bone Joint Surg Am. 2005;87:999-1006.
12. Carlsson LV, Albrektsson BE, Regner LR. Minimally invasive surgery versus conventional exposure using the Miller-Galante unicompartmental knee arthroplasty: a randomized radiostereometric study. J Arthroplasty. 2006;21:151-6.
13. Repicci JA, Eberle RW. Minimally invasive surgical technique for unicondylar knee arthroplasty. J South Orthop Assoc. 1999;8:20-7.
14. Argenson JN, Parratte S, Flecher X, Aubaniac JM. Unicompartmental knee arthroplasty: technique through a mini-incision. Clin Orthop Relat Res. 2007;464:32-6.
15. Gibson PH, Goodfellow JW. Stress radiography in degenerative arthritis of the knee. J Bone Joint Surg Br. 1986;68:608,609.
16. USFDA. Oxford™ meniscal unicompartmental knee system. FDA pre market approach. Summary of safety and effectiveness. P010014. Silver Spring, MD: USFDA, 2004. http://www.accessdata.fda.gov/scripts/cdrh/cfdocs/cftopic/pma/pma.cfm?num=p010014
17. Gleeson RE, Evans R, Ackroyd CE, et al. Fixed or mobile bearing unicompartmental knee replacement? A comparative cohort study. Knee. 2004;11:379-84.
18. Price AJ, Dodd CA, Svard UG, Murray DW. Oxford medial unicompartmental knee arthroplasty in patients younger and older than 60 years of age. J Bone Joint Surg Br. 2005;87(11):1488-92.
19. Argenson JN, Parratte S. The unicompartmental knee: design and technical considerations in minimizing wear. Clin Orthop Relat Res. 2006;452:137-42.
20. Fisher DA, Watts M, Davis KE. Implant position in knee surgery: a comparison of minimally invasive, open unicompartmental, and total knee arthroplasty. J Arthroplasty. 2003;18:2-8.
21. Hamilton WG, Collier MB, Tarabee E, et al. Incidence and reasons for reoperation after minimally invasive

unicompartmental knee arthroplasty. J Arthroplasty. 2006;21:98-107.

22. Pandit H, Jenkins C, Barker K, Dodd CA, Murray DW. The Oxford medial unicompartmental knee replacement using a minimally-invasive approach. J Bone Joint Surg Br. 2006;88:54-60.
23. Romanowski MR, Repicci JA. Minimally invasive unicondylar arthroplasty: eight-year follow-up. J Knee Surg. 2002;15:17-22.
24. Repicci JA. Mini-invasive knee unicompartmental arthroplasty: bone-sparing technique. Surg Technol Int. 2003;11:282-6.
25. Repicci JA, Hartman JF. Minimally invasive unicondylar knee arthroplasty for the treatment of unicompartmental osteoarthritis: an outpatient arthritic bypass procedure. Orthop Clin North Am. 2004;35:201-16.
26. Romanowski MR, Repicci JA. Technical aspects of medial versus lateral minimally invasive unicondylar arthroplasty. Orthopedics. 2003;26:289-93.
27. Murray D, Goodfellow J, O'Connor J. The Oxford medial unicompartmental arthroplasty. J Bone Joint Surg Br. 1998;80B:983.
28. Price A, Wait J, Svärd U. Long-term clinical results of the medial Oxford unicompartmental knee arthroplasty. Clin Orthop Rel Res. 2005;435:171-80.
29. Vorlat P, Putzeys G, Cottenie D, et al. The Oxford unicompartmental knee prosthesis: an independent 10-year survival analysis. Knee Surg Sports Traumatol Arthrosc. 2005;14:40.
30. Confalonieri N, Manzotti A, Pullen C. Comparison of a mobile with a fixed tibial bearing unicompartmental knee prosthesis: a prospective randomized trial using a dedicated outcome score. Knee. 2004;11:357.
31. Parratte S, Pauly V, Aubaniac JM, Argenson JN. No long-term difference between fixed and mobile medial unicompartmental arthroplasty. Clin Orthop Relat Res. 2012;470:61-8.
32. Price AJ, Short A, Kellett C, et al. Ten-year *in vivo* wear measurement of a fully congruent mobile bearing unicompartmental knee arthroplasty. J Bone Joint Surg Br. 2005;87-B:1493-7.
33. Walton NP, Jahromi I, Lewis PL, et al. Patient-perceived outcomes and return to sport and work: TKA versus mini-incision unicompartmental knee arthroplasty. J Knee Surg. 2006;19:112-6.
34. Steele RG, Hutabarat S, Evans RL, Ackroyd CE, Newman JH. Survivorship of the St Georg Sled medial unicompartmental knee replacement beyond ten years. J Bone Joint Surg Br. 2006;88-B:1164-8.
35. Deshmukh RV, Scott RD. Unicompartmental knee arthroplasty for younger patients: an alternative view. Clin Orthop. 2002;404:108-2.
36. Ashraf T, Newman JH, Evans RL, Ackroyd CE. Lateral unicompartmental knee eplacement survivorship and clinical experience over 21 years. J Bone Joint Surg Br. 2002;84:1126-30.
37. Gunther T, Murray D, Miller R. Lateral unicompartmental knee arthroplasty with Oxford meniscal knee. Knee. 1996;3:33-9.
38. Sah AP, Scott RD. Lateral unicompartmental knee arthroplasty through a medial approach. Study with an average five-year follow-up. J Bone Joint Surg Am. 2007;89:1948-54.
39. Scott RD. Lateral unicompartmental replacement: a road less traveled. Orthopedics. 2005;28:983-4.
40. Argenson JN, Parratte S, Bertani A, Flecher X, Aubaniac JM. Long-term results with a lateral unicondylar replacement. Clin Orthop Relat Res. 2008;466:2686-93.
41. Dennis D, Komistek RD, Hoff WA, Gabriel SM, et al. *In vivo* anteroposterior femorotibial translation: a multicenter analysis. Clin Orthop. 1998;356:47-57.
42. Argenson JN, Komistek RD, Aubaniac JM, et al. *In vivo* determination of knee kinematics for subjects implanted with a unicompartmental arthroplasty. J Arthroplasty. 2002;17:1049-54.
43. Weidow J. Lateral osteoarthritis of the knee. Etiology based on morphological, anatomical, kinematic and kinetic observations. Acta Orthop Suppl. 2006;77:3-44.
44. Aglietti P, Insall JN, Buzzi R, Deschamps D. Idiopathic osteonecrosis of the knee: aetiology, prognosis and treatment. J Bone Joint Surg Br. 1983;65:588-97.
45. Ahlback S, Bauer GCH, Bohne WH. Spontaneous osteonecrosis of the knee. Arthritis Rheum. 1968;11:705-33.
46. Ecker ML. Spontaneous osteonecrosis of the distal femur. Instr Course Lect. 2001;50:495-8.
47. Mont MA, Baumgarten KM, Rifai A, et al. Atraumatic osteonecrosis of the knee. J Bone Joint Surg Am. 2000;82:1279-90.
48. Myers TG, Cui Q, Kuskowski M, Mihalko WM, Saleh KJ. Outcomes of total and unicompartmental knee arthroplasty

for secondary and spontaneous osteonecrosis of the knee. J Bone Joint Surg Am. 2006;88:76-82.

49. Marmor L. Unicompartmental arthroplasty for osteonecrosis of the knee joint. Clin Orthop Relat Res. 1993;294: 247-53.
50. Muheim G, Bohne WH. Prognosis in spontaneous osteonecrosis of the knee. J Bone Joint Surg Br. 1970;52:605-12.
51. Carro LP, Cimiano JG, Del Alamo GG, Suarez GG. Core decompression and arthroscopic bone grafting for avascular necrosis of the knee. Arthroscopy. 1996;12:323-6.
52. Mont MA, Tomek IM, Hungerford DS. Core decompression for avascular necrosis of the distal femur: long-term follow-up. Clin Orthop Relat Res. 1997;334:124-30.
53. Bergman NR, Rand JA. Total knee arthroplasty in osteonecrosis. Clin Orthop Relat Res. 1991;273:77-82.
54. Lotke PA, Battish R, Nelson CL. Treatment of osteonecrosis of the knee. Instr Course Lect. 2001;50:483-8.
55. Mont MA, Rifai A, Baumgarten KM, Sheldon M, Hungerford DS. Total knee arthroplasty for osteonecrosis. J Bone Joint Surg Am. 2002;84:599-603.
56. Atsui K, Tateishi H, Futani H, Maruo S. Ceramic unicompartmental knee arthroplasty for spontaneous osteonecrosis of the knee joint. Bull Hosp Jt Dis. 1997;56:233-6.
57. Lotke PA, Abend JA, Ecker ML. The treatment of osteonecrosis of the medial femoral condyle. Clin Orthop Relat Res. 1982;171:109-16.

Chapter 8

Patellofemoral Arthroplasty

Jess H Lonner, Joel Kolmodin, Carlos A Higuera

INTRODUCTION

Rates of total joint arthroplasty have risen remarkably over the past 40 years, and these rates are only projected to increase further as the population ages and the burden of arthritis increases. According to a recent study, the demand for total hip and total knee arthroplasty (TKA) in America is expected to grow by 174 and 673% respectively, by the year 2030.[1] Concordant with the overall progression of arthritis, an increasing number of young patients to develop isolated patellofemoral arthritis is expected. While this type of arthritis can often be treated nonoperatively, it will become progressively more imperative that conservative operative options are available as an alternative to TKA for this small cohort of patients. Herein lies the role of patellofemoral arthroplasty (PFA), which is becoming a mainstream management option as the implant design improves and surgical technique is refined. This chapter will cover the prevalence and epidemiology surrounding isolated patellofemoral arthritis, the typical evaluation of a patient with this condition, the history and evolution of PFA implants, and past and present clinical results.

EPIDEMIOLOGY

Patellofemoral arthritis is proving to be a much more common entity than was thought in the past. A 2002 study by Davies et al. evaluated knee radiographs of 206 knees in 174 consecutive patients, looking specifically for patellofemoral arthritis on weight bearing AP and skyline views.[2] The prevalence was striking 32.7% of men and 36.1% of women older than 60 years displayed the patellofemoral joint space narrowing to less than 3 mm. Obviously, a large percentage of these patients had patellofemoral joint arthritis in the setting of medial and lateral tibiofemoral compartment osteoarthritis. However, arthritis was actually isolated to the patellofemoral compartment in 13.6% of men and 15.4% women over 60 years of age. Moreover, it was found in 9.2% of patients over the age of 40.

Patellofemoral arthritis has been found to be much more prevalent in women than in men. In agreement with the above study, another notable analysis compared 273 patients with knee pain to 240 control subjects.[3] Radiographic evidence of arthritis was found in 53% of those with pain and 17% of those who were asymptomatic.

Isolated, symptomatic patellofemoral arthritis was found to be four times more common in women (8% versus 2% of the patients surveyed), while women were twice as likely (24% versus 11%) to have radiographic evidence of isolated anterior compartment arthritis. Though the cause has not yet been fully elucidated, it is thought that these differences in prevalence are due to slight dysplasia and malalignment that is seen more commonly in the female population.[4]

Evaluation

Patients with isolated patellofemoral arthritis often complain of anterior knee pain during activity. This pain is frequently exacerbated by active extension of the flexed knee—during activities such as stair climbing, squatting, or rising from a seated position. Patients may even report anterior knee pain when seated with the knee flexed for an extended period of time. Often, these symptoms are reproducible on examination by having the patient perform a simple squat. Physical exam may reveal tenderness to the palpation around the patellofemoral joint (particularly with patellar compression and inhibition testing), an abnormal Q-angle, a positive J-sign, and appreciable quadriceps weakness and/or atrophy. Patellofemoral crepitus will be noted with active quadriceps contraction and knee motion.

Radiographic evaluation of the patient with anterior knee pain should include four views—AP, midflexion PA, lateral and merchant (**Figures 8.1A to D**). The former are important to rule out tibiofemoral arthritis. In patients with isolated patellofemoral arthritis, marked narrowing of the patellofemoral joint is often seen, along with osteophyte formation. Abnormal patellar tilt or asymmetric patellar degeneration on the Merchant view may provide evidence for patellar maltracking. It cannot be stressed enough that any patient being considered for PFA must have limited evidence of medial or lateral compartment arthritis on the AP or midflexion PA views. For surgical candidates in whom PFA is being considered, preoperative MRI is often recommended, primarily in an effort to evaluate the medial and lateral tibiofemoral compartments for signs of arthritis—including such subtleties as edema of the subchondral bone or even overt chondral damage. Also helpful is the evaluation of any pictures from past arthroscopic surgery, as this gives a first-hand view of the status of the tibiofemoral articular cartilage.

Nonoperative management is the initial treatment of choice for most patients with isolated patellofemoral arthritis. Options include anti-inflammatory medications, injections (such as steroids and viscosupplementation), physical therapy, weight reduction and certain types of bracing. Each of these may have variable success, with more limited benefit in the advanced stages of patellofemoral arthritis. In surgical candidates with substantial quadriceps weakness and atrophy, physical therapy should be stressed preoperatively to overcome potential postoperative functional limitations.

When nonoperative measures fail to provide adequate relief, surgery is a viable option. Noteworthy nonarthroplasty options include simple arthroscopic debridement, microfracture, patellectomy, unloading procedures, or cartilage restoration procedures. These interventions often have limited success, in the range of 60–70% efficacy.[5] Thus, arthroplasty alternatives may provide the most reliable outcomes, including pain relief and functional improvement. While TKA is effective in treating patellofemoral arthritis, some may prefer PFA for this entity, as it preserves the healthy tissue and optimizes natural kinematics.[6,7]

INDICATIONS

Patellofemoral arthroplasty should be limited to those with isolated primary or secondary (due to dysplasia or trauma) patellofemoral arthritis. Contraindications for PFA are numerous and include tibiofemoral arthritis, inflammatory arthritis, chondrocalcinosis, and uncorrectable patellofemoral malalignment or maltracking (as evidenced by an abnormally large Q-angle and a positive J-sign). The latter problems can usually be addressed at the time of PFA with soft tissue realignment or tibial tubercle realignment. Relative contraindications include cruciate ligament deficiency, obesity, limited motion, and diffuse pain.[8]

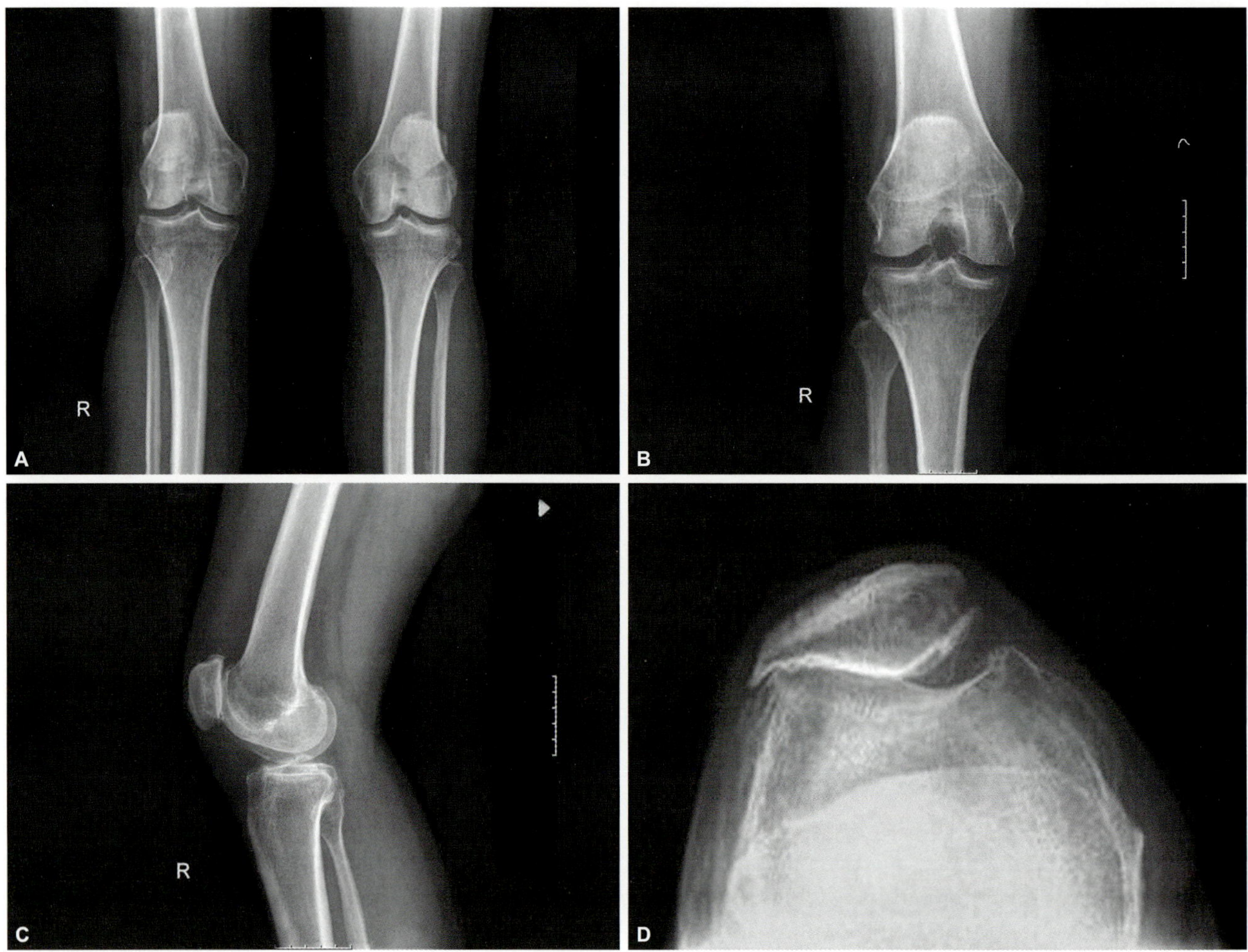

Figures 8.1A to D Standing anteroposterior, midflexion posteroanterior, lateral, and sunrise radiographs show arthritis localized to the patellofemoral compartment

DESIGN CONSIDERATIONS

Inlay-style Designs

A thorough discussion of PFA design is imperative to understand the progression from the generally unreliable first-generation implants to the more reliable second- and third-generation implants that are used today. Initial attempts at PFA were of an inlay-style, where the trochlear component was inset into the anatomic position of the patient's native trochlea. Some inlay-style designs still exist today, with less optimal results reported in national registries.[9] The prostheses were designed to be positioned flush with the surrounding trochlear articular cartilage—an effort to preserve the patient's native anatomy (**Figures 8.2A to D**). The error in this design was the failure to recognize that the patient's native anatomy is at times pathologic or dysplastic, and an attempt to recreate it forces the trochlear component to be internally rotated and can lead to prosthesis failure or more commonly patellar maltracking. Of particular importance is this tendency of the inlay designs to be placed in an overly internally rotated position, as the position is determined by the native trochlear rotation.[10] Internal rotation of the trochlear implant has three main effects: increasing the Q-angle, medialization of the trochlear groove, and placing abnormal tension on the lateral retinaculum.

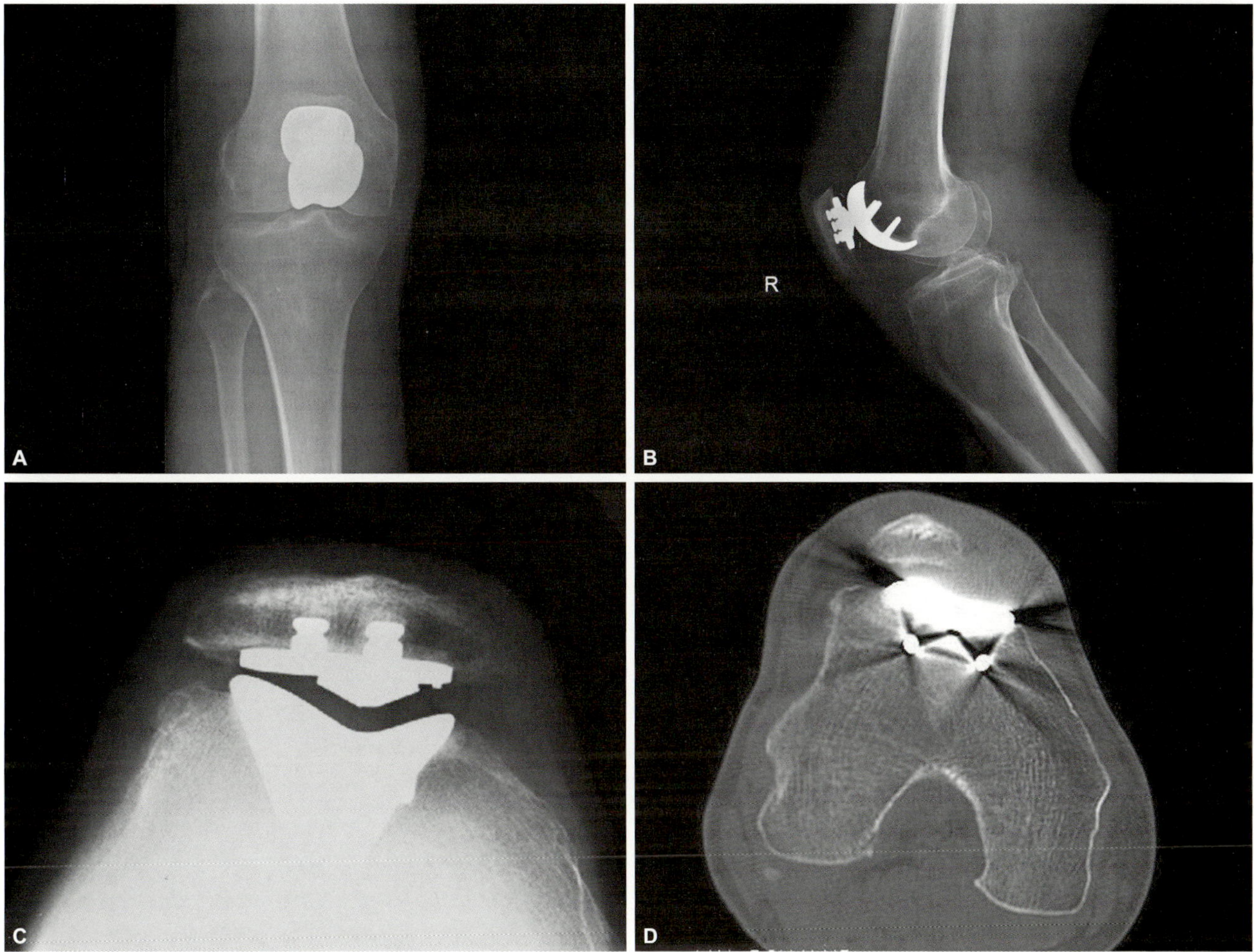

Figures 8.2A to D Postoperative AP, lateral and sunrise radiographs and computed tomography scan after PFA with an inlay-style trochlear component shows that it is internally rotated, causing lateral patellar subluxation and catching

This may predispose the prosthesis to excessively high rates of mechanical symptoms such as catching, patellar maltracking, and frank patellar subluxation.[5]

The trochlear inclination angles (TIAs) have recently been found to be of utmost importance in PFA. A complete understanding of the TIAs is imperative to be able to correctly perform a PFA and to understand the rationale for the transition from inlay-style implants to onlay-style trochlear implants. The TIA, defined as the angle formed by the line perpendicular to the AP axis (i.e. Whiteside's line) and a line connecting the peaks of the trochlear surfaces of the medial and lateral femoral condyles, is a measurement that can be made on any MRI. A recent study by Kamath et al. used MRI to evaluate the TIA of 329 knees—both normal and dysplastic.[10] They found that the TIA is normally internally rotated significantly: 11.4° for normal knees and 9.4° for dysplastic knees. Thus, when this natural trochlear internal rotation is not accounted for in the prosthesis design and surgical technique, patellar instability can occur.

Other design flaws are also commonly seen in the inlay-style prosthesis. As the prostheses are designed to sit flush with the surrounding trochlear cartilage, it was often unable to accommodate situations of severe trochlear dysplasia. This leads to a malpositioned, proud component that can cause catching. Additionally, several early prostheses had abnormally large radii of curvature. As one might expect, this would lead to the necessity for the implant to be positioned in a flexed position to avoid impingement on the ACL or tibia. In a component that is designed to sit flush with the trochlear cartilage, any implant flexion would cause the proximal aspect of the prosthesis to sit proud. In this way, the patella may have the propensity to catch or sublux in the initial phases of flexion.[11,12]

Finally, many inlay-style trochlear implants have inherent features that do not accommodate the patella effectively, such as a narrow body, a deep trochlear sulcus and limited extension. These features have contributed to the patellar catching or subluxation in the initial 30° of flexion that is common with inlay-style trochlear designs.[5]

Onlay-style Designs

In contrast, the onlay-style trochlear prostheses are designed to replace the entire anterior trochlear joint surface, and they are positioned perpendicular to the AP axis of the femur (**Figures 8.3A to D**). Unlike inlay-style designs, the onlay-style prostheses have almost eliminated the incidence of patellar instability. Additionally, due to the fact that this style of implant need not be influenced by the patient's native anatomy (which is often pathologic to begin with); the implant is

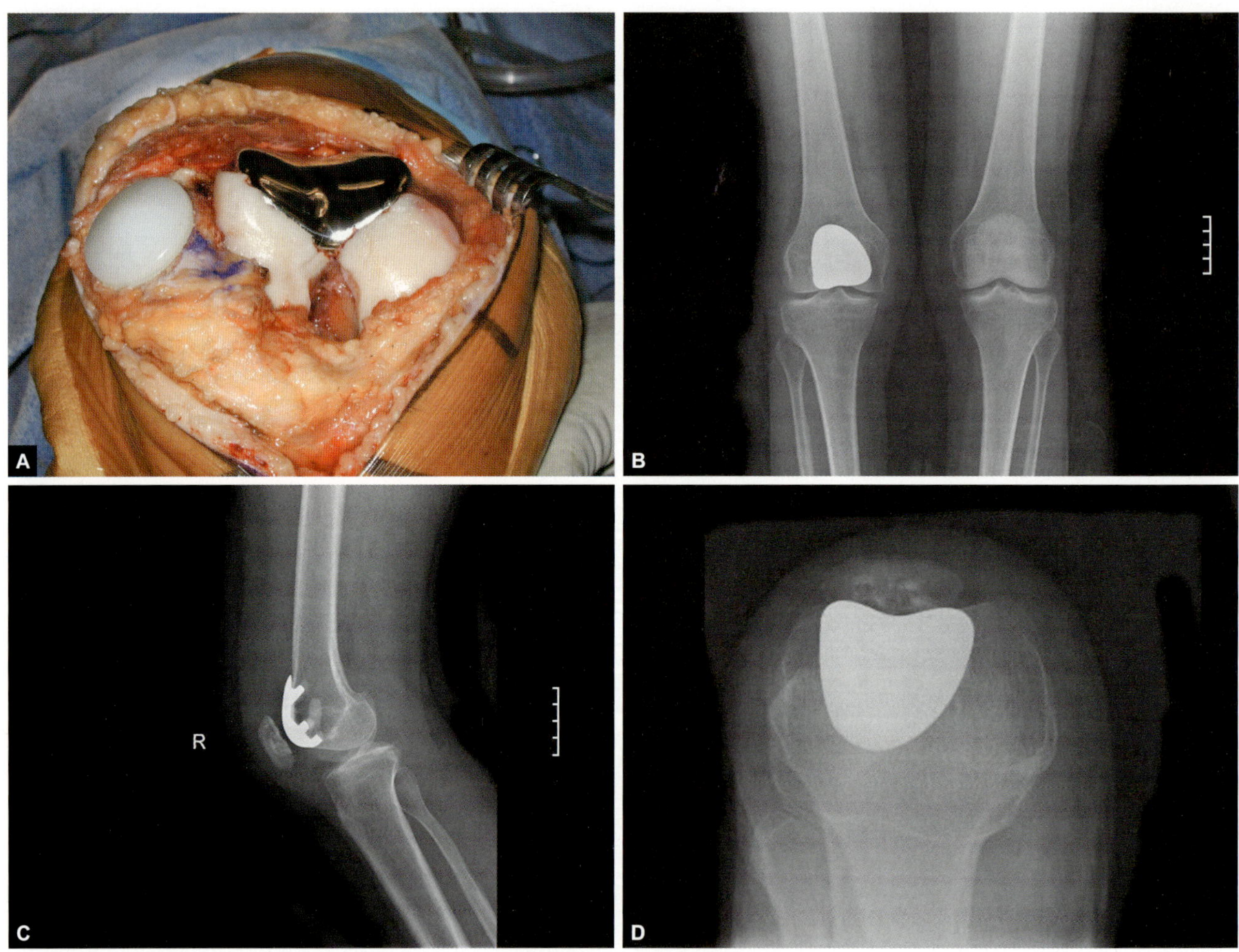

Figures 8.3A to D Intraoperative clinical photograph and postoperative AP, lateral, and sunrise radiographs after PFA with an onlay-style trochlear component positioned perpendicular to the AP axis of the femur, with good patellar tracking

much more versatile and accommodating of all trochlear morphologies.[5]

A variety of features have optimized outcomes. Notably, the rotation of the trochlear component is based on specific anatomic landmarks that are determined intraoperatively—the component is placed perpendicular to Whiteside's line (the anteroposterior axis of the knee) and parallel to the transepicondylar axis. By avoiding the tendency to be internally rotated, the trochlear component can better accommodate patellar tracking. Moreover, the onlay-style trochlear implants tend to be wider and less constraining than the inlay designs, accommodating variations in patellar tracking throughout the arc of motion. The onlay-style components are also made with more accommodating radii of curvature, permitting the prosthesis to sit flush with the anterior femoral cortex proximally and the intercondylar notch distally, and they tend to extend more proximally than inlay designs. These features enhance patellar tracking through the entire range of motion and account for the better outcomes with onlay compared to inlay designs.

The main differences between inlay and onlay generation designs are summarized in **Table 8.1**.

SURGICAL CONSIDERATIONS

Any standard TKA incision (medial parapatellar, subvastus, etc.) can be used to perform PFA. Since the goal of this procedure is to maintain healthy portions of the knee joint, extreme care should be taken to avoid injury to the articular cartilage, the menisci, and the ligamentous structures during the arthrotomy. After the joint is accessed, a thorough inspection should commence. At this point, any unanticipated joint derangement that was not identified preoperatively may signal the need to perform additional procedures such as the cartilage graft or TKA.

Though surgical techniques vary between systems, most protocols for onlay designs are centered on defining the anteroposterior axis of the knee joint (Whiteside's line). This is the landmark around which trochlear component rotation is set. Care is taken to position the trochlear component within the confines of the trochlear groove—not encroaching on weight-bearing condylar surfaces of the femur. The trochlear component is designed to sit flush with the surrounding articular cartilage; it should not be allowed to sit proud, and any cement used to secure the prosthesis must not be allowed to extrude from the cartilage-component interface. The patellar preparation is similar to that employed in TKA.

Trialling of the components allows for *in vivo* assessment of patellar tracking. Any abnormal patellar tilt or maltracking must be addressed intraoperatively, first by ensuring appropriate implant positioning, then with soft tissue procedures—most commonly a lateral retinacular release. Other more aggressive procedures (such as tibial tubercle transfer) may be necessary as well, but ideally the decision for a simultaneous procedure would be determined preoperatively and is based on a high Q-angle.

Postoperative management includes standard use of antibiotic prophylaxis and DVT chemoprophylaxis. Generally, full weight-bearing is allowed immediately after the procedure, with active and passive range of motion encouraged. Physical therapy is continued until reasonable quadriceps strength and range of motion return.

TABLE 8.1 Differences between inlay and onlay generation

	Trochlear position	*Trochlear rotation*	*Trochlear width*	*Trochlear proximal extension*	*Trochlear radius of curvature*
Inlay-style	Inset within the native trochlea	Identical to that of the native trochlea (Tendency is internal rotation)	Narrow	Identical to that of the native trochlea	Causes offset
Onlay-style	Perpendicular to the AP axis (Whiteside's line)	Determined by the surgeon; perpendicular to AP axis	Wide	Extending more proximal than the native trochlea	Articulation

RESULTS

Primary Patellofemoral Arthroplasty

Proper patient selection and proper surgical technique are important factors in determining the success of PFA. However, evaluation of the outcomes of PFA have shown a disparity in the short-term failures that occur as a result of maltracking and patellar instability, depending on which prosthesis is used—inlay- or onlay-style designs.[5] To this point there are no known studies which have directly compared the inlay- and onlay-style trochlear designs. A large majority of the evidence, however, shows improved outcomes with onlay-style designs, particularly as it relates to patellar maltracking, functional success rates and durability.

The results of studies involving the use of inlay- and onlay-style trochlear prosthesis designs are outlined in **Tables 8.2** and **8.3**.

It has become apparent that high reoperation and revision rates with inlay-style trochlear designs are attributed to component malposition, soft tissue imbalance and poor patient selection. In many series evaluating the inlay-style designs, failure most likely occurred due to improper trochlear component positioning that resulted in the prosthesis sitting proud in relation to surrounding articular surfaces (due to morphologic mismatches between the trochlear implant and surface

TABLE 8.2

Author (year)	*Implant type*	*Procedures performed*	*Average patient age (years)*	*Average follow-up (years)*	*Good/excellent results – (rating system) (%)*	*Revision rate (%)*
Blazina (1979)	Richards types I & II	57	39	2	—	35
Arciero (1988)	Richards type II (14); CFS-Knight (11)	25	62	5.3	85 (H&K)	28
Cartier (1990)	Richards types II & III	72	65	4	85 (MSS)	7
Argenson (1995)	Autocentric	66	57	5.5	84 (HSS)	15
Krajca (1996)	Richards types I & II	16	64	5.8	88 (H&K)	6
De Winter (2001)	Richards type II	26	59	11	76 (KSS)	19
Kooijman (2003)	Richards type II	45	50	17	86 (KSS)	22
Cartier (2005)	Richards types II & III	79	60	10	77 (KSS)	25
Argenson (2005)	Autocentric	66	57	16	—	42
van Jonbergen (2010)	Richards type II	185	52	13.3	—	25

Abbreviations: H&K – Hungerford and Kenna Knee Score, MSS – Mansat Scoring System, HSS – Hospital for Special Surgery Knee Score, KSS – Knee Society Score

TABLE 8.3

Author (year)	*Implant type*	*Procedures performed*	*Average patient age (years)*	*Average follow-up (years)*	*Good/excellent results – (rating system) %*	*Revision rate (%)*
Ackroyd (2007)	Avon	109	68	5.2	80 (BPS)	3.6
Starks (2009)	Avon	37	66	2	86 (KSS)	0
Leadbetter (2009)	Avon	79	58	3	84 (KSS)	6.3
Gao (2010)	Avon	11	54	2	100 (KSS)	0
Odumenya (2010)	Avon	50	66	5.3	—	4
Mont (2012)	Avon	43	29	7	—	12

Abbreviations: BPS – Bristol Pain Score, KSS – Knee Society Score

anatomy) and internally rotated due to the native trochlear inclination. Again, while poorly defined in studies to this point, these trochlear component design features likely lead to disproportionately low rates of satisfactory outcomes in the inlay-style designs.[13-26] These findings have been corroborated by the information published from the Australian National Joint Registry, showing a five-year revision rate that is over 20% for the inlay-style prostheses but less than 10% for the onlay-style designs.[9] To this point, the incidence of patellar maltracking has ranged from 17 to 36% in studies evaluating the results of inlay-style implants.[5,16,20,25,27] In contrast, series that have reviewed the outcomes of onlay-style trochlear designs have found much lower incidence of patellar maltracking, often less than 1%.[16,28-31] As a direct result of these finding, several of the inlay-style PFA systems are not being used presently. Nevertheless, as long as patella tracking is acceptable after PFA—even when inlay-style designs are used—acceptable outcomes can be achieved. In these circumstances the primary mode of failure is progressive tibiofemoral arthritis.

Many of the recent series regarding PFA have directly compared TKA to PFA for the treatment of isolated patellofemoral arthritis. A small study was published in the Chinese Medical Journal in 2010. Matched according to age, gender, bilaterality and body mass index, Gao et al. compared 11 patients who received Avon PFA implants with 23 patients who received TKA.[32] Outcomes were similar for both groups, but the PFA group had shorter operation times, decreased blood loss, and better post-operative range of motion. Additionally, Dahm et al. recently published results comparing PFA to TKA in patients with isolated patellofemoral arthritis.[6] At a mean follow-up of 29 months, significantly better results were seen in the PFA group regarding UCLA scores, blood loss, and hospital stay, while Knee Society Clinical Rating System scores were identical.

Revision

With the high rates of failure seen in the first-generation inlay-style PFAs, the need for revision can be a commonly encountered problem for the arthroplasty surgeon. Two options exist in this situation: revision to a second-generation onlay-style prosthesis or conversion to a TKA. In the short- to mid-term, both modalities have proven to be viable options.

Hendrix et al. published a series of 14 knees that were revised from first-generation (Lubinus) implants to second-generation (Avon) implants between 1996 and 2002.[33] Revision occurred in the setting of component malposition, patellar subluxation, or mechanical patellar problems. At a mean follow-up of 60 months, average Bristol knee scores improved from 58 preoperatively to 79 postoperatively. No radiographic evidence of loosening, malposition, or wear was seen in any revision patient.

Lonner et al. demonstrated in a recent study that revision to TKA can be a very successful option in patients with failed PFAs.[11] In their study, 12 failed patellofemoral replacements were revised to total knee arthroplasties. Indications for revision were progressive tibiofemoral arthritis (six knees), mechanical symptoms due to maltracking (three knees), or a combination thereof (three knees). Short-term follow-up demonstrated marked increase in the knee society functional and clinical scores, with no signs of persistent maltracking, wear, or loosening.

SUMMARY

Patellofemoral arthroplasty is emerging as a reliable method of treating isolated patellofemoral arthritis. Though early designs yielded inconsistent results, the development of improved implant designs, more standardized surgical instrumentation and techniques, and refinement of indications has improved all facets of PFA implementation. It should be noted, however, that though short-term follow-up studies regarding second-generation implants have been very encouraging, long-term studies are needed to verify that the prostheses remain a reliable and satisfactory mode of treatment. We anticipate that as our understanding of the patellofemoral joint and its pathology grows, instrumentation will only improve, which should lead to steadily improving outcomes. If this proves to be correct, PFA will become an increasingly mainstream alternative to total joint arthroplasty to address this complex clinical problem.

REFERENCES

1. Kurtz S, Ong K, Lau E, Mowat F, Halpern M. Projections of primary and revision hip and knee arthroplasty in the United States from 2005 to 2030. J Bone Joint Surg. 2007;89(4):780-5.
2. Davies AP, Vince AS, Shepstone L, Donell ST, Glasgow MM. The radiologic prevalence of patellofemoral osteoarthritis. Clin Orthop Relat Res. 2002;402:206-12.
3. McAlindon TE, Snow S, Cooper C, Dieppe PA. Radiographic patterns of osteoarthritis of the knee joint in the community: the importance of the patellofemoral joint. Ann Rheum Dis. 1992;51(7):844-9.
4. Grelsamer RP, Dejour D, Gould J. The pathophysiology of patellofemoral arthritis. Orthop Clin North Am. 2008;39(3):269-74.
5. Lonner JH. Patellofemoral arthroplasty: pros, cons, and design considerations. Clin Orthop Relat Res. 2004;428:158-65.
6. Dahm DL, et al. Patellofemoral arthroplasty versus total knee arthroplasty in patients with isolated patellofemoral arthritis. Am J Orthop. 2010;39(10):487-91.
7. Lonner JH. Patellofemoral arthroplasty. J Am Acad Orthop Surg. 2007;15(8):495-506.
8. Lonner JH. Patellofemoral arthroplasty. In: Lotke PA, Lonner JH (Eds), Master Techniques in Orthopaedic Surgery: Knee Arthroplasty, 2nd edn. Philadelphia, PA: Lippincott Williams and Wilkins; 2003. pp. 261-73.
9. Australian Orthopaedic Association National Joint Replacement Registry. Available at: http://dmac.adelaide.edu.au/aoanjrr/publications.jsp
10. Kamath AF, Slattery TR, Levack AE, et al. Trochlear inclination angles in normal and dysplastic knees. J Arthroplasty.2013;28(2):214-9.
11. Lonner JH, Jasko JG, Booth RE Jr. Revision of a failed patellofemoral arthroplasty to a total knee arthroplasty. J Bone Joint Surg. 2006;88(11):2337-42.
12. Lonner JH, Bloomfield MR. The clinical outcome of patellofemoral arthroplasty. Orthop Clin North Am. 2013;44(3):271-80.
13. Arciero RA, Toomey HE. Patellofemoral arthroplasty. A three- to nine-year follow-up study. Clin Orthop Relat Res. 1988;236:60-71.
14. Argenson JN, Guillaume JM, Aubaniac JM. Is there a place for patellofemoral arthroplasty? Clin Orthop Relat Res. 1995;321:162-7.
15. Argenson JN, Flecher X, Parratte S, Aubaniac JM. Patellofemoral arthroplasty: an update. Clin Orthop Relat Res. 2005;440:50-3.
16. Blazina ME, Fox JM, Del Pizzo W, Broukhim B, Ivey FM. Patellofemoral replacement. Clin Orthop Relat Res. 1979(144):98-102.
17. Cartier P, Sanouiller JL, Grelsamer R. Patellofemoral arthroplasty. 2–12-year follow-up study. J Arthrop. 1990;5(1):49-55.
18. Cartier P, Sanouiller JL, Khefacha A. Long-term results with the first patellofemoral prosthesis. Clin Orthop Relat Res. 2005;436:47-54.
19. Charalambous CP, Abiddin Z, Mills SP, et al. The low contact stress patellofemoral replacement: high early failure rate. J Bone Joint Surg. 2011;93(4):484-9.
20. de Winter WE, Feith R, van Loon CJ. The Richards type II patellofemoral arthroplasty: 26 cases followed for 1–20 years. Acta Orthop Scand. 2001;72(5):487-90.
21. Kooijman HJ, Driessen AP, van Horn JR. Long-term results of patellofemoral arthroplasty. A report of 56 arthroplasties with 17 years of follow-up. J Bone Joint Surg. 2003;85(6):836-40.
22. Krajca-Radcliffe JB, Coker TP. Patellofemoral arthroplasty. A 2- to 18-year follow-up study. Clin Orthop Relat Res. 1996;330:143-51.
23. Merchant AC. Early results with a total patellofemoral joint replacement arthroplasty prosthesis. J Arthrop. 2004;19(7):829-36.
24. Sisto DJ, Sarin VK. Custom patellofemoral arthroplasty of the knee. J Bone Joint Surg Am. 2006;88:1475-80.
25. Tauro B, Ackroyd CE, Newman JH, Shah NA. The Lubinus patellofemoral arthroplasty. A five- to ten-year prospective study. J Bone Joint Surg Br. 2001;83(5):696-701.
26. van Jonbergen HP, Werkman DM, Barnaart LF, van Kampen A. Long-term outcomes of patellofemoral arthroplasty. J Arthrop. 2010;25(7):1066-71.
27. Odumenya M, Costa ML, Parsons N, et al. The Avon patellofemoral joint replacement: five-year results from an independent centre. J Bone Joint Surg. 2010;92(1):56-60.

28. Ackroyd CE, Newman JH, Evans R, Eldridge JD, Joslin CC. The Avon patellofemoral arthroplasty: five-year survivorship and functional results. J Bone Joint Surg Br. 2007;89(3):310-5.
29. Leadbetter WB, Kolisek FR, Levitt RL, et al. Patellofemoral arthroplasty: a multi-centre study with minimum 2-year follow-up. Int Orthop. 2009;33(6):1597-601.
30. Mont MA, Johnson AJ, Naziri Q, Kolisek FR, Leadbetter WB. Patellofemoral arthroplasty: 7-year mean follow-up. J Arthrop. 2012;27(3):358-61.
31. Starks I, Roberts S, White SH. The Avon patellofemoral joint replacement: independent assessment of early functional outcomes. J Bone Joint Surg. 2009;91(12):1579-82.
32. Gao X, Xu ZJ, He RX, Yan SG, Wu LD. A preliminary report of patellofemoral arthroplasty in isolated patellofemoral arthritis. Chin Med J. 2010;123(21):3020-3.
33. Hendrix MR, Ackroyd CE, Lonner JH. Revision patellofemoral arthroplasty: three- to seven-year follow-up. J Arthrop. 2008;23(7):977-83.

Chapter 9

Cruciate Retaining Total Knee Arthroplasty: Technique and Results

Ashok Rajgopal, Attique Vasdev, Vivek Dahiya, Vipin Tyagi

INTRODUCTION

The debate on whether to preserve or sacrifice the posterior cruciate ligament (PCL)[1,2] has been going on ever since the polycentric knee[3] was described in 1971. Surgeons from the Massachusetts General Hospital preferred to save the PCL because it resulted in better flexion ranges allowing the patients with rheumatoid arthritis [85% of patients undergoing total knee arthroplasty (TKA)] to easily get up from a chair and negotiate stairs. Surgeons who preserve the PCL during TKA (**Figures 9.1A and B**) believe that it results in better function, range of motion, strength, and stability when compared with the cruciate sacrificing designs. The PCL transmits all the forces directly to the bone thereby minimizing stress between the implant and the bone.[4]

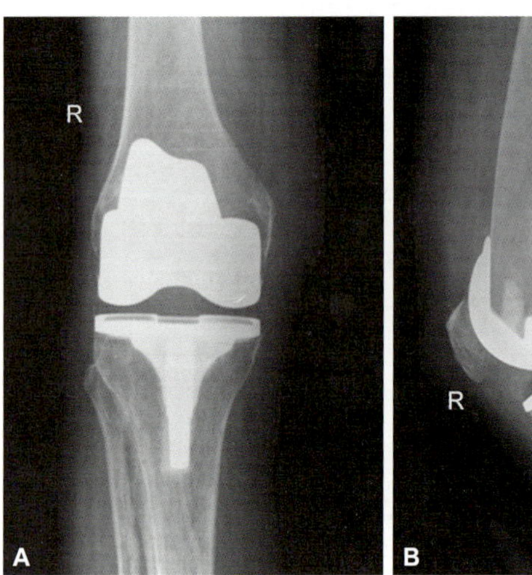

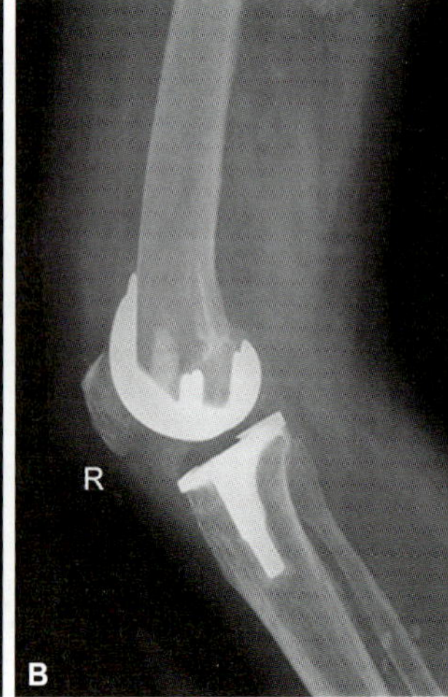

Figures 9.1A and B Cruciate retaining total knee arthroplasty

Studies have shown that PCL preservation leads to a normal and efficient gait pattern.[5-7] Proprioception from the knee is perceived to be better when the PCL is preserved because of the mechanoreceptors present within its substance.[8-11] Patients with a cruciate retaining total knee arthroplasty (CR TKA) find it easier to indulge in activities wherein knee stability in flexion is required, e.g. gardening, stair climbing, and so on.[12]

In this chapter, we endeavor to present the surgical technique and results of CR TKA. CR TKA aims to achieve normal knee kinematics in an effort to improve the function and longevity of the TKA.

HISTORY

Gluck described the first implantation of an artificial knee joint in 1890. He used a hinge fixed to stems made of ivory and bone glue to enhance fixation to the bone. He also coined the term 'arthroplasty'. This was followed by the technique of interpositional arthroplasty that was advocated by Murphy from Chicago. He used fascia lata interpositional arthroplasty in 1905. This was modified by Campbell in 1925.

The next stage of evolution encompassed the use of knee mold which was advocated by Smith Peterson at the Massachusetts General Hospital and subsequently by Campbell in 1940. The 1950s saw the introduction of tibial molds using metallic and acrylic materials to surface the tibial plateau. McKeever in 1952 and MacIntosh in 1958 were the pioneers of this technique. These implants worked as fillers correcting the deformity and providing stability by pulling out the collateral ligaments to their normal tension. This decade also saw the emergence of the hinged knee replacement popularized by Walladius (1951), Shiers (1953), Stanmore (1954), and Guepar (1970). Understanding of the kinematics of the knee and the forces acting across the joint established the need to relook the design rationale of knee replacement implants. Freeman et al. described the design rationale of knees, the surgical technique, and soft tissue balancing.

The first example of a cruciate retaining implant was the polycentric knee by Gunston,[3] which attempted to reproduce normal knee kinematics. The design allowed a polycentric pathway of motion. However, ligamentous laxity, instability, and tibial loosening were the most common modes of failure for the polycentric knee with a little over 50% of the knees surviving at 10 years.

The duocondylar prosthesis developed in the early 70s by Walker, Insall, and Ranawat[13] matched the shape of the normal femoral condyles aiming to reproduce the polycentric motion pattern. The tibial components were flat in the sagittal plane but had upward sloping curves towards the intercondylar eminence to provide mediolateral stability. Instability, tibial component loosening, and anterior knee pain were the predominant causes of failure of the duocondylar knee. A patellar flange was added onto the femoral component and the duopatellar total knee[13,14] was born. This reduced the incidence of patellofemoral pain from 20% to 5% when compared with the duocondylar knee. The other design change incorporated was that the tibial components were made curved in the sagittal plane. This led to a twofold increased incidence of tibial lucent lines at 2 years.

By 1979, it was proven in laboratory tests that a one-piece tibial component with a short stem enhanced tibial component fixation through an increased surface contact area. The tibial components were also made flat in the sagittal plane to allow femoral rollback in flexion. Duocondylar and duopatellar implants were a historical landmark in the development of the CR TKA as three major design issues were sorted out; the use of an anterior femoral flange, flat tibial surface geometry in the sagittal plane, and a one piece tibial component with a short central stem.[14,15]

The kinematic knee incorporated a valgus aligned patellar groove in the anterior flange and a flat metal backed tibial component with a short stem in its design. These two modifications corrected anterior knee pain and provided good range of motion.[16]

Townley[17] and Cloutier[18] prostheses were of similar design and philosophy. They aimed to reproduce the normal anatomy and kinematics of the knee joint. The tibial component was 'U' shaped which helped preserve both the cruciate ligaments.

The Miller-Galante prosthesis[19] was the first to be available in cemented and uncemented variants. The modularity of the system with seven femoral sizes and five tibial sizes was an improvement over the previous implants and aided in providing adequate coverage of the native bone. This was the prosthesis that helped shape and guide the implant systems available today.

POSTERIOR CRUCIATE LIGAMENT

Anatomy

The posterior cruciate ligament (PCL) is the strongest ligament in the body. It is 13 mm wide and approximately 38 mm long. The PCL arises from the anterolateral aspect of the medial femoral condyle in the region of the intercondylar notch. Its origin is much anterior to that of the anterior cruciate ligament (ACL). The PCL consists of two bundles named by the relative position of origin on the femur and insertion on the tibia. The anterolateral bundle arises from the anterior aspect of the femur and inserts on the lateral aspect of the intercondylar tibial eminence. The posteromedial bundle originates posterior to the anterolateral bundle on the femur and inserts medial to the anterolateral bundle on the tibia. The anterolateral bundle represents about 65% of the substance of the ligament. The tibial insertion of the PCL is posterior and distal on the tibia approximately 10 mm distal to the joint line. The tibial attachment site is smaller than the femoral origin site.[20-23]

The PCL is enveloped by a synovial envelope originating from the posterior aspect of the joint capsule. Both the ACL and the PCL are intra-articular but extrasynovial. The PCL is twice as strong as the ACL. It has a higher tensile strength and a greater cross-sectional area. Its fibers are oriented more vertically than the more oblique fibers of the ACL.

Function and Kinematics in a Normal Knee

The PCL is the primary restraint in preventing posterior translation of the tibia relative to the femur during flexion. The posterior fibers prevent hyperextension. In extension, the posteromedial bundle is tight. As the knee flexes to 90° the anterolateral bundle tightens and provides 95% of the resistance to posterior tibial translation. These fibers also help prevent hyperflexion. The PCL resists internal tibial rotation during flexion by winding around the ACL. The PCL also stabilizes the knee against excess varus or valgus angulation. The presence of mechanoreceptors in the substance of the PCL points toward a significant proprioceptive function, leading to better gait and confidence levels with the knee.[7,8]

The PCL plays a vital role in guiding the kinematics[23] of the knee during the arc of motion. It is considered as the collateral ligament for the medial compartment of the knee.[24] Flexion and extension of the knee are not simple hinge movements that occur in the elbow joint. Flexion and extension occur about a constantly changing center of rotation, i.e. polycentric rotation. This path of changing center of rotation describes a 'J' shaped curve about the femoral condyles. As the knee extends from a flexed position the shorter more highly curved lateral femoral condyle exhausts its articular surface and is checked by the ACL, whereas the larger and less curved medial condyle continues it's forward roll and skids backwards, assisted by the tightening of the PCL. This results in medial rotation of the femur that tightens the collateral ligaments and the joint is screwed home (screw home mechanism).[25]

Kinematics of a CR TKA

Retention of the PCL is believed to preserve the normal kinematics of a knee after a total knee replacement. As the knee flexes, the PCL tightens allowing for a normal femoral rollback thereby increasing the quadriceps efficiency and range of motion. This was perceived to be advantageous in negotiating stairs and other activities for which knee flexion is needed.[11] Fluoroscopic analysis has revealed that the CR knees exhibit better ranges of flexion and femoral rollback[26,27] is consistently observed. In a small percentage of knees, there is a paradoxical anterior translation of the femur as the knee flexes. The reason for this paradoxical movement is considered to be inadequate balancing of the PCL.[27] Studies[28] have shown that the ranges of motion achieved with CR and PS knees are similar but the gain in flexion relative to the preoperative status was greater in PS knees. This is due to greater posterior translation of the femur on the tibia aided by the post and cam mechanism that in turn leads to greater stresses on the insert and hence greater potential for early wear.[28]

Gait analysis[5,6] has ascertained that anteroposterior translation of the knee influences the ability of patients to ascend stairs in a normal manner. During early swing phase the femur moves forward because of the hamstring pull. At 45° of flexion the femur begins to move posteriorly as the PCL tightens. In a PS design it is only at 70° of flexion that the post and cam come into play to posteriorly displace the femur. This results in a reduced lever arm of the quadriceps muscle. As a result there is an increased flexion at the hip joint and the patient leans forward to compensate for reduced quadriceps efficiency. Patients with a CR TKA are able to negotiate stairs more comfortably and do not have to stoop forward.

The retention of the PCL also helps with a greater proprioceptive input from the knee leading to better gait patterns. Reports from patients implanted with a CR knee in one knee and a PS knee in the other also indicate that they have a more normal feel in the CR knee.[29]

A lateral femoral condylar lift off[27] is seen as the knee goes into flexion from full extension. This leads to an increase in peak subchondral cancellous bone loads supporting the use of metal backed tibial components.

Asymmetric femoral condyles promote femoral roll back independent of the PCL. Because of the longer path of the lateral femoral condyle, the screw home mechanism of normal knees is replicated.[30,31]

Surgical Technique of CR TKA

The surgery is performed with the patient in a supine position. After cleaning and draping the leg, the tourniquet is inflated. The tourniquet is used in all cases except in those patients with calcified vessels or peripheral vascular disease. The knee is exposed in the flexion. A longitudinal midline skin incision is given from about 2-inches superior to the proximal pole of patella to the tibial tuberosity distally. A medial parapatellar arthrotomy is performed. It is important to open the infrapatellar bursa so that patellar retraction is made easy. Thereafter, the ACL and the lateral meniscus are excised. After excising the anterior horn of medial meniscus the plane between the proximal tibia and the deep medial collateral ligament is developed. A curved periosteum elevator, an osteotome, is slid subperiosteally in a posterior direction up to the semimembranosus bursa. This allows the proximal tibia to be delivered in front of the femur by hyperflexing and externally rotating the knee.

The distal extent of the medial soft tissue release is dictated by the severity of the deformity. In a severe varus deformity, it should be prolonged distally and all the way posteriorly so as to release the posteromedial corner of the tibia. This should correct the deformity when applying a valgus directed force on the extended knee joint. In a valgus deformity, only about 1 cm of the proximal tibial needs to

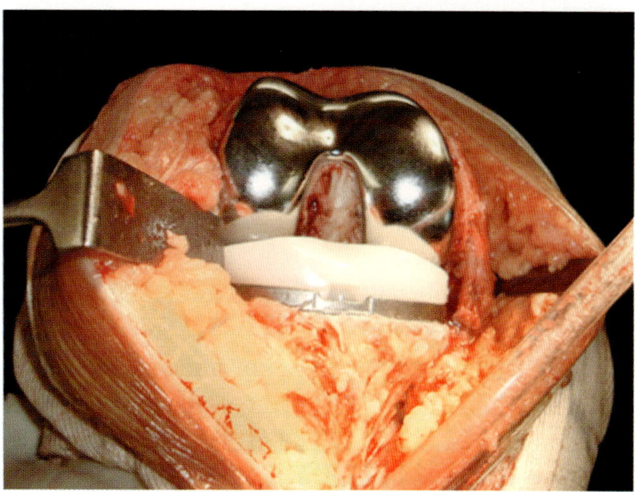

Figure 9.2 Intraoperative view of the PCL

released. Major attention is paid to an adequate lateral release. The adequacy of this valgus release is confirmed by the ability to internally rotate the tibial tuberosity past the midline.

The tibia is then cut at right angle to its axis using an extramedullary jig. We aim to remove approximately 10 mm of bone from the lesser-deformed condyle (lateral in a varus knee and medial in a valgus knee). Proximally the resection guide is centered over the medial third of the tibial tuberosity. Distally the midpoint of the bimalleolar line is taken as a reference point. Posterior tibial slope is a critical component of a CR TKA. A posterior slope of 7° is used. An attempt is made to reproduce the natural posterior slope of the tibia. It helps to open up the flexion space hence making it easier to adequately balance the PCL.

Intercondylar osteophytes are then removed with a thin curved osteotome freeing the PCL (**Figure 9.2**). The medullary canal of the femur is entered 1 cm above the origin of the PCL and a few millimeters medial to the center of the intercondylar notch. Using an intramedullary rod, the anterior surface of the femur is cut in 3° of external rotation. The amount of distal femoral resection is based on the premise that the thickness of bone and cartilage removed is equal to the thickness of the implant. The aim in a CR TKA is restoration of the joint line and avoiding a knee that is tighter in flexion than in extension. In the event of the extension space being tight, additional amount of distal femur is resected. Preoperative templating determines the valgus angle chosen for the distal resection. It is generally kept between 3° and 7°. After sizing the femur using an anterior referencing system, the femoral cuts are made. A laminar spreader is used to distract the cut surfaces of the tibial and femur to access the posterior aspect of the femoral condyles to remove osteophytes.

Once the femoral and tibial cuts are made a trial reduction is performed assessing the stability in an anteroposterior and mediolateral planes. Anteroposterior stability is checked by applying an anteriorly and posteriorly directed force on the proximal tibia in 90°, 60°, and 30° of flexion. A valgus and varus strain at the knee in extension allows the surgeon to check the mediolateral stability. A 1–2 mm jog of movement is acceptable during the stress test. The knee should come up to full extension and the patella should track centered in the femoral groove throughout the range of motion.

The next step addresses the balancing of the PCL that constitutes the most important step in a CR TKA. Scott[32] is credited with the description of the pullout lift off (POLO) test. The pullout test assesses the knee stability in flexion. In this test the knee is held in flexion, and an attempt is made to pull out the tibial component from under the femur. Scott used an insert with a posterior lip that was 3.5 mm higher than the anterior lip. If the tibial insert is easily pulled out then progressively thicker inserts are used to achieve stability in flexion. The lift off test (**Figures 9.3A and B**) then ascertains whether or not the knee is too tight in flexion. It is evidenced by lifting up of the anterior part of the insert. The tight PCL pulls the femur posteriorly on the tibia and the posterior condyles then push down upon the posterior part of the tibial insert making the anterior part to lift off. A tight PCL is often visualized and palpable. Usually the anterior and lateral fibers are tight. They are released in a sequential manner from the femur until the lift off disappears. One must make sure that the patella is not everted while assessing the lift off and all posterior osteophytes have been removed from the femur. Both of these situations are capable of eliciting a false positive lift off test.

All the bone surfaces are cleaned with a pulsatile lavage system. The surfaces are made dry and the definitive implants are cemented in place. The tibial component is placed first, followed by the insert and then the femoral component. The knee is gradually brought out to full extension to pressurize the bone-cement interface. Excess cement is removed from around the implant. Loose cement particles are an important factor leading to early polyethylene wear. A drain is then placed and the arthrotomy is closed with interrupted absorbable sutures. The skin is sutured and a compression bandage is given. The tourniquet is then released.

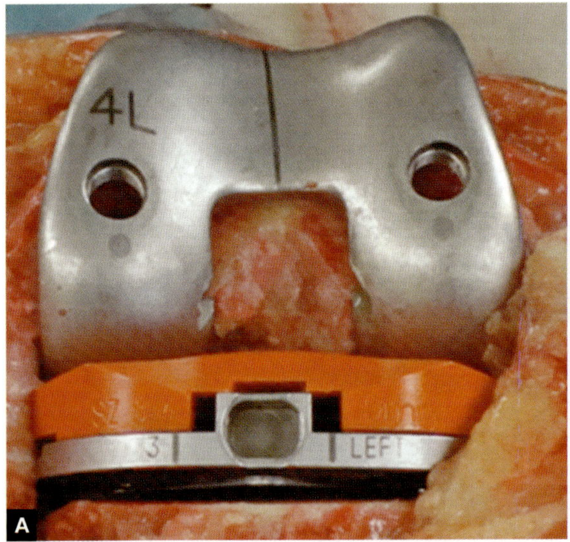

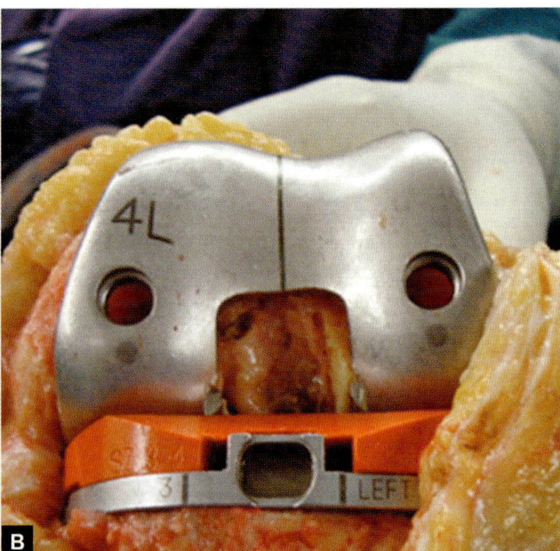

Figures 9.3A and B Tibial tray lift off

Scope of CR TKA

The PCL being a biological structure, its preservation makes sense so as to utilize its function as a primary restraint against posterior translation of the tibia. It allows for predictable femoral rollback, which in turn leads to enhanced proprioception from the replaced knee. This translates to better confidence levels while climbing stairs and other activities wherein knee flexion stability is brought into play.

Moreover, PCL retention allows for preservation of the joint line at normal levels. Resection of the PCL leads to an increased flexion space, which needs a thicker insert to achieve stability; additional distal femoral resection is needed to allow for full extension of the knee. Both of these raise the joint line distorting the collateral ligament kinematics resulting in mid-flexion laxity. The stresses borne by the ligament are directly transmitted to the bone.

In a cruciate sacrificing design, all the stress is taken up by the post of the insert, which potentially puts greater stress at the tibial component-cement interface. This may lead to premature loosening. The conforming design of the insert in PS knees potentially increases the wear rates as stresses across the metal and insert are increased. Cruciate retaining knees do well with a flat insert minimizing these stresses.

It makes sense to preserve the PCL in patients with smaller bones. The preserved bone stock helps prevent intraoperative fractures and is useful in revision situations.

The literature is awash with numerous articles citing the use and results of the CR TKA in severe varus (**Figures 9.4A and B**) and valgus deformities, ankylosed knees, and post high tibial osteotomy knees.

Scott[32], Ritter[33], Politi[34], McAuley[35] and Engh[36] have reported on excellent results by the use of cruciate retaining knee arthroplasty in case of valgus deformities. Their results are comparable to those achieved by cruciate sacrificing designs.

Rajgopal et al.[37] have reported on the presence of an intact and functional PCL in ankylosed knees. The long-term results in no way differ from the studies that used the cruciate sacrificing design.

Post high tibial osteotomy knees (**Figures 9.5A to D**) present with its peculiar problems of increased tibial slope, retained hardware, bone defects, and scarred soft tissues. Adhering to meticulous soft tissue detail and properly balancing the PCL gives good results in the long-term.[38,39]

The CR TKA also affords the surgeon the choice of cementless options (**Figures 9.6A to F**).

Results of CR TKA

Early cruciate retaining knees had encouraging results in the short-term but with time their longevity was brought into question because of design constraints. These initial

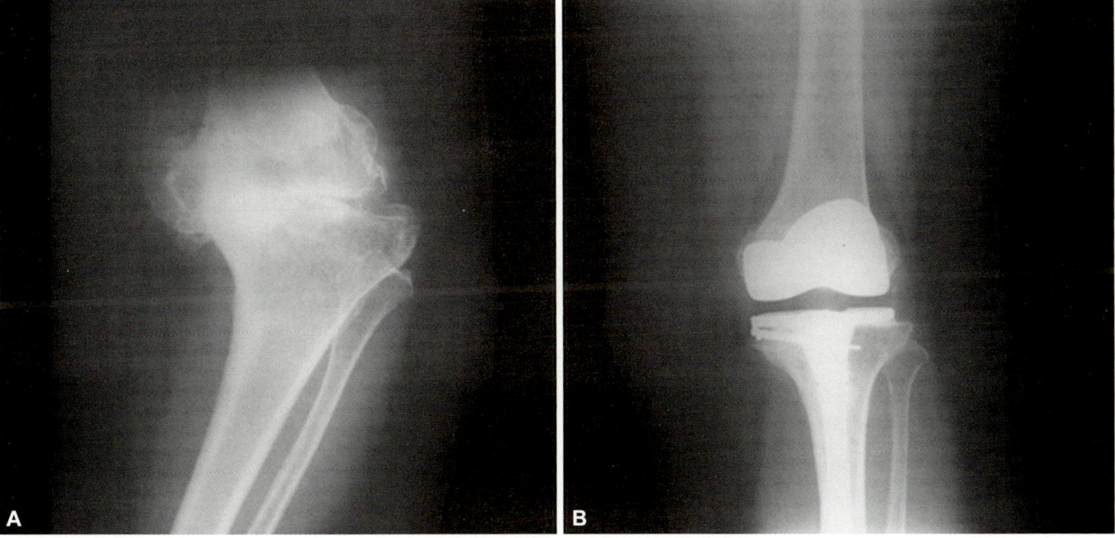

Figures 9.4A and B Ten-year follow-up of X-ray of CR TKA for severe varus deformity

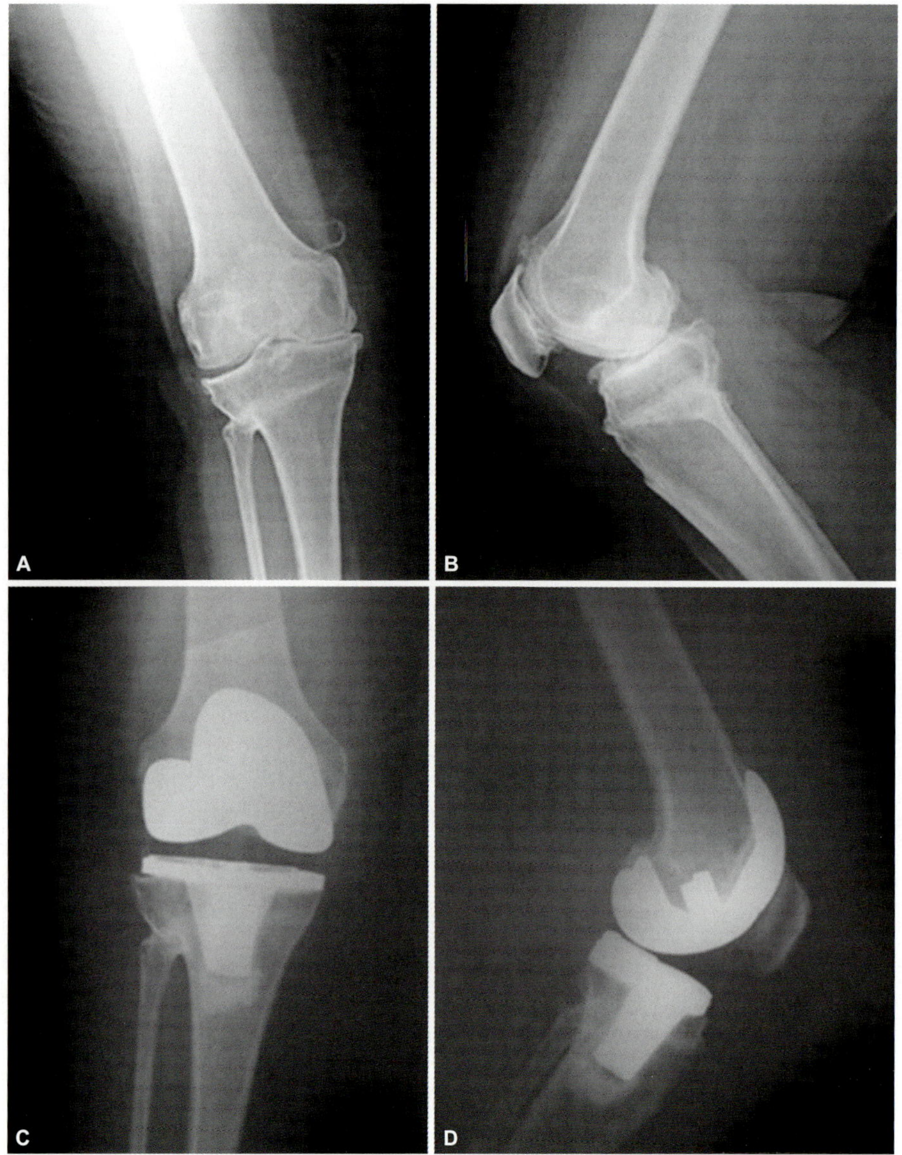

Figures 9.5A to D CR TKA after high tibial osteotomy

attempts to replicate normal knee kinematics were the precursors of modern day implants and aided the design refinements we observe today.

Early results of the polycentric knee[40] were promising wherein the patients had excellent pain relief and the average range of motion was greater than 90°. Lewallen et al.[41] in 1984 reported on the 10 years results and found that the probability of having a functional polycentric TKA was only 66%. This was calculated based on the Kaplan-Meir survival curve. Malalignment leading to ligamentous instability (13%) was the most common mode of failure. Loosening of the tibial component (7%) and deep infection (3%) were the other modes of failure. Out of the 209 knees studied 74 knees (34%) failed and required revision surgery.

The geometric knee developed by Coventry[42-44] aimed to better the results of TKA by avoiding the deficiencies of the hinge prostheses and provide increased stability when compared with the polycentric knee. It was a partially constrained implant with a single axis of rotation and preserved the cruciate ligaments. Skolnick et al.[45] reported that at two years of follow-up 93% of the patients were

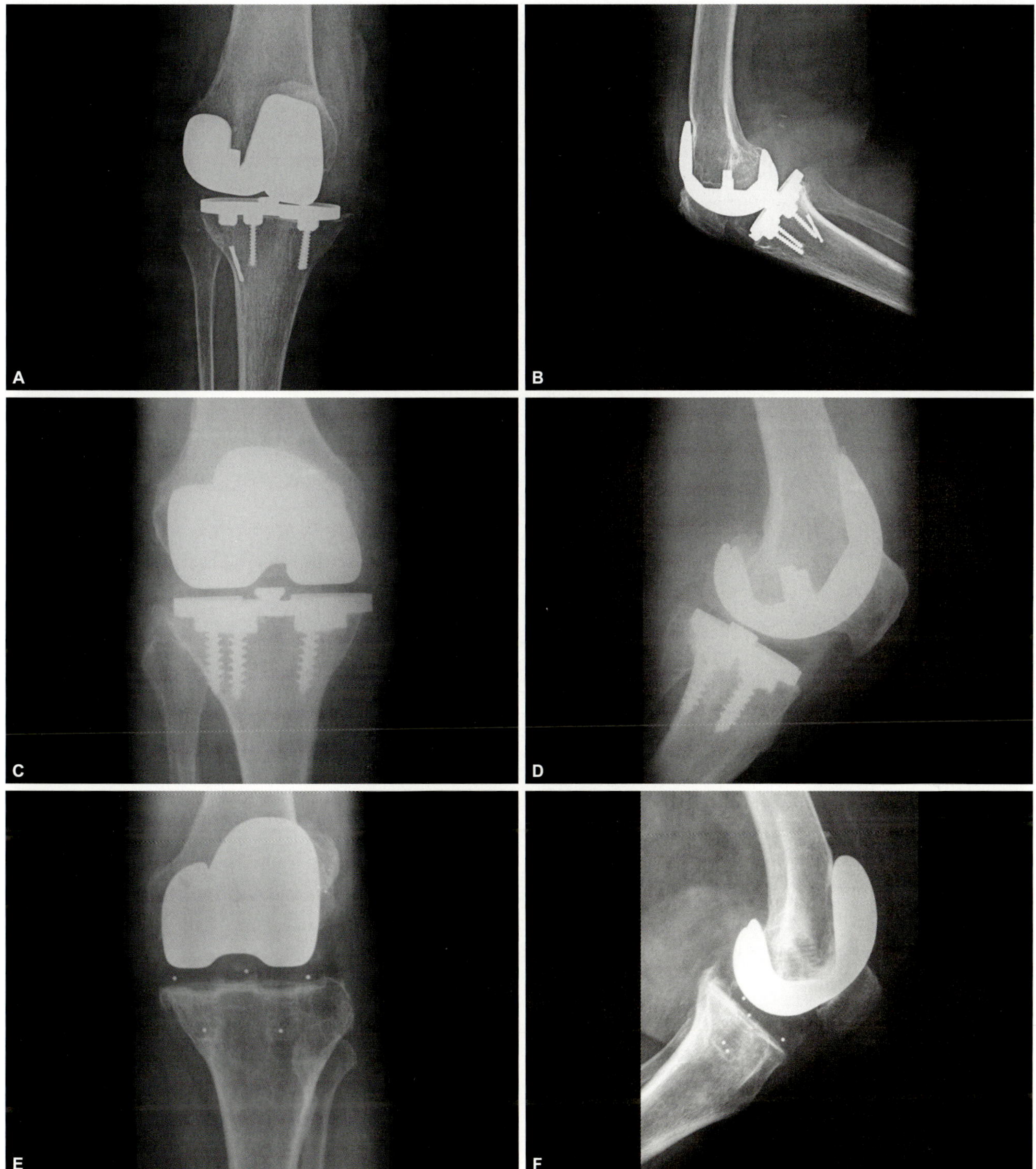

Figures 9.6A to F (A to D) Cementless "CR TKA" (E and F) Cementless "CR TKA"—27 years follow-up

satisfied with their knees. There were no cases of instability in contrast to the polycentric knee. Rand and Coventry[46] reported the results of 193 knees followed for an average of 10.8 years (minimum 8 years). Using revision surgery and pain as the endpoint the survival was calculated to be 69% at 10 years.

Seventy-five percent of the duocondylar knees[13,14] showed good or excellent results at a three-year follow-up. 9.3% of the knees showed evidence of instability and 5.3% had loosening. Patellofemoral pain was noted to be the most common cause of discomfort to the patients. An anterior patellar flange was added on the femur to result in the duopatellar knee. Scott[15] in 1982 reported on the two-year follow-up results of 100 duopatellar knees and found that 95% of the patients had excellent pain relief. The average range of motion was 106°. Two reoperations were necessary for patellar resurfacing. There was no incidence of tibial loosening.

The posterior cruciate condylar knee had a central posterior cruciate cut out section that allowed preservation of the PCL. The design aimed to provide better stability in activities requiring stability in flexion. Ritter[47] et al. in their study at five years follow-up reported 96.8% excellent or good results. The average postoperative range of motion was 101°. Only one knee out of the 94 studied had tibial loosening. At nine years follow-up study, there were 94.5% good or excellent results.[48] Using revision as an end point the estimated survivorship at 10 years was 95%. These studies revealed that with cruciate retaining knees excellent range of motion can be achieved and the deformity can be completely corrected. Ritter opined that changing the tibial insert to a flatter profile would help in better kinematics of this knee.

A flat polyethylene insert in the sagittal plane, metal backed short stemmed tibial component, and valgus alignment of the patellar groove were the design hallmarks of the kinematic total knee. Ewald[16] in a short-term study (2.25 years) reported 90% excellent or good results. The average range of motion was 106°. Two knees (1.6%) were revised on account of patellar dislocation and tibial component loosening. At 6 years, the range of motion improved to 109° and 88% of the patients had good or excellent results. Radiolucent lines were present in 40% of tibial, 30% of the femoral and 60% of the patellar components. At 10 years follow-up, Malkani[49] reported a mean range of motion of 105°. Complications were loosening of the patellar component in four knees, loosening of the femoral, and tibial component in two knees, supracondylar fracture in one, and deep infection in one knee. Using revision as an endpoint the survival was 96% at 10 years.

Townley[17] and Cloutier[18] implants were similar in the sense that both had a 'U' shaped tibial component to allow for preservation of both the cruciate ligaments. Early results of the Townley prosthesis were good to excellent in 89% of the knees. In a study of 360 knees that were evaluated for a mean follow-up of 8 years, 29 knees were revised (18 for loosening, 6 for instability and 5 for deep infection). A survivorship of 89% at 10 years was predicted. The Cloutier[50,51] knee showed good to excellent results in 79% of the knees when evaluated at 10 years postoperatively.

The Miller-Galante total knee was the first knee to be available in cemented and uncemented variants. Modularity of the components was the highlight of this design. Early results by Rosenberg[52] and Rorabeck[53] showed 90% of good to excellent results.

Schai and Scott[54] in 1999 published a study evaluating the long-term (11 years, range 10–13) results of TKA in patients with rheumatoid arthritis. The knee society scores averaged 95 points and the average postoperative flexion was 112°. There were no instances of symptomatic instability. Two knees were revised, one on account of patellar component loosening (metal backed) and the second for recurrent synovitis. Thirteen years survivorship based on need for revision surgery was 97%. Archibeck and Berger[55] found a 93% survival rate at 10.5 years (range 8 to 14 years) in rheumatoid patients. Seventy-two knees in 51 patients were studied prospectively. Six knees were revised on account of failure of metal backed patellar components. There was no incidence of aseptic loosening. Posterior instability was identified in 2 knees (2.8%).

Sextro, Berry, and Rand[56] from the Mayo clinic reported on the 15 years study of the kinematic I condylar prosthesis. Survivorship, taking revision as an end point, was 88.7%. Ritter[57] et al. evaluated the AGC knee at 15 years and found a survival rate of 98.86%.

Dixon and Scott[58] reported a 92.6% survival rate at 15 years using revision as an end point. The mean knee society and functional scores were 96 and 78 points respectively.

Rand et al.[59] evaluated the factors that influence the durability of primary total knee prosthesis. They carried out a survivorship analysis of 11,606 primary total knee arthroplasties carried out between 1 January 1978 and 31 December 2000. Prosthetic survivorship at 10 years was 91% for cruciate retaining implants and 76% for those with cruciate substitution. They concluded that for a woman above 70 years of age with inflammatory arthritis the ideal implant would be of a cruciate retaining design, cemented and with an all-polyethylene patellar component. The estimated 10-year survivorship was calculated to be 98%. Watanabe[60] reported on the excellent results with the uncemented CR TKA. Watanabe reported that the survivorship of uncemented cruciate retaining implants at the 10th year was 100% and at the 13th year was 96.7%.

Rodricks et al.[61] presented the 14–15 years survivorship of the PFC cruciate retaining knee. The 97.2% of the knees survived at this period using aseptic loosening as the end point.

Kubiak et al.[62] evaluated the 10-year results of CR knees in severe deformity (at least 15° in coronal plane). A 93% revision free survivorship was found. None of the knees demonstrated any instability or loosening.

PERSONAL EXPERIENCE

The senior author is a strong advocate of retaining the PCL in the TKA. The PCL is present in most cases needing knee replacements. It is our belief that the PCL retaining implants can be used to treat the vast majority of knees even those with severe deformities. Attention to detail in terms of appropriate soft tissue releases can ensure appropriate correction of deformities in most of the cases. Carefully removing posterior femoral condylar osteophytes and clearing the intercondylar area helps to balance the PCL. Posterior soft tissue clearance is critical to achieve good stability and facilitate good rollback. The PCL may need to be fractionally lengthened at its femoral attachment in cases where it is tight. Our experience with the conversion of ankylosed knees has shown that even in these knees a functional PCL is present. Knees with a severe varus deformity (greater than 20°), valgus deformity or post-high tibial osteotomy are amenable to a good correction. Evaluation of the long-term results of TKA in these severely deformed knees has shown a negligible incidence of late onset instability.

A number of CR TKA that need revision due to polyethylene wear 12 to 14 years after their surgery also demonstrate a viable PCL intraoperatively. Use of a cruciate retaining implant in these cases during revision surgery has given us excellent results.

CONCLUSION

The CR TKA is a technically demanding surgery wherein proper balancing of the deformity and the ligaments are essential to achieve a well-balanced knee that will perform well in the long term. The long-term results are similar for CR and cruciate substituting knees. The future will help quantify the degree of comfort the patient has with a CR knee and improved understanding of the kinematics may well lay the controversy of CR versus cruciate substituting knees to rest. Arthroplasty surgeons of the future will continue to carry forward the improvements in surgical techniques and stretch the indications for a CR knee.

REFERENCES

1. Andriacchi TP, Galante JO. Retention of the posterior cruciate in total knee arthroplasty. J Arthrop. 1998;3.
2. Freeman MA, Railton GT. Should the posterior cruciate ligament be retained or resected in condylar nonmeniscal knee arthroplasty: the case for resection. J Arthrop. 1988;3:83.
3. Gunston FH. Polycentric knee arthroplasty: prosthetic stimulation of normal knee movement. J Bone Joint Surg Br. 1971;53:272.
4. Scott RD, Volatile TB. Twelve years' experience with posterior cruciate retaining total knee arthroplasty. Clin Orthop. 1986;205:100.
5. Andriacchi TP, Galante JO, Fermier RW. The influence of total knee replacement design on walking and stair climbing. J Bone Joint Surg Am. 1982;64:1328.
6. Kelman GJ, Biden EN, Wyatt MP, Ritter MA, Colwell CW Jr. Gait laboratory analysis of a posterior cruciate-sparing total

knee arthroplasty in stair ascent and descent. Clin Orthop. 1989;248:21.

7. Swanik CB, Lephart SM, Rubash HE. Proprioception, kinesthesia, and balance after total knee arthroplasty with cruciate retaining and posterior stabilized prostheses. J Bone Joint Surg Am. 2004;86(2):328-34.
8. Simmon S, Lephart SM, Rubash HE, Pifer GW, Barrack R. Proprioception after unicondylar knee arthroplasty versus total knee arthroplasty. Clin Orthop. 1996;331:179.
9. Warren PJ, Olanlokun TK, Cobb AG, Bentley G. Proprioception after total knee arthroplasty: the influence of prosthetic design. Clin Orthop. 1993;297:182.
10. Cash RM, Gonzales MH, Garst J, Barmada R, Stern SH. Proprioception after arthroplasty: role of the posterior cruciate ligament. Clin Orthop Rel. 1996;331:172.
11. Conditt MA, Noble PC, Bertolusso R, Woody J, Parsley BS. The PCL significantly affects the functional outcome of total knee arthroplasty. J Arthrop. 2004;19:107.
12. Leslie Klenerman. The Evolution of Orthopedic Surgery. Chapter 3: RSM Press, London; 2002.
13. Ranawat CS, Shine JJ. Duocondylar total knee arthroplasty. Clin Ortop. 1973;94:185.
14. Ewald FC, et al. Duopatellar total knee arthroplasty in rheumatoid arthritis. Orthop Trans. 1978;2:202.
15. Scott RD. Duopatellar total knee replacement: the Brigham experience. Orthop Clin North Am. 1982;13:89.
16. Ewald FC, Jacobs MA, Miegel RE, et al. Kinematic total knee replacement. J Bone Joint Surg Am. 1984;66:1032.
17. Townley CO. The anatomic total knee resurfacing arthroplasty. Clin Orthop. 1985;192:82.
18. Cloutier JM. Results of total knee arthroplasty with a nonconstrained prosthesis. J Bone Joint Surg Am. 1983;65:906.
19. Landon GC, Galante JO, Maley MM. Noncemented total knee arthroplasty. Orthop Clin North Am. 1986; 205:49.
20. Covey DC, Sapega AA. Anatomy and function of the posterior cruciate ligament. Clin Sports Med. 1994;13(3): 509-18.
21. Gray's anatomy 36th edition.
22. Campbell's Operative Orthopedics. 11th edition. Elsevier, United States.
23. Fu FH, Harner DC, Johnson DL, Miller MD, Woo SL. Biomechanics of knee ligaments. Instructional course lecture. J Bone Joint Surg Am. 1993;75:11.
24. Elias SG, Freeman MA, Gokcay EI. A correlative study of the geometry and anatomy of the distal femur. Clin Orthop. 1990;260:98.
25. Kapandji IA. The Physiology of the Joints: The lower Limb, Vol. 2. London: Churchill Livingstone; 1970.p.120.
26. Most E, Zayontz S, Li G, et al. Femoral rollback after cruciate-retaining and stabilizing total knee arthroplasty. Clin Orthop. 2003;410:101-13.
27. Komistek RD, Denis DA. Fluoroscopic analysis of total knee replacement. Surgery of the Knee. 3rd edn. Vol 2. Chap 78. London: Churchill Livingstone.
28. Kim YH, Choi Y, Kwon OR, Kim JS. Functional outcome and range of motion of high-flexion posterior cruciate-retaining and high-flexion cruciate-substituting total knee prosthesis. J Bone Joint Surg Am. 2009;91:753.
29. Cates HE, Komistek RD, Mahfouz MR, Schmidt MA, Anderle M. *In vivo* comparison of knee kinematics for subjects having either a posterior stabilized or cruciate retaining high-flexion total knee arthroplasty. J Arthrop. 2008;23(7):1057.
30. Komistek RD, Mahfouz MR, Bertin KC, Rosenberg A, Kennedy W. *In vivo* determination of total knee arthroplasty kinematics—a multicentre analysis of an asymmetrical posterior cruciate retaining total knee arthroplasty. J Arthrop. 2008;23(1):41.
31. Bertin KC, Komistek RD, Denis DA, et al. *In vivo* determination of posterior femoral rollback for subjects having a Nexgen posterior cruciate retaining total knee arthroplasty. J Arthrop. 2002;17(8):1040.
32. Scott RD, Chmell MJ. Balancing the posterior cruciate ligament during cruciate-retaining fixed and mobile bearing total knee arthroplasty: description of the pull-out lift-off and slide-back tests. J Arthrop. 2008;4:605-8.
33. Ritter MA, Faris GW, Faris PM, Davis KE. Total knee arthroplasty in patients with angular varus or valgus deformities of > or = 20 degrees. J Arthrop. 2004;19(7):862-6.
34. Politi J, Scott R. Balancing severe valgus deformity in total knee arthroplasty using a lateral cruciform retinacular release. J Arthrop. 2004;19(5):553-7.

35. McAuley JP, Collier MB, Hamilton WG, Tabaraee E, Engh GA. Posterior cruciate retaining arthroplasty for valgus osteoarthritis. Clin Orthop Relat Res. 2008;466:2644-9.
36. Engh GA. The difficult knee: severe varus and valgus. Clin Orthop Relat Res. 2003;416:58-63.
37. Rajgopal A, Ahuja N, Dolai B. Total knee arthroplasty in stiff and ankylosed knees. J Arthrop. 2005;20(5):585-90.
38. Meding JB, Keating EM, Ritter MA, Faris PM. Total knee arthroplasty after failed high tibial osteotomy. J Bone Joint Surg Am. 2000;82:1252.
39. Staeheli JW, Cass JR, Morrey BF. Condylar total knee arthroplasty after failed proximal tibial osteotomy. J Bone Joint Surg Am. 1987;69:28.
40. Ilstrup DM, Combs JJ Jr, Bryan RS, Peterson LF, Skolnick MD. A statistical evaluation of polycentric total knee arthroplasties. Clin Orthop. 1976;120:18.
41. Lewallen DG, Bryan RS, Peterson LF. Polycentric total knee arthroplasty: a ten-year follow-up study. J Bone Joint Surg Am. 1984;66:1211.
42. Coventry MB, Upshaw JE, Riley LH, Finerman JA, Turner RH. Geometric total knee arthroplasty. I. Conception, design, indications and surgical technique. Clin Orthop. 1973;94:171.
43. Coventry MB, Upshaw JE, Riley LH, Finerman JA, Turner RH. Geometric total knee arthroplasty. II. Patient data and complications. Clin Orthop. 1973;94:171.
44. Ilstrup DM, Coventry MB, Skolnick MD. A statistical evaluation of Geometric total knee arthroplasties. Clin Orthop. 1976;120:37.
45. Skolnick MD, Coventry MB, Ilstrup DM. Geometric total knee arthroplasty: a two-year follow-up study. J Bone Joint Surg Am. 1976;58:749.
46. Rand JA, Coventry MB. Ten year evaluation of geometric total knee arthroplasty. Clin Orthop. 1988;232:168.
47. Ritter MA, Campbell E, Faris PM, Keating EM. Long-term survival analysis of the posterior cruciate condylar total knee arthroplasty: a 10-year evaluation. J Arthrop. 1989;4:293.
48. Lee JG, Keating EM, Ritter MA, Faris PM. Review of the all polyethylene tibial component in total knee arthroplasty. Clin Orthop. 1990;260:87.
49. Malkani AL, Rand JA, Bryan RS, Wallrichs SL. Total knee arthroplasty with the kinematic condylar prosthesis. A ten-year follow-up study. J Bone Joint Surg Am. 1995;77:423.
50. Cloutier JM. Long term results after nonconstrained total knee arthroplasty. Clin Orthop. 1991;273:63.
51. Cloutier JM. Long term results of total knee arthroplasty with retention of both cruciate ligaments. J Bone Joint Surg. 1998.
52. Rosenberg AG, Barden R, Galante JO. A comparison of cemented and cementless fixation with the Miller-Galante total knee arthroplasty. Orthop Clin North Am. 1989;20:97.
53. Rorabeck CH, Bourne RB, Lewis PL, Nott L. The Miller-Galante knee prosthesis for the treatment of osteoarthrosis. J Bone Joint Surg Am. 1993;75:402.
54. Schai PA, Thornhill TS, Scott RD. Total knee arthroplasty with the PFC system: results at a minimum of 10 years and survivorship analysis. J Bone Joint Surg Br. 1998;80: 850.
55. Archibeck MJ, Berger RA, Barden RM, et al. Posterior cruciate ligament retaining total knee arthroplasty in patients with rheumatoid arthritis. J Bone Joint Surg Am. 2001;83:1231.
56. Sextro GS, Berry DJ, Rand JA. Total knee arthroplasty using cruciate retaining Kinematic condylar prosthesis. Clin Orthop Relat Res. 2001;388:33-40.
57. Ritter MA, Berend ME, Meding JB, et al. Long-term follow-up of anatomic graduated components posterior cruciate retaining total knee replacement. Clin Orthop Relat Res. 2001;388:51-7.
58. Dixon MC, Brown RR, Parsch D, Scott RD. Modular fixed-bearing total knee arthroplasty with retention of the posterior cruciate ligament. J Bone Joint Surg Am. 2005;87:598.
59. Rand JA, Trousdale RT, Ilstrup DM, Harmsen WS. Factors affecting the durability of primary total knee prosthesis. J Bone Joint Surg Am. 2003;85(2):259-65.
60. Watanabe H, Akizulki S, Takizawa T. Survival analysis of a cementless, cruciate retaining total knee arthroplasty: clinical and radiographic assessment 10 to 13 years after surgery. J Bone Joint Surg Br. 2004;86(6):824-9.
61. Rodricks DJ, Patil S, Pulido P, Colwell CW Jr. Press-fit condylar design total knee arthroplasty: fourteen to seventeen year follow-up. J Bone Joint Surg Am. 2007; 89(1):89-95.
62. Kubiak P, Archibeck MJ, White RE Jr. Cruciate retaining total knee arthroplasty in patients with at least fifteen degrees of coronal plane deformity. J Arthrop. 2008;23(3):366-70.

Chapter 10

Posterior Cruciate Substituting Total Knee Arthroplasty

Giles R Scuderi, Ajit J Deshmukh, Joseph W Greene

INTRODUCTION

Total knee arthroplasty (TKA) has been one of the most successful orthopedic procedures over the last few decades. Excellent long-term results have been reported with multiple implant designs including cruciate retaining (CR), cruciate sacrificing and cruciate substituting prosthesis. Advocates of posterior CR TKA argue that it maintains proprioception, allows for joint line restoration, better knee kinematics, more normal stair climbing and gait pattern and better anteroposterior stability. However, advocates of posterior cruciate ligament (PCL) substituting designs (PS) have reported improved and reproducible results with PS implants, especially in cases with severe deformity and prior patellectomy. With consistent femoral rollback and axial rotation, improvement in postoperative knee range of motion (ROM) has been documented in several randomized controlled trials with the use of the PCL substituting TKA design.[1,2] In addition, when implanted with appropriate gap-balancing, the occurrence of flexion instability is less frequent with a PS TKA when compared to the CR designs.[3-7]

HISTORICAL PERSPECTIVE AND DESIGN FEATURES

The evolution of the PS TKA began with the total condylar prosthesis (TCP) that was introduced in 1974. This was a PCL sacrificing tricompartmental prosthesis and stability was achieved by soft tissue balance in extension and flexion as well as a relatively conforming tibiofemoral articulation.[8] In 1978, the TCP was modified to the Insall-Burstein (IB-I) posterior stabilized prosthesis, which included a tibial spine and femoral cam to function as a mechanical PCL. The original tibial component was all polyethylene, and metal backing was later introduced in 1981. Further modifications to the design in 1987 resulted in the modular IB-II prosthesis. The IB-I was the first PS TKA prosthesis and served as the predicate implant from which most present-day PS designs are derived (**Figure 10.1**). In the following paragraphs, we will discuss the salient characteristics of the PCL substituting the TKA and the rationale for its use.

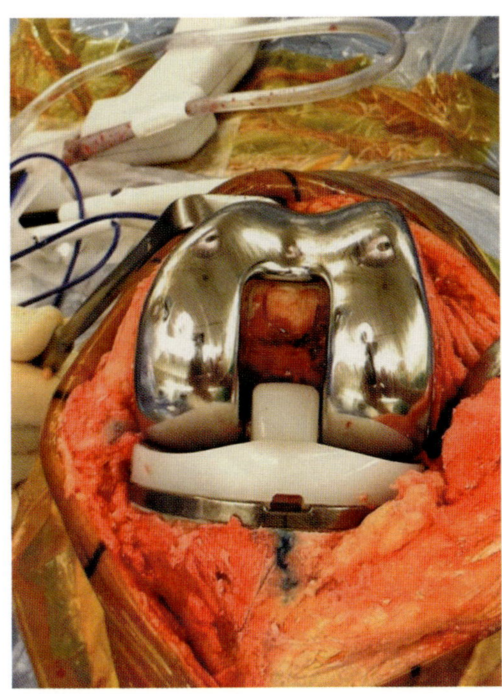

Figure 10.1 Fixed-bearing posterior stabilized knee prosthesis

In Vivo Kinematics

One of the primary goals of TKA is to restore painless ROM, which is a complex activity with flexion, rotation, and rollback. Overall, the restoration of knee kinematics has been more predictable with the PS TKA.[9,10] The tibial postarticulating with the femoral cam allows for femoral rollback while maintaining flexion stability. In a recent randomized trial using intraoperative computer navigation, femoral rollback was noted in both CR and PS knee designs, however, the femoral rollback significantly increased following surgery in the PS group.[11] Udomkiat et al. demonstrated by fluoroscopy that the anteroposterior femorotibial translation of PS TKA during gait and deep knee flexion was more similar to the native knee.[12] Furthermore, when compared to the CR and PCL sacrificing knee designs, more femoral rollback and better extensor mechanism efficiency has been reported with PS TKA.[13] In this study, Mahoney noted that both CR and PS TKA did not truly replicate knee kinematics compared to a normal knee but the PS TKA had a better femoral rollback and better quadriceps efficiency compared to a CR design.[13] Consequently, no significant difference could be found when spatiotemporal gait parameters, isokinetic muscle strength, and stair climbing ROM were compared between normal native knees and PS TKA.[14]

Proprioception

It has been suggested that PCL retention would improve proprioception following the TKA. However, it is possible that the degree of arthritis in the joint would actually determine proprioception as marked neurologic degeneration occurs in the PCL as part of the arthritic process.[15] It is not clear from the published literature which implant design has better postoperative proprioception. Warren et al. reported that proprioception improved after the TKA with either design but greater improvement occurred in CR knees.[16] Contrary to this, Simmons et al. noted that in patients with severe arthritis, proprioception was better with the PS TKA.[17] In another study, patients with the bilateral paired CR and PS TKA were compared and the authors found that 50% were unable to express a preference for either knee design. The remaining 50% had an equal preference for the two designs.[18] Lastly, Swanik et al., in a prospective randomized study comparing the CR and PS TKA reported that PS TKA reproduced joint position more accurately when the knee was extended from a flexed position and concluded that there is no proprioception and balance benefit with the CR knees.[19]

Range of Motion

The range of motion (ROM) is an important outcome variable and has a significant impact on the subjective outcome of the TKA.[20] Chaudhary et al., in a level 1 study, reported no statistically significant difference in the ROM between the CR and PS knees.[21] Similar results between the CR and PS TKA have been reported with the use of a so-called high-flex design.[22] However, in a recent meta-analysis comparing the CR and PS TKA, Bercik et al. found a statistically significant difference in flexion and the ROM favoring of PS TKA.[23] In another meta-analysis, postoperative ROM for PS TKA was 11.1° higher than for CR TKA.[24] Jacobs et al. analyzed eight randomized controlled trials and found that the ROM was 8° greater (105° versus 113°) in the PS TKA.[25] This difference may be due to the different pattern of gap kinematics between

TABLE 10.1 ROM data on the PS knees

Study and publication year	Prosthesis	Preoperative maximum passive flexion (degrees)	Postoperative maximum passive flexion (degrees)
Huang et al. 2005[56]	HF PS fixed	112.0	126.0
Kim et al. 2005[57]	HF PS fixed	126.0	136.0
Kim et al. 2008[58]	HF PS fixed	117.3	135.0
Ng et al. 2008[59]	HF PS fixed	104.0	106.0
Nutton et al. 2008[60]	HF PS fixed	119.0	127.0
McCalden et al. 2010[61]	HF PS fixed Std PS fixed	109.4 109.9	119.6 116.7
Tanavalee et al. 2011[62]	HF PS fixed	137.9	134.8
Scuderi et al. 2012[63]	HF PS fixed HF PS mobile	114.8 114.7	127.7 127.4
Meftah et al. 2012[55]	Std PS fixed all poly	113.1	115.0
Meftah et al. 2012[52]	Std PS mobile	111.2	119.0

Abbreviations: HF, high flex knee; Std, standard knee (not high flex); PS, posterior stabilized knee; fixed, fixed-bearing; mobile; mobile-bearing

the two designs.[26,27] Another reason could be the failure to appropriately balance the PCL in the CR TKA resulting in a tight PCL and resultant flexion gap tightness and therefore poorer flexion.[28] The ROM data on the PS knees has been summarized in **Table 10.1**.

Clinical Function

Kim et al. and Lozano-Calderon et al. prospectively compared functional outcomes of CR and PS TKA and reported no difference in pain, the ROM and function between the two designs.[22,29] Multiple clinical studies have demonstrated equivalent outcome measures when the CR and PS TKA were compared.[24] In another recent meta-analysis, no clinical differences were reported between the PS and CR TKA, despite better ROM in the PS group.[30] Hence, PCL retention did not appear to enhance clinical function after TKA.

Wear

Polyethylene insert wear was the leading etiology necessitating revision surgery about a decade ago.[31] With improvements in the quality of polyethylene, wear related complications seem to be on the decline. The PS knees utilize more conforming polyethylene articulation that helps maximize the contact area and decreases stresses on the polyethylene. This helps minimize wear, therefore improving implant longevity. A mobile-bearing prosthesis (**Figure 10.2**) was introduced to help minimize tibial polyethylene wear, osteolysis and aseptic loosening.[32] However, these purported advantages have not been proven.[33-35] Colizza et al. observed no evidence of marked polyethylene wear in a consecutive series of 165 PS knees at 10–14 year follow-up.[36] In contrast, the CR knees with less conforming articulation may be subjected to more wear of the polyethylene insert.[37,38] Additionally, if the PCL

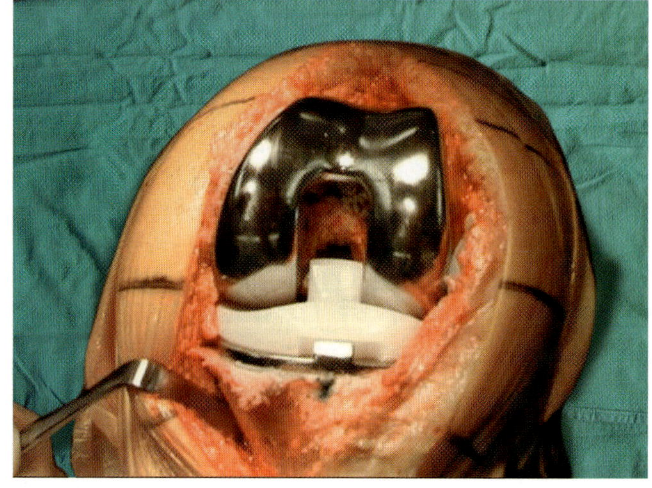

Figure 10.2 Mobile-bearing posterior stabilized knee prosthesis

is left too tight, asymmetric posterior polyethylene wear may occur. In PS TKA, the tibial-post and femoral cam can be another source of polyethylene wear.[39] However, the cam-post mechanism is variable amongst different manufacturers in terms of postlocation and geometry, leading to differences in the wear pattern.[39,40] Incidental cases of postfracture have also been documented. With the introduction of highly cross-linked polyethylene in the TKA, better wear, fatigue strength and tibial postdurability compared to conventional polyethylene have been reported in the laboratory.[41,42] In a prospective randomized trial, based on synovial fluid analysis, the reduction in wear of highly cross-linked polyethylene *in vivo* was not statistically significant compared to conventional polyethylene.[43] Long et al. studied 108 PS TKAs with highly cross-linked polyethylene at a mean follow-up of 52 months and reported excellent clinical and radiographic results.[44] However, further well-powered long-term studies are needed to determine long-term durability and mechanical properties of this material.

Surgical Exposure and Deformity Correction

Excision of the tight, contracted PCL during surgery not only makes tibial exposure and visualization easier, but also allows deformity correction and ligamentous balancing to be performed in a reproducible manner.[45,46] It also eliminates reliance on the abnormal PCL morphology for kinematic function. Ritter et al. recommended partial release of the PCL when using a CR knee in a knee with fixed angular deformity.[47] When the preoperative varus deformity was more than 15°, Laskin et al. reported more pain, less ROM, more radiolucencies and lower survivorship for the CR knees compared to PS knees.[48]

Stability

Biomechanical studies have reported that it is difficult to restore the normal strain pattern in the PCL after CR TKA, therefore over tightening is frequent, leading either to reduced flexion or postoperative PCL rupture.[13] The PCL can also become incompetent due to excessive proximal tibial resection, postoperative trauma or progression of inflammatory disease process. The PCL rupture may lead to flexion instability in the CR knees, resulting in pain and patient dissatisfaction. Pagnano et al. reported on the 25 CR knees with flexion instability and found the PCL to be grossly incompetent in all knees, requiring revision to the PS TKA with an appropriate balance in flexion and extension.[4] In a recent study utilizing intraoperative computer navigation to compare CR and PS knees, condylar lift-off was observed with CR implants between 20° and 60° of flexion, which was absent with PS knees.[11]

Bone Loss

Resection of additional bone (box cut) to accommodate the femoral cam- and tibial-post mechanism is needed in the PS TKA. Although this may be considered a potential disadvantage, no studies have found it to compromise the results of TKA. In fact, stress shielding has been shown to occur beneath the anterior flange of both the CR and PS knees.[49] This means that the bone in the notch region of the CR knees is of poor quality and a PS TKA is always used at the time of revision, thereby making the bone loss from the intercondylar notch inconsequential.

Aseptic Loosening and Implant Survivorship

Despite the constraint offered by the presence of cam and post in PS TKA, there appears to be no difference in the long-term risk of aseptic loosening compared with CR knees.[50] Survivorship at 10 and 16.4 years using revision for aseptic loosening as end-point has been 97.7% and 94.8% respectively.[50] Another study reported 98.4% survival rate of PS TKA at 14 years.[36] Rasquinha et al. reported 98.3% survival rate at 12 years for mechanical failure as an end-point and 94.6% survival rate for failure for any reason as an end-point.[51] Similarly, Meftah et al. reported on 106 PS mobile-bearing knees with a mean 10-year follow-up. There were no cases of aseptic loosening or osteolysis with a survival rate of 100% with revision due to mechanical failure as the end point, 97.7% with revision for any reason as the end-point and 95% with any reoperation as the end-point.[52] In a 30-year follow-up of the PS TKA, 82.7% survival for revision for aseptic loosening was documented.[53] The survivorship of PS TKA has been summarized in **Table 10.2**.

TABLE 10.2 Survivorship of posterior stabilized implants

Investigator and publication year	*PS prosthesis design*	*Survivorship % with mechanical failure as end-point*
Scuderi et al. 1989[63]	IB all poly tibia	97.3 at 10 years
Scuderi et al. 1989[63]	IB metal backed tibia	98.7 at 10 years
Stern et al. 1992[64]	IB all poly tibia	94 at 13 years
Colizza et al. 1995[36]	IB metal backed tibia	96.4 at 11 years
Font-Rodriguez et al. 1996[65]	IB all poly tibia	94 at 16 years
Font-Rodriguez et al. 1996[65]	IB metal backed tibia	98 at 14 years
Emmerson et al. 1996[66]	Kinematic stabilizer	95 at 10 years
Diduch et al. 1997[54]	IB all poly/ metal backed	94 at 18 years
Ranawat et al. 1997[67]	PFC modular PS	97 at 6 years
Rasquinha et al. 2006[51]	PFC modular PS	98.3 at 12 years
Meftah et al. 2012[55]	PFC/Sigma all poly tibia	97.7 at 12.4 years
Meftah et al. 2012[52]	PFC rotating platform	100 at 10 years
Wing et al. 2012[50]	IB-II	94.8 at 16.4 years
Bryce et al. (unpublished data)[53]	IB-I and II metal backed	82.7 at 30 years

Abbreviations: IB, Insall-Burstein posterior stabilized knee; PFC, press-fit condylar posterior stabilized knee

The Young and Active Patient

Several studies have reported that PS TKA in the young and active patient is a durable option. Diduch et al. reported 87% survival at 18 years in patients who were less than 55 years of age.[54] Meftah et al. reported on 44 all poly cemented PS TKA's implanted in 32 patients with a mean age of 56.1 years. At a mean follow-up of 12.4 years (range: 10–18 years), 96% knees had good to excellent results. 62% patients were still participating in sporting activities like running, gym exercises, tennis and golf. No cases of aseptic loosening, poly-wear or osteolysis were observed. Survivorship at 10 years due to mechanical failure was 97.7% and for all failures was 95.5%.[55] In a recent study performed at our center, 30-year survivorship (**Figures 10.3A and B**) of 114 knees implanted in patients 55 years or younger, with revision for aseptic loosening as the end-point, was 82.7%.[53] To our knowledge, this is the longest follow-up of the PS TKA ever reported in literature and demonstrates the durability of the PS TKA in this young and active patient population.

CONCLUSION

On the basis of the aforementioned advantages of the PS TKA, it is our belief that it is the prosthesis of choice for primary and the TKA. Potential benefits over the CR

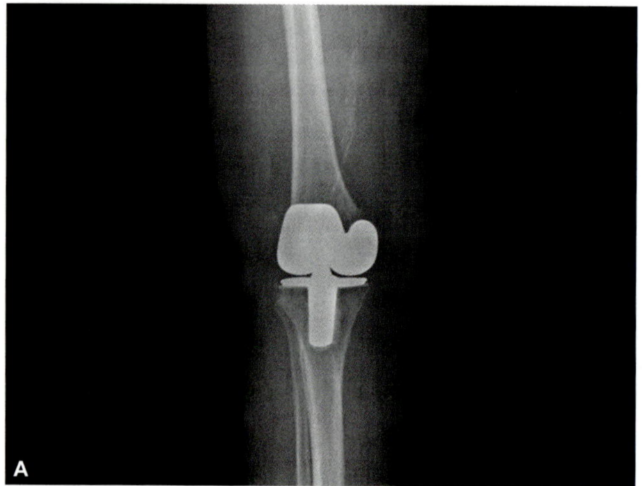

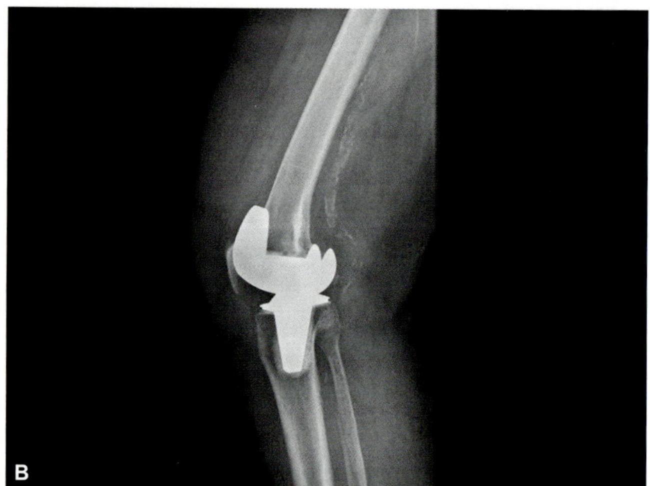

Figures 10.3A and B Radiographs of posterior stabilized total knee arthroplasty at 30 years. Anteroposterior (AP) view (A) and lateral view (B)

prosthesis include ease of surgical exposure and gap-balancing, predictable restoration of joint kinematics, the better ROM and knee flexion, less wear and instability. Additionally, in knees with a fixed angular deformity, rheumatoid arthritis and with patellectomy, the PS TKA provides superior results. Consequently, in the United States, there has been a marked increase in the use of the PS prosthesis. At one of the largest orthopedic centers in the country, the Mayo Clinic, the use of PCL substitution in the primary TKA increased from 10% in 1990 to 75% in 1997. The ROM after the PS TKA averages 112°–115° and is more reliably attained compared to CR TKA.[36,46] The incidence of instability, including flexion instability is less compared to the CR knees. Kinematically also, the PCL substitution appears to be superior to the PCL retention and there is no proven proprioceptive benefit to the use of the CR prosthesis. Biomechanical studies also do not show a significant difference between the CR and PS knees in spatiotemporal gait parameters and stair climbing. Finally, the PS designs have a proven track-record in terms of performance and longevity (**Figures 10.3A and B**). Based on all these findings, we strongly recommend the use of a cemented PS prosthesis in the primary TKA.

REFERENCES

1. Harato K, Bourne RB, Victor J, et al. Midterm comparison of posterior-cruciate retaining versus-substituting total knee arthroplasty using the Genesis II prosthesis: a multicenter prospective randomized trial. Knee. 2008;15(3):217-21.
2. Maruyama S, Yoshiya S, Matsui N, Kuroda R, Kurosaka M. Functional comparison of posterior cruciate-retaining versus posterior stabilized total knee arthroplasty. J Arthroplasty. 2004;19(3):349-53.
3. Scuderi GR, Pagnano MW. The rationale for posterior cruciate substituting total knee arthroplasty. J Orthop Surg. 2001;9(2):81-8.
4. Pagnano MW, Hanssen AD, Lewallen DG, Stuart MJ. Flexion instability after primary posterior cruciate retaining total knee arthroplasty. Clin Orthop Relat Res. 1998;356:39-46.
5. Laskin RS, O'Flynn HM. Total knee replacement with posterior cruciate ligament retention in rheumatoid arthritis: Problems and complications. Clin Orthop Relat Res. 1997;345:24-8.
6. Montgomery RL, Goodman SB, Congradi J. Late rupture of the posterior cruciate ligament after total knee arthroplasty. Lowa Orthop. 1993;13:167-70.
7. Ochsner Jr JL, Kostman WC, Dodson M. Posterior cruciate ligament avulsion in total knee arthroplasty. Orthop Rev. 1993;22:1121-24.
8. Insall JN, Hood RW, Flawn LB, Sullivan DJ. The total condylar prosthesis in gonarthrosis: a five to nine year follows up of the first one-hundred consecutive replacements. J Bone Joint Surg. 1983;65 A:619-28.
9. Dennis DA, Komistek RD, Hoff WA. *In vivo* knee kinematics derived using an inverse perspective technique. Clin Orthop Relat Res. 1996;331:107-17.
10. Ranawat CS, Komistek RD, Rodriguez JA, Dennis DA, Anderle M. *In vivo* kinematics for fixed and mobile-bearing posterior stabilized knee prosthesis. Clin Orthop Relat Res. 2004;418:184-90.
11. Baier C, Springorum HR, Gotz J, et al. Comparing navigation-based *in vivo* kinematics pre-and postoperatively between a cruciate-retaining and a cruciate-substituting implant. Int Orthop. 2013;37:407-14.
12. Udomkiat P, Meng BJ, Dorr LD, Wan Z. Functional comparison of posterior cruciate retention and substitution knee replacement. Clin Orthop Relat Res. 2000;378:192-201.
13. Mahoney OM, Noble PC, Rhoads DD, Alexander JW, Tullos HS. Posterior cruciate function following total knee Arthroplasty: a biomechanical study. J Arthroplasty. 1994;9:569-78.
14. Wilson SA, McCann PD, Gotlin RS, et al. Comprehensive gait analysis in posterior stabilized knee arthroplasty. J Arthroplasty. 1996;11:359-67.
15. Kleinbart FA, Bryk E, Evangelista J, Scott WN, Vigorita VJ. Histologic comparison of posterior cruciate ligaments from arthritic and age-matched knee specimens. J Arthroplasty. 1996;6:726-31.
16. Warren PI, Olanlokun TK, Cobb AG, Bentley G. Proprioception after knee arthroplasty: the influence of prosthetic design. Clin Orthop Relat Res. 1993;297:182-7.
17. Simmons S, Lephart S, Rubash H, Pifer GW, Barrack R. Proprioception after unicondylar knee arthroplasty versus total knee arthroplasty. Clin Orthop Relat Res. 1996;331:179-184.
18. Becker MW, Insall JN, Faris PM. Bilateral total knee arthroplasty: one cruciate retaining and one cruciate substituting. Clin Orthop Relat Res. 1990;271:122-4.

19. Swanik CB, Lephart SM, Rubash HE. Proprioception, kinesthesia and balance after total knee arthroplasty with cruciate retaining and posterior stabilized prosthesis. J Bone Joint Surg Am. 2004;86A:328-34.
20. Ritter MA, Campbell E. Effect of range of motion on the success of a total knee arthroplasty. J Arthroplasty. 1987;2:95.
21. Chaudhary R, Beaupre LA, Johnston DWC. Knee range of motion during the first-two years after use of posterior cruciate—stabilizing or posterior cruciate-retaining total knee prosthesis: a randomized clinical trial. J Bone Joint Surg Am. 2008;90:2579-86.
22. Kim YH, Choi Y, Kwon OR, Kim JS. Functional outcome and range of motion of high-flexion posterior cruciate-retaining and high-flexion posterior cruciate-substituting total knee prosthesis: a prospective randomized study. J Bone Joint Surg Am. 2009;91:753-60.
23. Bercik MJ, Joshi A, Parvizi J. Posterior cruciate-retaining versus posterior-stabilized total knee arthroplasty: a meta-analysis. J Arthroplasty. 2013;28:439-44.
24. Li N, Tan Y, Deng Y, Chen L. Posterior cruciate-retaining versus posterior stabilized total knee arthroplasty: a meta-analysis of randomized controlled trial. Knee Surg Sports Traumatol Arthrosc. 2012. (Epub ahead of print).
25. Jacobs WC, Clement DJ, Wymenga AB. Retention versus removal of the posterior cruciate ligament in total knee replacement: a systematic literature review within the Cochrane framework. Acta Orthop. 2005;76:757-68.
26. Matsumoto T, Kuroda R, Kubo S, et al. The intra-operative joint gap in a cruciate-retaining compared with posterior-stabilized total knee replacement. J Bone Joint Surg Br.2009;91:475-80.
27. Matsumoto T, Murats H, Kubo S, et al. Soft tissue tension in cruciate retaining and posterior-stabilized total knee Arthroplasty. J Arthroplasty. 2011;26:788-95.
28. Takayama K, Matsumoto T, Kubo S, et al. Influence of intra-operative joint gaps on post-operative flexion angle in posterior cruciate-retaining total knee arthroplasty. Knee Surg Sports Traumatol Arthrosc. 2012;20:532-7.
29. Lozano-Calderon SA, Shen J, Doumato DF, Greene DA, Zelicof SB. Cruciate-retaining versus posterior-substituting inserts in total knee arthroplasty: functional outcome comparison. J Arthroplasty. 2013;28:234-42.
30. Luo S, Zhao JM, Su W, Li X, Dong G. Posterior cruciate substituting versus posterior cruciate retaining total knee prosthesis: a meta-analysis. Knee. 2012;19:246-52.
31. Sharkey PF, Hozack WJ, Rothman RH, Shastri S, Jacoby SM. Insall award paper: why are total knee arthroplasties failing today? Clin Orthop Relat Res. 2002;404:7-13.
32. Insall JN. Adventures in mobile-bearing knee design: a mid-life crisis. Orthopedics. 1998;21:1021-23.
33. Ranawat AS, Rossi R, Loreti I, et al. Comparison of PFC sigma fixed-bearing and rotating-platform total knee arthroplasty in the same patient: short-term results. J Arthroplasty. 2004;19:35-9.
34. Bhan S, Malhotra R, Kiran EK, Shukla S, Bijjawara M. A comparison of fixed-bearing and mobile-bearing total knee arthroplasty at a minimum follow-up of 4.5 years. J Bone Joint Surg Am. 2005;87:2290-96.
35. Gioe TJ, Glynn J, Sembrano J, et al. Mobile and fixed-bearing (all polyethylene tibial component) total knee arthroplasty designs: a prospective randomized trial. J Bone Joint Surg Am. 2009;91:2104-12.
36. Colizza W, Insall JN, Scuderi GR. The posterior stabilized knee prosthesis: assessment of polyethylene damage and osteolysis after a minimum ten-year follow-up. J Bone Joint Surg. 1995;77A:1713-20.
37. Kilgus DJ, Moreland JR, Finerman GA, Funahashi TT, Tipton JS. Catastrophic wear of tibial polyethylene inserts. Clin Orthop Relat Res. 1991;273:223-31.
38. Waslewski GL, Marson BM, Benjamin JB. Early, incapacitating instability of posterior cruciate ligament-retaining total knee arthroplasty. J Arthroplasty. 1998;13:763-67.
39. Puloski SK, McCalden RW, MacDonald SJ, Rorabeck CH, Bourne RB. Tibial post wear in posterior stabilized total knee arthroplasty: an unrecognized source of polyethylene debris. J Bone Joint Surg Am. 2001;83:390-97.
40. Dolan MM, Kelly NH, Nguyen JT, Wright TM, Haas SB. Implant design influences tibial post wear damage in posterior stabilized knees. Clin Orthop Relat Res. 2011;469:160-7.
41. Laurent MP, Yao JQ, Bhambri S, et al. High cycle wear of highly cross-linked UHMWPE tibial articular surfaces evaluated in a knee wear simulator: 28th annual meeting transactions. Society of Biomaterials. 2002.p.712.
42. Popoola OO, Yao JQ, Johnson TS, Blanchard CR. Wear, delamination, and fatigue resistance of melt-annealed highly cross-linked UHMWPE cruciate-retaining knee inserts under activities of daily living. J Orthop Res. 2010;28:1120-26.

43. Hinarejos P, Pinol I, Torres A, et al. Highly cross-linked polyethylene does not reduce wear in total knee arthroplasty: *in vivo* study of particles in synovial fluid. J Arthroplasty. 2013.
44. Long WJ, Levi GS, Scuderi GR. Highly cross-linked polyethylene in posterior stabilized total knee arthroplasty: early results. Orthop Clin N Am. 2012;43:e35-8.
45. Barnes CL, Sledge CB. Total knee arthroplasty with posterior cruciate ligament retention designs. In: Insall JN (Ed.), Surgery of the knee, 2nd edn. New York: Churchill Livingstone; 1993. pp. 815-27.
46. Hirsh HS, Lotke PA, Morrison LD. The posterior cruciate ligament in total knee surgery: save, sacrifice, or substitute. Clin Orthop Relat Res. 1994; 309:64-8.
47. Ritter MA, Faris PM, Keating EM. Posterior cruciate ligament balancing during total knee arthroplasty. J Arthroplasty. 1988;3:323-6.
48. Laskin RS. Total knee replacement with posterior cruciate ligament retention in patients with a fixed varus deformity. Clin Orthop Relat Res. 1996;331:29-34.
49. Mintzer CM, Robertson DD, Rackemann S, et al. Bone loss in the distal anterior femur after total knee arthroplasty. Clin Orthop Relat Res. 1990;260:135-43.
50. Wing CK, Kwok-Hing C. Sixteen years' result of posterior-stabilized TKA. J Knee Surg. 2012;25:245-48.
51. Rasquinha VJ, Ranawat CS, Cervieri CL, Rodriguez JA. The press-fit condylar modular total knee system with a posterior cruciate-substituting design: a concise follow-up of a previous report. J Bone Joint Surg Am. 2006;88A:1006-10.
52. Meftah M, Ranawat AS, Ranawat CS. Ten-year follow-up of a rotating-platform, posterior stabilized total knee arthroplasty. J Bone Joint Surg Am. 2012;94:426-32.
53. Bryce CD, Long WJ, Scott WN, et al. Long-term (35 years) outcome analysis of the young total knee patient: minimum 20 years. Annual Meeting 2013; American Academy of Orthopaedic Surgeons (AAOS), March 2013.
54. Diduch DR, Insall JN, Scott WN, Scuderi GR, Font-Rodriguez D. Total knee replacement in young, active patients: long-term follow-up and functional outcome. J Bone Joint Surg Am. 1997;79:575-82.
55. Meftah M, Ranawat AS, Sood AB, Rodriguez JA, Ranawat CS. All-Polyethylene tibial implant in young, active patients: a concise follow-up, 10 to 18 years. J Arthroplasty. 2012;27:10-4.
56. Huang HT, Su JY, Wang GJ. The early results of high-flex total knee arthroplasty: minimum of 2 years of follow-up. J Arthroplasty. 2005;20:674-9.
57. Kim YH, Sohn KS, Kim JS. Range of motion of standard and high-flexion posterior stabilized total knee prostheses. A prospective, randomized study. J Bone Joint Surg Am. 2005;87:1470-75.
58. Kim TH, Lee DH, Bin SI. The NexGen LPS-flex to the knee prosthesis at a minimum of three years. J Bone Joint Surg Br. 2008;90:1304-10.
59. Ng FY, Wong HL, Yau WP, Chiu KY, Tang WM. Comparison of range of motion after standard and high-flexion posterior stabilized total knee replacement. Int Orthop. 2008;32:795-8.
60. McCalden RW, MacDonald SJ, Charron KD, Bourne RB, Naudie DD. The role of polyethylene design on postoperative TKA flexion: an analysis of 1534 cases. Clin Orthop Relat Res. 2010;468:108-14.
61. Tanavalee A, Ngarmukos S, Tantavisut S, Limtrakul A. High-flexion TKA in patients with a minimum of 120 degrees of pre-operative knee flexion: outcomes at six years of follow-up. Int Orthop. 2011;35:1321-26.
62. Scuderi GR, Hedden DR, Maltry JA. Early clinical results of high-flexion, posterior-stabilized, mobile-bearing total knee arthroplasty: a US investigational device exemption trial. J Arthroplasty. 2012;27:421-9.
63. Scuderi GR, Insall HN, Windsor RE, Moran MC. Survivorship of cemented total knee replacements. J Bone Joint Surg. 1989;71:798-803.
64. Stern SH, Insall JN. Posterior stabilized prosthesis. Results after follow-up of nine to twelve years. J bone Joint Surg. 1992;74A:980-6.
65. Font-Rodriguez DE, Scuderi GR, Insall JN. Survivorship of cemented total knee arthroplasty. Clin Orthop Relat Res. 1997;345:79-86.
66. Emmerson KP, Moran CG, Pinder IM. Survivorship analysis of the kinematic stabilizer total knee replacement: a ten to fourteen year follow-up. J Bone Joint Surg. 1996;78:441-5.
67. Ranawat CS, Luessenhop CP, Rodriguez JA. The press-fit condylar modular total knee system. Four-to-six year results with a posterior-cruciate-substituting design. J Bone Joint Surg Am. 1997;79:342-8.

Chapter 11

Mobile-bearing Total Knee Arthroplasty

Samih Tarabichi, Mohamed Elfekky, Azam Badar Khan

INTRODUCTION

In 1996 scientists discovered a 2600-year-old mummy of an Egyptian priest "Usermontu" belonging to the Rosicrucian Egyptian Museum which educed worldwide attention when an X-ray betrayed an ancient 9" metal screw connecting the mummys thigh and lower leg. According to Dr Richard Jackson, the pin was a biomechanical precursor to the fixing and stabilizing concepts we use today in orthopedic surgery.[1]

The first chronicled knee surgery was performed in 1891 by German surgeon Theophilus Gluck, who experimented with harvested muscle fat, nylon and pig bladders to cushion the knee joint. He is also believed to have performed the first true knee replacement surgery employing plastic/metal hinged ivory to simulate the knee joint structure. Glucks technique was ameliorated during the early 19th century, using metal and plastic components, but the hinge type device was inflexible and was prone to complications and failure.[2]

In 1974, a group of researchers at the Massachusetts General Hospital developed a round plastic component that intently allegorized the natural knee structure and allowed for total knee replacement and the design came to be known as "Total condylar knee."

The total condylar knee or fixed bearing total knee arthroplasty proved successful in long-term outcome studies with 95% good to excellent result 10–15 years[3] after surgery in the elderly patients. It however could not simulate the kinematics of the natural knee. The natural menisci provide conformity and mobility, while conforming to the femoral condyles the menisci are able to rotate, to some degree on the tibial plateau. This combination of conformity and mobility acquiesces for stability and load distribution, not only in the neutral position but also when the femur is rotated in relation to the tibia. In fixed bearing total knee arthroplasty (TKA) conformity of the menisci and femoral condyles can be equated by increasing the conformity of the articulating surfaces but by introducing superfluous constraint. Largely because of its inherent lack of physiological rotation of the menisci, the fixed bearing TKA remains a compromise between conformity and mobility, which in turn leads to component loosening and polyethylene wear. Good long-term results in older patients, however, has fuelled patient expectations and have encouraged surgeons to consider performing TKA on younger patients, who have higher activity appetite.

INDICATIONS AND DESIGN RATIONALE

From a 9" long pin in a 2600-year-old mummy, to fixed bearing TKA, it was a long odyssey for orthopedic science to cover, and the inquest was far from over.

The mobile/menisci bearing knee replacement was first designed by Goodfellow and O'Conner, in 1976. Almost simultaneously Dr Fred Beuchel and Michael Pappas designed the low contact stress knee in 1977, which continues to hold unflinching popularity. The rationale behind mobile bearing designs is to increase survival of the prosthesis by reducing the rate of aseptic loosening and improving the range of motion. This theoretically is achieved by lowering the rate of polyethylene wear as compared to fixed designs, due to lower contact and constraint forces. A better range of motion is achieved as a result of an additional moving surface between two fixed planes, allowing mobility with congruency. With rotating mobile bearing TKA maximum conformity between articulating components was possible with minimum constraint. Optimal stability was thus present at any degree of rotation while diminishing the risk of loosening and wear. Load was distributed over a large surface regardless of the rotational position of the femur in relation to the tibia. The bicondylar contact area of a mobile bearing knee may exceed 1000 sq mm, which is approximately 5 times the contact area of a standard, partially conforming fixed bearing design. Accordingly the decrease in contact stress is reduced from approximately 25 MPa in fixed bearing to less than 5 MPa in mobile bearing. Anteroposterior (AP) translation was also a feature of several meniscal-bearing designs. A combination of rotation and AP translation mimics physiological meniscal function more closely.[4]

These advantages of the mobile bearing design may cause higher rates of breakage and disengagement of the polyethylene inserts, if the implantation technique is not strictly adhered to leading to the development of the rotating platform mobile prosthesis.[5]

BIOMECHANICAL AND CLINICAL REVIEW OF A MOBILE-BEARING TOTAL KNEE ARTHROPLASTY

Biomechanical studies have demonstrated that the contact stress on the tibial polyethylene component is closely related to polyethylene wear.[6,7] This was measured by Matsuda et al.[8] who measured the contact pressures on the upper and under-surface of the tibial polyethylene insert with a neutral and malrotated tibial tray of three different mobile-bearing designs and one fixed-bearing design. Their study showed that mobile-bearing designs had an advantages over the fixed-bearing design in the presence of moderate rotational malalignment of the tibial component. Stukenborg-Colsman et al.[9] using electronic resistive pressure sensors to measure tibiofemoral contact stresses of fixed and mobile-bearing TKP under dynamic loading conditions in internally and externally rotated positions showed that there was an increase in the contact stresses in a malrotated tibial component with fixed-bearing designs. These increases were not demonstrated with mobile-bearing designs. They also suggested that mobile-bearing designs allowed the tibial insert to translate on the tibial base plate permiting the component to align itself with the femoral component reducing contact stress by maximizing the contact area. This feature also reduces the likelihood of cold flow and stress-peak damage. The contact stresses in tibial polyethylene component of fixed- and mobile-bearing knee prostheses under medial-lateral, anterior-posterior maltranslations and in internal-external malrotations of tibiofemoral joint were measured by Cheng et al.[10] who demonstrated that the mobile-bearing design could reduce maximum contact pressure more significantly than the fixed-bearing design when malalignment conditions of the tibiofemoral joint occured, especially in the internal/external malrotation offering the advantage of self-adjustment over the fixed-bearing design to accommodate surgical malalignment.

Gait analysis also have shown an increased sagittal plane conformity with better control of anteroposterior translation, with reduced paradoxical anterior femoral translation.[11,12] Increased coronal plane conformity as seen in mobile-bearing TKA, increases the contact area and lessens the contact stresses that are present in case of femoral condylar liftoff.[13-16] as observed on Tech Scan analysis.[17] In a well aligned flat-on-flat design which allows equal loading of each condyle, approximately 16 MPa of peak polyethylene stresses are reached whereas if the same design is loaded in 3 degrees of varus malalignment, with shifting of load to one condyle, as seen in femoral condylar liftoff, peak stresses increase to 38 MPa which exceeds the yield strength of polyethylene (20 to 22 MPa). The increased conformity as seen with mobile-bearing designs increase contact area and reduce contact stresses, reducing the rate of polyethylene wear.[18-22]

Greenwald and Heim[19] demonstrated that the contact areas of mobile-bearing TKA during gait range from approximately 400 to 800 mm^2, which minimizes contact stresses to 14 MPa or less. This contact area is significantly greater than what is seen in most fixed-bearing TKA designs (200 to 250 mm^2) other studies have shown similar results.[22-24] McNulty et al.[25] and McEwen et al.[26] in separate laboratory evaluations demonstrated diminished polyethylene wear rates (94% and Four fold reduction respectively) with highly conforming rotating platform designs when compared with similarly designed fixed-bearing systems.

In vivo fluoroscopic kinematic studies by Dennis et al.[27] demonstrated that the polyethylene mobility occurred following mobile-bearing TKA and this mobility probably resulted in low contact stresses thus reducing poly wear. Komistek et al.[28] in an earlier *in vivo* kinemetic study showed that the polyethylene bearing rotated primarily relative to the tibia in contrast to the femur thereby causing the bearing to rotate in the same magnitude as in the axial rotation of the femur resulting in reduced shear stresses reducing wear. D'Lima et al.[29] analyzed the knee kinematics of mobile-bearing knees in closed chain knee extension model with posterior cruciate retaining designs and substituting designs with high and low conformity and with or without rotational constraint respectively. Their results showed that mobile bearing inserts rotated with the femur and increasing conformity or rotational constraint did not affect knee kinemetics in mobile-bearing designs.

Central patellar tracking due to self aligning may be an advantage in the rotating platform knee TKA system. In a retrospective analysis of 1318 consecutive primary TKAs, Yang et al.[30] studied the incidence of lateral retinacular release using the moble-bearing or the fixed-bearing prosthesis. The incidence of lateral release was 5.3% in mobile-bearing as compared to 14.3% in the fixed-bearing group. They concluded that the incidence of fewer lateral releases in the mobile-bearing group may be the result of better extension mechanism centralization due to bearing rotation.

Axial rotation occurring during deep flexion activities is an important factor in knee implant designs. *In vivo* fluoroscopic femorotibial axial rotation evaluation of over 1000 knees analyzed by Dennis et al.[31] atleast 19% patients following TKA had a reverse axial rotational pattern during deep knee bending. Normal axial rotation patterns are essential for attaining maximum knee flexion, reducing patellofemoral shear forces and for a good patellar tracking. Therefore, mobile-bearing TKA designs that provide more freedom of rotation should reduce rotational polyethylene impingement, with the potential for reduction of polyethylene wear. In the posterior cruciate-substituting (PS) knees, polyethylene post wear leading to TKA failure has been often attributed to excessive axial rotation leading to premature polyethylene wear and compromise of the central post.[32] This is attributed to the lateral and medial postimpingement on attempted excessive rotation of a fixed tibial polyethylene post in a fixed femoral intercondylar housing. The freedom of rotation present in rotating platform designs allows for greater range of axial rotation without causing rotational impingement and wear on posterior cruciate-stabilizing posts.

The generation of polyethylene particles and accelerated polyethylene wear on the undersurface of the polyethylene over the polyethylene-metal interface has raised concerns about rotating platform knees. However in fixed-bearing TKA systems, backside polyethylene motion against a rough tibial tray not designed to accommodate motion has also shown significant polyethylene wear leading to subsequent periprosthetic osteolysis.[33-35] A rotating yet flat polyethylene bearing is matched against a highly polished, cobalt-chromium surface with extremely low surface roughness in rotating platform kness and in present data backside polyethylene wear has not emerged as a clinically significant issue. Retrieval studies examining backside wear on the bearing surface of rotating platform polyethylene inserts have not reported significant undersurface wear.[36,37]

The lack of clinically significant backside polyethylene wear may be due to the decoupling of multidirectional motions occurring at the articular interfaces with rotating designs,[27,38] whereas in fixed-bearing systems, all rotational, translational, and flexion-extension motion patterns happen on the superior articular surface. This leads to multidirectional motion pathways causing increased wear. In rotating platform designs allowing no anteroposterior translation, the inferior surface, is designed to experience purely rotational (reciprocal-unidirectional) motion patterns whereas mobile-bearing designs in which the polyethylene bearing tracks with the femoral component,[28,29] the superior articular surface (femoral component–polyethylene interface) primarily experiences flexion-extension (reciprocal-unidirectional) motion due to rotation occurring on the inferior aspect of the bearing. When high-density polyethylene is subjected to unidirectional sliding, molecules tend to align along the direction of sliding, leading to lowering of the coefficient of friction, reducing wear of the material.[39] Conversely, polyethylene wear is accelerated when the material is exposed to multidirectional wear pathways due to a rise in cross-shear stresses. Multidirectional shear stresses experienced at the single polyethylene interface in fixed-bearing systems contribute to 4 to 10 times the polyethylene wear compared to that experienced by unidirectional interfaces in rotating platform designs.[40,41] Rotating platform TKA designs reduce polyethylene wear by decoupling multidirectional motions to more monodirectional motion patterns at two differing interfaces, reducing cross-shear stresses and wear occurring on both interfaces.

Analysis of wear debris created in fixed-bearing and rotating platform TKA designs by Fisher et al.[42] in a knee simulator analysis under high kinematic conditions showed no differences in microparticulate size, though the osteolytic potential was considered much higher in fixed-bearing designs because of substantially more debris particle generation.

Certain mobile-bearing TKA systems that permit rotation and anteroposterior translation to occur on the inferior aspect of the polyethylene bearing exposing the inferior aspect of the polyethylene bearing to multidirectional motion patterns. In a comparative wear analysis of a rotating platform TKA (LCS RP; DePuy) in a knee simulator by Jennings et al.[43] at 5 million cycles, twice the amount of polyethylene wear in the LCS AP Glide TKA was observed meriting close follow-up of such systems.

There are many mobile-bearing knee prostheses today. Although most rotating-platform knees look alike, there are major differences in design, and classification is needed as proposed by Greenwald and Heim.[19] This may be based on the femorotibial contact area which may be big or small or on the movement at the distal surface between the polyethylene bearing and tibial tray which may be unidirectional or multidirectional. They can also be classified based on the way the bearing surface is controlled as in the form of metal cylinders, slots, or stops. These often lead to suboptimal kinematics and stress on the polyethylene leading to damage and wear.

Mobile-bearing knee devises may be devided into those with:

- Multidirectional platform
- Rotating platform
- Meniscal bearing
- A combination of rotating platform and meniscal bearing implants.

MULTIDIRECTIONAL PLATFORM

A multidirectional platform is one where a single polyethylene bearing allows both rotation and antero-posterior motion in the transverse plane.

Seventy-four knees implanted with the accord total knee arthroplasty were reviewed by Duffy and Phillipson.[44] Twenty-five knees required revision or further surgery. The mean knee score was 60 and the mean function score was 42. Of the 25 failed knees, 19 had been revised due to instability. Survivorship at 10 years was 58% with an average follow-up of 5 years 4 months. These results are poor compared with more conventional TKAs.

Kaper et al.[45] reported the results of 141 patients who were implanted with the self aligning 1 knee for osteoarthritis with an average follow-up for 5.6 years. Patient satisfaction of good or very good at last follow-up was 94%. They reported a survivorship of 91.7% with revision as the end point.

In a prospective study conducted by Morgan-Jones et al.[46] of 62 patients (75 knees) with a mean follow-up of 2.5 years no mobile bearing dislocation, subluxation, or breakage was reported. Radiologically, there was no evidence of subsidence or osteolysis. Polyzoides et al.[47] in a retrospective study involving 170 knees (161 patients) who received a Rotaglide total knee reported no mechanical implant failures and no platform bearing dislocations.

ROTATING PLATFORM

A single polyethylene bearing that rotates in the transverse plane without anteroposterior motion constitutes a rotating platform.

Callaghan et al.[48] in 119 consecutive cemented LCS rotating platform TKAs reported their results in 114 knees. No knees required resurgery and no dislocations were seen. They also reported no evidence of periprosthetic osteolysis on radiographs in this study. No implant loosening was reported at final follow-up. They attributed avoidance of a loose flexion gap for the absence of platform dislocation and osteolysis from backside wear.

Grodzki et al.[49] in their series of 38 patients (12 PFC and 26 LCS) followed for a period of 1 year. They reported improved Knee Society Scores at 6 weeks with the rotating tibia component compared to the fixed polyethylene inlay with the same rehabilitation and mobilization techniques.

MENISCAL BEARING DEVICES

Separate medial and/or lateral mobile polyethylene bearings that slide independently in tracks that run anteriorly and posteriorly in the fixed metal tibial component comprises a meniscal bearing device.

Bert[50] in his study of 43 consecutive TKAs using a mobile-bearing low contact stress (LCS) implant reported 91% good to excellent results at 1 year. They reported dislocation and/or subluxation of the meniscal bearing elements in four patients with three dislocating within 2 weeks of surgery. All 4 cases needed revision surgery. The author (Bert JM 1990)[50] were of the opinion that proper measurement of the flexion-tension of the tibiofemoral gap was critical in preventing dislocation/subluxation of the meniscal bearing elements.

Hartford et al.[51] reported a survivorship of 93% at an average of 7.8 years of 139 mobile-bearing knees in 104 patients. They had a 27% incidence of radiolucency for the femur and 31% for the tibia in their series. They reported a higher incidence of aseptic loosening where uncemented components were used.

Kim et al.[52] in their study of 120 simultaneous bilateral TKRs with the LCS mobile-bearing knee was implanted on one side and an AMK fixed-bearing knee on the other reported similar results for the LCS and AMK groups with 2 revisions from each group. Survivorship with revision as an endpoint for any reason in their series was 98% for both groups at 7.4 years.

COMBINATION OF ROTATING PLATFORM AND MENISCAL BEARING

In a twenty-year evaluation of the initial series of 373 New Jersey Low Contact Stress knee replacements performed by Buechel et al.[53] in 282 patients who survived at least 10 years, excellent outcomes were seen in 68.1% of the primary PCR meniscal bearing knees. Osteolysis was observed in 1.8% requiring bearing exchange and bone grafting.

Buechel and Pappas[54] in multiple evaluations of the New Jersey Low Contact Stress-Knee Replacement system including 357 knees (149 cemented and 208 uncemented) with an average follow-up of 91.2 months for cemented and 52.4 for the noncemented group reported 95.1% good to excellent for the primary cemented group and 91.8% for the cementless group. They reported a 85.2% excellent to good result in revision cases with an dislocation rate of 3.2% predominately in revision cases.

Callaghan et al.[48] in their evaluation of 119 consecutive TKAs in 86 patients operated upon by a single surgeon concluded that the cemented LCS rotating platform knee had durable clinical and radiological results at a 20-year follow-up. However osteolysis continued to increase as the duration of follow-up became longer.

Stiehl et al.[55] in a prospective nonrandomized study of consecutive 290 knees reported an overall survivorship 97.5% for meniscal-bearing knees and 100% rotating platform knees at 7 years follow-up. They postulated that with careful IM alignment and flexion-extension gap balancing most bearing failures could be avoided.

Surgical Technique

The surgical technique for the implantation of a mobile-bearing TKA is no different from that of fixed-bearing TKA systems. Soft tissue balancing, creation of equal flexion and extension gaps, and accurate component positioning are extremely important in both.

Extension and flexion gap balance is paramount with the use of a mobile-bearing TKA to prevent bearing dislocation or spin-out. Gap balance may be achieved by the use of spacer blocks to evaluate and balance the extension gap and the flexion gap. Femoral component rotation is also essential to obtain a balanced flexion gap. Correct femoral component rotation may be achieved with the help of cutting jigs that automatically externally rotate the femoral component three or more degrees relative to the posterior condylar axis or by placing the femoral component parallel to the trans-epicondylar axis or perpendicular to the anteroposterior axis and by placing the femoral component parallel to the tibial resection, with each collateral ligament equally tensioned.

It is advised to use a combination of femoral component rotational methods to prevent femoral component internal rotation. The Authors recommend the use of the gap balancing method with some type of tensioning device (e.g. laminar spreaders, spacer blocks, specific gap-tensioning device) to tension the flexion gap while femoral component rotation is determined with the use of mobile-bearing TKA systems. 1 to 2 mm of medial and lateral laxity in flexion is desireable with the use of mobile-bearing TKA systems. Any inability to obtain flexion-extension gap balance or collateral incompetence should prompt consideration of using a fixed-bearing TKA to avoid polyethylene bearing instability.

OUR EXPERIENCE WITH MOBILE-BEARING TOTAL KNEE REPLACEMENT

Patients have different needs after total knee replacement. The activity of daily living for Asian and Middle-Eastern is different from that of the European. The Asian require full flexion to continue on with their lifestyle and they spent sometimes long hours kneeling on the ground and sitting comfortably on the ground with knee fully flexed without any difficulty. It was of concern that in patients who acquired full flexion after total knee replacement (**Figures 11.1A and B**) with regular nonflex implant the lateral condyle may actually spin off the tibial tray in deep

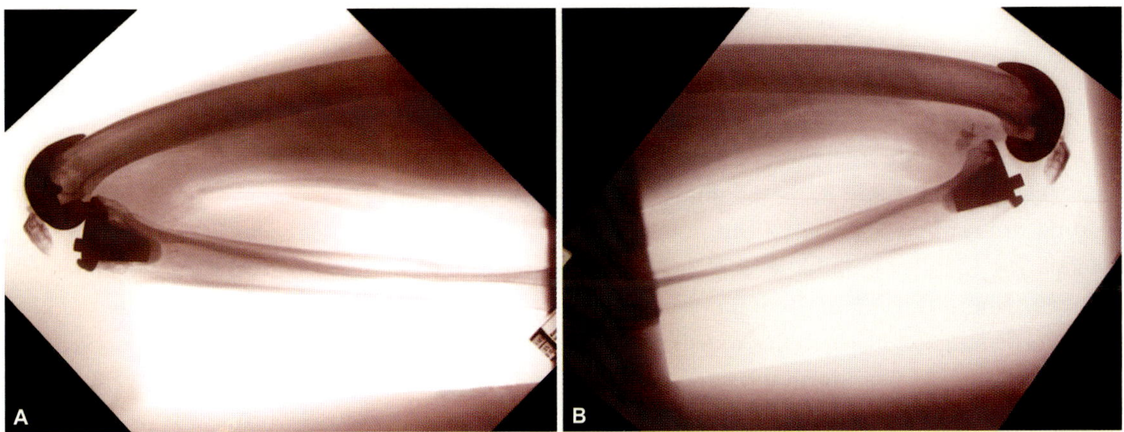

Figures 11.1A and B A 70-year-old patient acquired full flexion after bilateral total knee replacement using LPS flex

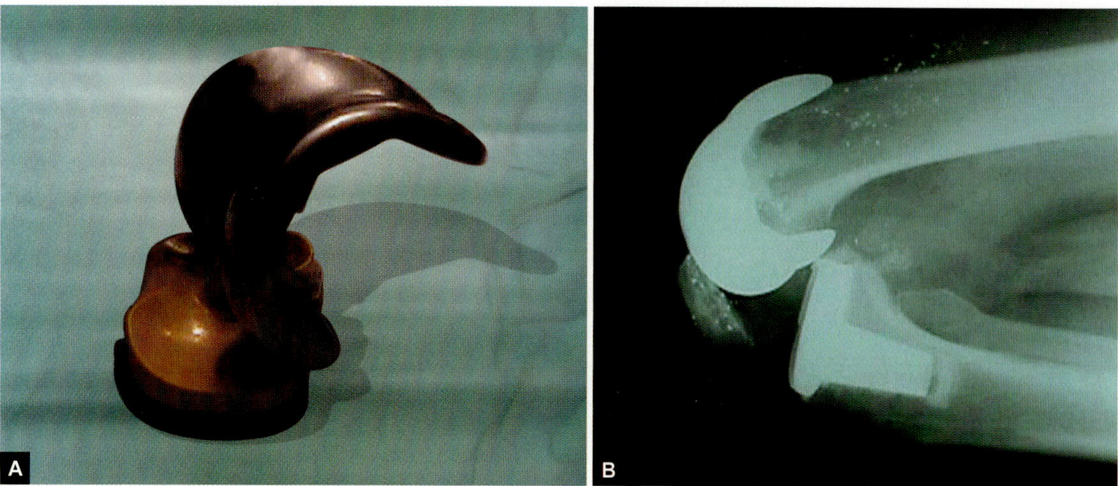

Figures 11.2A and B (A) Lateral femoral condyle spinning around the tibial tray; (B) X-ray of post TKA in patient obtained full flexion with a normal fixed bearing LPS implant. The X-ray clearly shows that the lateral condyles spinning off the tibial tray when the patient kneels fully

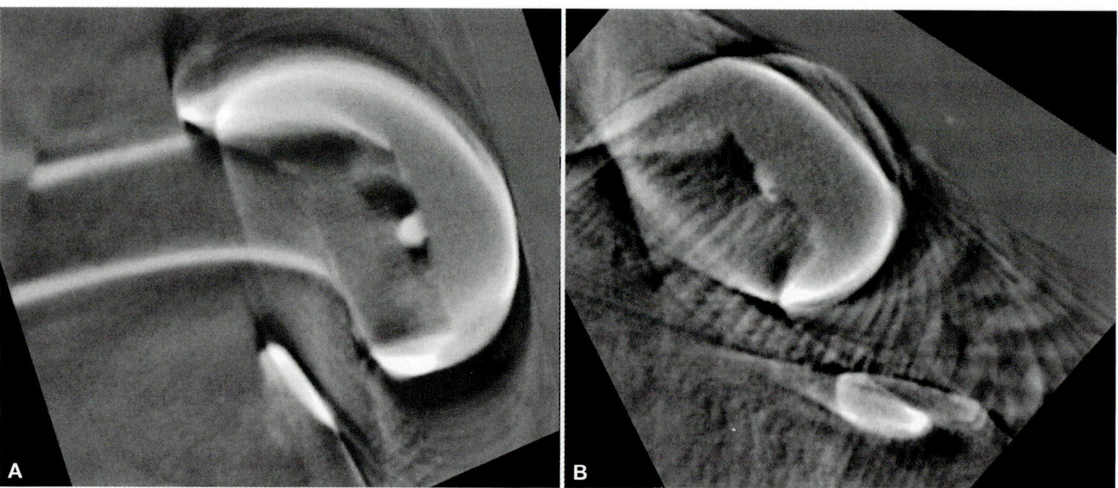

Figures 11.3A and B Section through 3D images showing lateral condyle spin off

flexion (**Figures 11.2 and 11.3**). The philosophy of Dr Insall was that the Asian patients who kneel frequently on the ground would require freedom to rotate the tibia on the femur (**Figures 11.4A and B**). Based on that need, I started doing the mobile-bearing LPS-implant in all of our patients. The LPS-flex mobile-bearing has a fixed version as well, where the femoral component is the same, however, the surgeon has a choice of using either a mobile-bearing or a fixed-bearing on the same implant. We presented our study at the American Academy Meeting in 2006. We matched the fixed-bearing group to that of the mobile-bearing group as far as age and body mass. The results of both the group were the same as far as the knee score and we focused on our study on full flexion and frequent kneeler.

We defined full flexion as the ability of the patient to kneel down on the ground with a calf-touching thigh for at least one minute. We defined frequent kneeler as the patients who at least kneel on the ground at least five times a day. This new definition reflects the activity of daily living for our population. The result was the same as far as the knee score and we had more full range of motion 68%

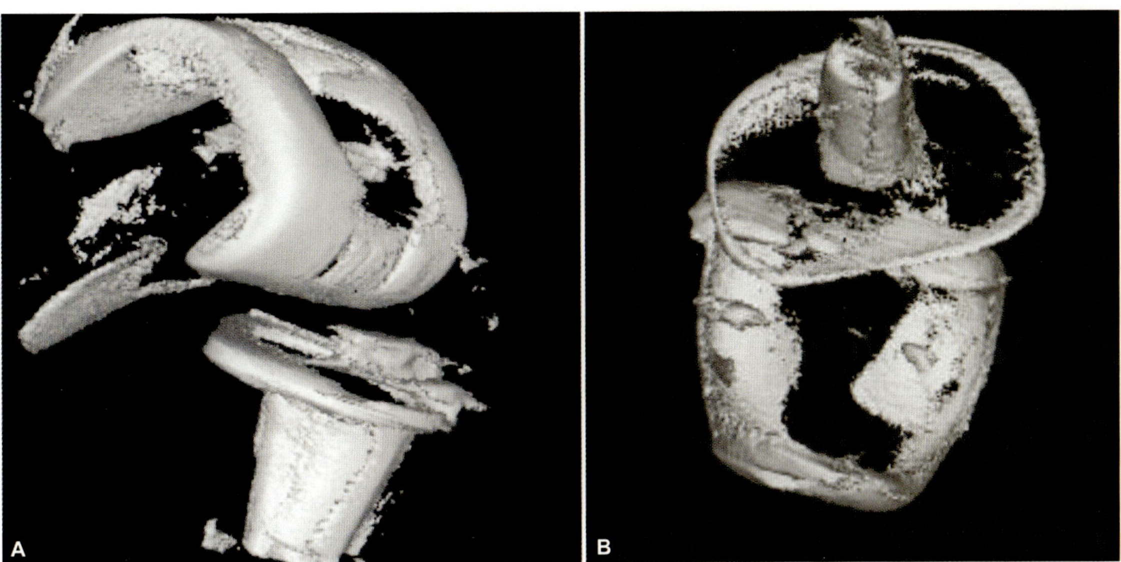

Figures 11.4A and B 3D picture of the knee in deep flexion showing the extent of internal tibial rotation

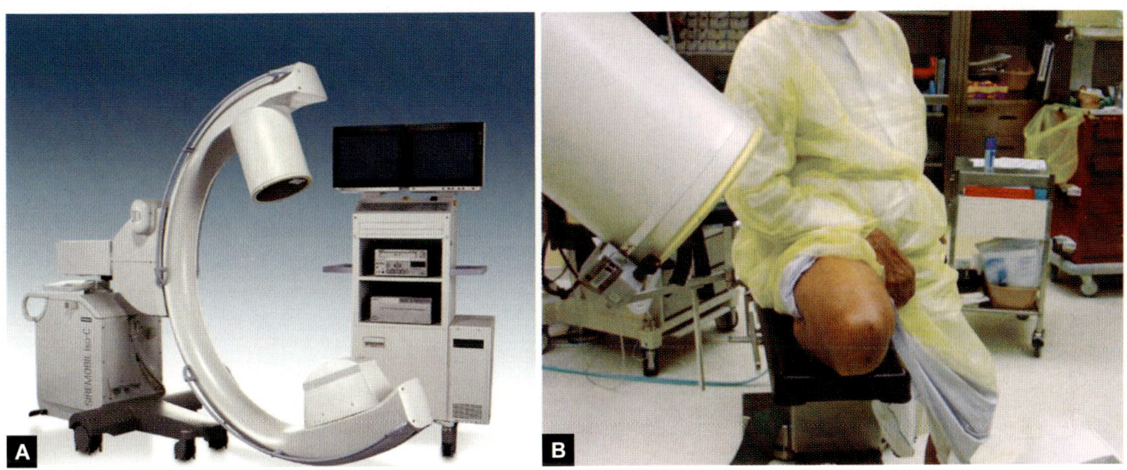

Figures 11.5A and B C-arm by Siemen's Siremobil to visualize the tibia and the femur used to scan the knee in full flexion

with a mobile-bearing versus the 55% of the fixed-bearing group, which was not significantly higher, however, when we compared the frequent kneeler, we discovered that we have higher rate of a frequent kneeler in the mobile-bearing group of 61% as compared to 48% with a fixed-bearing for the frequent kneeler. Our explanation for this finding was the fact that probably mobile-bearing implant allows some rotation of the tibia on the femur to make the patient more comfortable as compared to fixed-bearing where the soft tissue sleeve around the knee could be tight not allowing the tibia to rotating freely.

To further study the tibiofemoral movement in the full flexion patients, we selected a group of a frequent kneeler and we asked him to kneel on the knee fully with their weight. Using a 3D C-arm by Siemen's Siremobil to visualize the tibia and the femur (**Figures 11.5A and B**) our finding showed that although the tibiofemoral movement for the mobile-bearing implant is paradoxical in deep flexion, all of our patients had excessive external rotation as shown in **Figures 11.6 and 11.7**.

It should be understood that the mobile-bearing has a slightly higher complication as far as the knee dislocation

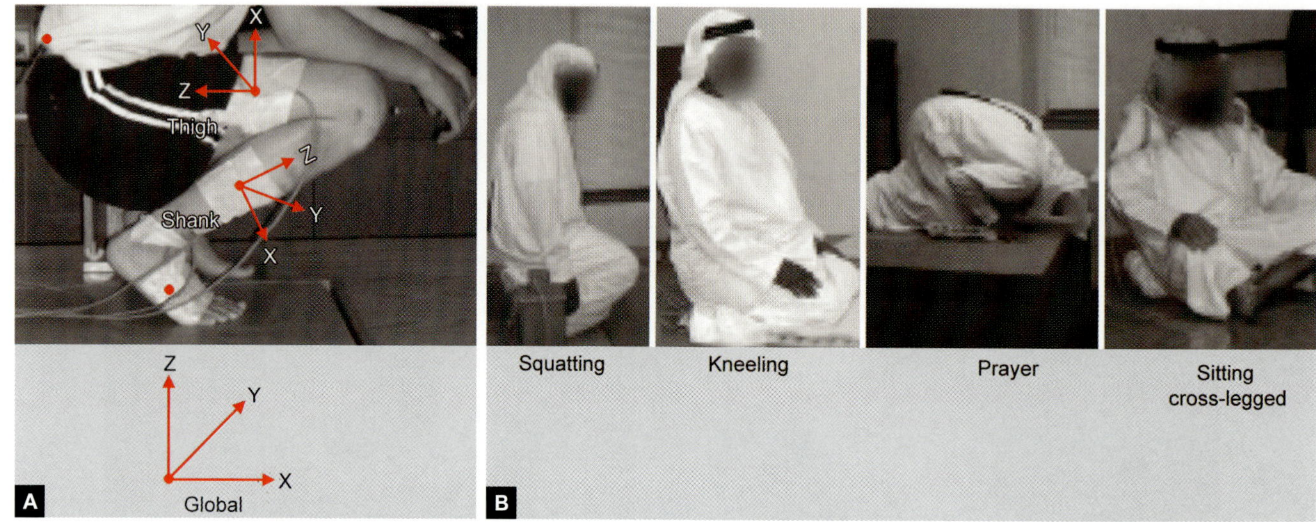

Figures 11.6A and B (A) Fastrak attached to patient leg; (B) Graph showing degrees of different motions in different groups

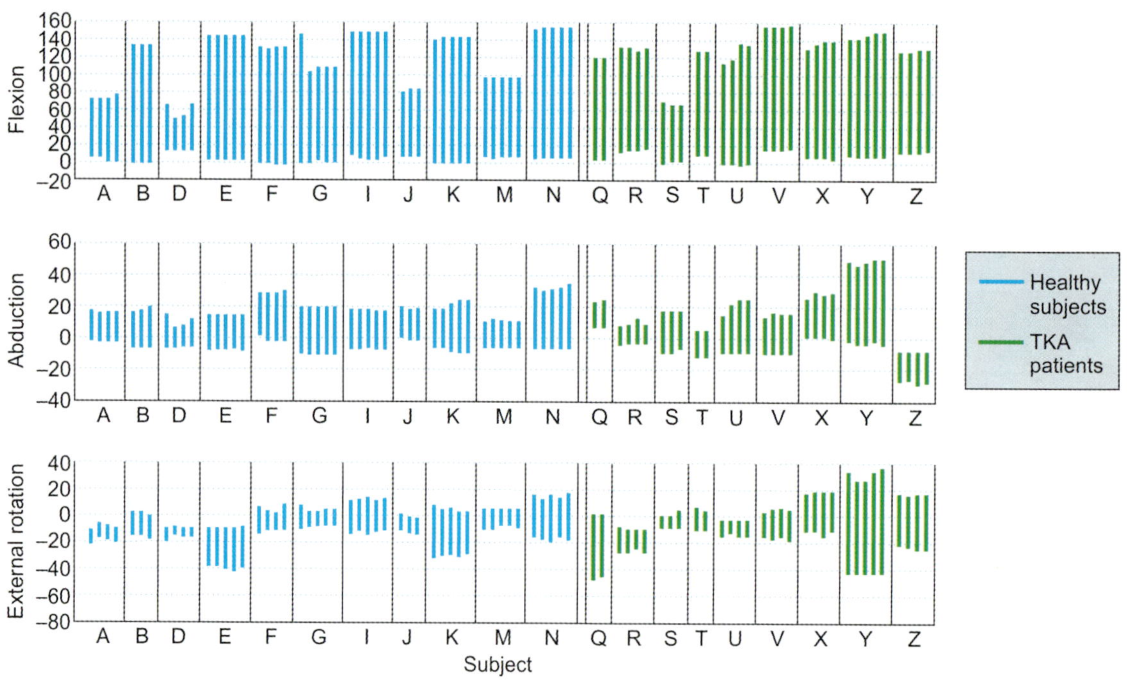

Figure 11.7A

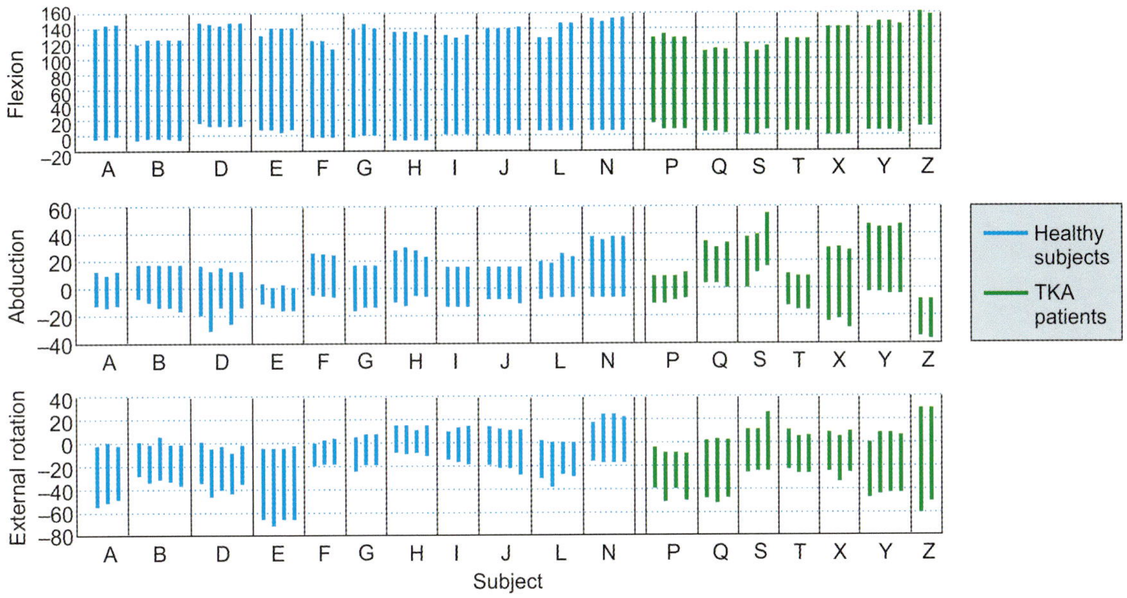

Figure 11.7B

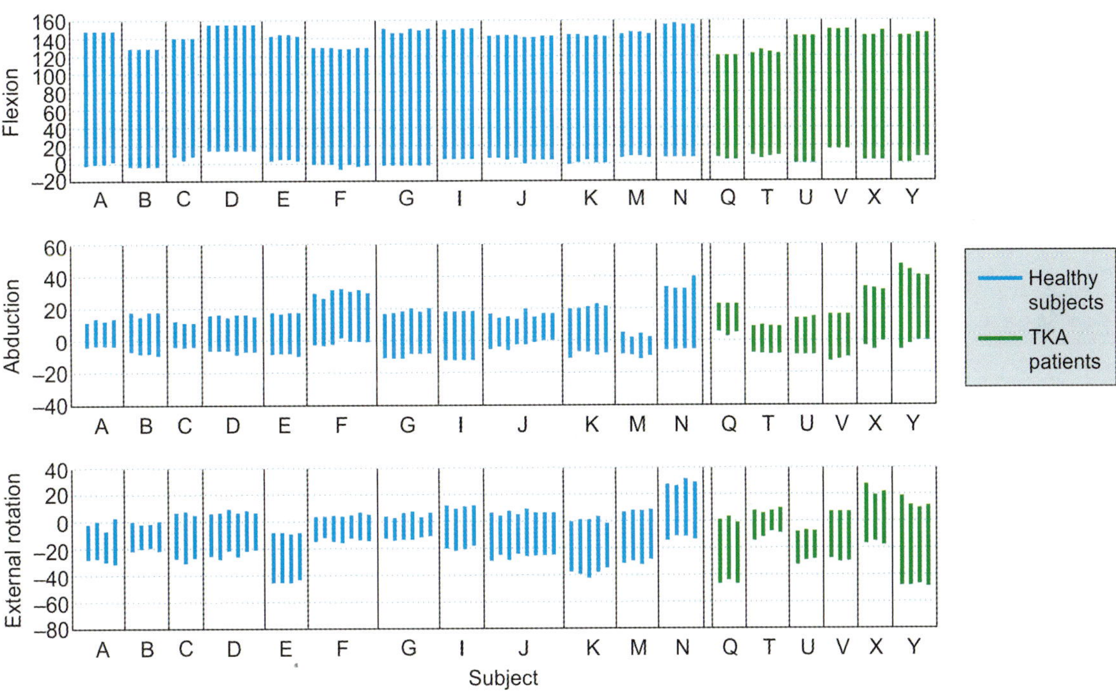

Figure 11.7C

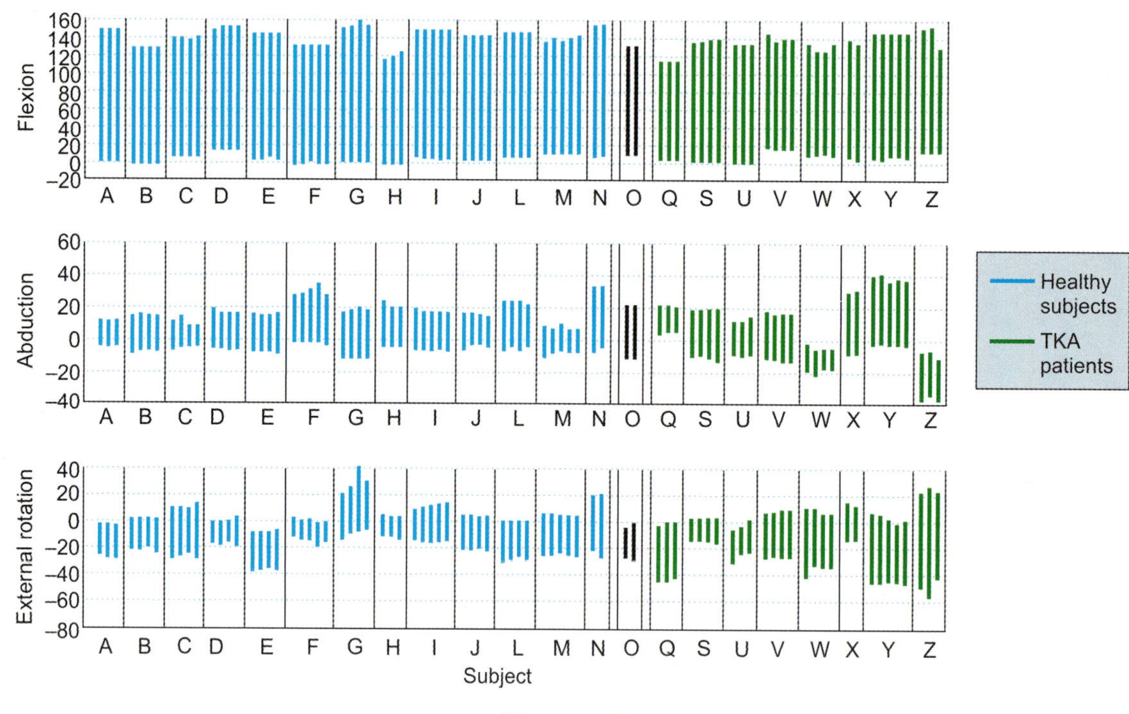

Figure 11.7D

Figures 11.7A to D (A) Individual squatting trials; (B) Individual SCL trials; (C) Individual kneeling trials; (D) Individual prayer trials

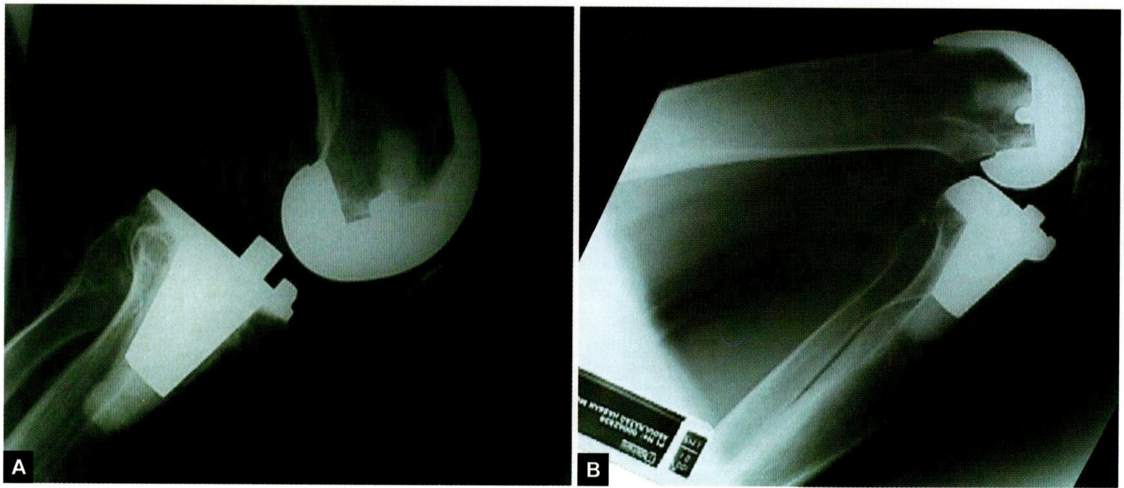

Figures 11.8A and B Mobile-bearing total knee replacement showing dislocation of the components reduced closed

(**Figures 11.8A and B**). In our series that we have presented at the American Academy meeting, we confirmed having total of a three knee dislocation all of which were for patients with gross deformity preoperatively and they needed extensive soft tissue release intraoperatively and were not preceded by trauma. Our fixed-bearing group had zero dislocation. In another words, the using of mobile-bearing has the same complication rate as compared to fixed-bearing except for knee dislocation which could happen and the surgeon has to accept some higher risk incidence in the mobile-bearing. This incidence of dislocation in the mobile-bearing group for gross deformity patients has added one selective criterion for not using the mobile-bearing in patients with preoperative gross deformity. Our current practice at this point is to use mobile only in active patients with body mass index of less than 30 and who have full flexion preoperatively. Patients who have a high flexion pre-operatively, can benefit greatly from the mobile-bearing and they are usually much happier with their activity of daily living. Our practice at this point is to limit mobile- bearing knees to these patients and intraoperatively focus on perfect soft tissue balance. Also it has been very helpful to us in our practice to use the LPS which has the freedom to go between fixed and mobile-bearing intraoperatively even after femoral and tibial preparation so the decision to choose between mobile and fixed-bearing is left to the surgeon according to the situation of the soft tissue sleeve and the soft tissue release to be performed.

CONCLUSION

The mobile-bearing TKA has limitations and will probably never duplicate physiological knee function. Even though the rotational platform accedes for greater conformity of the articular surfaces to reduce contact stresses, the artificial materials cannot duplicate the complex properties of shock absorption of the viscoelastic meniscus. Failure and dislocation of the bearing still remains a concern and the prospect of durable TKA in younger patients a galvanizing challenge.

REFERENCES

1. *info@ancient.wisdom.co.uk*
2. *E.How.com*
3. Introduction, meniscal bearing knee replacement—John N Insall, Paola Aglietti, A Baldini Mark E Easley, Surgery of the Knee, 3rd edn, Insall and Scott, Churchill Livingstone, Philadelphia.
4. Introduction, Mobile Bearing Concept in Knee Arthroplasty, Nahum Rosemberg, Aarnan greentala and Michael Soudry, Orthopedic surgery "A" Dept., Rambam - Health Care Campus, Haifa Ruth and Bruce Rappaport Faculty of Medicine, Technion – Israel Institute of Technology, Haifa Israel.
5. Dennis DA, Komistek RD, Kim RH, Sharma A. Gap balancing versus measured resection technique for total knee arthroplasty. Clin Orthop Relat Res. 2010;468:102-7.
6. Bartel DL, Bicknell VL, Wright TM. The effect of conformity, thickness, and material on stresses in ultra-high molecular weight components for total joint replacement. J Bone Joint Surg Am. 1986;68(7):1041-51.
7. Rose RM, Goldfarb HV, Ellis E, Crugnola AM. On the pressure dependence of the wear of ultra-high molecular weight polyethylene. Wear. 1980.pp.181-3, 250-7.
8. Matsuda S, White SE, Williams VG 2nd, McCarthy DS, Whiteside LA. Contact stress analysis in meniscal bearing total knee arthroplasty. J Arthroplasty. 1998;13(6):699-706.
9. Stukenborg-Colsman C, Ostermeier S, Hurschler C, Wirth CJ. Tibiofemoral contact stress after total knee arthroplasty: comparison of fixed and mobile-bearing inlay designs. Acta Orthop Scand. 2002;73(6):638-46.
10. Cheng CK, Huang CH, Liau JJ, Huang CH. The influence of surgical malalignment on the contact pressures of fixed and mobile bearing knee prostheses: a biomechanical study. Clin Biomech. 2003;18:231-6.
11. Dennis DA, Komistek RD, Mahfouz MR, et al. Multicenter determination of *in vivo* kinematics after total knee arthroplasty. Clin Orthop Relat Res. 2003;416:37-57.
12. Stiehl JB, Dennis DA, Komistek RD, et al. *In vivo* kinematic analysis of a mobile bearing total knee prosthesis. Clin Orthop Relat Res. 1997;345:60-6.
13. Bartel DL, Bicknell VL, Ithaca MS, et al. The effect of conformity, thickness and material on stresses in ultra-high molecular weight components for total joint replacement. J Bone Joint Surg Am. 1986;68:1041-51.
14. D'Lima DD, Chen PC, Colwell Jr CW. Polyethylene contact stress, articular congruity, and knee alignment. Clin Orthop Relat Res. 2001;392:232-8.
15. Liau JJ, Cheng CK, Huang CH, et al. The effect of malalignment on stresses in polyethylene component of total knee prostheses—a finite element analysis. Clin Biomech. 2002;17:140-6.
16. Scuderi GR, Komistek RD, Dennis DA, et al. The impact of femoral component rotational alignment on condylar lift-off. Clin Orthop Relat Res. 2003;410:148-54.

17. Sharma A, Komistek RD, Ranawat CS, et al. *In vivo* contact pressures in total knee arthroplasty. J Arthroplasty 2007;22:404-16.
18. Blunn GW, Walker PS, Joshi A, et al. The dominance of cyclic sliding in producing wear in total knee replacements. Clin Orthop Relat Res. 1991;273:253-60.
19. Greenwald AS, Heim CS. Mobile-bearing knee systems: ultra-high molecular weight polyethylene wear and design issues. Instr Course Lect. 2005;54:195-205.
20. Otto JK, Callaghan JJ, Brown TD. Gait cycle finite element comparison of rotating-platform total knee designs. Clin Orthop Relat Res. 2003;410:181-8.
21. Stukenborg-Coleman C, Ostermeier S, Hurschler C, et al. Tibiofemoral contact stress after total knee arthroplasty: comparison of fixed and mobile-bearing inlay designs. Acta Orthop Scand. 2002;73:638-46.
22. Bartel DL, Rawlinson JJ, Burstein AH, et al. Stresses in polyethylene components of contemporary total knee replacements. Clin Orthop Relat Res. 1995;317:76-82.
23. Miller GJ, Petty W, Goll C. Congruency and varus/valgus loading effect on prosthetic knee contact stress. Presented at the Combined Orthopaedic Research Society Meeting, San Diego, Calif, 1995.
24. Otto JK, Callaghan JJ, Brown TD. Mobility and contact mechanics of a rotating platform total knee arthroplasty. Clin Orthop Relat Res. 2001;392:24-37.
25. McNulty D, Swope SW, Auger DD, Smith T. The effect of crosslinking UHMWPE on *in vitro* wear rates of fixed and mobile bearing knees. Presented at the ASTM Symposium on Crosslinked and Thermally Treated UHMWPE for TJR, 2002.
26. McEwen HM, Barnett PI, Bell CJ, et al. The influence of design, materials and kinematics on the *in vitro* wear of total knee replacements. J Biomech. 2005;38:357-65.
27. Dennis DA, Komistek RD, Mahfouz MR, et al. Mobile-bearing total knee arthroplasty: do the polyethylene bearings rotate? Clin Orthop Relat Res. 2005;440:88-95.
28. Komistek RD, Dennis DA, Mahfouz MR, et al. *In vivo* polyethylene-bearing mobility is maintained in posterior stabilized total knee arthroplasty. Clin Orthop Relat Res. 2004;428:207-13.
29. D'Lima DD, Trice M, Urquhart AG, et al. Tibiofemoral conformity and kinematics of rotating-bearing knee prostheses. Clin Orthop Relat Res. 2001;386:235-42.
30. Yang CC, McFadden LA, Dennis DA, et al. Lateral retinacular release rates in mobile-versus fixed-bearing TKA. Clin Orthop Relat Res. 2008;466:2656-61.
31. Dennis DA, Komistek RD, Mahfouz MR, et al. A multicenter analysis of axial femorotibial rotation following total knee arthroplasty. Clin Orthop Relat Res. 2004;428:180-9.
32. Puloski SKT, McCalden RW, MacDonald SJ, et al. Tibial post wear in posterior stabilized total knee arthroplasty. J Bone Joint Surg Am. 2001;83:390-7.
33. Engh GA, Lounici S, Rao AR, et al. *In vivo* deterioration of tibial baseplate locking mechanisms in modular total knee components. J Bone Joint Surg Am. 2001;83:1660-5.
34. Rao AR, Engh GA, Collier MB, et al. Tibial interface wear in retrieved total knee components and correlations with modular insert motion. J Bone Joint Surg Am. 2002;89:1849-55.
35. Wasielewski RC, Parks N, Williams I, et al. Tibial insert undersurface as a contributing source of polyethylene wear debris. Clin Orthop Relat Res. 1997;345:53-9.
36. Huang CH, Ma HM, Liau JJ, et al. Late dislocation of rotating platform in New Jersey low-contact stress knee prosthesis. Clin Orthop Relat Res. 2002;405:189-94.
37. Huang CH, Ma HM, Liau JJ, et al. Osteolysis in failed total knee arthroplasty: a comparison of mobile-bearing and fixed-bearing knees. J Bone Joint Surg Am. 2002;84:2224-9.
38. McNulty DE, Liau YS, Haas BD. The influence of sterilization method on wear performance of the low contact stress total knee system. Orthopaedics. 2002;25:243-6.
39. Pooley C, Tabor D. Friction and molecular structure: the behavior of some thermoplastics. Proc R Soc Lond. 1972;3A29:251.
40. Jones VC, Barton DC, Fitzpatrick DP, et al. An experimental model of tibial counterface polyethylene wear in mobile bearing knees: the influence of design and kinematics. Biomed Mater Eng. 1999;9:189-96.
41. Murray DW, Goodfellow JW, O'Connor JJ. The Oxford unicompartmental arthroplasty: a ten-year survival study. J Bone Joint Surg Br. 1998;80:983-9.
42. Fisher J, McEwen H, Tipper J et al. Wear-simulation analysis of rotating-platform mobile-bearing knees. Orthopedics. 2006;29(Suppl):S36-S41.
43. Jennings LM, Galvin AL, McEwen HM, Fisher J. The influence of design on the wear of mobile bearing total knee replacements. ORS poster no. 2002. Presented at the

54th Annual Meeting of the Orthopaedic Research Society, San Francisco, March 2–5, 2008.

44. Duffy PJ, Phillipson AP. Long-term results of the accord total knee replacement in the Countess of Chester Hospital. Knee. 2000;7(3):175-8. PubMed PMID: 10927212.
45. Kaper BP, Smith PN, Bourne RB, Rorabeck CH, Robertson D. Medium-term results of a mobile bearing total knee replacement. Clin Orthop Relat Res. 1999;(367):201-9. PubMed PMID: 10546616.
46. Morgan-Jones RL, Roger GJ, Solis G, Parish EN, Cross MJ. Meniscal bearing uncemented total knee arthroplasty: early clinical results at a minimum 2-year review. J Arthroplasty. 2003;18(1):41-4. PubMed PMID: 12555181.
47. Polyzoides AJ, Dendrinos GK, Tsakonas H. The Rotaglide total knee arthroplasty. Prosthesis design and early results. J Arthroplasty. 1996;11(4):453-9. PubMed PMID: 8792253.
48. Callaghan JJ, Wells CW, Liu SS, Goetz DD, Johnston RC. Cemented rotating-platform total knee replacement: a concise follow-up, at a minimum of twenty years, of a previous report. J Bone Joint Surg Am. 2010;92(7):1635-9. doi: 10.2106/JBJS.I.01012. PubMed PMID: 20595570.
49. Grodzki T, Haak H, Behrendt R, Merk H, Krauspe R. Prospective randomized comparative study of early functional outcome of 2 knee joint endoprosthesis systems--rotation plateau versus fixed polyethylene inlay. Z Orthop Ihre Grenzgeb. 2001;139(5):393-6.
50. Bert JM. Dislocation/subluxation of meniscal bearing elements after New Jersey low-contact stress total knee arthroplasty. Clin Orthop Relat Res. 1990;254:211-5. PubMed PMID: 2323133.
51. Hartford JM, Hunt T, Kaufer H. Low contact stress mobile bearing total knee arthroplasty: results at 5 to 13 years. J Arthroplasty. 2001;16(8):977-83. PubMed PMID: 11740751.
52. Shaw JA. The definitive answer: fixed-bearing versus mobile-bearing TKA: commentary on an article by Young-Hoo Kim, MD, et al. Long-term comparison of fixed-bearing and mobile-bearing total knee replacements in patients younger than fifty-one years of age with osteoarthritis. J Bone Joint Surg Am. 2012;94(10):e69. doi: 10.2106/JBJS.K.01725. PubMed PMID: 22617935.
53. Buechel FF Sr, Buechel FF Jr, Pappas MJ, D'Alessio J. Twenty-year evaluation of meniscal bearing and rotating platform knee replacements. Clin Orthop Relat Res. 2001; 388:41-50.
54. Buechel FF, Pappas MJ. New Jersey low contact stress knee replacement system. Ten-year evaluation of meniscal bearings. Orthop Clin North Am. 1989;20(2):147-77. Erratum in: Orthop Clin North Am. 1989;20(4):preceding 519. PubMed PMID: 2922189.
55. Stiehl JB, Hamelynck KJ, Voorhorst PE. International multi-centre survivorship analysis of mobile bearing total knee arthroplasty. Int Orthop. 2006;30(3):190-9. Epub 2006 Mar 18. PubMed PMID: 16547718; PubMed Central PMCID: PMC2532087.

Chapter 12

Patellar Resurfacing in Total Knee Arthroplasty

Alfred J Tria Jr, William Baione, Brian Culp

INTRODUCTION

Resurfacing of the patella as a part of the total knee arthroplasty (TKA) has been a controversial topic since its inception in 1974.[1] It was first introduced as an answer to the residual anterior knee pain (AKP) that patients experienced with the earliest TKA designs that failed to account for the symptoms generated by patellofemoral joint arthritis.[2] Acknowledgment of the role of patellofemoral disease led to the development of a prosthesis that aimed to replace the worn patellar articular surface.[3]

Patellar resurfacing was well supported in the early 1980s as an adjunct to knee arthroplasty because it appeared to appropriately address the issue of AKP and it essentially completed the 'total' knee replacement by offering a solution to tricompartmental disease of the knee.[4,5] As with many new innovations the initial enthusiasm waned with the emergence of numerous patellar resurfacing related complications. These included patellar instability, component failure, component loosening, patellar clunk syndrome, osteonecrosis, patellar fracture, and extensor mechanism rupture.[6-10] The rise in incidence of failures and revisions led many surgeons to question the resurfacing technique and reconsider the indication for its routine use.

Historically, poor outcomes where associated with inadequate implant designs and inferior implantation techniques. Recent advances in prosthetic design and refinement of component insertion techniques has led to an overall decline in the complication rates associated with patellar resurfacing.[11,12] However, many surgeons have opted to avoid resurfacing the patella as a means of reducing the risk of complications.

Patellar resurfacing as a part of TKA still remains controversial. The lack of consensus has led to subdivisions within the international orthopedic community. There are those who always resurface, those that never resurface, and those that selectively resurface the patella during TKA.[13,14] Modern day patellar resurfacing has a very low complication rate and helps to decrease some of the AKP that is often seen in total knee replacements after surgery.

HISTORICAL PERSPECTIVE

In 1955, McKeever proposed an isolated patellar resurfacing.[15] The prosthesis was a metallic device that was screwed into the patellar bed creating a new articular surface to track on the femoral sulcus. The sulcus, itself, was not changed. The early results were encouraging, but a long-term follow-up by Levitt showed deterioration with time.[16] In 1974, Insall, Ranawat and Walker reported on the total condylar knee that included resurfacing of the patella as a standard part of the surgery.[1,2] The dome-shaped polyethylene (PE) prosthesis was designed to articulate with the metallic femoral sulcus and offered the first 'total' knee resurfacing to address the AKP associated with early TKAs.

During the course of the 1980s, most of the development for the TKA was directed at the femoral tibial articulation with little change for the patella. The early femoral components were symmetric with no consideration for a right versus left design and had shallow trochlear grooves that often led to maltracking of the patella. The introduction of cementless designs led to metal backing with porous coating for the patellar PE.[17,18] This allowed bony ingrowth, but limited the available thickness for the PE. The combination of thinner PE and lateral tracking exposed the patellar button to large forces at the location where it was thinnest. The early wear exposed the metal skeleton and the metal-on-metal articulation produced debris, synovitis, and destruction of components.[19-21] Revision of the patella was difficult if bony ingrowth was good and it often led to fracture of the underlying bed, further compromising the result.[12]

The posterior cruciate substituting knee arthroplasties were initially designed with a deep box on the femoral side to accommodate the post.[22] The resurfaced patella could develop a scar tissue around its superior rim that could catch in the femoral box as the knee moved from flexion to extension producing a visible and sometimes audible 'clunk.'[8,23]

Lateral retinacular releases to address patellar maltracking were very common and led to a significant incidence of avascular necrosis of the underlying patellar bed.[24,25] Fracture was often thought to be a result of the division of the superior lateral geniculate vessel during a lateral release that compromised the remaining blood supply to the patella after the standard medial arthrotomy.[26-29] Conventional surgical approaches for TKA include the medial parapatellar approach and straight arthrotomy. Several surgical approaches have been developed in an attempt to decrease devascularization of the patella and enhance tracking. Subvastus and midvastus arthrotomies preserve the superomedial blood supply to the patella. Some series have demonstrated a relationship between avascularity and fracture, while others have failed to do so. There is no evidence that patellar tracking is superior with either of these approaches.

The issues of metal backing, patellar clunk, and avascular necrosis brought disfavor upon patellar resurfacing. The concept of the 'total' knee resurfacing was brought into question and the argument remains similar up to this date.

COMPONENT DESIGNS

There are many anatomic and mechanical factors that influence patellofemoral kinematics and they are not merely limited to the patellar surface. The patellofemoral articulation is exposed to stresses as high as 20× body weight.[30] The patellar contact with the femur varies with the position of the knee. The patella contact area is small and distal in early flexion, and increases in area and progresses proximally throughout increasing flexion. The maximal patellofemoral contact occurs at 120° of flexion.[31] When these high patellofemoral loads are paired with small patellofemoral contact areas the resultant high stresses indicate the need for caution in the design and development of a patellofemoral component for total joint replacement.[32]

Increased patellofemoral complications and extensor mechanism failures raised awareness of the shortcomings of the available knee components that failed to provide for normal patellofemoral function. Modern prostheses were designed to incorporate the patella in a way that reduced contact stress between them, so that they interacted like normal patellofemoral joints, consequently reducing postoperative AKP. Many femoral component alterations were designed to be 'patella-friendly'; improving function as well as patient satisfaction. These designs allowed the patella to articulate with the femoral component throughout the whole range of flexion and spread the forces out more equally across the surface to avoid edge wear.[2] Whiteside used an experimental model to demonstrate that specific femoral design changes including deepening and distal extension of the trochlea groove improved patella tracking compared with an unmodified femoral component.[33] Prostheses related factors play an important role in the success of a TKA.

Changes to the femoral component design have had a profound effect on the success and performance of the patella in TKA regardless of resurfacing. Theiss noted a fourteen fold decrease in patella-related complications when using a patella-friendly design with an extended anterior flange, and a deeper and wider trochlea groove.[34] The more proximal capture of the patella in a deeper groove with more gradual proximal-to-distal transition appeared advantageous in reducing patella morbidity. The box of the femoral component for the posterior stabilized knees was modified by shallowing it out and the sulcus was shaped to blend more with the superior aspect of the box to avoid the patellar clunk. The proximal extent of the anterior flange minimized the chance that the patella could ride off the implant proximally in terminal extension. Changing the shape of the lateral femoral flange from a linear design to a more curved one helped to improve patellar tracking and congruence; especially for the anatomic nonresurfaced patellas.[35,36] Alterations to the height and shape of the anterior femoral flange in nonanatomic patellar trochlear grooves improved stability and tracking of the patellar buttons. Abrupt changes in sagittal radius of the trochlea have been shown to create abnormal patellar kinematics and increase the risk of patellar maltracking.[12] This may account for the reported increase in AKP in nonresurfaced patellae with patella 'unfriendly' femoral components.

There are two basic patellar implant designs—inlay or onlay buttons. The inlay design has the proposed benefit of better shear stress resistance and a smaller reduction in patellar strength because there is less bone removal. The onlay designs can be all PE or metal backed to allow for bony ingrowth. Metal backing was mostly abandoned due to mixed results and cementless designs became much less common.[18,19,37] The second generation metal-backed mobile bearing patellar implant with anatomic facets theoretically improved tracking and contact stress, but implantation techniques are more challenging and revision of these implants has a high risk of fracture. Longevity of cemented all PE patellar buttons has been surprisingly good.[9,38] The three post design is favored over the single large central post to reduce the stress riser in the center of patella with less intraosseous vascular disruption and risk of fracture.[39] However, there is a risk of fatigue failure and peg fracture with the three-peg design. Most current femoral components, however, present a surface geometry designed to articulate with a designated patellar component (domed, offset, mobile bearing, and anatomic), but are not equipped to accommodate the native patella.

Despite these advances and modifications to the TKA components to improve patellofemoral resurfacing outcomes, it is very important to stress surgical technique and to avoid implant malpositioning. Malrotation of components is often the root of most patellar complications and careful attention to rotation will produce a centrally tracking patella with low risk for fracture, wear, or loosening.

Surgical Techniques

The surgical techniques have been improved to address the problems of patellar fracture, patellar wear, patellar clunk, and patellofemoral pain. The goals of the patellar resurfacing include preservation of blood supply, appropriate component positioning, restoration of the patellar thickness and tilt, and balanced soft tissues to allow for central patellar tracking.[40,41]

Adequate exposure is important in all aspects of orthopedic surgery. Removal of the patellar fat pad expedites the exposure and does not affect the blood supply to the patellar bed.[42] All of the facets should be clearly visualized; however, all of the soft tissues around the patellar margin should not be removed in order to preserve the circular ring of blood vessels.[25,43] The synovium above the patella along the quadriceps tendon should be removed to eliminate any opportunity for a patellar clunk. While it is entirely possible to cut the patellar surface by freehand or by 'eye,' instruments make the procedure more precise.

Onlay Technique

The onlay surgical technique removes the bone from the surface of the patella and places the implant directly onto the newly created surface (**Figure 12.1**). The thickness of the resurfaced patella remains controversial with some surgeons recommending a reduction in the thickness by 2 mm and others recommending maintenance of the original measurement or even an increase by 2 mm. The average thickness of the male patella is 25 mm and the female patella is 22 mm. The goal of measuring and cutting is to maintain the anatomical thickness. A caliper is used to measure the central patellar thickness. There is general agreement that the remaining patellar bone should not be reduced below 10–12 mm to avoid fracture of the remaining bone given the high mechanical pressures it is subjected to.[44] In the case of a thin and sclerotic patella, it may be advisable to avoid patellar resurfacing altogether. Under resection or a thick button can lead to 'overstuffing' of the patellofemoral joint. The increased thickness elevates the patella away from the sulcus of the femur and increases the joint reactive forces resulting in decreased knee flexion and AKP.[45]

The resection of the patella should leave the remaining bed with a symmetric surface through all areas. Excess tilt of the surface cut or a 'facetized' resurfacing should be avoided, and the goal should be a flat cut. This common error occurs when equal amounts of bone are resected from both facets. The medial facet is usually thicker than the lateral facet, so taking too much bone from the lateral facet creates an abnormal tilt to the patella. Tilting the cut may lead to abnormal wear or tracking. If the patella is placed on only the medial or lateral facet because the exposure is inadequate, the tracking and thickness will again be affected. A good technique to avoid this is to 'under-resect' the lateral facet, removing only subchondral bone, and continuing the cut into the substance of the medial facet.

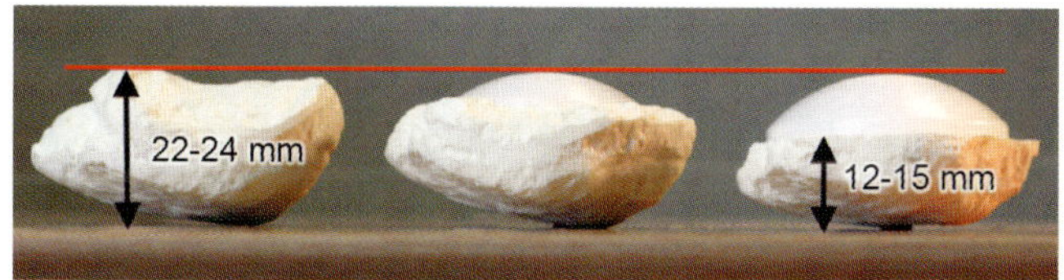

Figure 12.1 Patellar thickness measurement with the inlay technique in the middle and the onlay technique on the right (with permission from Insall and Scott, Surgery of the Knee, Chapter 113, 'Patellar resurfacing in total knee arthroplasty,' figure 113–23, page 1178, Elsevier Publishing, Philadelphia, PA, 2012)

After the patella is resurfaced, the tracking must be evaluated. Evaluating the tracking without touching the patella throughout the range of motion with the medial capsule open (so-called 'no thumbs' technique) is misleading and will contribute to excess use of the lateral release. The normal patella does not track across the front of the femur with the capsule open. It is best to check the tracking either with a slight longitudinal traction force on the quadriceps tendon proximally or with two towel clips holding the medial capsule closed. If the patella stays well in the midline and, then, moves centrally down the sulcus throughout the range of motion, the tracking is normal and does not require any alignment.

If the patella does track laterally with either the longitudinal traction or the towel clip technique, the entire arthroplasty must be re-evaluated. It is extremely important to return to the primary components first before addressing the extensor mechanism. The femoral component must be aligned with the anatomical axes of the femur. The rotation should be confirmed with the epicondylar, anteroposterior, and the posterior condylar axis. The flexion gap technique will also help confirm the femoral positioning but is not as accurate as the anatomic axes. Internal rotation of the femoral component will allow the patella to track or subluxate laterally through the range of motion. The femoral component should be place centrally on the end of the femur; however, if there is a slight variation, the component should be placed more laterally than medially. This adjustment favors the tracking of the patella.

The tibial component must be aligned with the tibial tubercle and not internally rotated. Once again, internal rotation of the tibia will lead to maltracking of the patella as the knee is brought from extension to flexion. The patellar component should cover the entire surface of the patellar bed. Many authors believe that the remaining uncovered bone surfaces encourage increased scar formation with increased crepitation after the operation.[46] If the patellar cut surface is oval and not circular, the component should be positioned medially and slightly superior. Medial placement favors better articulation with the femoral sulcus and superior positioning helps to avoid patella baja with the associated AKP and possible loss of range of overall motion.[34]

If the patella does track laterally and the femur and tibial alignments are normal, it may be necessary to realign the extensor mechanism. The initial balancing of the extensor mechanism begins with release of the lateral capsule, either from inside out or from outside in. Some surgeons try to complete the release of the lateral capsule with preservation of the superolateral geniculate vessel to preserve the blood supply to the patella. This is difficult and not always successful. An alternative described technique is the mesh expansion release which uses multiple stab-like incisions.[47] This helps to maintain the lateral capsule integrity and preserve the lateral geniculate blood supply to the patella. If the lateral release is not sufficient to correct the tracking, if may be necessary to add a proximal realignment or a distal tubercle transfer.

Inlay Technique

This technique is less commonly used and often constitutes the final resurfacing option when the native patella is too small to accommodate the standard onlay resection. The inlay technique drills the original surface to a prespecified remaining thickness (**Figures 12.2A and B**). The position is determined right from the start in terms of medial to lateral and inferior to superior. The goal is to insert the prosthesis so that it is flush with the remaining articular surface bone on the medial and lateral sides.

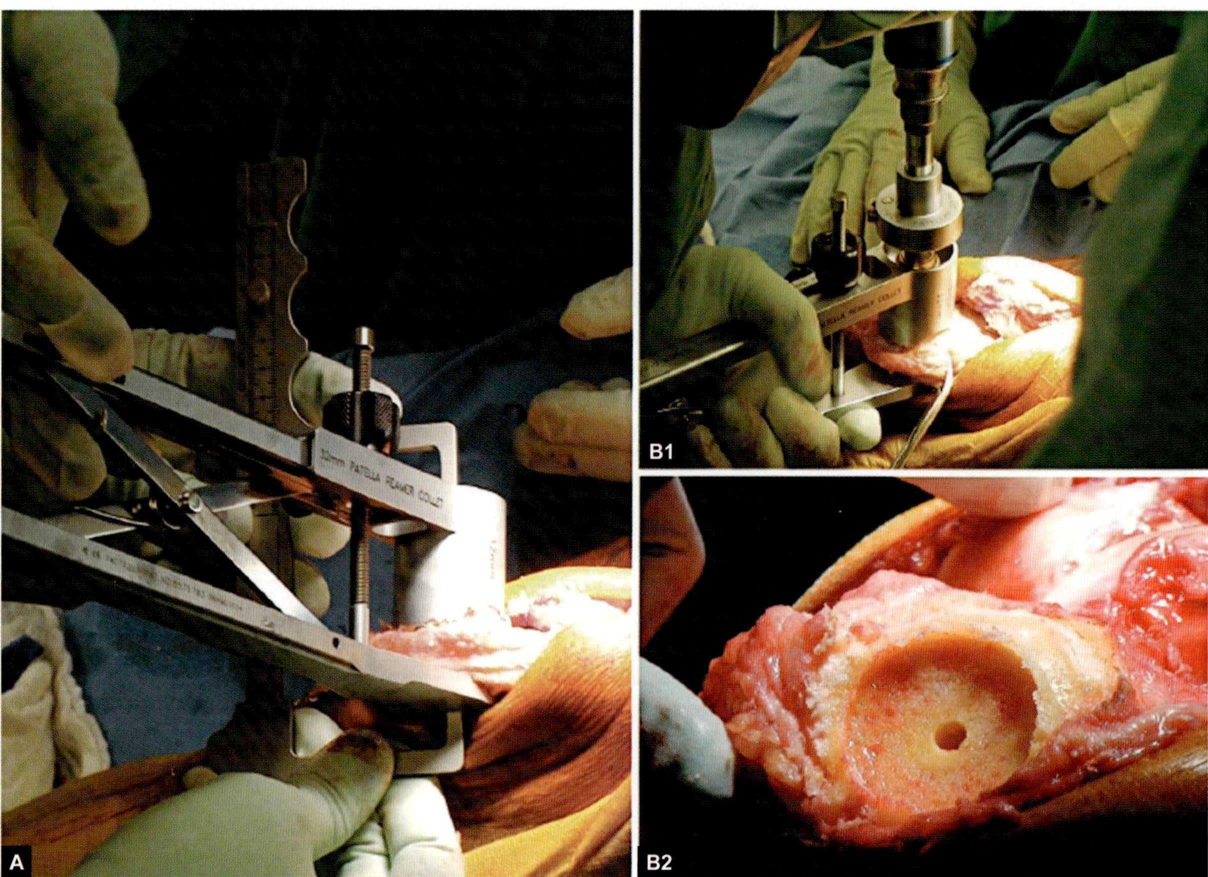

Figures 12.2A and B The inlay technique of inserting the prosthesis into the patella (with permission from Insall and Scott, Surgery of the Knee, Chapter 113, 'Patellar resurfacing in total knee arthroplasty,' figure 113–26, page 1179, Elsevier, Philadelphia, PA, 2012)

The technique aims to reconstitute the same thickness of the patella and to preserve as much bone as possible. The concepts of tracking, balance, and extensor alignment remain the same as with the onlay techniques.

Revision Techniques

As the number of TKAs continues to increase around the world and the replacements continue to age, there will be an ever-increasing number of revisions. While every revision does not necessarily require revision of the patellar component, the surgeon must always be prepared to consider this during the course of a revision. A thorough inspection must be completed before making a final decision. It is not uncommon for the PE surface to appear smooth and completely intact but the underlying bone interface may be invaded secondary to advancing PE disease with hidden loosening. Removal of the all PE patellar component is not difficult and a wide oscillating saw blade will often cut across the base of the pegs and permit simple extraction. If the remaining bone bed is 10 mm or more in thickness, the bone can be resurfaced with care. It is possible to remove one of the three pegs from the standard implant and still obtain good cement fixation with two remaining pegs. The well-fixed metal backed component is a challenge to remove without injuring the underlying bone.[37,48] It is best to have high speed instruments with modified diamond type surfaces to facilitate cutting beneath the metal back.

After removal of the implant, a decision must be made about the remaining bone surface. If the patellar shell of bone is 10 mm or more in thickness, it may be possible to cement a pegged component into the remaining bone. If the bone is thinner than 10 mm, it may be necessary to leave the shell unresurfaced. This may lead to a slight increase in AKP but may represent the only viable solution. The gull wing osteotomy proposed by Vince[49] (**Figures 12.3A and B**) or the patelloplasty proposed by Hanssen[50] (**Figures 12.4A to D**) are alternate solutions for the unresurfaced bone. It is most important to preserve the extensor mechanism at all costs and to confirm its integrity before closing the knee.

Patelloplasty (Tiding Up)

Even if the surgeon chooses not to resurface the patella, there is often a patelloplasty or 'tidy up' procedure performed. Patellar reshaping includes resecting the partial lateral facet of the patella and the osteophytes surrounding the patella, trimming the patella to match the trochlea of the femoral component. In addition, some authors advocate smoothing any fibrillated cartilage and drilling eburnated bone in the patella.[51] Others describe a more extensive preparation that includes a soft tissue release laterally, division

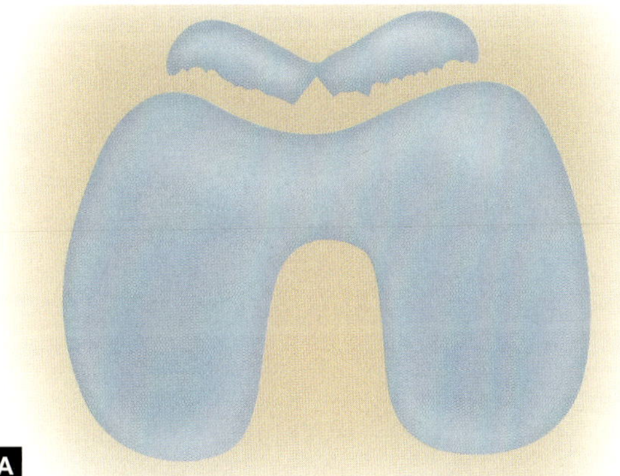

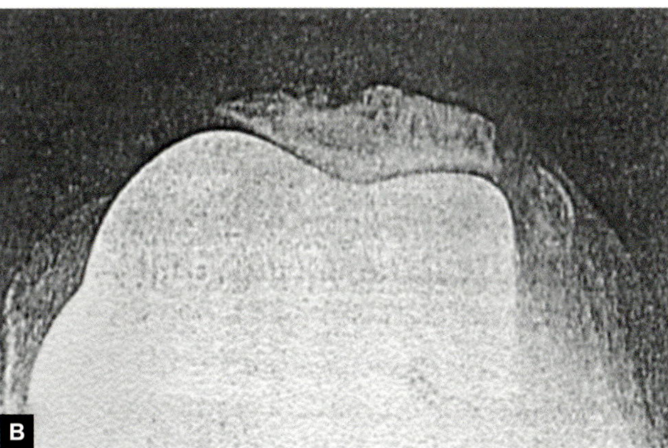

Figures 12.3A and B The gull-wing osteotomy (with permission from Klein GR, Levine HB, Ambrose JF, Lamothe HC, Hartzband MA. Gull-wing osteotomy for the treatment of the deficient patella in revision total knee arthroplasty. J Arthrop. 2010;25(2):252. Elsevier, New York, NY)

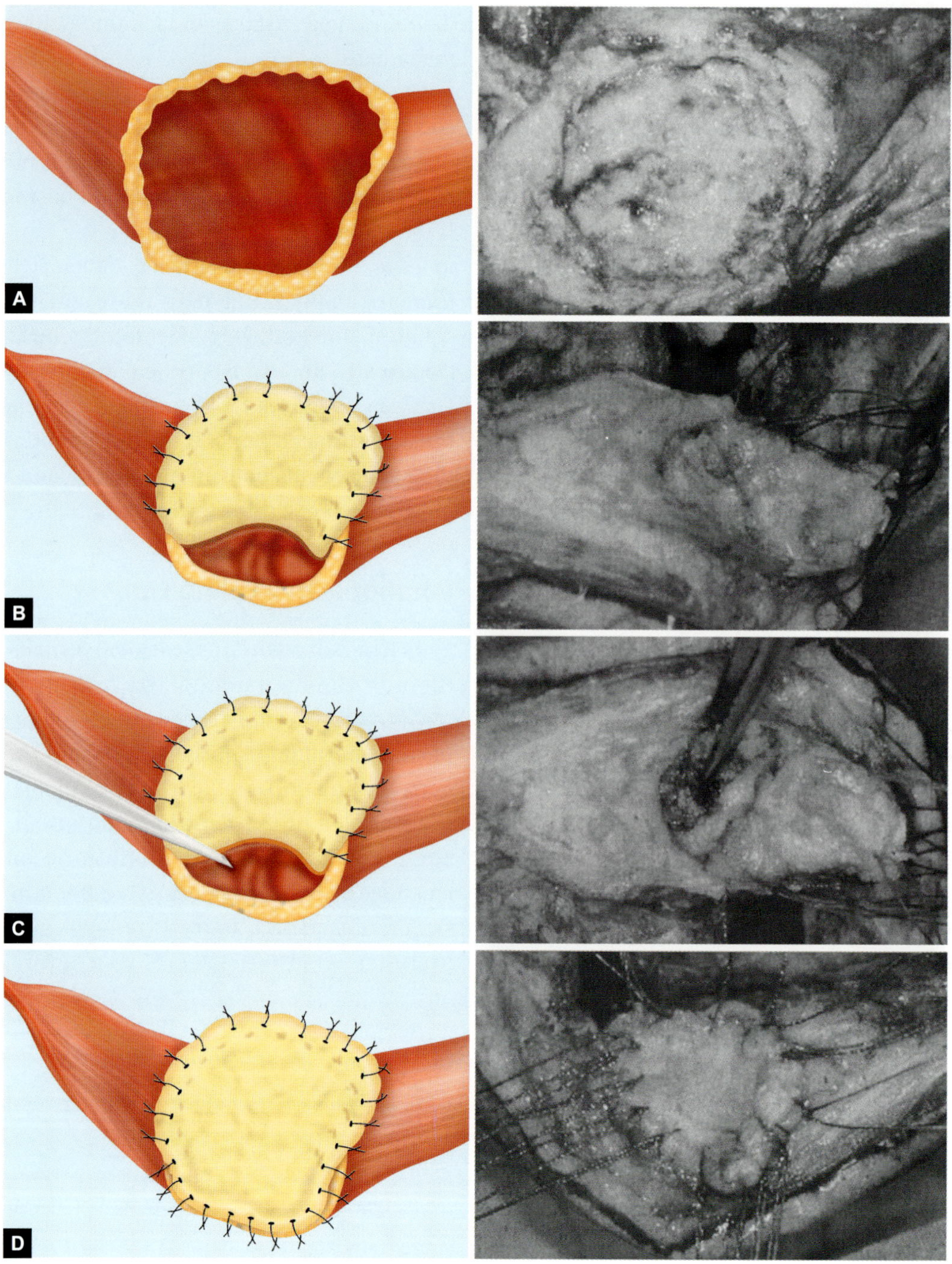

Figures 12.4A to D Patelloplasty to reconstruct the deficient patellar bed in revision TKA (with permission from Hanssen AD. Bone-grafting for severe patellar bone loss during revision total knee arthroplasty. J Bone Joint Surg. 2001;83A,174)

of the patellofemoral ligament, denervation by electrocautery of the patellar rim, and subchondral decompression via drill holes.[52] Prior to component cementing a trial reduction should be performed to assess tracking. If the tracking is unsatisfactory, the primary components should be evaluated first as noted above; and, after that, the extensor mechanism can be rechecked.

COMPLICATIONS

Implant Failure

The PE prosthesis can occasionally fail with fracture of the underlying pegs. This was slightly more common years ago with some of the single peg designs. Revision is not difficult because the base can be cut with a wide oscillating saw blade and a new implant inserted. Some of the mobile bearing designs will have a dissociation of the mobile PE bearing from the underlying metal base. If the base is still normal and the tibiofemoral component rotations are correct, the PE can be replaced. If there is an associated failure of the underlying metal base, the entire prosthesis will need to be removed. In most cases if it is possible to resurface the patella again, the implant will need to be cemented.

Implant Loosening

The rate of loosening of the patellar component with or without displacement is reported to be 0.6–4.8%.[38,53] The patellar implant can loosen over time either as a primary event or as a result of other involvement in the knee. Factors that can lead to loosening include poor remaining bone stock, asymmetric patellar resection, small fixation pegs, inadequate implant fixation, and patellar maltracking secondary to component malalignment, osteonecrosis, and osteolysis secondary to PE wear or infection. It is necessary to make proper diagnosis for the failure and, then, proceed to the revision. The incidence of loosening has decreased significantly since 1990s when most metal backed patellas were withdrawn. Meding reviewed 8531 TKAs and identified the risk factors for patellar loosening. Obesity placed the patella at 6.3x the risk of loosening, followed by lateral release at 3.8x, elevated joint line at 2.2x, and flexion greater than 100° at 2.1x.[38] The thickness of the patella combination should be evaluated in case there has been a great increase in the thickness with the resurfacing. Such an increase will lead to 'over stuffing' of the patellofemoral joint with subsequent increased pressure leading to wear or loosening along with a decrease in the range of motion. The shape of the patellar surface has been improved to articulate better with the underlying femoral sulcus.[17] Recognition of the detrimental effects of gamma sterilization techniques in air and shelf life affecting poststerilization oxidation and degradation has also improved outcomes.

Patella Fracture (Osteonecrosis)

Fracture of the patella can occur during the course of resurfacing or it may present as a finding much later after the surgery. If it occurs during the surgical procedure, the key factor is to confirm that the extensor mechanism of the knee is intact. A transverse fracture can lead to compromise of extension and requires internal fixation with screws or wires. If there is doubt about the quality of the fracture fixation, a tibial bolt with a cerclage wire above the proximal pole of the patella should be incorporated for additional protection.

A nontraumatic, late fracture of the resurfaced patella is usually a result of avascular necrosis (**Figures 12.5A and B**). The patient will present with gradually increasing AKP associated with motion of the knee. The pain does not typically appear acutely. The fracture may be difficult to visualize in some cases and a technetium bone scan can often be helpful to confirm the diagnosis. Early surgery can be fraught with difficulty because the remaining bone will fragment easily. In the majority of cases, the fracture can be treated symptomatically and will heal over a period of six to eight weeks. The patella does tend to fragment slightly through the healing period and will appear to be enlarged on both the AP and lateral X-rays as a result of this process. Sometimes the patient will present with a vague history of AKP over a period of months and the only finding may be the enlarged patellar bed that will suggest the diagnosis of AVN.[29] Occasionally, the implant may break free from the underlying bone and will need to be removed surgically. It is difficult to resurface the remaining patellar bed and probably best to leave it unresurfaced.

Patellar Instability

The patellar tracking can be unstable whether there is resurfacing or not. Patellar instability is the most common reason for secondary revision surgery.[53] Patients' symptoms range from mild discomfort to weakness or the sensation

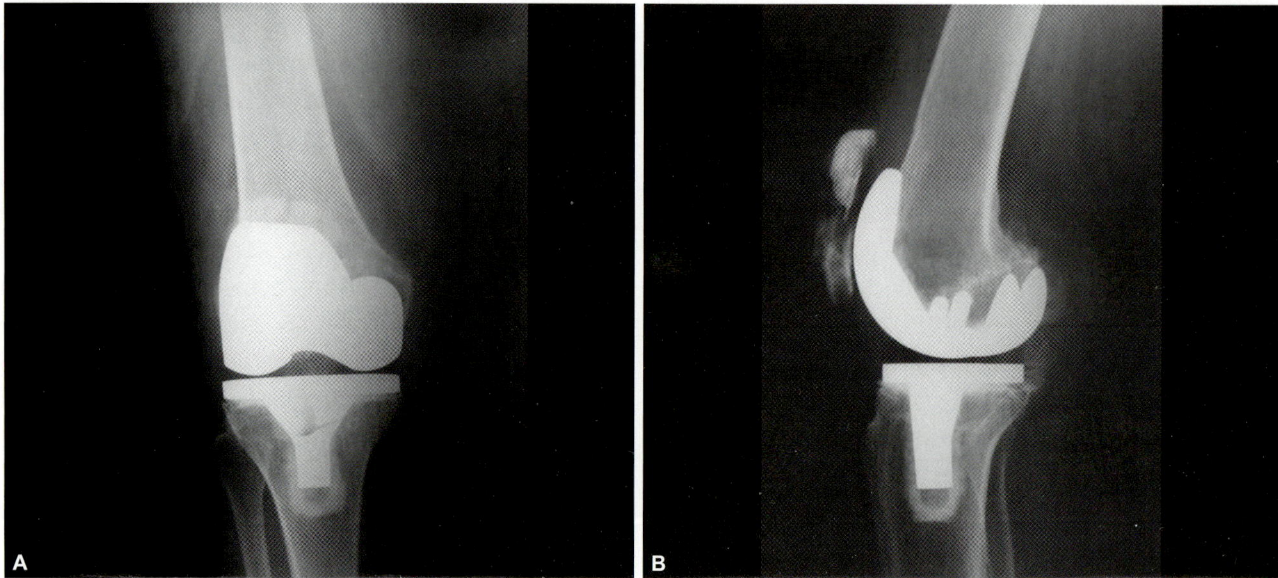

Figures 12.5A and B Lateral X-ray of an avascular patella with a resultant displaced fracture in a patient with no history of trauma

of locking or giving way. The entire arthroplasty should be evaluated to identify factors that contribute to instability before the extensor mechanism is modified. It is important to rule out internal rotation of components, residual valgus malalignment of the leg, a medially translated femoral component, asymmetric patellar button placement or resection, or soft tissue imbalancing. In the absence of these factors a lateral patellar retinacular release is considered (with lateral advancement of the vastus medialis obliquus muscle) or tibial tubercle transfers have been used. Surgical procedures on the patellar tendon itself may risk rupture of the extensor mechanism.[54]

Extensor Mechanism Disruption

During the course of patellar resurfacing, the extensor mechanism can be placed under tension. Excessive retraction may lead to avulsion of the insertion into the tibial tubercle or to fracture of the remaining patellar bed. Patellar tendon disruption associated with TKA is an uncommon, but potentially disastrous complication. Repair with isolated suture fixation is insufficient, and autograft and allograft tendon reconstruction techniques have variable results.[55,56] Repositioning the avulsed tendon at the tubercle with simple sutures or staples is often inadequate and must be augmented with a bolt and wire technique or with the semitendinosus tendon. The wire or the tendon must be brought around the superior pole of the patella and attached to the tibia on either side of the tubercle to protect the primary repair. Tejwani found that there were no significant differences with regard to outcome when he compared the operative treatment of patella fractures with those of quadriceps tendon and patella tendon ruptures.[57]

Patellar Clunk

Patellar clunk is unique to the posterior stabilized designs and occurs from flexion to extension. Scar tissue that forms at the superior pole of the patella catches in the femoral box and snaps out as the patella moves from flexion to extension.[8,23] As the prostheses have been modified, this phenomenon is much less common. The initial treatment is isometric exercises in full extension. If the symptoms persist, arthroscopic synovectomy is effective and usually solves the problem without recurrence.[58,59]

OUTCOMES

The controversy over whether or not to routinely resurface the patella during a TKA has persisted despite three decades of successful joint replacement procedures. Although, historically it was thought by some surgeons that resurfacing of the patella carried with it an unacceptable increase in the risk of patella specific complications with worse outcomes, the recent literature seems to suggest otherwise. Many early studies have tried to address this question, but most were retrospective and nonrandomized. There was often selection bias and it was difficult to compare results with completely different prosthetic designs.

Resurfacing is supported by numerous studies that have shown lower rates of reoperation following TKA. Patellar resurfacing patients have shown high satisfaction and a decreased risk of reoperation with less AKP. One of the largest retrospective comparisons comes from the Swedish knee register that compared resurfaced patellae versus nonresurfaced patellae during primary TKA. Patients seemed to have a higher satisfaction rate with resurfacing regardless of the etiology of arthritis (12,298 for osteoarthritis and 3021 for RA).[60] Many surgeons also argue that the procedure is relatively inexpensive and not time consuming when performed during a standard TKA. Advocates of resurfacing may argue that it is better to address the patella during the primary TKA than to subject the patient to potentially another anesthetic, infection risk and extensive rehabilitation. The articulation between cartilage and metal is considered nonphysiologic,[61] and prolonged exposure to high compressive forces is believed to cause cartilage erosion.

Data from several national registries suggests a diminished revision risk in knees that had primary patellar resurfacing during their index procedure. The 2004 annual report from the Swedish registry showed an increased 10 year cumulative revision rate of 1.4 for nonresurfaced TKAs.[62] Much of the cumulated revision rate was caused by secondary patellar resurfacing. The Australian National Joint Registry showed a similar trend with a 7 year cumulative percent revision rate of 4.7% for nonresurfaced TKAs , compared to 3.8% and an adjusted hazard ratio of 1.32.[63] The proportion of revisions attributable to the resurfaced patella has dropped over the past 25 years from almost 50 % in the 1980s to 12% today. This is largely attributed to changes in prosthetic design and improvement of surgical techniques.

The proponents of nonresurfacing frequently cite the fact that the studies comparing postoperative knee scores after TKA in patella resurfacing and nonresurfacing groups have been inconclusive. Even though there is a slight trend in the overall literature that seems to favor resurfacing, there are clearly patients who are not disadvantaged by leaving the patella nonresurfaced. In addition, surgeons that leave the patella nonresurfaced, cite avoidance of complications that include patellar stress fracture,[10,26,64] avascular necrosis,[24,25,42,65] patellar tendon injury and instability.[10,66] Patients with postoperative pain and a nonresurfaced patella have the option of undergoing the resurfacing as a remedial procedure to address AKP should it arise. The patient with the resurfaced patella and AKP is often treated conservatively with no further intervention.

Isolated patellar component revision for AKP in TKA is associated with some improvement in pain and overall knee scores; however, there is a substantial risk (26% in some series) of secondary revision and further patellofemoral complications.[48] In a 2010 report from the Australian Orthopaedic Association National Joint Replacement Registry, revisions for patellofemoral pain were more common in the nonresurfaced patellae group (17%), than in the resurfaced patellae group (1%), and ‘patella only’ revisions were more common in the nonresurfaced patellae group (29%) than in the resurfaced patellae group (6%). However, 15% of nonresurfaced knees that are revised for patellar resurfacing go on to another revision within 4 years. This seemed to suggest an early beneficial outcome for patella resurfacing at primary arthroplasty based on revision rates up to 5 years. It would, then, appear reasonable to suggest that failure of patients to improve following secondary resurfacing may point to either a multifactorial etiology or a different cause for pain other than a problem pertaining to the patellofemoral joint.

A meta-analysis by Pakos in 2005 included 10 randomized control trials with a minimum follow-up of 1 year. The best quality and largest trials favored patellar resurfacing with a calculated relative risk (RR) of revision

(RR = 0.48)/CI(0.3–0.75) and AKP (RR = 0.40)/CI 0.19–0.85 when the patella was left nonresurfaced. In studies with less than 5 years follow-up, there was no difference between groups.[67] Parvizi looked at 14 randomized and bilateral pseudorandomized control trials of patients with osteoarthritis and rheumatoid arthritis. There was no difference in reoperation between patellar resurfaced and nonresurfaced groups. The resurfaced group had a lower (RR = 0.35)/CI 0.26–0.48 for AKP postoperatively. Knee score improvement remained unchanged between groups.[68] Nizard showed similar results in his analysis of 12 randomized and pseudorandomized control trials with at least 1-year follow-up. The overall risk for patellar-related reoperation was less in the patella resurfaced group with (RR = 0.43)/CI 0.27–0.71. AKP was decreased with patellar resurfacing, (RR = 0.39),CI 0.20–0.75.[69] Fu analyzed 10 trials and showed that the absolute risk of reoperation was reduced by 4% (95%CI, 1–7%) with patellar resurfacing. Quantitative data from seven of the included studies showed that there was no difference between the two groups in terms of AKP.[41,70] Interestingly in Pilling's 2012 meta-analysis of the 16 RCTs that included 3465 TKAs the knee component of the knee society score was significantly higher in the resurfacing group ($p = 0.005$). However, no significant difference was observed for the functional component of the knee society score or for any other reported knee score. There were 93 reported patellofemoral complications in the resurfacing group and 205 in the nonresurfacing group. The resultant rate of reoperation because of AKP ($p = 0.00001$) and the rate of reoperation because of any patellofemoral complication ($p = 0.002$) were significantly higher in the nonresurfaced group. No differences were found in the analyses of the infection rate, operative time, or radiographic appearance.[71]

The debate stems from the lack of clear indications for patellar resurfacing and the avoidance. The natural history of the patella that is left unresurfaced during primary TKA is of central importance in determining if resurfacing is warranted routinely. Shih et al. retrospectively looked at 227 TKAs with patellae left nonresurfaced. At 9 year follow-up 60% had no significant progression of patellofemoral arthritis or maltracking. It was observed that those patients who had preoperative maltracking most often went on to develop progressive symptoms. This raises the question that maybe only these 'higher risk' patients should be resurfaced.[72] Selective patellar resurfacing would be the ideal solution if sound preoperative criteria could be established.

Patient Selection

Some surgeons consider patellar resurfacing as an all or nothing option. They either resurface all of their cases or none, while a smaller percentage of surgeons selectively resurface the patella according to the patient's habitus or the underlying diagnosis. Insall originally suggested that all knees should include patellar resurfacing, but later modified his approach and excluded the knees with an extremely small patella and knees in the markedly obese. The smaller patella may not afford enough thickness to allow for the peg fixation into the underlying bone. The obese patient may subject the patellar surface to exceptionally high forces that may lead to fracture and/or premature wear. Occasionally, the younger patient may present with advanced femorotibial arthritis with minimal involvement of the patellofemoral joint. It may be advisable to leave the patella alone in that setting where the forces across the joint may be higher than in the knee of an older patient.

Commonly accepted indications for patellar resurfacing are rheumatoid arthritis, patellar cysts, hard patellar bone, and loss of congruence between the patella and the trochlear design of the prosthesis. Other indications are patients with osteoarthritis over 65 kg in body weight and those over 160 cm tall.[73] Resurfacing the patella in inflammatory arthritis limits the amount of remaining exposed cartilage in the knee that may act as a source for the autoimmune reaction. Sledge postulated continued release of sequestered antigen as a cause for recurrent pain and inflammation.[74]

Some studies have reported no clinical difference in outcome of resurfaced versus nonresurfaced patellae in TKA based on intraoperative grading of patellar chondromalacia.[75,76] The outerbridge classification of cartilage defects in the patella is commonly used in the literature as a predictive tool for whether or not the patella should be resurfaced.[77] The classification looks at the gross patella: (i) softening and swelling of articular cartilage, (ii) fragmentation and fissuring of articular cartilage affecting an area of <0.5 inches, (iii) Fragmentation and fissuring of articular cartilage affecting an area >0.5 inches, and (iv) cartilage erosion to bone. In a 2009 study from Spain, Rodriguea-Merchan compared two cohorts of patients undergoing TKA. Group A with Outerbridge (i-iii), and Group B Outerbridge (iv) patella, assessed intraoperatively. Then each group was divided in two, where half had the patella resurfaced and half did not. Revision surgery to resurface the patella because of patellar pain was required more often in Group B than Group A ($p = 0.001$). The risk (odds ratio) of needing a revision for patellar, resurfacing resulting from AKP was 21.5 times greater than in Group A.[78]

Bourne formulated a clinical algorithm that took a systematic approach to evaluate whether or not to resurface the patella during TKA. It combined objective patient specific parameters including history, physical exam, intraoperative assessment of the patellar cartilage integrity, congruency, and tracking. If these findings were poor, then a resurfacing could be performed. In addition, if these parameters were good or acceptable then the etiology of disease (inflammatory versus noninflammatory), age, and habitus could also be considered.[79,38] According to the algorithm, patellar resurfacing could be avoided in patients that are younger than 60-years-old with knee osteoarthritis, but without patellofemoral disease on history or examination and intraoperative assessment that shows preserved patellar cartilage on a well articulating and centrally tracking patella. Selective resurfacing appears as an ideal solution, but evidence regarding the validity of selection criteria remains elusive.

CONCLUSION

Patellar resurfacing as a part of TKA still remains controversial. When it comes to the patella during TKA, a surgeon has three options. Always resurface, never resurface and selectively resurface. All options have potential risks and benefits that need to be assessed and balanced based on a surgeon's experience, preference, and patient expectations. Most of the objections to resurfacing are based on earlier complications that have now been addressed and corrected through superior implant design and fixation, better surgical technique, and more anatomical extensor mechanism alignment.

Modern day patellar resurfacing has a very low complication rate and helps to reduce postoperative AKP and effectively reduces the risk of patellar-related secondary revision. However, the surgeon and patient will need to be prepared for potential complications related to the resurfacing itself.

There are instances where it may make sense to leave the patella nonresurfaced; however, the authors believe that these cases are rare and unique in their nature. Based on the evidence to date, it appears that patellar resurfacing is the better option.

REFERENCES

1. Aglietti P, Insall JN, Walker PS, Trent P. A new patella prosthesis. Design and application. Clin Orthop Relat Res. 1975;107:175-87.
2. Ranawat CS, Insall J, Shine J. Duo-condylar knee arthroplasty: hospital for special surgery design. Clin Orthop Relat Res. 1976;120:76-82.
3. Insall J, Tria AJ, Aglietti P. Resurfacing of the patella. J Bone Joint Surg Am. 1980;62(6):933-6.
4. Amstutz HC, Finerman GA. Knee joint replacement-development and evaluation. Clin Orthop Relat Res. 1973;94:24-41.
5. Ranawat CS, Sculco TP. History and development of the total knee prosthesis at the Hospital of Special Surgery. Total Condylar Knee Arthroplasty. 1985.pp.3-6.
6. Ritter MA, Campbell ED. Postoperative patellar complications with or without lateral release during total knee arthroplasty. Clin Orthop Relat Res. 1987;219:163-8.
7. Ritter MA, Pierce MJ, Zhou H, Meding JB, Faris PM, Keating EM. Patellar complications (total knee arthroplasty). Effect of lateral release and thickness. Clin Orthop Relat Res. 1999;367:149-57.
8. Beight JL, Yao B, Hozack WJ, Hearn SL, Booth RE, Jr. The patellar 'clunk' syndrome after posterior stabilized total knee arthroplasty. Clin Orthop Relat Res. 1994;299:139-42.
9. Berend ME, Ritter MA, Keating EM, Faris PM, Crites BM. The failure of all-polyethylene patellar components in total knee replacement. Clin Orthop Relat Res. 2001; 388:105-11.

10. Clayton ML, Thirupathi R. Patellar complications after total condylar arthroplasty. Clin Orthop Relat Res. 1982;170:152-5.
11. Boyd AD, Jr., Ewald FC, Thomas WH, Poss R, Sledge CB. Long-term complications after total knee arthroplasty with or without resurfacing of the patella. J Bone Joint Surg Am. 1993;75(5):674-81.
12. Campbell DG, Mintz AD, Stevenson TM. Early patellofemoral revision following total knee arthroplasty. J Arthrop. 1995;10(3):287-91.
13. Burnett RS, Bourne RB. Indications for patellar resurfacing in total knee arthroplasty. Instr Course lect. 2004;53:167-86.
14. Bourne RB. To resurface the patella or not? Better assessments needed to address the benefits for total knee replacement: commentary on an article by George Pavlou, BSc, MRCS, et al. Patellar resurfacing in total knee arthroplasty: does design matter? A meta-analysis of 7075 cases. J Bone Joint Surg Am. 2011;93(14):e82.
15. McKeever DC. Patellar prosthesis. J Bone Joint Surg Am. 1955;37-A(5):1074-84.
16. Levitt RL. A long-term evaluation of patellar prostheses. Clin Orthop Relat Res. 1973;97:153-7.
17. Hsu HP, Walker PS. Wear and deformation of patellar components in total knee arthroplasty. Clin Orthop Relat Res. 1989;246:260-5.
18. Laskin RS, Bucknell A. The use of metal-backed patellar prostheses in total knee arthroplasty. Clin Orthop Relat Res. 1990;260:52-5.
19. Bayley JC, Scott RD, Ewald FC, Holmes GB, Jr. Failure of the metal-backed patellar component after total knee replacement. J Bone Joint Surg Am. 1988;70(5):668-74.
20. Stulberg SD, Stulberg BN, Hamati Y, Tsao A. Failure mechanisms of metal-backed patellar components. Clin Orthop Relat Res. 1988;236:88-105.
21. Piraino D, Richmond B, Freed H, Belhobek G, Schils J, Stulberg B. Total knee replacement: radiologic findings in failure of porous-coated metal-backed patellar component. AJR Am J Roentgenol. 1990;155(3):555-8.
22. Insall JN, Lachiewicz PF, Burstein AH. The posterior stabilized condylar prosthesis: a modification of the total condylar design. Two to four-year clinical experience. J Bone Joint Surg Am. 1982;64(9):1317-23.
23. Hozack WJ, Rothman RH, Booth RE, Jr., Balderston RA. The patellar clunk syndrome. A complication of posterior stabilized total knee arthroplasty. Clin Orthop Relat Res. 1989;241:203-8.
24. Scuderi G, Scharf SC, Meltzer L, Nisonson B, Scott WN. Evaluation of patella viability after disruption of the arterial circulation. Am J Sports Med. 1987;15(5):490-3.
25. Brick GW, Scott RD. Blood supply to the patella. Significance in total knee arthroplasty. J Arthrop. 1989;4:S75-79.
26. Scott RD, Turoff N, Ewald FC. Stress fracture of the patella following duopatellar total knee arthroplasty with patellar resurfacing. Clin Orthop Relat Res. 1982;170:147-51.
27. Scuderi G, Scharf SC, Meltzer LP, Scott WN. The relationship of lateral releases to patella viability in total knee arthroplasty. J Arthrop. 1987;2(3):209-14.
28. Kayler DE, Lyttle D. Surgical interruption of patellar blood supply by total knee arthroplasty. Clin Orthop Relat Res. 1988;229:221-7.
29. Tria AJ, Jr., Harwood DA, Alicea JA, Cody RP. Patellar fractures in posterior stabilized knee arthroplasties. Clin Orthop Relat Res. 1994;299:131-8.
30. Schindler OS, Scott WN. Basic kinematics and biomechanics of the patello-femoral joint. Part 1: the native patella. Acta Orthop Belg. 2011;77(4):421-31.
31. Hehne HJ. Biomechanics of the patellofemoral joint and its clinical relevance. Clin Orthop Relat Res. 1990;258:73-85.
32. Matthews LS, Sonstegard DA, Henke JA. Load bearing characteristics of the patello-femoral joint. Acta Orthop Scand. 1977;48(5):511-6.
33. Yoshii I, Whiteside LA, Anouchi YS. The effect of patellar button placement and femoral component design on patellar tracking in total knee arthroplasty. Clin Orthop Relat Res. 1992;275:211-9.
34. Theiss SM, Kitziger KJ, Lotke PS, Lotke PA. Component design affecting patellofemoral complications after total knee arthroplasty. Clin Orthop Relat Res. 1996;326:183-7.
35. Hwang BH, Yang IH, Han CD. Comparison of patellar retention versus resurfacing in LCS mobile-bearing total knee arthroplasty. Knee Surg Sports Traumatol Arthrosc. 2012;20(3):524-31.
36. Ma HM, Lu YC, Kwok TG, Ho FY, Huang CY, Huang CH. The effect of the design of the femoral component on the conformity of the patellofemoral joint in total knee replacement. J Bone Joint Surg Br. 2007;89(3):408-12.
37. Milliano MT, Whiteside LA, Kaiser AD, Zwirkoski PA. Evaluation of the effect of the femoral articular surface

material on the wear of a metal-backed patellar component. Clin Orthop Relat Res. 1993;287:178-86.
38. Meding JB, Fish MD, Berend ME, Ritter MA, Keating EM. Predicting patellar failure after total knee arthroplasty. Clin Orthop Relat Res. 2008;466(11):2769-74.
39. Larson CM, McDowell CM, Lachiewicz PF. One-peg versus three-peg patella component fixation in total knee arthroplasty. Clin Orthop Relat Res. 2001; 392:94-100.
40. Pagnano MW KM. The intraoperative assessment of patellar tracking. In: Scuderi GR TAJ (Ed.) Surgical techniques in total knee arthroplasty. New York: Springer; 2002.
41. Liu ZT, Fu PL, Wu HS, Zhu Y. Patellar reshaping versus resurfacing in total knee arthroplasty—Results of a randomized prospective trial at a minimum of 7 years' follow-up. Knee. 2012;19(3):198-202.
42. McMahon MS, Scuderi GR, Glashow JL, Scharf SC, Meltzer LP, Scott WN. Scintigraphic determination of patellar viability after excision of infrapatellar fat pad and/or lateral retinacular release in total knee arthroplasty. Clin Orthop Relat Res. 1990;260:10-6.
43. Scapinelli R. Blood supply of the human patella. Its relation to ischaemic necrosis after fracture. J Bone Joint Surg Br. 1967;49(3):563-70.
44. Reuben JD, McDonald CL, Woodard PL, Hennington LJ. Effect of patella thickness on patella strain following total knee arthroplasty. J Arthrop. 1991;6(3):251-8.
45. Mihalko W, Fishkin Z, Krackow K. Patellofemoral overstuff and its relationship to flexion after total knee arthroplasty. Clin Orthop Relat Res. 2006;449:283-7.
46. Dennis DA. Principles of total knee arthroplasty. Semin Arthrop. 1991;2(1):2-11.
47. Healy WL, Iorio R, Warren P. Mesh expansion release of the lateral patellar retinaculum during total knee arthroplasty. J Bone Joint Surg Am. 2004;86-A(Pt 2):193-200.
48. Berry DJ, Rand JA. Isolated patellar component revision of total knee arthroplasty. Clin Orthop Relat Res. 1993;286:110-5.
49. Klein GR, Levine HB, Ambrose JF, Lamothe HC, Hartzband MA. Gull-wing osteotomy for the treatment of the deficient patella in revision total knee arthroplasty. J Arthroplasty. 2010;25(2):249-53.
50. Parvizi J, Seel MJ, Hanssen AD, Berry DJ, Morrey BF. Patellar component resection arthroplasty for the severely compromised patella. Clin Orthop Relat Res. 2002;397:356-61.
51. Barrack RL, Schrader T, Bertot AJ, Wolfe MW, Myers L. Component rotation and anterior knee pain after total knee arthroplasty. Clin Orthop Relat Res. 2001;392:46-55.
52. Keblish PA, Varma AK, Greenwald AS. Patellar resurfacing or retention in total knee arthroplasty. A prospective study of patients with bilateral replacements. J Bone Joint Surg Br. 1994;76(6):930-7.
53. Brick GW, Scott RD. The patellofemoral component of total knee arthroplasty. Clin Orthop Relat Res. 1988;231: 163-78.
54. Malo M, Vince KG. The unstable patella after total knee arthroplasty: etiology, prevention, and management. J Am Acad Orthop Surg. 2003;11(5):364-71.
55. Roidis N, Varitimidis S, Poultsides L, Liakou P, Karachalios T, Malizos K. A 'biologic technique' for the treatment of a disruption of the extensor mechanism after revision total knee arthroplasty: a case report. Knee Surg Sports Traumatol Arthrosc. 2008;16(7):661-5.
56. Burnett RS, Berger RA, Paprosky WG, Della Valle CJ, Jacobs JJ, Rosenberg AG. Extensor mechanism allograft reconstruction after total knee arthroplasty. A comparison of two techniques. J Bone Joint Surg Am. 2004;86-A(12):2694-9.
57. Tejwani NC, Lekic N, Bechtel C, Montero N, Egol KA. Outcomes after knee joint extensor mechanism disruptions: is it better to fracture the patella or rupture the tendon? J Orthop Trauma. 2012;26(11):648-51.
58. Dajani KA, Stuart MJ, Dahm DL, Levy BA. Arthroscopic treatment of patellar clunk and synovial hyperplasia after total knee arthroplasty. J Arthrop. 2010;25(1):97-103.
59. Lucas TS, DeLuca PF, Nazarian DG, Bartolozzi AR, Booth RE, Jr. Arthroscopic treatment of patellar clunk. Clin Orthop Relat Res. 1999;367:226-9.
60. Robertsson O, Dunbar M, Pehrsson T, Knutson K, Lidgren L. Patient satisfaction after knee arthroplasty: a report on 27,372 knees operated on between 1981 and 1995 in Sweden. Acta Orthop Scand. 2000;71(3):262-7.
61. Forster H, Fisher J. The influence of continuous sliding and subsequent surface wear on the friction of articular cartilage. Proc Inst Mech Eng H. 1999;213(4):329-45.
62. Knutson K, Robertsson O. The Swedish Knee Arthroplasty Register (www.knee.se). Acta Orthop. 2010;81(1):5-7.

63. AJNRR. Australian Arthroplasty Register 2011 Annual Report. http://*www.dmac.adelaide.edu.au/aoanjrr/publications.jsp?section=reports2011*.
64. Grace JN, Sim FH. Fracture of the patella after total knee arthroplasty. Clin Orthop Relat Res. 1988;230:168-75.
65. Ritter MA, Keating EM, Faris PM. Clinical, roentgenographic, and scintigraphic results after interruption of the superior lateral genicular artery during total knee arthroplasty. Clin Orthop Relat Res. 1989;248:145-51.
66. Insall J, Goldberg V, Salvati E. Recurrent dislocation and the high-riding patella. Clin Orthop Relat Res. 1972;88:67-9.
67. Pakos EE, Ntzani EE, Trikalinos TA. Patellar resurfacing in total knee arthroplasty. A meta-analysis. J Bone Joint Surg Am. 2005;87(7):1438-45.
68. Parvizi J, Rapuri VR, Saleh KJ, Kuskowski MA, Sharkey PF, Mont MA. Failure to resurface the patella during total knee arthroplasty may result in more knee pain and secondary surgery. Clin Orthop Relat Res. 2005;438:191-6.
69. Nizard RS, Biau D, Porcher R, et al. A meta-analysis of patellar replacement in total knee arthroplasty. Clin Orthop Relat Res. 2005;432:196-203.
70. Fu Y, Wang G, Fu Q. Patellar resurfacing in total knee arthroplasty for osteoarthritis: a meta-analysis. Knee Surg Sports Traumatol Arthrosc. 2011;19(9):1460-6.
71. Pilling RW, Moulder E, Allgar V, et al. Patellar resurfacing in primary total knee replacement: a meta-analysis. J Bone Joint Surg Am. 2012;94(24):2270-8.
72. Shih HN, Shih LY, Wong YC, Hsu RW. Long-term changes of the nonresurfaced patella after total knee arthroplasty. J Bone Joint Surg Am. 2004;86-A(5):935-9.
73. Lynch AF, Rorabeck CH, Bourne RB. Extensor mechanism complications following total knee arthroplasty. J Arthrop. 1987;2(2):135-40.
74. Sledge CB, Walker PS. Total knee arthroplasty in rheumatoid arthritis. Clin Orthop Relat Res. 1984;182:127-36.
75. Barrack RL, Bertot AJ, Wolfe MW, et al. Patellar resurfacing in total knee arthroplasty. A prospective, randomized, double-blind study with five to seven years of follow-up. J Bone Joint Surg Am. 2001;83-A(9):1376-81.
76. Burnett RS, Haydon CM, Rorabeck CH, Bourne RB. Patella resurfacing versus nonresurfacing in total knee arthroplasty: results of a randomized controlled clinical trial at a minimum of 10 years' followup. Clin Orthop Relat Res. 2004;428:12-25.
77. Outerbridge RE. The etiology of chondromalacia patellae. J Bone Joint Surg Br. 1961;43-B:752-7.
78. Rodriguez-Merchan EC, Gomez-Cardero P. The outerbridge classification predicts the need for patellar resurfacing in TKA. Clin Orthop Relat Res. 2010;468(5):1254-7.
79. Bourne RB, Burnett RS. The consequences of not resurfacing the patella. Clin Orthop Relat Res. 2004;428:166-9.

Chapter 13

Patient-specific Instrumentation in Total Knee Arthroplasty

Francesco Benazzo, Stefano Marco Paolo Rossi, Matteo Ghiara, Alberto Combi

INTRODUCTION

In the last decade, there has been an increasing requirement of developing a system that improves the results following a total knee arthroplasty (TKA). The procedure has a survival rate from 91 to 95% from 15 to 23 years,[1-5] but the rate of satisfaction of the patients reported in literature is between 75% and 89%. Though the technical issue of the surgical instruments has improved considerably, the identification of the surgical reference points for component sizing and positioning can induce some mistakes. It is well demonstrated that adequate patient satisfaction is related to patient expectations, ligament tension, rehabilitative program and component position in the three dimensions. The coronal plane alignment influences the outcome in terms of early loosening and polyethylene wear in case of malalignment (+/– 3°); internal rotation of the femoral and/or tibial component induces patellar instability, pain and stiffness. In the sagittal plane an overstuffing can induce pain and stiffness and an over-resection of the posterior condyles can provoke a midflexion instability. Furthermore, soft tissue impingement of the components can induce pain and undersizing can provoke a subsidence. So, the correct position and the adequate size of the components are crucial to obtain a good outcome. Conventionally, the surgeons utilize intra- or extramedullary rods guide, but in the interest of obtaining better alignment and positioning the industry developed a system that allows saving intraoperative time and increasing precision: patient-specific instrumentation.

PATIENT-SPECIFIC INSTRUMENTATION

The origin of the technique dates back to 1980s[6] with the introduction of the rapid prototyping and the stereolithography, a manufacturing technology that is a process of fusing materials from three-dimensional data. This technology gained success in dental surgery[7] and then was introduced in knee surgery. The PSI involves the use of preoperative advances in imaging techniques: computed tomography (CT) with limited cuts of the hip and the ankle, magnetic resonance imaging (MRI) and full-length radiographs. These images, combined with the rapid prototyping techniques, allow to create 'custom-made' cutting guides; these patient-specific bone resections guides can be used to locate pins of the conventional instrumentation (pinning system) or they can be used to make the cuts by themselves (cutting system). By algorithms specific for every industry the preoperative images allow to create guides that by reproducing specific anatomic landmarks of the knee, assist the surgeon to locate the pins in the three-dimensional position. There are some differences between CT or MRI technique: in a study on ten ovine knees (2008), White et al. demonstrated that CT scans are more predictable of the measurements (however, slightly larger than the real measurements) and the surfaces boundaries of the models generated were smooth, continuous and free from distorting artifacts,[8] but it has the limits of the delineation of the articular cartilage. MRI, on the other hand, gives models that are smaller and less free of distorting artifact.[6] The radiation dose generated by CT is comparable with the dose of the traditional long-leg X-rays, if specific protocols are followed.[9]

Patient-specific instrumentation (PSI) theoretically improves surgical accuracy and reproducibility and reduces the number of operative steps and the number of instrumentation trays. So if each surgical procedure lasts for a lesser time, we have a possible increase in the total number of the surgical interventions, and it means that there is an overall reduction of the costs, despite the cost of the preoperative images (CT or MRI). A review shows that this preoperative study can reduce the surgical procedure by as many as 21 steps and the femoral preparation by 12 steps.[10] Follow-up studies are needed to evaluate the benefit in terms of survivorship of the implant (better position means better and longer outcomes) and the possible effects such as reduction of blood loss and elimination of the fat emboli (no violation of the femoral canal).

SURGICAL TECHNIQUE

The surgery starts much before the skin incision because accurate preoperative planning is very important to achieve good results. The surgeon reviews the plan obtained by radiological images and, when it is needed, (and it is always), he makes the modifications needed. Then patient-specific guides are produced by rapid prototyping technology and carried to the surgical procedure. The sterilization process can be done by the industry or in some cases by the hospital. After the surgical approach preferred by the surgeon, the fabricated guide can be placed on the femur. It is of paramount importance to leave the osteophytes because they are considered in the radiological planning as part of the supporting surface of the guide, to give the orientation of the components, so the removal can produce mistakes in not providing the correct adaptation of the guide to the bone. At this point, the surgeon using the manufactured guide places the pins and checks the distal resection angle, the rotation, the level of resection and the sizes. The distal femoral cuts can be made using the conventional cutting jig or through the slot of the guide. The tibial resection is also made using the customized jig again avoiding the elimination of the osteophytes. The rotation, the slope, and the level of resection are checked before making the cuts. As mentioned before, the procedure allows to save 21 surgical steps.[10] The time saved as well as the cost, are also due to the fact that number of instrumentation and cutting blocks can be minimized by keeping only blocks of the predetermined size.

LITERATURE EVIDENCE

In the literature, there is no agreement in the judgment of this novel technique, because different studies show different results.

In 2012, Ng et al.[11] published the comparison of a series of 105 TKAs performed with PSI (planning made with MRI) with a series of 55 TKAs performed with manual instrumentation showing that the overall mechanical axis passed through the central third of the knee more with PSI guides (88%) rather than with manual instrumentation (78%). Also in the first group, there are less outliers (patient with +/- 3° hip-knee-ankle angle) rather than manual instrumentation, so they concluded that PSI assists in achieving a neutral mechanical axis with reduction in outliers.

In 2013, Chareancholvanich et al.[12] directed a prospective and randomized trial on 80 patients undergoing TKA to evaluate the difference in the mechanical axis deviation in the coronal plane between PSI (planning made by CT) and conventional instrumentation, showing no significant difference in terms of the tibiofemoral angle or femoral component alignment (89.8° versus 90.5°; $p = 0.030$). The author also evaluated the skin incision length, blood loss, blood transfusion and length of the hospital stay, and the results were similar for both groups. The use of PSI reduced slightly the bone cutting time (mean 3.6 minutes) and operative time (5.1 minutes).

In 2013, Victor et al.[13] enrolled 128 patients in a prospective and randomized trial with a planning for PSI based on CT scan. They concluded that not only did PSI not improve accuracy in TKA, but also there were more outliers in terms of coronal tibial alignment and sagittal tibial alignment than the conventional cohort. In the PSI group, there were frequent changes made in the level of the distal femoral and proximal tibial cut and in component size; the authors allocated this fact to the difficulty in assessing resection levels and flexion—extension gaps without clinical information on the patient's ligament status.

In 2013, Issa et al.[14] enrolled a cohort of 84 patients undergoing 89 primary TKAs and showed excellent outcome using preoperative templating with PSI. The plan, made by MRI, was able to predict the tibial size in 93% of the cases and femoral size in 95.5% of the cases; finally, 73% of the prosthesis was implanted without any intraoperative changes.

In 2013, Stronach et al.[1] evaluated the plan (made by MRI) and surgery in 60 patients with 66 TKAs performed with PSI and they recorded 161 intraoperative changes with a mean of 2.4 changes for any knee. The majority of the knee had one, two or three intraoperative changes. PSI predicted the correct size in only 23% of the femurs and in 47% of the tibias. The problem regarding the femur was that the planned component would have been too large in the sagittal plane, whilst the tibial component was frequently undersized with the subsequent risk of subsidence and instability. They also observed that patient-specific guides did not always obtain a secure intraoperative fit.

The disagreement between the different authors and the preoperative study shows that there is no consensus favoring MRI or CT method for preoperative planning.

However, the methods seem to improve the efficiency in the operating room turn-around time by the efficient use of the gained surgical time. There is a time saving of 30 minutes for procedure, subdivided in 10 minutes for cutting time and 20 minutes for preparation.[15] An analysis based on activity-based costing model, including different parameters (price of the knee prosthesis, personnel costs, diagnostics cost, hospital costs) suggests that the use of PSI in TKA is economically effective and gives additional revenues compared to conventional instrumentation.

In the last year, Kerens et al.[16] proposed the use of this novel technique also in revision surgery of unicondylar knee arthroplasty to TKA. They enrolled 10 patients with previous medial UKA and planned by CT scan preoperative and software analysis of the images. The guides were created to fit on both components of the UKA and used native bony reference points. The surgeon positioned the guide on the UKA and he placed three pins, the last one was placed after the UKA removal. This new technique gave good results and it allowed accurately predicting the need for an augmentation or for a long-stem prosthesis.

OUR EXPERIENCE

MRI Registration

Before starting to perform preoperative MRIs the radiological center must create a specific MRI protocol based on the indications given by the manufacturer. This is needed to get standardized images that can be elaborated by the computer to create a 3D model of the knee and to produce the proper preoperative planning.

The creation of this protocol is not always that easy and to have a certified radiological center is not always a straightforward option.

The second problem with the MRI images is that once these are collected, they need to be uploaded to the center of elaboration for approval before the planning starts to be generated. Approval is not immediate, and if, for any reason, the images are rejected the patient needs to be called back for another scan.

In case of major deformities, MRI does not seem to be able to provide a correct evaluation.

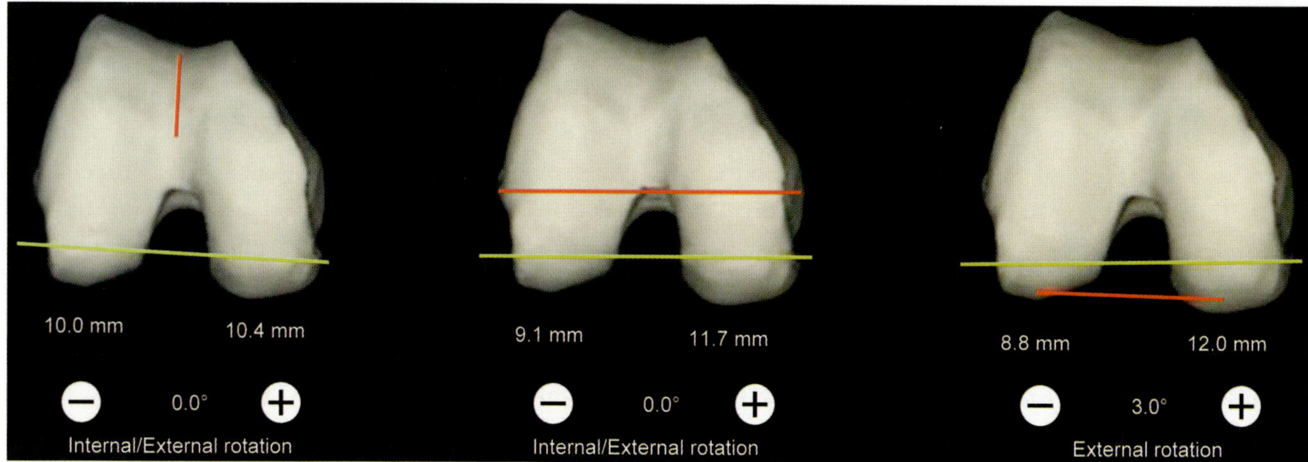

Figure 13.1 Femoral rotational landmarks

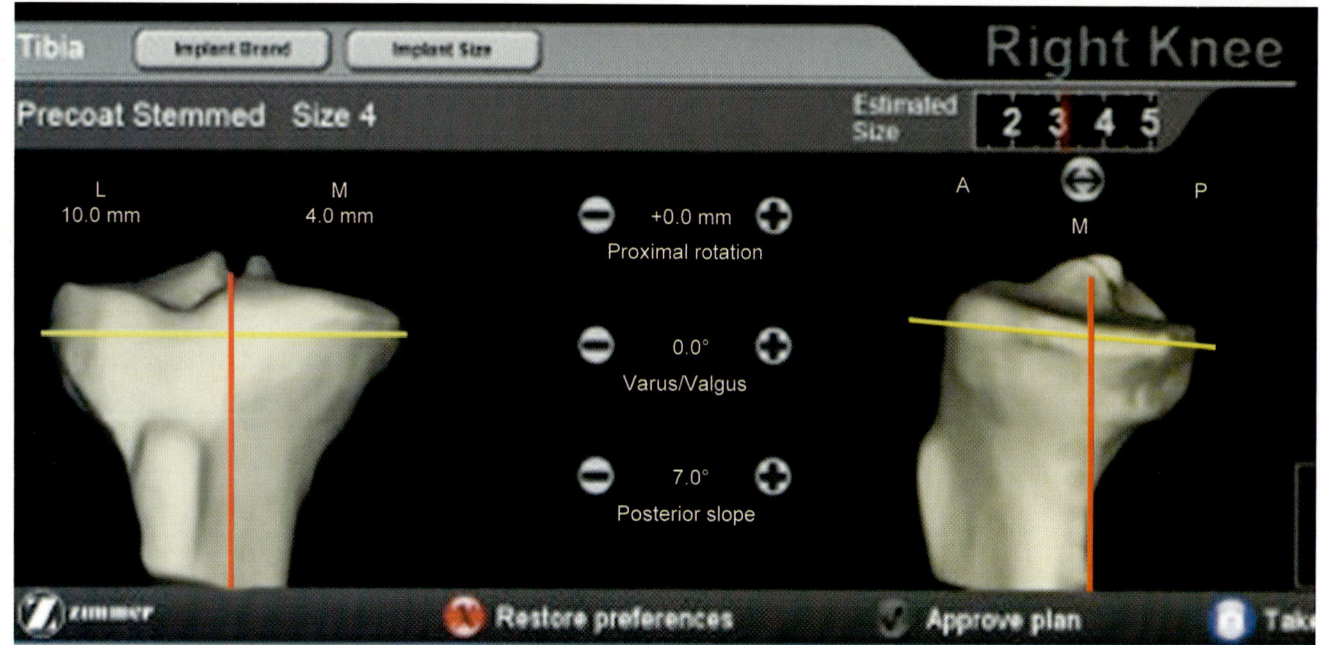

Figure 13.2 Tibial cut planning

Planning

The possibility of a 3D preoperative planning has very important advantages. First of all concerning the sizing of the components; it can show the need of sizes that are not immediately available, or also the need to get compromises for discrepancy between the sizes of the two components. The 3D-reconstruction of the femur can also give the possibility to choose accurately the reference for rotation and to understand the relationship between the different landmarks (**Figure 13.1**). On the tibial side, slope can be accurately planned as well as the sizing and positioning of the tibial plate to avoid overhanging (**Figure 13.2**).

Another advantage of the preoperative planning is the possibility of verify the cuts removing the implant, looking for signs such as the 'grand piano' that allow to validate your planning.

The main disadvantage of this kind of planning is that is made on images that are taken with the patient laying on a supine position and not under weight-bearing (**Figure 13.3**).

Intraoperative Experience

We always found that the guides are perfectly adaptable on the articular surface.

In the system, we have experience with, the guiding blocks are not the actual cutting blocks, but they guide the placing of the pins for the cutting blocks. This is for us the best solution because they do not lose stability and accurately reproduce the precision of the original cutting blocks (**Figures 13.4A and B**).

A problem that we found was the necessity, several times, of a recut on the femoral or on the tibial side probably for an underestimation of the thickness in the preoperative planning.

A limitation of this system comes from the impossibility to take into consideration in preoperative planning the possible soft tissue laxity(ies) of the joint that may be found intraoperatively.

It is important to record as precisely as possible the clinical issues of the knee to be operated, in order to overcome the problem of the lack of information on ligaments in the PSI system.

Another point that has to be stressed, is the time and importance the surgeon should dedicate to the verification and correction of the planning provided by the manufacturer of the guides. As a matter of fact, it is the transposition of the intraoperative navigation, where the decisions have to be made in a bloody field, and in a short time frame, to a comfortable, surgeon-chosen time, and on a computer screen, where the decisions can be made with all the time needed, and revisited before the final approval.

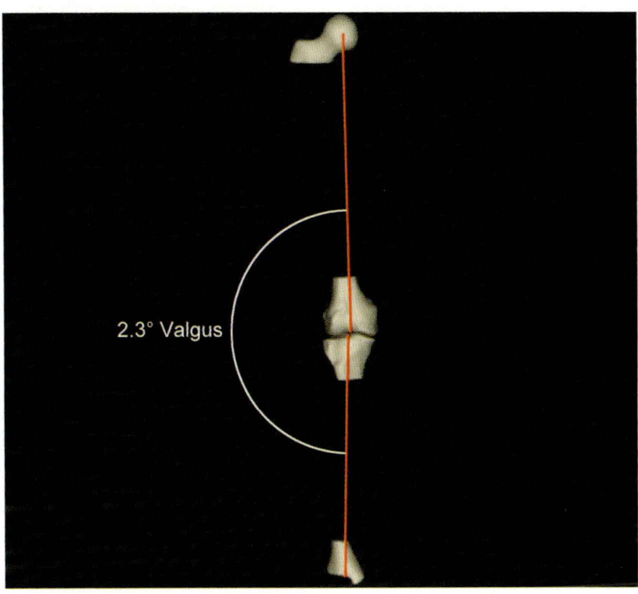

Figure 13.3 Planning based on a nonweight-bearing imaging (MRI scan)

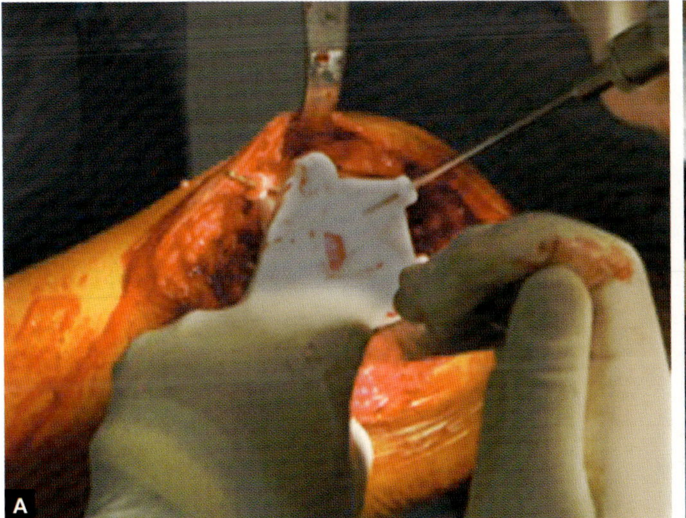

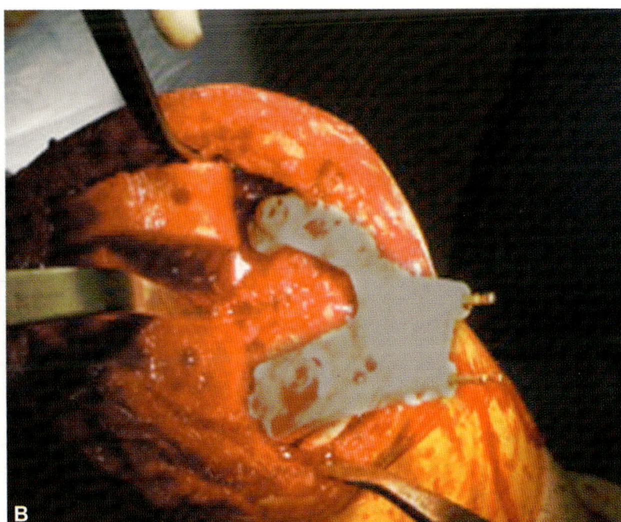

Figures 13.4A and B Guides in place on surgical field

The last important consideration that needs to be made is that with these techniques the normal surgical mentality and flow are limited, firstly because checks and verification can be done only intraoperatively and secondly because it becomes very difficult once you believe in the system to do intraoperative changes from the planning.

CONSIDERATIONS

We believe that this system is very precise and helpful. It provides several advantages both on the surgical side, as well as on the economical side.

On the other hand, it has limitations, especially on the planning side not considering the problems related to the soft tissues and also the possible modifications given by the weight bearing.

In some ways, this kind of techniques has the potential advantage of reducing the outliers especially in less experienced surgeons who can take advantage of this solutions especially to enrich their learning curve. Concerning the more experienced surgeons we do not see the need for this kind of techniques unless, they are used in consideration of their economical advantage.

REFERENCES

1. Stronach BM, Pelt CE, Erikson J,Peters CL, et al. Patient-specific total knee arthroplasty required frequent surgeon-directed changes. Clin Orthop Relat Res. 2013;471:169-74.
2. Ecker ML, Lotke PA, Windsor RE, Cella JP, et al. Long-term results after total condylar knee arthroplasty: significance of radiolucent lines. Clin Orthop Relat Res. 1987;216:151-8.
3. Ma HM, Lu YC, Ho FY, Huang CH. Long-term results of total condylar knee arthroplasty. J Arthroplasty. 2005;20:580-4.
4. Nafei A, Kristensen O, Knudsen HM, Hvid I, Jensen J. Survivorship analysis of cemented total condylar knee arthroplasty: a long-term follow-up report on 348 cases. J Arthroplasty. 1996;11:7-10.
5. Pavone V, Boettner F, Fickert S, Sculco TP. Total condylar knee arthroplasty: a long-term follow-up. Clin Orthop Relat Res. 2001;388:18-25.
6. Krishnan SP, Dawood A, Richards R, Henckel J. A review of rapid prototyped surgical guides for patient-specific total knee replacement. J Bone Joint Surg Br. 2012;94(11):1457-61.
7. Lal K, White GS, Morea DN, Wright RF, et al. Use of stereolithographic templates for surgical and prosthodontic implant planning and placement. Part I. The concept. J Prosthodont. 2006;15:51-8.
8. White D, Chelule KL, Seedhorn BB, et al. Accuracy of MRI versus CT imaging with particular reference to patient specific templates for total knee replacement surgery. Int J Med Robot. 2008;4:224-31.
9. Holme TJ, Henckel J, Cobb J, Hart AJ, et al. Quantification of the difference between 3D-CT and plain radiograph for measurement of the position of medial unicompartmental knee replacement. Knee. 2011;18:300-5.
10. Ast MP, Nam D, Haas SB, et al. Patient-specific instrumentation for total knee arthroplasty: a review. Orthop Clin North Am. 2012:43:e17-22.
11. Ng VY, DeClaire JH, Berend KR, et al. Improved accuracy of alignment with patient-specific positioning guides compared with manual instrumentation in TKA. Clin Orthop Relat Res. 2012;470:99-107.
12. Chareancholvanich K, Narkbunnam R, Pornrattanama-neewong C, et al. A prospective randomised controlled study of patient-specific cutting guides compared with conventional instrumentation in total knee replacement. Bone Joint J. 2013;95-B(3):354-9.
13. Victor J, Dujardin J, Vandenneucker, et al. Patient-specific guides do not improve accuracy in total knee arthroplasty. Clin Orthop Relat Res. 2013.
14. Issa K, Rifai A, McGrath MS, et al. Reliability of templating with patient-specific instrumentation in total knee arthroplasty. J Knee Surg. 2013;26(6):429-33.
15. Tibesku CO, Hofer P, Portegies W, et al. Benefits of using customized instrumentation in total knee arthroplasty: results from an activity-based costing model. Arch Orthop Trauma Surg. 2013;133:405-11.
16. Kerens B, Boonen B, Schotanus M, Kort N, et al. Patient-specific guide for revision of medial unicondylar knee arthroplasty to total knee arthroplasty: beneficial first results of a new operating technique performed on 10 patients. Acta Orthop. 2013;84(2):165-9.

Chapter 14

Technique of Navigated Total Knee Arthroplasty

Arun Mullaji

INTRODUCTION

With rapid advancement in technology and materials in total knee arthroplasty (TKA), long-term survival and function of the total knee is now increasingly dependent on a proper surgical technique. Every step of the surgical technique needs to be well thought of before execution. The aim of the author, like that of most surgeons, has been to ensure a well-aligned, well-balanced, and well-fixed TKA. Ligament balancing is an integral part of TKA and the soft-tissue release should follow a functional and anatomic rationale to achieve correct alignment and ligament balance in flexion and extension.

The two basic techniques commonly used in TKA are the measured resection technique and the gap balancing technique. The author has used the gap balancing technique in all cases. This technique has proved reliable across various types and severity of knee deformity. Only posterior cruciate-substituting (CS) TKAs have been used by the author. The rationale of using only CS knees is based on the finding that the posterior cruciate ligament may undergo marked structural and functional deterioration in arthritic knees especially in severe grades of arthritis[1] and that the functional outcome may be more predictable with a CS knee. Tibial preparation is performed as the first step in the majority of the knees. Ligament and gap balancing is done first in extension and is followed by femoral sizing and creating a flexion gap equal to the extension gap. Only cemented components have been used in all knees and all knees have undergone patellar resurfacing. Medial parapatellar arthrotomy has been used in all knees. The author uses computer navigation for all cases not only to ensure accurate limb and component alignment but also to quantify ligament balancing and the amount of bone resection and soft-tissue release performed. Hence, navigation is used more as a tool for verification wherein it provides real-time feedback of various surgical steps. It is important to note that when computer navigation is being used the surgeon needs to be aware about its limitations and may have to over-ride some of its recommendations whenever required. It may be unwise to use computer navigation on an 'auto-pilot mode' with the surgeon's experience and clinical judgment taking a back seat. Although it does involve a learning curve and may add to the surgical time initially, in the author's experience the surgical time during computer-assisted TKA becomes

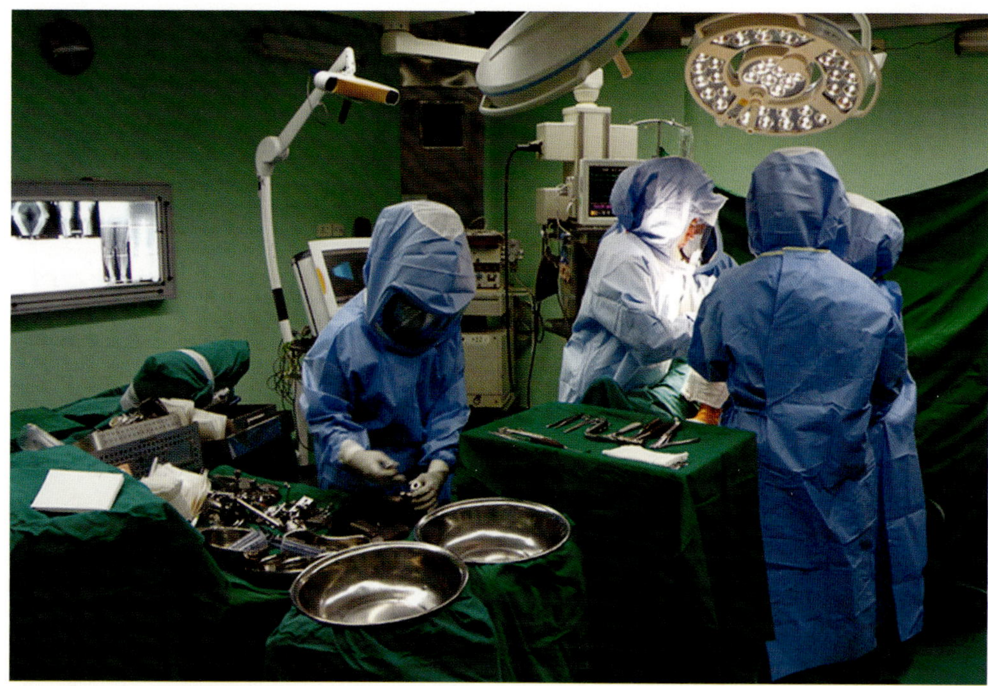

Figure 14.1 Shows the typical arrangement of computer monitor and camera. The author always prefers to operate from the patient's right side. So the monitor and camera are behind the surgeon while he is operating on the left knee. The camera and monitor are kept facing the surgeon (to the patient's left) when operating on the right knee

equivalent to the conventional TKA technique with experience. This section gives a brief overview of the basic set-up of computer navigation and its use during TKA (**Figure 14.1**). We have used the image-free Ci navigation system with its software (BrainLab, Munich, Germany) for all cases. The computer navigation system consists of a camera unit, a computer screen and the arrays. The Ci navigation system is based on infrared technology where the infrared light emitted by the camera unit is reflected back by tibial and femoral reflective array of spheres as well as two other devices (the pointer tool and the plane verification tool) and is detected by two cameras.

SURGICAL APPROACH AND EXPOSURE

We use the classical anterior skin incision with the medial parapatellar arthrotomy to approach the knee in most cases. Rare exceptions include a knee with severe valgus arthritis and patellar maltracking that requires a lateral parapatellar arthrotomy and a very stiff arthritic knee where a tibial tubercle osteotomy may be performed to improve exposure. After arthrotomy, the following seven sequential steps are performed to adequately expose the knee for TKA.

1. **Patella:** Division of the patellofemoral ligament, excision of the infrapatellar fat pad and removal of patellar osteophytes and peripatellar synovium to facilitate displacement of the extensor apparatus and eversion of patella when patella needs to be prepared for resurfacing.
2. **Anterior surface of femur:** Elevation of the synovium and soft-tissue from over the anterior surface of distal femur, especially along the medial surface and anteromedial border of the distal femur. This helps in accurate registration and mitigates the possibility of notching of the femur.
3. **Cruciates:** Excision of both cruciate.
4. **Osteophytes:** Removal of osteophytes around the distal end of the femur and the proximal tibia.

5. **Knee dislocation:** The knee is now flexed maximally and the tibia gently externally rotated with an assistant gently applying downward pressure on the distal femur while the surgeon simultaneously releases the deep MCL and along the medial and posteromedial edge of the tibial articular surface using diathermy. This safely dislocates the knee and brings the tibia fully forward. A Hohmann's retractor then applied to the posterolateral aspect of the tibia adjacent to the patella, helps to completely expose the tibial articular surface.
6. **Menisci:** Excision of both menisci with cauterization of the lateral genicular vessels.
7. **Posterior osteophytes:** Excision of posteromedial tibial osteophytes with a broad flat osteotome and removal of posterior femoral osteophytes using a curved osteotome. Removal of the medial meniscus beforehand improves access to the posterior surface of the femoral condyle for removal of these osteophytes.

After completing these seven basic exposure steps, the knee is now extended and checked for the amount of correction achieved with these preliminary soft-tissue releases and the amount of soft-tissue laxity present on the opposite side.

Fixation of arrays: The tibial and femoral arrays, each with three reflective spheres, are fixed to the bone using two 4 mm Schanz pins placed unicortically. The position of the pins is usually confined to the proximal 1/3 of tibia and distal 1/3 of femur. The arrays may be fixed within the surgical wound or outside it using small stab incisions. When placed within the surgical wound, care should be taken that the pins do not come in way of the cutting blocks or the components. For the tibial pins, we fix the first pin one thumb's width below the medial tibial articular surface with both the pins directed away from the position of the tibial stem (**Figure 14.2**). For the femur, the distal-most pin is placed midway between the articular cartilage margin and the medial epicondyle (**Figure 14.3**) if through the wound otherwise in the suprapatellar region.

The spheres reflect infrared beams from the camera back to the camera that communicates with the computer in real-time.

Registration: Registration is the process of providing data to the computer by indicating certain landmarks, lines and surfaces so that the software prepares a 3D model of the bones and the limb. The accuracy of this can be verified and then the data are used by the surgeon to perform cuts, check alignment, gaps, and determine the sizes and placement of components. Registration starts by the kinematic identification of the center of the femoral head, mapping of the lower femur, upper tibia and bony

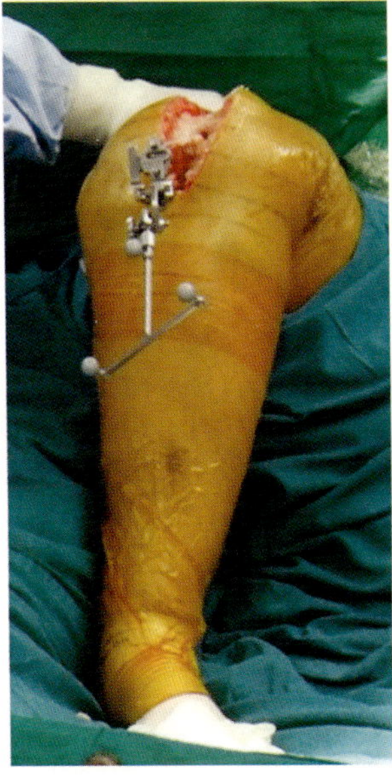

Figure 14.2 The T-shaped tibial array with three reflecting spheres fixed with two unicortical Schanz screws inside the wound

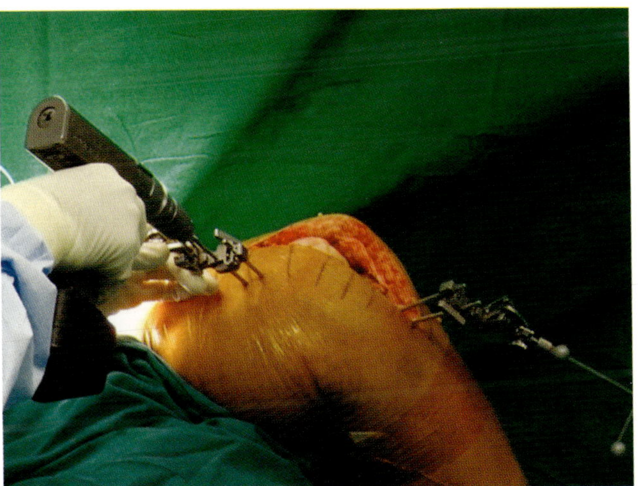

Figure 14.3 The two Schanz screws for the femoral array being introduced through stab incisions on the medial side outside of the wound

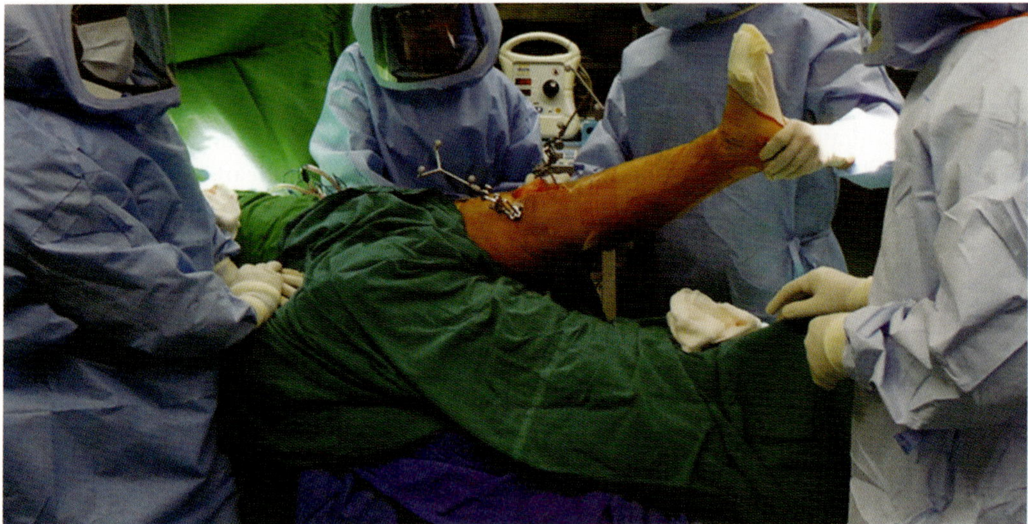

Figure 14.4 The leg being pivoted while the pelvis is steadied for computing the femoral head center

landmarks of the ankle. The center of the femoral head is computed by rotating the entire limb in a circular fashion within the free range of motion of the hip joint (**Figure 14.4**). The computer calculates the center of the femoral head as the apex of a cone described in space by the arrays as the leg is pivoted. The computer accepts the data only if the accuracy is within 3 mm else one needs to repeat the process. It is important to steady the pelvis while the leg is being pivoted to ensure accuracy.

This is followed by the surgeon performing registration of bony landmarks, lines and planes on the distal femur and tibia using the pointer tool that also has reflective spheres on it (**Figure 14.5**). The computer screen prompts the surgeon with a diagram to indicate each step. As it receives enough data points provided by the pointer it moves to the next step. The sequence is as follows: the center of the distal femur, medial epicondyle, lateral epicondyle, anterior cortex, Whitesides' line, medial femoral condyle, lateral femoral condyle and the anterior surface of distal femur. On the tibial side the malleoli are registered, followed by the center of tibial plateau, medial, lateral and anterior margin of the tibia, the AP direction of tibia and anterior cortex of the tibia. The initial mechanical axis of the lower limb is then computed using the center of the femoral head, the center of the knee and the center of the ankle (computed from the malleoli).

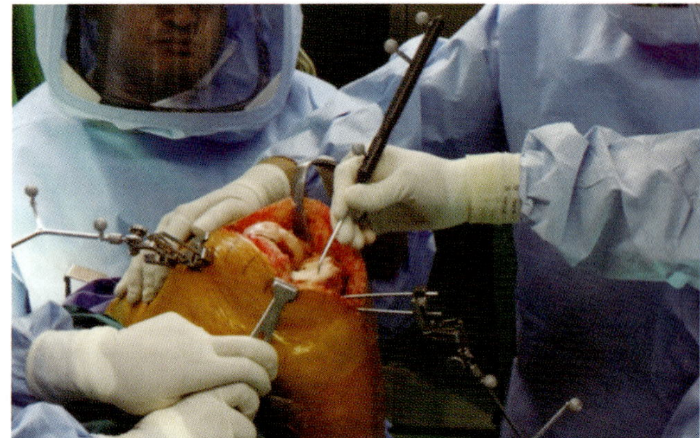

Figure 14.5 The pointer tool being used to provide data points to the computer from the medial tibial plateau

Navigating cutting blocks: Conventional or navigation-specific cutting blocks for the tibial, distal femoral, and anteroposterior femoral cuts can be navigated in position to obtain the desired cuts. The positions of these cutting blocks are verified using the flat verification tool that also has spheres affixed to it (**Figure 14.6**).

Tibial resection: The tibial cut affects both the extension and the flexion gaps. The minimum thickness of tibia that needs to be resected is governed by the type and severity of the knee deformity and the knee prosthesis design. The standard tibial cut involves resecting the minimum insert

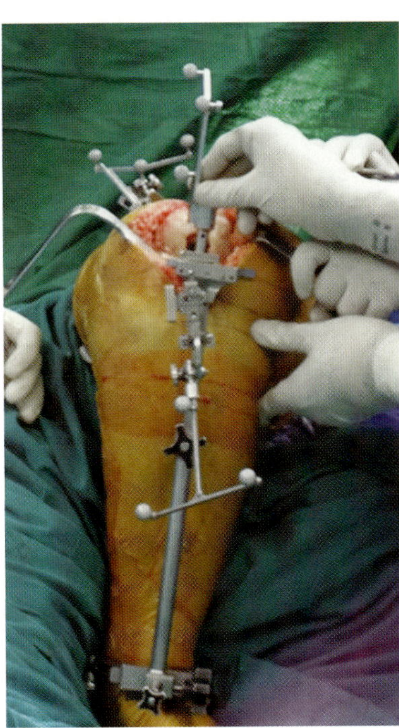

Figure 14.6 The plane verification tool being used to check position of the tibial jig prior to tibial resection

thickness available with an implant system (i.e. 8 mm or 10 mm from the less involved side). However, this needs to be varied depending on the type and severity of the deformity. More severe the coronal plane deformity (varus or valgus), less should be the amount of tibial resection. Similarly, less bone needs to be resected in knees with severe ligamentous instability or in a hyperextending knee. The coronal plane of tibial resection has been classically recommended to be perpendicular to the mechanical axis of the tibia. Slope of the tibial cut is governed by the implant being used and the design and instrumentation of that implant. Certain designs have a built-in slope in the polyethylene insert. The tibia should be cut at neutral with respect to the sagittal plane if the implant polyethylene already has an inbuilt slope.

The default setting can be modified by the surgeon by adjusting the settings on the computer screen to alter the plane of the cut and the amount of resected bone. The amount and plane of the tibial cut is then verified and may be fine-tuned if needed.

Gap balancing in extension and flexion: In extension, navigation allows the quantification of medial and lateral gaps and the limb alignment for a given spacer. It also allows visualizing the degree of mediolateral laxity present for a given spacer. In flexion, the mediolateral gap balance can be assessed with respect to the position of distal femoral bony landmarks such as the transepicondylar line, Whiteside line and the posterior condylar axis. The optimized version of the Ci navigation software allows the surgeon to simulate the effect of change in rotation, flexion or extension, upsizing or downsizing of the femoral component on the flexion gap vis-a-vis the extension gap.

BALANCING IN EXTENSION AND DISTAL FEMORAL RESECTION

The distal femoral cut affects only the extension gap. After the tibial cut, a soft-tissue tensioning device or laminar spreaders are used to tension the medial and lateral soft-tissues so as to achieve equal medial and lateral ligament tension and the limb mechanical axis is determined in full extension (**Figure 14.7**). It is important to remove all osteophytes especially from the posterior aspect of femoral condyle before this step as their presence may lead to an underestimation of the extension gap. If either the medial-lateral gap or the limb alignment in full extension is suboptimal, then additional soft-tissue release needs to be performed to achieve a balanced extension gap and a satisfactory limb alignment.

The default setting enables the distal femoral cut to be made perpendicular to the mechanical axis of the femur. Conventionally, this is performed using intramedullary guides that are commonly set at an angle of 5°–7° valgus. A recent prospective study done by the author has shown wide variations in this angle among patients with the distal femoral valgus correction angle (VCA) varying from 2° to 11° and almost 45% of limbs having a VCA outside the conventional 5°–7° range.[2] This is commonly due to femoral bowing of the femoral shaft in the coronal plane that is frequently encountered in Asian patients undergoing TKA.[3] Evaluation of femoral bowing in our patients undergoing TKA revealed that one in five varus limbs had significant femoral bowing in the coronal plane. Using an intramedullary guide (straight rod) in a bowed femur (curved canal) will lead to displacement of the cutting jig and an inaccurate cut vis-a-vis the mechanical axis of the femur. Hence, to avoid malalignment of femoral component in the

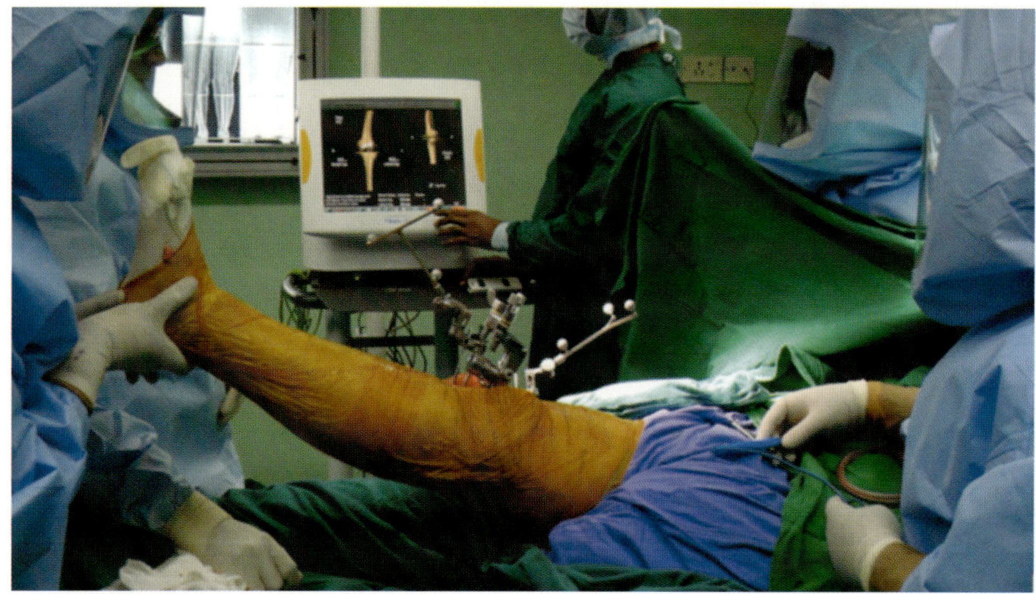

Figure 14.7 Checking alignment and gap balance in extension with a tensioner in place

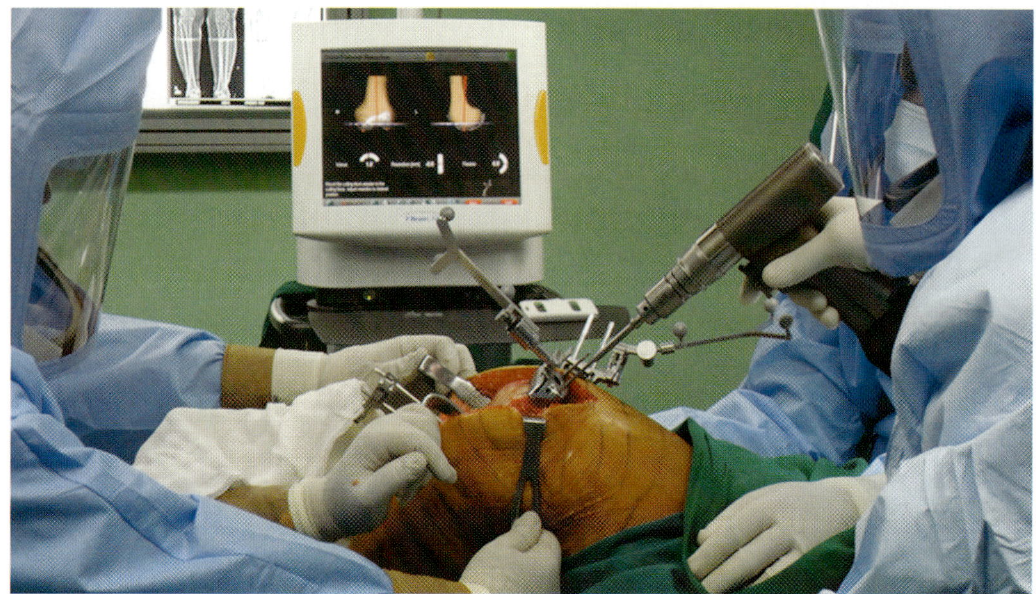

Figure 14.8 The distal cutting block being navigated into position with the plane verification tool in the cutting slot

coronal plane during conventional surgery, the distal femoral cut should be tailored in each limb based on the VCA determined on preoperative full-length hip-to-ankle radiographs. Of course, with navigation this problem is taken care of! However, the surgeon can alter this angle (almost never required), as well as the slope and thickness of resected distal femur. The plane verification tool is inserted in the slot of the distal cutting block, navigated into position and held by two pins (**Figure 14.8**). The distal cut is performed and verified.

BALANCING IN FLEXION, FEMORAL SIZING, AND ROTATION

After achieving a well-balanced extension gap, the flexion gap is assessed using a soft-tissue tensioner or laminar spreaders. The aim is to achieve a flexion gap equal to the previously created extension gap. Mediolateral soft-tissue tension is assessed at 90° flexion with an assistant supporting the thigh. Ideally the medial and the lateral gaps should have equal tension at 90° flexion. However, arthritic knees in general, based on the authors' experience, tend to be more lax laterally beyond 100°–110°. Hence, 2–3 mm of disparity between the medial and lateral gaps (lateral more lax than the medial side in varus knees) may be accepted in deeper flexion and does not seem to affect the overall function of the knee. In varus knees, in the presence of excessive medial tightness there is a risk of the femoral component being placed in excessive internal rotation.

Based on the soft-tissue tension in extension, flexion and the resected amount of bone, the optimized setting of the software allows gaps to be balanced by adjusting the size and placement of the femoral component. The computer will provide a femoral size it has computed to balance gaps. The size and position of the femoral component can be manipulated on the computer screen till it meets the surgeon's approval. Ensure with a stylus or angel wing that notching will not occur. Also check on the computer screen that it is parallel to the epicondylar axis and perpendicular to the Whiteside's line. After pinning the AP cutting block to the distal femur under navigation control (**Figure 14.9**), the flexion gap balance is assessed using a spacer block. If the flexion gap seems too tight compared to the extension gap, the femur can be downsized or vice versa. This is the author's concept of 'combined referencing' to determine the position, size, and rotation of the femoral component. Preparation of the distal femur is then completed using a notch-cutting block of appropriate size to perform the notch and chamfer cuts.

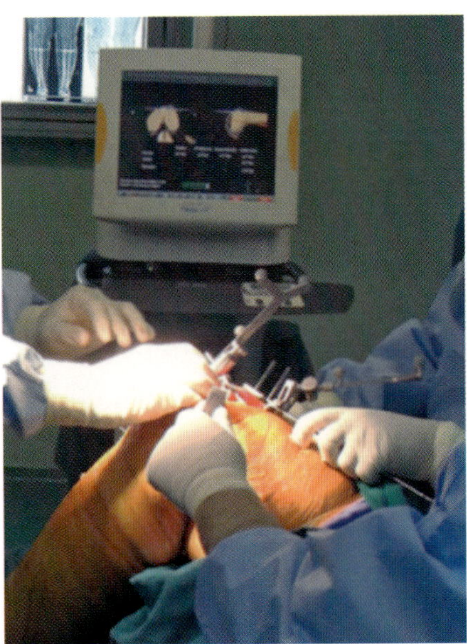

Figure 14.9 The AP cutting block being navigated into position to determine rotation of femoral component and the absence of notching

TIBIAL SIZING AND ROTATION

After the femoral chamfer and notch cuts, limb alignment, extension and flexion gap balance are assessed using trial components. In varus knees showing excessive medial tightness and/or excessive lateral laxity, additional soft-tissue release with or without a reduction osteotomy and downsizing of the tibial component may be needed. Use one size thicker and thinner inserts to assess the range of motion and soft-tissue stability.

Tibial component rotation is determined by putting the knee through an arc of flexion and extension and the most optimum position of the tray is marked using cautery on the anterior aspect of the tibia. The tibial tray is placed on the lateral cortex of the tibial cut surface to determine the size of the tray relevant to the femoral component size used. Any medial uncapped bone is removed with an osteotome to prevent tenting of the medial soft-tissue sleeve. Final trial reduction is performed and the alignment of the limb and stability throughout the range of motion are assessed with navigation (**Figure 14.10**).

PATELLA

The authors resurface the patella in all cases of TKA. Navigation is not deployed for this step by the author although a separate patellar array is available that has to be drilled into the anterior cortex of the patella. Preparation is otherwise done in a routine manner.

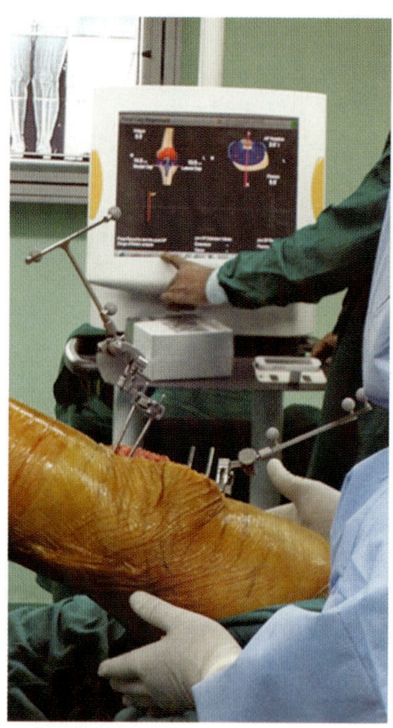

Figure 14.10 Final alignment, range of motion, and gap balance being checked with trial components in place

CEMENTING

The authors use cemented components in all TKAs. A thorough preparation of the femoral, tibial and patellar cancellous bone surfaces and pressurization are essential to ensure good penetration of bone cement and fixation of the components.

Final alignment: the final alignment of the limb and gaps can be confirmed after implantation of the prosthesis especially when the cement is setting. Holding the limb in the right position while the cement is setting is crucial to avoid malalignment of the tibial and femoral components due to an uneven cement mantle. Navigation allows for real-time continuous visualization of the limb position in both the coronal and sagittal planes while the cement is curing.

CLOSURE

We deflate the tourniquet after the cement has hardened. While the cement is setting, excessive cement around the components is scraped out and the periarticular soft-tissue sleeve is infiltrated with an analgesic 'cocktail'. Once the cement has hardened, the tourniquet is deflated and the knee is put through a range of flexion and extension to check patellar tracking. Any sign of lateral maltracking or patellar component lift-off is dealt with by a lateral retinacular release. The final alignment is noted right through the range of motion and the computer also displays the medial and lateral gaps through the entire range. Throughout the surgery, the software automatically records the key steps and the surgeon can also take additional screenshots when desired. The entire navigation record can be burnt onto a CD and this is done at the end of the procedure by the computer. The arrays and Schanz screws are removed. After thorough hemostasis, the incision is closed in layers over a negative suction drain.[4]

Advantages of CAS

Navigation for TKA is of immense benefit to many key ingredients that contribute to the performance of TKA.[5] Orthopedic surgeons are not accurate in visually assessing alignment as they would have themselves believe![6] Navigation ensures predictable alignment and we showed in a prospective study that we were able to substantially reduce outliers in terms of alignment of component and the overall limb alignment as well when compared to conventional surgery where we used image intensification to determine the hip and ankle centers intraoperatively.[7] There is a wide variation in the VCA[2] and routine use of a fixed distal femoral cutting angle of 5°, 6°, or 7° can lead to a large error in alignment due to the significant coronal bowing of the femur often seen in our patients.[3] Computer-assisted surgery (CAS) ignores the diaphyseal bowing and ensures accurate femoral component placement. In a more recent study we looked at the reasons for outliers in 1500 computer-assisted TKAs and found that preoperative varus deformity of more than 20° and femoral bowing of more than 5° were associated with increased risk of placing the limb mechanical axis outside the acceptable ± 3° range.[8] Significant hindfoot deformity (flatfoot) can cause a lateral deviation of the weight-bearing axis of the limb even if the hip-knee-ankle axis is perfectly restored by CAS.[9] Using navigation, one can accurately alter the alignment (i.e. slight over- or under-correction) to ensure that the weight-bearing axis passes through the center of the implant rather than eccentrically either medially or laterally to prevent overload of bone, implant or ligaments.

Navigation facilitates soft-tissue balancing and we have quantified the effect of release of various posteromedial structures that are sequentially released in correction of varus deformity to determine the effect on alignment and medial and lateral gaps in flexion and extension.[10] CAS also helps in accurate restoration of joint line and posterior femoral offset.[11] Many of our patients have significant tibial intorsion[12] and a wide variation in the distal femoral landmarks[13] and CAS helps to take into account all the landmarks, so the surgeon can see all these on the screen and better judge rotational placement of both tibial and femoral components.

The greatest value of navigation is the correction of deformity that can often be extremely challenging[14,15] (**Figures 14.11 and 14.12**). We have shown how CAS helps

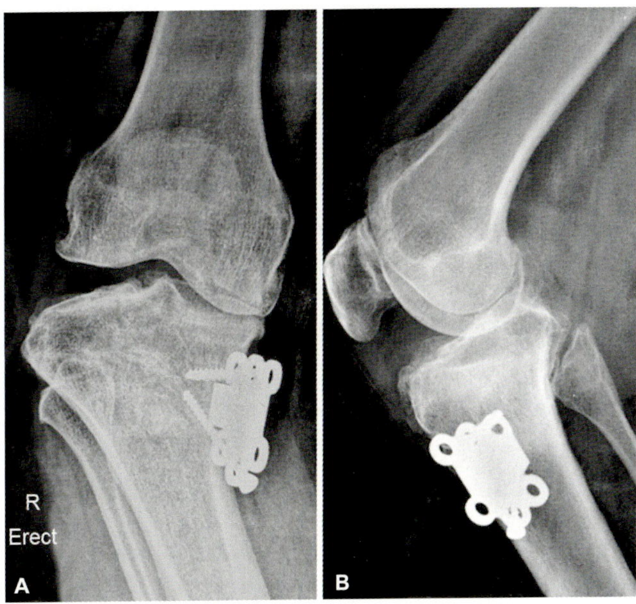

Figures 14.11A and B Preoperative radiographs of severe varus deformity after high tibial osteotomy

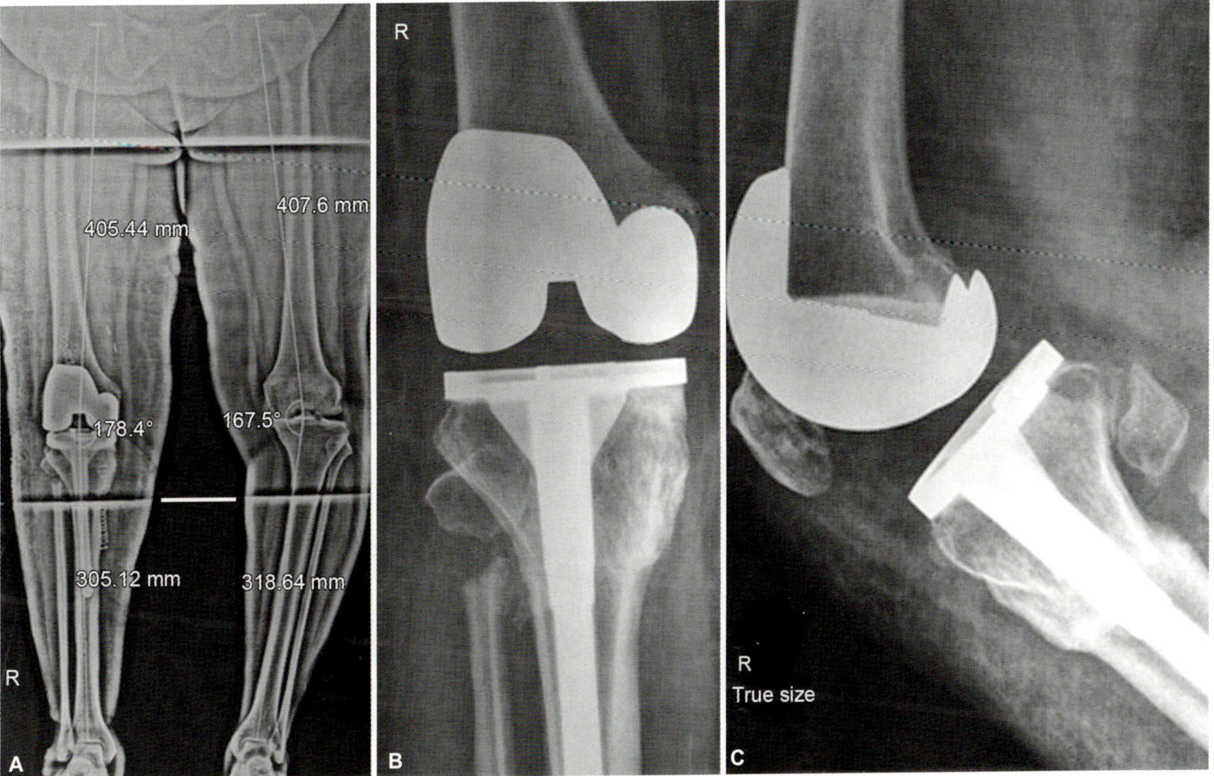

Figures 14.12A to C Postoperative radiographs after CAS TKA with tibial osteotomy and use of a long-stem tibial component

in correction of severe deformity whether it is varus,[16,17] valgus,[18,19] recurvatum,[20] or extra-articular deformity.[21] We have classified stress fractures that may often be present in patients undergoing TKA and presented a treatment algorithm,[22] and CAS is of great value in ensuring the alignment. Moreover, if there is an altered hip center (due to prior hip surgery), CAS helps to restore accurate alignment.[23] It is of great value in patients with hardware in the femur that may prevent use of intramedullary jigs used in conventional TKA.

Navigation enables bilateral simultaneous TKAs to be performed and we have reported the functional recovery of bilateral TKAs being no different from that of the unilateral TKA thus putting to rest concerns about longer hospital stay and lengthier recovery.[24] Use of modern pain control methods[25,26] along with CAS has ensured speedy and painless recovery in our patients and more than makes up for the disadvantages of CAS that include an initial learning curve, few extra minutes of registration and the initial cost of the equipment.

REFERENCES

1. Mullaji AB, Marawar S, Simha M, Jindal G. Cruciate ligaments in arthritic knees: a histological study with radiological correlation. J Arthroplasty. 2008;23(4):567-72.
2. Shetty GM, Mullaji A, Kanna R, Vadapalli R. Variation in valgus correction angle and factors affecting it: analysis of 503 navigated total knee arthroplasties. J Arthroplasty. 2013;28:20-7.
3. Mullaji AB, Marawar SV, Mittal V. A comparison of coronal plane axial femoral relationships in Asian patients with varus osteoarthritic knees and healthy knees. J Arthroplasty. 2009;24(6):861-7.
4. Prasad N, Padmanabhan V, Mullaji A. Comparison between two methods of drain clamping after total knee arthroplasty. Arch Orthop Trauma Surg. 2005;125(6):381-4.
5. Mullaji A, Shetty GM. Computer-assisted TKA: greater accuracy, doubtful clinical efficacy: opposes. Orthopedics 2009;32(9):1-4.
6. Shetty GM, Mullaji A, Lingaraju AP, Bhayde S. How accurate are orthopaedic surgeons in visually estimating lower limb alignment? Acta Orthop Belg. 2011;5:638-43.
7. Mullaji A, Kanna R, Marawar S, Kohli A. Comparison of limb and component alignment using computer-assisted navigation versus image intensifier-guided conventional total knee replacement: a prospective randomised single-surgeon study of 467 knees. J Arthroplasty. 2007;22(7):953-9.
8. Mullaji AB, Shetty GM, Lingaraju AP, Bhayde S. Which Factors Increase Risk of Malalignment of the Hip-Knee-Ankle Axis in TKA? Clin Orthop Relat Res. 2013;471(1):134-41.
9. Mullaji A, Shetty GM. Persistent hindfoot valgus causes lateral deviation of weight-bearing axis after total knee arthroplasty. Clin Orthop Relat Res. 2011;469:1154-60.
10. Mullaji A, Sharma A, Marawar S, Kanna R. Quantification of Effect of Sequential Posteromedial Release on Flexion and Extension Gaps: A computer-assisted study in cadaveric knees. J Arthroplasty. 2009;24(5):795-805.
11. Shetty GM, Mullaji A, Bhayde S. Computer guided restoration of joint line and femoral offset in cruciate substituting total knee arthroplasty. Knee. 2012;19(5):611-6.
12. Mullaji AB, Sharma AK, Marawar S, Kohli A. Tibial torsion in non-arthritic Indian adults: a computer tomography study of 100 limbs. Indian J Orthop. 2008:42(3):309-13.
13. Mullaji AB, Sharma AK, Maravar S, Kohli A, Singh DP. Distal femoral rotational axes in Indian knees. J Orthop Surg. 2009;17(2):295-8.
14. Mullaji AB, Padmanabhan V, Jindal G. Total knee arthroplasty for profound varus deformity: technique and radiological results in 173 knees with varus more than 20 degrees. J Arthroplasty. 2005;20(5):550-61.
15. Mullaji AB, Marawar S, Sharma A. Correcting varus deformity. J Arthroplasty. 2007;22(4):15-9.
16. Mullaji A, Shetty GM. Correction of varus deformity during TKA with reduction osteotomy. Clin Orthop Relat Res. 2014;472:126-32..
17. Mullaji A, Shetty GM. Surgical technique: computer-assisted sliding medial condylar osteotomy to achieve gap balance in varus knees during TKA. Clin Orthop Relat Res. 2013;471:1484-91.
18. Mullaji A, Shetty GM. Lateral epicondylar osteotomy using computer navigation in total knee arthroplasty for rigid valgus deformities. J Arthroplasty. 2010;25(1):166-9.
19. Shetty GM, Mullaji A. Alignment in computer-navigated versus conventional total knee arthroplasty for valgus deformity. South African Orthop J. 2009;41-6.

20. Mullaji A, Shetty GM, Lingaraju AP. Computer-assisted total knee replacement in patients with arthritis and a recurvatum deformity. J Bone Joint Surg Br. 2012;94(5):642-7.
21. Mullaji A, Shetty G. Computer-assisted total knee arthroplasty for arthritis with extra-articular deformity. J Arthroplasty. 2009;24(8):1164-9.
22. Mullaji A, Shetty G. Total knee replacement for arthritic knees with tibio-fibular stress fractures: classification and treatment guidelines. J Arthroplasty. 2010;25(2):295-301.
23. Mullaji A, Lingaraju AP, Shetty GM. Alignment of computer-assisted total knee arthroplasty in patients with altered hip center. J Arthroplasty. 2011;26:1072-7.
24. Shetty G, Mullaji A. Simultaneous bilateral versus unilateral computer-assisted total knee arthroplasty: a prospective comparison of early postoperative pain and functional recovery. Knee. 2010;17:191-5.
25. Shetty GM, Mullaji A, Bhayde S, Desai D, Sathe M. Effect of periarticular clonidine on postoperative pain and function after total knee arthroplasty. J Orthrop Rehab. 2011;1:44-50.
26. Mullaji AB, Kanna R, Chawda V, Singh DP. Efficacy of periarticular injection of bupivacaine, fentanyl and methylprednisolone in TKA: a prospective, randomised trial. J Arthroplasty. 2010;25:851-7.

Chapter 15

Cementless Total Knee Arthroplasty

Aaron G Rosenberg

INTRODUCTION

The initial application of bone ingrowth technology to the fixation of total knee arthroplasty (TKA) components without bone cement was based on the premise that bone cement was 'not biologic,' and so over time it would undergo fatigue failure with subsequent loosening. It was hoped that this problem could be obviated by cementless fixation by bone ingrowth that would lead to biologic fixation that would remodel over time and not fatigue. In addition, it was anticipated that the failed cementless TKA might be easier to revise and leave the surgeon with more bone to work with.[1] Whether or not cementless fixation of TKA components was justified on any of these counts was uncertain through the first decade of their use. Much of the data accumulated during that perio poorly supported these contentions, while cemented TKA was increasingly reported as a reliable, consistent and less complicated form of TKA fixation.[2-6] However, over the past decade, new evidence has accumulated demonstrating greater success with this technology. This chapter will review the underlying basic and clinical science behind the design and clinical use of cementless TKA components, the early clinical history of cementless TKA, as well as more recent clinical data supporting the cementless fixation of TKA components.

BASIC SCIENCE OF CEMENTLESS FIXATION

The Ingrowth Process

Cementless ingrowth fixation refers to fixation of an implant by virtue of the host's bone growing into a porous surface on the implant. The majority of knee implants placed without cement involve porous materials in which bone actually bridges from the host and into the pores of the implanted substrate.

The requirements for bone ingrowth into a porous surface have been thoroughly studied for several decades.[1,7,8] These basic requirements involve the osteogenic potential of the bone, the intrinsic material properties of ingrowth surface (porosity and biocompatibility), as well as the proximity and stability of the materials at the interface. Three requirements must specifically be met: (1) the interface must involve biologically viable bone and a biocompatible material with adequate porosity characteristics; (2) the interface must place the two materials in sufficient proximity for the biological process to take place; and (3) under physiologic loading conditions there must be sufficiently little relative motion at the interface to allow the biologic process to occur. These requirements are interactive in the sense that when optimized they increases the extent of ingrowth, and when any factor is less than optimal, reduce ingrowth.[1]

While surface interactions between bone and implant may provide clinical fixation, particularly with osteophilic materials that have had appropriate surface treatments (either material or chemical), the actual degree of contact between the implants surface and the new bone that forms has been categorized as a function of the distance between the bone and the surface of the metal at a microscopic level.[9] In contact osteogenesis, bone forms directly on the implant surface and is seen with titanium and cobalt chrome alloys if the implant surface displays appropriate topography. In distance osteogenesis, observed with stainless steel, the bone grows from the bone surface toward the implant. Bond osteogenesis occurs in the presence of bone stimulating materials such as calcium—phosphate ceramics like hydroxyapatite (**Figures 15.1A to D**).

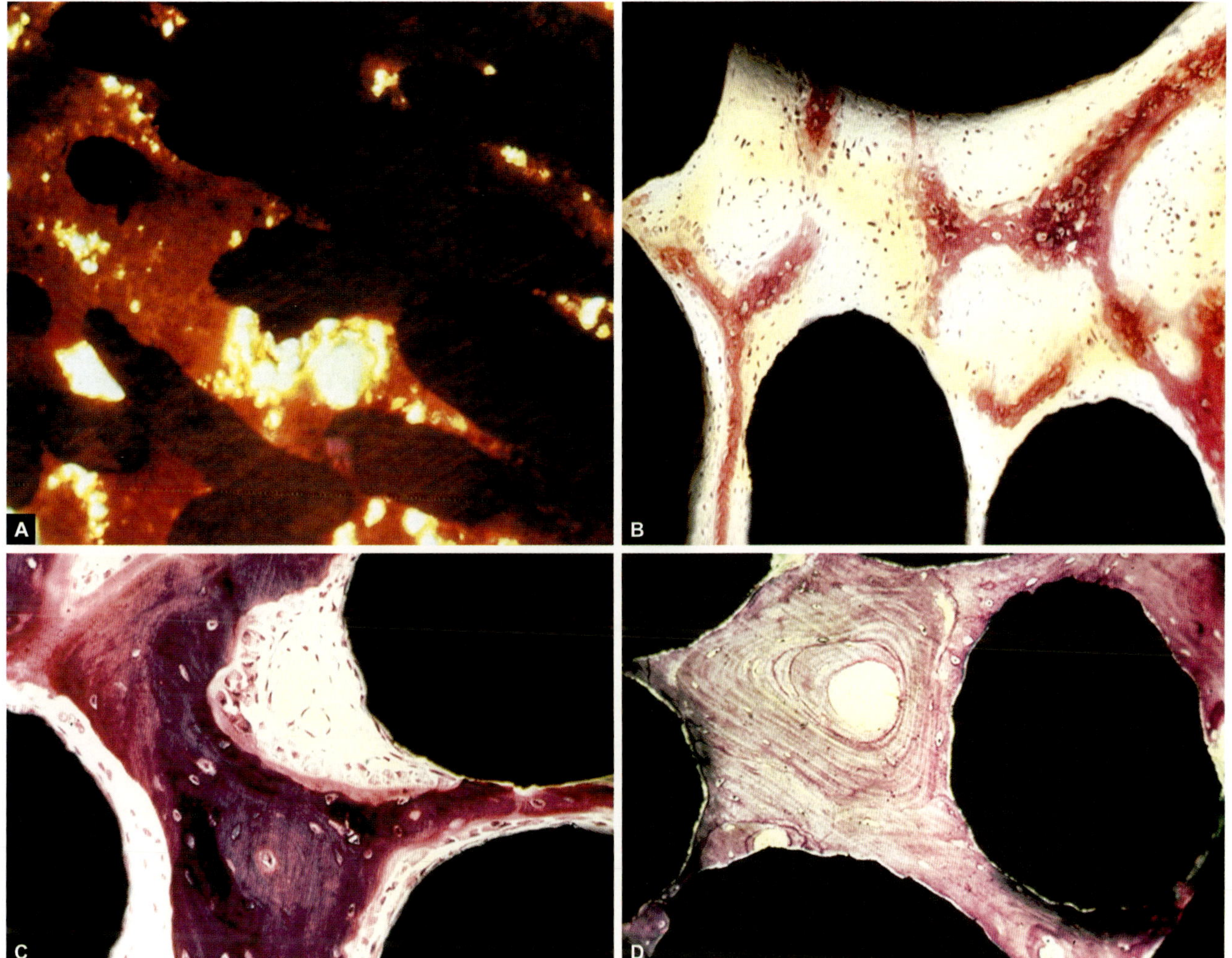

Figures 15.1A to D (A) Cross-sectional microscopy of titanium fiber metal mesh implant 3 days postimplantation. Hematoma fills the porous space between the kinked, sintered metal wire seen in black; (B) At 3 weeks postimplantation pluripotential mesenchymal cells fill the pore spaces and osteoblasts lay down seams of osteoid that are beginning to calcify; (C) By 6 weeks mature ostenal systems are seen within the porous substrate with osteoclasts and osteoblasts engaged in remodeling of bone; (D) By 6 months mature bone fills the pore space with no cellular intermediary between the ingrown bone and the porous substrate

The biologic process of ingrowth has been likened to fracture healing. A common sequence of events can be seen in multiple animal models with the main differences seen in the time interval over which the process occurs.[1] Rat models appear to demonstrate a significantly more rapid process than canines and primates, which are most commonly used for investigation of the parameters affecting bone growth into the porous surface. The trauma of implantation damages the bone and subsequent bleeding from the traumatized bone leads to formation of a hematoma, which occupies the porous structure remaining contiguous with the damaged bone. The hematoma is gradually replaced by mesenchymal tissue, which is gradually transformed by woven bone similar to the response seen in primary fracture healing. In the porous material intramembranous bone begins to appear within a week. With adequate interface proximity and stability, woven bone is abundant by 3 weeks and lamellar bone remodeling is well under way by 6 weeks.[8-11] Over time further remodeling and maturation of bone is noted. However, micromovement at the interface can be associated with areas of enchondral bone formation and with a fibrocartilaginous intermediate (**Figures 15.2A to E**).[12]

Stability at the interface is achieved by ingrowth of bone and to some extent by the formation of a fibrous tissue rather than a bony interface. In some cases function with a fibrous interface may be clinically successful, but ingrowth of bone over a significant portion of the interface provides a more reliable and consistent clinical result. The degree of ingrowth may be measured by histological evaluation of the extent to which the interface substrate is occupied by bone as well as by evaluating the strength of fixation under mechanical testing conditions.[13-15]

Surface Characteristics

The primary material characteristics that determine the degree of actual ingrowth are related to pore size, degree (percentage of the space unoccupied by the material also called porosity) as well interconnectivity, the size and extent of the connections from one pore to another. These characteristics are determined by the manufacturing process and material properties of the elements used to create the ingrowth substrate. Commonly used technologies have included plasma spraying or sintering of titanium or cobalt chrome microspheres (beaded surfaces), diffusion bonding of kinked titanium wire (fiber mesh), and more recently the creation of ultraporous metals (heat deposition tantalum).[16]

While the absolute minimal pore size required for ingrowth would be the minimum size of a typical osteon (10 μm), and structural organization of the bone would require pores of 100 microns, the pore size that provides optimal ingrowth is between 150 and 400 microns. At greater sizes the tendency is for the bone to form surface attachment or ongrowth, rather than actual ingrowth into the pores.[1]

The degree of porosity (interconnectivity) in the materials commonly used for cementless TKA, cobalt microspheres or titanium mesh, is dependent on manufacturing technology and has ranged from 30% to 50%. Newer ultraporous metals such as heat deposition tantalum have been noted to have up to 80% porosity.[16]

The Interface: Contact and Motion

The distance between the bone and ingrowth surface after implantation, as well as the stability of this interface (the amount of motion which occurs at the interface under the loading conditions experienced after implantation) determines the type and extent of ingrowth. Animal models of ingrowth consistently demonstrate that as the gap between bone and porous surface increases, the quantity and quality of ingrowth declines. Beyond 50 microns distance the ingrowth is increasingly fibrous and not bone. However, implant-bone interface stability, as measured by relative interfacial motion under load clearly influences this relationship.[1,8]

Multiple studies involving a variety of models have sought to determine the upper bounds for acceptable motion in the ingrowth setting. The findings are consistent that increasing interface motion decreases ingrowth fixation histologically, as well as strength of fixation testing. In some settings increased motion results in bone formation in the porous material but without a bony connection to the adjacent skeleton.[10,12] Excessive motion inhibits bone formation and can result in fibrous

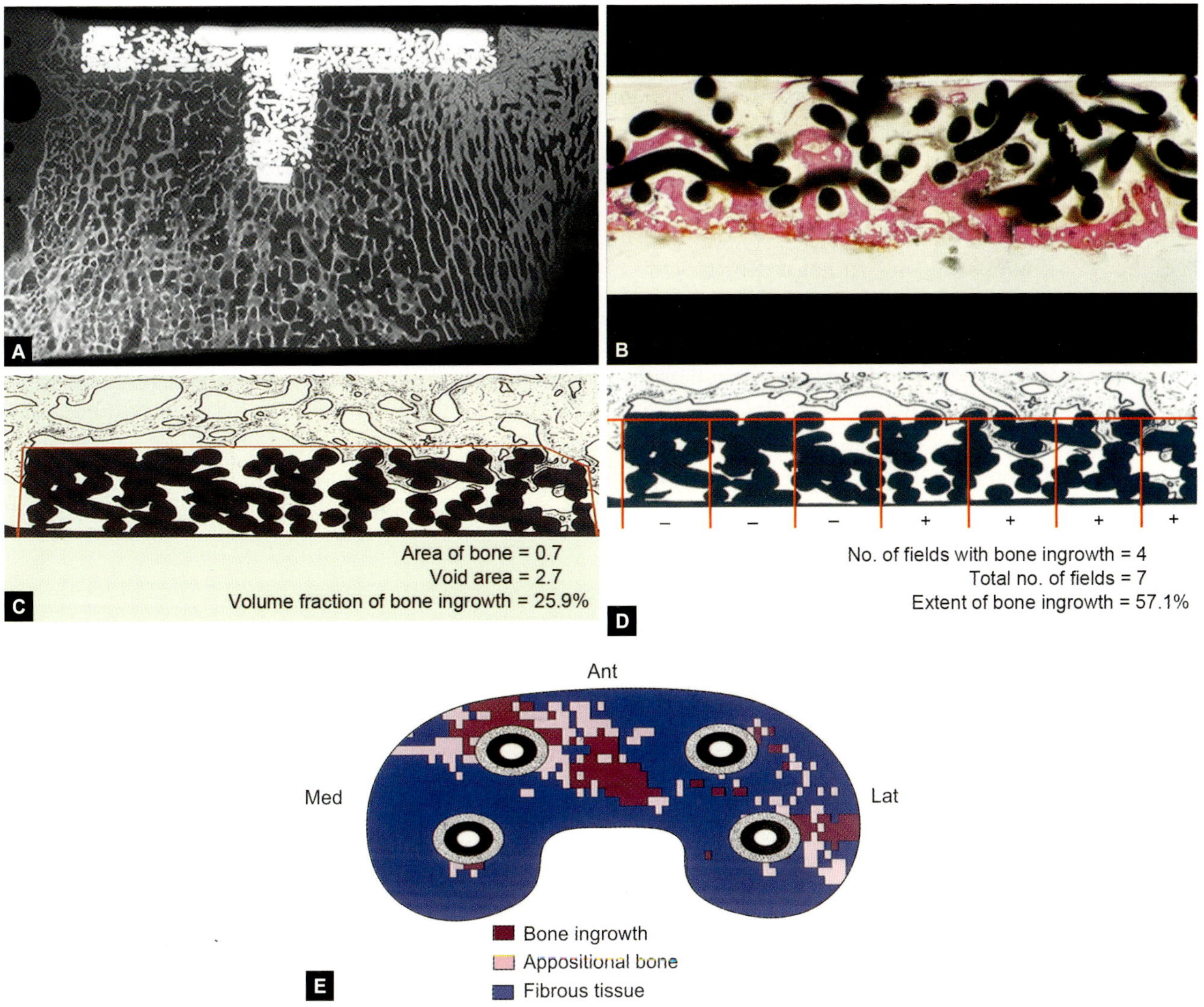

Figures 15.2A to E (A) Thin section slab radiograph of canine ingrowth TKA component retrieved at 3 months; (B) Histologic section demonstrating bone ingrowth into the porous structure; (C) Measuring ingrowth by evaluating a segment of interface and determining the void area and the percentage of that area occupied by bone; (D) Measuring ingrowth by evaluating a number of fields at the interface and determining the percentage of fields that demonstrate some bone ingrowth; (E) Topological mapping of the bone/porous substrate interface

or a fibrocartilaginous attachment at the interface along with areas of enchondral bone formation. The ideal upper bound of motion appears to be approximately 20 microns with 40 microns being considered excessive. Given the importance of interface contact and implant stability, the early studies of bone ingrowth into TKA components focused much attention on the surgical techniques required to insure the components were accurately seated and that the implants were designed to minimize interfacial motion.[17-21]

Component Design

Achieving adequate implant stability after implantation under the loading conditions of motion and weight bearing is challenging, and substantial effort has gone into developing methods to enhance the initial fixation achieved with ingrowth components. Initially based on creation a frictional interference 'press' fit, continuing adequate stability to allow for robust ingrowth depends on the magnitude of the loading forces as well as on the intrinsic stability of the implant conferred by the geometry of the implant and its relationship to the corresponding bones surface configuration. The design features required for successful ingrowth must focus on achieving intimate implant bone contact and adequate interface stability while the ingrowth process takes place. Adequate initial bone implant interface contact has been shown to be achievable but does require careful attention to surgical technique and appropriate bone cutting techniques.[12, 17-21]

The femoral component is generally considered to be more stable in its intrinsic configuration. In resurfacing the distal femur the component has a box like configuration that resists anteroposterior translation and flexion/extension as well as varus valgus rotation. The degree of interference fit along the anterior and posterior aspects of the implant resists cephalocaudal as well as medial/lateral translation and rotation in all planes. The addition of pegs on the femoral component increases the intrinsic resistance to rotation and translation in several planes imparted by the box like configuration of the component.[1,21-23]

The tibial component is essentially a 'flat-on-flat' configuration and is less intrinsically stable than the femoral. Thus, there has been much effort to enhance fixation of the cementless tibial component. Most tibial components have required some method of improving initial stability, and almost all initially had screws through the baseplate that greatly increased initial stability. Additional adjuncts have included modifications of the traditional tibial keel as well as the addition of pegs, stems, and sleeves (**Figures 15.3A to D**).[1,24-26] However, clinical studies have shown that screws are not needed if

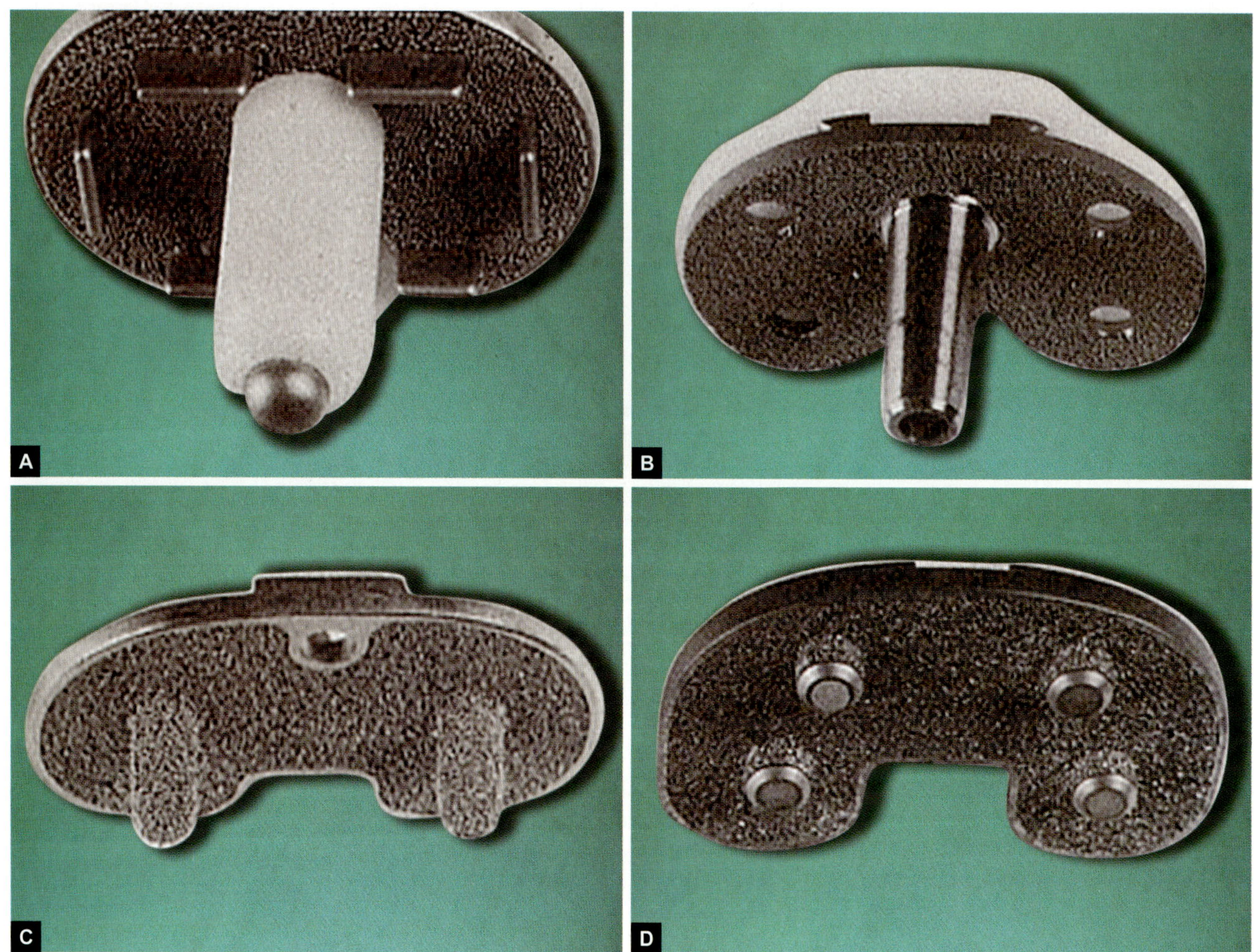

Figures 15.3A to D Improving tibial component stability: variations on a theme (A) Fins + sleeve added to keel; (B) Screws + large central keel; (C) 2 porous pegs; (D) Four shorter pegs + screws

other modalities enhance stability sufficiently. Schepers reported on a randomized prospective study comparing tibial fixation with and without screws in 154 prostheses that had a large keel and four adjunctive pegs at a mean follow-up of 5 years. The prosthesis seemed to provide adequate stability to allow ingrowth as no significant differences in radiologic results or revision rates were noted.[27]

ASSESSING INGROWTH: RETRIEVAL STUDIES

Histologic and radiographic analysis of retrieved TKA components allows for precise analysis of the bone ingrowth that may occur *in vivo*. Unfortunately, variation in the clinical situation that eventuated in the components removal may prejudice conclusions reached in such studies. Typical of the mix of diagnoses in retrievals can be seen in a study by Cook et al. on 85 porous-coated knee components (26 femoral, 34 tibial, and 25 patellar) retrieved from 45 patients for malposition, instability, unexplained pain, late infection, postmortem or postamputation, and post-trauma.[13] No component was clinically or radiographically loose at the time of removal. The average time *in situ* was 12 months (2 weeks to 53 months) and preretrieval radiographs were available for two-thirds of the components. Overall, 52% of the components showed no evidence of bone ingrowth, 29% showed minimal (less than 2%), 12% showed moderate (2–5%), and 7% showed extensive (5–10%) ingrowth. In no component was bone present in more than 10% of the available pore volume. There were no significant differences in the incidence or extent of bone ingrowth among femoral, tibial, and patellar components, nor in the extent of ingrowth in comparing different implant designs, materials, or porous coating types. When bone ingrowth was observed the anatomic location was consistent in each type of component.

In a more focused review of 13 retrievals of one implant type (titanium fiber mesh) (**Figures 15.4A and B**) tibial components removed for reasons unrelated to fixation or infections were quantitatively described.[28] The average length of implantation was 15.3 months (3–30). While all components had supplemental ingrowth pegs, all but one also had four supplemental screws. The average extent of bone ingrowth within the tray was 27.1 +/- 16.1%, and the average volume fraction was 9.5 +/- 7.5%. There was significantly more bone ingrowth within the fixation pegs than within the tray and also more bone ingrowth in the anterior half of the tray than posteriorly. There was no correlation between the amount of bone ingrowth and the length of implantation, age, or sex of the patient; however, the depth and orientation of the resection plane were found to correlate with the topographic distribution of bone ingrowth. Particulate debris appeared to gain access to the interface via soft tissue pathways both at the periphery and through the holes for adjuvant screw

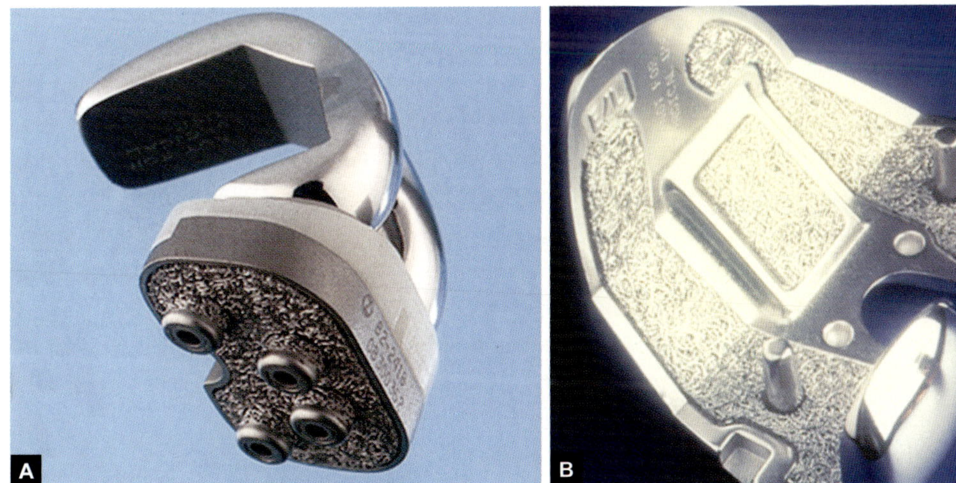

Figures 15.4A and B (A) Modular tibial component with titanium fiber mesh ingrowth pegs and holes for supplemental screws; (B) Titanium fiber mesh ingrowth surface on a femoral component

fixation. Similar postmortem analysis of 8 porous-coated asymmetric tibial components secured with four pegs and two screws where the autograft bone chips were applied to the resected tibia during implantation.[29] Time *in situ* averaged 47+/–36 months. Backscattered electron imaging showed that the bone ingrowth averaged 6%+/–2%.

Early Clinical Findings

Several investigators found higher survival rates at intermediate length follow-up in their cemented compared to their cementless total knees.[2,30-33] While other investigators found better results in the cementless fixation groups, these were almost all reported by the implant developers.[25,26] During this decade roentgen stereophotogrammetric analysis (RSA) became available and has since been commonly used to assess the stability of cementless components.[23,34] As retrieval studies became available, they revealed large numbers of components showing little or no ingrowth into the porous surface. Because tibial component fixation appeared more difficult to achieve clinically and radiographically,[2,32] and was noted to be consistently less impressive in retrieval studies,[9,13] the concept of 'hybrid fixation,' cementing the tibia and patella and using a cementless femoral component, became popular.

It was generally acknowledged, from mechanical considerations, increased surface area and intrinsically greater component stability, that ingrowth would be easier to obtain on the femoral side of the articulation. Indeed Huddleston et al. noted fewer radiolucent lines along the posterior condylar regions of cementless femoral components compared to cemented components.[35] However, several studies have found this construct less than satisfactory. Campbell, Duffy and Trousdale at the Mayo Clinic [36] evaluated 74 consecutive Hybrid TKA using the J&J Press Fit Condylar TKA at a mean 7 year follow-up (5–10). They noted a failure rate of 14%, with 8 of 9 knees requiring revision because of femoral component failure (loosening in 6, and fracture with underlying osteolyisis in 2). Chockalingam and Scott[22] reported on a comparison of 150 cemented and 201 cementless femoral components using the Freeman Samuelson Modular Prosthesis (Sulzer). At 6 years the cementless femoral component failure rate was 9.8% versus 0.6% for cemented components. Carlsson et al.[37] compared porous coated, hydroxyapatite coated, and cemented tibial components over 5 years comparing component fixation in a randomized radiostereometric study finding that cement provided more stable bone-implant contact. While a randomized study of the cementless versus cemented J&J PFC TKA at 5 years [38] showed similar survival and knee scores between cemented and cementless groups.

In light of multiple series documenting excellent long-term follow-up of cemented TKA in the younger population with 10 year survivals of 99% and 15-year survivals of 95%,[5,6,39-41] there was little data in the first two decades of cementless TKA to support the premises under which cementless TKA fixation was introduced or which would justify its continued application. However, over the past decade more persuasive data has accumulated.

Contemporary Results

Contemporary reports of the cementless TKA include long term studies of cementless TKA implantation performed with first generation implants (many of which are no longer available), mid-term reports of more contemporary designs, meta-analyses, and the findings of national registry studies.

Eriksen et al. reported on a 20-year follow-up of a consecutive series of porous-coated AGC cementless TKA.[42] With prosthesis revision as a failure criterion, the cumulative survival rate of all prosthetic components at 20 years was 84.4%. The fall in success rate was primarily due to early tibial and late patellar component failure. The cumulative survival rate at 20 years of the tibial component was 97.2% and the femoral component 100%. Survival of the cementless Miller-Galante I at 14–17 years in 124 consecutive cases was reported by Goldberg and Kraay.[43] The overall knee survival rate was 87% because of the high failure rate of the original metal backed patella; however, survival of the ingrowth tibial component was 99% with only one tibial tray revised.

Park and Kim reported on a randomized study evaluating clinical and radiological results in 50 patients with cemented and cementless NexGen (Zimmer, Warsaw,

USA) total knees implanted bilaterally in the same patient and followed 13 to 14 years.[44] All clinical and radiographic measures were similar as was the 14 survival of the femoral components at 100%. Survival of the cemented tibial component was 100% and 98% in the cementless and cemented tibial component. No osteolysis was identified in either group. Gao et al. evaluated 41 knees randomized to receive a NexGen (Zimmer, Warsaw, USA) CR TKA with either a cemented or uncemented non HA-coated femoral component. Found that no differences at 2 years were noted by clinical and radiological evaluation as well as by RSA, suggesting that uncemented non HA-coated femoral component may perform equally as well as a cemented in the long-term.[45]

Long-term studies of the use of adjuvants such as hydroxylapatite to improve the ingrowth process have also been reported. Cosetto et al. reported on 175 cementless fixed bearing tibial trays with a hydroxyapatite augmented beaded surface.[46] The average knee score at final follow-up using the knee society score was 92 with 96.6% scoring in the excellent range. None of the patients had significant polyethylene wear or osteolysis; and all but one case had bone ingrowth in the tibial tray. Survivorship at an average of 5 years and 7 months was 98.85%. Similarly, in a prospective, randomized series of hydroxyapatite-coated, uncoated, and cemented tibial components followed for 11 to 16 years clinically with RSA to evaluate migration, Pijls and coinvestigators found no statistically significant differences between the fixation groups regarding clinical or radiographic scores.[47] However mean migration at 10 years was 2.25 mm for uncoated components and 1.66 mm for HA-coated components. The cemented group averaged 0.79 mm for ($p < 0.001$).

Posteriorly stabilized (PS) TKA with ingrowth fixation has not been widely attempted because of the unpredictable results noted in multiple early series and concern about the degree of micromotion at the fixation interface induced by cam/postinteractions. Harwin et al. reported on a prospective consecutive series of 114 cementless, tricompartmental periapatite-coated PS implants in 110 patients with a mean age 62 years to determine if initial stability and biologic fixation could be achieved.[48] At a mean follow-up of 36 months, all implants demonstrated radiographic evidence of stable biologic fixation with no evidence of loosening, osteolysis, stress shielding, or progressive radiolucent lines.

Other Diagnoses and Comorbidities

Most series of cementless TKA restrict the procedure to patients with degenerative arthritis. Thus, there are few series evaluating this technique in the inflammatory arthritis patient. However, Woo et al. reported on a series of 112 rheumatoid arthritis patients treated with cementless total knees followed for a mean of 10 years with a final implant survival of 96.8%.[49] Viganó and Whiteside reported on a consecutive series of 47 patients with 64 knees for an average of 83 months (61–124). Survivorship was 98.4% at 10 years postoperatively and there were no failures due to loosening.[50]

Two reports on cementless TKA in obese patients demonstrated survival comparable to cement. Zicat and his colleagues[51] have reviewed a series of obese patients (BMI > 30) undergoing cementless TKA and compared them to a case matched non obese group and found comparable survival rates and no difference in the radiographic appearance of the implant fixation interfaces. Whiteside compared a consecutive series of 122 patients with 167 knees who were younger than 55 with weight greater than 90 kg, and compared them to a gender-matched consecutive series of 122 patients (167 knees) 65 or older and who weighed less than 80 kg.[52] At a follow-up mean of 7.3 years (5–10), mean knee society and pain scores were similar while function scores were better for the young, heavy patients at each interval. None of the knees in either group loosened, while one patient in the young, heavy group underwent poly revision for wear.

Meta-analysis and Registry Results

Despite the large number of papers published on ingrowth fixation of TKA there are relatively few high quality meta-analyses. Gandhi et al. reviewed randomized controlled trials as well as observational studies comparing cemented and uncemented TKA fixation.[53] The primary outcome was implant survival free of aseptic loosening with a secondary outcome of joint function measured by the knee society score. 15 studies met the eligibility criteria.

The combined odds ratio for failure of the implant due to aseptic loosening for the uncemented group was 4.2 (95% confidence interval (CI) 2.7 to 6.5) ($p < 0.0001$). However, subgroup analysis of only randomized trials showed no differences between the groups for odds of aseptic loosening (odds ratio 1.9, 95% CI 0.55 to 6.40, $p = 0.314$). There was no difference in the mean knee society score between groups for all pooled data.

A systematic literature review conducted by Arnold et al. found only 11 randomized trials published between 1980 and January 2011 comparing differences in clinical outcome scores between groups allocated to either cemented or uncemented fixation for TKR.[54] Nine of the 11 studies included in the review reported no significant differences in clinical outcomes. Critical appraisal of methodological bias revealed consistent shortcomings in study design and execution.

Nakama et al. performed a systematic literature review and meta-analysis of comparative randomized studies using RSA to evaluate cemented and cementless TKA components for the Cochrane database.[55] Five randomized controlled trials (RCTs) and 297 participants were included. Cemented fixation of the tibial components demonstrated smaller displacement in relation to cementless fixation (with and without hydroxyapatite) after a follow-up of 2 years. However, the risk of future aseptic loosening with uncemented fixation was approximately half that of cemented fixation, according to the arthroplasty instability classification from RSA with a 16% absolute risk difference between groups. Meta-analysis on patient related outcomes and adverse events was not possible, but the authors of each study reviewed independently found no significant difference between groups.

Registries from other countries have not published data that select out and report on specific implant types, but rather reports on more undifferentiated data. The Australian registry[56] reported the number of revisions out of 100 patient years of observation (95% CI) to be similar between cemented 0.72 (0.70–0.74), cementless 0.81 (0.78–0.85), and Hybrid at 0.66 (0.64–0.69). The results in other registries have been less comparable. The registry of England and Wales[57] found cement at 0.98 (90.93–1.03) revisions out of 100 patient years of observation, all uncemented at 1.99 (1.74–2.28), and hybrid fixation at 1.31 (0.96–1.80), while New Zealand[58] reported cement at 0.48 (0.46–0.51), cementless 0.98 (0.82–1.16), and hybrid 0.52 (0.42–0.63).

However, Niemeläinen et al.[59] did review a separate cohort of 1143 porous tantalum monoblock tibial components in the Finnish arthroplasty registry implanted from 2003 to 2010. Seven-year survivorship of these TKAs was 100% (95% CI 99–100) with revision for aseptic loosening of the tibial component, and 97% (95% CI 96–98) with revision for any reason as the respective end points. Other reports from individual investigators support these findings as noted below.

Trabecular Metal

Traditionally, porous fixation surfaces of either mesh or beads were affixed to a relatively rigid substrate and had relatively low volumetric porosity available for ingrowth with only moderate frictional characteristics to aid in initial implant stability. Newer porous structural biomaterials have been developed and introduced to address these limitations. The earliest of these materials is tantalum. Developed with a structure resembling the cancellous bone, it is marketed as trabecular metal (TM) and offers potential advantages over conventional materials used for ingrowth by the virtue of its uniformity, structural continuity, strength, elasticity, high porosity, and high coefficient of friction along with outstanding biocompatibility.[16,60] Early reports on its use in primary TKA became available in 2009. These implants were nonmodular and achieved initial stability by virtue of multiple large pegs driven into undersized holes drilled out in the metaphyseal bone (**Figures 15.5A to D**).

O'Keefe et al. reported on minimum 5 year outcomes for 125 TM monoblock tibial components.[61] No patients were lost to follow-up and clinical and radiographic follow-up showed all components to be stable with no implants at risk of loosening, no observable osteolysis, and no observed change in bone density. Survivorship free of revision for tibial component loosening was 100% at 5 years. At a short-term follow-up Unger et al. noted no tibial loosening in 108 TM tibias.[62] Ghalayini and Helm et al.[63,64] reported on a series of 109 TM tibias followed for 3–5 years with only one tibial revision (for trauma). At a minimum

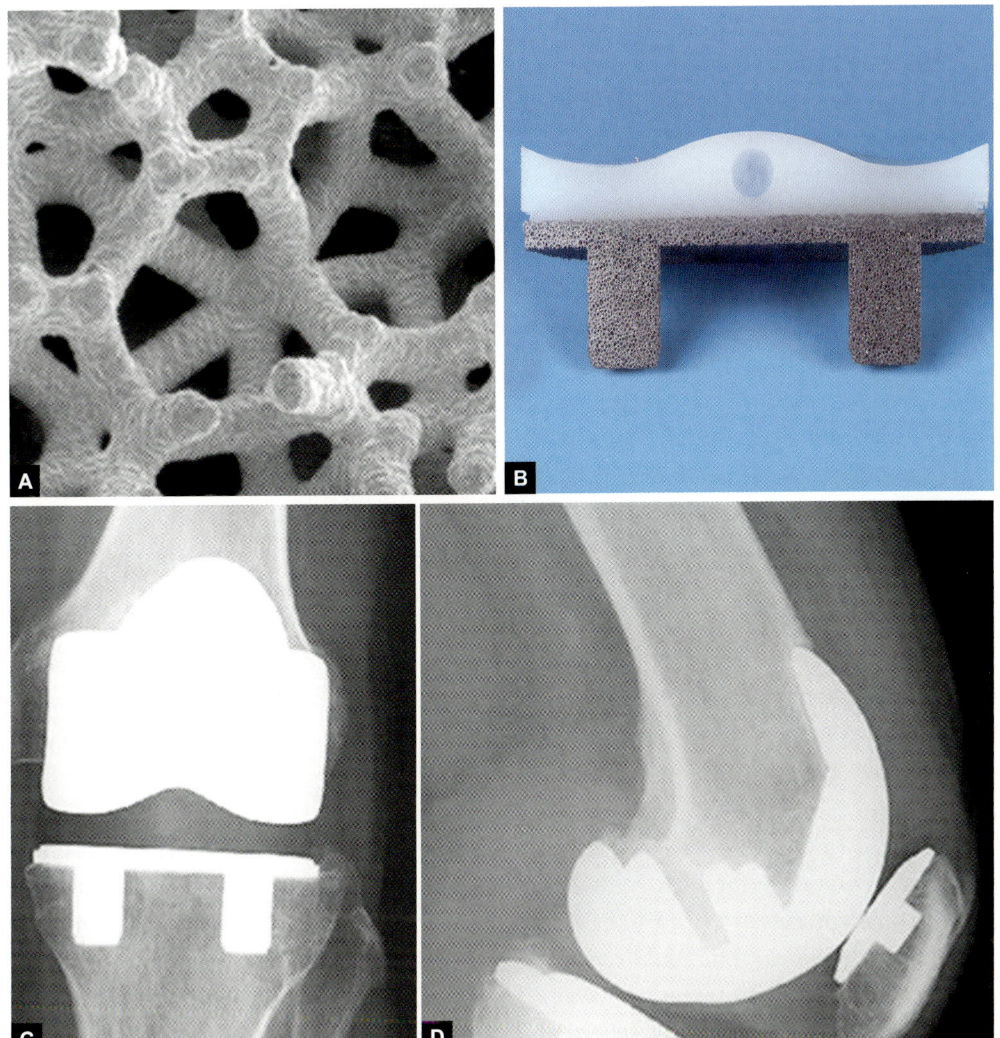

Figures 15.5A to D (A) Porous tantalum. Note high degree of interconnecting porosity, void space and roughened edges of tantalum struts which increase frictional interference fit; (B) Cross-section of porous tantalum monoblock tibial component; (C and D) Anteroposterior and lateral radiograph of ingrowth TM cementless femoral, tibial, and patellar components at 5-year follow-up

of 6 years there was no radiographic evidence of loosening in any implant but one was revised for unexplained pain.

Kamath reported on 100 consecutive TM components with a traditional posterior stabilized cam and post in patients 55 years of age or less compared with 312 concurrent cemented implants at a minimum of 5 years.[65]

Knee society scores were excellent and equivalent beyond six months with no significant difference in blood loss, complication rates, or cost. Radiographs revealed no failures of ingrowth at last follow-up. While there were three uncemented failures, none were due to fixation failure.

Stilling et al. reported on randomized study using RSA to compare TM pegged baseplates with a titanium mesh tibial implant fixed with supplemental screws.[66] While all tibial components migrated initially, most of the TM components migration occurred within three months of surgery whereas Ti components appeared to stabilize after 1 year. Overall the TM components were also noted to migrate less than the Ti components at 1 ($p = 0.01$) and 2 years ($p = 0.004$).

Dunbar et al.[67] evaluated a group of 70 TKAs randomized to receive either the TM or the cemented tibial component followed by RSA. A subset of the TM components migrated extensively in the postoperative period, but all stabilized by 1 year and the proportion considered to be at risk for early aseptic loosening was 0.0, while four cemented components were considered to be at risk for early aseptic loosening. At further follow-up of the same cohort at 5 years the TM components had significantly greater subsidence than the cemented components (p = 0.001) but the mean total point migration values were similar in the two groups and the proportion of components deemed 'at risk' was 2 of 18 in the cemented group and 0 of 27 in the TM group.[68]

Fernandez-Fairen followed a cohort of 145 patients randomized to receive TM or cemented CR tibial components for a minimum of 5 years with radiographs, knee society and Western Ontario and McMaster Universities Index (WOMAC) scores noting complications, reoperations, and radiographic failures. Complications, reoperations, and radiographic failures were recorded and no difference in the frequency of complications or in aseptic loosening between the two groups was found.[69]

Revision of Cementless TKA

What about revision of the failed cementless versus the failed cemented TKA? Fehring and Griffin[70] reviewed their series of 268 TKA revisions and found 63 revisions for aseptic loosening. 36 were originally cemented and 27 cementless. While they did not find any difference in the end result of these revisions, nor did they comment on differences in revision difficulty or bone loss as a result of fixation differences, they did note a substantially shorter time from implantation to revision in the cementless group and a substantially higher proportion of patients in this group who never had pain relief. While removal of 'loose' implants is substantially easier than removal of well fixed implants, it has been the author's impression based on a large number of revisions including well fixed cementless implants that: (1) well fixed cementless implants are more difficult to remove without taking significant amounts of bone, (2) the underlying bone stock is less supportive than under loose or well fixed cemented components. That said, multiple studies have looked at bone density under cemented and cementless femoral components with the majority showing no significant differences.[65,71-73]

Finally, there is the issue of osteolysis. This issue remains debated and because of the multifactorial nature of particle generation, the addition of modularity, backside wear and new articular surface geometries to the earlier generation of cementless knees introduced in the 1980s, it is difficult to point at the interface as the primary source of increased reports of osteolysis in the cementless TKA literature. Nonetheless, there is a substantially higher incidence of osteolysis (without component loosening) noted in multiple reports.[74,75]

The large number of earlier studies finding a higher failure rate in cementless TKA, the findings of registry studies, and the higher degree of surgical precision required in cementless fixation would suggest that cemented fixation will remain the routine for most surgeons performing TKA. However, the results achieved with more contemporary designs, suggest that a very low failure rate of cementless TKA can be achieved using innovative ingrowth surfaces.

REFERENCES

1. Rosenberg AG. Basic science of bone ingrowth in total knee arthroplasty. Am J Knee Surg. 1991;4:209-19.
2. Rosenberg AG, Barden RM, Galante JO. A comparison of cemented and cementless fixation of the Miller-Galante prosthesis. Clin Orthop. 1990;260:71-9.
3. Berger RA, Lyon JH, Jacobs JJ, et al. Problems with cementless total knee arthroplasty at 11 years follow-up. Clin Orthop Relat Res. 2001;392:196-207.
4. Duffy GP, Berry DJ, Rand JA. Cement versus cementless fixation in total knee arthroplasty. Clin Orthop. 1998;356:66-72.
5. Ranawat CS, Padgett DE, Ohasi Y. Total knee arthroplasty for patients younger than 55 years. Clin Orthop. 1989;248: 27-33.
6. Gill GS, Chan KC, Mills DM. Five to eighteen year follow-up study of cemented total knee arthroplasty for patients fifty five years old or younger. J Arthroplasty. 1997;12:49-54.
7. Rosenberg AG, Silverton C. Editorial-cementless TKA fixation: an issue for the '90s. Am J Knee Surg. 1993;6:133-4.
8. Tompkins GS, Rosenberg AG. Porous ingrowth and implant fixation. Sem Arthrop. 1993;4:223-37.
9. Kienapfel H, Sumner DR, Jacobs JJ, et al. A quantitative topographic evaluation of bone ingrowth in tibial

components removed from human patients. In: Heimke G, Slotesa U, Lee AGC (Eds). Clinical Implant Materials. Amsterdam: Elsevier; 1990: pp. 415-20.

10. Sumner DR, Berzins A, Turner TM, Igloria R, Natarajan RN. Initial *in vitro* stability of the tibial component in a canine model of cementless total knee replacement. J Biomech. 1993;27(7):929-39.
11. Turner TM, Urban RM, Sumner DR, Skipor AK, Galante JO. Bone ingrowth into the tibial component of a canine total condylar knee replacement prosthesis. J Orthop Res. 1989;7(6):893-901.
12. Aspenberg P, Goodman S, Toksvig-Larsen S, Ryd L, Albrektsson T. Intermittent micromotion inhibits bone ingrowth. Titanium implants in rabbits. Acta Orthop Scand. 1992;63(2):141-5.
13. Cook SD, Barrack RL, Thomas KA, Haddad RJ. Quantitative histologic analysis of tissue growth into porous total knee components. J Arthroplasty. 1989;4:s33-s43.
14. Lee TQ, Barnett SL, Kim WC. Effects of screw types in cementless fixation of tibial tray implants: stability and strength assessment. Clin Biomech. 1999;14(4):258-64.
15. Ramamurti BS, Orr TS, Bragdon CR, et al. Factors influencing stability at the interface between a porous surface and cancellous bone: a finite element analysis of a canine *in vivo* micromotion experiment. J Biomed Mater Res. 1997;36(2):274-80.
16. Cohen R. A porous tantalum trabecular metal: basic science. Am J Orthop. 2002;31(4):216-7.
17. Fadda M, Marcacci M, Toksvig-Larsen S, Wang T, Meneghello R. Improving accuracy of bone resections using robotics tool holder and a high speed milling cutting tool. J Med Eng Technol. 1998;22(6):280-4.
18. Toksvig-Larsen S, Ryd L. Surface flatness after bone cutting. A cadaver study of tibial condyles. Acta Orthop Scand. 1991;62(1):15-8.
19. Toksvig-Larsen S, Ryd L, Lindstrand A. Temperature influence in different orthopedic saw blades. J Arthroplasty. 1992;7(1):21-4.
20. Toksvig-Larsen S, Ryd L. Surface characteristics following tibial preparation during total knee arthroplasty. J Arthroplasty. 1994;9(1):63-6.
21. Macdonald W, Styf J, Carlsson LV, Jacobsson CM. Improved tibial cutting accuracy in knee arthroplasty. Med Eng Phys. 2004;26(9):807-12.
22. Chockalingam S, Scott G. The outcome of cemented vs. cementless fixation of a femoral component in total knee replacement with the identification of radiological signs for the prediction of failure. Knee. 2000;7:233-8.
23. Nilsson KG, Kärrholm J, Linder L. Femoral component migration in total knee arthroplasty: randomized study comparing cemented and uncemented fixation of the Miller-Galante I design. J Orthop Res. 1995;13(3):347-56.
24. Sumner DR, Turner TM, Dawson D, et al. Effect of pegs and screws on bone ingrowth in cementless total knee arthroplasty. Clin Orthop Relat Res. 1994;309:150-5.
25. Hungerford DS, Krackow KA, Kenna RV. Cementless total knee replacements in patients 50 years old and younger. Orthop Clin North Am. 1989;20:131-7.
26. Whiteside LA. Four screws for fixation of the tibial component in cementless total knee arthroplasty. Clin Orthop Rel Res. 1994;299:72-6.
27. Schepers A, Cullingworth L, van der Jagt DR. A prospective randomized clinical trial comparing tibial baseplate fixation with or without screws in total knee arthroplasty: a radiographic evaluation. J Arthroplasty. 2012;27(3):454-60.
28. Sumner DR, Kienapfel H, Jacobs JJ, et al. Bone ingrowth and wear debris in well-fixed cementless porous-coated tibial components removed from patients. J Arthroplasty. 1995;10(2):157-67.
29. Bloebaum RD, Bachus KN, Jensen JW, Hofmann AA. Postmortem analysis of consecutively retrieved asymmetric porous-coated tibial components. J Arthroplasty. 1997;12(8):920-9.
30. Rorabeck CH, Bourne RB, Nott L. The cemented Kinematic II and the non-cemented porous coated anatomic prosthesis for total knee replacement-a prospective study. J Bone Joint Surg. 1988;70A:483-90.
31. Moran CG, Pinder IM, Lees TA, Midwinter MS. Survivorship analysis of the uncemented porous coated anatomic knee replacement. J Bone Joint Surg. 1991;73(8):848-57.
32. Collins DN, Heim SA, Nelson CL, Smith P 3rd. Porous-coated anatomic total knee arthroplasty. A prospective analysis comparing cemented and cementless fixation. Clin Orthop Relat Res. 1991;267:128-36.
33. Ritter MA, Campbell E, Faris PM, Keating EM. The AGC 2000 total knee arthroplasty with and without cement. Am J Knee Surg. 1989;2:160-3.

34. Ryd L. Micromotion in knee arthroplasty. A roentgen stereophotogrammetric analysis of tibial component fixation. Acta Orthop Scand Suppl. 1986;220:1-80.
35. Huddleston JI, Wiley JW, Scott RD. Zone 4 femoral radiolucent lines in hybrid versus cemented total knee arthroplasties: are they clinically significant? Clin Orthop Relat Res. 2005;441:334-9.
36. Campbell MD, Duffy GP, Trousdale RT. Femoral component failure in hybrid total knee arthroplasty. Clin Orthop Relat Res. 1998:356;58-65.
37. Carlsson A, Björkman A, Besjakov J, Onsten I. Cemented tibial component fixation performs better than cementless fixation: a randomized radiostereometric study comparing porous-coated, hydroxyapatite-coated and cemented tibial components over 5 years. Acta Orthop. 2005;76(3): 362-9.
38. McCaskie AW, Deehan DJ, Green TP, et al. Randomized, prospective study comparing cemented and cementless total knee replacement: results of press-fit condylar total knee replacement at five years. J Bone Joint Surg Br. 1998;80(6):971-5.
39. Dalury DF, Ewald FC, Christie MJ, Scott RD. Total knee arthroplasty in a group of patients less than 45 years of age. J Arthroplasty. 1995;10:598-602.
40. Duffy GP, Trousdale RT, Stuart MJ. Total knee arthroplasty in patients 55 years old or younger. 10–17 year results. Clin Orthop. 1998;356:22-7.
41. Diduch DR, Insall JN, Scott WN, Scuderi GR, Font-Rodriguez D. Total knee replacement in young active patients. J Bone Joint Surg. 1997;79(4):575-82.
42. Eriksen J, Christensen J, Solgaard S, Schrøder H. The cementless AGC 2000 knee prosthesis: 20-year results in a consecutive series. Acta Orthop Belg. 2009;75(2):225-33.
43. Goldberg VM, Kraay M. The outcome of the cementless tibial component: a minimum 14-year clinical evaluation. Clin Orthop Relat Res. 2004;428:214-20.
44. Park JW, Kim YH. Simultaneous cemented and cementless total knee replacement in the same patients: a prospective comparison of long-term outcomes using an identical design of NexGen prosthesis. J Bone Joint Surg Br. 2011;93(11):1479-86.
45. Gao F, Henricson A, Nilsson KG. Cemented versus uncemented fixation of the femoral component of the NexGen CR total knee replacement in patients younger than 60 years: a prospective randomized controlled RSA study. Knee. 2009;16(3):200-6.
46. Cosetto DJ, Gouda AD. Uncemented tibial fixation in total knee arthroplasty. J Arthroplasty. 2011;26(1):41-4.
47. Pijls BG, Valstar ER, Kaptein BL, Fiocco M, Nelissen RG. The beneficial effect of hydroxyapatite lasts: a randomized radiostereometric trial comparing hydroxyapatite-coated, uncoated, and cemented tibial components for up to 16 years. Acta Orthop. 2012;83(2):135-41.
48. Harwin SF, Kester MA, Malkani AL, Manley MT. Excellent fixation achieved with cementless posteriorly stabilized total knee arthroplasty. J Arthroplasty. 2013;28(1): 7-13.
49. Woo YK, Kim KW, Chung JW, Lee HS. Average 10.1-year follow-up of cementless total knee arthroplasty in patients with rheumatoid arthritis. Can J Surg. 2011;54(3):179-84.
50. Viganó R, Whiteside LA, Roy M. Clinical results of bone ingrowth TKA in patients with rheumatoid arthritis. Clin Orthop Relat Res. 2008;466(12):3071-7.
51. Jackson MP, Sexton SA, Walter WL, Walter WK, Zicat BA. The impact of obesity on the mid-term outcome of cementless total knee replacement. J Bone Joint Surg Br. 2009;91(8):1044-8.
52. Whiteside LA, Viganò R. Young and heavy patients with a cementless TKA do as well as older and lightweight patients. Clin Orthop Relat Res. 2007;464:93-8.
53. Gandhi R, Tsvetkov D, Davey JR, Mahomed NN. Survival and clinical function of cemented and uncemented prostheses in total knee replacement: a meta-analysis. J Bone Joint Surg Br. 2009;91(7):889-95.
54. Arnold JB, Walters JL, Solomon LB, Thewlis D. Does the method of component fixation influence clinical outcomes after total knee replacement? A systematic literature review. J Arthroplasty. 2013;28(5):740-6.
55. Nakama GY, Peccin MS, Almeida GJ, et al. Cemented, cementless or hybrid fixation options in total knee arthroplasty for osteoarthritis and other non-traumatic diseases. Cochrane Database Syst Rev. 2012.
56. Hip and Knee Arthroplasty Registry, Australian Orthopedic Association, Annual Report, 2012. *http://aoanjrr.dmac.adelaide.edu.au/*
57. National Joint Registry For England and Wales, 9th Annual Report, pg. 165 www.njrcentre.org.uk

58. New Zealand Joint Registry Thirteen Year Report. *http://www.cdhb.govt.nz/NJR/reports/A2D65CA3.pdf*
59. Niemeläinen M, Skyttä ET, Remes V, Mäkelä K, Eskelinen A. Total knee arthroplasty with an uncemented trabecular metal tibial component: a registry-based analysis. J Arthroplasty. 2013.
60. Levine B, Sporer S, Della Valle CJ, Jacobs JJ, Paprosky W. Porous tantalum in reconstructive surgery of the knee: a review. J Knee Surg. 2007;20(3):185-94.
61. O'Keefe TJ, Winter S, Lewallen DG, Robertson DD, Poggie RA. Clinical and radiographic evaluation of a monoblock tibial component. J Arthroplasty. 2010;25(5):785-92.
62. Unger AS, Duggan JP. Midterm results of a porous tantalum monoblock tibia component - clinical and radiographic results of 108 knees. J Arthroplasty. 2011;26(6):855-60.
63. Ghalayini SR, Helm AT, McLauchlan GJ. Minimum 6 year results of an uncemented trabecular metal tibial component in total knee arthroplasty. Knee. 2012;19(6):872-4.
64. Helm AT, Kerin C, Ghalayini SR, McLauchlan GJ. Preliminary results of an uncemented trabecular metal tibial component in total knee arthroplasty. J Arthroplasty. 2009;24(6):941-4.
65. Kamath AF, Lee GC, Sheth NP, et al. Prospective results of uncemented tantalum monoblock tibia in total knee arthroplasty: minimum 5-year follow-up in patients younger than 55 years. J Arthroplasty. 2011;26(8):1390-5.
66. Stilling M, Madsen F, Odgaard A, et al. Superior fixation of pegged trabecular metal over screw-fixed pegged porous titanium fiber mesh: a randomized clinical RSA study on cementless tibial components. Acta Orthop. 2011;82(2):177-86.
67. Dunbar MJ, Wilson DA, Hennigar AW, et al. Fixation of a trabecular metal knee arthroplasty component. A prospective randomized study. J Bone Joint Surg Am. 2009;91(7):1578-86.
68. Wilson DA, Richardson G, Hennigar AW, Dunbar MJ. Continued stabilization of trabecular metal tibial monoblock total knee arthroplasty components at 5 years-measured with radiostereometric analysis. Acta Orthop. 2012;83(1):36-40.
69. Fernandez-Fairen M, Hernández-Vaquero D, Murcia A, Torres A, Llopis R. Trabecular metal in total knee arthroplasty associated with higher knee scores: Clin Orthop Relat Res. 2013. [Epub ahead of print]
70. Fehring TK, Griffin WL. Revision of failed cementless total knee implants with cement. Clin Orthop. 1998;356:34-38.
71. Seki T, Omori G, Koga Y, et al. Is bone density in the distal femur affected by use of cement and by femoral component design in total knee arthroplasty? J Orthop Sci. 1999;4(3):180-6.
72. Abu-Rajab RB, Watson WS, Walker B, et al. Peri-prosthetic bone mineral density after total knee arthroplasty. cemented versus cementless fixation. J Bone Joint Surg Br. 2006;88(5):606-13.
73. Kamath S, Chang W, Shaari E, et al. Comparison of peri-prosthetic bone density in cemented and uncemented total knee arthroplasty. Acta Orthop Belg. 2008;74(3):354-9.
74. Gustafson A, Clark IC, Saha S, Campbell P. Catastrophic peri-implant bone loss caused by polyethylene and metallic wear in total knees. J Long Term Effects Med Implants. 1993;3:91-104.
75. Peters PC, Engh GA, Dwyer KA, Vinh TN. Osteolysis after total knee arthroplasty without cement. J Bone Joint Surg. 1992;74(6):864-76.

Chapter 16

Minimally Invasive Approach to Total Knee Arthroplasty

Alfred J Tria Jr, William Baione, Brian Culp

EVOLUTION OF APPROACHES

The standard midline approach to the knee has led to very acceptable clinical results over the past 20 years for total knee arthroplasty (TKA).[1,2] However, there has been a movement toward minimally invasive surgery (MIS) in the appropriately selected patient. Accordingly, surgeons are increasingly faced with the challenge of implanting prostheses with long-term survival through a smaller surgical wound. As the results of joint replacements are more critically evaluated, patient satisfaction and short-term outcome have become significant components of the review process.

Today's patients present to the office setting more knowledgeable and with high expectations for their surgeon. Their concerns may not always directly align with the surgeon's concerns. Patients are often worried about cosmetic, postoperative pain, and the total recovery time.[3,4] Many patients associate their postoperative outcome with the incision length and compare their wounds to those of their friends. Furthermore, the internet has become a major source of information and minimally invasive procedures are commonly included in the discussions.[5] The surgeon must find a way to balance the patients' concerns with the surgical goals of long-term durability and minimal complications.

While the traditional techniques correctly emphasized the importance of exposure and visualization, they included a significant skin incision of 20–25 cm in length and violation of the quadriceps mechanism.[6] Disruption of the quadriceps mechanism has been associated with higher pain, increased blood loss, slower postoperative recovery, and extensor mechanism weakness after surgery.[7-10] The midvastus and subvastus approaches were advocated as a way to find a less traumatic 'intermuscular plane' with decreased insult to the vastus medialis obliquus (VMO).[11-13] These approaches are still extensile, and gain access to the knee by a complete eversion of the patella. This requires significant dissection to achieve mobilization, and can place stress on the patellar tendon insertion leading to patella baja,[14,15] loss of motion, and increased anterior knee pain.[10,16,17] While these novel approaches addressed some of the concerns, they still required significant soft tissue dissection and were often difficult to perform.

As surgical instrumentation and protocols advance, so too must the surgical technique. Patient satisfaction has definitely become a major part of the equation for the results of the TKA. The perception of pain and the postoperative function are now evaluated from both the surgeon's and patient's perspective. Extensive soft tissue dissection undertaken in extensile approaches leads to a high level of inflammation and pain.[10,18] This slows recovery, and prolongs hospitalization in the postoperative period.[19] With the ever common goal of decreased inpatient stay versus outpatient surgery, a novel technique might allow for a more mobile and comfortable patient immediately after the surgery[20,21] and one eventually is more satisfied with their outcome. More limited approaches were introduced to address these issues and hopefully maintain the same or better results.

HISTORY

John Insall recommended adequate exposure for the TKA and the median parapatellar approach became the gold standard for the surgery.[6] Other authors appreciated the risk to the extensor mechanism and created variations that included the midvastus and subvastus approaches.[11-13,22] All three options were extensile in order to provide the proper visualization for the implant with a well aligned and balanced knee. In the 1990s, novel minimalist approaches for unicondylar arthroplasty showed excellent success.[23,24] Repicci was able to implant the partial knee replacement with minimal invasion of the quadriceps mechanism and excellent early function. This led arthroplasty surgeons to question whether the same techniques could be applied to TKA.[7,25]

Several approaches were trialed during this time, including the 'quadriceps sparing,'[26] the mini midvastus,[10] and the mini subvastus approaches.[27] Each held the same principal of minimal violation to the quadriceps tendon, subluxation rather than eversion of the patella, and decreased soft tissue trauma. They depended upon proper patient selection and a new way of visualizing the anatomy at the time of the surgery. The incision was used as a 'mobile window' with movement in different directions to aid in the visualization. Simple static positioning of the retractors was no longer helpful and the knee was placed in different degrees of flexion throughout the procedure to improve the view. The instruments were modified to accommodate the smaller incisions and the techniques began to flourish around the world.

PATIENT SELECTION

While many of these developing techniques relied on surgeon skill, paramount to their success was appropriate patient selection. Not every patient's anatomy will permit these less invasive techniques; therefore, it is critical to observe strict selection criteria in order to avoid complications.

The pre-existing level of deformity will have an effect upon the surgical procedure. It may not be possible to perform proper surgical corrections with all deformities using these minimalist approaches. Patients with a varus deformity greater than 10° or a valgus deformity greater than 15° may not be suitable candidates.[28] A flexion contracture greater than 10° will be difficult to correct using a limited approach. Patients should have preoperative range of motion of 110°, demonstrating that they have adequately mobile soft tissue.[9,28]

Patient body habitus has also been a frequent consideration. While patient weight greater than 180 lbs or a BMI above 33 has been cited as a contraindication, this is not a universal rule.[28,29] The shape of the lower limb is probably more significant in predicting the level of difficulty of the operation rather than the patient's absolute weight or BMI. Alternatively, the surgeon can calculate the ratio by comparing the length of the thigh to the circumference of the knee [anterior-superior iliac spine (ASIS) to the middle of the patella with the leg in full extension divided by the circumference of the knee at the level of the patella]. Patients with a ratio above three are the best candidates for an MIS approach.[26] Muscular men may have large VMOs and this may also limit MIS approaches. Patients with a large femur or tibia require a larger femoral and/or tibial component that may be difficult to insert into the knee with a limited arthrotomy. Patella baja makes it difficult to subluxate the patella laterally and is a relative contraindication. Proper patient selection will make the surgical procedure more predictable and minimize component malposition and complications.

PREOPERATIVE PLANNING

Preoperative planning is essential for the limited approach surgery. Patients should be examined for scars around the planned surgical site. Range of motion and soft tissue should be assessed to ensure the knee is supple and mobile. The ligamentous examination should document the status of all four of the major ligaments. As with any TKA, it is best to plan for the appropriate design of the prosthesis (either posterior substituting or cruciate retaining). Both are viable options with this approach. Overall alignment of the knee should be checked, and it should be determined if the deformity can be corrected. Routine standing knee radiographs are important to aid in the assessment of deformity and bone stock. Mechanical axis X-rays of the leg are not necessary, but certainly are helpful. Templating is not an absolute requirement, but will help to warn the surgeon, if the implant is going to be very large.

The preoperative planning should also include the choice of the operative approach and the plan for extension of the exposure, if visualization becomes difficult. The component and instrumentation considerations must be made before surgery. The MIS approaches do not permit all standard instrumentation to be used for bone cuts.[30] Especially designed instruments that are low profile make the most sense. Computer-navigated instruments or patient specific cutting blocks may provide a useful alternative, if the surgeon is familiar with the techniques and has made the proper preoperative evaluations.

The operative procedure should be well outlined before beginning and the appropriate steps should be sequenced to facilitate the exposure. The first bone cut either on the tibial or the femoral side is usually the most difficult. After the resected bone is removed the subsequent steps are made slightly easier because of the increased space within the joint capsule.

TRANSITIONING TO THE MIS TECHNIQUE

The transition to MIS procedures involves the incorporation of the smaller incisions and the use of smaller, sometimes less familiar, instruments. The newer instruments can be incorporated into the standard operative procedure. The patellar subluxation can be included at this stage and once the surgeon is comfortable with these steps, the operative approach can be added. The limited visualization of standard landmarks will be challenging at first, and so careful consideration of necessary exposure should always be remembered. Once the MIS procedure is completed in its entirety, it is probably best to extend the approach and confirm that all of the alignment and balancing has been fully accomplished. Every approach should have a simple extension so that the surgeon has the opportunity to convert the technique at any time.

The learning curve can be steep. Many of the reported complications occur when surgeons are transitioning to MIS technique. It is best to learn in a controlled setting and to select 'easy' patients in the initial period.

Surgical Technique

The MIS approaches begin with a limited skin incision that is approximately 10–14 cm in length (**Figure 16.1**).

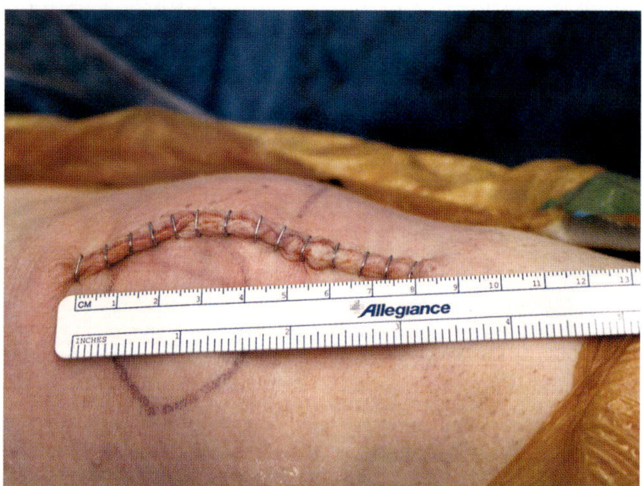

Figure 16.1 Medial MIS incision

This should extend from the superior border of the patella along the medial border to the superior aspect of the tibial tubercle.[7] Soft tissue flaps should be raised medially and laterally, as well as proximally and distally. This will permit mobilization of the skin to provide a 'window' to see the needed exposures.

The superior aspect of the capsular incision is extended up to the level of the superior border of the patella in the quadriceps sparing technique (**Figure 16.2**). The mini midvastus curves the incision at the border of the distal one-third and the proximal two-thirds of the vastus medialis and extends 2 cm into the muscle, but not further (**Figure 16.3**).[25] The mini subvastus curves the incision just beneath the vastus medialis muscle belly and extends 2 cm proximally, but once again not further (**Figure 16.4**).[27] The further the capsular incision is carried, the more similar it will become to the standard approaches, leading to the loss of benefit of the MIS.[9]

After the capsule has been opened, the patella can then be subluxed laterally to enable good visualization of the notch (**Figure 16.5**). At this point, removal of any excessively large osteophytes or constraining capsular reflections may afford better excursion. This should provide a 'mobile window' to sufficiently visualize the necessary

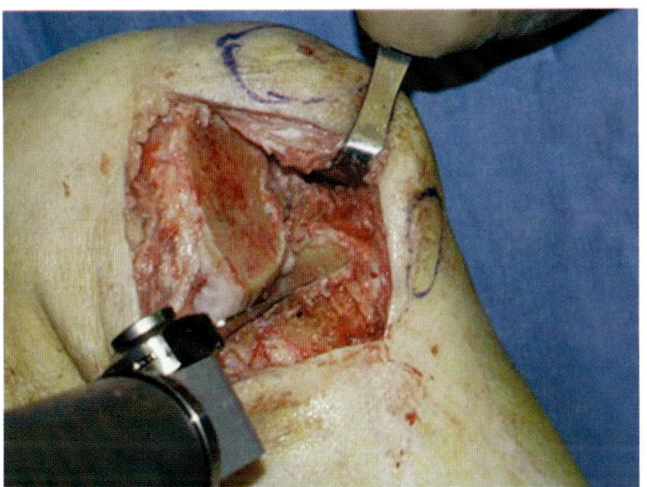

Figure 16.2 The quadriceps sparing arthrotomy from the superior pole of the patella extending to 2 cm below the tibiofemoral joint line

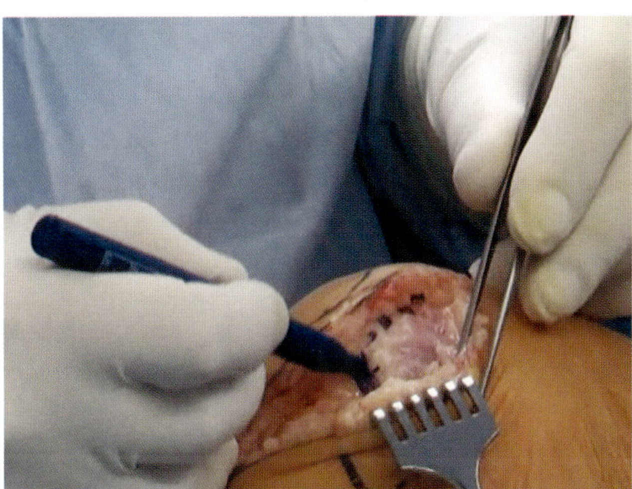

Figure 16.4 The blue marking identifies the inferior border of the vastus medialis for the subvastus approach

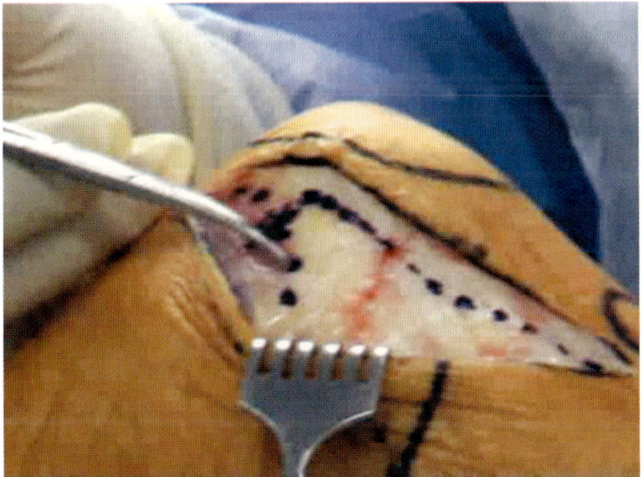

Figure 16.3 The mini-midvastus incision with the 2 cm extension into the vastus medialis at the junction of the distal one third-proximal two-thirds of the muscle

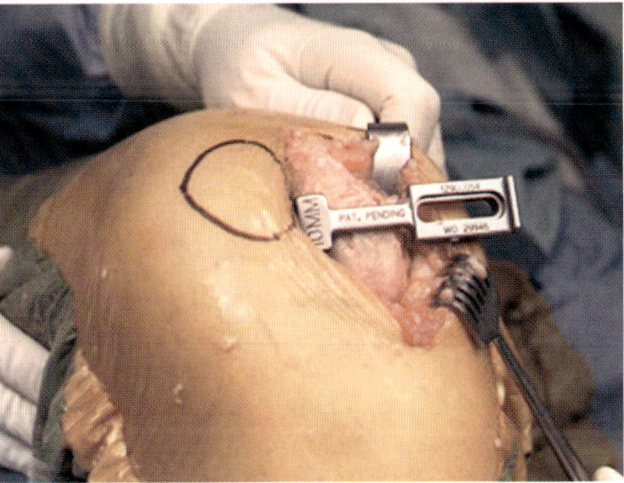

Figure 16.5 The intramedullary guide for the distal resection of the femoral condyles subluxes the patella to the lateral side of the knee without eversion

landmarks and starting points to place instrumentation. It is important to avoid undue tension throughout the entire operation in order to avoid soft tissue complications. If the cruciate ligaments are to be sacrificed, this can be completed at this stage to allow the tibia to translate forward.

The surgery may begin on either the femoral or tibial side. A measured resection of the femur using anatomic axes and landmarks removes the bony prominences and facilitates the tibial exposure. Initial tibial resection permits flexion/extension balancing before attempting the femoral preparation.

The authors prefer to complete the femoral preparation first and use intramedullary referencing as a guide. It is possible to use patient specific instrumentation for this step and this avoids the intramedullary instrument. Most systems have modified the four-in-one cutting blocks so that they are smaller and can be inserted into the wound without excessive retraction of the soft tissues. After the femur is prepared, the tibia can be brought slightly forward and an extramedullary guide can be positioned. The knee can be moved from the 90° flexion position to a midrange of flexion that will allow easier positioning of the guide within the mobile window. The extramedullary jig is applied and the plateau is cut perpendicular to the anatomic axis of the tibia. Throughout the procedure, it is important to monitor the position of the retractors so that they are moved together and not pulled harshly in opposite directions. Moving the mobile window facilitates the exposure and excessive retraction in two opposite directions actually shortens the total length of the incision for visualization. Slightly extend the leg, if necessary, and remove the tibial bone carefully releasing soft tissue attachments as the segment is removed.

If the tibial resection is completed first, the same instrumentation can be used and the resected tibial bone should be removed with care by flexing and extending the knee to facilitate the exposure. After the tibial resection is completed, the flexion and extension gaps can be evaluated before proceeding to the femoral side.

With either of the two techniques, spacer blocks (modified to a smaller size) and/or tensioning instruments can be inserted to confirm alignment and balance. Traditional ligament releasing or tightening can be used without difficulty once the bony resections have been completed. The medial releases on the tibial side are facilitated by flexing the knee to 45° and moving the mobile window over the tibial metaphyseal area. The lateral releases (either the pie crusting technique or the sequential anatomic release) are best performed with the knee again flexed to 45° and with gentle retraction upon the noneverted, subluxed patella. The posterior capsular release on the femoral side for a pre-existing flexion contracture is best completed with the knee in 90° of flexion and with slight distraction from an inserted laminar spreader or with external distraction from the first assistant.

Patellar resurfacing can be included in the procedure without difficulty after the resections are completed on the femoral and tibial side. It is best to complete this without any of the trials in position because there is more soft tissue laxity and minimal retraction is necessary. The resurfacing is at the discretion of the surgeon and is not a mandatory part of the MIS procedures.

The trial components are inserted at this point and this can be difficult in some cases depending upon the prosthetic design. Cruciate retaining femoral components usually have a tibial tray with abbreviated undersurface pegs that can be easily inserted on the tibia and, then, the femoral component can be slide onto the femoral cut surface using the tibial prosthetic surface for a guide. Posterior cruciate substituting designs usually have a longer intramedullary keel on the tibial tray and will require more facility with the mobile window positioning. Once again, mid flexion of 45° for the insertion is typically preferred.

After the trialing is completed, the surfaces can be prepared for the final implant. The tibial tray should be inserted first and, if cemented, the remaining cement can be removed without difficulty. It is not difficult to insert the femoral component on top of the tibial trays, but cement removal can be challenging. Therefore, it is best to place the cement on the component and not on the exposed bony surfaces. This technique limits the amount of cement that is extruded behind the femoral runners.

COMPONENT CONSIDERATIONS

Some companies did proceed to make modified prostheses that were slightly smaller in size and enabled easier insertion of the device. The majority of the changes were made on the tibial side because of the keels. The tibial changes never gained much popularity and many surgeons were concerned about the possibility of loosening with the abbreviated tibial keel.[31] The senior author (Alfred J Tria Jr) did consider the possibility of inserting the femoral component in two or three pieces to accommodate the smaller incision but this proved to be difficult to design and would have complicated the overall procedure.

While some surgeons attempted to perform the procedures with standard instruments, the results were not as acceptable and led to malalignment and an increased number of surgical outliers. The senior author initially designed completely novel instruments for the quadriceps sparing technique. These instruments complemented each of the surgical steps and facilitated a precise technique through a smaller window.[32] Unfortunately, the instruments were not familiar to most surgeons and required a more significant learning curve.[33] It has made much more sense to modify the pre-existing designs and just decrease their overall size. This allows the surgeon to use the approach with a more familiar system.

Computer navigation may help the surgeon to identify the anatomic landmarks with greater ease within the limited incision. However, navigation may add time to the procedure with a considerable expense and a distinct learning curve.[34] The combination of MIS and computer navigation may be more than a surgeon should attempt when beginning to use these limited approaches.

Patient-specific cutting blocks are still in the early phases of development, but they are compatible with the MIS techniques and they have been shown to increase accuracy and to decrease operative time by eliminating many repetitive steps. These cutting blocks may definitely have a place in the future of MIS surgery.[32]

COMPLICATIONS

Some authors note a higher complication rate with MIS techniques as opposed to the classically described approach.[35,36] Most of the complications associated with the MIS procedures are related to the difficulty of visualizing the entire joint through a limited incision. It is best to review these from the start to the finish of the operative procedure. Skin compromise has been cited as a complication of MIS knee surgery.[35] The mobile window is critical for the surgery and there is a tendency for the assistants to over retract the skin. This complication can be more common in patients with fragile skin, such as the elderly or patients with rheumatoid arthritis. The incision should be moved medial to lateral and inferior to superior throughout the case to avoid skin necrosis.[37] The brevity of the skin incision, while an attractive component of MIS TKA, has less of an impact on the proposed postoperative benefits than the capsular incision.

Extensor mechanism injury is a dreaded complication and can be a concern in MIS techniques.[35] This is especially true for patients who might be at the extremes of the recommended patient selection guidelines. After the arthrotomy is completed, it is important to keep sight of the patellar tendon insertion throughout the operation. The patella should be subluxed to the lateral side and not everted to avoid excess tension. Ultimately, if this cannot be accomplished safely, the capsular incision should be extended.

Component malalignment has also been cited as a concern for minimal incision approaches.[17,30] This mistake was more common as the technique was being newly developed and before the modified instrumentation was available. Each of the bone cuts should be monitored and confirmed with the traditional landmarks. Femoral valgus should be adjusted with intramedullary referencing and/or extramedullary confirmation with the ASIS of the pelvis. Femoral rotation should reference the AP-axis. The epicondylar axis is more difficult to visualize, but is a good addition. The tibial cut is usually difficult because of the limited access to the posterolateral plateau. This can often lead to a varus cut and early failure. The newer cutting blocks and instrumentation systems have largely solved these problems with the majority of recent studies indicating that there is no difference in component alignment between MIS and standard approaches.[10,35,38]

Another concern is failure of fixation and therefore, higher rates of loosening.[31] Most implants are cemented and it is critical to establish a good mantle around both the femoral and tibial prostheses. On occasion, residual debris in the knee from cement that has not been completely removed from the margins of the prostheses may lead to surface wear of the polyethylene and subsequent loosening. Striking a balance between enough and too much cement can prove more difficult in this limited approach. Alternatively, the MIS procedures are amenable to cementless designs; however, it is critical to establish perfect surfaces to insure solid contact between the implants and the bone.

In general, it is not a good principle to attempt a revision TKA through a limited incision. Revisions are fraught with a multitude of decisions and a requirement for excellent exposure. Although some have successfully used this technique, these are exceptions and not the rule.[39] It is not wise to limit the exposure in such a setting.

Intraoperative fractures are a rare occurrence, but they must be treated expeditiously and with a definite extension of the exposure. When recognized and properly internally fixed, they can yield similar results to the uncomplicated procedure. A more common occurrence than fracture with the MIS technique is femoral notching. While this is not always associated with fracture, it is often due to incomplete visualization of the cut.[35,36]

With the higher level of surgical difficulty, some surgeons have noted an increase in operative time or tourniquet time to complete the MIS TKA.[17,40] The reports vary from no difference to a 15% increase in the time requirement. With experience, the time requirement will certainly decrease, but the surgeon should certainly consider this factor during the surgery and be prepared to change the approach, if the time becomes a major factor.

All of the above complications can be either avoided or corrected with proper extension of the exposure. MIS surgery does have definite benefits, but should not compromise the basic principles of TKA.

OUTCOMES

The early outcomes of the MIS procedures for TKA were a reflection of the inexperience of the surgeons and the novelty of the operation. The initial flurry of enthusiasm led to complications and early failures.[7,27] It took time and training to learn how to choose the proper patients and the proper approach. Initially, the instruments were radically changed to accommodate the smaller environment (**Figure 16.6**). These instruments were more useful for the smaller incisions, but were too foreign to the surgeon. Standard instruments were then modified and these proved to be the correct answer. More recent reports document the value of the MIS procedures in the correct patients.[9,20,41]

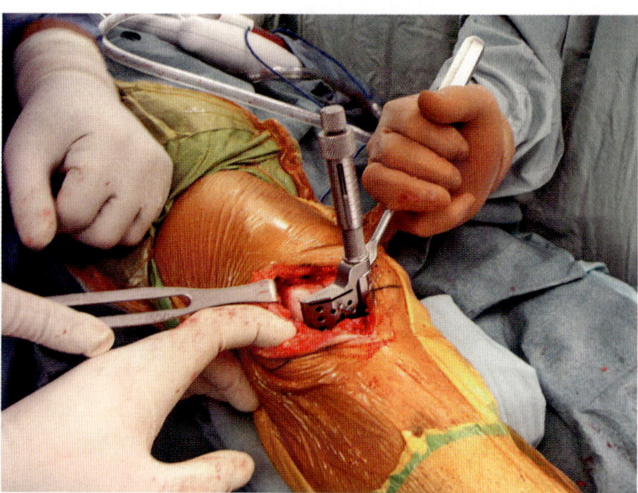

Figure 16.6 An MIS specific instrument designed to resect the anterior surface of the femur

Many of the proposed benefits would seem logical given the decreased amount of injury to the soft tissue. Several authors have cited reduced intraoperative blood loss and lower needs for transfusion. Others note that patients have less pain in the immediate postoperative period.[10,17,42] Still more say that the patients have better function in postoperative recovery, including a better range of motion and higher quadriceps strength.[17,43] These proposed advantages lead to a shorter postoperative stay.[7,10,32,44]

While these positive outcomes have been shown in a number of papers, they have not been reported in all of the subsequent studies.[35,38] There are reports of longer operative time, a higher incidence of complications, and a lack of the proposed advantages of the procedures. The reason why these results are not consistently achieved has yet to be determined. As indicated, the learning curve for the procedure is steep, and may lead to difficulty in the transition period.[45] The optimum number of cases needed for a surgeon to develop a comfort level is not clear, and may vary between surgeons. The definition of MIS also shows some variability in the literature. Authors use MIS to describe anything from the length of the skin incision itself to the capsular incision. They also variably mention suprapatellar pouch dissection, avoidance of hyperflexion, or patellar subluxation rather than eversion.[39] This inconsistency of the definition of MIS TKA may also provide some insight as to why the results are not all the same.

CONCLUSION

The debate over the value of MIS TKA is still ongoing. The actual solution and perfect indications still remain to be defined. Most surgeons agree that the soft tissues should be respected during the surgical approach. Ultimately, MIS TKA is not meant for every patient or every surgeon. In the right setting, however, the result can be very gratifying for both.

REFERENCES

1. Stern SH, Insall JN. Posterior stabilized prosthesis: results after follow-up of nine to twelve years. J Bone Joint Surg Am. 1992;74(7):980-6.
2. Ranawat CS, Flynn WF Jr, Saddler S, Hansraj KK, Maynard MJ. Long-term results of the total condylar knee arthroplasty: a 15-year survivorship study. Clin Orthop Relat Res. 1993;286:94-102.
3. Moran M, Khan A, Sochart DH, Andrew G. Evaluation of patient concerns before total knee and hip arthroplasty. J Arthrop. 2003;18(4):442-5.
4. Trousdale RT, McGrory BJ, Berry DJ, Becker MW, Harmsen WS. Patients' concerns prior to undergoing total hip and total knee arthroplasty. Mayo Clin Proc. 1999;74(10):978-82.
5. Callaghan JJ, Warth LC, Liu SS, Hozack WJ, Klein GR. Internet promotion of MIS and CAOS in TKA by knee society members. Clin Orthop Relat Res. 2006;452:97-101.
6. Insall J. A midline approach to the knee. J Bone Joint Surg Am. 1971;53(8):1584-6.
7. Tria AJ Jr, Coon TM. Minimal incision total knee arthroplasty: early experience. Clin Orthop Relat Res. 2003;416:185-90.
8. Goble EM, Justin DF. Minimally invasive total knee replacement: principles and technique. Orthop Clin North Am. 2004;35(2):235-45.
9. Tanavalee A, Thiengwittayaporn S, Itiravivong P. Progressive quadriceps incision during minimally invasive surgery for total knee arthroplasty: the effect on early postoperative ambulation. J Arthrop. 2007;22(7):1013-8.
10. Laskin RS, Beksac B, Phongjunakorn A, et al. Minimally invasive total knee replacement through a mini-midvastus incision: an outcome study. Clin Orthop Relat Res. 2004;428:74-81.
11. Engh GA, Holt BT, Parks NL. A midvastus muscle-splitting approach for total knee arthroplasty. J Arthrop. 1997;12(3):322-31.
12. Hofmann AA, Plaster RL, Murdock LE. Subvastus (Southern) approach for primary total knee arthroplasty. Clin Orthop Relat Res. 1991;269:70-7.
13. Roysam GS, Oakley MJ. Subvastus approach for total knee arthroplasty: a prospective, randomized, and observer-blinded trial. J Arthrop. 2001;16(4):454-7.
14. Weale AE, Murray DW, Newman JH, Ackroyd CE. The length of the patellar tendon after unicompartmental and total knee replacement. J Bone Joint Surg Br. 1999;81(5):790-5.
15. Floren M, Davis J, Peterson MG, Laskin RS. A mini-midvastus capsular approach with patellar displacement decreases the prevalence of patella baja. J Arthrop. 2007;22:51-7.
16. McAllister CM, Stepanian JD. The impact of minimally invasive surgical techniques on early range of motion after primary total knee arthroplasty. J Arthrop. 2008;23(1):10-8.
17. Tashiro Y, Miura H, Matsuda S, Okazaki K, Iwamoto Y. Minimally invasive versus standard approach in total knee arthroplasty. Clin Orthop Relat Res. 2007;463:144-50.
18. Bonutti PM, Mont MA, McMahon M, Ragland PS, Kester M. Minimally invasive total knee arthroplasty. J Bone Joint Surg Am. 2004;86-A(2):26-32.
19. Lombardi AV, Jr., Viacava AJ, Berend KR. Rapid recovery protocols and minimally invasive surgery help achieve high knee flexion. Clin Orthop Relat Res. 2006;452:117-22.
20. Huang HT, Su JY, Chang JK, Chen CH, Wang GJ. The early clinical outcome of minimally invasive quadriceps-sparing total knee arthroplasty: report of a 2-year follow-up. J Arthrop. 2007;22(7):1007-12.
21. Stevens-Lapsley JE, Bade MJ, Shulman BC, Kohrt WM, Dayton MR. Minimally invasive total knee arthroplasty

improves early knee strength but not functional performance: a randomized controlled trial. J Arthrop. 2012;27(10):1812-19 e1812.
22. Cooper RE Jr, Trinidad G, Buck WR. Midvastus approach in total knee arthroplasty: a description and a cadaveric study determining the distance of the popliteal artery from the patellar margin of the incision. J Arthrop. 1999; 14(4):505-8.
23. Repicci JA, Eberle RW. Minimally invasive surgical technique for unicondylar knee arthroplasty. J South Orthop Assoc. 1999;8(1):20-27.
24. Romanowski MR, Repicci JA. Minimally invasive unicondylar arthroplasty: an eight-year follow-up. J Knee Surg. 2002;15(1):17-22.
25. Haas SB, Cook S, Beksac B. Minimally invasive total knee replacement through a mini midvastus approach: a comparative study. Clin Orthop Relat Res. 2004;428:68-73.
26. Chen AF, Alan RK, Redziniak DE, Tria AJ Jr. Quadriceps sparing total knee replacement. The initial experience with results at two to four years. J Bone Joint Surg Br. 2006;88(11):1448-53.
27. Boerger TO, Aglietti P, Mondanelli N, Sensi L. Mini-subvastus versus medial parapatellar approach in total knee arthroplasty. Clin Orthop Relat Res. 2005;440:82-7.
28. Laskin RS. Minimally invasive total knee arthroplasty: the results justify its use. Clin Orthop Relat Res. 2005;440:54-9.
29. Haas SB, Manitta MA, Burdick P. Minimally invasive total knee arthroplasty: the mini midvastus approach. Clin Orthop Relat Res. 2006;452:112-6.
30. Dalury DF, Dennis DA. Mini-incision total knee arthroplasty can increase risk of component malalignment. Clin Orthop Relat Res. 2005;440:77-81.
31. Foran JR, Whited BW, Sporer SM. Early aseptic loosening with a precoated low-profile tibial component: a case series. J Arthrop. 2011;26(8):1445-50.
32. Tria AJ, Jr. Minimally invasive total knee arthroplasty: the importance of instrumentation. Orthop Clin North Am. 2004;35(2):227-34.
33. Martin A, Sheinkop MB, Langhenry MM, et al. Comparison of two minimally invasive implantation instrument-sets for total knee arthroplasty. Knee Surg Sports Traumatol Arthrosc. 2010;18(3):359-66.
34. Bonutti PM, Dethmers D, Ulrich SD, Seyler TM, Mont MA. Computer navigation-assisted versus minimally invasive TKA: benefits and drawbacks. Clin Orthop Relat Res. 2008;466(11):2756-62.
35. Kim YH, Kim JS, Kim DY. Clinical outcome and rate of complications after primary total knee replacement performed with quadriceps-sparing or standard arthrotomy. J Bone Joint Surg Br. 2007;89(4):467-70.
36. Gandhi R, Smith H, Lefaivre KA, Davey JR, Mahomed NN. Complications after minimally invasive total knee arthroplasty as compared with traditional incision techniques: a meta-analysis. J Arthrop. 2011;26(1):29-35.
37. Scuderi GR, Tenholder M, Capeci C. Surgical approaches in mini-incision total knee arthroplasty. Clin Orthop Relat Res. 2004;428:61-7.
38. Wulker N, Lambermont JP, Sacchetti L, Lazaro JG, Nardi J. A prospective randomized study of minimally invasive total knee arthroplasty compared with conventional surgery. J Bone Joint Surg Am. 2010;92(7):1584-90.
39. Bonutti PM, Seyler TM, Kester M, McMahon M, Mont MA. Minimally invasive revision total knee arthroplasty. Clin Orthop Relat Res. 2006;446:69-75.
40. Cheng T, Liu T, Zhang G, Peng X, Zhang X. Does minimally invasive surgery improve short-term recovery in total knee arthroplasty? Clin Orthop Relat Res. 2010;468(6):1635-48.
41. Karpman RR, Smith HL. Comparison of the early results of minimally invasive vs standard approaches to total knee arthroplasty: a prospective, randomized study. J Arthrop. 2009;24(5):681-8.
42. Laskin RS. Mini-incision: occasionally desirable, rarely necessary in opposition. J Arthrop. 2006;21:19-21.
43. Kim JG, Lee SW, Ha JK, Choi HJ, Yang SJ, Lee MY. The effectiveness of minimally invasive total knee arthroplasty to preserve quadriceps strength: a randomized controlled trial. Knee. 2011;18(6):443-7.
44. Bonutti PM, Mont MA, Kester MA. Minimally invasive total knee arthroplasty: a 10-feature evolutionary approach. Orthop Clin North Am. 2004;35(2):217-26.
45. Lee MS, Yim MC, Wages JJ, Nakasone CK. Component alignment after minimally invasive total knee arthroplasty: results of the first 100 cases performed. J Arthrop. 2011;26(6):926-30.

Chapter 17

Defect Management in Total Knee Arthroplasty and Role of Trabecular Metal in TKA

Hemant Wakankar, Sinukumar Bhaskaran

INTRODUCTION

Bone defect management is one of the major challenges in total knee arthroplasty (TKA). In revision TKA, bone defects are very common; however, sometimes bone defects are encountered in complex primary TKA as well. Delayed presentation of knee arthritis is usually associated with significant deformities and bone loss from the concave side of the deformity. The management of such bone loss as well as the correction of the deformity is therefore an important surgical challenge.

In a complex primary case, the resected bone can be used as a bone graft and hence a biological solution is feasible. However, in revision TKA, such an option is not available and unless allografts from the bone bank are available, one has to look for bone substituting options.

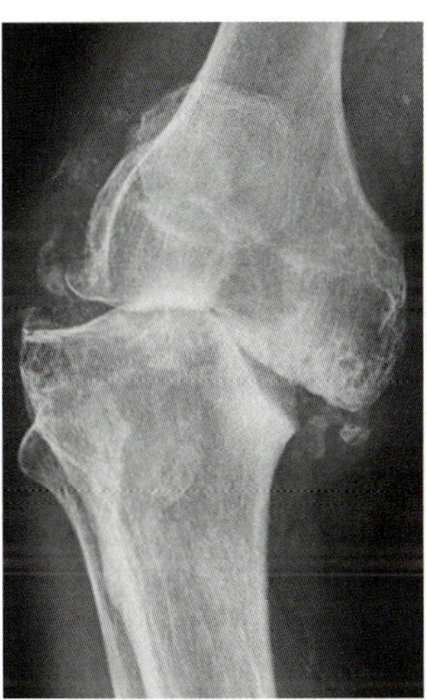

Figure 17.1 Severe varus with large defect involving the major part of the medial tibial plateau. Note: minimal lateral stretching secondary to subluxation

BONE DEFECTS IN COMPLEX PRIMARY TOTAL KNEE ARTHROPLASTY

Bone defects are a consequence of progressive wear on the concave side of the deformity. In a varus knee, the defects are primarily seen on the medial tibial plateau (**Figure 17.1**).

With minimal varus, the location of this defect is usually on the posteromedial side and is consistently seen in knees that have anterior cruciate ligament insufficiency. In knees

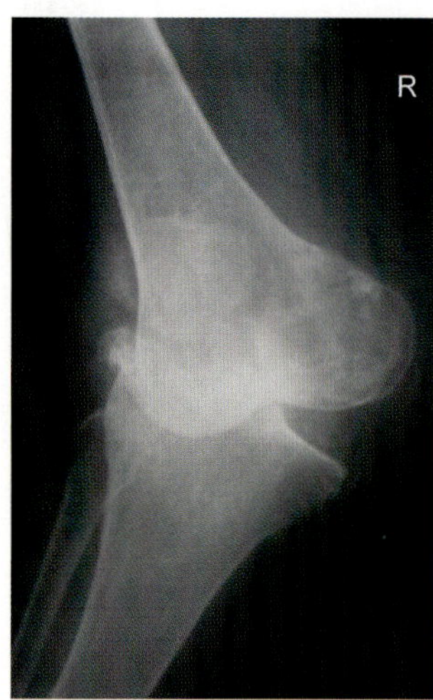

Figure 17.2 Severe valgus deformity with contained defect involving the lateral tibial plateau. Note hypoplastic/worn lateral femoral condyle

that have anterior cruciate ligament intact, the defect tends to be in the central part of the medial tibial plateau. Rarely, when a varus is associated with the hyperextension deformity, the defect is seen on anteromedial aspect. In severe varus, the defect can involve almost entire medial tibial plateau as shown in (**Figure 17.1**). The wear on the femoral side is usually not severe enough and is usually accounted for in the resection of the distal femur.

In valgus knee, the lateral side of the knee shows variable bone defects. The lateral femoral condyle tends to be hypoplastic and both the distal and posterior aspects of lateral femoral condyles tend to be deficient. The defect is also seen on the lateral tibial plateau and can vary (**Figure 17.2**). The defects may be accounted for in the resection of both the femur and tibia, but in some cases with advanced wear, the deficiency has to be dealt with.

BONE DEFECTS IN REVISION TOTAL KNEE ARTHROPLASTY

Bone loss is probably the biggest challenge in revision TKA. Bone loss is usually secondary to aseptic loosening and osteolysis. It is therefore important to avoid any further bone loss during implant removal. It is useful to classify the extent and location of bone defects while planning for a revision surgery. The severity of the bone defect would decide the type of implant to be used and also the need for structural allografts and/or metallic augments. It also gives the surgeon an approximation of the complexity of the surgery.

True anteroposterior (AP) and lateral view X-rays help in classifying the defects; however, the bone defects are usually much worse than those seen on the X-ray. Oblique views are sometimes useful in certain cases to view distal femoral osteolytic lesions, especially with posterior stabilized prosthesis. CT scan is highly accurate in estimating the extent of the osteolytic defects. One must remember that the defects are always underestimated in plain radiographic examination.

AORI BONE DEFECT CLASSIFICATION

Engh et al. from the Anderson Orthopedic Research Institute (AORI) described a very practical method of classifying bone defects.[1]

AORI Classification

Type 1 defect (intact metaphyseal bone): Minor bone defects that do not compromise the stability of the component.

Type 2 defect (damaged metaphyseal bone): Loss of cancellous bone in the metaphyseal segment that necessitates an area of cement fill, augments, or bone graft to restore a reasonable joint line level. Type 2 defects can occur in one femoral condyle or tibial plateau (2A) or both the condyles and plateaus (2B).

Type 3 defect (deficient metaphyseal segment): Bone loss that compromises a major portion of either condyle or plateau. These defects are occasionally associated with collateral or patellar ligament detachment and usually require bone grafts or custom implants.

GUIDELINES FOR CLASSIFYING DEFECTS USING RADIOGRAPHS

F1 and T1 Defects

- No component subsidence or osteolysis
- *Femur:* Normal joint line with full condylar profile

- *Tibia:* Component above the fibular head and a full metaphyseal segment.

F2 and T2 Defects

- *Femur:* Joint line elevation and a reduced condylar profile
- *Tibia:* Component is at or below the tip of the fibular head and the tibial flare is reduced.

F3 and T3 Defects

A deficient metaphyseal segment of the femur or tibia.

PRINCIPLES OF BONY RECONSTRUCTION

The most important aspect of reconstruction is the extent of host bone contact with the prosthesis and the extent of shear forces at the cement bone interface. If the primary stability is not adequate, the cement bone interface can fail early. Therefore, the addition of the intramedullary extension stem is very useful in such a scenario. The addition of a stem reduces the stress at the cement bone interface by almost 50%. Whenever the defect involves more than one-third of the tibial plateau, which needs either bone graft or wedges, one has to add the stem.

Restoration of the bone stock is also critical especially in younger patients who may require further revision surgery in their lifetime. In a primary knee, resected bone is readily available as autograft, but in revision TKA, one has to rely on the bone bank for the supply of allografts. If allografts are not available, one has to use metal augments, so that the extent of cement filling can be minimized. The advent of newer bone substitution options like trabecular metal (TM) has reduced the need for the allograft.

OPTIONS FOR MANAGEMENT OF BONE DEFECTS IN COMPLEX PRIMARY TOTAL KNEE ARTHROPLASTY

- Increased resection to cover defect
- Cement only

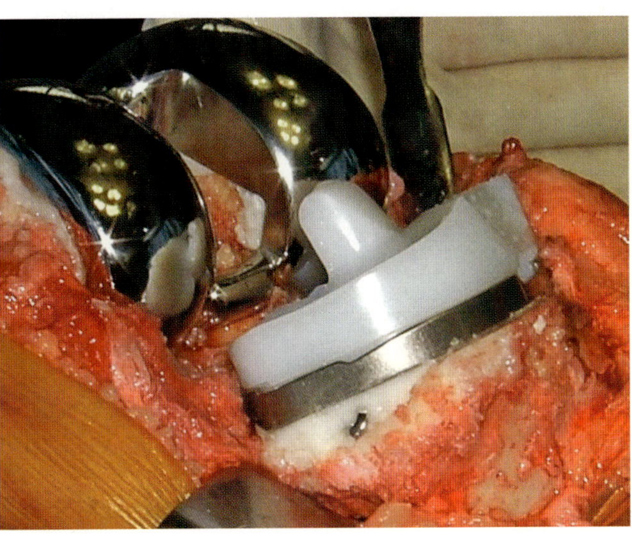

Figure 17.3 Posteromedial tibial defect is filled with cement reinforced with a screw

- Cement with screw (**Figure 17.3**)
- *Bone grafting:* Autologous or allografts (**Figures 17.4A to D**)
- *Metal augments:* Wedges, blocks, etc. (**Figure 17.5**)
- *Bone substitution options:* TM cones.

Increased Resection to Cover Defect

This option is possible only on the tibial side in a primary TKA, if the defect is small and there is no significant laxity of soft tissues. If by increasing the level of tibial resection, one is able to cover the defect completely, one can obliterate the defect completely. However, if there is significant stretching of the collateral ligament, one needs to restrict the resection level of the tibia, since after balancing the knee with soft tissue releases on the concave side of deformity, the required polyethylene thickness may be very large.

Cement Only

In the defect is up to 1 cm deep and less than one-third of the involved tibial plateau, the defect may be filled up only with cement. Multiple anchoring holes are made into the defect prior to cementing.

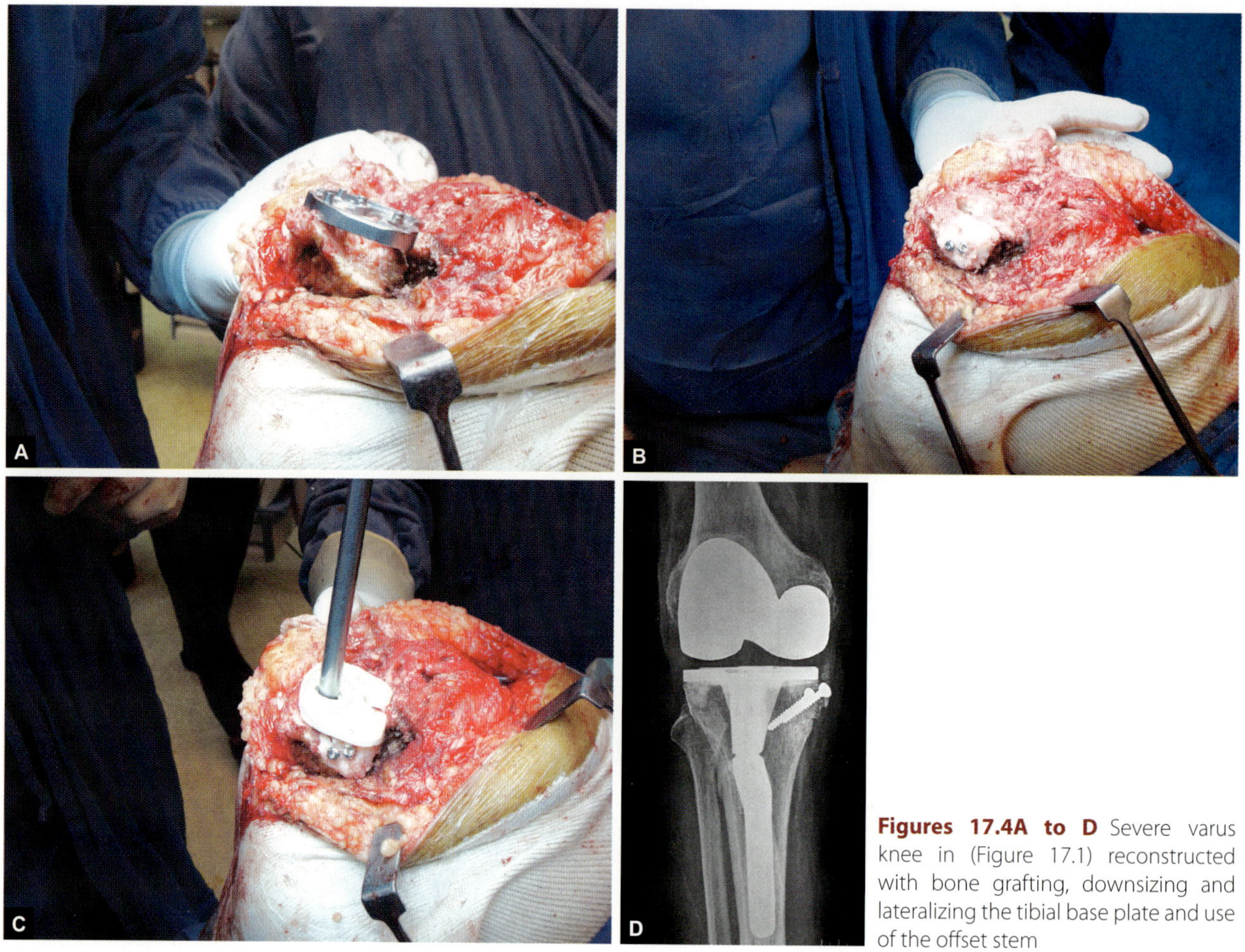

Figures 17.4A to D Severe varus knee in (Figure 17.1) reconstructed with bone grafting, downsizing and lateralizing the tibial base plate and use of the offset stem

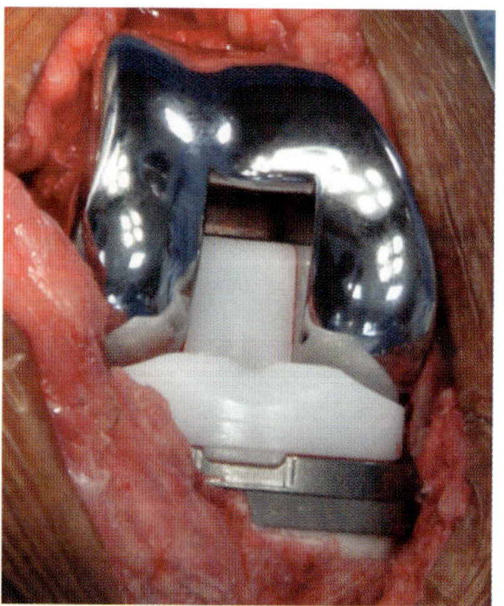

Figure 17.5 Medial tibial block augment for medial tibial defect

Cement with a Screw

Methyl methacrylate cement alone is very poor in shear stress. Therefore, the addition of a screw within the cement mantle adds to the strength of the construct. This is possible only for defects up to 1 cm depth (**Figure 17.3**).

Bone Grafting

In primary TKA, the autologous bone graft is readily available from the resected bone. The configuration of the defect needs to be assessed and the available resected bone is shaped to fill the defect. A resected tibial cut surface may be used for a flat defect surface or a resected femoral condyle may be shaped to fit in the concave defect. It is important that all the soft tissue and cartilage is removed from the graft, and multiple drill holes made in a sclerotic hard surface of the defect. The graft is fixed in a place secured with screws. It is important to make sure that the screw heads are not in contact with the tibial base plate, since dissimilar metals in contact can induce galvanic corrosion. If the area of the bone defect is large and involves more than one-third of the medial or lateral tibial plateau, it is mandatory to supplement the tibial base plate with an extension stem. The use of the offset stem allows downsizing and lateralization of the tibial baseplate, thereby reducing the area of the bone defect to be covered in a varus knee (**Figures 17.4A to D**).

Metal Augments

The use of metal augments is another attractive option to cover the bone defects. The augments are available in various forms, such as wedges and blocks. The metal augments are fixed to the implants and cemented in place with the component. The defect needs to be modified and sometimes extended to accommodate the augment. In primary knee arthroplasty, the most common instance where the augment may be needed is for the severe varus knee with the medial tibial defect. The defect is usually sloping and may be suitable for the use of a metal wedge augment. With the use of an augment, it is necessary to add an extension stem to the tibial base plate. If the defect configuration is appropriate, the metal block augment is preferred to the wedge, as there is no shear stress with the rectangular block (**Figure 17.5**).

Bone Substitution Options

The advent of newer metals for bone substitution is an exciting prospect. Until recently, metallic augments were used as an adjunct to the prosthesis to cover the bone defects and establish the host bone contact. However, the host bone contact can be limited and, as a result, the stress transfer to the host bone can exceed the physiological limit, leading to the early failure. The advent of tantalum as bone substituting 'trabecular metal' promises to revolutionize the management of bone defects (**Figure 17.6**).

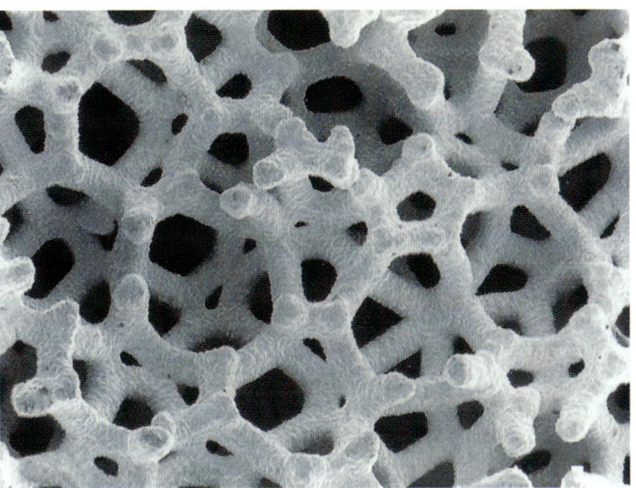

Figure 17.6 Trabecular metal: microscopic view

TANTALUM: TRABECULAR METAL

Tantalum (atomic no 73) was discovered by Swedish chemist Anders Gustav in 1802. It was named after the *Tantalus* the invincible Greek god since its oxide was undissolvable in acids. Tantalum has excellent biocompatibility and has been used to produce implantable devices for more than 50 years. The proprietary manufacturing process developed by Zimmer (Warsaw, IN, USA) creates porous tantalum with 80% porosity. The tantalum TM has an open cell structure of repeating dodecahedrons with a regular array of highly interconnected pores, closely approximates the structure of the cancellous bone.[2] The chemical vapor deposition technique is used in the manufacturing process. For any material to allow for bone ingrowth and neovascularization, the pore size has to be at least 300 μm.[3] The TM has an average porosity of 430 ± 270 μm helping in providing a framework supporting bone ingrowth.

The advantages of this metal include:

- Excellent bone ingrowth, which encourages stable long-term fixation
- Property of the 'scratch fit' allows for excellent primary fixation and hence immediate load bearing
- Various sizes available to match the defect anatomy
- Provides a stable base upon which the components irrespective of the type or make can be supported

- Easier to use and lower infection risk when compared to structural allografts (**Figures 17.6 to 17.9**).

Surgical Technique

After the extraction of previous implants and thorough debridement, bone defects are assessed. The bone defects are then classified as per the previously described AORI system. The types 2 and 3 defects are usually suited for the use of TM cones (**Figure 17.7**). The conical central metaphyseal defects are most suited for the use of the TM cone where it provides an independent stable foundation for the prosthesis.

The trial cones are placed in the canal to assess the size required. The host bone may be trimmed or burred to accommodate the cone but as far as possible avoid removing the host bone. The trial cone augment is then gently tapped into place assessing the fit and stability. The cones can accommodate the medullary stem attached to any type of prosthesis. Once the trial reduction is done, and implant size is determined, the appropriate TM cone is readied for implantation (**Figure 17.8**).

The TM cones have an excellent scratch fit with a host bone and are very rigid once implanted within the host cavity. Any space between the host bone and the TM cone is packed with the cancellous bone graft. The TM has to be considered to be a bone substitute and hence no cement should get in the interface between the TM and the host bone. The revision TKR implants are then cemented within the cone. On the femoral side, one must be on the watch for diaphyseal fractures while impacting the cone in. It is advisable to prophylactically use the cerclage wire in the case of the extremely tight distal femur to offset the hoop stresses. The femoral cones are available in various sizes to match the bone defects (**Figure 17.9**).

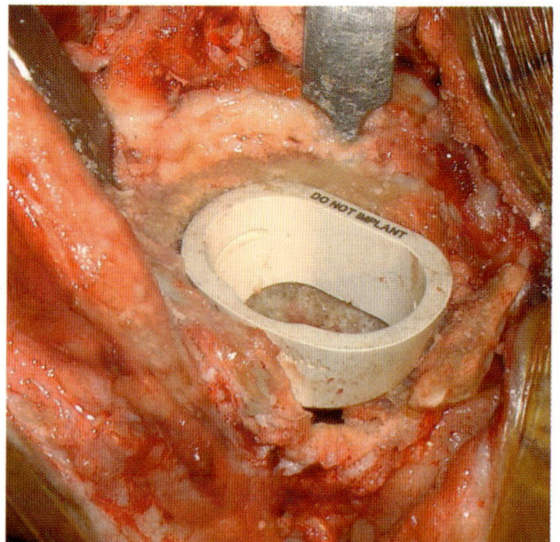

Figure 17.7 Trial tibial cone in place. Note: large tibial metaphyseal defect

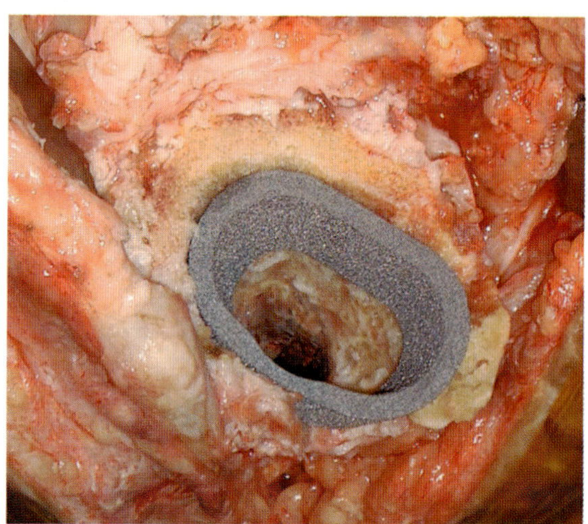

Figure 17.8 Tibial TM cone implanted

Though there have been excellent long-term results of the use of TM in hip replacement surgery, published long-term data regarding TM cone usage in bone defects in knee arthroplasty are awaited. Numerous mid-term to short-term studies in TKR have shown encouraging results. Meneghini et al.[4] presented their results in 15 patients with types 2 and 3 tibial defects and reported good bone ingrowth without any evidence of loosening or migration at 2–3 years of the follow-up. Another retrospective study by Scuderi and Long[5] published results of the follow-up of 16 patients, of which 13 were the cases of aseptic loosening and 3 were the cases of infected revisions. At 31 months, they found that in 14 cases the reconstructions were functioning well with good osseointegration, while two cases required the removal of well-fixed cones due to reinfection. More recently Villenueva-Martinez et al.[6] evaluated 36-month follow-up in 21 patients who needed TM cones; all of them showed good evidence of stable osseointegration and only one cone had to be removed due to persistent infection.

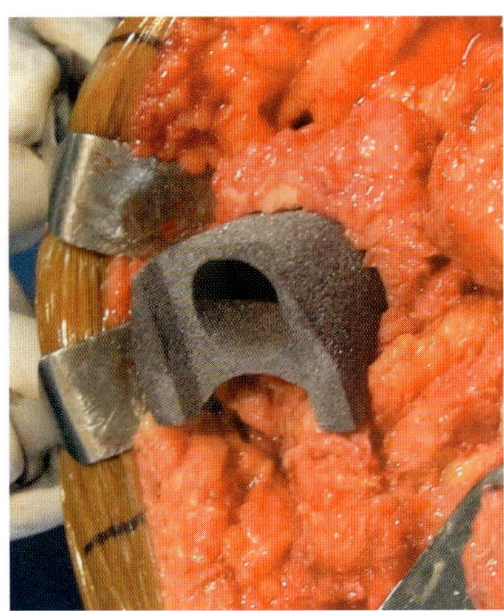

Figure 17.9 TM femoral cone impacted in the diaphysis to reconstruct distal femur. Rotating hinge TKR prosthesis cemented onto the cone

Most of these studies proved successful osseo-integration into the cones even in the face of severely damaged bone in these situations. There are distinct advantages of TM cones over structural allografts such as better primary fixation, quicker to use and reduced infection risk. The only foreseeable disadvantage is the extreme difficulty anticipated in the removal of the well-integrated cone augment for infection, as not many studies have reported on ease or otherwise of implant removal.

TM holds great promise as a bone substituting material, especially in situations where allografts are not available. More surgical options using this metal continue to be developed.

REFERENCES

1. Engh GA, Ammeen DJ. Bone loss with revision total knee arthroplasty: defect classification and alternatives for reconstruction. Instr Course Lect. 1999;48:167-75.
2. Bobyn JD, Hacking SA, Chan SP, et al. Characterization of a new porous tantalum biomaterial for reconstructive orthopaedics. Annual meet of AAOS edition, Anaheim; CA; 1999.
3. Karageorgious V, Kaplan D. Porosity of 3D biomaterial scaffolds and osteogenesis. Biomaterials. 2005;26(27):5474-91.
4. Meneghini RM, Lewallen DG, Hanssen AD. Use of porous tantalum metaphyseal for severe tibial bone loss during revision total knee replacement. J Bone Joint Surg Am. 2008;90:78-84.
5. Long WJ, Scuderi GR. Porous tantalum cones for large metaphyseal tibial defects in revision total knee arthroplasty. J Arthroplasty. 2009;24(7):1086-94.
6. Villenueva-Martinez M, De la Torre-Escudero B, Rojo-Manaute, et al. Tantalum cones in revision total knee arthroplasty. A promising short-term result with 29 cones in 21 patients. J Arthroplasty. 2013;28(6):988-93.

Chapter 18

Instability Following Total Knee Arthroplasty

Andrew A Freiberg, Matthew J Dietz

INTRODUCTION

Addressing the complexities of instability after total knee arthroplasty can be a substantial challenge given the multitude of variables that play a part in the etiology of this, often under diagnosed, postoperative complication. Multiple studies have found that tibiofemoral instability occurs in less than 1–2% of patients undergoing total knee arthroplasty.[1] Symptomatic instability accounts for 10–20% of all revisions with many of these occurring within 5 years of the primary arthroplasty.[2,3]

Other early failures of total knee arthroplasty can result from aseptic loosening, infection, complications involving the patella or the extensor mechanism, stiffness or fracture. However, it is in the domain of preventing postoperative instability that the surgeon can have the greatest effect in patient selection, surgical technique and selection of the prosthesis.[4] Both the techniques and implants used can be greatly influenced by the patient's medical and surgical history and the surgeon must be aware of those patients who are at increased risk for postoperative instability.

RISK FACTORS FOR POSTOPERATIVE INSTABILITY

Numerous factors can play a role in the potential for postoperative instability after a total knee arthroplasty (**Table 18.1**). Patients prone to instability after total knee arthroplasty are those with large preoperative deformities, both intra- and extra-articular, that can require large corrections including aggressive soft tissue releases. Outside of inherent anatomical abnormalities these situations can be seen in patients with a history of trauma, revision surgeries, prior knee arthrodesis, or significant bone loss. Patients with gait abnormalities due to generalized or regional neuromuscular pathology are also at risk for postoperative instability. Severe quadriceps weakness, which can often be seen in postpolio patients, can lead to genu recurvatum, while abductor weakness can lead to medial thrust to the knee. Foot deformities such as those seen in posterior tibial tendon dysfunction or pes planus can impart a valgus moment on the knee. Valgus neck-shaft angles after total hip arthroplasty can

TABLE 18.1 Causes of knee instability

Patient factors	*Technique/surgical factors*
Connective tissue disorders (Ehlers–Danlos)	Ligament imbalance
Diabetes mellitus	Component alignment or size
Obesity	Implant design
Quadriceps weakness (postpolio, spinal stenosis)	Bone loss
Gait abnormalities	Collateral ligament disruption
Hind foot disorders	Prosthetic breakage
Prior hip surgeries	Surface wear

also lead to valgus moments at the knee.[5,6] Obesity is also a risk factor for knee instability. The body habitus in these patients complicates surgical exposure that can lead to component malposition and puts the collateral ligaments at risk as evidence by the 8% incidence of avulsion of the medial collateral ligament as described by Winiarsky et al. when outlining the complications of total knee arthroplasty in the morbidly obese.[5-7] The weight of the extremity can also make it difficult to assess intraoperative stability. These patients also tend to walk with a wide-based gait due to thigh circumference that imparts a large stress on the medial collateral ligament.[5,7]

PCL insufficiency can lead to posterior instability and therefore implant selection is very important in the subset of patients such as those at risk to have an incompetent PCL. These can include rheumatoid arthritis, previous patellectomy, PCL recession, flexion contractures, or prior tibial osteotomies.[6]

History

A patient's complaint of 'knee instability' should not be taken as a diagnosis. They will often misinterpret a 'buckling' knee due to quadriceps weakness or patella maltracking as a dislocating or unstable knee. It is important to obtain a thorough history and physical examination and radiographs to accurately diagnose potential causes of instability.

Occasionally patients will present with obvious tibiofemoral dislocations or subluxations usually due to acute trauma. In these situations the diagnosis is fairly obvious. However, it is the patient in which subtle instability has led to continued discomfort and pain in which an accurate diagnosis relies upon a thorough history and physical examination. These patients will often complain of recurrent effusions, restricted motion, a 'giving way' or even a locking of the knee. Flexion instability can lead to anterior knee pain. These feelings of instability can manifest itself when flexing the knee between 30° and 60° such as when rising from a chair.[2] It is also important to inquire as to the reasons for their primary total knee arthroplasty and to try and obtain the preoperative and postoperative radiographs as well as the operative reports from that surgery to provide additional insight into their current clinical situation.

Clinical Examination

Physical examination of the knee should begin with evaluation of the patient's gait, stair climbing, and the overall limb alignment while standing and in the supine position. The examination also includes an assessment of knee range of motion, the integrity of the extensor mechanism, and the presence of an effusion. Sagittal deformities such as flexion contractures or genu recurvatum should be noted. Any anterior or posterior instability can be found by an anterior (posterior) drawer test, or by a posterior sag test (**Figure 18.1B**). The quad active test, in which the foot is placed on a table with knee flexed to 90° and active firing of the quadriceps mechanism leads to a reduction of the knee joint also assesses anteroposterior stability.[8] Patella tracking should also be assessed, as a maltracking patella can often be mistaken for instability. Coronal instability should be carefully assessed at full extension, 30° of flexion and 90° of flexion. It is important to assess midflexion stability because at full extension varus/valgus instability is masked and only becomes evident with relaxation of the posterior capsule during increased flexion. It is important to be aware of pseudolaxity that may be present due to bone loss or correction of the joint to normal alignment. It is critical to assess the competence of the collateral ligaments as part of the diagnosis and treatment of instability.

Radiographic Examination

Radiographic examinations of the unstable total knee arthroplasty should include full-length weight-bearing films to assess lower limb alignment as well as component position. Lateral radiographs with the knee in full extension may demonstrate recurvatum, while full flexion lateral knee radiographs may demonstrate posterior subluxation of the tibia that can be seen when increased tibial slope is present (**Figure 18.2D**). Stress (varus, valgus, anterior and posterior drawer) radiographs or even fluoroscopy may provide additional information regarding the integrity of collateral ligaments and flexion/extension gap balance. These examinations can be time consuming in clinic and often difficult to reproduce consistently.[9,10] Serial radiographs can also be useful for documenting the movement of loose implants or progressive bone loss. CT scans are useful for documenting rotational alignment of components that may be a significant factor in patellofemoral maltracking.[11,12] Radionucleotide bone scanning can be used to exclude loosening or infection but has a very low sensitivity (33%) and can remain positive in 65–90% of asymptomatic knees even 1 year after implantation.[9,13]

Many patients with instability have recurrent effusions. Fehring et al. reported that repeated synovial trauma caused by instability will lead to recurrent hemarthrosis. In the evaluation of knees with documented instability that have undergone an aspiration were found to have an average of 64,000 rbc/mm.[3,2] Knee aspiration is not typically used in the diagnosis of instability, but in conjunction with erythrocyte sedimentation rate and C-reactive protein can be useful in excluding infection as a cause for the failed total knee arthroplasty.

CATEGORIZATION OF TOTAL KNEE INSTABILITY

Postoperative instability of the knee can be defined by its temporal relationship to the primary arthroplasty, or by the type of instability and causative factors. Both definitions are important as they help us determine why the knee failed and can provide answers as to how to best treat the patient.

Early versus Late Instability

Early instability occurring in the weeks to months after the primary knee arthroplasty is most commonly the result of ligament loss, technical issues, or soft tissue laxity. Instability in the early postoperative period can be caused by malalignment of the components, failure to restore the mechanical axis, improper balancing of the flexion and extension spaces, or a liner that is not thick enough. Also intraoperative assessment of stability may have changed with postoperative stretching or laxity. Laceration of the lateral or medial collateral ligaments, rupture of the posterior cruciate ligament, or patellar tendon or fracture of the patella can also lead to early instability of the knee.[6] Late instability following total knee arthroplasty is most commonly associated with polyethylene wear but can also be in combination with ligamentous instability (**Figures 18.1A to E**). Wear can be due to malalignment or poor polyethylene quality. However, wear is most frequently seen medially or posteromedially as a result of unreleased MCL contracture and resulting varus deformity.[6,14] Rotating platform designs can have prosthetic instability early or late depending on the cause.

EXTENSION INSTABILITY

Instability in extension after total knee arthroplasty can be defined as symmetric or asymmetric. Symmetric extension instability is also called 'instability due to bone resection'[4,15] (**Figures 18.2A to F**). This occurs when the thickness of the components is less than the extension gap between bone ends. Excessive removal of bone from the distal femur can lead to extension instability but addressing this can be challenging. A thicker polyethylene does not solve the problem of pure extension instability due to excessive distal femoral resection. This would tighten the flexion space and elevate the joint line, potentially limit flexion, affect patellar tracking and lead to midflexion instability.[6,16] The simplest solution to correct symmetric extension instability is through the addition of distal femoral augments. If flexion instability exists at the same time this is likely due to excessive proximal tibial resection that then leads to instability in both flexion and extension. If the combined flexion/extension instability is identified

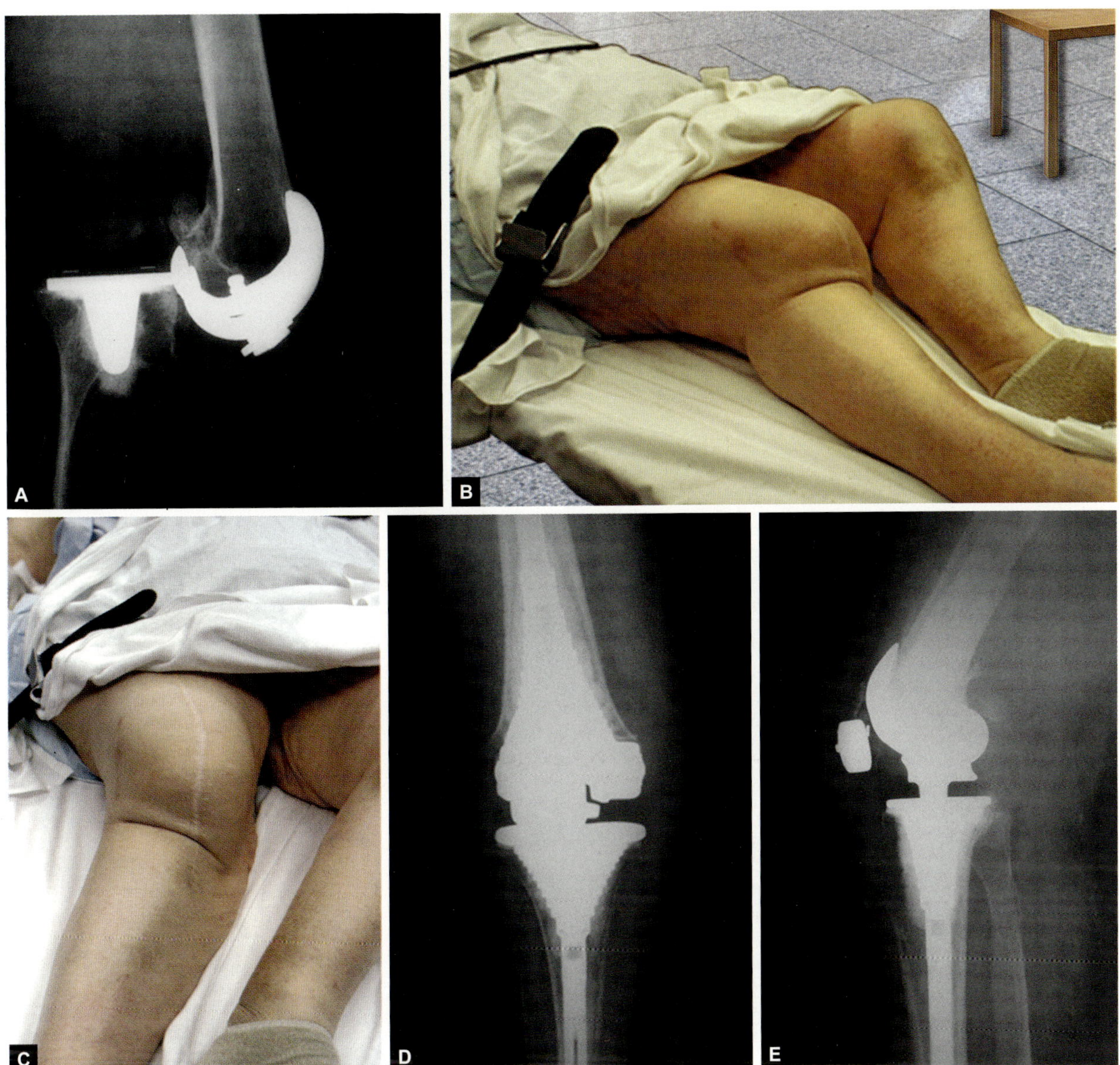

Figures 18.1A to E (A) This patient presented with a chronic dislocation that became incapacitating. The posterior sag of the tibia on the femur is evident in these clinical photos; (B and C) Due to the attrition of soft tissues and concern for prolonged stability the patient was revised to a rotating hinge prosthesis (D and E)

at the time of surgery, this can be corrected with a thicker polyethylene insert. One concern with this larger tibial resection is that the tibial tray is now seated on more distal and weaker bone. In addition, a smaller tibial surface can force the use of smaller femoral implant because of size compatibility.[4,6,15,17]

Asymmetric Extension Instability

Asymmetric extension instability is much more common and is typically related to a preoperative angular deformity and is caused by persistent or intraoperative ligamentous instability.[6,15,17] Undercorrection of a fixed angular

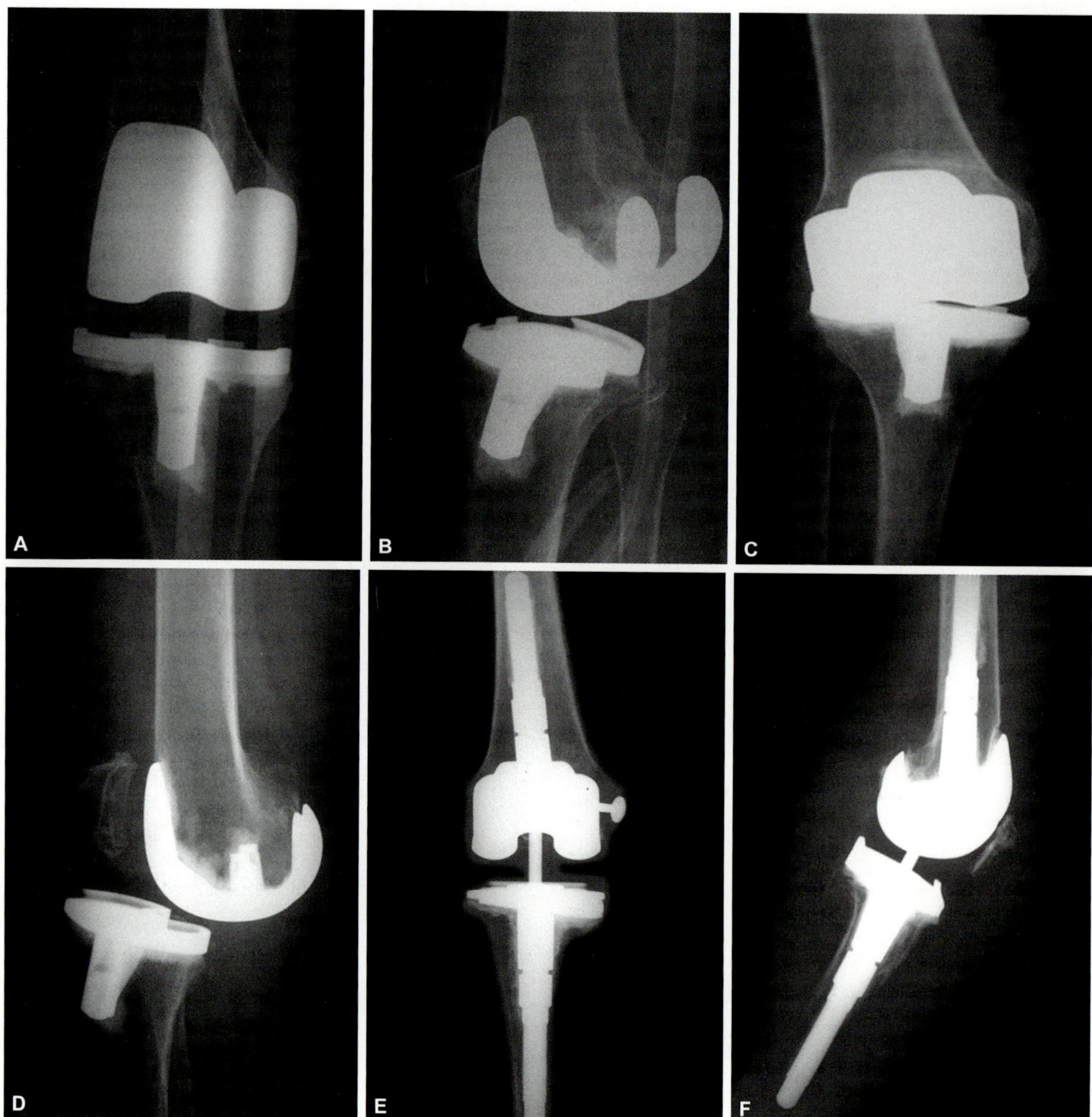

Figures 18.2A to F (A and B) Postoperative total knee arthroplasty X-rays for primary osteoarthritis. These demonstrate a varus cut on the tibia and excessive posterior slope. Both of these factors lead to flexion instability and eventual loss of competence of the PCL; (C and D) Demonstrate radiographs at 6 weeks. The patient had complaints of instability, weakness and recurrent effusions. The patient underwent a revision to a constrained condylar device (E and F)

deformity is often due to a concern of creating instability on the opposite side. As an example a varus knee that is undercorrected at the time of surgery will lead to a knee that is tight on the medial side. This is fact is compounded if the overall alignment remains in varus. The combination of the malalignment and tension on the medial side leads to stretching of the tissues on the lateral side and wear of the polyethylene medially.[4,15]

Similarly, undercorrection of a valgus knee will leave the knee still tight laterally and with some laxity in the medial collateral ligament. The MCL will not tighten over time, which will lead to a progressively worsening valgus deformity. Only minimal medial laxity should be accepted and therefore Insall et al. advocated sequential lateral releases starting with the lateral collateral ligament, the popliteus, and the lateral head of the gastrocnemius.[18]

This technique, however, led to the over-release of the lateral ligaments and instability that led to several reports of dislocations of posterior stabilized total knee prostheses due to mismatched flexion gaps.[19] This led to the development of the pie-crusting technique in which multiple punctures are used to release lateral structures that feel tight. During this series of horizontal perforations the popliteus tendon is protected and all the lateral structures are lengthened in continuity and not divided.[19,20] During pie-crusting the depth of the blade penetration should be kept < 5 mm to minimize the risk of injury to the peroneal nerve according to anatomical and *in vivo* studies performed by Clarke et al.[21] Care must be taken when a preoperative valgus deformity of >20° exists as there is a risk of stretching the peroneal nerve with correction.[20] Easley et al. reported good clinical and radiographic results at a mean follow up of 8 years in 44 primary constrained condylar knee implants used to treat valgus knees. The deformity was left undercorrected and the increased constraint compensated for the residual laxity of the medial side.[22]

Iatrogenic causes of asymmetric instability can be due to malalignment of the femoral or tibial components or due to damage of the medial collateral ligament during surgery. Injury to the medial collateral ligament most commonly occurs when cutting the proximal tibia or the posterior condyles of the femur or during vigorous attempts at testing varus-valgus stability.[17,23] MCL insufficiency is a known complication when performing total knee arthroplasty in the obese with reported rates of intraoperative injury to the MCL as high as 8%. This is most likely due to avulsion of the ligament during hyperflexion of the knee. The hyperflexion leads to the tibia being forced against a large amount of adipose tissue placing excessive tension on the ligament. The authors of this study recommend the removal medial osteophytes and limiting the amount of hyperextension during the surgery to maintain the competence of the ligament.[7] Leopold et al. reported on successful results of end-to-end repair of midsubstance lacerations and suture anchor (or screw/washer) reattachment of MCL avulsions.[23] This is in contrast to other reports that found lower Knee Society Scores and higher rates of revision for instability when components with increased varus/valgus constraint were not used.[24] It has been our practice to use a more constrained device to treat MCL loss or dysfunction.

Flexion Instability

Instability in flexion results from a relatively larger flexion gap than extension gap. This can often be a subtle problem and is often underdiagnosed. The first cause of under filling the flexion gap can be due to downsizing of the femoral component. To correct this, a larger femoral component could be used, with posterior augments if needed. A knee with excessive tibial slope can also lead to flexion instability. A PCL rendered incompetent during surgery can present late (months) after surgery, leading to recurrent effusions and anterior knee pain especially with climbing stairs or rising from a seated position.[3] These complaints can be manifested as vague symptoms or even as a frank tibiofemoral dislocation.

Removal of the PCL can disproportionately increase the flexion gap. The amount of flexion space opening with removal of the PCL is variable. This variation can create an imbalance that lends itself towards instability.[6] To improve flexion stability in posterior stabilized knee changes to the cam-post design have increased the 'jump distance' to the point where dislocations are much less frequent (less than 0.5%).[25,26] When the posterior stabilized knee dislocates it most frequently occurs in deep knee flexion with a varus stress (such as when placing the ankle of the operated limb on the contralateral knee to put on a shoe or sock). When a frank dislocation does occur it often can be reduced with the patient relaxed under anesthesia. A first time dislocation can be treated with closed reduction and bracing. Any recurrent dislocations should be addressed with revision surgery, to increase the thickness of the polyethylene insert or convert to a more constrained device.[25]

Flexion instability in the cruciate retaining knee is an under diagnosed problem.[8] These patients usually have well fixed and aligned knees that can be stable in extension, but will present with similar complaints as outlined before. Important in this physical examination is the posterior drawer or posterior sag, best seen with the patient sitting and relaxed. The goal is to have less than

5 mm of anterior translation of the tibia when the knee is tested intraoperatively at 90°of flexion with the patella reduced.[15]

Failure of the PCL can occur late as a function of chronic attrition, but may also be due tibial resection or exposure (**Figure 18.2**).[8,15,27] Unrecognized direct injury to the PCL can cause a significant increase in the flexion gap.[8] Another cause of PCL disruption can occur when a knee is left too tight during flexion. In attempts to improve their flexion patients will work aggressively to increase their range of motion. This can lead to a rupture of the posterior cruciate ligament. These patients can often recall a specific pop followed by a dramatic increase in their range of motion. This may then be followed by progressive instability.[27,28]

Midflexion Instability

Midflexion instability can occur in multiple scenarios. The most common of which is during a primary total knee arthroplasty when a large distal femoral cut is made to address a preoperative flexion contracture.[15,29] The cut allows the knee to achieve full extension, and while in extension the contracted posterior capsule will provide varus/valgus stability. As the knee is brought to 30° of flexion the posterior capsule is no longer taut, the collateral ligaments become loose due to elevation of the joint line, and the knee will demonstrate increased varus/valgus instability.[5] Midflexion instability is best addressed by avoiding an overly large distal femoral resection and improving a preoperative flexion contracture through posterior capsular release and removal of posterior osteophytes. Revision for midflexion instability requires the restoration of the joint line and balancing of the flexion and extension spaces. If one must accept an elevated joint line, a prosthesis with additional constraint should be considered (**Figures 18.3A to D**).[29]

Genu Recurvatum

Genu recurvatum after total knee arthroplasty is a condition that can be anticipated based on the patients preoperative comorbidities and should give the surgeon great caution when undertaking a total knee arthroplasty. Recurvatum or anterior subluxation of the tibia is typically seen in patients suffering from rheumatoid arthritis, neuromuscular conditions, and some connective tissue disorders (i.e. Ehlers-Danlos syndrome). Dysfunction of the extensor mechanism usually exists that causes the patient to force the knee into hyperextension during the stance phase of gait for increased stability. This can lead to worsening of the deformity increased instability and failure of the joint.[30] Patients who have antigravity functions of their extensor mechanism tend to have the best outcomes from total knee arthroplasty and preoperative recurvatum deformity. Making the joint line as distal as possible and consideration of a rotating hinged implant with a hyperextension stop can provide reliable results. In the revision setting, a hinged device with an extension stop or an arthrodesis may be the most viable options.[29,30] Some authors report successes with advancing collateral ligaments by moving the femoral origins of the medial and lateral collateral ligaments proximally and posteriorly to recreate a tightening action during extension.[31] These techniques can be challenging and difficult to reproduce and are not used in the authors' practice.

GLOBAL INSTABILITY

Global instability is a pattern of instability that exists in multiple planes. This is typically a combination of loose flexion and extension gaps. The primary causes of global instability can be due to polyethylene wear, which leads to laxity of the surrounding soft tissue envelope, implant migration, motor dysfunction, and extensor mechanism disruption. Global instability is generally treated through revision of all components to a more constrained device as treatment with bracing or insert exchange only is typically unsuccessful.[15,32]

Treatment Options

Treatment options for instability are isolated polyethylene insert exchange, single component revision, full component revision or even the use of a hinged total knee arthroplasty. Nonoperative treatment includes strengthening of the surrounding musculature and local modalities can improve some symptoms, but is less

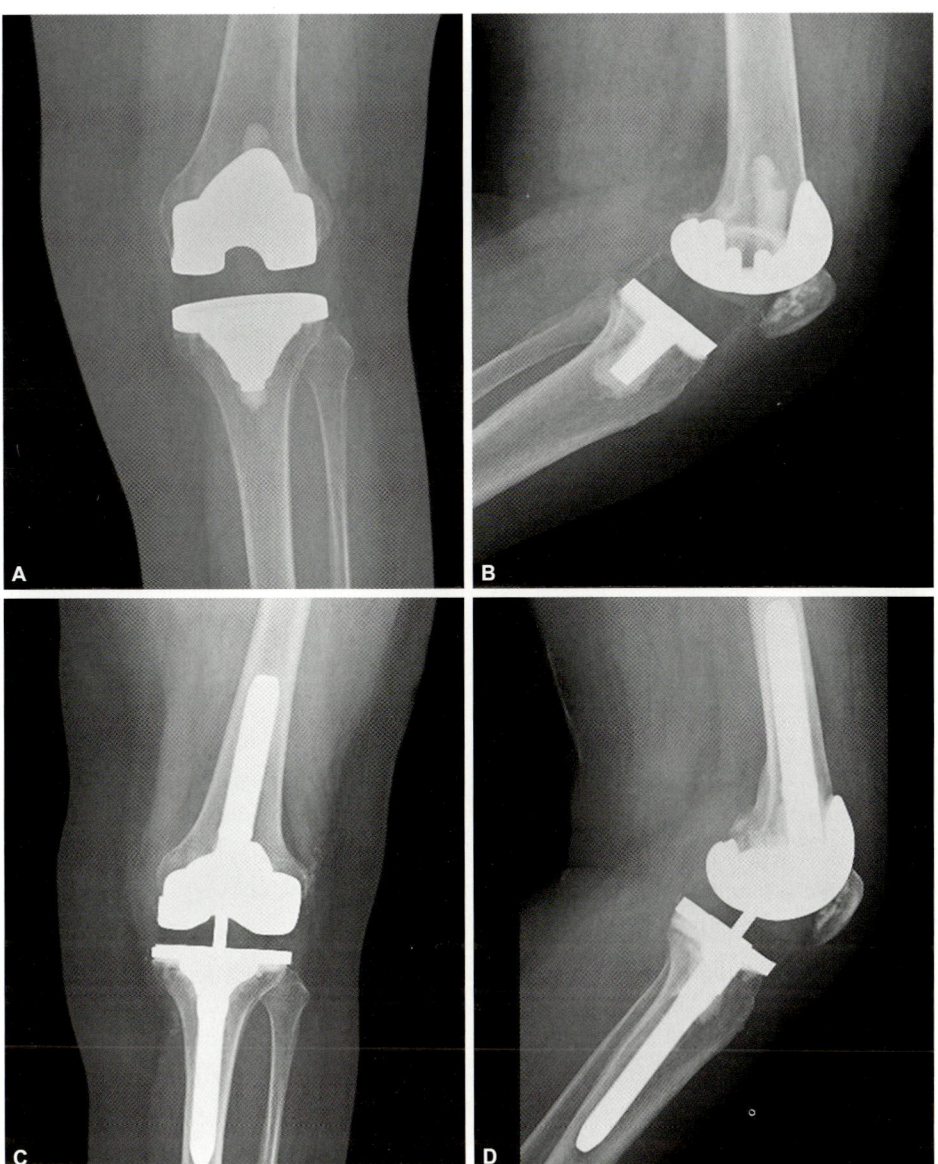

Figures 18.3A to D This patient presented 2 years after total knee arthroplasty with complaints of a buckling knee and unable to climb stairs. She was found to have a large tibial polyethylene insert and small femoral component with flexion instability. (A and B) She underwent a revision total knee arthroplasty in which a constrained condylar device was used along with 10 mm distal femoral augment and 5 mm posterior augments. The patient had been found to have large flexion and extension gaps approximately 30–35 mm. The polyethylene was downsized to size 16 mm. This created increased stability in both flexion and extension and lowered the joint line correcting prior patella baja (C and D). (*Radiographs courtesy:* John Siliski, MD)

successful when patients have more marked disability due to flexion instability.[8] Lombardi et al. reported successful results with conservative treatment for initial dislocation of a posterior stabilized total knee arthroplasty.[33] Conservative management includes closed reduction, brace or cast immobilization and physical therapy and rehabilitation. Patient compliance is a major issue in this treatment regimen.[10]

Most symptomatic instabilities require revision surgery of one or all components. It is imperative to determine the type of instability prior to proceeding with any surgical intervention. Categorization of the instability as well as determining the competence of the collateral ligaments can greatly impact the chances of a successful revision.[10] Preoperative planning and evaluation can give an indication as to the required constraint at the time of revision.[34]

LIGAMENT ADVANCEMENT AND TIGHTENING PROCEDURES

In the presence of an attenuated MCL in valgus knees medial ligament advancement has been found useful by some authors.[35,36] This should be used in concert with a constrained condylar implant as treating instability through soft tissue advancement alone can be quite challenging. The patient's age, quality of soft tissue, quality of bone, ability to rehabilitate, as well as technical concerns such as competence of repair, presence of adjacent femoral stems, and intercondylar hardware can increase the difficulty of these procedures.[10,37]

Isolated Polyethylene Exchange

Exchange of the polyethylene insert is an attractive option given its simplicity and low morbidity, but is only acceptable in certain situations. A well-fixed well-aligned total knee arthroplasty that develops late polyethylene wear and subsequent instability may benefit from isolated exchange. Another occasion may be when there is global postoperative instability due to a liner that was not thick enough to fill the flexion and extension gaps[38,39] (**Figures 18.4A to D**). Brooks et al. reported on 14 knees that had undergone revision of polyethylene liner only for instability with 10 of those (71%) achieving clinical stability and improvement of their HSS knee scores. This, however, meant that 30% of the patients failed at an average of 3 years. Most failures were seen in those knees with an incompetent ligament treated with isolated liner exchange.[38] When PCL insufficiency occurs in a cruciate retaining implant, conversion of the polyethylene insert to an highly congruent or AP constrained insert is an option. Hoffman et al. reported on 53 primary and 47 revision total knee arthroplasties in which an ultracongruent component was used with no revisions due to instability at an average follow up of 5 years.[40]

Single Component Revision

Another option if a cruciate retaining knee develops an incompetent PCL is a revision of one component (typically the femoral component). This requires that the tibial modular component be well fixed and in proper axial alignment. The femoral component can then be revised to a posterior stabilized construct. Revision of the femoral component may also be beneficial in the setting of asymmetric flexion instability caused by rotational malalignment of the femur. Isolated femoral revision allows for changes to the joint line elevation, rotational alignment of the femur, an opportunity to balance flexion and extension gaps and adjust the level of constraint for the prosthesis as needed. In contrast, isolated revision of the tibial component provides little benefit other than adjusting the thickness of the tibial insert, tibial rotation, and slope.[39] In a retrospective review of all revisions performed for purposes other than infection, Fehring et al. found the greatest outcome discrepancies in partial versus full component revisions in those knees treated for instability. They found that those undergoing full revision had Knee Society Scores that were on average 22 points higher ($p = 0.0001$).[41]

Full Component Revision

Full component revision is necessary when the current implants are malaligned, have historically poor track record, or unsatisfactory constraint options available. Isolated polyethylene exchange or single component exchange does not always address the underlying imbalance between the flexion and extension gaps. A revision surgery in which the tibial slope can be adjusted and surgery that allows for a larger femoral component with posterior augmentation if needed can provide reproducible results. Pagnano et al. reported that 19 of 22 knees that were revised to a posterior stabilized design saw significant improvements as opposed to those that only underwent tibial insert exchange.[8] An important principle in treating instability is to use the least constrained implant possible to solve the identified problems. Posterior stabilized implants provide some

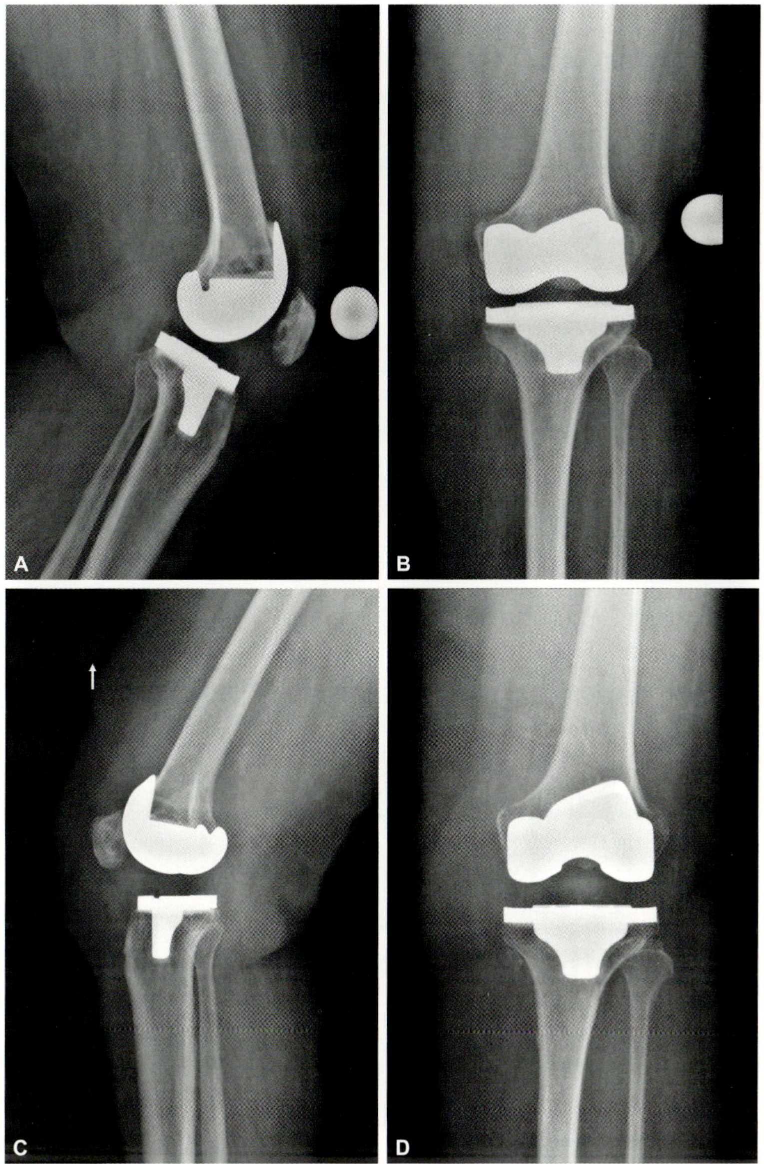

Figures 18.4A to D This patient had undergone a posterior stabilized knee 5 years ago. (A and B) She had multiple episodes of dislocation in which the cam jumped the post. She initially could reduce the knee herself but eventually required assistance from the emergency department over the last several episodes. She was found to have global instability with 20° of recurvatum and flexion instability. Her polyethylene was exchanged from size 13 mm to 19 mm and was found to be quite stable (C and D). (*Radiographs courtesy:* Hany Bediar, MD)

anteroposterior stability but have little stability in the coronal plane. The post can vary between manufacturers and account for different levels of varus/valgus constraint and rotational constraint due to different post heights and widths. A constrained insert provides improved varus/valgus constraint and augments deficient collateral ligaments. Theoretically increased constraint can result in loosening and wear; however, there has been no clinical difference in failure rates between posterior stabilized and condylar constrained prosthesis.[42,43]

Hinged arthroplasties provide a linked constraint between the tibia and femur. Most hinged arthroplasties now have a rotational component to decrease shear forces across the implant and has led to more satisfactory results than prior designs that did not allow for axial rotation.[12,44,45] Indications for a hinged arthroplasty include severe distal femoral bone loss with loss of collateral ligament attachments, large flexion gaps, or complete disruption of an MCL in an elderly patient. Care must be taken when compensating for large flexion gaps as rotating hinge knee prosthesis can dislocate when a large enough gap exists.[46]

Surgical Pearls

Revision of one or both components is a primary technique for addressing instability and correcting any flexion/extension gap imbalance. In some cases anatomical landmarks for assessing the joint line may not exist. Therefore, the use of reference points according to the prosthetic joint line marked prior to the removal of implants may be beneficial.

When revising both components the first step is safe removal of implants preserving as much bone stock as possible. A flat tibial surface should then be established that is perpendicular to the mechanical axis of the tibia. The recreation of this tibial surface can include intramedullary stems, augments, allograft, or trabecular metal cones along with the tibial tray and a modular polyethylene tray insert. The flexion gap should then be recreated by sizing a femoral trial with the knee flexed at 90°. Here one can assess if the flexion gap is loose requiring larger femoral component or perhaps posterior augmentation. If distal femoral deformities exists the use of offset stems allow for of the use of intramedullary stems while maximizing the femoral component position. In the revision setting the flexion gap is rarely tight but if this is the circumstance then downsizing the femoral component may be of benefit.

The extension gap should then be assessed. This can be done using previously made reference marks or via anatomical landmarks. If the knee is found to be loose in extension the surgeon can add distal femoral augmentation or change to a thicker tibial polyethylene insert. Care must be taken as to the effects this can have of the joint line and location of the patella relative to this. If the knee is found to be tight in extension additional distal femoral resection can be performed.[6,10] In older patients or those with substantial instability the use of constrained devices may be indicated.

SUMMARY

Instability after total knee arthroplasty is a common problem. Surgeons can have a direct impact on outcomes if they can identify those patients who are at risk for postoperative instability. Careful attention must be paid to balancing flexion and extension gaps at the time of primary surgery. Proper evaluation and identification of the causes of an unstable total knee arthroplasty will lead to better results when trying to correct their problems. Correction of the instability often leads to increasing the degree of constraint but should also focus on balancing the flexion and extension gaps and restoration of alignment.

REFERENCES

1. Clarke HD, Scott WN. Knee: axial instability. Orthop Clin North Am. 2001;32(4):627-37.
2. Fehring TK, Valadie AL. Knee instability after total knee arthroplasty. Clin Orthop Relat Res. 1994;299:157-62.
3. Fehring TK, Odum S, Griffin WL, Mason B, Nadaud M. Early failures in total knee arthroplasty. Clin Orthop Relat Res. 2001;392:315-18.
4. Yercan HS, Ait Si Selmi T, Sugun TS, Neyret P. Tibiofemoral instability in primary total knee replacement: a review, Part 1: basic principles and classification. Knee. 2005;12: 257-66.
5. Vince KG, Abdeen A, Sugimori T. The unstable total knee arthroplasty: causes and cures. J Arthroplasty. 2006;21(4):44-9.
6. Rodriguez-Merchan EC. Instability following total knee arthroplasty. HSS J. 2011;7:273-8.
7. Winiarsky R, Barth P, Lotke P. Total knee arthroplasty in morbidly obese patients. J Bone Joint Surg Am. 1998;80:1770.
8. Pagnano MW, Hanssen AD, Lewallen DG, Stuart MJ. Flexion instability after primary posterior cruciate retaining total knee arthroplasty. Clin Orthop Relat Res. 1998;356:39-46.
9. Saleh KJ, Clark CR, Sharkey PF, et al. Mode of failure and preoperative evaluation. J Bone Joint Surg Am. 2003;85-A Suppl 1:S21-5.
10. Yercan HS, Selmi TA, Sugun TS, Neyret P. Tibiofemoral instability in primary total knee replacement: a review. Part 2: diagnosis, patient evaluation, and treatment. Knee. 2005;12:336-40.

11. Berger RA, Crosset LS, Jacobs JJ, Rubash HE. Malrotation causing patellofemoral complications. Clin Orthop Relat Res. 1998;356:144-53.
12. Barrack RL. Evolution of the rotating hinge for complex total knee arthroplasty. Clin Orthop Relat Res. 2001;392:292-9.
13. Levitsky KA, Hozack WJ, Balderston RA, et al. Evaluation of the painful prosthetic joint. Relative value of bone scan, sedimentation rate, and joint aspiration. J Arthroplasty. 1991;6:237-44.
14. Wasliewski RC, Galante JO, Leighty RM, Natarajan JN, Rosenber AG. Wear pattern on retrieved polyethylene tibial inserts and their relationship to technical consideration during total knee arthroplasty. Clin Orthop Relat Res. 1994;299:31-43.
15. Parratte S, Pagnano MW. Instability after total knee arthroplasty. J Bone Joint Surg. 2008;90(1):184-94.
16. Martin JW, Whiteside LA. The influence of join line position on knee stability after condylar knee arthroplasty. Clin Orthop Relat Res. 1990;259:146-56.
17. Brassard MF, Insall JN, Scuderi GR, Faris PM. Complications of total knee arthroplasty. In: Scott WN, (Ed). Insall and Scott Surgery of the Knee. Vol 2. 4th edn. Philadelphia: Churchill Livingstone/Elsevier; 2006. p. 1716-60.
18. Insall JN, Binazzi R, Soudry M, Mestriner LA. Total knee arthroplasty. Clin Ortho Relat Res. 1985;192:13-22.
19. Mihalko WM, Krackow KA. Anatomic and biomechanical aspects of pie crusting posterolateral structures for valgus deformity correction in total knee arthroplasty: a cadaveric study. J Arthroplasty. 200;15:347-53.
20. Clarke HD, Fuchs R, Scuderi GR, Scott WN, Insall JN. Clinical results in valgus total knee arthroplasty with the 'pie crust' technique of lateral soft tissue releases. J Arthroplasty. 2005;20:1010-4.
21. Clarke HD, Schwartz JB, Math KR, Scuderi GR. Anatomic risk of peroneal nerve injury with the 'pie crust' technique for valgus release in total knee arthroplasty. J Arthroplasty. 2004;19:40-4.
22. Easley ME, Insall JN, Scuderi GR, Bullek DD. Primary constrained condylar knee arthroplasty for the arthritic valgus knee. Clin Orthop Relat Res. 2000;380:58-64.
23. Leopold SS, McStay C, Klafeta K, et al. Primary repair of intraoperative disruption of the medial collateral ligament during total knee arthroplasty. J Bone Joint Surg Am. 2001;83(1):86-91.
24. Lee GC, Lotke PA. Management of intraoperative medial collateral ligament injury during TKA. Clin Orthop Relat Res. 2011;469(1):64-8.
25. Schwab JH, Haidukewych GJ, Hanssen AD, Jacofsky DJ, Pagnano MW. Flexion instability without dislocation after posterior stabilized total knees. Clin Orthop Relat Res. 2005;440:96-100.
26. Kocmond JH, Delp SL, Stern SH. Stability and range of motion of Insall-Burstein Condylar prostheses: a computer simulation study. J Arthroplasty. 1995;10:383-8.
27. Montgomery RL, Goodman SB, Congradi J. Late rupture of the posterior cruciate ligament after total knee arthroplasty. Iowa Orthop. 1993;13:167-70.
28. Pagnano MW, Hanssen AD, Lewellen DG, Stuart MJ. Flexion instability after primary posterior cruciate retaining total knee arthroplasty. Clin Orthop Relat Res. 1998;356:39-46.
29. Del Gaizo DJ, Della Valle CJ. Instability in primary total knee arthroplasty. Orthopaedics. 2011;34(9):e519-21.
30. Giori NJ, Lewallen DG. Total knee arthroplasty in limbs affected by poliomyelitis. J Bone Joint Surg Am. 2002;84:1157-61.
31. Krackow KA, Weiss AP. Recurvatum deformity complicating performance of total knee arthroplasty. A brief note. J Bone Joint Surg Am. 1990;72(2):268-71.
32. Babis GC, Trousdale RT, Morey BF. The effectiveness of isolated tibial insert exchange in revision total knee arthroplasty. J Bone Joint Surg Am. 2002;84:64-8.
33. Lombardi AV, Mallory FH, Vaugh BK, et al. Dislocation following primary posterior-stabilized total knee arthroplasty. J Arthroplasty. 1993;8:633-9.
34. Gustke KA. Preoperative planning for revision total knee arthroplasty: avoiding chaos. J Arthroplasty. 2005;20:37-40.
35. Healy WL, Iorio R, Lemos DW. Medial reconstruction during total knee arthroplasty for severe valgus deformity. Clin Orthop Relat Res. 1998;356:161-9.
36. Krackow KA, Jones MM, Teeny SM, Hungerford DS. Primary total knee arthroplasty in patients with fixed valgus deformity. Clin Orthop Relat Res. 1991;273:9-18.
37. Krackow KA. Revision total knee replacement ligament balancing for deformity. Clin Orthop Relat Res. 2002;404:152-7.
38. Brooks DH, Fehring TK, Griffin WL, Mason JB, McCoy TH. Polyethylene exchange only for prosthetic knee instability. Clin Orthop Relat Res. 2002;405:182-8.

39. Dennis D, Berry D, Engh G, et al. Revision total knee arthroplasty. J Am Acad Orthop Surg. 2008;16(8):442-54.
40. Hofmann AA, Tkach TK, Evanich CJ, Camargo MP. Posterior stabilization in total knee arthroplasty with use of an ultracongruent polyethylene insert. J Arthroplasty. 2000;15(5):576-83.
41. Fehring TK, Odum S, Griffin WL, Mason JB. Outcome comparison of partial and full component revision TKA. Clin Orthop Relat Res. 2005;440:131-4.
42. Scuderi G. Revision total knee arthroplasty: how much constraint is enough? Clin Orthop Relat Res. 2001;392:300-5.
43. Nelson CL, Gioe J, Cheng EY, Thompson Jr RC. Implant selection in revision total knee arthroplasty. J Bone Joint Surg Am. 2003;85:43-51.
44. McAuley JP, Engh GA. Constraint in total knee arthroplasty: when and what? J Arthroplasty. 2003;18(3):51-4.
45. Springer BD, Hanssen AD, Sim FH, Lewallen DG. The kinematic rotating hinge prosthesis for complex knee arthroplasty. Clin Orthop Relat Res. 2001;392:283-91.
46. Ward WG, Haight D, Ritchie P, Gordon S, Eckardt JJ. Dislocation of rotating hinge prosthesis. J Bone Joint Surg Am. 2003;85:448-63.

Chapter 19

Osteolysis in Total Knee Arthroplasty

Douglas A Dennis, Justin Duke

INTRODUCTION

Arthroplasty of the knee is a common and prolific procedure that brings relief to millions of patients worldwide. The number of total knee arthroplasty (TKA) procedures is predicted to increase significantly as the population ages.[43] The long-term success rates and survivorship of TKA are well documented, but there are modes of failure that orthopedic surgeons must identify and strive to reduce.[18,27] The reasons for failure of TKA are varied and have been described as early and late. This chapter focuses on periprosthetic osteolysis following TKA, a condition that occurs most commonly in failures that occur 5 or more years from the index surgical procedure.

The incidence of osteolysis is widely variable with rates ranging from 3% to 27% in some series.[12,18,26,40,44,54,61] The incidence of osteolysis may be decreasing due to improvements in implants and operative technique, but the significant increase in number of procedures being performed will ensure that osteolysis remains a significant concern. Kurtz projected that the number of primary TKA procedures will increase from 450,000 cases (performed in 2005) to 3.48 million by 2030.[43] Osteolysis is a condition that is characterized by structural changes in bone and is predominantly caused from the generation of microparticulate wear particles from years of TKA use.[30] These lesions may or may not be symptomatic clinically, but can become problematic if enough bone is destroyed leading to loss of implant fixation, pain, or discomfort, and in some cases result in catastrophic failure of the joint arthroplasty with periprosthetic fracture (**Figure 19.1**).[37]

The earliest knee replacements achieved the goal of providing pain relief but lacked in qualities such as range of motion and ease of traversing stairs. These early designs had high levels of congruency between components, which provided large contact areas between implant interfaces and reduced contact stresses (**Figure 19.2**). Surgeons and engineers strove to increase the functional performance of knee replacements by design changes that incorporated less implant conformity and created different kinematic patterns (**Figure 19.3**). While these less conforming designs improved knee flexion, they exhibited reduced contact area that increased the polyethylene contact stresses. This also decreased the inherent stability of the joint and increased the cross shear forces on the bearing surface, which resulted in an increased incidence of failure due to

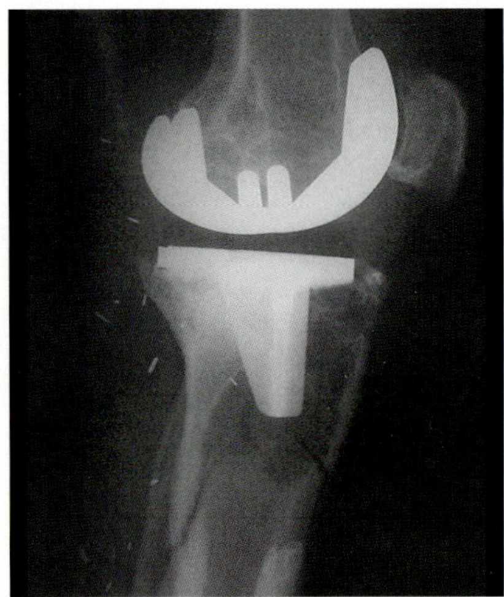

Figure 19.1 Lateral knee radiograph demonstrating extensive proximal tibial osteolysis resulting in a proximal tibial periprosthetic fracture

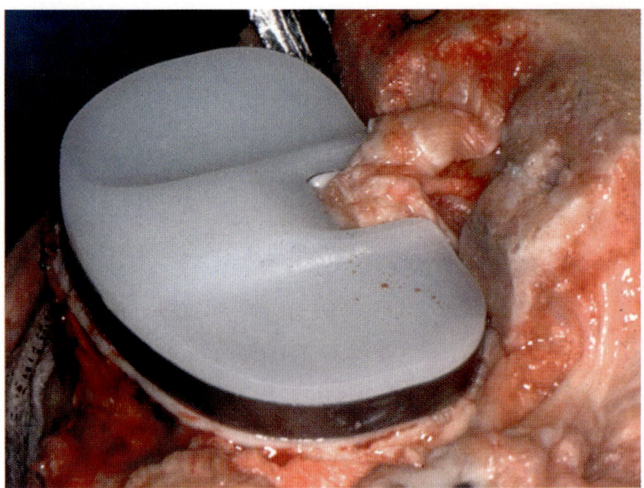

Figure 19.3 Intraoperative photograph of a tibial component with limited articular conformity

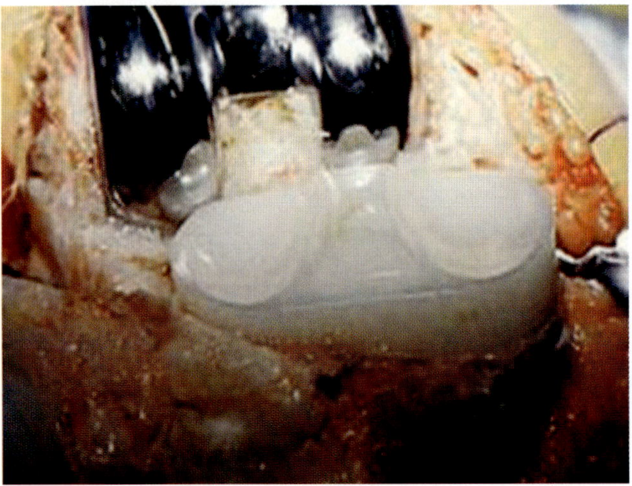

Figure 19.2 Intraoperative photograph of an early condylar total knee arthroplasty design demonstrating increased articular conformity

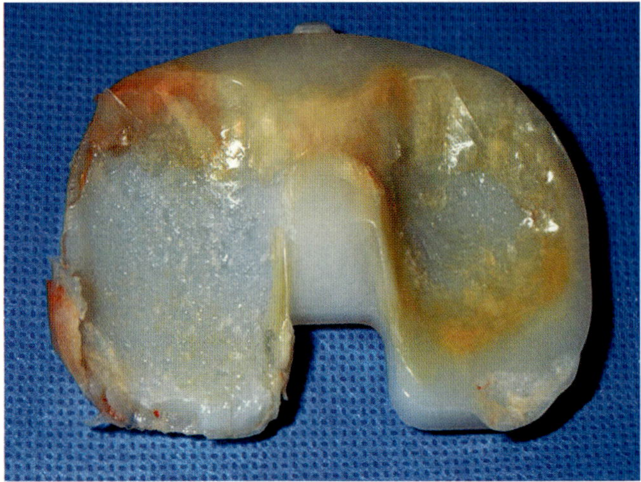

Figure 19.4 Photograph of a retrieved tibial polyethylene insert with limited conformity and demonstrating premature delaminating polyethylene wear

premature polyethylene wear (**Figure 19.4**). In addition to changes in articular surface geometry, other changes such as the introduction of modular tibial components occurred. This design feature provided surgeons with more flexibility to fine-tune the fit and stability of the implant and to facilitate possible bearing changes without removal of the entire tibial component. Some characteristics of tibial tray modularity have contributed to increased rates of osteolysis. Modularity resulted in a second polyethylene interface from which wear particles could be generated and osteolysis secondary to 'backside wear' due to motion between the tibial tray and undersurface of the polyethylene insert was observed.[12] Having the implants made of metal and polyethylene also reduced the nominal thickness of the polyethylene, negatively affecting the wear characteristics of this material.[63]

This chapter will discuss the pathogenesis, etiologic factors, diagnosis, and treatment of periprosthetic osteolysis following TKA.

PATHOGENESIS

Osteolysis is the result of a biologic process that is initiated from a myriad of conditions. For osteolytic destruction of bone to occur, there has to be an inflammatory insult. This most commonly occurs as a sequelae of polyethylene wear, but there are other documented initiators of inflammation. The extent of osteolysis is related to the volume and size of the foreign body microparticulate debris and the inherent inflammatory properties of the foreign substance.[66]

Metallic debris has been shown to induce osteolysis, which can result from either direct metal-to-metal articulations, junctions, or by inadvertent metal contact from implant failure that results in metal-metal contact. Metal particles can also induce soft tissue reactions including pseudocyst formation, necrosis, as well as osteolysis.[65] The type of metal is also significant to the type and extent of the osseous reaction. Particles of cobalt chromium (CoCr) are toxic to macrophages and thus attenuate their potential to create osteolytic lesions. Titanium particles are less toxic to macrophages and stimulate a greater tissue response and elevated levels of interleukin-6 release.[35] Other foreign substances have been shown to induce osteolysis such as synthetic ligament materials and other implants used in arthroscopic procedures.[55,68] It is important to identify potential sources of particle generation as these must be addressed and removed at time of TKA to prevent future osteolysis.

The majority of osteolysis in TKA is initiated by microscopic particles of polyethylene that are generated by various mechanisms. The size of the debris particle is important to understanding the response to that particle. Osteolysis has been observed more extensively in total hip arthroplasty (THA). The prosthetic hip articulation is highly conforming and the polyethylene wear generated comes from abrasive and adhesive wear mechanisms. The majority of the wear particles subsequently created in hip replacements are small (< 1 micrometer) and therefore more reactive.[36,66] In contrast, the TKA articulation is less conforming and can lead to higher peak contact stresses that can exceed the yield strength of the polyethylene. The kinematic motion patterns in TKA are complex with rotation, rolling, and sliding that result in wear patterns that are distinctly different from THA and include delamination, pitting, and fatigue cracking, in addition to some abrasive and adhesive wear. The wear particles generated in TKA are typically three times larger and less reactive than those created in THA.[66]

To initiate the inflammatory response of osteolysis, the wear particles initiate an inflammatory cascade by activating macrophages and giant cells and by stimulating the production of degradative chemicals such as stromelysin, prostaglandin E2, interleukin-1, and tumor necrosis factor. The activated macrophages induce osteolysis by inhibiting the mobility of osteoclasts resulting in localized bone resorption.[2] Indirect osteolysis is the more destructive type and is mediated by the activation of osteoclasts through cytokines that are produced by synovial tissue that has been stimulated to release the cytokines. These same cytokines have also been shown to inhibit the osteoblast from forming bone.[76]

FACTORS AFFECTING POLYETHYLENE WEAR

The polyethylene in TKA is subject to fatigue, adhesive, abrasive, and oxidative wear. The majority of wear observed at the articular surface is fatigue related that creates delamination of the polyethylene from subsurface cracks that propagate. As previously stated, the particles created from this mode of wear are larger and usually relatively inert in regard to the inflammatory response that triggers osteolysis. Adhesive wear can also occur on the articular surface and will create small bioactive particles as the femoral component pulls away particles from the polyethylene articular surface. Abrasive wear can occur on the articular surface and will be increased with the presence of any third body particles that enter the articulation such as stray bone cement (polymethylmethacrylate) fragments or bone chips. Third bodies can be generated from a number of sources such as unremoved osteophytes, bone debris generated from resection of bone, or particles of bone cement that were not removed at the time of the operative procedure. Careful operative technique including meticulous trimming and removal of excessive bone cement and copious pulsatile irrigation at completion of the TKA is imperative to reduce the volume of third body debris particles.

The type or style of implant can also greatly influence the potential for osteolytic lesions. Prior to modular tibial baseplates, there were few instances of osteolysis recognized with monoblock metal-backed designs or with all-polyethylene tibial components. When O'Rourke examined the incidence of osteolysis at mid-term follow-up duration, he observed a 16% incidence of osteolysis in the group of knees that utilized a modular tibial baseplate versus an absence of osteolysis in a group of patients who had received knee arthroplasties performed during the same time period implanted with an all-polyethylene tibial component.[60] The increased conformity introduced in some TKA designs in the 1990s exacerbated the issues of backside wear, as these more conforming designs transmitted higher torque loads to the modular insert-tibial tray interface, thus creating a higher potential for backside wear on the inferior aspect of the polyethylene bearing.[73]

Motion at the interface between the modular baseplate and the polyethylene insert generates backside wear debris that is typically microparticulate in size with a substantial potential to result in osteolysis. Due to the sizable surface area of polyethylene bearing that is in contact with the tibial tray, insert-tray micromotion can generate enormous numbers of microscopic wear particles that can dramatically increase the risk of osteolytic lesions (**Figure 19.5**).[12,74]

The style and type of tibial tray-insert locking mechanism affects the magnitude of wear. There are numerous variations and iterations of locking mechanisms available. All locking mechanisms attempt to rigidly secure the insert to the modular baseplate, but the method by which this occurs usually has some compromises. Locking mechanisms cannot be grouped into discrete categories as many manufactures use a combination of locking styles including peripheral capture, partial capture, central dovetail style, locking pins, and rails. The task of creating a secure locking mechanism is a challenge as it must resist the complex multidirectional motion of the knee joint. When

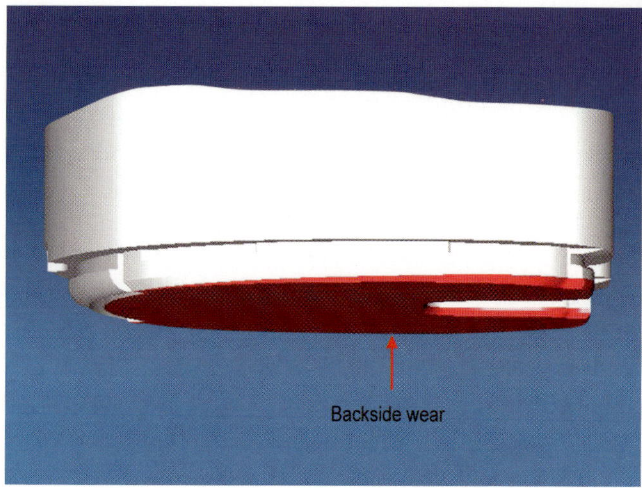

Figure 19.5 Diagram demonstrating that a small amount of linear wear over a larger surface area results in a large volume of microparticulate debris

Jayabalan et al. investigated three TKA tibial tray designs with different locking mechanisms, they found that the stout anteroposterior (AP) mechanism of the Insall-Burstein II design (Zimmer, Inc.; Warsaw, IN) restrained AP motion, but medial-lateral motion was excessive and allowed backside wear.[39] The most volumetric wear that was observed in backside wear was in the locking mechanism that did not limit rotational motion in the transverse plane.[39] Ideally the locking mechanism needs to limit motion in the coronal, sagittal, and transverse planes. Engh and Ammeen showed that a locking mechanism that is initially secure can lose effectiveness and allow increased micromotion over time. This creates a design challenge to develop locking mechanisms that are not only secure, but that maintain rigid fixation of the modular polyethylene insert after years of *in vivo* use.[21,22]

The material and surface finish used in modular tibial baseplates will also influence the amount of wear that occurs at that interface (**Figure 19.6**).[7,74] Use of CoCr material due to superior material hardness and scratch resistance as well as polishing the modular baseplate reduces the abrasive wear on the backside of the polyethylene insert.[7,12,26] Berry et al. analyzed the wear of various modular tibial polyethylene inserts retrieved from fixed-bearing tibial trays manufactured from titanium, which had a rougher surface finish, versus those

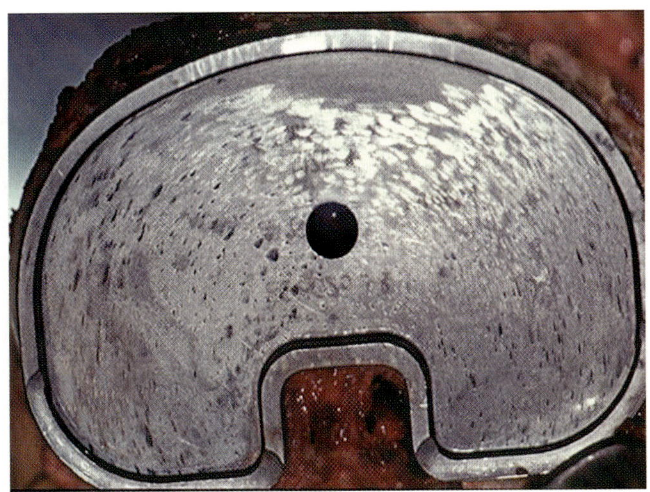

Figure 19.6 Photograph of retrieved titanium modular tibial tray demonstrating stippling of the surface indicative of surface abrasion and subsequent backside wear of the polyethylene insert

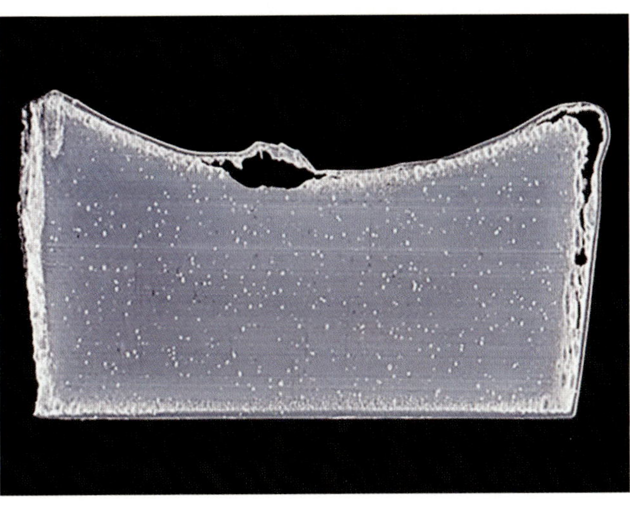

Figure 19.7 Photograph of a retrieved tibial polyethylene insert demonstrating a white line at the periphery and delamination consistent with polyethylene oxidation

retrieved from trays made of polished CoCr. The wear of these designs was further compared with retrievals from rotating platform designs with a polished CoCr tibial tray. They observed the least wear in mobile-bearing retrievals. Fixed-bearing inserts from polished CoCr trays demonstrated less wear than insert retrievals from titanium trays. The wear rate of inserts associated with a polished CoCr surface did not appear to increase over time.[7]

Polyethylene quality is important in determining wear rate of the material. The type of resin used in the manufacture of the polyethylene affects the length of the molecular chains of the polymer, and high molecular weight resin formulations are favored. Currier et al. reported that resin type and shelf life influenced the amount of oxidation found in polyethylene inserts that were gamma radiated in the presence of oxygen. They found that inserts manufactured from GUR 415/412 resin exhibited more oxidation than Himont 1900 and often displayed a thin subsurface white band (**Figure 19.7**), which was not typically observed in inserts made with the Himont 1900 resin.[15] They showed the white band occurs secondary to high levels of polyethylene oxidation and embrittles the material resulting in an increased incidence of material cracking and delamination. The amount of cross-linking, manufacturing process, method of sterilization, and shelf life have all been demonstrated to be significant factors affecting the wear characteristics of polyethylene.[11,12,26] Once the resins are mixed into liquid form, they can be shaped into either bars by ram extrusion, compressed into sheets, or by direct shape compression molding into the final implant. Use of ram-extruded bars is the most commonly used method today. The final polyethylene inserts are then machined from the ram extruded bars, much as they are from compression sheets. In direct compression molding, each insert is formed individually in a mold. Lombardi et al. showed that compression molded polyethylene had a greater resistance to wear than similar inserts manufactured by machining.[47] Others have shown through retrieval data that compression molding the polyethylene insert imparts the best wear characteristics to the implant[6,9] but is used less frequently due to the increased cost of manufacture.

Sterilization has substantial effects on the properties of polyethylene and certain methods can adversely affect polyethylene properties. Chemical sterilization methods such as use of gas plasma and ethylene oxide do not impart any alterations in the innate physical properties of polyethylene. Retrieved polyethylene inserts sterilized with ethylene oxide demonstrate very limited oxidation levels, no evidence of subsurface white bands, and substantially lower wear rates when compared with inserts sterilized with gamma irradiation in the presence of oxygen.[75] Use of ethylene oxide, however, does not enhance cross-linking of polyethylene that can impart favorable wear characteristics.

Gamma irradiation as a form of sterilization can be useful as it induces a dose-dependent effect of increasing the number of cross-linked bonds between the long chains of polyethylene. Cross-linking can improve the yield strength of polyethylene and potentially improve wear of the material. Gamma irradiation, however, can induce unfavorable effects on polyethylene by creation of free radicals leading to increased rates of oxidation and thus fatigue delamination, especially if the polyethylene was sterilized in an oxygen-rich environment. The free radicals actively bond with oxygen molecules (oxidation) as they infuse into the material resulting in chain scission, reduced molecular weight, and increased wear rates.[75] The amount of free radicals generated is dose-dependent with increasing levels of free radicals, oxidation, and wear observed with increasing radiation dose in an oxygen-rich environment. Polyethylene sterilized with gamma radiation in the presence of oxygen has been shown to have the highest wear rates.[7,10,75] Another adverse effect of use of gamma irradiation sterilization in oxygen is the effect of shelf life. Researchers have shown that inserts packaged with the presence of oxygen oxidize within the package due to the presence of free radicals.[14,26] A longer shelf life of the insert before implantation correlated with more rapid *in vivo* wear rates due to increased oxidation levels.[50]

Subsequently, numerous methods have been developed that utilize the cross-linking ability of gamma radiation while reducing the creation of free radicals.[28,32] These involve irradiating polyethylene in an inert gas or vacuum, remelting, annealing, and including a free-radical scavenger such as an antioxidant in the material. Irradiating polyethylene in an inert environment without oxygen and use of barrier packaging to prevent exposure to oxygen has been shown to limit shelf oxidation before implantation. It does not, however, prevent oxidation after *in vivo* implantation.[7] Remelting is a process in which polyethylene is heated above its melt temperature, which 'frees' free radicals entrapped within the crystalline region and allows them to recombine with each other, thereby reducing the amount of free radicals available to oxidize the material.[48,51] Annealing is a process where the polyethylene is heated below the melting point and has the advantage of having less effect on material strength than remelting. It similarly reduces the amount of free radicals, but less so than remelting and therefore higher oxidation levels have been observed in retrieved annealed tibial inserts.[16,52]

The latest generation of polyethylene seeks to reduce *in vivo* oxidation and wear by addition of an antioxidant chemical to the material.[58,59,69] The antioxidant can then bond with the oxygen present after implantation and lessen free radical production and subsequent *in vivo* oxidation.[31,53] Artificial aging of antioxidant polyethylene and subsequent knee simulator wear analysis has shown no oxidation or changes in mechanical properties of the material and a substantial reduction in wear when compared with traditional polyethylene.[53] Lastly, Green et al. have demonstrated antioxidant polyethylene microparticulate debris to be less reactive in an animal evaluation.[31]

The thickness of the polyethylene insert has also been described as relevant to the wear characteristics and longevity. Historically, Bartel et al. performed a finite element analysis evaluating the effect of polyethylene thickness on contact stresses and recommended an absolute minimum polyethylene thickness of 4 mm for highly conforming THA articulations and 6 mm for less conforming TKA articulations. They found the contact stresses increased exponentially as the thickness decreased below these recommended levels.[3,4] More recently, Pijls et al. similarly observed the association of polyethylene thickness with wear in an evaluation of 84 TKA (168 half bearings) followed for 11–16 years. They compared the need for polyethylene-bearing exchange in 6 mm bearings versus those measuring 8 mm or thicker.[63] They found a significantly higher risk of revision for polyethylene wear in the 6 mm thick cohort and subsequently recommended a minimum thickness of 8 mm for all primary TKA inserts.

The surface finish of the femoral component can affect the amount and type of particle wear created in TKA. Lancaster et al. performed a pin on disk wear test and observed the magnitude of polyethylene wear was proportional to the roughness of the surface regardless of the material.[45] Lancaster also found no difference in wear between various materials when the differing materials had the same surface roughness.[45] An independent laboratory evaluation compared wear with use of an oxidized zirconium femoral component versus a traditional femoral component manufactured from CoCr and observed a 42% reduction in wear with the ceramized femoral component.[25] Essner et al. demonstrated that during stair climbing, a ceramized femoral component did not outperform a conventional CoCr implant with regard to wear.[24] The reduced wear observed may be more related to the scratch resistance of the implant surface and the minimization of the ridge height created from the scratch than the actual surface finish of the implant.[29] Despite the favorable wear reduction observed in laboratory studies, a short-term registry evaluation did not demonstrate superiority in clinical results with use of oxidized zirconia femoral components.[38] In addition to the surface finish of the weight-bearing articular surfaces, surface finish of the cam of posterior cruciate substituting femoral components is important. Puloski et al. noticed inconsistencies in surface finish of the cam among differing designs that affected subsequent polyethylene post wear.[64]

With cemented implants, well-interdigitated bone cement can act as seal to the ingress of wear particles and provide a protective effect against osteolysis. Cementless implants have been shown to have higher rates of osteolysis.[23] Holes in modular tibial trays for cementless fixation screws or augment fixation provide a direct pathway for ingress of microparticulate material deep into the cancellous bone. When these conditions are combined with the hydrostatic fluid pressures present around the knee, the pressurized fluid can drive particulate debris through these channels deep into the bone where osteolysis can occur.[71]

In addition to improvements in articular surface geometry and knee kinematics to reduce polyethylene wear, use of mobile-bearing technology offers a potential for further reduction in polyethylene wear. Mobile-bearing TKA designs have the advantage of allowing increased implant conformity and contact area, reducing cross shear stresses, without dramatically increasing stresses transmitted to the polyethylene material or fixation interface. This is reflected in clinical reports of mobile-bearing TKA, which demonstrate a very low incidence of osteolysis.[1,41] One explanation for the limited incidence of osteolysis is the decoupling of multidirectional motions occurring at the articular interfaces with rotating platform TKA designs.[49] In fixed-bearing systems, all rotational, translational, and flexion-extension motion patterns are experienced at a single (superior) articular surface, resulting in multidirectional motion pathways. In rotating platform designs that allow no AP translation, the inferior, or tibial tray-polyethylene articulation, experiences purely rotational (unidirectional) motion patterns. Since the polyethylene bearing primarily tracks with the femoral component, the superior articular surface (femoral component-polyethylene bearing interface) primarily experiences flexion-extension (unidirectional) motion since rotation is occurring on the inferior aspect of the bearing.[19,42] Pooley and Tabor reported when polyethylene is subjected to unidirectional sliding, the molecules align along the direction of motion, lowering the coefficient of friction and reducing wear of the material.[62] Conversely, when polyethylene is exposed to multidirectional wear patterns, increased cross shear stresses are created, which enhance wear. Therefore, use of rotating platform TKA designs can reduce polyethylene wear by decoupling multidirectional motions to more unidirectional motion patterns occurring at two differing interfaces, thus reducing cross shear stresses and wear at both interfaces.

OSTEOLYSIS DIAGNOSIS

The initial evaluation of a painful TKA should include osteolysis as a potential source of pain.[8] Knees with osteolysis as a source of knee pain will likely demonstrate an effusion and synovitis secondary to the chronic inflammatory response. The presenting symptom may also be a popliteal cyst presenting late after TKA.[21] Many knees with osteolysis will demonstrate some degree of instability that results in increased polyethylene shear forces, which increase the potential of polyethylene wear. Dalury recently documented that osteolysis was the reason for late TKA revision in 8% (greater than 5 years from the index procedure). In this same group of over 800 revisions, osteolysis was implicated in less than 2% of early revisions—TKA failures requiring revision within the first 5 years from index procedure.[18]

Many subjects with periprosthetic knee osteolysis will be asymptomatic and the lesions are discovered on routine follow-up radiographs. Symptoms may be associated with a loose prosthesis, if the lesion is significant enough to lead to implant instability, or even fracture.[34] Review of the operative report may aid in the evaluation as you can determine if the implants used have a track record of premature failure and osteolysis.

Imaging of TKA is the most definitive method utilized to diagnosis osteolysis. Standard radiographs have been shown to have limitations when investigating for osteolytic lesions, especially when they are small or when occurring in association with posterior cruciate substituting femoral component designs, since the intercondylar box blocks visual access of distal condylar osteolytic lesions. Nadaud et al. demonstrated that medial and lateral oblique views were quite reliable in detecting lesions that were obscured on standard AP and lateral views with posterior cruciate substituting femoral components (**Figure 19.8**).[57] Critical evaluation of the posterior condylar region of the femur and peripheral regions of the proximal tibia is important as osteolytic lesions frequently initially present in those areas, possibly due to inferior bone cement penetration in those areas. Since small osteolytic lesions may not be apparent on plain radiographs, additional imaging methods are often required. Magnetic resonance imaging (MRI) and computed topography (CT) have both been shown to be quite accurate at detecting lytic lesions around total knee prostheses (**Figure 19.9**).[56,67,78] When compared with MRI, radiographic evaluation identified osteolytic lesions, but consistently underestimated the extent of osteolysis. Additional lesions not visible on radiographs are often identified on MRIs.[72]

OSTEOLYSIS TREATMENT

The method of treatment of osteolysis following TKA is dependent on numerous factors including lesion size, rate of enlargement, associated patient symptoms, and historical success of the current TKA design. If a small asymptomatic lesion is discovered on routine radiographs, it is often appropriate to observe the lesion although more frequent radiographic surveillance every 6-12 months is wise to assess if the osteolytic lesion is rapidly progressive. The pathogeneses previously discussed creates opportunities for treatment modalities that may reduce the incidence of osteolysis by affecting the immune response and blunting the effect of inflammatory pathways.[77] Limited evaluations of pharmacological therapies have been performed in animal models. In a murine model,

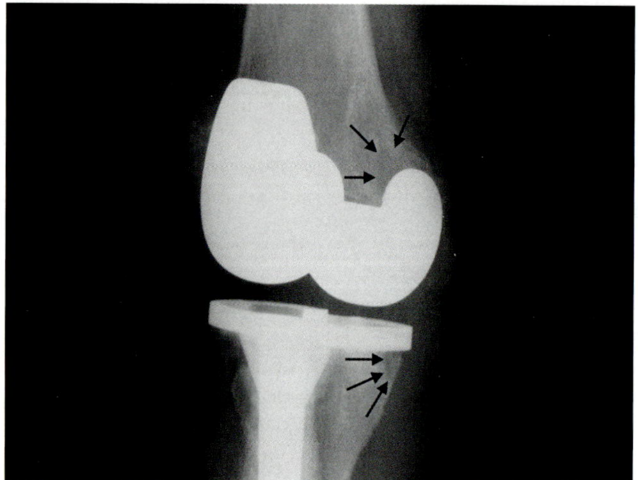

Figure 19.8 Oblique radiograph demonstrating osteolysis of the posterior femoral condyle and proximal tibia (arrows)

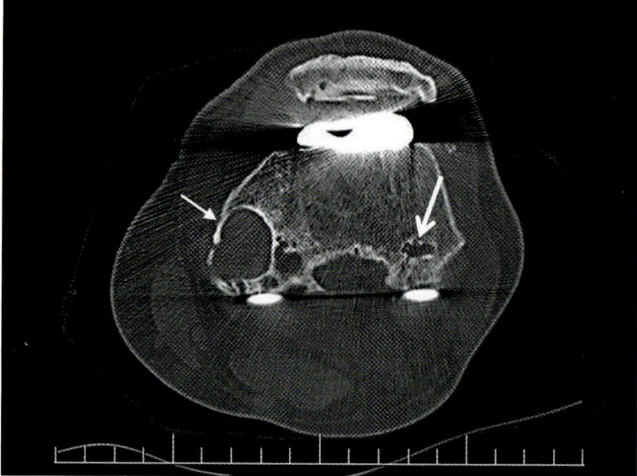

Figure 19.9 CT scan image of a failed total knee arthroplasty demonstrating distal femoral osteolytic lesions (arrows)

Zhang et al. used osteoprotegerin gene transfer to modulate the activation of osteoclasts and attenuate the osteolysis created by a titanium pin prosthesis failure model. In the modified mice, the osteoclastic activity was decreased and peri-implant bone density was increased compared with the untreated mice, thus inhibiting the osteolysis.[77] Clinically, there is a report of successful treatment of osteolytic lesions around THAs treated with oral bisphosphonates in a few human patients.[70] More extensive clinical data is required to recommend use of bisphosphonates for osteolysis management, but may be a viable medical therapy for the patient who is not a surgical candidate.

If the implant is known to have a track record of premature failure and yielding catastrophic osteolytic lesions, the osteolytic lesion is large (≥ 1–2 cm), progressively enlarging on serial radiographs, or if there is an associated periprosthetic fracture, substantial instability, excessive polyethylene wear, or loss of implant fixation, revision TKA is indicated. When preparing for knee revision surgery, it is paramount to determine all factors that have resulted in failure of the arthroplasty as all must be corrected at the time of revision TKA. Revision options include polyethylene liner exchange or component removal. If there are no obvious deficiencies with the index TKA and the source of osteolysis can be attributed to long-term polyethylene wear or to the presence of low quality polyethylene, an isolated polyethylene liner exchange can be performed.[33] If the associated osteolytic lesions are contained and well defined, localized grafting of the lesions can be performed using autologous, allogeneic, or synthetic bone graft substitutes.[5,13,17]

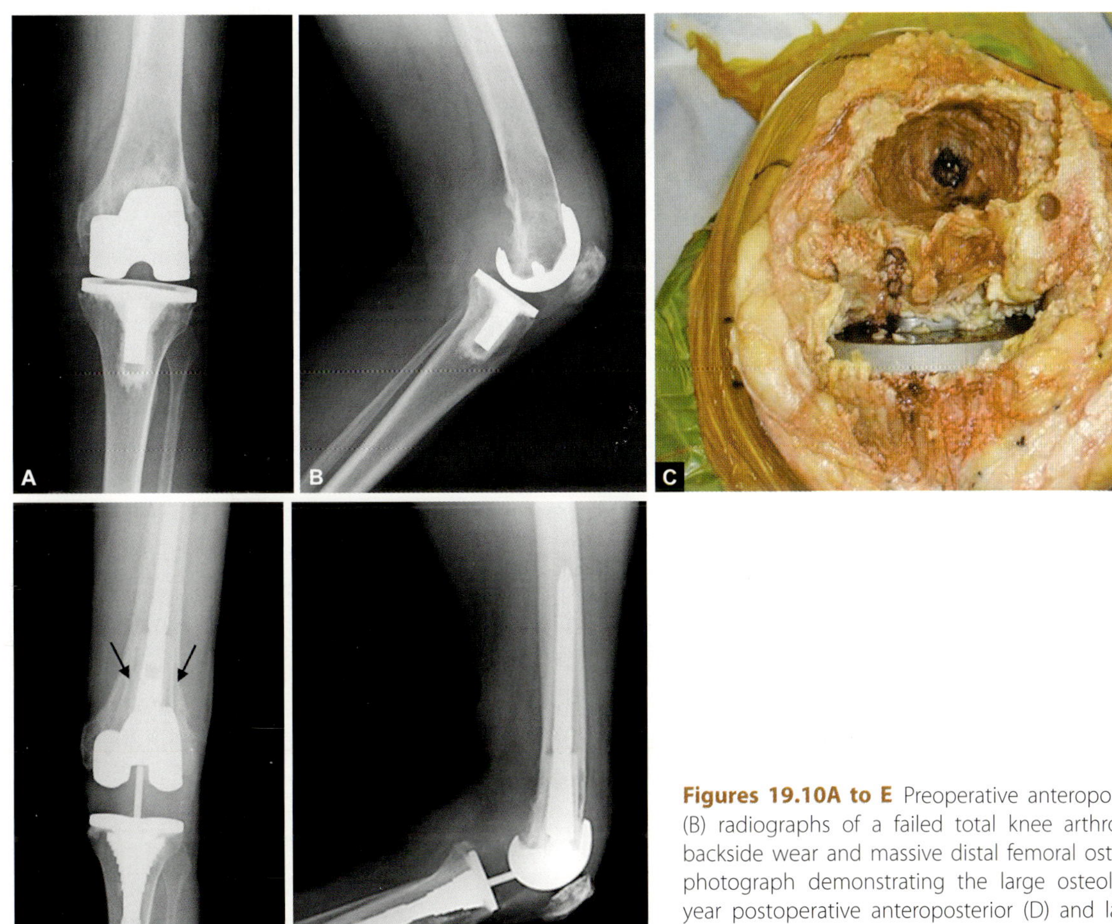

Figures 19.10A to E Preoperative anteroposterior (A) and lateral (B) radiographs of a failed total knee arthroplasty (TKA) due to backside wear and massive distal femoral osteolysis. Intraoperative photograph demonstrating the large osteolytic defect (C). Five-year postoperative anteroposterior (D) and lateral (E) radiographs following revision TKA utilizing in intramedullary structural distal femoral allograft (arrows)

In cases where osteolysis and other associated failure modes such as instability, loss of fixation, or component malposition are present, complete revision of components is necessary. In these cases, extra care must be applied during component removal since the risk of fracture is enhanced due to weakened osteolytic bone. After components are removed, excellent access to osteolytic lesions is typically obtained. Treatment of osteolytic lesions is based on size and location. Numerous treatment options are available including use of particulate or structural bone graft, cement ± screws, augmentation, metaphyseal sleeves, or metaphyseal cones (**Figures 19.10A to E**).[17,20,46] Principles of revision surgery should be followed to obtain restoration of bone stock, stable fixation of implants, neutral mechanical limb alignment, knee stability, and a central tracking extensor mechanism.

SUMMARY

The etiology of periprosthetic osteolysis following TKA is multifactorial but usually associated with conditions that create excessive creation of microparticulate polyethylene wear debris such as femoral–tibial instability or poor quality polyethylene. Wear of the inferior aspect of the polyethylene bearing (backside wear) due to breakdown of modular tibial tray locking mechanisms has been a major source of wear debris and subsequent osteolysis. Smaller osteolytic lesions are often asymptomatic and invisible on routine radiographs. Advance imaging with either MRI or CT scanning may be required for diagnosis. Treatment is based on lesion size and location, rate of lesion growth, associated patient symptoms, and historical success of the current TKA implant. Treatment options include observation, pharmacological management, isolated polyethylene liner exchange, or full-component revision.

REFERENCES

1. Aggarwal AK, Agrawal A. Mobile vs fixed-bearing total knee arthroplasty performed by a single surgeon: a 4- to 6.5-year randomized, prospective, controlled, double-blinded study. J Arthroplasty. 2013;13:0130-7.
2. Athanasou NA, Quinn J, Bulstrode CJ. Resorption of bone by inflammatory cells derived from the joint capsule of hip arthroplasties. J Bone Joint Surg Br. 1992;74(1):57-62.
3. Bartel DL, Bicknell VL, Wright TM. The effect of conformity, thickness, and material on stresses in ultra-high molecular weight components for total joint replacement. J Bone Joint Surg Am. 1968;68(7):1041-51.
4. Bartel DL, Burstein AH, Toda MD, Edwards DL. The effect of conformity and plastic thickness on contact stresses in metal-backed plastic implants. J Biomech Eng. 1985;107(3):193-9.
5. Benson ER, Christensen CP, Monesmith EA, Gomes SL, Bierbaum BE. Particulate bone grafting of osteolytic femoral lesions around stable cementless stems. Clin Orthop Relat Res. 2000;381:58-67.
6. Benson LC, DesJardins JD, LaBerge M. Effects of *in vitro* wear of machined and molded UHMWPE tibial inserts on TKR kinematics. J Biomed Mater Res. 2001;58(5):496-504.
7. Berry DJ, Currier BH, Mayor MB, Collier JP. Gamma-irradiation sterilization in an inert environment: a partial solution. Clin Orthop Relat Res. 2012;470(7):1805-13.
8. Berry DJ. Recognizing and identifying osteolysis around total knee arthroplasty. Instr Course Lect. 2004;53:261-4.
9. Berzins A, Jacobs JJ, Berger R, et al. Surface damage in machined ram-extruded and net-shape molded retrieved polyethylene tibial inserts of total knee replacements. J Bone Joint Surg Am. 2002;84-A(9):1534-40.
10. Collier JP, Sutula LC, Currier BH, et al. Overview of polyethylene as a bearing material: comparison of sterilization methods. Clin Orthop Relat Res. 1996;333:76-86.
11. Collier MB, Engh CA Jr, Engh GA. Shelf age of the polyethylene tibial component and outcome of unicondylar knee arthroplasty. J Bone Joint Surg Am. 2004;86-A(4):763-9.
12. Collier MB, Engh CA Jr, McAuley JP, Ginn SD, Engh GA. Osteolysis after total knee arthroplasty: influence of tibial baseplate surface finish and sterilization of polyethylene insert. Findings at five to ten years postoperatively. J Bone Joint Surg Am. 2005;87(12):2702-8.
13. Cuckler JM. Bone loss in total knee arthroplasty: graft augment and options. J Arthroplasty. 2004;19(4 Suppl 1):56-8.
14. Currier BH, Currier JH, Collier JP, Mayor MB, Scott RD. Shelf life and *in vivo* duration. Impacts on performance of tibial bearings. Clin Orthop Relat Res. 1997;342:111-22.
15. Currier BH, Currier JH, Collier JP, Mayor MB. Effect of fabrication method and resin type on performance of tibial bearings. J Biomed Mater Res. 2000;53(2):143-51.

16. Currier BH, Van Citters DW, Currier JH, et al. *In vivo* oxidation in retrieved highly crosslinked tibial inserts. J Biomed Mater Res B Appl Biomater. 2013;101(3):441-8.
17. Daines BK, Dennis DA. Management of bone defects in revision total knee arthroplasty. J Bone Joint Surg Am. 2012;94(12):1131-9.
18. Dalury DF, Pomeroy DL, Gorab RS, Adams MJ. Why are total knee arthroplasties being revised? J Arthroplasty. 2013;28 (8 Suppl):120-1.
19. Dennis DA, Komistek RD. Kinematics of mobile-bearing total knee arthroplasty. Instr Course Lect. 2005;54:207-20.
20. Dennis DA, Berry DJ, Engh G, et al. Revision total knee arthroplasty. J Am Acad Orthop Surg. 2008;16(8):442-54.
21. Engh GA, Ammeen DJ. Periprosthetic osteolysis with total knee arthroplasty. Instr Course Lect. 2001;50:391-8.
22. Engh GA, Lounici S, Rao AR, Collier MB. *In vivo* deterioration of tibial baseplate locking mechanisms in contemporary modular total knee components. J Bone Joint Surg Am. 2001;83-A(11):1660-5.
23. Engh GA, Parks NL, Ammeen DJ. Tibial osteolysis in cementless total knee arthroplasty. A review of 25 cases treated with and without tibial component revision. Clin Orthop Relat Res. 1994;309:33-43.
24. Essner A, Herrera L, Hughes P, Kester M. The influence of material and design on total knee replacement wear. J Knee Surg. 2011;24(1):9-17.
25. Ezzet KA, Hermida JC, Colwell CW Jr, D'Lima DD. Oxidized zirconium femoral components reduce polyethylene wear in a knee wear simulator. Clin Orthop Relat Res. 2004;(428):120-4.
26. Fehring TK, Murphy JA, Hayes TD, et al. Factors influencing wear and osteolysis in press-fit condylar modular total knee replacements. Clin Orthop Relat Res. 2004;428:40-50.
27. Fehring TK, Odum S, Griffin WL, Mason JB, Nadaud M. Early failures in total knee arthroplasty. Clin Orthop Relat Res. 2001;392:315-8.
28. Ferroni D, Quaglini V. Thermal stabilization of highly crosslinked UHMWPE: a comparative study between annealed and remelted resins. J Appl Biomater Biomech. 2010;8(2):82-8.
29. Galetz MC, Fleischmann EW, Konrad CH, Schuetz A, Glatzel U. Abrasion resistance of oxidized zirconium in comparison with CoCrMo and titanium nitride coatings for artificial knee joints. J Biomed Mater Res B Appl Biomater. 2010;93(1):244-51.
30. Gallo J, Goodman SB, Konttinen YT, Wimmer MA, Holinka M. Osteolysis around total knee arthroplasty: a review of pathogenetic mechanisms. Acta Biomater. 2013;9(9):8046-58.
31. Green JM, Hallab NJ, Liao YS, et al. Anti-oxidation treatment of ultra high molecular weight polyethylene components to decrease periprosthetic osteolysis: evaluation of osteolytic and osteogenic properties of wear debris particles in a murine calvaria model. Curr Rheumatol Rep. 2013;15(5):325.
32. Greulich MT, Roy ME, Whiteside LA. The influence of sterilization method on articular surface damage of retrieved cruciate-retaining tibial inserts. J Arthroplasty. 2012;27(6):1085-93.
33. Griffin WL, Scott RD, Dalury DF, et al. Modular insert exchange in knee arthroplasty for treatment of wear and osteolysis. Clin Orthop Relat Res. 2007;464:132-7.
34. Han CD, Han CW, Yang IH. Femoral component fracture due to osteolysis after cemented mobile-bearing total knee arthroplasty. J Arthroplasty. 2009;24(2):323.e7-12.
35. Haynes DR, Rogers SD, Hay S, Pearcy MJ, Howie DW. The differences in toxicity and release of bone-resorbing mediators induced by titanium and cobalt-chromium-alloy wear particles. J Bone Joint Surg Am. 1993;75(6):825-34.
36. Horikoshi M, Macaulay W, Booth RE, Crossett LS, Rubash HE. Comparison of interface membranes obtained from failed cemented and cementless hip and knee prostheses. Clin Orthop Relat Res. 1994;309:69-87.
37. Huang CH, Yang CY, Cheng CK. Fracture of the femoral component associated with polyethylene wear and osteolysis after total knee arthroplasty. J Arthroplasty. 1999;14(3):375-9.
38. Inacio MC, Cafri G, Paxton EW, Kurtz SM, Namba RS. Alternative bearings in total knee arthroplasty: risk of early revision compared to traditional bearings: an analysis of 62,177 primary cases. Acta Orthop. 2013;84(2):145-52.
39. Jayabalan P, Furman BD, Cottrell JM, Wright TM. Backside wear in modern total knee designs. HSS J. 2007;3(1):30-4.
40. Kasahara Y, Majima T, Kimura S, Nishiike O, Uchida J. What are the causes of revision total knee arthroplasty in Japan? Clin Orthop Relat Res. 2013;471(5):1533-8.
41. Kim YH, Kim JS, Choi Y. Osteolysis after unidirectional and multidirectional mobile-bearing total knee arthroplasty in young patients. J Arthroplasty. 2009;24(4):586-93.

42. Komistek RD, Dennis DA, Mahfouz MR, Walker S, Outten J. *In vivo* polyethylene bearing mobility is maintained in posterior stabilized total knee arthroplasty. Clin Orthop Relat Res. 2004;428:207-13.
43. Kurtz S, Ong K, Lau E, Mowat F, Halpern M. Projections of primary and revision hip and knee arthroplasty in the United States from 2005 to 2030. J Bone Joint Surg Am. 2007;89(4):780-5.
44. Lachiewicz PF, Soileau ES. Fixation, survival and osteolysis with a modern posterior-stabilized total knee arthroplasty. J Arthroplasty. 2013;(13)373-2.
45. Lancaster JG, Dowson D, Isaac GH, Fisher J. The wear of ultra-high molecular weight polyethylene sliding on metallic and ceramic counterfaces representative of current femoral surfaces in joint replacement. Proc Inst Mech Eng H. 1997;211(1):17-24.
46. Lewallen DG, Fehring TK, Dennis DA, Scuderi GR. Revision total knee arthroplasty: surgical techniques. J Bone Joint Surg Am. 2009;91(Suppl 5):69-71.
47. Lombardi AV Jr, Ellison BS, Berend KR. Polyethylene wear is influenced by manufacturing technique in modular TKA. Clin Orthop Relat Res. 2008;466(11):2798-805.
48. Maher SA, Furman BD, Babalola OM, Cottrell JM, Wright TM. Effect of crosslinking, remelting, and aging on UHMWPE damage in a linear experimental wear model. J Orthop Res. 2007;25(7):849-57.
49. McEwen HM, Barnett PI, Bell CJ, et al. The influence of design, materials and kinematics on the *in vitro* wear of total knee replacements. J Biomech. 2005;38(2):357-65.
50. McGovern TF, Ammeen DJ, Collier JP, Currier BH, Engh GA. Rapid polyethylene failure of unicondylar tibial components sterilized with gamma irradiation in air and implanted after a long shelf life. J Bone Joint Surg Am. 2002;84-A(6):901-6.
51. Medel FJ, Peña P, Cegoñino J, Gómez-Barrena E, Puértolas JA. Comparative fatigue behavior and toughness of remelted and annealed highly crosslinked polyethylenes. J Biomed Mater Res B Appl Biomater. 2007;83(2):380-90.
52. Medel FJ, Kurtz SM, Hozack WJ, et al. Gamma inert sterilization: a solution to polyethylene oxidation? J Bone Joint Surg Am. 2009;91(4):839-49.
53. Micheli BR, Wannomae KK, Lozynsky AJ, Christensen SD, Muratoglu OK. Knee simulator wear of vitamin E stabilized irradiated ultrahigh molecular weight polyethylene. J Arthroplasty. 2012;27(1):95-104.
54. Mikulak SA, Mahoney OM, dela Rosa MA, Schmalzried TP. Loosening and osteolysis with the press-fit condylar posterior-cruciate-substituting total knee replacement. J Bone Joint Surg Am. 2001;83-A(3):398-403.
55. Miller MD, Peters CL, Allen B. Early aseptic loosening of a total knee arthroplasty due to Gore-Tex particle-induced osteolysis. J Arthroplasty. 2006;21(5):765-70.
56. Mosher TJ, Davis CM 3rd. Magnetic resonance imaging to evaluate osteolysis around total knee arthroplasty. J Arthroplasty. 2006;21(3):460-3.
57. Nadaud MC, Fehring TK, Fehring K. Underestimation of osteolysis in posterior stabilized total knee arthroplasty. J Arthroplasty. 2004;19(1):110-5.
58. Oral E, Christensen SD, Malhi AS, Wannomae KK, Muratoglu OK. Wear resistance and mechanical properties of highly cross-linked, ultrahigh-molecular weight polyethylene doped with vitamin E. J Arthroplasty. 2006;21(4):580-91.
59. Oral E, Malhi AS, Muratoglu OK. Mechanisms of decrease in fatigue crack propagation resistance in irradiated and melted UHMWPE. Biomaterials. 2006;27(6):917-25.
60. O'Rourke MR, Callaghan JJ, Goetz DD, Sullivan PM, Johnston RC. Osteolysis associated with a cemented modular posterior-cruciate-substituting total knee design: five to eight-year follow-up. J Bone Joint Surg Am. 2002;84-A(8):1362-71.
61. Peters PC Jr, Engh GA, Dwyer KA, Vinh TN. Osteolysis after total knee arthroplasty without cement. J Bone Joint Surg Am. 1992;74(6):864-76.
62. Pooley CM, Tbaor D. Friction and molecular structure: the behavior of some thermoplastics. Proc R Soc Lond A. 1972;329:251-74.
63. Pijls BG, Van der Linden-Van der Zwaag HM, Nelissen RG. Polyethylene thickness is a risk factor for wear necessitating insert exchange. Int Orthop. 2012;36(6):1175-80.
64. Puloski SK, McCalden RW, MacDonald SJ, Rorabeck CH, Bourne RB. Tibial post wear in posterior stabilized total knee arthroplasty. An unrecognized source of polyethylene debris. J Bone Joint Surg Am. 2001;83-A(3):390-7.
65. Sansone V, Pagani D, Melato M. The effects on bone cells of metal ions released from orthopaedic implants. A review. Clin Cases Miner Bone Metab. 2013;10(1):34-40.

66. Schmalzried TP, Jasty M, Rosenberg A, Harris WH. Polyethylene wear debris and tissue reactions in knee as compared to hip replacement prostheses. J Appl Biomater. 1994;5(3):185-90.
67. Solomon LB, Stamenkov RB, MacDonald AJ, et al. Imaging periprosthetic osteolysis around total knee arthroplasties using a human cadaver model. J Arthroplasty. 2012;27(6):1069-74.
68. Sonnery-Cottet B, Mortati R, Gadea F, et al. Osteolysis of the tibial plateau after meniscal repair with hybrid suture anchor. Knee Surg Sports Traumatol Arthrosc. 2013;21(9):2137-40.
69. Teramura S, Sakoda H, Terao T, et al. Reduction of wear volume from ultrahigh molecular weight polyethylene knee components by the addition of vitamin E. J Orthop Res. 2008;26(4):460-4.
70. Trevisan C, Nava V, Mattavelli M, Parra CG. Bisphosphonate treatment for osteolysis in total hip arthroplasty. A report of four cases. Clin Cases Miner Bone Metab. 2013; 10(1):61-4.
71. Van der Vis HM, Aspenberg P, Marti RK, Tigchelaar W, Van Noorden CJ. Fluid pressure causes bone resorption in a rabbit model of prosthetic loosening. Clin Orthop Relat Res. 1998;350:201-8.
72. Vessely MB, Frick MA, Oakes D, Wenger DE, Berry DJ. Magnetic resonance imaging with metal suppression for evaluation of periprosthetic osteolysis after total knee arthroplasty. J Arthroplasty. 2006;21(6):826-31.
73. Wasielewski RC, Galante JO, Leighty RM, Natarajan RN, Rosenberg AG. Wear patterns on retrieved polyethylene tibial inserts and their relationship to technical considerations during total knee arthroplasty. Clin Orthop Relat Res. 1994;299:31-43.
74. Wasielewski RC. The causes of insert backside wear in total knee arthroplasty. Clin Orthop Relat Res. 2002;404:232-46.
75. Williams IR, Mayor MB, Collier JP. The impact of sterilization method on wear in knee arthroplasty. Clin Orthop Relat Res. 1998;356:170-80.
76. Yao J, Cs-Szabó G, Jacobs JJ, Kuettner KE, Glant TT. Suppression of osteoblast function by titanium particles. J Bone Joint Surg Am. 1997;79(1):107-12.
77. Zhang T, Yu H, Gong W, et al. The effect of osteoprotegerin gene modification on wear debris-induced osteolysis in a murine model of knee prosthesis failure. Biomaterials. 2009;30(30):6102-8.
78. Zotti MG, Campbell DG, Woodman R. Detection of periprosthetic osteolysis around total knee arthroplasties an *in vitro* study. J Arthroplasty. 2019;27(2):317-22.

Chapter 20

Extensor Mechanism Reconstruction for Ruptures or Deficiencies after Total Knee Arthroplasty

Andrea Baldini, Francesco Traverso, Caterina Guarducci, Pierpaolo Summa

INTRODUCTION

Extensor mechanism (ExtMech) disruption in total knee arthroplasty (TKA) is a severe complication that compromises both the joint function and the implant longevity. Reported rate in the literature, combining the different sites including the patellar bone, varies from 0.1 to 2.5% of the TKAs.[1,2] Most of the time the damage of the ExtMech has a chronic degenerative pattern. For this reason, it is quite uncommon for the surgeon to be able to repair these lesions with a direct suturing type of technique. Multiple techniques have been attempted, including primary repair with wire,[3] sutures,[4] or staples,[2] and internal fixation of the avulsed osseous fragments[5] with fair or poor results. New tissue needs to be fixed in place reinforcing or substituting the damaged or deficient quadriceps or patellar tendon.

Augmentation with autogenous tissue such as a free fascia lata graft,[5] a gracilis tendon,[2] a semitendinosus tendon,[2,6] or a gastrocnemius muscle flap[7] has been described. Reconstruction of a patellar tendon lesion in TKA with autologous tissue is the classic technique described by Cadambi and Engh using the semitendinosus tendon directly harvested from the injured limb of the patient and looped proximally around or inside the patellar bone (**Figure 20.1**). This technique is applicable only to the patellar tendon lesions and it showed suboptimal results having a significant residual extensor lag in all the patients.[6] This was related to the quality of the harvested tissue and to the difficulty to apply the right amount of ExtMech tension with this type of suture.

Emerson et al. described in 1990 an alternative technique using a complete ExtMech allograft (EMA).[8,9] Few years later, Crosset et al. described a successful technique using the Achilles tendon allograft (ATA) for the ExtMech repair.[10] In the following years, alternatives with synthetic ligaments or hernia meshes have been successfully reported too.[11,12]

PREOPERATIVE PLANNING

Treatment of ExtMech lesions depends on a number of parameters including the size and site of the lesion, the TKA implant type and status, the viability of the skin layer, and the general status of the patient. In case of concomitant infection, the allograft cannot be implanted

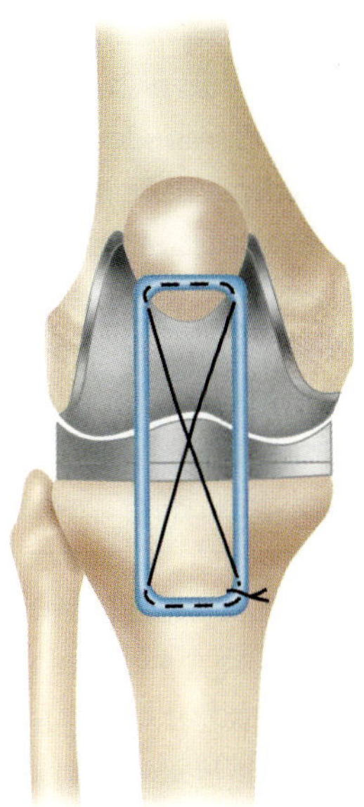

Figure 20.1 Augmentation of patellar tendon with autologous tissue

as it represents a large heterologous tissue, easy ground for germs. Nevertheless, the results of the study by Nazarian and Booth suggests the possibility of using these grafts in postinfection cases treated with two-stage technique, with acceptable rates of reinfection, not different from other series of septic revision TKA without allografts.[13] The ExtMech can be damaged in combination with a failed TKA for septic or mechanical reasons. These cases of combined revision of the implant and EM must be planned carefully and the time devoted to the revision of the prosthesis must be minimized.

In the clinical examination, particular attention should be paid to the study of the skin layer. Previous incisions are often present in these cases. Poorly vascularized skin areas or skin adherence around old scars should be identified and treated in advance. In fact, one of the most frequent causes of failure of the EM reconstruction is the skin dehiscence with infection of the underlying graft. Any plastic surgery reparative skin procedure should be scheduled prior to the EM reconstruction.

ExtMech lesions invariably cause a deficiency of active extension (extensor lag). It will be necessary to distinguish this deficit from a fixed flexion contracture with extension loss, as this will not be resolved by restoring the quadriceps extension power but by a revision TKA procedure involving the tibiofemoral joint.

The patient type and comorbidities are another important factor that can influence the result of the reconstruction. The ideal patient is relatively old, with enough quadriceps muscle mass preserved. Relatively young patients (below 65 years old) have a higher frequency of re-ruptures, accelerated resorption of the graft's bone portions, and a lack of compliance in the long recovery period.

GRAFT CHOICE CRITERIA

There is yet no clear choice criteria based on the results in the literature. Grafts should be fresh frozen and accompanied by a description of the size of their components (**Figures 20.2A and B**). There are a number of factors that should be considered in choosing the type of graft between an ATA and a total ExtMech allograft (EMA) (**Table 20.1**).

The ATA is preferable if the surgeon wishes to preserve the autologous tissues to the maximum, in the presence of a still acceptable patella.[10,14,15] The ATA is mostly used in case of patellar tendon's lesions. The ATA has a higher elasticity, not containing the patella, and consisting of a lower amount of tissue. In addition to that, the ATA is more readily available at the bone banks, and it does not need a matching side or sex. The ATA must be accompanied by a minimum 3 × 4 cm calcaneal bone block. In case the surgeon has to restore an ExtMech where the patella is absent or comminuted and/or there is extensive damage of the quadriceps tendon, it is preferable to use an EMA. This type of allograft must match the side of the involved knee (to maintain the proper direction of the 'Q angle' and prevent patellar maltracking). The matching of sex is less necessary and mostly related to the dimensions of the patellar bone. A small lady cannot accept a 30 mm thick patella of a male graft. Some minimal dimensional features such as a sufficient size of the tibial bone block (at least 6–7 × 3 cm) and length of the limb quadriceps (at least 7–8 cm) must be respected (**Figures 20.3A and B**).

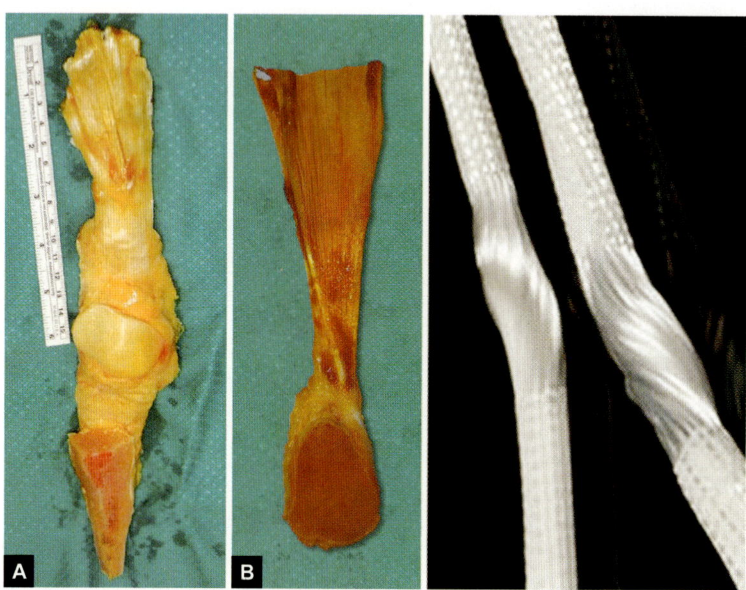

Figures 20.2A and B Different graft options: (A) Extensor tendon allograft (ETA) and (B) Achilles tendon allograft (ATA)

TABLE 20.1 Factors that should be considered while selecting the type of graft for extensor mechanism reconstruction

Parameters	*EMA*	*ATA*
Site of lesion	Proximal	Distal
Patella status	Not important	Possibly intact
Timing	Chronic lesions	Chronic lesions
Patients' age	Older	Younger
Graft availability	Difficult	Easier

Abbreviations: EMA, extensor mechanism allograft; ATA, Achilles tendon allograft.

SURGICAL TECHNIQUE

Incision

During the exposure, it is necessary to take special care of the superficial layers in order to avoid skin devascularization and possible necrosis. The subcutaneous layer should be undermined including all the fat tissue down to the fascia in order to include the skin blood supply. Subcutaneous dissection over the lateral side of the wound should be limited being that this side is less perfused than the medial side. Skin incision should be extensive (approximately 25-30 cm), possibly using a previous incisions, if appropriate. The skin incision is considered adequate when myotendinous transition point of the quadriceps rectum is exposed. Distally, the skin incision should be extended for about 10-15 cm to the joint line to ensure sufficient space for the tibial bone block positioning. The capsulotomy should be exactly anterior-central in order to create two symmetric layers of capsular margins medially and laterally. If the patellar bone is present, it should be removed by cutting it longitudinally with a sawblade and then removed from both sides with subperiosteal dissection.[16]

Tibial Preparation for Total Extensor Mechanism Allograft

The EMA is placed over the replaced joint in full extension to calculate the ideal patellar height. Final adjustments will depend on graft size and on patient size. Ideally, the tibial bone block of the graft should rest at 15-20 mm from the tibial component baseplate in order to leave a sufficiently strong bony bridge. The optimal patellar position should be checked in full extension. The proximal patellar pole of the graft should sit slightly proximal to the beginning of the trochlea of the femoral component.

When preparing the tibial trough, the proximal line of tibial osteotomy should have an obliquity of approximately 30°-40° to create a dovetail engagement with the tibial bone block of the graft (**Figures 20.3 and 20.4**).[16] The next step is to perform a longitudinal osteotomy with a sagittal saw on the lateral side of the tibial tubercle of the patient in order to keep a lateral cortical layer that will represent the lateral

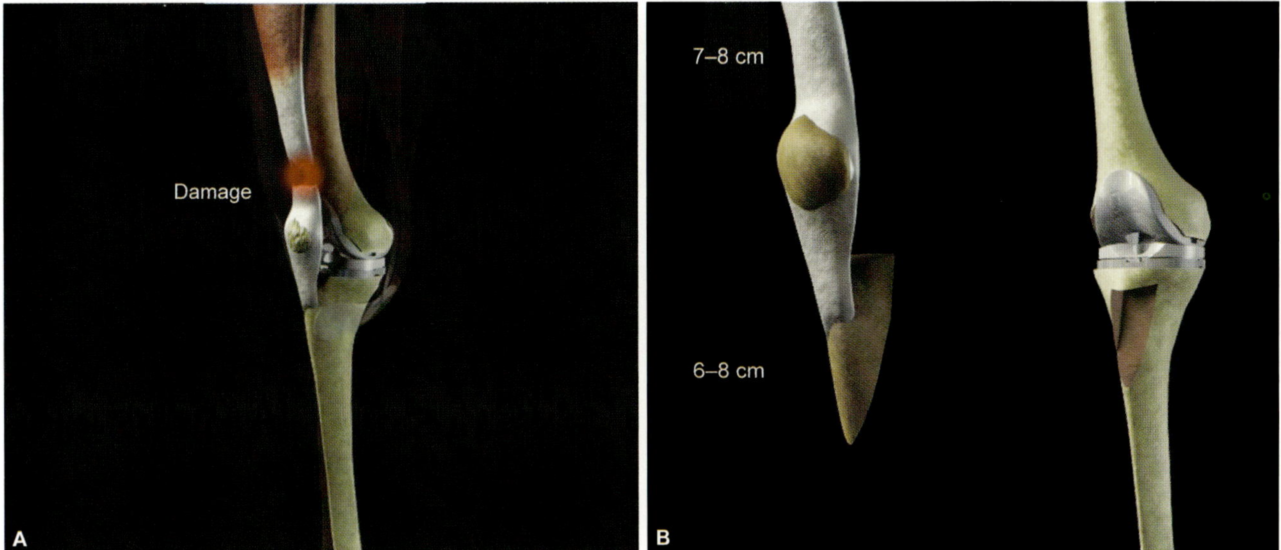

Figures 20.3A and B Extensor mechanism allograft for extensive damage to quadriceps mechanism. While preparing the tibial trough, the proximal line of tibial osteotomy is at an obliquity of approximately 30°–40° to create a dovetail engagement with the tibial bone block of the graft

margin of the trough. The presence of this residual lateral longitudinal bone will also serve to relatively medialize the implanted tuberosity in order to facilitate the final patellar tracking. The distal osteotomy resection from medial to lateral, in the coronal plane, has also an oblique direction. Distally, it emerges superficially without creating steps to reduce the risk of fracture at that level (**Figure 20.4C**). This possible complication is facilitated by a step cut on the tibia that represents a dangerous stress riser particularly in the absence of a tibial stem extension. The shape of the tibial trough is then reproduced on a sterile paper template that will be used to quickly prepare the tibial portion of the graft on a back-table. Further adjustments are carried out employing a high-speed burr (**Figures 20.5A and B**). The graft should be encased as deeply as possible up to the contact to the underlying implant in order to maintain adequate thickness of the bone block of the graft and simultaneously to facilitate skin closure at that level.[16] The proximal portion of the tibial bone block is prepared with a bevel cut to engage with a dovetail shape in the tibial trough. This will ensure immediate resistance to proximal traction of the ExtMech. The additional fixation has the sole purpose of avoiding the lifting of the distal portion of the tuberosity and to maintain a close contact to facilitate the marginal integration for creeping substitution as demonstrated by Burnett et al.[17] The fixation devices that can be used are wires cerclage or screws (**Figures 20.6 and 20.7**). Failure of fixation at this level or breakage of the tibial block is one of the most common complications with this technique.[16,18] Our method of choice is with two self-threading acetabular screws. The advantage of this fixation is that the self-threading profile of the screws does not pose the risk of graft's fracture; they have a good grip in the cancellous tibial metaphysis, and the low-profile flathead does not protrude from the surface. Two screws are inserted while holding the graft firmly in place and with predrilling their path with a 3.2 mm diameter drill-bit (enlarging the entry point to 6.5 mm). Drilling direction, and consequently screws direction, is from anterior to posterior, from medial to lateral, and from the caudocranial pointing toward the proximal tibiofibular syndesmosis.

Proximal Fixation for Total Extensor Mechanism Allograft

The quadriceps tendon part of the graft is prepared with Krackow sutures on the medial and lateral sides using Ethibond #5 sutures (Ethicon, Johnson & Johnson, Somerville, NJ) (**Figure 20.8A**). The same preparation is also carried out on both the medial and lateral sides of the residual autologous quadriceps tissue (**Figure 20.8B**). These ends will be used to exert distal traction of the

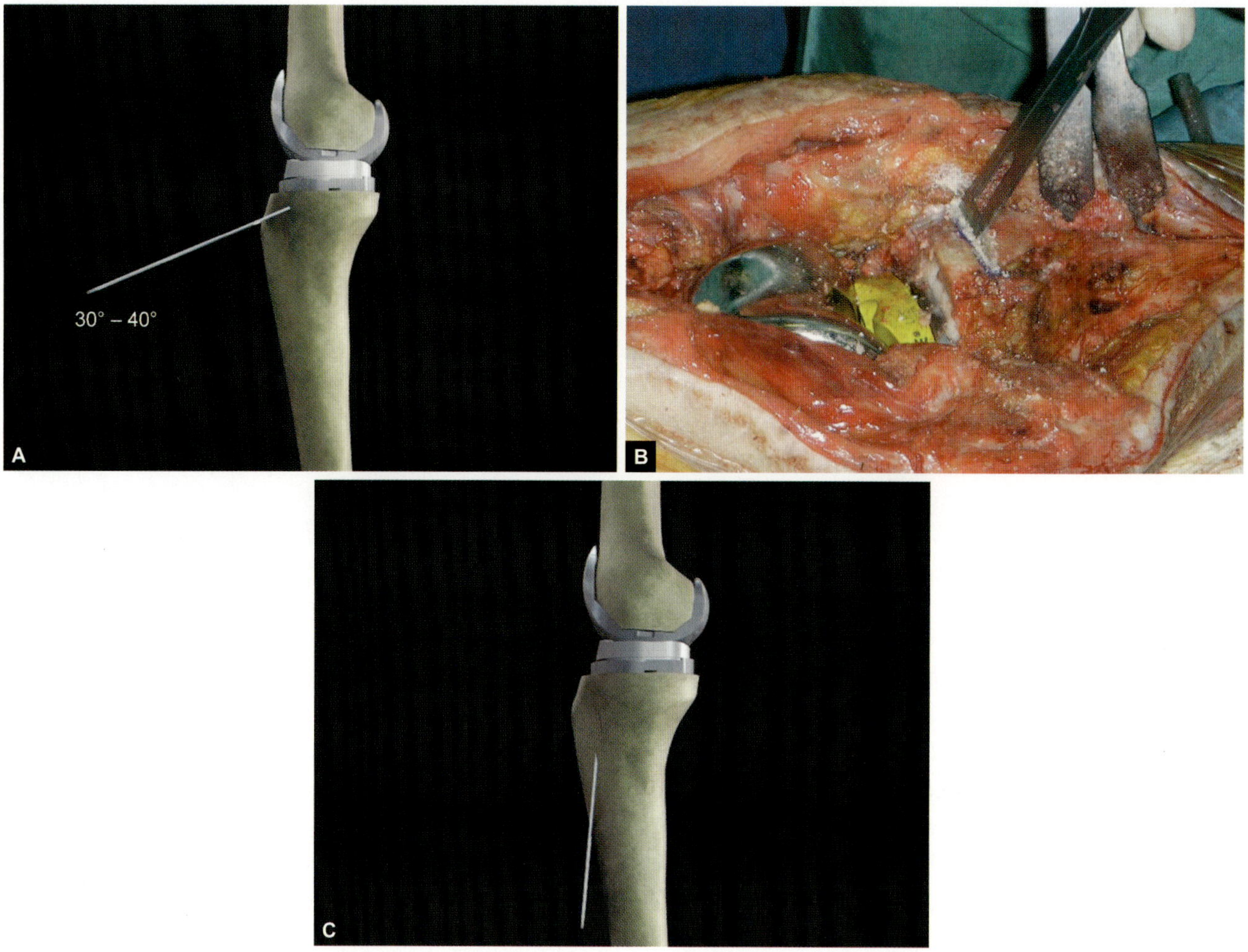

Figures 20.4A to C While preparing the tibial trough, the proximal line of tibial osteotomy is at an obliquity of approximately 30°–40° to create a dovetail engagement with the tibial bone block of the graft

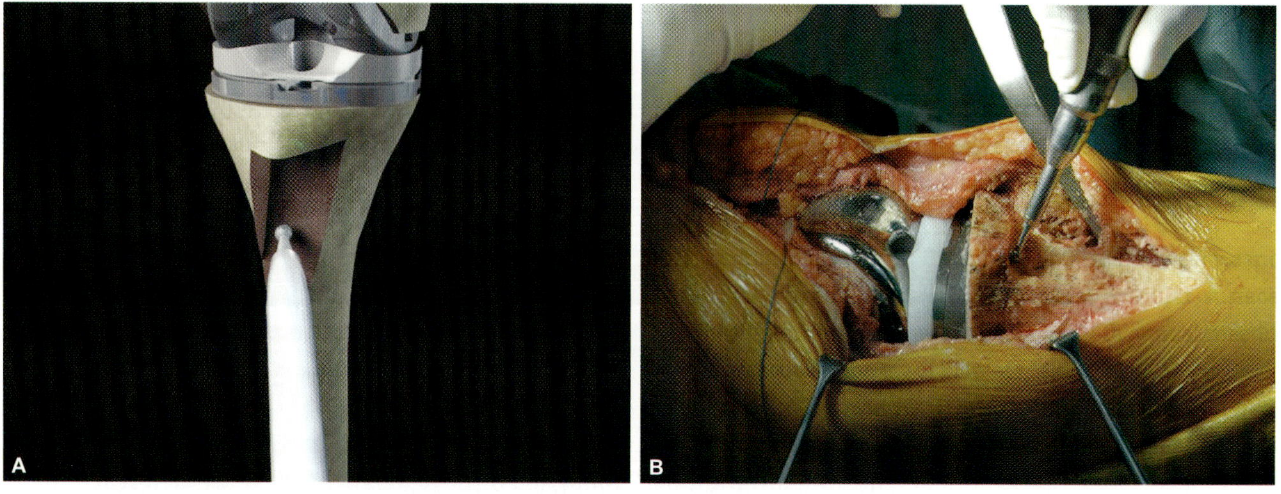

Figures 20.5A and B A high-speed burr is used to exactly shape the tibial trough to match that of the allograft

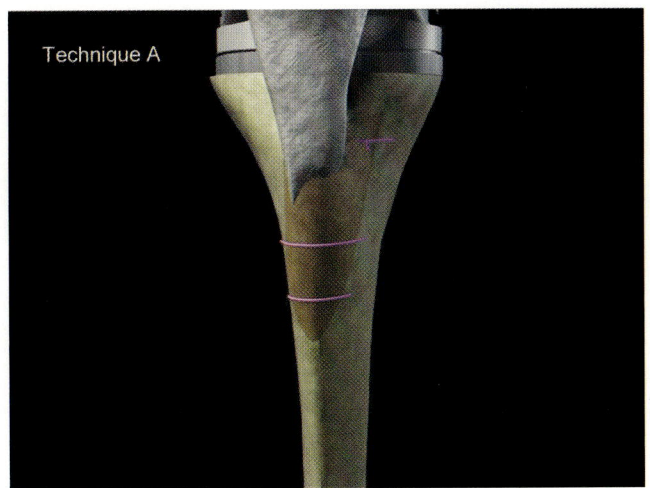

Figure 20.6 Cerclage wires used to fix the draft into the tibial trough

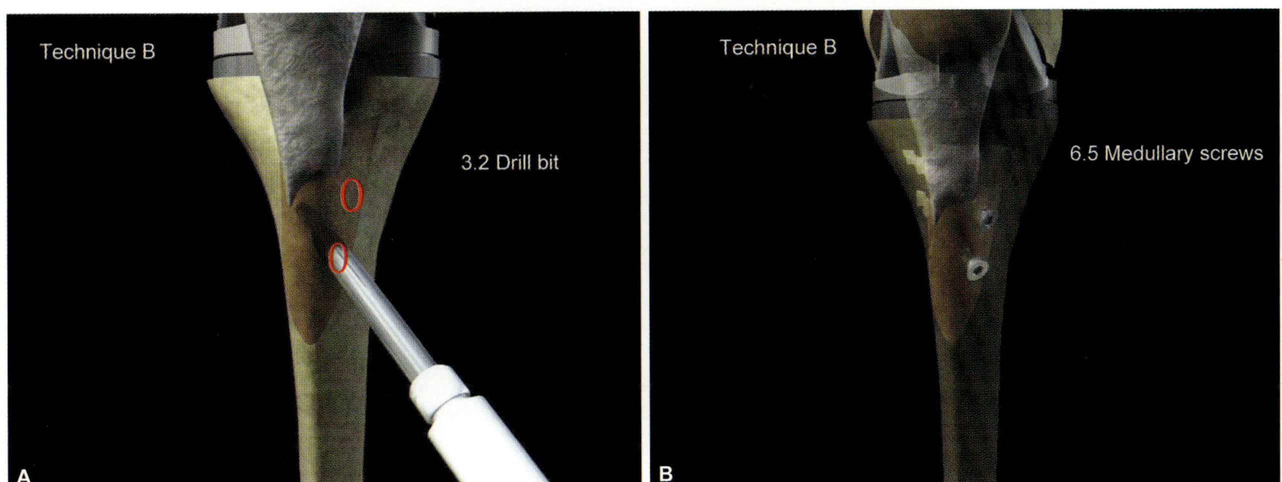

Figures 20.7A and B Screws used to fix the draft into the tibial trough

quadriceps medial and lateral margins of the patient. The graft is then passed below the quadriceps and the sutures are retrieved through two interruptions of approximately 2 cm each performed longitudinally at the myotendinous transition of the quadriceps tendon on the medial and lateral margins of the tendon (**Figure 20.8C**). The sutures are then tractioned proximally and the quadriceps distally with the other pairs of sutures while maintaining the limb in full extension (**Figure 20.9A**). In this phase, the overlapping portions of autologous tissue and graft are sutured with full-thickness Ethibond #5 and #2 nonabsorbable sutures (Ethicon, Johnson & Johnson, Somerville, NJ) (**Figure 20.9B**). Finally, the two proximal ends used for the graft's traction are joined together to reinforce the proximal suture. The residual tissues are then sutured with absorbable sutures, trying to cover the graft as much as possible with the autologous tissue to limit its subcutaneous exposure (**Figures 20.10 and 20.11**). It is important that the knee not be flexed after graft fixation.[19] Subcutaneous tissue and skin closure are completed over a drain, and a compression dressing is applied.

Patella Management and Technique Using Achilles Tendon Allograft

In case of an EMA reconstruction, the patella or its remnants must be removed from the EM. If the patella is largely present and undamaged, it can simply be

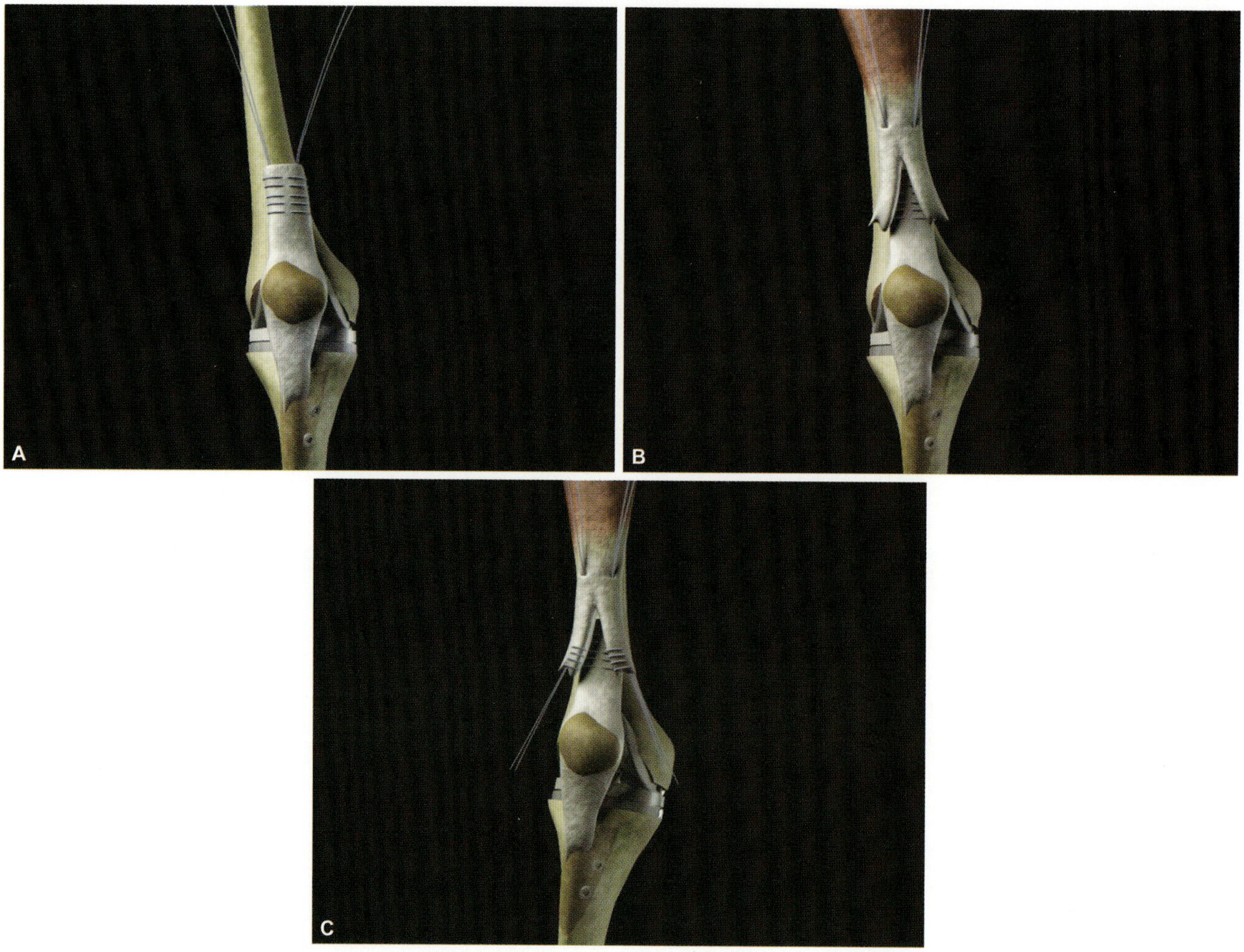

Figures 20.8A to C (A) Quadriceps tendon part of the graft prepared with Krackow sutures on the medial and lateral sides using Ethibond #5 sutures; (B) The same preparation is also carried out on both the medial and lateral sides of the residual autologous quadriceps tissue; (C) The graft is then passed below the quadriceps and the sutures are retrieved through two interruptions of approximately 2 cm each performed longitudinally at the myotendinous transition of the quadriceps tendon on the medial and lateral margins of the tendon

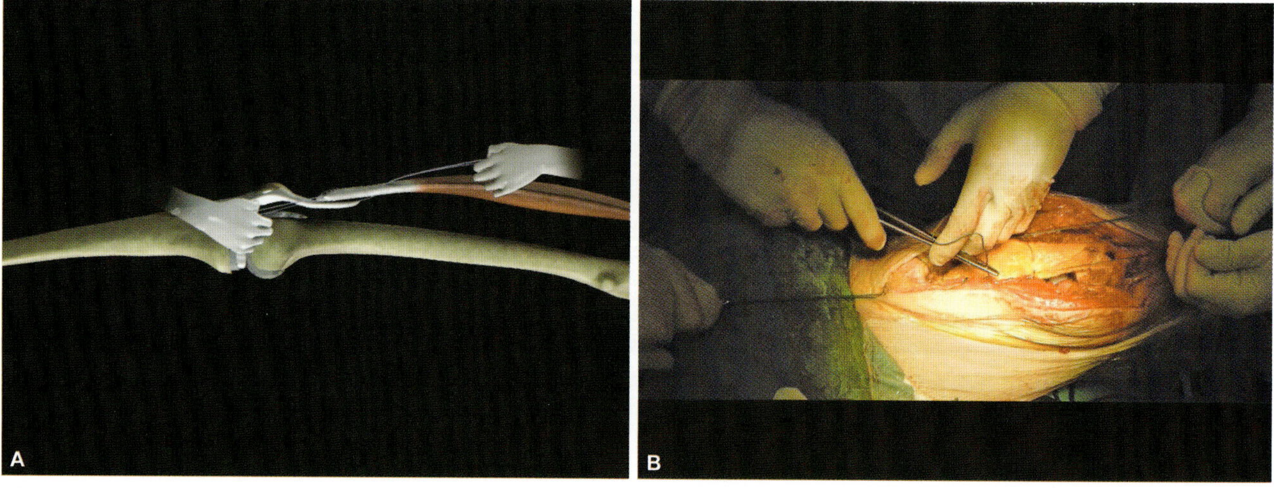

Figures 20.9A and B (A) Sutures tractioned proximally and the quadriceps distally with the other pairs of sutures while maintaining the limb in full extension; (B) Overlapping portions of autologous tissue and graft are sutured

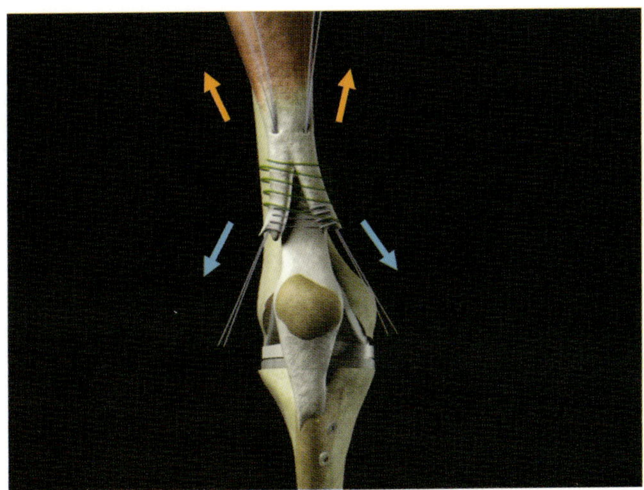

Figure 20.10 Graft fixed with a screw into the tibial trough and all the residual tissues sutured with absorbable sutures, to cover the graft as much as possible with the autologous tissue to limit its subcutaneous exposure

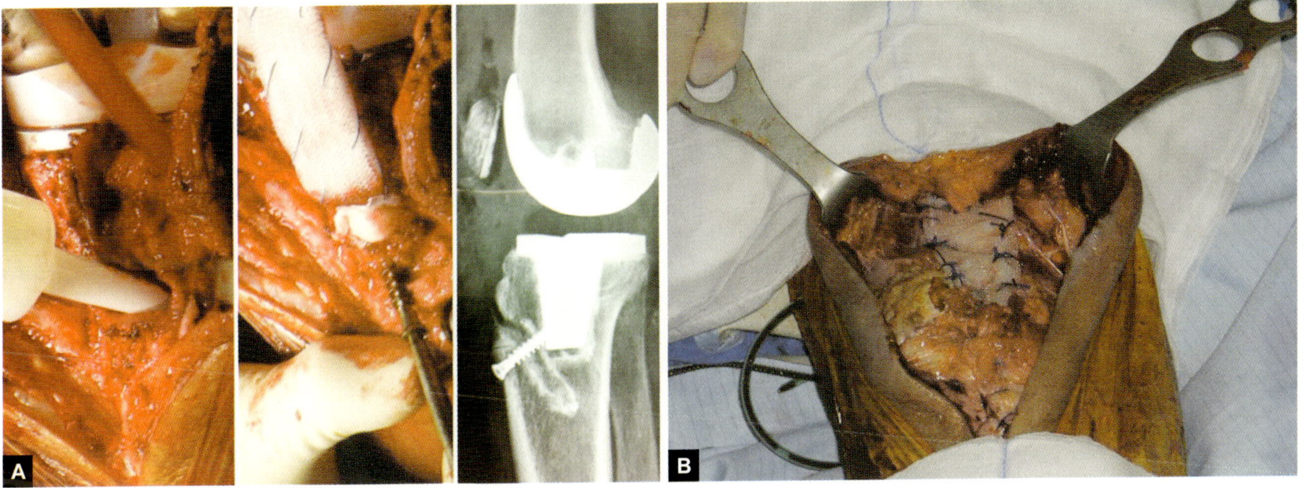

Figures 20.11A and B Graft fixed with a screw into the tibial trough and all the residual tissues sutured with absorbable sutures, to cover the graft as much as possible with the autologous tissue to limit its subcutaneous exposure

subperiosteally enucleated from the tendon's portion as previously described.[16] In this way, the greatest possible amount of autologous tissue remains available to be put on the graft. In the case of extremely low patella, it is recommended to remove it and use EMA.

In case of an intact patella and a distal lesion, if a reconstruction with ATA is chosen, it is recommended to perform a standard anteromedial longitudinal parapatellar incision. The ATA graft can be implanted maintaining the tendon's portion in single band, passed beneath the patellar tendon (or what remains of it), then passed above the patella, medially crossing it, and finally sutured under tension to the edge of the capsulotomy.[14,15] This path of the graft will ensure a resultant force on the ExtMech with a medially directed vector that prevents against patellar maltracking. Some authors leave the whole intra-articular part of the tendon graft directly in contact with the trochlear groove of the femoral component. Our preferred technique includes the fixation of the calcaneus bone block approximately 2–3 cm distally to the tibial component platform. The calcaneus bone is shaped to be encased in a tibial bone recess at the level of the tibial tuberosity. The deepness of the tibial trough should be maximized and will depend from the distance of the tibial stem to the anterior surface of the bone. The calcaneus bone is then fixed in place either using two acetabular screws directed superolaterally in the tibia, or using two cerclage wires. The tendinous portion of the graft will then be divided into two strips, which penetrate into the patella and merge under the quadriceps tendon. To allow this passage of the graft though the patella, a double parallel tunnel is performed in the patella. An cruciate ligament tibial guide is used to insert K-wires caudocranially, which will serve as a guide for cannulated reamers that will ream the patella tunnels with a various diameter from 7 to 9 mm depending on the native patellar thickness. The tendinous portion of the graft will then be divided into two strips, which will penetrate into the patella double parallel tunnels and will merge under the quadriceps tendon. At the quadriceps tendon level, the two parts of the allograft tendon can be retrieved extra-articularly and sutured under tension in full extension on the quadriceps tendon of the patient, while a second assistant is tractioning the patellar bone distally.

If the patella is relatively small, we suggest to perform a single hole that will accept only one of the two graft tendon branches, while the other will be in a medial position along the capsulotomy controlling the lateral tilt of the patella while suturing.

It is author's opinion that this technique with intraosseous passage of the graft allows a higher degree of area contact between the host and the graft tissue, while the graft is kept far from the superficial skin layer with a better protection from possible septic contaminations.

Surgical Tips for Implant Revision Technique with Simultaneous ExtMech Allograft

When a revision TKA is performed in the same stage of ExtMech reconstruction, a few technical details should be considered. In fact, the procedure is performed without the normal tension and traction exerted by the ExtMech on the tibiofemoral joint. This tends to overestimate the size of the flexion gap especially, if the collateral ligaments are deficient. In this case, it is important to reach full extension and bridge the flexion gap as much as possible accepting a residual laxity within 5–6 mm that will then be neutralized by the presence of valid ExtMech. It will be possible to bridge the larger flexion gap avoiding the use of large polyethylene inserts with two technical adaptations: use the largest femoral component size possible without medial-lateral overhang and posteriorly direct the component with a femoral offset stem extension. It will then necessitate the need for femoral posterior augments in order to fill the flexion gap. It is also convenient to use a higher constraint degree than the one considered necessary for the same articulation with a valid ExtMech (if PS → CCK, if CCK → hinge), both for the inability to completely test the stability of the joint with reduced EM, and as a protection in case of incomplete recovery of extensor strength. Another technical detail in the reconstruction phase is to take into account for the need of housing space for the tibial bone block of the graft. For this purpose, the tibial component could be driven few millimeters posteriorly by modifying the tibial canal reaming technique or by using a tibial stem extension with a posterior offset.

Once cemented, the joint is positioned in extension and this position should be maintained until the ExtMech implant is in place, and it is important not to test the tension by trying to flex the knee intraoperatively.[19,20]

REHABILITATION PROTOCOL

Different protocols have been described in the literature. In the past 10 years, all the literature on ExtMech reconstruction agrees to keep the knee joint in extension for a minimum of 6 weeks after these procedures (**Table 20.2**).[10,13,15,16,18,19]

Postoperatively, the knee is immobilized in a hinged brace locked in full extension. If the patient is not fully compliant, we recommend to manufacture a plaster tubular cast. Touch-down weight-bearing is allowed immediately. Isometric quadriceps muscle activation is encouraged immediately. We recommend to withhold both flexion exercises and straight leg raise (SLR) exercises for 6 weeks. At this term, the brace or cast is removed twice a day for additional 3 weeks to allow passive and active knee flexion exercise with caution but no restriction up to 90°. For every degree of flexion gained, ensure the maintenance of full extension during SLR. After 9 weeks, flexion beyond 90° is allowed; if the patient can tolerate it and extension strength is monitored, SLR is now allowed.

TABLE 20.2 Rehabilitation protocols described by various authors in literature

	Emerson	*Booth*	*Crossett*	*Emerson*	*Garvin*	*Barrack*	*Berger*	*Ries*	*Barrack*	*Rajesh*	*Lewullis*	*Baldini*
Postoperative immobilization	Yes	Yes	Yes	Yes	–	Yes	Yes	–	Yes	Yes	Yes	Yes
Immobilization period	4 weeks	6 weeks	4 weeks	6 weeks	–	4 weeks	8 weeks	–	4 weeks	8 weeks	6–12 weeks	6 weeks
Modalità immobilization	Knee bent at 60°	Complete extension	Complete extension	Complete extension	–	Complete extension	Complete extension	–	Complete extension	Complete extension	Complete extension	Complete extension
Tipologia immobilization	Tutore mobile	Gesso	Gesso		–	Tutore	Gesso	–	–	Gesso	Gesso	Tutore nonarticolato
Postoperative flexion	0°–60° in the first 4 weeks	0°–30° after 6 weeks	0°–40° after 4 weeks	0°–90° after 6 weeks	–	0°–45° in the first 4 weeks	Not allowed	–	0°–45° after 4 weeks	Not allowed	Not allowed	Free after 6 weeks controlling lag
Flexion progresses	60°–90° after 4 weeks	30°–90° after 3 months	40°–90° after 8 weeks		–	45°–90° after 2 months	0°–30° after 8 weeks	–	45°–90° after 8 weeks	0°–90° after 12 weeks	0°–30° after 6–12 weeks	Depending on pain tolerance
Postoperative muscular exercises	Yes	Yes	Yes		–	Yes	30°–90° after 12 weeks	–	90°– >90° after 16 weeks		30°–90°after 18 weeks	Yes
Isometric contractions	In the first 4 weeks	After 3 months			–	In the first 4 weeks	Yes	–	Yes	Yes	Yes	Yes
Esercizi di rafforzamento	In the first 4 weeks	After 3 months			–	In the first 4 weeks	In the first 8 weeks	–	In the first 4 weeks	In the first 8 weeks	After 18 weeks	After 12 weeks
Deambulation	5 = crutches	2 = walker	2 = walker	4 = no assistance	–	5 = crutches			6 = crutches	3 = no assistance	2 = no assistance	All = no assistance
	1 = no assistance	10 = crutches	1 = no assistance	6 = walker	–	2 = walker			6= walker	1= assistance	1 = crutches	
	2 = walker		6 = crutches	5 = crutches	–	7 = no assistance			7= no assistance		3 = walker	
				3 = wheelchair	–							

The patient should refrain from doing isokinetic leg extension type of exercises. Close-chain exercises should be preferred but performed with caution.

RESULTS

From January 2005 to the present, we performed 42 ExtMech repairs or substitutions in patients with TKA. In 37 patients, the procedure was performed because of a chronic rupture of the patellar tendon (53% of the cases), quadriceps tendon (22%), patella (8%), or for a patellar plus quadriceps rupture (17%). In additional five patients, an ExtMech allograft procedure was performed not because of a rupture but because of recurrent ankylosis after multiple procedures with nonfunctional calcified ExtMech. In the series of the 37 ruptures, we employed an EMA in 25 cases, an ATA in 8 cases, a hernia mesh in 2 cases (**Figures 20.12A and B**) and an artificial tendon in two cases.

We tend to use the artificial tendons and the hernia mesh as a rescue procedure in case we find an unexpected lesion during revision TKA and the allograft is not available. This may happen, for instance, after revising an infected TKA treated with a static spacer where the ExtMech function cannot be assessed. Our rationale on graft selection (EMA versus ATA) is: we prefer to use EMA, if the lesion is proximal (quadriceps) or if it is extensive, if the patient is older than 70 years, or if the patella of the TKA has been already replaced. Our selective indications for ATA include a patellar tendon lesion, a patient younger than 70 years (in order to keep as much as possible tissue from the host), patella not replaced (**Table 20.1**). All reconstructions were performed with solid distal fixation of the graft (tubercle or calcaneus) with medullary screws and/or wires. Proximal fixation was performed in full extension using both number 5 and 2 nonabsorbable sutures. Immobilization in a brace or cast in full extension was maintained for 6 weeks.

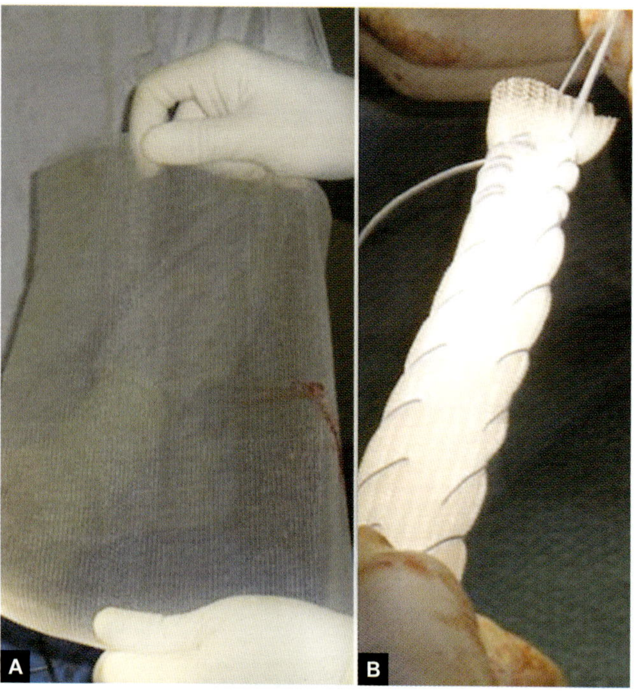

Figures 20.12A and B (A) Hernia mesh and (B) Artificial tendon

The average time from ExtMech disruption to surgery was 10 months (range, 1–120 months). At a mean follow-up of 40 months (range, 6–96 months), all patients were community ambulators.

Average postoperative maximum flexion was 106° (80–130°) for the ruptured group and 80° (75–90°) for the ankylosed group. All patients thought their functional status had improved, and 70% were very satisfied, 17% were satisfied, and 13% not satisfied (this represented 3 of the patients with complications), with the results of the allograft reconstruction. All the patients preoperatively had a lag greater than 30°. Average postoperative extensor lag was 3.5° ± 4.5°. The majority of the patients did not show any extensor lag (excluding five patients with complications). Nine patients had lag up to 10°, only two patients had lag over 10°. There were five complications in this cohort. One patient had a recurrence of the infection after the two-stage reconstruction (of the total 14 infected TKA cases treated in this cohort) with the allograft. This patient was already a 'two-time' looser, for this reason, we decided to perform a revision with arthrodesis. Three cases had failure of the tibial tuberosity with patellar tendon graft avulsions. Two of them were successfully revised with another allograft (one patient is waiting for the revision procedure). One patient had a failure of the hernia mesh with recurrent lag. He was successfully revised with an EMA (**Table 20.3**). Of the five multiply operated ankylosed patient treated with EMA and TKA revision, two were able to reach 90° of flexion (very satisfied), one reached 60° of

TABLE 20.3 Results in literature following extensor mechanism reconstruction

	Emerson	*Booth*	*Crossett*	*Emerson*	*Garvin*	*Barrack*	*Berger*	*Ries*	*Barrack*	*Rajesh*	*Lewullis*	*Baldini*
Publication year	1990	1999	2002	2003	2003	2003	2004	2005	2006	2008	2010	Current
Number of cases	13	38	9	27	3	14	13	9	19	4	8	33
Allograft: ATA Allograft: EMA	13 EMAs	38 EMAs	9 ATAs	27 EMAs		8 ATAs 6 EMAs	13 EMAs	9 EMAs	10 ATAs 9 EMAs	4 EMAs	8 EMAs	6 ATAs 23 EMAs
												2 LARS 2 Hernia Mesh
Average follow-up (months)	6-51	42	28	48	56	42	37	44	56	21	36	38
Range follow-up		3.6 years (range 2–10 months)	2.4 years (range 16–36 months)	3.8 years (range 1–14 months)		3.5 years (range 24–60)			2 years (range 24–96 months)	1.9 years (range 14–30)	3.1 years (range 2–6.3 years)	3.2 years (range 6–96 months)
Postoperative flexion	103°	98°	107°	All > 90°	–	98°	104°	–	98°			106°
Extensor lag	6 = 0°	15 = 13° Average (Av)	1 = 20°	3 = 40°		1 = 45°	Av 4°		3 > 30°	3 = 0°	2 = 10°	18 = 0°
									1 = 15°			
	1 = 10°	21=0°	2 = 5°	5 = 20°		1 = 30°			5 = 10°	1=10°	4 ≥ 20°	8 ≤ 10°
	1 = 15°		6 = 0°	10 = 0°		2 = 15°		Av = 5°	7 = 5°			2 ≥ 10°
	1 = 20°		Av 3°	Av 8°		10 ≤ 10°			3 = 0°			
									Av 11°			
Complications	2 fractures	2 avulsion	1 avulsion	4 fractures		1 fracture	1 avulsion	1 fracture	1 avulsion	1 infection	2 infections	4 fractures
		8 fractures	1 tibia fx	2 infections			1 fracture	2 infection	1 fracture			1 infection
		2 infection	1 infection	1 patellar loosening			1 MUA					
							1 swelling					
							1 CPRS					

Abbreviations: EMA, extensor mechanism allograft; ATA, Achilles tendon allograft.

flexion (moderately satisfied), and two had a recurrence of arthrofibrosis with very limited motion (unsatisfied).

The total EMA and ATA both were successful in the treatment of the failed ExtMech (**Figures 20.13 to 20.16**). Results for the treatment of the ankylosed knee are still under investigation (**Figures 20.17A and B**).

CONCLUSION

In the last decade, a patient suffering from ExtMech rupture after TKA was condemned to either an unfunctional repair with residual extensor lag or to perform a knee arthrodesis.[13] With the reconstructive option given by the

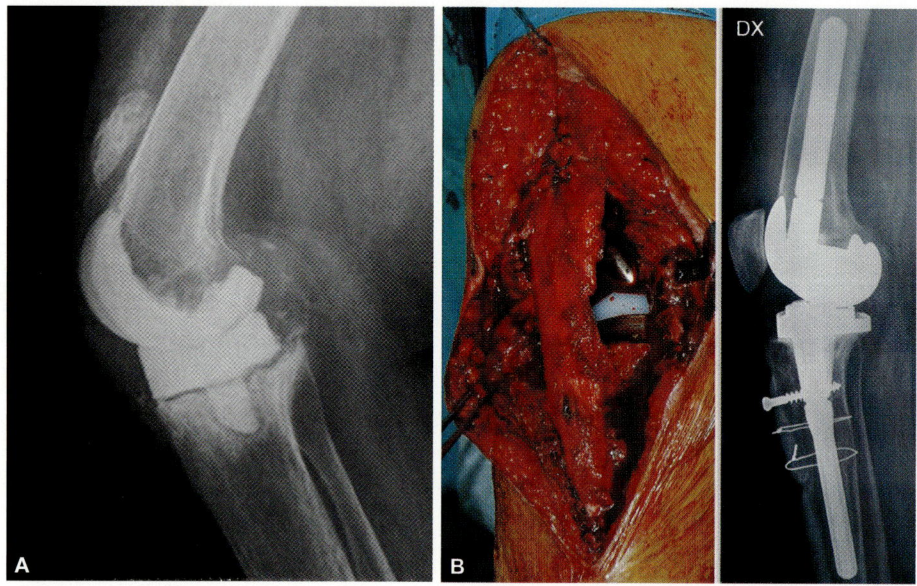

Figures 20.13A and B Infected TKR with failed extensor mechanism treated with an antibiotic spacer followed by revision TKR with a extensor mechanism allograft reconstruction

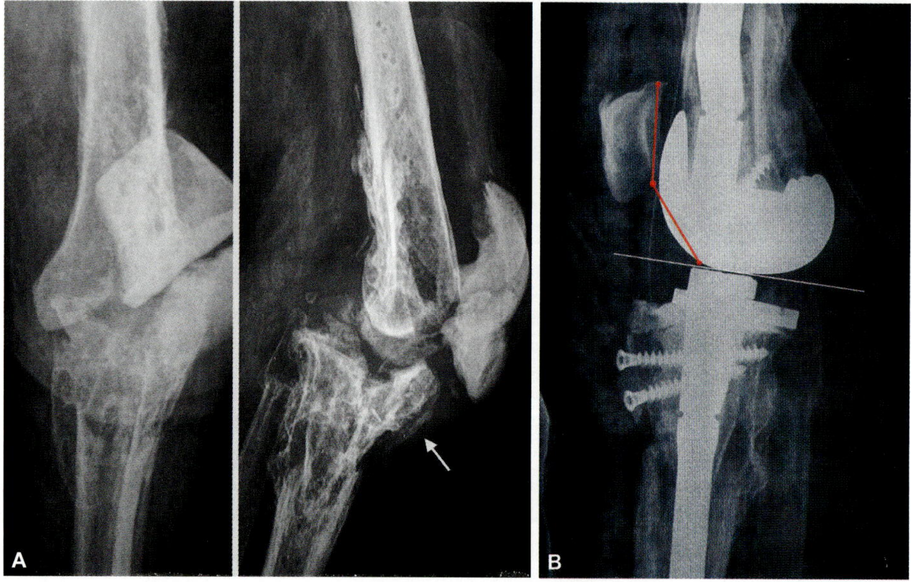

Figures 20.14A and B Revision TKA following infected TKA with extensor mechanism failure treated with an extensor mechanism allograft

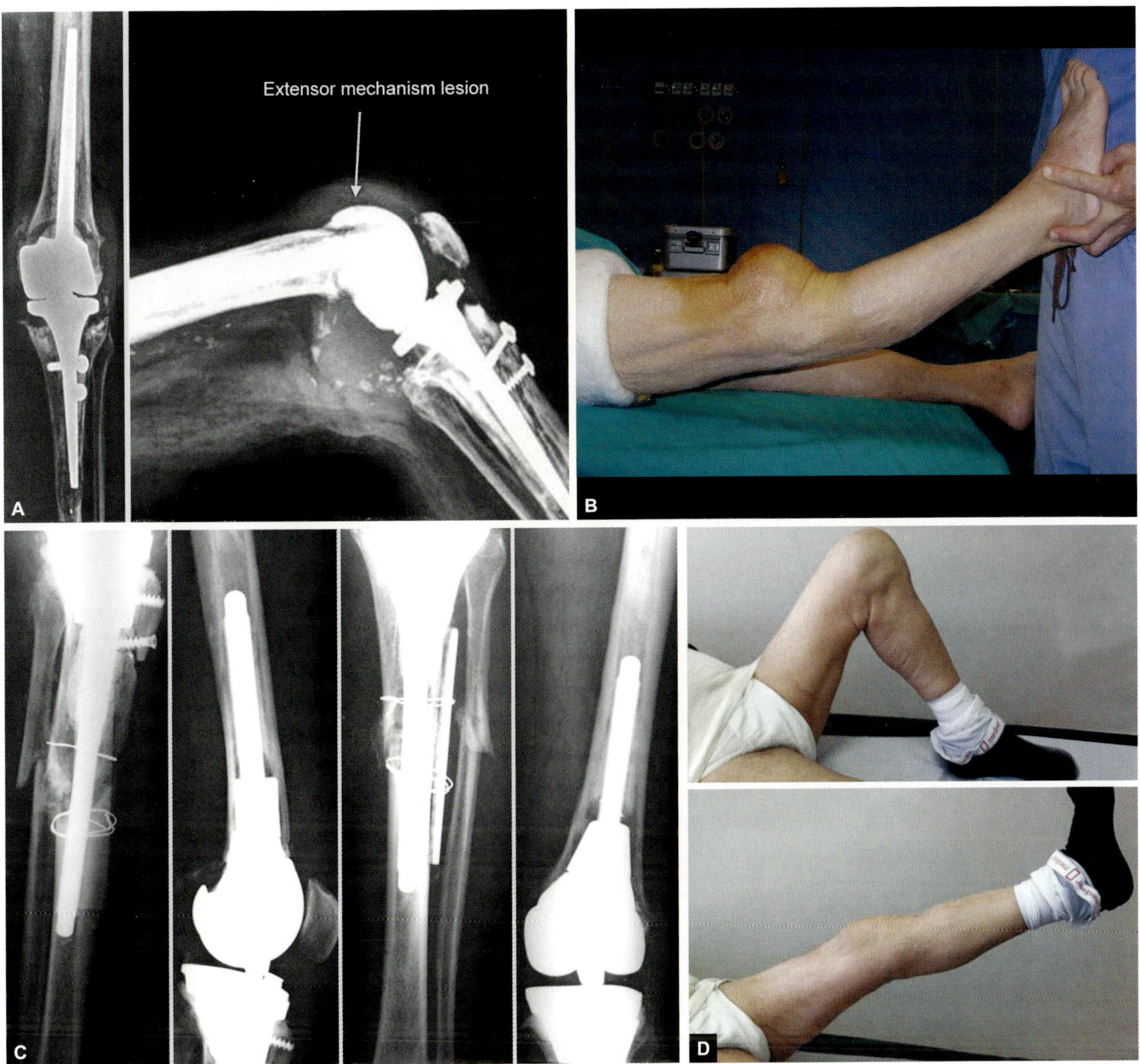

Figures 20.15A to D Revision for infected TKR. Extensor mechanism disruption treated with an extensor mechanism allograft with good clinical outcomes

use of allografts, and more recently by the use of synthetic scaffolds, there is a consistent possibility to offer function back to the patients with a chronically interrupted ExtMech. These reconstructive options should be considered as an extra step of 'salvage' procedure for the knee joint. The surgeon indicating this type of reconstruction should keep in mind that the ExtMech allografts, in the form of both ATA and EMA, are an additional foreign body for the patient, and in case of septic contamination the proximity to the skin layers makes another attempt of reconstruction very unlikely. Revision of a deficient ExtMech plus skin layer has been described using extended gastrocnemius flaps but their functional results in term of lag are definitely not ideal.[7,21] Jaureguito et al. used a medial gastrocnemius muscle flap to reconstruct a ruptured ExtMech in six patients. At an average of 26 months postoperatively, the average range of motion was 100° and the average extensor lag was 24°.[7]

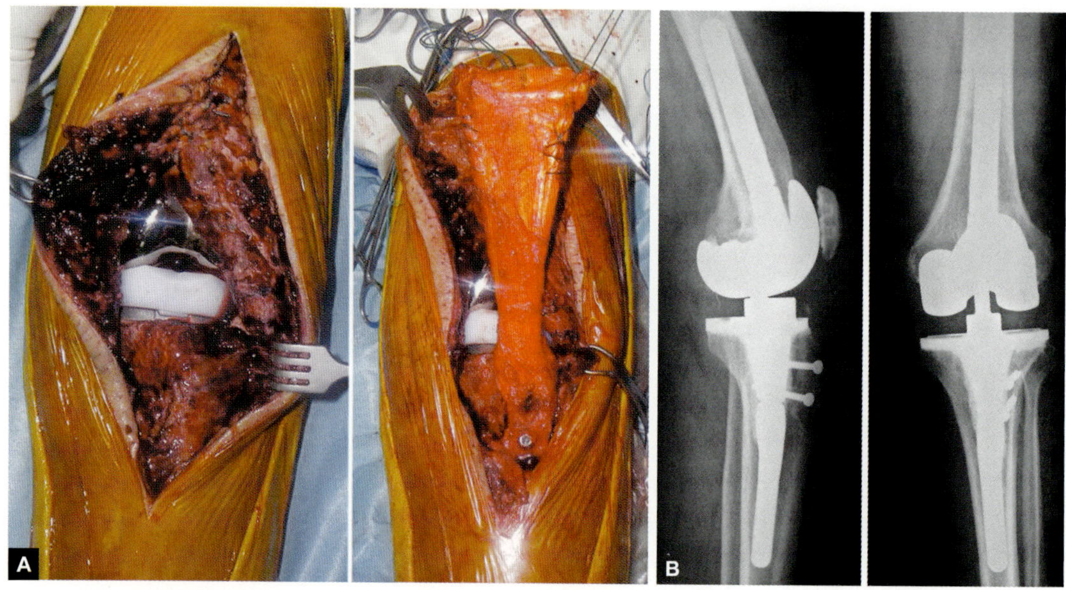

Figures 20.16A and B Extensor mechanism treated with an Achilles tendon allograft

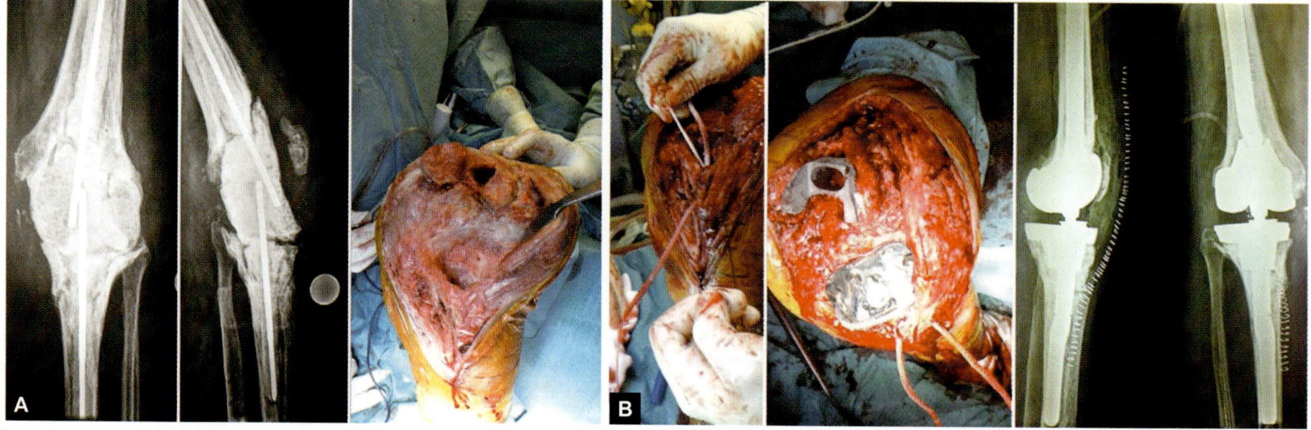

Figures 20.17A and B Revision TKA with extensor mechanism reconstruction following a failed arthrodesis

The use of a synthetic scaffold in the form of a ligament or of a tubularized hernia mesh is appealing because they are always available, easier to be managed, and they may be easier to be embedded in the host tissue.[11,12] There are some enthusiastic reports in the literature with these materials, but in the authors limited experience the patients with this type of reconstruction were experiencing more extensor lag than those patients reconstructed with an allograft.

In conclusion, ExtMech reconstruction now provides a standardized technique with steps that are now established. Compliance with the proper indications and technical details offers the possibility of excellent clinical and functional results. The use of allografts in the form of EMA or ATA has improved the results obtained from direct or autologous tissue repair. The functional validity of these grafts does not seem to deteriorate in the medium term. It should be expected that some functional deterioration at a longer follow-up will occur, since graft resorption of its osseous components has been described.[22] For this reason, their function in the long-term and in the relatively young and active patient remains to be evaluated. More extensive case studies and comparative studies are needed to assess what is the most suitable graft, although both types seem to have peculiar indications.[6,8,10,15-17,20-22]

REFERENCES

1. Lynch AF, Rorabeck CH, Bourne RB. Extensor mechanism complications following total knee arthroplasty. J Arthroplasty. 1987;2:135-40.
2. Rand JA, Morrey BF, Bryan RS. Patellar tendon rupture after total knee arthroplasty. Clin Orthop Relat Res. 1989;244:233-8.
3. Abril JC, Alvarez L, Vallejo JC. Patellar tendon avulsion after total knee arthroplasty: a new technique. J Arthroplasty. 1995;10:275-9.
4. Grace JN, Rand JA. Patellar instability after total knee arthroplasty. Clin Orthop Relat Res. 1988;237:184-9.
5. Gustilo RB, Thompson R. Quadriceps and patellar tendon ruptures following total knee arthroplasty. In: Rand JA, Dorr LD (Eds). Total arthroplasty of the knee: proceedings of the knee society 1985-1986. Rockville, MD: Aspen; 1987. pp. 41-70.
6. Cadambi A, Engh GA. Use of a semitendinosus autogenous graft for rupture of the patellar ligament after total knee arthroplasty. J Bone Joint Surg. 1992;74A:974-9.
7. Jaureguito JW, Dubois CM, Smith SR, Gottlieb LJ, Finn HA. Medial gastrocnemius transposition flap for the treatment of disruption of the extensor mechanism after total knee arthroplasty. J Bone Joint Surg Am. 1997;79(6):866-73.
8. Emerson RH Jr, Head WC, Malinin TI. Reconstruction of patellar tendon rupture after total knee arthroplasty with an extensor mechanism allograft. Clin Orthop Relat Res. 1990;260:154-61.
9. Emerson RH Jr, Head WC, Malinin TI. Extensor mechanism reconstruction with an allograft after total knee arthroplasty. Clin Orthop Relat Res. 1994;303:79-85.
10. Crossett LS, Sinha RK, Sechriest VF, Rubash HE. Reconstruction of a ruptured patellar tendon with Achilles tendon allograft following total knee arthroplasty. J Bone Joint Surg Am. 2002;84:1354-61.
11. Browne JA, Hanssen AD. Reconstruction of patellar tendon disruption after total knee arthroplasty: results of a new technique utilizing synthetic mesh. J Bone Joint Surg Am. 2011;93(12):1137-43
12. Dominkus M, Sabeti M, Toma C, et al. Reconstructing the extensor apparatus with a new polyester ligament. Clin Orthop Relat Res. 2006;453:328-34.
13. Nazarian DG, Booth RE Jr. Extensor mechanism allografts in total knee arthroplasty. Clin Orthop Relat Res. 1999;367:123-9.
14. Barrack RL, Stanley T, Butler AR. Treating extensor mechanism disruption after total knee arthroplasty. Clin Orthop Relat Res. 2003;416:98-104.
15. Burnett RS, Butler RA, Barrack RL. Extensor mechanism allograft reconstruction in TKA at a mean of 56 months. Clin Orthop Relat Res. 2006;452:159-65.
16. Burnett RS, Berger RA, Della Valle CJ, et al. Extensor mechanism allograft reconstruction after total knee arthroplasty. J Bone Joint Surg Am. 2005;87A:175-94.
17. Burnett RS, Berger RA, Paprosky WG, et al. Extensor mechanism allograft reconstruction after total knee arthroplasty: a comparison of two techniques. J Bone Joint Surg Am. 2004;86:2694-9.
18. Emerson RH Jr. Extensor mechanism allografting in revision total knee replacement. Techniques in Knee Surgery. 2003, 2(2):91-8.
19. Burnett RS, Fornasier VL, Haydon CM, et al. Retrieval of a well-functioning extensor mechanism allograft from a total knee arthroplasty: clinical and histological findings. J Bone Joint Surg Br. 2004;86:986-90.
20. Leopold SS, Greidanus N, Paprosky WG, Berger RA, Rosenberg AG. High rate of failure of allograft reconstruction of the extensor mechanism after total knee arthroplasty. J Bone Joint Surg Am. 1999;81:1574-9.
21. Busfield BT, Huffman GR, Nahai F, Hoffman W, Ries MD. Extended medial gastrocnemius rotational flap for treatment of chronic knee extensor mechanism deficiency in patients with and without total knee arthroplasty. Clin Orthop Relat Res. 2004;(428):190-7.
22. Busfield BT, Ries MD. Whole patellar allograft for total knee arthroplasty after previous patellectomy. Clin Orthop Relat Res. 2006;450:145-9.

Chapter 21

Complications Following Total Knee Arthroplasty

Jack W Shilling, Robert E Booth

Total knee arthroplasty (TKA) is one of the most common and successful surgeries done throughout the world. Each year, advances in implant design, materials, and surgical technique speed postoperative recovery and improve patient outcomes. In 2010, it was estimated that 243,802 TKAs were performed in the United States alone. While the incidence of complications is exceedingly low, the financial and human costs associated with complications cannot be understated. The diagnosis and management of common causes of morbidity and mortality remain paramount to overall success of the procedure. This chapter hopes to shed some light on common complications after TKA and their current treatment plans.

PERIPROSTHETIC FRACTURES

Periprosthetic fractures of the femur, tibia and patella are relatively uncommon complications after TKA. Their incidence has been reported as '0.3-5.5% for primary TKA, and as high as 30% in revision TKA.' These percentages are small, but as the number of TKA procedures increases over time, their absolute numbers are sure to rise. Risk factors may include increased age, obesity, osteoporosis, dementia, balance disorders and surgical technique. Multiple classification systems have been described to help define patterns of injury. These fractures almost always require surgical intervention and their treatment can be quite complex. Often the patients who incur these injuries are of elevated age and with significant medical comorbidities. Perioperative morbidity and mortality can be quite high for even the most experienced surgeons. Thankfully, improvements in implants and surgical techniques have improved our ability to resolve these challenging problems.

Distal Femur

Fractures of the distal femur represent the most common of all periprosthetic TKA fractures. Often, the patient's bone quality is poor due to osteoporosis, and fixation of the fracture fragments may be very difficult to achieve. These fractures generally fall into two classes. In the first group, the fracture involves the distal femoral shaft or metaphyseal region, and the femoral implant remains stable. In this instance, the injury is usually treated with lateral plate fixation of the involved fragments using a

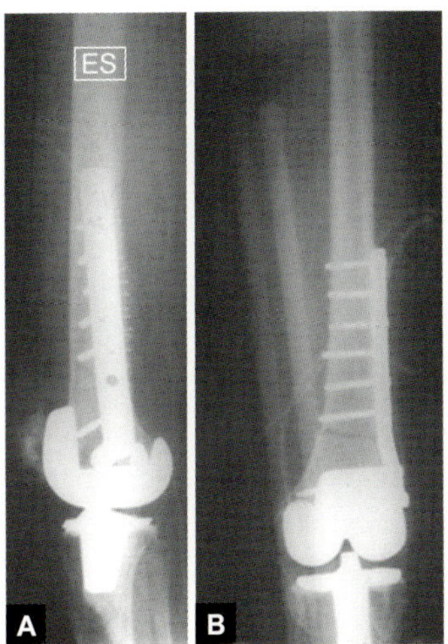

Figures 21.1A and B Open reduction and internal fixation of distal femoral periprosthetic fracture with distal femoral plate and screws

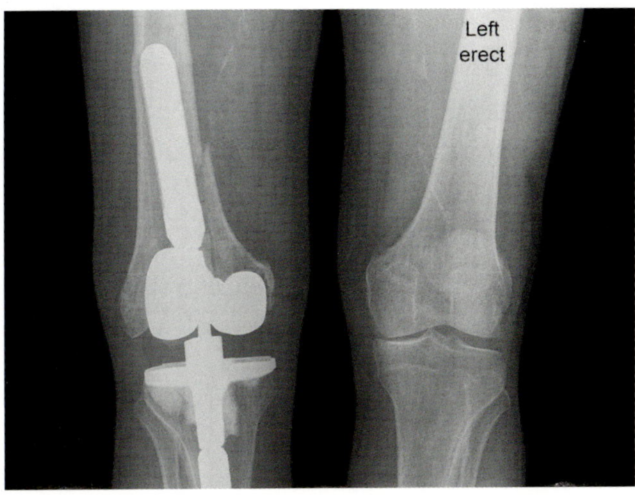

Figure 21.2 Comminuted distal femoral periprosthetic fracture around stemmed femoral component

laterally based incision and approach. Recent advances in locking plate technology have increased the number of fractures that can be successfully treated with open reduction and internal fixation. These devices typically work best with noncomminuted fractures of the distal femoral shaft or metaphysical area where reduction is readily achieved (**Figures 21.1A and B**).

An alternative treatment for comminuted or extremely osteoporotic fractures is retrograde femoral nailing. This technique requires that the knee joint be exposed and the femoral implant be allowed access to the femoral notch. In a posterior cruciate ligament (PCL) retaining (CR) design, careful attention to the PCL origin is essential when creating the starting hole, lest the knee be destabilized. Most modern PCL sacrificing (CS) knee designs utilize a femoral component design with an 'open box' to allow access to the notch. A 'closed box' design is typically a contraindication to the use of a retrograde nail. The osteoporotic distal bone often compromises screw purchase of the distal locking screws. Proximal locking screws are often needed to help stabilize comminuted metaphyseal fractures. Both of these fixation techniques have demonstrated good clinical results in the literature. For the unstable implant, the injury typically requires revision. In many cases, a 'mega' prosthesis, or distal femoral replacement is required to deal with poor bone quality and overall distal femoral bone loss

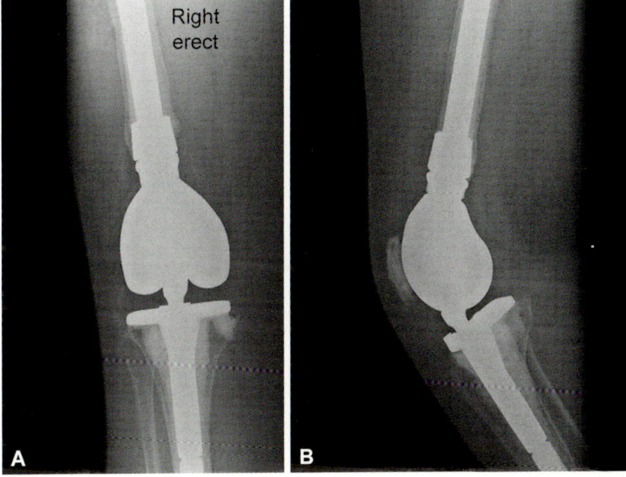

Figures 21.3A and B Distal femoral replacement for comminuted distal femoral periprosthetic fracture with bone loss

(**Figures 21.2 and 21.3**). This technique almost always requires revision of the tibial component to a constrained implant that mates with the new distal femur. Revision to a constrained TKA construct often has the benefit of immediate weight-bearing and patient mobility that may not be possible with fracture fixation techniques. Extensile knee approaches may be necessary to handle these fractures, and will be covered in later chapters in this book.

Tibial Fracture

Periprosthetic tibial fractures typically involve a high-energy mechanism of injury in healthy bone, or may occur with lower demand activities in osteoporotic bone. Typically, these fractures involve the tibial implant and cement mantle, if present. While fractures of the proximal tibial shaft below a well-fixed implant do occur, they are in the minority. When these fracture types are seen, they are often fixed with lateral tibial plate fixation, with bicortical distal screws and a proximal screw construct that includes or goes around the tibial cement construct. In the past several years, several companies have released implants specifically designed to aid in the fixation of periprosthetic femur and tibia fractures. These implants typically have holes in multiple planes, and offer variable angle and locking screws to allow very precise screw placement and improved screw purchase.

More often than not, however, the tibial component is loose and will require revision to a stemmed implant that bypasses the fracture line. Augments may be added to the tibial base plate as needed to fill the bone void created by the injury. If significant proximal tibial bone is lost, a proximal tibial replacement may be required. This type of implant requires revision of the femoral component to a constrained implant that will link to the tibia. As mentioned previously, revision of the TKA construct often allows earlier postoperative weight bearing and range of motion that fracture fixation would not allow.

Patella Fracture

Periprosthetic fractures of the patella are uncommon, but can have very debilitating consequences. These injuries are usually caused when a patient stumbles or falls on a flexed knee. In addition, avascular necrosis or osteolysis of the previously operated patella may play a role in weakening the patellar bone stock. Fractures that do not compromise the extensor mechanism or do not result in loosening of the implants can be treated nonsurgically. If pain persists after this type of injury, partial patellectomy can be considered.

Unfortunately, 'stable' fractures make up a very small portion of periprosthetic patella fractures. More commonly, the implant is jarred loose at the time of the injury and requires surgical correction. If the fracture pattern is too comminuted or the bone quality does not allow placement of a new patellar implant, partial or total patellectomy may need to be considered. Regardless of the ability to repair or revise the patella, if the extensor mechanism is disrupted, it must be repaired to allow for ambulation and appropriate knee stability. In recent years, patellar replacement implants made from porous metals have become available as alternatives to total patellectomy. These devices, as well as patellar allografts, may have a role in treating these complicated fractures.

INFECTION AND WOUND HEALING CONCERNS

Infection after primary knee replacement remains one of the biggest challenges in orthopedic surgery today. For that reason, a separate chapter in this book is dedicated to the diagnosis, and management of periprosthetic TKA infection. While the reported incidence rates of 1–2% remain low, the functional and financial consequences of this problem can be staggering. For these reasons, infection should always be at the top of the list when it comes to differential diagnosis of the painful or unstable TKA.

The effective treatment of periprosthetic infection requires an appropriate diagnosis. As mentioned above, details of an appropriate infection work-up will be provided elsewhere in this book. We would like to mention that genetically based advances in the diagnosis and treatment of infection are becoming available to help combat this difficult problem. Recently techniques have been described in the orthopedic literature that adds to the surgeon's armamentarium when combating periprosthetic infection. The work of Deirmengian et al. has shown promise in the identification of the presence of bacteria in a synovial sample, using an mRNA marker. Early data have shown rapid, sensitive and specific results. In addition, Parvizi et al. have suggested the use of a DNA 'data bank' for specific bacterial strains. Additional work is needed, but as the catalog of pathogen DNA signatures grows, we can imagine a day where the imperfections of culture growth may be a relic of the past.

Paramount to the prevention of postoperative infection is wound healing. Clearly, a sterile operating environment is necessary for surgical success with any proposed procedure. Excellent surgical technique and appropriate implant placement are imperative for the expected functional patient outcomes to be achieved. However, a 'perfect' postoperative radiograph does not guarantee surgical success, if the soft tissues around the knee do not heal properly. Patients with medical histories containing obesity, smoking, diabetes, malnutrition, lymph edema, renal failure, chronic skin conditions and peripheral vascular disease, all harbor increased risks of delayed wound healing. In addition, patients with immunocompromised states such as inflammatory arthritic conditions, autoimmune disorders, HIV and chronic steroid use also pose significant wound healing challenges. During the preoperative work-up, these conditions must be recognized and optimized. The surgeon must be willing to discuss the increased risks these conditions present for the patient, and also assure that nutritional parameters, correctable laboratory results and blood glucose levels are optimized before proceeding with elective TKA.

Persistent early wound drainage can have several causes. These include hematoma, seroma, fat necrosis and infection. Post-TKA hematoma drainage typically represents the egress of 'old' blood lost at the time of surgery. Active bleeding and its causes must always be considered. This will be covered later in this chapter. The authors advocate the use of drains in the immediate postoperative period to minimize the risk of hematoma formation, although the orthopedic literature is divided on this topic. Aggressive postoperative anticoagulation therapy, aimed at decreasing the risk of deep venous thrombosis (DVT) can also play a role in hematoma formation and postoperative wound drainage. All anticoagulants, including the commonly used low molecular weight heparin preparations, warfarin and aspirin can create or exacerbate postoperative bleeding or seroma formation after TKA. In our practice, we favor the use of low-dose warfarin therapy, combined with a short low molecular weight heparin bridge, to obtain appropriate DVT and pulmonary embolism (PE) protection, while minimizing the risk of hematoma formation.

In recent years, vacuum-assisted closure (VAC) has proven to be a useful tool in the treatment of postoperative wound drainage. A 'skin VAC' is typically placed over the incision line and removes the subcutaneous fluid while also hastening skin closure. Multiple techniques for its use have been described in the literature, and new applications are being investigated as this chapter is written. If drainage persists beyond 4–5 days of VAC use or beyond 7–14 days from surgery, an operative irrigation and debridement may be necessary to diagnose and eradicate the source of the problem.

DEEP VENOUS THROMBOSIS AND PULMONARY EMBOLISM

The risk of DVT and PE after primary TKA has been well documented in the orthopedic literature. The incidence of DVT is reported between 1% and 5% in various articles. PE rates are typically less than 1%. 'Virchow's triad' of stasis, activation of the clotting cascade and endothelial damage, has long been felt to be the pathophysiologic platform for developing a DVT after surgery. TKA provides an environment where procoagulants such as fat and other tissue fragments are injected into the bloodstream, while endothelial injury occurs from leg manipulation, retractor placement, venous enlargement secondary to anesthesia, or laceration during the procedure. After surgery, mobility is encouraged but periods of decreased mobility are unavoidable. Thus, the risk of venous stasis, and subsequent venous thromboembolism is increased for 2–7 days postoperative. Certain patient groups also carry their own increased risks. A previous history of DVT, PE, obesity, as well as protein C and protein S deficiencies present an even more concerning clinical picture when preparing for TKA.

After surgery patients should be examined for excessive calf pain, erythema, or swelling. These signs are often seen after TKA, but must alert the physician and patient to the possibility of DVT. If appropriate clinical concern is present, an ultrasound of the calf and leg can be done to rule out the presence of a clot. The 'D-Dimer' blood test has also become available in many institutions over the past several years to aid in the diagnosis. If a DVT is diagnosed, anticoagulation target levels are shifted from prophylactic to therapeutic levels, and treatment length is extended. Patients with DVT for any reason have increased long-term risks of recurrent DVT, postphlebitic syndrome and PE. It is PE that presents the greatest immediate danger after DVT development. Virchow postulated over 150 years ago that peripheral blood clots and acute pulmonary failure events were linked. Presenting signs and symptoms can include acute shortness of breath, chest pain, decreased oxygen saturation levels, rapid onset supraventricular tachycardia and sudden death. 'Lateral strain patterns' can be seen on EKG. An arterial blood gas typically reveals significantly decreased oxygen levels and an increased 'A-A gradient.' For years, diagnosis confirmation was done with ventilation/perfusion scans that provided results with varying probability. Pulmonary angiography has been considered the diagnostic 'gold standard' for years. More recently, this was combined with helical or spiral CT, and this is now considered state-of-the-art. The sensitivity of these tests is a significant improvement over V/Q scans, but they also detect much smaller clots than previous tests. This could increase the rates of PEs reported over the next several years.

NERVE AND VASCULAR INJURY

Vascular injury after primary TKA is an uncommon complication. The most commonly injured vessel is the popliteal artery. Occlusion of the popliteal artery by thrombus is the most common mechanism. Laceration of an arterial structure is second. Risk factors for these injuries include smoking, diabetes mellitus, peripheral vascular disease and previous knee surgery. The most common mechanism is perforation of the posterior capsule of the knee with a saw or retractor while cutting or exposing the tibia. With a tourniquet in place, the injury may not be noted until the end of the case when it is let down. If a significant injury is suspected during surgery, we recommend finishing the arthroplasty where able, and consulting a vascular surgeon while in the OR. Postoperative signs and symptoms include excessive drainage or blood pressure liability, decreased peripheral pulses in the affected extremity, pseudoaneurysm and compartment syndrome. Diagnosis is confirmed with angiography and treatment is with emergent surgical repair of the injured vessel. Failure to diagnose this problem can be catastrophic and result in limb loss, or death. While a rare complication, the surgeon must be vigilant for its occurrence.

Neurologic injury is also very rare after TKA. The peroneal nerve (PN) is the most common neurologic structure involved in these cases. Risk factors include a significant valgus knee deformity, with or without the presence of a knee flexion contracture. Often, the damage occurs with a stretching mechanism, either by manipulation during the procedure, or by the placement of retractors. Knees at greatest risk for PN injury are those with a chronic 15° valgus deformity, combined with a flexion contracture of over 10°. The incidence of PN injury with correction of this combination of deformities has been reported as high as 50%. Direct postoperative pressure can also create significant neurologic problems after surgery. Improper leg placement in a continuous passive motion (CPM) machine and tight postoperative bandages has also been implicated as the source of injuries to the PN. If an abnormal neurologic finding is noted in the immediate postoperative period, release all bandages and remove the leg from the CPM. All possible pressure-related sources of injury must be discontinued. If the signs and symptoms of nerve injury do not improve, neurologic consultation to define the extent of injury and supportive care are appropriate. Often an electromyogram and nerve conduction study are used to monitor nerve recovery. If the patient is noted to have predominantly sensory deficits, the use of supportive medications including gabapentin or pregabalin can be considered. If functional weakness of the leg is demonstrated, supportive bracing such as a modified ankle foot orthosis may be necessary while the nerve recovers. These complications can have significant long-term functional consequences and must be avoided. Patients at increased risk of injury must be educated to this fact prior to surgery. Once injury is seen however, a teamed approach with neurologic, physical medicine and pain management colleagues often yields the best results.

STIFF TOTAL KNEE

Patients undergoing TKA have several goals in mind as they prepare for the surgery. Decreased pain levels and improved knee function are high on that list. There are several factors that contribute to successful outcomes in these areas. First, it is the surgeon's responsibility to place the implants correctly. The femoral, tibial and patellar components must be appropriately sized and rotated with regard to the bones in question. The implants and bone must be well-fixed, either with a variety of bone cements, or with the use of appropriate ingrowth-encouraging cementless materials. In addition, the flexion and extension gaps must be appropriately balanced. Failure to complete any of these tasks appropriately can result in a stiff and painful TKA.

If a patient is having difficulty achieving full extension after TKA, it must be considered that an inadequate resection of the distal femur was undertaken. Conversely, a knee that will not appropriately flex, can suggest a tight flexion gap due to an under-resection of the posterior femoral condyles. An 'overstuffed' patellofemoral joint, caused by an oversized patellar implant or an inappropriately thin patellar bone resection, can also contribute to knee flexion issues after TKA. Lastly, if both the flexion and extension gaps seem tight and the patient is struggling in both planes, an inadequate proximal tibial bone resection may well be to blame. All of these issues are to be avoided as their only correction is likely through revision of the implants.

Providing the patient with a well balanced, appropriately sized, and positioned TKA, creates the platform for a successful surgical outcome. However, the effort put forth by the patient and physical therapist to assure the return of function range of motion, strength and gait is every bit as critical. Generally speaking, there is a 6–8 week window after the surgery to get the knee to full extension and beyond 90° of flexion. If these goals are not achieved during this initial time frame, manipulation under anesthesia (MUA) can be considered. Typically, flexion is easier to correct than extension with an MUA. MUA should not be considered beyond 12 weeks postoperative as it is unlikely to improve range of motion and the risk of complications increases significantly.

To perform this procedure, the patient is given intravenous sedation by the anesthesia service. Muscle relaxation is the key for successful manipulation without complication. Gentle pressure is placed on the ankle with one hand and the knee is supported with the other. The knee is then placed in a progressively flexed position. It is not uncommon to feel and hear arthrofibrotic bands breaking down as the knee is flexed. The amount of force applied to the knee and leg during the manipulation must be carefully calculated. An overly aggressive technique can certainly result in a tendinous or ligamentous injury. In extreme cases, fractures of the femur, tibia, and patella have been reported. Postmanipulation radiographs are recommended to help rule out these potential complications.

Patients with a preoperative flexion contracture are at greatest risk of developing a postoperative extension problem due to continued tightness in the posterior knee capsule. In these patients, a knee immobilizer will sometimes be placed after surgery to help achieve and maintain full extension. Regardless of the risk factors, extension of the knee should be encouraged when in bed after surgery and the placement of pillows behind the knee for postoperative comfort is to be avoided. During the first several weeks, if a significant extension deficit is identified, the addition of a knee immobilizer should be considered to help correct this issue.

After TKA, the patient range of motion and function will improve for months. A significant portion of the recovery will occur in the first 6–8 weeks after surgery, but improvements can be noted for over a year. However, if a patient has not achieved functional improvement and continues with poor motion, strength and function beyond 6 months from surgery, a work-up to exclude occult periprosthetic infection should be undertaken. Typically, an erythrocyte sedimentation rate and C-reactive protein (CRP) levels are sent for analysis and if abnormally high, the knee is aspirated. Positive results for infection need to be addressed with likely resection arthroplasty and cement spacer placement, as well as an appropriate course of antibiotics. If infection is not suspected after the testing has been completed, continued aggressive physical therapy efforts to improve motion, strength and ambulation should be pursued. If unacceptable functional results remain after 1 year, revision TKA may need to be considered.

INSTABILITY

The 'unstable' TKA is a very common cause of aseptic total knee revision. Like 'stiffness,' the causes can be multifactorial. The authors typically divide instability issues into 'early' and 'late' categories of causation. Early causes are often iatrogenic and include intraoperative issues such as component malposition or sizing, inadequate restoration of mechanical axis, improper soft tissue or 'gap' balancing and ligamentous injuries. Late instability is often due to polyethylene wear or component loosening, but can also be associated with postoperative soft tissue failure, or injury. Risk factors for instability of all types include infection, obesity, neuromuscular disorders, inflammatory arthritides, severe preoperative knee deformities, preoperative knee instability, as well as prior knee surgery.

When TKA instability occurs early or late, several classes or patterns are seen. Coronal plane or 'varus/valgus' issues are often seen when either the collateral ligaments are compromised, the femoral component is malpositioned, the tibial component is malpositioned, or all of the above. The most common causes of this type of instability include intraoperative MCL injury, or undercorrection of a significant valgus knee ligamentous deformity, resulting in residual MCL laxity. While bracing and physical therapy for quadriceps strengthening may be successful for mild laxity, correction often requires revision to a high postimplant to improve coronal balance.

Anterior-posterior instability (API) can be seen in flexion and/or extension and often results from improper gap balancing. If the extension gap is too large, the knee may fall into recurvatum when fully extended. This posterior thrust may also be seen with a very weak extensor mechanism and quadriceps-strengthening exercises may help to decrease symptoms of instability. More often than not, this imbalance is created by over-resection of the distal femur during the index surgery. Patella baja may also be seen in this instance that decreases the mechanical advantage of the patella in active extension. Surgical correction of this issue requires femoral revision and distal femoral augmentation to properly restore the joint line and patellar position.

If the flexion gap is larger than the extension gap, API will be seen when the knee is placed in the flexed position. Over-aggressive posterior femoral bone resection or PCL laxity in a cruciate retaining TKA construct are common causes of this scenario. Patients may have complaints of 'giving way' when ambulating on flat ground, but problems are more often noted when going from a seated to standing position, or vice versa. Stair climbing with power can also be a challenge. Again, bracing and therapy can be considered for mild symptoms, but femoral component revision with posterior femoral condylar augmentation is often necessary.

These patterns can also be seen in combination. Multidirectional instability can occur early and result from issues in all of the planes mentioned above. Often, however, it is seen months or years after the index surgery is completed. Polyethylene wear, with or without osteolysis and component loosening, is commonly seen. Infection, causing soft tissue damage or implant subsidence, is another frequently seen source. As with any painful or unstable TKA, a diagnostic infection work-up must be completed prior to proceeding with a treatment plan. Correction of multiplane TKA instability almost always includes implant revision to a constrained construct. Two-stage correction must be considered when infection dictates its use.

Patellar instability will be addressed by itself. It can be related to the previous topics, but often occurs alone. Through the years, many authors have reported that patellar complications are among the most common in TKA and often result in the need for surgical revision. Preoperative risk factors for patellar instability after TKA include prior instability or lateral patellar tilt, obesity, severe valgus deformity, neuromuscular disorders and previous knee surgery. Lateral subluxation or dislocation is most commonly seen. Component position is very often to blame for patellar maltracking. If the femoral component is internally rotated or medialized on the distal femur, lateral subluxation can occur. An internally rotated tibial component can have similar effects, as can a laterally placed or improperly sized patellar implant. A simple lateral retinacular release can help to correct intraoperative patellar tracking issues, but avoiding the implant placement issues mentioned above is critical for success after TKA.

BIBLIOGRAPHY

1. Adams AL,Paxton EW,Wang JQ, et al. Surgical outcomes of total knee replacement according to diabetes status and glycemic control, 2001-2009. J Bone Joint Surg Am. 2013;95(6):481-7.
2. Asp J, Rand JA. Peroneal nerve palsy after total knee arthroplasty. Clin Orthop Relat Res. 1990;261;233-7.
3. Beer K, Lombardi AV Jr, Mallory TH. The efficacy of suction drains after routine total joint arthroplasty. J Bone Joint Surg Am. 1991;73(5):584-7.
4. Butt U, Samuel R, Sahu A, et al. Arterial injury in total knee arthroplasty. J Arthroplasty. 2010;25(8):1311-8.
5. Calligaro KD, DeLaurantis DA, Booth RE, et al. Acute arterial thrombosis associated with total knee arthroplasty. J Vasc Surg. 1994;20(6):927-32.
6. Calligaro KD, Dougherty MJ, Ryan S, et al. Acute arterial complications associated with total hip and knee arthroplasty. J Vasc Surg. 2003;38(6):1170-7.
7. Clarke HD, Scuderi GR. Flexion instability in primary total knee arthroplasty. J Knee Surg. 2003;16(2):123-8.
8. Colwell CW Jr. What is the state-of-the-art in orthopedic thromboprophyl axis in lower extremity reconstruction? Instr Course Lect. 2011;60:283-90.
9. Cram P, Lu X, Kates SL, et al. Total knee arthroplasty volume, utilization, and outcomes among medicare beneficiaries, 1991-2010 knee arthroplasty volume, use, and outcomes. JAMA. 2012;308(12):1227-36.
10. Della Rocca G, Leung KS, Pape HC, et al. Periprosthetic fractures: epidemiology and future projections. J Orthop Trauma. 2011;2:66-70.
11. Della Valle CJ, Haidukewych GJ, Callaghan JJ. Periprosthetic fractures of the hip and knee: a problem on the rise but better solutions. Instr Course Lect. 2010;59:563-75.
12. Deirmengian C, Hallab N, Tarabishy A, et al. Synovial fluid biomarkers for periprosthetic infection. Clin Orthop Relat Res. 2010;468:2017-23.
13. Fering TK, Valadie AL. Knee instability after total knee arthroplasty. Clin Orthop Relat Res. 1994;299:157-62.
14. Gandhi R, deBeer J, Leone J, et al. Predictive risk factors for stiff knees in total knee arthroplasty. J Arthroplasty. 2006;21(1):46-52.
15. Gollwitzer H, Dombrowski Y, Prodinger PM, et al. Antimicrobial peptides and proinflammatory cytokines in periprosthetic joint infection. J Bone Joint Surg Am. 2013;95(7):644-51.
16. Gill GS, Mills D, Joshi AB. Mortality following primary total knee arthroplasty. J Bone Joint Surg Am. 2003;85(3):432-5.
17. Haidukewych GJ. Innovations in locking plate technology. J Am Acad Orthop Surg. 2004;12(4):205-12.
18. Haidukewych GJ, Langford JR, Liporace FA. Revision for periprosthetic fractures of the hip and knee. Instr Course Lect. 2013;62:333-40.
19. Heit JA, Silverstein MD, Mohr DN, et al. Risk factors for deep vein thrombosis and pulmonary embolism. JAMA. 2000;160(6):809-15.
20. Hull R, Roskob G, Pineo G, et al. A comparison of subcutaneous low-molecular-weight heparin with warfarin sodium for prophylaxis against deep vein thrombosis after hip or knee implantation. N Engl J Med. 993;329(19): 1370-6.
21. Jacovides CL, Kreft R, Adeli B, et al. Successful identification of pathogens by polymerase chain reaction-based electron spray ionization time-of-flight mass spectrometry (ESI-TOF-MS) in culture-negative periprosthetic joint infection. J Bone Joint Surg Am. 2012;94(24):2247-54.
22. Katz J, Barrett J, Mohomed NN, et al. Association between hospital and surgeon procedure volume and the outcomes of total knee replacement. J Bone Joint Surg Am. 2004;86(9):1909-16.
23. Kumar SN, Chapman JA, Rawlins I. Vascular injuries in total knee arthroplasty. A review of the problem with special reference to the possible effects of the tourniquet. J Arthroplasty. 1998;13(2):211-6.
24. Lane GJ, Hozack WJ, Shah S, et al. Simultaneous bilateral versus unilateral total knee arthroplasty: outcomes analysis. Clin Orthop Relat Res. 1997;345:106-12.
25. Lachiewicz P. Comparing and contrasting current guidelines for venous thromboembolism prophylaxis after total hip and knee arthroplasty. Instr Course Lect. 2011;60:301-10.
26. Lemos MJ, Sutton D, Hozack WJ, et al. Pulmonary embolism in total hip and knee arthroplasty. Risk factors in patients on warfarin prophylaxis and analysis of the prothrombin time as an indicator of warfarin's prophylactic effect. Clin Orthop Relat Res. 1992;282:158-63.
27. Liporace FA, Donegan DJ, Lanford JR, et al. Contemporary internal fixation techniques for periprosthetic fractures of the hip and knee. Instr Course Lect. 2013;62:317-32.

28. Moleney WJ. The stiff total knee arthroplasty: evaluation and management. J Arthroplasty. 2002;17(4):71-3.
29. Moojen DJ, Spijkers SN, Schot CS, et al. Identification of orthopedic infections using broad-range polymerase chain reaction and reverse line blot hybridization. J Bone Joint Surg Am. 2007;89(6):1298-305.
30. Mahomed NN, Barrettj, Katz JN, et al. Epidemiology of Total Knee Replacement in the United States Medicare Population. J Bone Joint Surg Am. 2005;87(6):1222-8.
31. Paiement G, et al. Thromboembolic disease in hip and knee replacement patients. AAOS OKU Hip and Knee Reconstruction, 1995.pp.1-7.
32. Parratte S, Pagnano MW. Instability after total knee arthroplasty. Instr Course Lect. 2008;57:295-304.
33. Parvizi J, Jain N, Schmidt AH. Periprosthetic knee fractures. J Orthop Trauma. 2008;22(9):663-71.
34. Parvizi J, Kim KL, Oliashirazi A, et al. Periprosthetic patellar fractures. Clin Orthop Relat Res. 2006;446:161-6.
35. Parvizi J, Jacovides C, Adeli B, et al. Synovial c-reactive protein: a prospective marker for periprosthetic knee joint infection. Clin Orthop Relat Res. 2012;470:54-60.
36. Patel J, Ries MD, Bozic KJ. Extensor mechanism complications after total knee arthroplasty. Instr Course Lect. 2008;57:283-94.
37. Patel VP, Walsh M, Sehgal B, et al. Factors associated with prolonged wound drainage after primary total hip and knee arthroplasty. J Bone Joint Surg Am. 2007;89(1): 33-8.
38. Rand JA. Vascular complications of total knee arthroplasty: report of three cases. J Arthroplasty. 1987;2:89-93.
39. Rand JA. Management of nerve and vascular injuries associated with total knee arthroplasty. AAOS Advanced Reconstruction Knee, Chapter 33. 2011:pp.283-92.
40. Ritter MA, Faris PM, Keating EM. Anterior femoral notching and ipsilateral femur fracture in total knee arthroplasty. J Arthroplasty. 1988;3(2):185-7.
41. Rush JH, Vidovich JD, Johnson MA. Arterial complications of total knee replacement: the Australian experience. J Bone Joint Surg Br. 1987;69(3): 400-2.
42. Schinsky M, Macaulay W, Parks ML, et al. Nerve injury after primary total knee arthroplasty. J Arthroplasty. 2001;16(8):1048-54.
43. Sharkey PF, Hozack WJ, Rothman RH, et al. Why are total knee arthroplasties failing today? Clin Orthop Relat Res. 2002;404:7-13.
44. Weinstein AM, Rome BN, Reichmann WM, et al. Estimating the burden of total knee replacement in the United States. J Bone Joint Surg Am. 2013;95(5):385-92.
45. Wstrich Gh, Haas SB, Mosca P, et al. Meta-analysis of thromboembolic prophylaxis after total knee arthroplasty. J Bone Joint Surg Br. 2000;82(6):795-800.
46. Zarin J, et al. Complications after total knee arthroplasty, adult reconstruction. Lippincott: Williams and Wilkins, Chapter 26: 177-187.

Chapter 22

Principles of Revision Total Knee Arthroplasty

Kelly G Vince, Michel Malo

THOUGHTS EXPERIMENTAL

Consider the challenge of revision knee arthroplasty realistically, by visualizing a failed knee replacement with all the components removed. Indeterminate amounts of bone have gone from a highly variable soft tissue environment. From one revision to the next, the surgeon cannot predict what will be available and what must be reconstructed. To assume otherwise is to pretend and be caught unprepared, especially by the most challenging cases.

Imagine our theoretical case; stabilizing soft tissues may be lax or stretched to the point of failure. Alternately, they may be scarred and leathery stiff. Though easy to evaluate at surgery, the condition of the soft tissues may be difficult to anticipate accurately. Take our case in the mind's eye and magically restore all the original bone- and even the articular cartilage. The anterior cruciate ligament will have disappeared and the posterior cruciate, even if conserved at the primary will probably have changed structurally and mechanically. We expect the posterior capsule to remain but with how much scarring? The collateral ligaments may be present but are just as likely to have deformed plastically or contracted tightly.

The defining question is: after you magically restored the normal bone, and with it the vaunted joint line, to its original three-dimensional morphology, can you expect that knee to function normally? Will there be stability and motion, through all positions? Most would say 'unlikely'; but all must agree, 'not dependably.'

KEYS TO REVISION TKA SURGICAL TECHNIQUE

There can be no successful revision surgery without extensive preoperative assessment and planning, as described below. Once surgery begins, simple keys prevail:

- The femoral component controls the soft tissues
- The flexion gap is largely a function of the size of the femoral component
- The extension gap is controlled by the proximal-distal position of the femoral component
- Because the tibial component constitutes one side of both the flexion and the extension gaps, it cannot be used to control the kinematics of the arthroplasty,

but only to establish a well-positioned, 'platform' as a reference for the surgical reconstruction, and eventually, to support the patient physically.

These keys are infallible guides no matter how complex the case and comprise the essence of the principles that follow.

Before Surgery: Make a Diagnosis

The importance of a diagnosis before treatment seems embarrassingly self-evident. Unfortunately revision surgery is often performed as a 'repeat' or 'redo' with little attention paid to the essence of 'revision': changing or correcting underlying faults. Any facile or superficial diagnosis made from a quick first impression is dangerous. Noncircumferential radiolucencies at the interface, for example, do not constitute loosening. And, the symptom of 'pain' is neither a diagnosis nor an indication for revision. Any diagnosis made from an initial 'heuristic' impression as described by Groopman[1] must then be subjected to analysis and deduction. The ways that cognitively difficult problems may be dangerously reduced to more simple questions are well catalogued.[2]

The process of diagnosis, as in all branches of medicine, is based on the 'differential diagnosis' or list of possible explanations for a set of symptoms and physical findings. This list can be anatomically oriented, in an approach originally suggested by Moreland[3] and later modified by Vince[4,5] (**Table 22.1**). *Systematic* evaluation, meaning a thorough and focused clinical history plus a physical exam, followed by a standard set of investigations, is necessary for every patient. The classic questions that characterize pain (location, duration, quality, exacerbating and ameliorating features) must be put to all patients. Painful arthroplasties can usefully be separated into those that were once successful and are now painful versus those that never provided pain relief. Something has deteriorated in the first group (infection, ruptured extensor mechanism, late instability, loosening/component breakage or periprosthetic fracture). The latter group can be further divided into those with the same pain that was present prior to arthroplasty (implying that something like radicular spine pain, radiating pain from an arthritic hip remains uncorrected) from those who developed new symptoms immediately after the arthroplasty, where something in the arthroplasty or healing has never been right (infection, stiffness, patellar tracking problems and rotational positioning issues). A *systematic* approach must be complemented by *comprehensive* analysis. This means that once a systematic evaluation yields a diagnosis, all other possible diagnoses must still be considered. Unlike conventional clinical problems, the failed revision may well defy the principle established by 'Ockham's Razor', (*'Numquam ponenda est pluralitas sine necessitate' or, 'Plurality ought never be posed without necessity')* that generally supports a single causation for all given phenomenon.[6] When arthroplasties come loose, for example, they might also have been infected or stiff or internally rotated. A stiff arthroplasty may be infected or loose or even infected and loose. As all problems in the arthroplasty will have to be corrected, all problems must be identified.

TABLE 22.1 Modes of failure

1.	Sepsis
2.	Extensor rupture
3.	Stiffness
4.	Instability
5.	Patella and malrotation
6.	Loosening
7.	Periprosthetic fracture
8.	Component breakage
9.	PAIN without diagnosis

Disciplined Diagnosis of Infection

Infection must be suspected in all failed knee replacements and probably 'assumed' in all failed revisions. Recent collaborations produced superb guidelines for the diagnosis[7,8] and definition[9] of periprosthetic infections. This extensive work can be summarized by the following principles. Patients with a problem knee arthroplasty should be stratified according to the level of clinical suspicion for infection and should have synovial fluid aspirated from the knee if a peripheral blood erythrocyte sedimentation rate (ESR) or 'C' reactive protein (CRP) value is elevated or if clinical suspicion is high. This fluid should be quantified for white blood cells (WBCs), for the differential (or types of WBCs) and sent for bacterial culture and sensitivity. If infection is suspected clinically, but the results of the initial aspiration are negative, another aspiration is recommended. Aspirations should be performed with the patient off of antibiotic medication for a minimum of 2 weeks. Others have suggested that a third aspiration should be performed if the situation is unclear after two.[10]

The remaining guidelines from the AAOS committee may be summarized. They acknowledge that radioisotope imaging is often equivocal, but may be useful if sepsis is suspected but not diagnosed by aspiration, and if surgery is not planned. While a bone scan is a strong predictor of the absence of infection if negative, scans will be positive for a multitude of reasons. No recommendations are given regarding the usefulness of CT or MR scans to diagnose infection. At surgery, gram stains are unreliable, but counting the numbers of leukocytes per high-powered frozen section may be used if the diagnosis of sepsis has neither been established nor excluded prior to surgery, remembering that this method can be subject to sampling error. Multiple intraoperative cultures may be useful for the patient who is being assessed for infection, especially when a component is being removed but not revised. Whenever possible, the diagnosis of infection should be made prior to surgery. The review panel opposes antibiotic treatment in 'suspicious' cases unless an aspiration has been performed. They strongly recommend against withholding prophylactic antibiotics at revision surgery, as the diagnosis should be established before surgery[8] and delays in the administration of antibiotic prophylaxis compromise their efficacy, which is particularly dangerous in revision surgery. In cases where a two-stage reimplantation protocol is being initiated for infection, but the quality of the preoperative culture material is uncertain, withholding antibiotics is reasonable, as neither metal nor plastic are being reimplanted at that time.

The Center for Disease Control classifies surgical infections as: superficial incisional, deep incisional or organ space.[11] For arthroplasty wounds, this effectively translates into the simpler, but tremendously important distinction between superficial and periprosthetic infections.[12,13] Wound problems and superficial infections require aggressive surgical management to prevent deep infection.[14-17] Periprosthetic infections require definitive surgical treatment, either with a one[18] or two stage protocol.[19] The Musculoskeletal Infection Society criteria for the diagnosis of periprosthetic infection[9] include a draining sinus tract communicating with the joint *or* two positive intraoperative cultures from the inside of the joint (aspiration or intraoperative specimen). Alternately, four of six lesser criteria constitute infection: (1) elevated ESR and CRP (2) elevated synovial fluid WBC counts (3) elevated percentage of polymorphonucleocytes (PMN) (4) purulence in the joint (5) a micro-organism in one culture of joint fluid or periprosthetic tissue or (6) more than five WBC/hpf in periprosthetic tissue at 400 power magnification on a frozen section. Even so-called 'low-grade' infections cannot be diagnosed without these criteria.

Do a 'Revision' not a 'Repeat Surgery'

The patient is unhappy with their knee replacement and the obliging surgeon says: 'fine, let's give you another one.' This approach may satisfy the retail consumer, but is a disaster in arthroplasty surgery. Revision surgery must be an opportunity to *identify and correct* the problems that have led to trouble. Revisions performed without a coherent explanation for the failure are at great risk of failure for exactly the same reason as the primary.

The differential diagnosis scheme modified from Moreland's original scheme[4] begins with the consideration of sepsis. Any number of sequences for the 8 diagnoses can be envisaged, (actually 8 of 40,320 sequences) but the order in **Table 22.1** begins with the most important (sepsis) and then considers several that are very easy to diagnose or discard (extensor rupture and stiffness) followed by those that are slightly more complex (instability and patellar complications associated with rotational position). Loosening, because so many surgeons seem to associate it synonymously with pain, is well down on the list to prevent 'jumping to conclusions.' Periprosthetic fractures and broken components, as they occur less frequently and are usually obvious, comprise the balance. Pain without a diagnosis is a 9th option and an indication for trepidation and further evaluation, but definitely not surgery.[20]

Performing a corrective revision as opposed to a 'repeat' surgery also means understanding the etiology of that failure. Ruptures of the extensor mechanism are frequently associated with surgical approaches that inadvertently transected or inexpertly avulsed a majority of longitudinal fibers of the quadriceps or patellar tendon[21] and like all problems of the extensor may be associated with rotational positioning of the tibial and femoral components. Sometime the extensor mechanism is the last substantive structure holding an unstable TKA together and concurrent revision for instability will be essential. As with many ligamentous failures of the knee, simple repair is generally inadequate and tissue substitution will be necessary—generally with an extensor mechanism allograft.[22,23]

The stiff total knee arthroplasty (TKA) is an obvious diagnosis but a thorny clinical proposition. The problem is almost invariably multifactorial and not amenable to simple interventions[24,25] (**Figure 22.1**). One of the main, though often unappreciated features of the stiff TKA is rotational positioning of the tibial and femoral components. CT scanning in advance of revision is recommended.[25] Only a small minority of cases will have become stiff primarily as the result of scarring or arthrofibrosis.[26] In most cases, scarring will be the inevitable sequel to immobility, not the cause of stiffness. If true 'arthrofibrosis' is felt to be at the heart of the problem, then revision should be resisted; what will protect the revision from the same fate as the primary- failure from inordinate scar?

Tibial-femoral instability yields the best results of any revision procedures assuming that the mode and causes of instability are identified accurately.[27-30]

The arthroplasty in extension may suffer instability in the sagittal (plane of motion or intersection of 'z' and 'y' axes) or the frontal (varus-valgus) planes. Alternately, or additionally, arthroplasties may be unstable in the flexed position (**Figure 22.2**). Instability in the plane of motion inexorably results from malfunction of the static posterior stabilizing structures and the extensor mechanism. For example, patients with compromised extensor function suffer buckling, which they usually report as instability. This may result from obesity where the extensor strength is inadequate to support body weight or prior surgical removal of the patella. If extensor insufficiency is advanced, then the patient will lock the knee in hyperextension to prevent buckling. Eventually this may lead to recurvatum

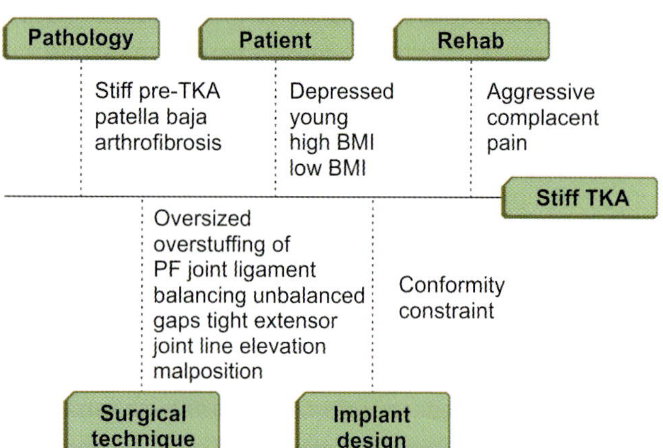

Figure 22.1 A fish diagram used to illustrate and analyze situations where numerous factors contribute to the causation of complex outcome. This diagram argues against the likelihood of single causation of 'stiffness' and accordingly against limited surgical interventions

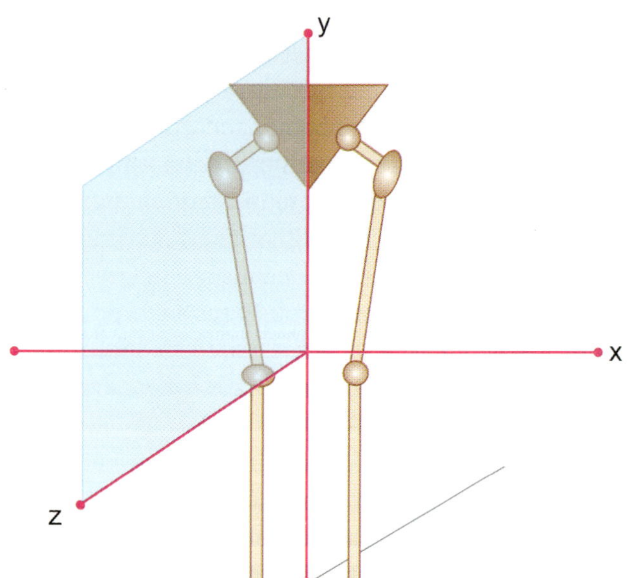

Figure 22.2 Three-dimensional axes (x, y, and z) mapped onto a stick figure of the lower extremity. While the precise location of an object in space can be specified by its rotational and translational orientation on each axis, planes of instability can also be specified as the intersection of two axes

instability, much like the polio patient. In those cases, recurvatum instability is directly secondary to extensor malfunction. Unless both the instability and the causative extensor insufficiency are addressed revision surgery will likely fail. In these cases, it is wise to remember that Insall identified recurvatum from neurologic causes and also significant quadriceps weakness as two of four relative contraindications to arthroplasty.[31] Hinged devices with hyperextension stops are often recommended but cannot address the actual problem, and arthrodesis must be discussed with the patient. With the similar result of buckling, the patient with a fixed flexion contracture requires superior quadriceps strength to walk or stand as they are never able to lock the knee in full extension. The moment the quadriceps becomes exhausted and fails, the knee collapses.

Varus-valgus instability is the archetype when surgeons consider 'instability.' The usual thought is for a constrained implant, but this addresses only part of the problem.[32] Inevitably there are destructive forces at the heart of the failure, most notably the axial alignment and gait abnormalities. It is important to correct or improve these problems whenever possible.

Flexion instability is easily corrected with revision if it has been diagnosed. The classic descriptions[33,34] remind us that these patients usually begin their rehabilitation as dramatic successes with rapid achievement of full flexion, because the flexion gap is lax or indeed unstable. The same patient progresses to trouble with stair climbing and rising from a chair, persistent effusions and periarticular tenderness from a stressed soft tissue capsule and ligaments. This surprisingly common problem originates in failure to balance the flexion and extension gaps. Every patient who presents for arthroplasty with a fixed flexion deformity (FFD) is at risk. When TKA is performed in the presence of a FFD and the standard bone cuts are made but no soft tissue releases or additional removal of distal femoral bone is performed, the extension gap will be smaller and tighter than the flexion gap, whether the surgeon recognizes it or not. The articular polyethylene is usually selected to give full extension, and with the knee locked fully straight, there may be the impression of excellent varus valgus stability. In fact, if that knee is flexed only a few degrees to relax the posterior structures, the lack of balance in the collateral ligaments manifest (**Figures 22.3A to D**). This phenomenon has been described as a new entity by some surgeons: 'mid flexion instability.' In fact, it is invariably simple flexion instability that results from unbalanced flexion and extension gaps, a problem as old as knee arthroplasty surgery itself. Some have posited a sophisticated theory of joint line height as an explanation for mid-flexion instability in primary arthroplasty,[35] that others have disputed.[36] An abstruse theory, no widely accepted, has been forwarded to explain 'mid-flexion' instability specifically in revision arthroplasty as a function of anterior medial collateral ligament attenuation and component design.[37] Revision to balance the gaps, following the principle that the femur controls the soft tissues and that femoral component size and position control the flexion and extension gaps respectively will be successful (We can provide a case of flexion instability/ posterior dislocation after revision TKA, illustrating a too-small revised femoral component with no stem that was mistakenly chosen with reference to the residual deficient bone—another important revision principle).

In all cases with patellar complications, rotational position of the tibial and femoral components should be quantified, ideally with a CT scan following the protocol as described by Berger et al.[38] This includes cases of maltracking, but also of patellar fracture. The longitudinal fracture often occurs because the patellar bone wants to dislocate as a result of maltracking, while the patellar button is confined in the groove. They part company in the form of a fracture. Similar mechanisms underlie patellar component loosening and breakage. Revision with rotational realignment will be successful. Sometimes, if the extensor has been dislocated for an extended period of time, it will have shortened and scarred. While the extensor may be returned to the femoral trochlear groove at revision, it prefers the 'short cut' position of dislocation, once the knee flexes. This force may be strong enough to externally rotate or spin the tibia, displace the tubercle laterally and reproduce the dislocation, especially with a revision implant system that permits rotation of the tibia under the femur either due to a nonconforming articulation or a mobile bearing. In cases such as this, rotational constraint may be essential (To the case I provided, we should add the reference to our article on

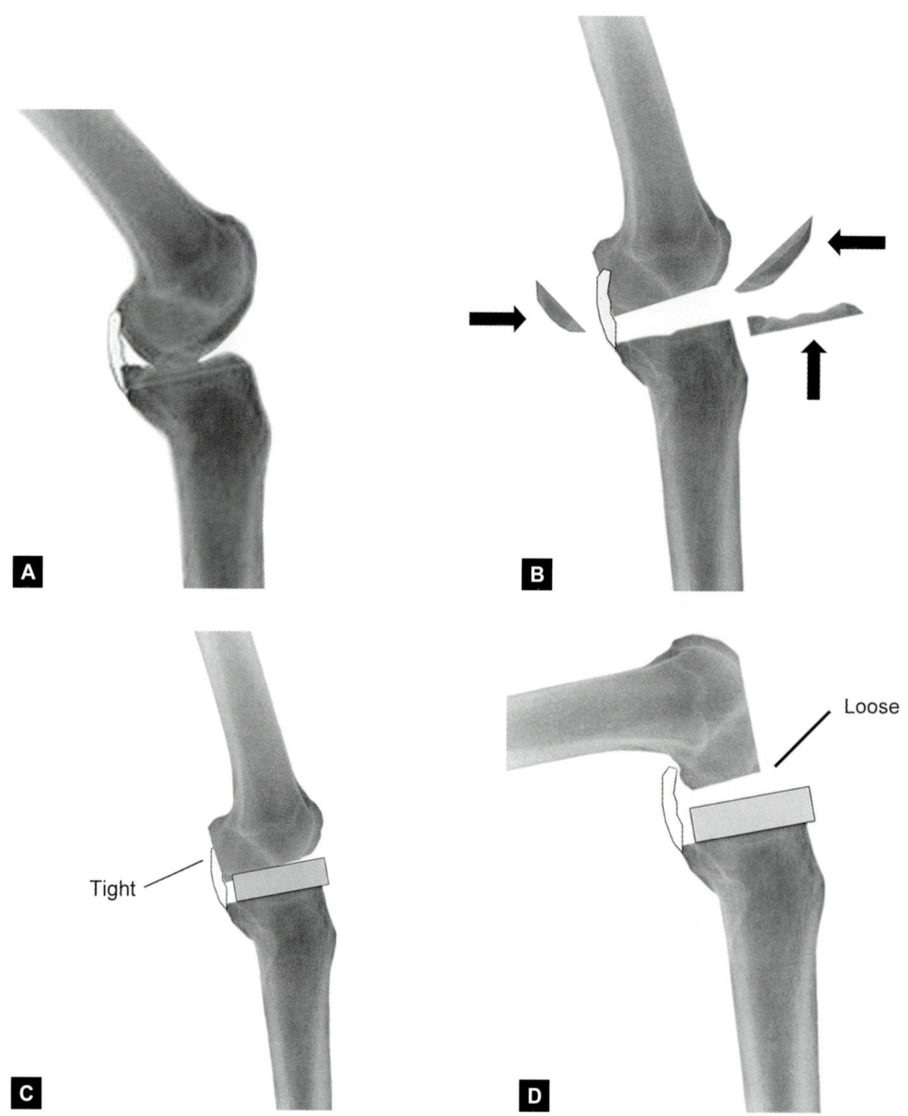

Figures 22.3A to D A common though infrequently recognized phenomenon: the original of flexion instability with measured resection arthroplasty technique. (A) Patient presents with fixed flexion deformity. The posterior structures (and perhaps more) are contracted; (B) If standard bone cuts are performed with neither release of the posterior capsule nor additional corrective bone removal from the distal femur, the knee comes easily to full extension, but the extension gap is probably smaller than it would be without the flexion contracture pathology; (C) Full extension in this situation necessitates a relatively smaller 'spacer' block, the equivalent later in the procedure of a thinner polyethylene insert; (D) Unless the flexion space is critically assessed, it will not be appreciated that the thin spacer permitting full extension has left the knee unstable in flexion. This is probably the pathophysiology of so-called: 'mid flexion' instability: the knee feels tight to varus and valgus forces in full extension when the posterior structures are tight. Once the knee is flexed slightly, the posterior structures relax and laxity (or imbalance) in the collateral structures can be appreciated. This laxity was always present, but masked in full extension. The discrepancy may be quite subtle, but has been exaggerated in these diagrams for clarity

Patella Instability—Malo M, Vince KG. The Unstable Patella after Knee Replacement: Etiology, Prevention and Management. AAOS. 2003;11(5):364-71).

Periprosthetic fractures are usually best treated with open reduction and internal fixation[39] and only occasionally with revision arthroplasty. If revision is appropriate, given patient age and debility, then it is best to proceed directly to this surgery rather than fixing the fracture, only to have it fail and become infected. Failed surgery for periprosthetic fractures, especially when complicated by infection is a common scenario in catastrophic failures that result in amputation.[40]

Loosening in often invoked by surgeons even when the necessary data to support the diagnosis are incomplete. Aseptic loosening can only be demonstrated by circumferential radiolucencies or change in position of a component. Isolated radiolucencies or osteolysis alone are insufficient to make this diagnosis. Infection must always be ruled out. Early loosening is fortunately rare, and associated with failure of bone ingrowth, subsidence of soft bone or very poor cementing technique. A fashion of cement fixation, with methacrylate applied only to the cut proximal surface and omitted from the medullary canal in primary arthroplasties has increasingly been identified with this mode of failure. Late loosening is almost always a biological phenomenon,[41,42] resulting from accumulated wear debris of dangerous sized particles that are phagocytosed by monocytes in a process that ends in osteolysis and loosening. Improvement in polyethylene quality and in the locking mechanism of modular tibial inserts[43] will decrease this mode of failure. Wear rates are affected by patient weight and activity, plus overloading (usually medial) from a varus mechanical alignment. Revision arthroplasty should improve a mechanical axis that has been overloading the medial side. Occasionally, internal rotation of a tibial component will accelerate wear in the posterolateral tibial, as the femoral component will not track congruently in the polyethylene and wear will accelerate (**Figure 22.4**).

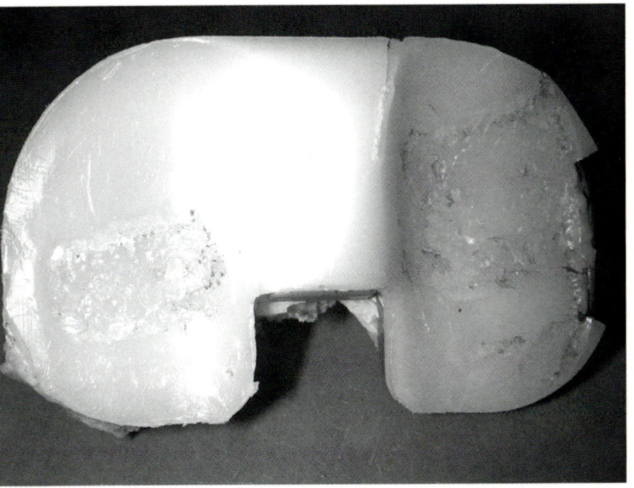

Figure 22.4 Retrieved left tibial component at revision for wear, osteolysis and loosening. The typical delamination features are apparent but on the left side, corresponding to the lateral tibial plateau, the wear is considerably more posterior, the result of an internal rotation position. The medial plateau opposite has more uniform and extensive wear corresponding to the greater loads that typically pass though this side

Component breakage is fortunately rare as most modern implant designs are resistant structural failure. Clearly, revision arthroplasty has to remove all susceptible components and reconstruct the joint to minimize the effect of damaging forces.[44]

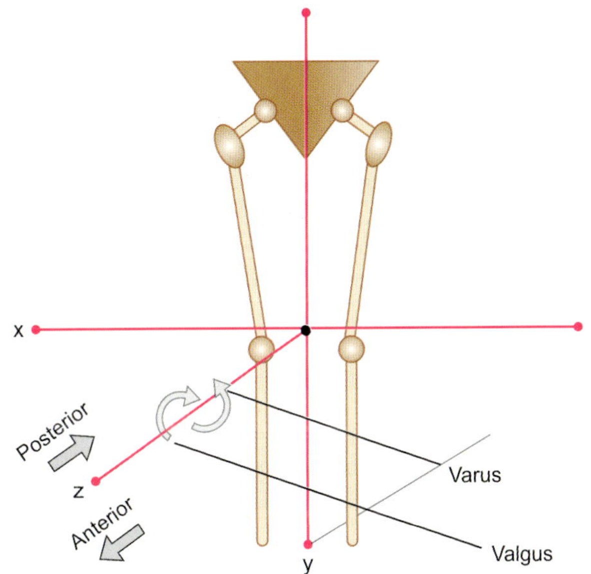

Figure 22.5 The three axes x, y z mapped onto a stick figure of the lower extremities, illustrating the concept of 'six degrees of freedom' that define any object in space. Here, translation and rotation are depicted about the 'z' axis. Translation correlates to the surgical nomenclature of 'anterior-posterior' positioning and rotation to 'varus-valgus' angulation. Translation is always expressed in units of length and rotation in degrees

A REVISION ARTHROPLASTY IS NOT A PRIMARY KNEE REPLACEMENT

Revision knee arthroplasty can be easy and gratifying, but not if the surgeon insists on adapting concepts, techniques, instruments and implants from primary arthroplasty. Only the basic concepts of alignment, component position in all six degrees of freedom (**Figure 22.5**), and balanced gaps are common to primary and revision surgery. The anatomic landmarks offered by articular cartilage, the ability to cut to flat surfaces and a familiar ligamentous environment are not reliably part of the revision, where

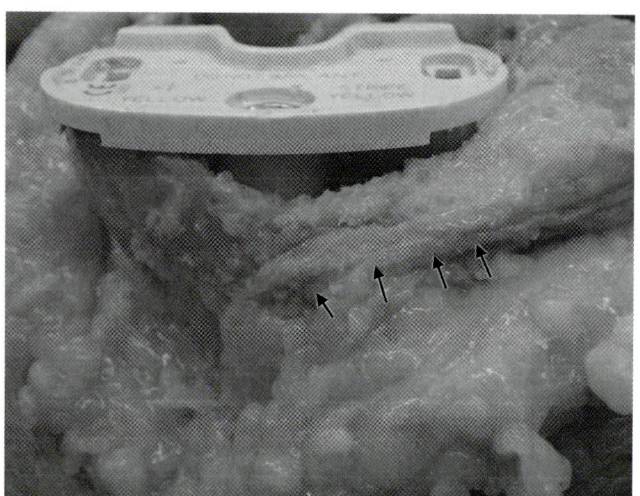

Figure 22.6 A stemmed trial tibial component sitting in a cadaver specimen after a TKA (total knee arthroplasty) prosthesis has been removed. This simulates the first step in revision TKA—'Re-establishment of the tibial platform.' The patellar tendon (arrows) has been dislocated to the lateral side of the knee (right side of the figure). There is scant space for a conventional extra-medullary tibial cutting guide to be applied proximal to the patellar tendon attachment and yet be expected to resect any bone. Indeed bones already gone and should be preserved not resected further. Additionally, the bone that would be expected to hold pins is thin sclerotic and likely to fracture. This illustrates the fallacy of trying to perform revision knee arthroplasty with conventional primary style instrumentation

the articular surface is long gone, bone may be grossly deficient and soft tissues are stretched or scarred unpredictably. Primary instruments don't usually work. Most tibial resection guides will not fit between any level of bone that can be cut and the attachment of the patellar tendon (**Figure 22.6**). The ubiquitous and effective 'measured resection' instruments[45] have no osseous points of reference in revision surgery. The damaged residual bone at revision surgery is vulnerable to pins that secure primary instruments.

The vicissitudes of bone quality and shape after arthroplasty failure demand entirely new strategies for component fixation-usually with stems extending into the canal. Even the bone surface,[46] sclerotic and dense, rather than cancellous and permeable, makes direct cementing inutile. As a result, revision surgery with primary style implants does not reliably produce good results.[47] Many revision knee prosthesis systems, some better than others, provide useful instruments, intramedullary fixation, varying degrees of constraint[32] and augments to reconstruct deficient bone as well as to control kinematics.

Despite the importance of revision systems for revision surgery, if a surgeon's first question on encountering a failed arthroplasty is: 'what implant should I use', that surgeon is asking the wrong question. We cannot expect implant systems to address all the challenges of revision surgery. The initial requirements for revision knee arthroplasty are a diagnosis and an explanation for the underlying causes of failure. Subsequent planning should be a mental facsimile of the surgery itself, with the surgeon visualizing every step from exposure to removal and reconstruction.[48]

Provide Additional Fixation

Fixation in primary arthroplasty depends on close matching of the cut bone surfaces and the implant, management and reduction of forces so that components are forced against the bone in manageable intensity and some medium of fixation-either ingrowth or bone cement. A congruent bone surface cannot be ensured in revision arthroplasty, where failure may have led to considerable bone loss. It will not be constructive to remove bone, in the presence of an asymmetric defect, simply to create a flat tibial.

Revision surgery requires a different and more robust approach to fixation than primary arthroplasty, especially if an arthroplasty has failed form loosening. This generally means fixation into the medullary canal with either fully cemented stem extensions of modest length or longer stems that engage the diaphysis without cement use in the canal. The intermediate option of metaphyseal length stem extensions without bone cement has proven unsatisfactory.[49] Primary components for revision arthroplasty may work in occasional cases but will not generally be reliable. In addition, as we have seen, press fit diaphyseal engaging trial components can facilitate the surgical technique by maintaining the position of trial components during revision arthroplasty.[50] A newer strategy of very short, fully cemented stem extensions with fixation augmented by tantalum, porous metal cones has been proposed.[51, 52] These tantalum cones have had a profound effect on revision arthroplasty surgery functioning both as fixation devices and as augments for bone defects with uniformly encouraging results[53,54] including the experience of independent surgeons not involved in the development of the products.[55]

Porous metals promise to revolutionize fixation and bone reconstruction in revision arthroplasty.[56] Reliable immediate fixation is followed by durable ingrowth into materials that are more porous than older surface coatings. These devices, originally introduced as augments for bone defects, have seen their real advantage as modular fixation devices. Laboratory research suggests that the complex surface geometry of these materials may also inhibit bacterial proliferation,[57] highlighting a substantive advantage over structural bone graft material.

Get Exposure Safely

Asking the right questions also applies to surgical exposure. Surgeons have been conditioned to ask, when the exposure is difficult: is a proximal soft tissue intervention (patellar tendon snip or 'turndown') or tibial tubercle osteotomy (TTO) best?[58] This is quite possibly the wrong question. Neither option is usually necessary, if close attention is paid to the details of surgical exposure: (1) synovectomy, (2) removal of scar from the deep surface of the patellar tendon, (3) re-establishment of the para-femoral gutters, (4) liberation of the scar that binds the quadriceps to the femur, (5) a lateral patellar retinacular release and (6) a gentle manipulation or flexion of the arthroplasty before failed components are removed to stretch the freed extensor.[50,59] In the most difficult cases, such as stiff or infected TKAs, a proximal, posteromedial release that includes the insertion of semimembranosus (as is used to correct varus deformities) permits 90° of external rotation of the tibia, dislocation of the knee, and effectively lateralizes the tubercle precisely to where it would be after a TTO, but without the need to cut bone or the risk of nonunion. The price paid for this maneuver may be a nonlinked constrained implant, which is frequently required in these cases anyway. Though increased skill can make tibial tubercle osteotomies unnecessary, they are still preferred over the catastrophic avulsion of the patellar tendon (**Figures 22.7A and B**).

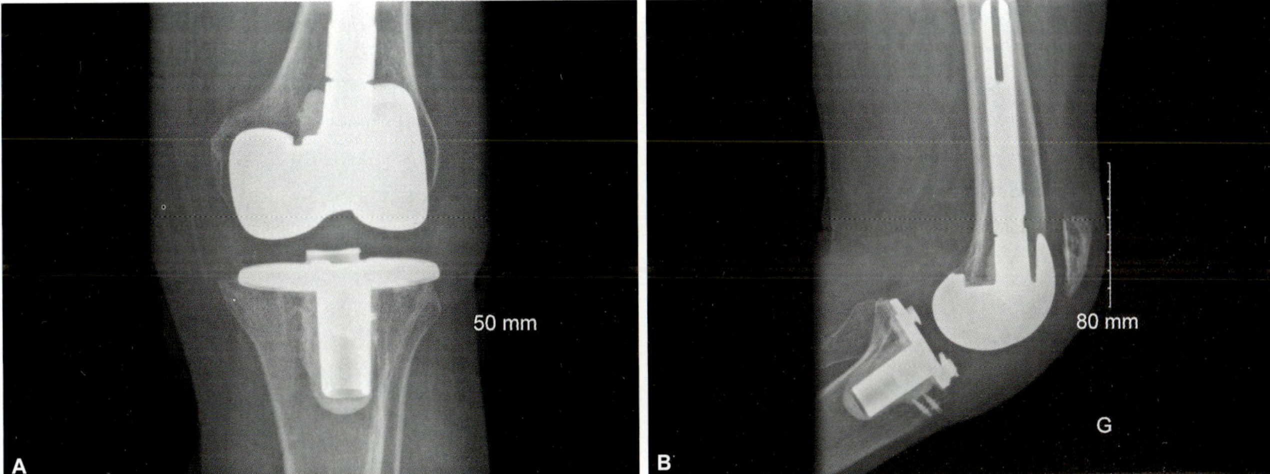

Figures 22.7A and B (A) Anteroposterior radiograph of an ill-advised technique for revision arthroplasty. Patient had a two-stage reimplantation for infection 6 months earlier, and presents with 'functional impairment of his knee.' Because instability is often a problem after effective debridement, failure to add a tibial stem extension means that a constrained implant was not an option at revision. In addition, the tibial component appears to be internally rotated: an observation that must be quantified by CT scan; (B) The associated features of two suture anchors in the region of the tubercle and extreme patella alta indicate avulsion of the patellar tendon at revision surgery. While this could be avoided with tibial tubercle osteotomy, that is a maneuver that itself is associated with increased infection rates[74] and can be avoided with attention to the details of surgical dissection[59] plus a large posteromedial release and external rotation of the tibia. This patient will require an extensor mechanism allograft

Avoid Partial Revisions

Why are the results of partial revision generally regarded as poor[60,61] and those of isolated tibial insert exchange even worse?[62, 63] By revisiting the 'keys to revision surgery' we acknowledge that if we do not revise the femoral component we will neither be able to manipulate the flexion-extension gap balance nor have the option of a constrained implant (unless of course the failed arthroplasty already included a constrained femoral implant). Surgical exposure for isolated revision of the tibia, tempting in cases of tibial component loosening, is usually hampered by the retained femoral prosthesis. A levered retractor placed behind the tibia to force it out in front of the femur may stretch the collateral ligaments to the point of being nonserviceable, assuming they were correctly balanced in the failed arthroplasty. If the femur is not revised, those changes cannot be corrected with manipulation of the gaps or constraint. In addition, the results of partial revision are poor because problems like a varus mechanical axis that overloaded the medial compartment and lead to tibial component loosening, may have originated in the femoral component position. A femoral component will be left untouched by the unsuspecting surgeon if it is well fixed, even though it may be mal-positioned.[64] Internal rotation can be a subtle problem, often at the root of patellar complications, stiffness, pain or instability that may be ignored if the component is well fixed (**Figure 22.8**). Simply put, single component revisions often treat the effect and neglect the cause.

When can a single component revision be recommended? Exchange of the modular polyethylene is mandatory in cases of acute infection when the surgeon hopes to save an arthroplasty with 'open debridement and poly exchange' (ODPE).[65] Failure to remove the modular insert means that pus and an incipient slime layer or glycocalyx biofilm will be left unmolested between the metal baseplate and the modular insert. Arthroscopic debridement of infected arthroplasties must be condemned for this reason, except in patients who are physiologically unstable because of the abscess in their arthroplasty. Dire toxicity may be reversed by flushing the joint with arthroscopic fluid but the infection will likely recur some mechanical failures may reasonably be treated with isolated modular polyethylene exchange; the older patient who, after many years of good performance from an arthroplasty, has worn through the polyethylene, may be a candidate for isolated exchange.

Stiffness is almost always a multifactorial problem.[25] It is tempting and arguably sensible to treat stiff knees with an isolated poly exchange to a thinner insert, but the results have been poor.[63] Stiff TKAs appropriate for poly insert exchange are rare, because multiple factors contribute to motion (femoral component size, patellar thickness, femoral component flexion angle, tibial slope and importantly component rotation) and usually all must be modified in favor of flexion, even at the expense of stability. Finally, most stiff arthroplasties were usually tight at the time of primary surgery, leading the surgeon to implant the thinnest polyethylene component when additional resection of proximal tibia for a globally stiff knee, or of distal femur for flexion contracture or of posterior femoral condyle with a smaller component for poor bending at surgery would have been more successful. When the thinnest component has been implanted then, there is no option of isolated revision to an even thinner component.

Overly optimistic surgeons sometimes suggest thicker polyethylene as a remedy for coronal plane instability thinking that it will 'tighten' the collateral ligaments. Most cases of frontal plane instability are driven by mal-alignment that requires correction and are accompanied by failure of the collateral ligament in tension on the convexity of the deformity requiring mechanical constraint.[28] Even if the ligament on the concavity of the deformity is released (lateral structures in the case of valgus instability) the thicker poly insert often creates a flexion contracture as the posterior structures are relatively shorter and tighter. Recurvatum and varus-valgus instability in conjunction with flexion instability, or 'global instability' might respond to thicker polyethylene, but these cases have usually suffered complete failure of the soft tissue environment that requires revision with larger, constrained implants in better positions. Isolated recurvatum, if treated with thicker polyethylene results in a knee with poor flexion, and flexion instability treated with thicker inserts limits extension. Isolated poly exchange may solve some mechanical failures but only if there is: (i) stable fixation of all components, (ii) neutral rotational position of femoral and tibial components, preferably confirmed by CT scan, (iii) ideal sizing and position of the femoral component, (iv) intact and balanced collateral ligaments, posterior capsule and extensor mechanism with (v) centrally tracking patella.

Isolated femoral component revision may be appropriate in rare cases, usually for kinematic failures related to flexion-extension gap imbalance. The globally stiff knee might be revised to a smaller, more proximally located femoral component, to widen both the flexion and extension gaps. This effect will be similar to reducing polyethylene thickness but with an effect on the joint line, and necessary when the thinnest insert has already been used. This strategy requires perfect rotational positioning of the retained tibial component and no anticipated need for constraint. Removal of the femur moreover, facilitates scar release. Isolated malrotation of the femoral component responsible for patellar tracking complications can be rectified with isolated femoral component exchange. Again, there must be no need for constrained articulations or the tibial component must already be suitable for a constrained implant. Any tibial component that is left must be well fixed and its rotational position should be confirmed, by a critical eye at surgery or a preferably with a CT scan prior to revision. A loose femoral component may be revised in isolation, but only in the unlikely event that osteolysis does not jeopardize the tibial component fixation.

Secondary patellar component resurfacing, a kind of isolated patellar revision surgery may work,[66,67] but not if performed without a very definite diagnosis. Not all painful TKAs with un-resurfaced patella are candidates for this procedure. Pain must be reproduced on physical examination by compression of the patella against the femoral component and moving it from side to side. These symptoms must be reproduced by maneuvers in the clinic that load the patella-femoral joint, such as stair ascent, descent and rising from a chair. A 'systematic and comprehensive' assessment must have eliminated all other sources of pain. Remember that anterior knee pain, as in the case in **Figures 22.8A to H**, may originate from internally rotated tibial and femoral components.[68] Accordingly, a CT scan to quantify rotational position[38] is important prior to isolated patellar surgery, emphasizing the principle of diagnosis.

Link Tibia and Femur through Soft Tissues

Most revision surgery is performed with what can be best described as 'independent tibial and femoral preparation.' The manufacturer's manuals, often prepared by engineers or technical writers with scant surgical experience, highlight tools that are useful to fit the products to the ends of bones after failed components have been removed. Recesses, angles and holes are created, sometimes with elaborate gadgets, to ensure that the femoral product fits on the femur and the tibial product fits on the tibia. These two procedures should be, but often are not, linked to each other by the patient's residual soft tissues in steps that are intrinsic to the surgical technique. The soft tissues that comprise the four sides of the knee joint will be in a highly unpredictable condition, depending on the mode and severity of failure.

The obeisant surgeon, after dutifully attaching the components, may be dismayed to find that they do not articulate as a stable joint. Most frequently, the flexion gap will be very much larger and constraint will save the day. If the extension gap is the larger, this will be difficult to reconfigure.

Three Step Technique

Numerous techniques for revision knee arthroplasty have been described. A procedure in three steps, that starts with the proximal tibia, then stabilizes the knee in flexion and finally balances the joint in extension, inherently acknowledges the state of the patient's soft tissues and accommodates them to the reconstruction.[50] This sequence starts with the tibia, which constitutes one side of both the flexion and extension gaps and so represents a common foundation from which each gap can be reconstructed. The flexion gap is stabilized, largely by the size of femoral component, followed by the extension gap as a function of its proximal-distal position. This technique is derived from the classic concepts of flexion and extension gaps pioneered for primary arthroplasty by Freeman,[69] Insall[31]

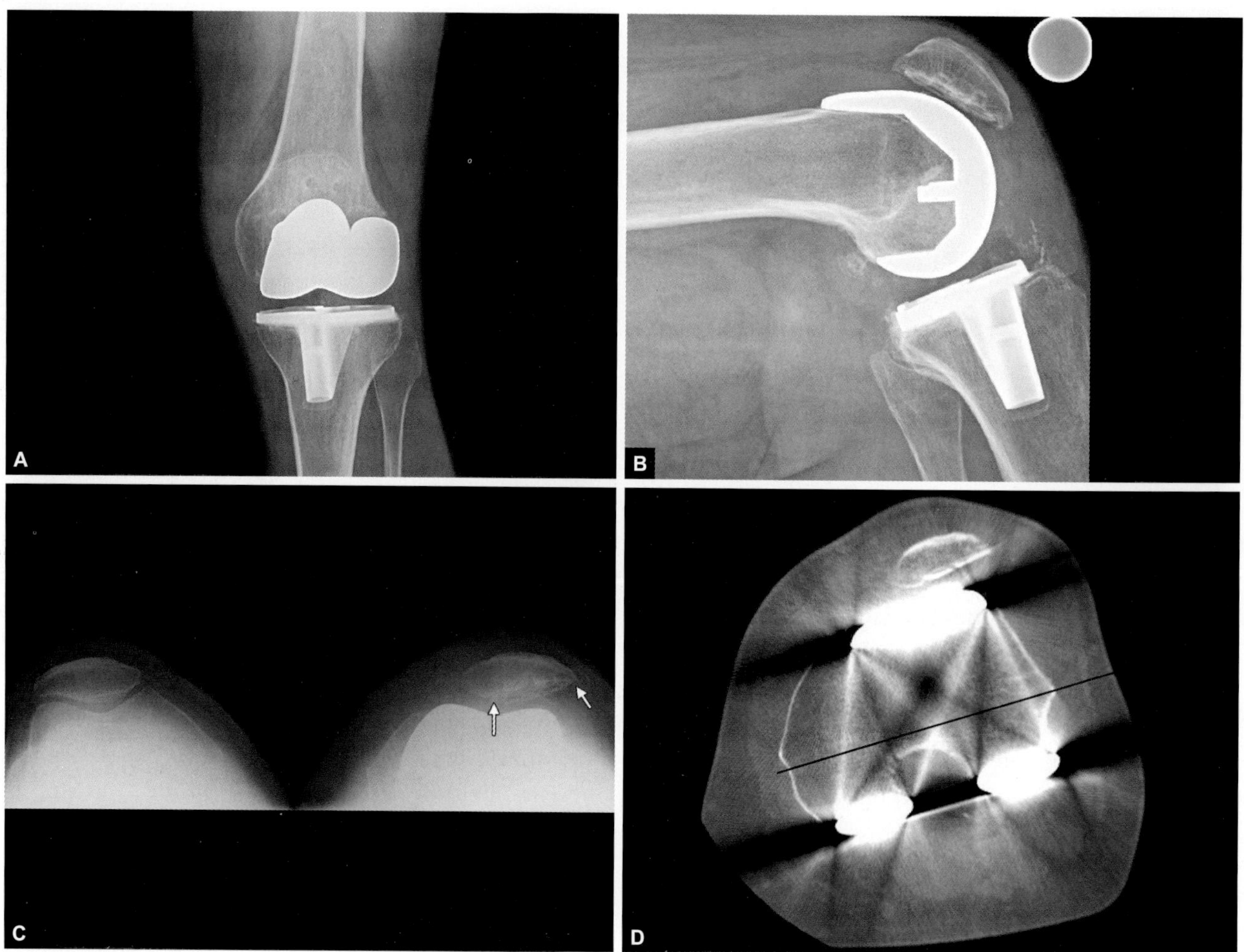

Figures 22.8A to D (A) Anteroposterior radiograph 1 year after TKA in a 55-year-old male who has been suffering anterior knee pain and buckling. These symptoms are different form the pain he had prior to the arthroplasty. Note the very asymmetric appearance of the components: we see the posterior lateral femoral condyle prominently and the entire lateral tibial fin but none of the medial tibial fin. These components are positioned internally relative to the X-ray beam and yet the limb itself, as indicated by the relationship between the fibular head and the proximal tibial is rotated correctly to the beam; (B) The patella had been resurfaced and flexion was limited to less than 90°. Both components are well fixed: the tibia sits with slight anterior slope and the femoral component is in a slightly flexed position, but not detrimental position. There is patellar alta, but no extensor lag; (C) Merchant patellofemoral radiograph—the patellar is tracking centrally, despite internal rotation noted in Figure 22.7A, probably because flexion is limited. If the knee were lax enough to flex further, the patella would probably dislocate due to internal rotation. The initial surgeon was considering an isolated patellar revision because of the asymmetric resection of the patella at the primary and sought a second opinion. The patellar revision would not be expected to improve motion or reduce pain or buckling all of which can be attributed to internal rotation; (D) CT scan to quantify rotational position of the femoral component, with one cut through the level of the femoral epicondyles (black line). This indicates satisfactory rotational position of the femoral component, aligned rotationally with the transepicondylar axis, (TEA)

and Ranawat[70] in the 1970s. These concepts were applied to a 'Three Step Revision Arthroplasty Technique' in the 1980s.[71]

The principle of this surgical algorithm includes getting the 'big picture' first. That means identifying component size and position, with provisional fixation achieved with diaphyseal engaging press-fit stem extensions, rather than depending on pins or screws that may damage poor quality revision bone and are unlikely to hold securely. Surgeons will save time by following these steps before reconstructing bone defects. If details, such as bone grafting or augmentation are performed prematurely, and then if the arthroplasty cannot be reduced or made stable, the basic steps and the details may have to be repeated.

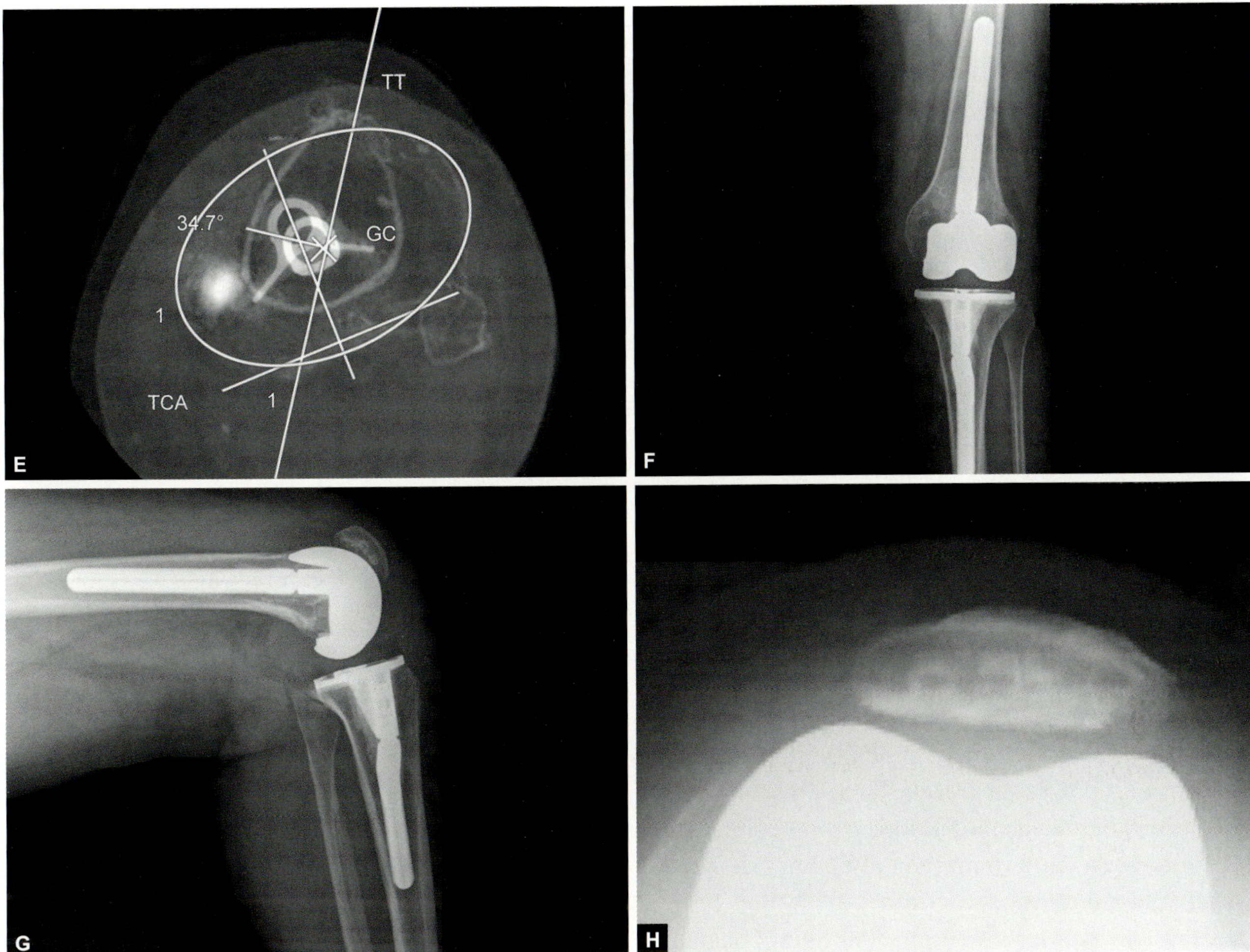

Figures 22.8E to H (E) Overlay of 3 CT scan cuts through the proximal tibia. One cut is through the component and establishes the 'Tibial Component Angle' (TCA). The second images the proximal tibial bone immediately distal to the component and establishes the 'Geometric Center' (GC) of the tibia. The third CT cut passes through the tibial tubercle (TT) and enables the surgeon to calculate the angle between: i. the line at right angles to the TCA and passing through the GC with, ii. The line joining GC and TT. In this case it is a disabling 37.4°; (F) AP radiograph after revision surgery according to a three-step technique, using diaphyseal engaging press fit stems with cementing of the metaphyseal areas in tibia and femur. Unusually in this case, the tibial offset stem has been placed laterally, a position that does not correlate with the usual anatomy. A full-length radiograph would indicate if this is an anatomic anomaly and whether the designed mechanical axis has been achieved. Note the same projection of the limb to the X-ray beam (relationship between fibular head and proximal tibia) plus the symmetric appearance of the revision components, demonstrating that the prior internal rotation has been corrected; (G) Lateral radiograph after revision demonstrating the same patella alta with modest improvements to motion. This is difficult as the quadriceps muscle is ultimately the limiting factor; (H) Merchant patella-femoral radiograph, showing revised patellar component that is tracking centrally. The prior anterior knee pain and buckling have been corrected as a result of correct rotational positioning

Surgical Technique Step 1: Re-establishment of Tibial Platform

Surgical reconstruction begins with the tibial 'platform' after surgical exposure and removal of components. The word 'platform' indicates a stable, level surface created by a trial component that is supported by part of the residual proximal tibia and to a great extent by an uncemented trial stem extension lodged into the diaphysis of the tibial canal. This is clearly not the 'joint line', but rather a foundation for the arthroplasty and a frame of reference from which to measure and reconstruct stable flexion and extension gaps. Bone defects should not be reconstructed yet. The only proximal tibial bone to have been resected at this stage is what was necessary to disrupt the fixation interface of the failed implant with a bone saw. So-called 'cleanup cuts' are usually overly aggressive and tend to sacrifice otherwise good bone unnecessarily. Removal of bone to eliminate defects and create a flat, 'primary like' surface, leads to the undesirable mating of a large femoral component with an inordinately small tibia.

The position of every object can be defined in space, by its translational and rotational orientation with respect to the x, y and z axes as described in **Figure 22.5**. Ideal tibial baseplate position in revision arthroplasty can be defined by a few important osseous landmarks, without concern for soft tissues and eventually 'fixed' to the tibial bone with respect to all six of these 'degrees of freedom.' The technique for orienting the femoral component spatially depends largely on osseous anatomy but must include significant considerations of the stabilizing soft tissues, especially for component size and proximal-distal position. A strong argument can be made, especially in revision arthroplasty, against rotating the femoral component to satisfy soft tissue tension, i.e. to create a 'rectangular gap.' This makes sense, remembering again that the femoral component enables the surgeon to control the soft tissue balance of the arthroplasty.

In the first step of a revision, the tibial baseplate will be oriented to the tibial bone and held temporarily by the diaphyseal engaging stem, with respect to: (1) medial-lateral, (2) flexion-extension, (3) proximal-distal, (4) internal-external rotational, (5) anterior-posterior and (6) varus-valgus positions. Neither the modular articular surface nor the joint line, are part of this step. The precise proximal-distal level of the tibial trial baseplate (its translational position on the 'y' axis) is immaterial at this preliminary stage, so long as it contacts a majority of the host tibia and is far enough from the posterior femoral condyle to eventually accommodate a modular insert. The tibia, as stated, is common to both the flexion and extension gaps so it does not affect kinematic balance. Ultimately, the effects of tibial bone, baseplate metal and articular polyethylene on stabilizing the arthroplasty are equivalent and interchangeable.

The right entry point for access to the tibial medullary canal initiates accurate tibial component position. Tibial implants that depend on intramedullary stem extensions for fixation will, if configured anatomically, have the attachment point for the stem extension located quite far anteriorly on the undersurface of the tray and require anterior entry point (**Figures 22.9A to C**). Surgical technique and component design will also require some accommodation for the fact that the center of the diaphyseal canal is generally 3–4 mm medial to the center of the proximal tibia[72] (**Figures 22.10A to C**). This adaptation may take the form of an asymmetric stem extension or a 'keel' for attachment of stems that is itself located medial of center. Then, if the tibial component is implanted in neutral alignment, the stem extension will be parallel to the mechanical axis of the tibia, but located a few millimeters medial to it in most cases, such that the tip of the stem extension will be lodged in the center of the diaphysis for secure fixation. Ideal anteroposterior and medial-lateral position will be compromised if the design of the component is not sufficiently asymmetric to fit the range of anatomical shapes. The amount of 'uncovered' bone or overhanging component will correlate with the sophistication of the design.

If the surgeon prefers fully cemented fixation, the longer and wider diaphyseal engaging trial stems may still be useful at this stage to guide position. As with the femoral preparation later, correct position of the trial component identifies where bone deficiencies will require augmentation or bone graft reconstruction. Bone defects should not guide the positioning of the components. Once a component is held in the proper position by trial press fit stem extensions and the augments have been fitted, the correct position will have been defined and maintained. Large stems intended for a press fit will not be required if full cementation (with smaller stems) is ultimately preferred.

Positioning the tibial component is challenging. The mechanical axis of the tibia, which extends from the center of the knee to the center of the ankle, does not usually pass though the center of the diaphysis, where a stem extension would be expected to find purchase. The mid-diaphyseal point is usually located about 4 mm more medially.[72] This means that a symmetric tibial component with a straight, diaphyseal engaging stem extension centered at the knee will usually be cocked into valgus. Alternately, when a

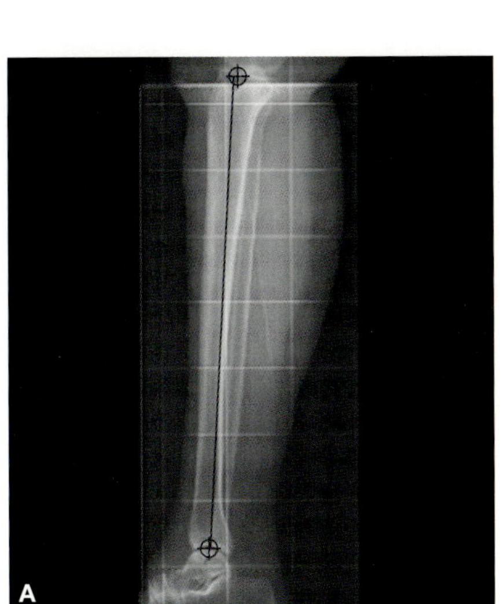

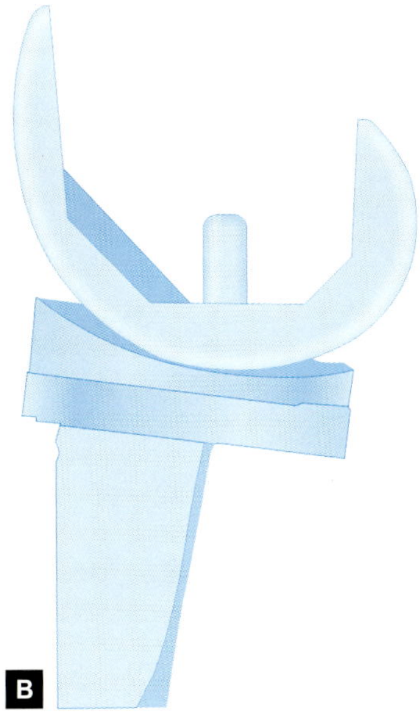

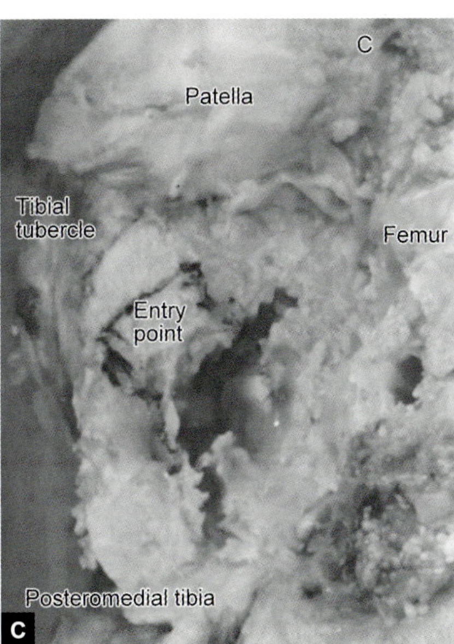

Figures 22.9A to C (A) Lateral radiograph of a tibia with a line from the anterior third of the joint to the center of the talus indicating the mechanical axis of the bone viewed in the sagittal plane. Even this more anterior entry point is problematic as the mechanical axis collides with the posterior endosteal cortex, indicating a challenge. A canal-filling stem introduced from this entry point will be deflected anteriorly at the tip resulting in unanticipated posterior slope; (B) Silhouette of a (NexGen) tibial component, as would be used for pre-op planning on a lateral radiograph, demonstrating the anterior location of the stem housing to attach modular stem extensions. This location is driven by tibial anatomy; (C) Intraoperative photograph of initial tibial preparation, looking down upon the proximal tibia after the failed component had been removed. The existing opening in the tibia corresponds to the component that was removed. The new opening has been marked with a pen as a rectangular (labeled 'entry point') to visualize the desired rotational position. It is as close to the anterior cortex as possible without jeopardizing the integrity of the cortical bone

straight stem extension is centered over the mid-diaphysis, the component will either be undersized or overhanging medially. The final option would be an undersized stem extension that dangles in the medullary canal, where it cannot contribute to fixation[73] (**Figures 22.11A to C**).

Once a trial tibial component has been satisfactorily inserted with solid, albeit temporary diaphyseal intramedullary fixation, the flexion gap can be stabilized. To reduce surgical time (and in turn surgical infection rates)[74] we can overlap Steps 1 and 2 when preparing the medullary canals with reamers. After a reamer is used on the tibia, it can be applied to the femur immediately. This saves progressing through the reamer sequence two times.

Surgical Technique Step 2A: The Flexion Gap and Femoral Component Rotation

The flexion gap, or the 'space between the proximal tibia (now defined by the trial tibial baseplate) and the posterior articular surface of the femoral component should be stabilized next. Different methods of determining the rotational position of the femoral component (rotation on the 'y' axis with the limb in the anatomic position) have been described. The proposed technique using the trans-epicondylar axis landmark for rotational positioning is predicated on the CT research data that shows problems with patellar tracking, anterior knee pain and stiffness when the femoral component deviates from the trans-epicondylar axis.[25,38,68] Rotational position derived as a function of soft tissue tensions (i.e. establishing a rectangular flexion gap) risks aberrant positioning, especially in revision surgery, because of soft tissue derangement. When soft tissue inadequacy is the problem, mechanical constraint is generally the answer. If some type of inter-condylar notch preparation is required for the revision implant system, that can be marked physically, even cut with the saw, as a visual reminder of desired femoral component rotation in this step.

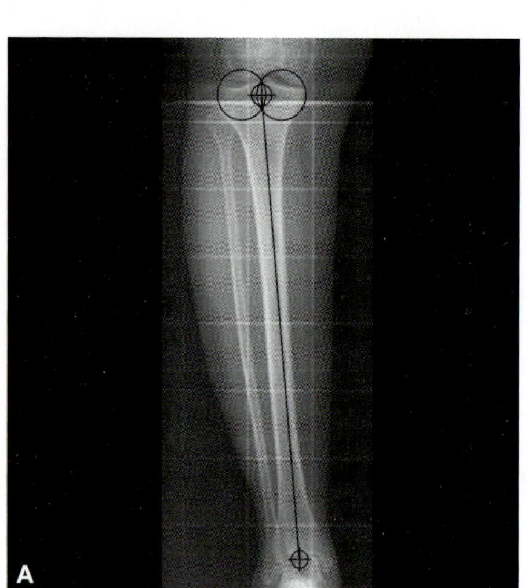

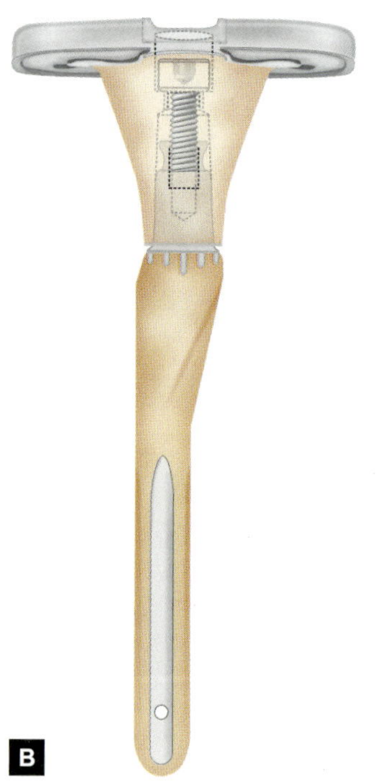

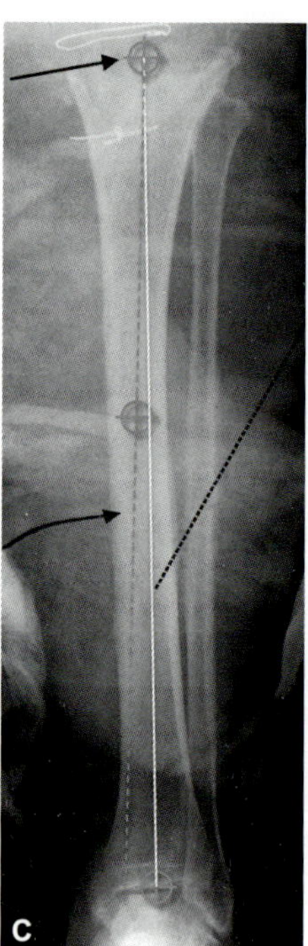

Figures 22.10A to C (A) AP radiograph of a tibia for anatomic evaluation. Bisected double circles at the knee joint locate the center of the knee and a line joining this to the center of the talus constitutes the mechanical axis of the tibia. The center of the diaphyseal canal is reliably about 4 mm medial to the center of the knee itself. This indicates that an entry point slightly medial to the center, with an offset stem should be an ideal combination; (B) Silhouette of a (NexGen) tibial component with a modular, offset 145 mm length stem extension attached, as would be used for preoperative planning on an AP radiograph. The offset stem was originally designed to be used in this position to accommodate the typical asymmetric anatomy of the tibia; (C) The typical anatomic challenge of canal filling, press fit diaphyseal length tibial stem extensions. The center of the knee is indicated by the top circle and cross hairs or 'target' (black arrow with straight shaft). The target indicates the resting point of a canal filling diaphyseal length stem and the lowest target indicates the center of the ankle. A solid vertical white line (indicated by dotted black line from right) represents the mechanical axis of the tibia. The dotted gray vertical line indicated by the curved solid black arrow is the typical position of a straight canal-filling stem: in several degrees of valgus

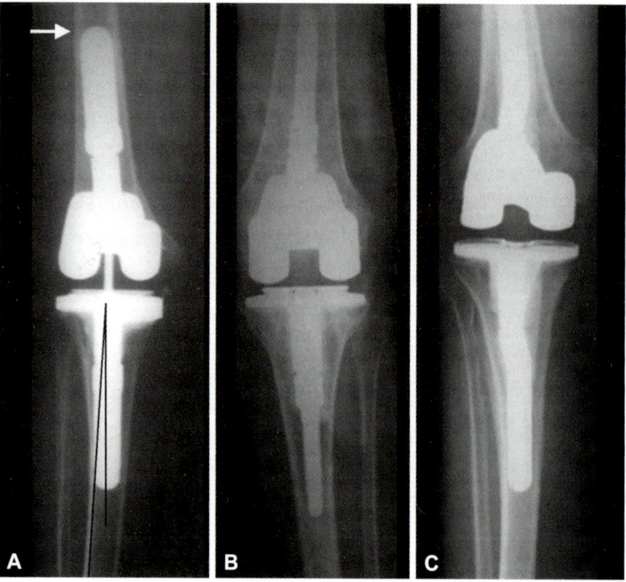

Figures 22.11A to C (A) Old style metaphyseal length press fit stem extensions. Canal fill has been achieved in this femur but with cortical reaction on the lateral side (arrow). The straight tibial stem fills the canal but at the expense of valgus alignment (Two fine black lines depict discrepancy between the tibial mechanical axis and the component position). This component failed from aseptic loosening; (B) So-called 'dangling stem' technique where undersized stem extensions are used and should not impede desired alignment. Without endosteal contact, it is difficult to understand how they can assist with fixation. Despite that, the tibial component is in valgus in this case; (C) Contemporary, favored approach, diaphyseal engaging, offset tibial stem of 145 mm length

Surgical Technique Step 2B: The Flexion Gap and Stability

The flexion gap is stabilized by femoral component size and position, plus the tibial baseplate and articular polyethylene insert. This combination can stabilize the knee only if the collateral ligaments have some structural integrity. Remembering that previous surgery and arthroplasty failure often change the entire stabilizing soft tissue envelope so that the femoral component size indicated by the radiographs prior to the primary surgery may or may not be the right size for the revision. The same knee joint may benefit from a different size of femoral component depending on the mode of failure and state of the ligaments. Imagine an arthroplasty having failed for stiffness versus instability. The former case requires a smaller component to restore function than the latter. Irrespective of the revision implant system, the *largest* femoral component that can be used for any knee is the one that has a medial-lateral dimension corresponding to the width of the distal femur. An implant so large that it hangs over the cortex medially or laterally would not be appropriate.

As with the tibia, the femoral technique is facilitated by diaphyseal engaging press fit stems that define and maintain component position. Begin by inserting the largest possible component, i.e. the one that extends from the medial to lateral cortex. The requisite modular articular polyethylene will stabilize the flexion gap when added to the trial tibial baseplate.

At this stage of the revision, five of the six degrees of freedom for the femoral component will be satisfied: varus-valgus (rotation on 'z') medial-lateral (translation on 'x'), flexion-extension (rotation on 'x') and anteroposterior (translation on 'z'). The best combination of femoral component size and tibial polyethylene thickness will be determined in the next step: 2c. Proximal-distal seating (translation on 'y') is reserved for the third and final step.

Surgical Technique Step 2C: Joint 'Line' in Flexion

The joint line has received considerable attention in revision knee arthroplasty,[75-85] all of which focuses narrowly on where the distal femur meets the polyethylene exclusively in full extension. This is a limited perspective, shaped by greater concern for the radiograph than the functioning knee itself.

The 'level of the articulation' should be recognized as a three dimensional construct and not simply a 'line.' This implies then, numerous joint lines, one for every degree of knee flexion. With our Three Step Technique, whatever joint line height the surgeon constructs in flexion during step 2c, will be replicated stably and accurately in Step 3, extension gap reconstruction.

During the preceding step, 2b, several combinations of decreasing femoral component size and increasing thickness of polyethylene may stabilize any flexion gap with intact collateral ligaments. The difference between each combination will be the level of the joint line, where the posterior femur contacts the tibia, in flexion and eventually in extension. Now, in Step 2c, the individual combination of femoral component size and tibial polyethylene thickness yielding both stability and the preferred joint line height will be selected.

The joint line position can be judged in several ways. An expedient method related to function will be the distance from the inferior pole of the patellar, after noting the state of the patellar tendon. After all, a tendon that has contracted will necessarily draw the patella more distally, known as 'patella infera' or 'patella baja' (**Figure 22.12**). Though clever techniques have been described to restore length to a contracted patellar tendon, (tibial tubercle osteotomy and proximal repositioning, 'Z' lengthening) they all risk rupture of the extensor.

Analysis of the joint line challenge leads to the logical conclusion that the best that can be accomplished in bringing a potentially elevated joint down maximally, will be the largest femoral component, i.e. the one that fits the femur from the medial to lateral cortex. A larger femoral component overhangs inappropriately and everything smaller means thicker polyethylene, a higher joint line in flexion, more resection of distal femur to accommodate that polyethylene in extension and *ergo,* a higher joint line in extension. If the flexion gap is stabilized with the correct joint line height, this will automatically follow in extension. The converse is not true.

One of two indications for constrained components will be inability to stabilize the knee in flexion (Step 2b) with the

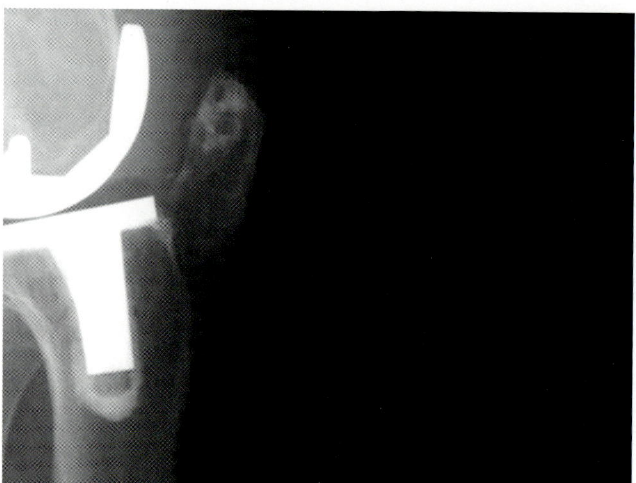

Figure 22.12 Lateral radiograph of a painful TKA performed for post-traumatic arthritis in a patient with an old femur fracture. The patella 'baja' or patella 'infera' could hardly be more extreme. The true pathology is that the patellar tendon is now a short, scarred, leathery hinge, not the supple flexible structure it should be. Elevation of the tibial tubercle will not treat that problem but may risk avulsion if the tip of the tubercle is situated above the base of the tibial cut. The patient also had significant malrotation of the tibial and femoral components that was corrected with revision. Pain was decreased and motion improved slightly. Patellar height was not addressed directly with tendon lengthening or tubercle osteotomy

largest femoral component and the thickest polyethylene insert, even when metal augments have been added to the tibia baseplate. This situation is a clear indication that the collateral ligaments have suffered plastic deformation and that the knee must be stabilized mechanically, with a nonlinked or linked (hinged) prostheses, depending on the degree of laxity and the preference of the surgeon[32]. At the completion of Step 2c all the difficult kinematic work has been accomplished:

- Tibial baseplate size and orientation for all 6 degrees of freedom
- Tibial articular polyethylene thickness plus consideration of one indication for constrained implants
- Femoral component size and position for 5 of 6 degrees of freedom.

Surgical Technique Step 3: The Extension Gap

The proximal-distal seating of the femoral component (translation on 'y') and consideration of the second indication for constraint (collateral ligament inadequacy in extension and 30 degrees of flexion) are the goals of Step 3, the extension gap. This step is extremely simple as a result of the work accomplished in the previous steps. With all the components selected and temporarily stabilized by diaphyseal engaging stems, which yet allow the femoral component to 'slide' proximally, the surgeon slowly and fully extends the knee, leaving neither recurvatum nor flexion contracture. This pushes the femoral component more proximally, though perhaps not far enough to contact the residual distal femoral condyle by the time the posterior soft tissues are tight. The residual space between the end of the femur and the inside of the prosthesis indicates the need for augmentation of the distal femur. In the unique case of revision for stiffness, it may be necessary to remove additional distal femur bone to achieve full extension even if the posterior capsular contraction has been released surgically.

Stabilizing the flexion gap first is efficient, by choosing between *incremental and discrete* sizes of components. The balance achieved in flexion can be matched precisely in extension, on a *continuum,* by sliding the femoral component to the right position—millimeter for millimeter.[86]

This returns to the 'keys' of revision TKA:

- The femoral component determines soft tissue balance
- The flexion gap is determined by femoral component size
- The extension gap is determined by femoral component position.

The indications for constraint are based on soft tissue integrity and the inability to stabilize the knee in flexion or extension. Constraint is not the best answer to bone loss.

REFERENCES

1. Groopman JE. How doctors think. Boston, MA: Houghton Mifflin; 2007.p. 307.
2. Wikipedia. Heuristic 2013. *http://en.wikipedia.org/wiki/Heuristic - cite_note-12.*
3. Moreland JR. Mechanisms of failure in total knee arthroplasty. Clin Orthop. 1988;226:49-64.

4. Vince K. Modes of Failure in Total Knee Arthroplasty. In: al BDe (Ed.), Advanced Reconstruction of the Knee: American Academy of Orthopedic Surgeons; 2011. pp. 341-54.
5. Vince KG. Why knees fail. J Arthroplasty. 2003;18:39-44.
6. Wardrop D. Ockham's razor: sharpen or re-sheathe? J R Soc Med. 2008;101(2):50-1.
7. Parvizi J, Della Valle CJ. AAOS Clinical Practice Guideline: diagnosis and treatment of periprosthetic joint infections of the hip and knee. J Am Acad Orthop Surg. 2010;18(12):771-2.
8. Della Valle C, Parvizi J, Bauer TW, et al. American academy of orthopedic surgeons clinical practice guideline on: the diagnosis of periprosthetic joint infections of the hip and knee. J Bone Joint Surg Am. 2011;93(14):1355-7.
9. Parvizi J, Zmistowski B, Berbari EF, et al. New definition for periprosthetic joint infection: from the workgroup of the musculoskeletal infection society. Clin Orthop Relat Res. 2011;469(11):2992-4.
10. Munjal S, Phillips MJ, Krackow KA. Revision total knee arthroplasty: planning, controversies, and management--infection. Instr Course Lect. 2001;50:367-77.
11. Mangram AJ, Horan TC, Pearson ML, Silver LC, Jarvis WR. Guideline for prevention of surgical site infection, 1999. Centers for disease control and prevention (CDC) hospital infection control practices advisory committee. Am J Infect Control. 1999;27(2):97-132.
12. Vince KG, Abdeen A. Wound problems in total knee arthroplasty. Clin Orthop Relat Res. 2006;452:88-90.
13. Vince K, Chivas D, Droll KP. Wound complications after total knee arthroplasty. J Arthroplasty. 2007;22:39-44.
14. Galat DD, McGovern SC, Larson DR, et al. Surgical treatment of early wound complications following primary total knee arthroplasty. J Bone Joint Surg Am. 2009;91(1):48-54.
15. Jaberi FM, Parvizi J, Haytmanek CT, Joshi A, Purtill J. Procrastination of wound drainage and malnutrition affect the outcome of joint arthroplasty. Clin Orthop Relat Res. 2008;466(6):1368-71.
16. Patel VP, Walsh M, Sehgal B, et al. Factors associated with prolonged wound drainage after primary total hip and knee arthroplasty. J Bone Joint Surg Am. 2007;89(1):33-8.
17. Weiss AP, Krackow KA. Persistent wound drainage after primary total knee arthroplasty. J Arthroplasty. 1993;8(3):285-9.
18. Parkinson RW, Kay PR, Rawal A. A case for one-stage revision in infected total knee arthroplasty? Knee. 2011;18(1):1-4.
19. Leone JM, Hanssen AD. Management of infection at the site of a total knee arthroplasty. Instr Course Lect. 2006;55:449-61.
20. Jacobs MA, Hungerford DS, Krackow KA, Lennox DW. Revision total knee arthroplasty for aseptic failure. Clin Orthop. 1988;226:78-85.
21. Hendel D, Weisbort M, Garti A. 'Wandering resident' surgical exposure for 1- or 2-stage revision arthroplasty in stiff aseptic and septic knee arthroplasty. J Arthroplasty. 2004;19(6):757-9.
22. Vince K. Extensor Mechanism Disruption After Total Knee Arthroplasty. In: N S (Ed.) Insall and Scott: Surgery of the Knee, 5th edn. Philadelphia: Elsevier - Churchill Livingstone; 2011. pp. 1386-410.
23. Vince K, Nakasone C. Extensor Mechanism Disruption after Total Knee Arthroplasty. In: Scott NW (Ed.) Surgery of The Knee. New York: Churchill-Livingstone; 2005.
24. Vince K EE. The Stiff TKA. In: Harner CFF, Vince K (Eds), Knee Surgery, 2nd edn. Baltimore: Lippincott Williams and Wilkins; 1994. pp. 1529-38.
25. Bedard M, Vince KG, Redfern J, Collen SR. Internal rotation of the tibial component is frequent in stiff total knee arthroplasty. Clin Orthop Relat Res. 2011;469(8):2346-55.
26. Parvizi J, Tarity TD, Steinbeck MJ, et al. Management of stiffness following total knee arthroplasty. J Bone Joint Surg Am. 2006;88:175-81.
27. Vince KG, Abdeen A, Sugimori T. The unstable total knee arthroplasty: causes and cures. J Arthroplasty. 2006;21:44-9.
28. Vince KG. Diagnosis and management of patients with instability of the knee. Instr Course Lect. 2012;61:515-24.
29. Berry P, Trousdale and Dennis (Eds), Revision of Total Hip and Knee Arthroplasty. Philadelphia: Lippincott Williams and Wilkins; 2006.
30. Malo MaVK. Laxités fémorotibiales des prothèses totales du genou. In: Burdin P HD (Ed), Reprises de prothèses totales du genou. Paris, France: Elsevier; 2003. pp. 129-43.
31. Insall J. Total Knee Arthroplasty. In: Insall J (Ed.), Surgery of the Knee. New York: Churchill Livingstone; 1984.pp. 1478-552.
32. Vince K, Bedard M, Ebramzedah E. Balancing the Revision TKA. Restraint with Constraint. In: Brown T (Ed),

Arthritis and Arthroplasty- The Knee: Elsevier; 2009. pp. 203-11.
33. Pagnano MW, Hanssen AD, Lewallen DG, Stuart MJ. Flexion instability after primary posterior cruciate retaining total knee arthroplasty. Clin Orthop. 1998;356:39-46.
34. Schwab JH, Haidukewych GJ, Hanssen AD, Jacofsky DJ, Pagnano MW. Flexion instability without dislocation after posterior stabilized total knees. Clin Orthop Relat Res. 2005 Nov;440:96-100. PubMed PMID: 16239790. Epub 2005/10/22. eng.
35. Martin JW, Whiteside LA. The influence of joint line position on knee stability after condylar knee arthroplasty. Clin Orthop. 1990;259:146-56.
36. Konig C, Matziolis G, Sharenkov A, et al. Collateral ligament length change patterns after joint line elevation may not explain midflexion instability following TKA. Medical engineering & physics. 2011;33(10):1303-8.
37. McPherson EJ, Cuckler J, Lombardi AV. Midflexion instability in revision total knee arthroplasty. Surg Technol Int. 2008;17:249-52.
38. Berger RA, Crossett LS, Jacobs JJ, Rubash HE. Malrotation causing patellofemoral complications after total knee arthroplasty. Clin Orthop Relat Res. 1998;356:144-53.
39. Tharani R, Nakasone C, Vince KG. Periprosthetic fractures after total knee arthroplasty. J Arthroplasty. 2005;20(4 Suppl 2):27-32. PubMed PMID: 15991125. Epub 2005/07/02. eng.
40. Vince K CR, Morgan-Jones R. The Knee Arthroplasty Endgame: Four Options in the Face of Calamity. In: Hirschmann M (Ed), The unhappy total knee replacement-a comprehensive review and management guide. in press. Zurich: Springer-Verlag.
41. Howie DW, Vernon-Roberts B. The synovial response to intraarticular cobalt-chrome wear particles. Clin Orthop. 1988;232:244-54.
42. Howie DW, Vernon-Roberts B, Oakeshott R, Manthey B. A rat model of resorption of bone at the cement-bone interface in the presence of polyethylene wear particles. J Bone Joint Surg Am. 1988;70(2):257-63.
43. Pagnano MW, Scuderi GR, Insall JN. Tibial osteolysis associated with the modular tibial tray of a cemented posterior stabilized total knee replacement: a case report. J Bone Joint Surg Am. 2001;83-A(10):1545-8.
44. Vince K. Revision Total Knee Arthroplasty and Arthrodesis of the Knee. In: Chapman M (Ed) Operative Orthopedics. Philadelphia: Lippincott Willimas & Wilkins; 2001. pp. 2897-952.
45. Krackow KA, Hungerford DS, Kenna RV. Results of Uncemented Total Knee Arthroplasty using the PCA System. Total Knee Replacement: Springer; 1991. pp. 183-92.
46. Bechtold JE, Kubic V, Soballe K. A controlled experimental model of revision implants: Part I. Development. Acta Orthop Scand. 2001;72(6):642-9.
47. Bugbee WD, Ammeen DJ, Engh GA. Does implant selection affect outcome of revision knee arthroplasty? J Arthroplasty. 2001;16(5):581-5.
48. Vince K. Planning revision total knee arthroplasty. Semin Arthroplasty. 1996;7(4):301-13.
49. Vince KG, Long W. Revision knee arthroplasty. The limits of press fit medullary fixation. Clin Orthop. 1995;317:172-7.
50. Vince K, Bedard M. Implanting the Revision Total Knee Arthroplasty. In: Lotke PA, Lonner J (Eds), Master Techniques in Orthopedic Surgery. Baltimore: Lippincott Williams and Wilkins; 2008. pp. 203-28.
51. Lachiewicz PF, Bolognesi MP, Henderson RA, Soileau ES, Vail TP. Can tantalum cones provide fixation in complex revision knee arthroplasty? Clinical Orthop Relat Res. 2011. http://www.ncbi.nlm.nih.gov/pubmed/21465329.
52. Lachiewicz PF, Bolognesi MP, Henderson RA, Soileau ES, Vail TP. Can tantalum cones provide fixation in complex revision knee arthroplasty? Clin Orthop Relat Res. 2012;470(1):199-204.
53. Howard JL, Kudera J, Lewallen DG, Hanssen AD. Early results of the use of tantalum femoral cones for revision total knee arthroplasty. J Bone Joint Surg Am. 2011;93(5):478-84.
54. Meneghini RM, Lewallen DG, Hanssen AD. Use of porous tantalum metaphyseal cones for severe tibial bone loss during revision total knee replacement. J Bone Joint Surg Am. 2008;90(1):78-84.
55. Derome P, Sternheim A, Backstein D, Malo M. Treatment of large bone defects with trabecular metal cones in revision total knee arthroplasty: short term clinical and radiographic outcomes. J Arthroplasty. 2013.
56. Jensen CL, Petersen MM, Schroder HM, Flivik G, Lund B. Revision total knee arthroplasty with the use of trabecular

metal cones: a randomized radiostereometric analysis with 2 years of follow-up. J Arthroplasty. 2012.
57. Schildhauer TA, Peter E, Muhr G, Koller M. Activation of human leukocytes on tantalum trabecular metal in comparison to commonly used orthopedic metal implant materials. J Biomed Mater Res A. 2009;88(2):332-41.
58. Satish BR, Ganesan JC, Chandran P, Basanagoudar PL, Balachandar D. Efficacy and mid term results of lateral parapatellar approach without tibial tubercle osteotomy for primary total knee arthroplasty in fixed valgus knees. J Arthroplasty. 2013.
59. Sharkey PF, Homesley HD, Shastri S, et al. Results of revision total knee arthroplasty after exposure of the knee with extensor mechanism tenolysis. J Arthroplasty. 2004;19(6):751-6.
60. Fehring TK, Odum S, Griffin WL, Mason JB. Outcome comparison of partial and full component revision TKA. Clin Orthop Relat Res. 2005;440:131-4.
61. Mackay DC, Siddique MS. The results of revision knee arthroplasty with and without retention of secure cemented femoral components. J Bone Joint Surg Br. 2003;85(4):517-20.
62. Babis GC, Trousdale RT, Morrey BF. The effectiveness of isolated tibial insert exchange in revision total knee arthroplasty. J Bone Joint Surg Am. 2002;84-A(1):64-8.
63. Babis GC, Trousdale RT, Pagnano MW, Morrey BF. Poor outcomes of isolated tibial insert exchange and arthrolysis for the management of stiffness following total knee arthroplasty. J Bone Joint Surg Am. 2001;83-A(10):1534-6.
64. Vince KG, Abdeen A. Revision TKA: four cases that taught me new things. Orthopedics. 2006;29(9):853-5.
65. Gardner J, Gioe TJ, Tatman P. Can this prosthesis be saved?: implant salvage attempts in infected primary TKA. Clin Orthop Relat Res. 2011;469(4):970-6.
66. Garcia RM, Kraay MJ, Goldberg VM. Isolated resurfacing of the previously unresurfaced patella total knee arthroplasty. J Arthroplasty. 2009.
67. Khatod M, Codsi M, Bierbaum B. Results of resurfacing a native patella in patients with a painful total knee arthroplasty. J Knee Surg. 2004;17(3):151-5.
68. Barrack RL, Schrader T, Bertot AJ, Wolfe MW, Myers L. Component rotation and anterior knee pain after total knee arthroplasty. Clin Orthop Relat Res. 2001;392:46-55.
69. Freeman MA, Insall JN, Besser W, Walker PS, Hallel T. Excision of the cruciate ligaments in total knee replacement. Clin Orthop. 1977;126:209-12.
70. Insall J, Ranawat CS, Scott WN, Walker P. Total condylar knee replacement: preliminary report. Clin Orthop Relat Res. 1976;120:149-54.
71. Vince KG. Revision knee arthroplasty technique. Instr Course Lect. 1993;42:325-39.
72. Nakasone CK, Abdeen A, Khachatourians AG, Sugimori T, Vince KG. Component alignment in revision total knee arthroplasty using diaphyseal engaging modular offset press-fit stems. J Arthroplasty. 2008;23(8):1178-81.
73. Haas SB, Insall JN, Montgomery W, 3rd, Windsor RE. Revision total knee arthroplasty with use of modular components with stems inserted without cement. J Bone Joint Surg Am. 1995;77(11):1700-7.
74. Namba RS, Inacio MC, Paxton EW. Risk factors associated with deep surgical site infections after primary total knee arthroplasty: an analysis of 56,216 knees. J Bone Joint Surg Am. 2013;95(9):775-82.
75. Iacono F, Lo Presti M, Bruni D, et al. The adductor tubercle: a reliable landmark for analysing the level of the femorotibial joint line. Knee Surg Sports Traumatol Arthrosc. 2012.
76. Tang Q, Zhou Y, Yang D, Tang J, Shao H. The knee joint line position measured from the tibial side in Chinese people. J Arthroplasty. 2011;26(7):989-93.
77. Romero J, Seifert B, Reinhardt O, Ziegler O, Kessler O. A useful radiologic method for preoperative joint-line determination in revision total knee arthroplasty. Clin Orthop Relat Res. 2010;468(5):1279-83.
78. Servien E, Viskontas D, Giuffre BM, Coolican MR, Parker DA. Reliability of bony landmarks for restoration of the joint line in revision knee arthroplasty. Knee Surg Sports Traumatol Arthrosc. 2008;16(3):263-9.
79. Havet E, Gabrion A, Leiber-Wackenheim F, et al. Radiological study of the knee joint line position measured from the fibular head and proximal tibial landmarks. Surg Radiol Anat. 2007;29(4):285-9.
80. Perlick L, Luring C, Tingart M, Grifka J, Bathis H. [Revision prosthetic of the knee joint. The influence of a navigation system on the alignment and reconstruction of the joint line]. Orthopade. 2006;35(10):1080-6.

81. Mason M, Belisle A, Bonutti P, et al. An accurate and reproducible method for locating the joint line during a revision total knee arthroplasty. J Arthroplasty. 2006;21(8):1147-53.
82. Mahoney OM, Kinsey TL. Modular femoral offset stems facilitate joint line restoration in revision knee arthroplasty. Clin Orthop Relat Res. 2006;446:93-8.
83. Hofmann AA, Kurtin SM, Lyons S, Tanner AM, Bolognesi MP. Clinical and radiographic analysis of accurate restoration of the joint line in revision total knee arthroplasty. J Arthroplasty. 2006;21(8):1154-62.
84. ten Ham AM, Wymenga AB, Jacobs WC. The use of the knee joint-line balancer to control patella position in revision total knee arthroplasty. Knee. 2005;12(2):89-92.
85. Partington PF, Sawhney J, Rorabeck CH, Barrack RL, Moore J. Joint line restoration after revision total knee arthroplasty. Clin Orthop. 1999;367:165-71.
86. Vince KG, Droll KP, Chivas D. Your next revision total knee arthroplasty: why start in flexion? Orthopedics. 2007;30(9):791-2.

Chapter 23

Current Practices in Diagnosing Periprosthetic Infection in Knee

Karthikeyan Chinnakkannu, Javad Parvizi

INTRODUCTION

Total knee arthroplasty (TKA) is one of the most successful surgeries performed worldwide. Periprosthetic joint infection (PJI) often compromises the result of TKA that is the most common cause in United States[1] and second most common complication of TKA worldwide.[2] It is devastating not only by affecting the lifestyle of the patient with significant mortality and morbidity and increasing his economic burden, it also impacts the healthcare burden of the community as a whole.[3-6] The current incidence of PJI in TKA is between 1.1% and 2.0%.[7,8] Although the percentage is low, the absolute numbers are expected to rise because of increasing number of TKAs each year.[9-12] Diagnosing periprosthetic infection is demanding and requires thorough clinical examination and combination of tests as there is no single gold standard test to do it. This chapter will discuss about systemic approach to diagnose PJI.

Definition of Periprosthetic Infection

International Consensus Meeting on Periprosthetic Joint Infection (ICM PJI 2013) modified Musculoskeletal Infection Society (MSIS) criteria and defined periprosthetic infection as two positive periprosthetic cultures with phenotypically identical organisms, or A sinus tract communicating with the joint, or having three of the following minor criteria:

- Elevated serum erythrocyte sedimentation rate (ESR) and C-reactive protein (CRP)
- Elevated synovial fluid white blood cell (WBC) count or ++ change on leukocyte esterase test strip
- Elevated synovial fluid neutrophil percentage (PMN %)
- Positive histological analysis of periprosthetic tissue
- A single positive culture.

HISTORY AND PHYSICAL EXAMINATION

The first and foremost step in any suspected case of PJI is complete history and clinical examination.[13] The history of persistent pain in the joint and stiffness should raise a high suspicion regarding PJI. It is suggested that in all the patients who are undergoing revision for aseptic failure, infection should be ruled out.[14]

Any focus of infection suggestive of recent bacteremia (urinary tract infection, infective endocarditis, dental procedure), multiple surgeries on the same joint, history of PJI, conditions predisposing to an immunocompromised state (e.g. diabetes mellitus, inflammatory arthropathy, malnourishment, steroid intake, and dialysis), smoking, obesity, intravenous drug use, wound insufficiency, psoriasis, chronic venous stasis, or skin ulceration, and superficial surgical site infection related to the joint also should arise the suspicion of PJI.[7,15,16]

During physical examination if there is sinus communicating with joint, it is pathognomonic sign of PJI. One also should look for joint warmth, redness, swelling, wound inflammation/dehiscence, pain during range of movements, and stiffness.

X-RAY

After clinical examination, plain radiographs of the corresponding joint should be obtained. At least two projections should be obtained to visualize all the areas around the implant. It is also necessary to check the exposure of the films because they may produce false results. Although plain radiographs may not show any changes, it is recommended to do plain radiographs as part of initial set of investigation to rule out other causes of failure.

Serial radiographs have more value than single one. Findings suggestive of PJI are subperiosteal bone formation, transcortical sinus tracts, erosion of the endosteal profile, and early loosening of well-fixed implant (**Figures 23.1A and B**). Plain radiographs are not only inexpensive they also help to rule out other apparent causes like wear, malposition.

It should be kept in mind that plain radiographs have poor sensitivity, and sometimes may take a few months from the onset of PJI to show visible radiological signs. Although plain radiographs give information about bone and implant interface, they are poor indicators of what is happening in the surrounding soft tissues.

SEROLOGY

After clinical examination and radiograph, the ESR and CRP form the initial set of investigations. They are excellent screening tests and American Academy of Orthopaedic Surgeons (AAOS) guidelines recommend these tests in any case of suspected PJI.[17] It is one of the minor criteria defining the periprosthetic infection.

ESR and CRP are nonspecific inflammatory markers; their levels rise immediately after surgery. In TKA patients,

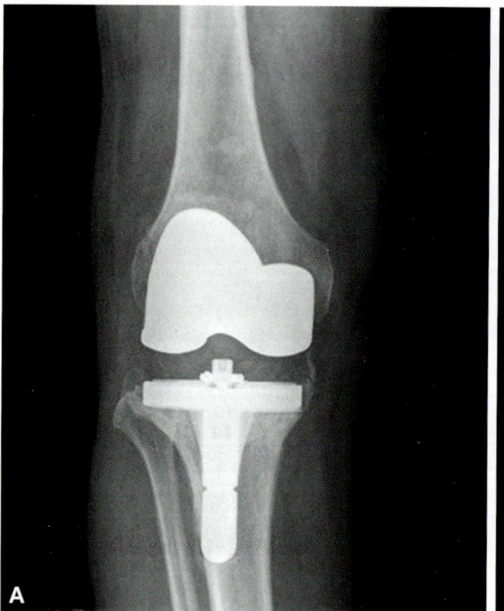

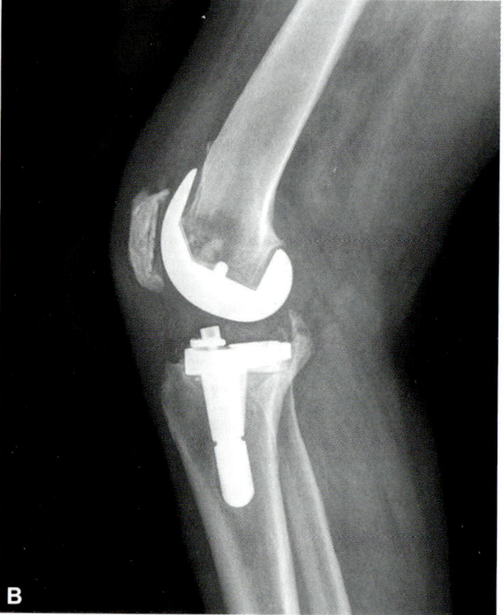

Figures 23.1A and B Loosening of femoral and tibial components in periprosthetic joint infection (Three-phase bone scintigraphy)

ESR and CRP reach their respective peak 5–7 days and 3 days after surgery and return to normal around 3 months and 3 weeks, respectively.

Although ESR and CRP are nonspecific, they have good sensitivity in detecting the PJI.[17-21] Both are good at ruling out infection, CRP is more reliable in 'ruling in' the infection than ESR.[21] Instead of using either test separately combination of both has good post-test probability of predicting the infection.[18] Spangehl et al. found no cases of periprosthetic infection in total hip arthroplasty (THA) patients with normal ESR and CRP.[22]

Advantages of these serological tests are that they are inexpensive and good in ruling out infection, although they are elevated in inflammatory disorders cutoff values for diagnosis of PJI remain same.[21] The disadvantages of these tests are not good at ruling in when either test is used alone (although CRP is somewhat better), their value may vary according to age and sex, and may be elevated in other infections, inflammatory diseases and in acute postoperative period. They are also not useful in determining the control of infection in the acute postoperative period.[23]

The currently accepted criteria for diagnosis of PJI greater than 6 weeks from most recent surgery are (approximately) ESR > 30 mm/h, CRP > 10 mg/L.[7] The threshold for diagnosing or ruling out PJI less than 6 weeks from most recent surgery is approximately CRP >100 mg/L. ESR is not used in acute postoperative period because of its nonreliability.

If all of these tests (history, clinical examination, X-ray, and serological tests) are normal, there is less likelihood of infection. If any of tests are positive, this indicates a high suspicion of infection and it should be followed by joint aspiration.

KNEE JOINT ASPIRATION

The suspicion of infection or abnormal X-ray/serology should lead to aspiration of the joint, as per the American Academy of Orthopaedic Surgeons guidelines on PJI. Normally knee aspiration is done under local/surface anesthesia.

Under aseptic precautions, knee joint is aspirated using the medial or lateral patellofemoral approach. One study that evaluated the accurate needle placement for injection suggested lateral midpatellar approach in the joints without swelling.[24] But its application in aspiration in compared with others has not been evaluated. It is recommended to stop the antibiotics at least 2 weeks before the aspiration to avoid false negative results.[25]

Dry tap can be encountered in small number of patients. If dry tap occurs, aspiration can be repeated by repositioning the needle without drawing it out of the skin. If the aspiration is still negative, few authors recommend aspiration following saline injection.

Aspirate should be evaluated for cell count, PMNs count, and culture. If saline is used, then aspirated fluid is not representative one, so WBC and neutrophil count has less value and likely to produce false negative results on culture.[26] Synovial fluid should be sent in blood culture tube to maximize the outcomes.[27]Alternatively similar results can be obtained using BACTEC and radiometric broth. If fluid is blood stained, it can be adjusted according to red blood cells (RBCs) present.[28]

Ultrasound can be used for aspiration and it helps to evaluate the location and quantity of fluid in addition to aiding needle placement for aspiration. But like other ultrasound-guided procedures, it is subject to variation depending on the person's expertise. Fluoroscopic guidance can be used to determine the accuracy of needle placement but is associated with radiation exposure.

Although aspiration of knee joint is a quick and easy procedure, the risk of introducing the infection into the joint always remains and is contraindicated in presence of superficial infection/cellulitis. Ultrasound may be of help in those situations by finding superficial collections and passing needle by avoiding them.

Although joint aspiration has been used in the diagnosis of native joint infection, and in the diagnosis of PJI for the past two to three decades, the consensus regarding criteria for diagnosing PJI based on synovial fluid analysis has been reached only recently.

The current recommendation for diagnosis of PJI is shown in **Table 23.1**.

But when either ESR or CRP is elevated, higher cutoff point is suggested. Schinsky et al. in analysis of perioperative markers in THA suggested cutoff of WBC>9000/μL in synovial fluid when either of these is elevated.[29]

TABLE 23.1 Test values or threshold for diagnosis of PJI

The thresholds for diagnosis of PJI within 6 weeks (acute PJI) from most recent surgery are as follows: • CRP > 100 mg/L • Synovial WBC count > 10,000 cells/μL • Synovial PMN% > 90%.
The thresholds for diagnosis of PJI greater than 6 weeks (chronic PJI) from most recent surgery are as follows: • ESR > 30 mm/h • CRP > 10 mg/L • Synovial WBC count > 3000 cells /μL • Synovial PMN% > 80%

It is recommended that synovial fluid analysis is performed within 6 hours. If there is delay, it should be collected in EDTA tubes. The cell count and neutrophil count are not affected for at least 24 hours, if EDTA has been used.[30] Automated counters produce accurate result rather than the manual ones in counting WBC and PMNs in synovial fluid.[30,31]

Aspiration should be repeated if there is a high suspicion of infection or only one positive culture is obtained with other criteria in cases of dry aspiration. The aspirated fluid should be sent for AFB and fungal culture in addition to the routine WBC, PMNs, and bacterial culture.

If cultures are negative or only one minor criterion is positive, then the surgeon should proceed to next step and perform other investigations to rule out infection.

SYNOVIAL CRP

Synovial CRP is normally elevated in periprosthetic infections and has been tried as a marker to detect infections. Synovial CRP is found to have good sensitivity, specificity, and accuracy in the diagnosis PJI. Synovial CRP as a marker for PJI has accuracy of 92–93% when using the cutoff value of 3.7 mg/dL.[32,33]

Leukocyte Esterase

Leukocyte esterase is an enzyme secreted by neutrophils, which migrate to sites of infection. When infected synovial fluid is exposed to leukocyte esterase strips, they produce color change and are in considered positive. It is included as one of the minor criteria in the definition of PJI.

Parvizi et al. first tested the ability of enzyme to differentiate between septic and aseptic PJI using leukocyte esterase strip in knees. They found this test has sensitivity, specificity, PPV, and NPV value of 80%, 100%, 100%, and 93%, respectively. The test also showed correlation with ESR, CRP, synovial fluid WBC count, and PMNs percentage. The advantage of the test is it is simple, cost-effective, and fast. Blood staining should be avoided during aspiration as it may potentially affect the results.[34] Overall this test has sensitivity and specificity of 80–100% and 87–100%, respectively.[34-36]

BIOPSY

Culture of the organism from periprosthetic tissue has been considered as standard by many for diagnosing PJI. Tissue biopsy for culture can be obtained preoperatively or intraoperatively during the surgery. If biopsy is obtained preoperatively, arthroscopic method is the preferred one. Alternatives to arthroscopic biopsy are mini-open or image-guided biopsy. If arthroscopy is used, it is done via routine portals to obtain tissue sample. Advantage of arthroscopic procedure is that it is as good as intraoperative samples in identifying inflamed areas, can identify the risk of wear particles, and debris can be removed during the same procedure. The disadvantage is scratching the implants and chance of infection during the procedure.

The biopsy tissue is normally obtained from femur, tibia, bone-implant interface, and periprosthetic tissue. It is advised to get three to five samples from representative areas to increase the probability of the growth of organisms in culture. The biopsy sample at the same time can be used for histopathological examination.

CULTURE

Culture of the infecting organism in two or more samples confirms the diagnosis of periprosthetic infection. Aspirated synovial fluid, intraoperative swabs, periprosthetic tissue, and sonicated fluid are commonly used for inoculation.

Cultures are usually kept for 5–14 days. In suspected cases of PJI with low virulent organisms or preoperative cultures that do not show any growth cultures can be extended for up to 14 days. Studies have shown that increasing the duration of culture up to 14 days does not compromise the results while improving the sensitivity[37-39] and chances to identifying the *Propionibacterium acnes*. There is chance of missing infection in 24% of culture negative cases if the duration is not extended.[39] When culture comes negative, it is better to discuss with concerned microbiologist regarding further steps in identifying the organism.

Current recommendation for AFB and fungal culture is only for those cases with high suspicion of PJI due to atypical organisms because the AFB and fungal organisms form less than 1% of periprosthetic infections.[40] In those cases, Lowenstein-Jensen medium, Middlebrook agar, BBL mycobacteria growth indicator tube for AFB and sheep blood agar, and Sabouraud agar for fungus can be used. It may be necessary to keep cultures up to 8 weeks to identify the organisms.

Despite best of efforts culture can be false negative due to use of prolonged antibiotics. But it is important to note that use of preoperative prophylactic antibiotic does not affect culture results.[41,42] In those culture negative cases, sonication of explanted implant and culture/polymerase chain reaction (PCR) may be useful.

Role of Sonication of Implants

Sonication is one of the techniques recommended to identify the organism in the PJI. It is based on the principle that organisms are released from the biofilm when they are subjected to ultrasound exposure. It is highly useful in identifying the biofilm forming organisms.[43]

From previously published results, sonication is superior in identification of organism than culture of preoperative aspiration or from the intraoperative tissue samples.[43,44] Sonication of implant is better than scraping in the detection of organisms.[45] Multiple sampling increases the detection of organism rather than a single one.[44] Sonication is useful in identifying the organism even if antibiotic was used within 2 weeks. Usually after sonication, sonicated fluid is subjected to culture or PCR.

The factors affecting sonication are type of organism, duration of exposure, temperature of the sonication fluid, and the type of sonication tube used. Through the literature different methods and settings have been used for sonication. Monsen et al.[46] suggested optimum condition for sonication of implants to be done in thin-walled glass tubes, at 22°C, for 7 minutes. Higher temperature or increased duration of exposure may result in death of organisms and result in negative growth. Gram-positive bacteria are more resistant to USG than gram-negative ones.[46]Using polyethylene bags may result in leakage and contamination of specimen.[47]

Current recommendation of sonication is to use it only for those cases in which preoperatively organism is not identified or the aspirated fluid did not show any results. Although it increases the detection of organism, the issues related to cost and availability are its disadvantages.

The rapidity of detection of organisms is increased when microcalorimetry is used instead of culture. It is based on measuring heat production during biological processes of microorganisms. Its sensitivity is higher because it can detect as low as 10 CFU/mL. The disadvantage is it cannot identify the specific organism, and so needs other methods to be performed subsequently to identify the organism. It can be useful in detection of antimicrobial resistance.[48] But further studies are needed to use this method routinely.

Histopathology and Frozen Section

Histopathology and frozen sections are used along with intraoperative cultures to diagnose the periprosthetic infection. They are more useful when preoperative investigations and culture fail to identify the infection. Although high number of surgeons believes it is confirmatory of periprosthetic infection, it is prone to false negative results.

Finding of 5–10 neutrophils/HPF in at least 5 fields is considered as indicative of infection. While counting, neutrophils entrapped in fibrin should not be included. They may give false positive results in diagnosing infection.

The suggested areas of sampling for histopathology and frozen section are from tibia, femur, bone-prosthesis interface, and surrounding tissue. Minimum of three and maximum of six samples can be sent for the evaluation. They should be sent immediately to the lab or in case of permanent section it should be stored in formalin.

The advantages are it is quick and simple and usually performed during the surgery. The disadvantages are false negative due to failure to obtain appropriate samples, delay in sending the samples to lab (delay may result in migration and perivascular extravasation), bacterial contamination, previous use of antibiotic within 2 weeks, and false positives due to other inflammations, fastidious organisms that fail to grow in culture and lymphocytes may resemble neutrophils and get counted. As with any other histopathology examination, it also requires an experienced pathologist to identify these changes. From meta-analysis by Tsaras et al., it should be noted that while frozen section is good for ruling in, it is poor in ruling out the infection.[49]

ALGORITHM FOR DIAGNOSIS OF PJI

Modified AAOS algorithm that has been adopted by the International Consensus Meeting on PJI is used for diagnosis of periprosthetic infections/septic failure (**Flow chart 23.1**).

OTHER IMAGING MODALITIES

Ultrasound

Role of ultrasound in periprosthetic infection of TKA is limited. Although they are used to diagnose effusion and guiding aspiration in THA, their application is limited in knee because most of the collections are visible or can be aspirated blindly. In spite of this they can be used in cases of dry aspiration and to rule out superficial collections before aspiration. By detecting/ruling out superficial abscess, they help in guiding the needle and thus prevent contamination of the joint.

Computed Tomography and Magnetic Resonance Imaging

Computed tomography (CT) is helpful in identifying and defining the sinus tracts, effusions, abscess, bony erosion, implant malpositioning, and loosening than plain radiographs. But the role of CT is limited in the diagnosis of PJI because of artifacts associated with implants and most of the time they do not add detail to the plain radiographs. So, CT is currently not recommended for routine evaluation.

MRI is better than CT in detecting periprosthetic collections and soft tissue abnormalities. But the images are affected by artifacts due to implants and their routine use has not been evaluated well in diagnosis of PJI.

Nuclear Imaging

Nuclear imaging studies are recommended for those patients who have high probability of infection, but repeated aspiration yields negative culture.

^{99m}Tc-bone scintigraphy, ^{67}gallium, ^{111}indium, or ^{99m}Tc-labeled WBCs, combined leukocyte marrow imaging, and 18-flurodeoxyglucose positron emission tomography (FDG-PET) are commonly used nuclear imaging modalities.[50-53] The major advantage of the nuclear imaging is that the results are not affected by metallic hardware.[54]

Bone scintigraphy/bone scan is done by measuring the activity of the radioactive marker after giving it to the patient. Its accumulation depends on blood flow and the rate of new bone formation. The advantage of bone scintigraphy is that it is available in many centers, easily performed, and can be completed quickly. Triphasic ^{99m}Tc-labeled diphosphonates scintigraphy is commonly used, and accumulation during blood flow, blood pool, and late phase (all three phases) is considered as indicative of infection (see **Figures 23.2 to 23.4**). The bone scintigraphy has sensitivity of 68–88% and specificity of 76–90%.[55] The disadvantages are its low specificity, uptake in conditions of increased bone turnover like fracture, heterotopic ossification, and physiological remodeling, and it may accumulate in areas of particle debris and aseptic loosening, radiation, and is not useful within first few years of surgery as postsurgical inflammatory changes may persist.

^{67}Gallium that is derived from gallium citrate or nitrate is handled in the body like ferric iron. ^{67}Gallium scintigraphy when used alone has very low specificity. ^{67}Gallium scintigraphy that is done sequential to ^{99m}Tc triphasic bone scan improves the specificity in identifying

Flow chart 23.1 Algorithm for diagnosis of periprosthetic joint infection (PJI)

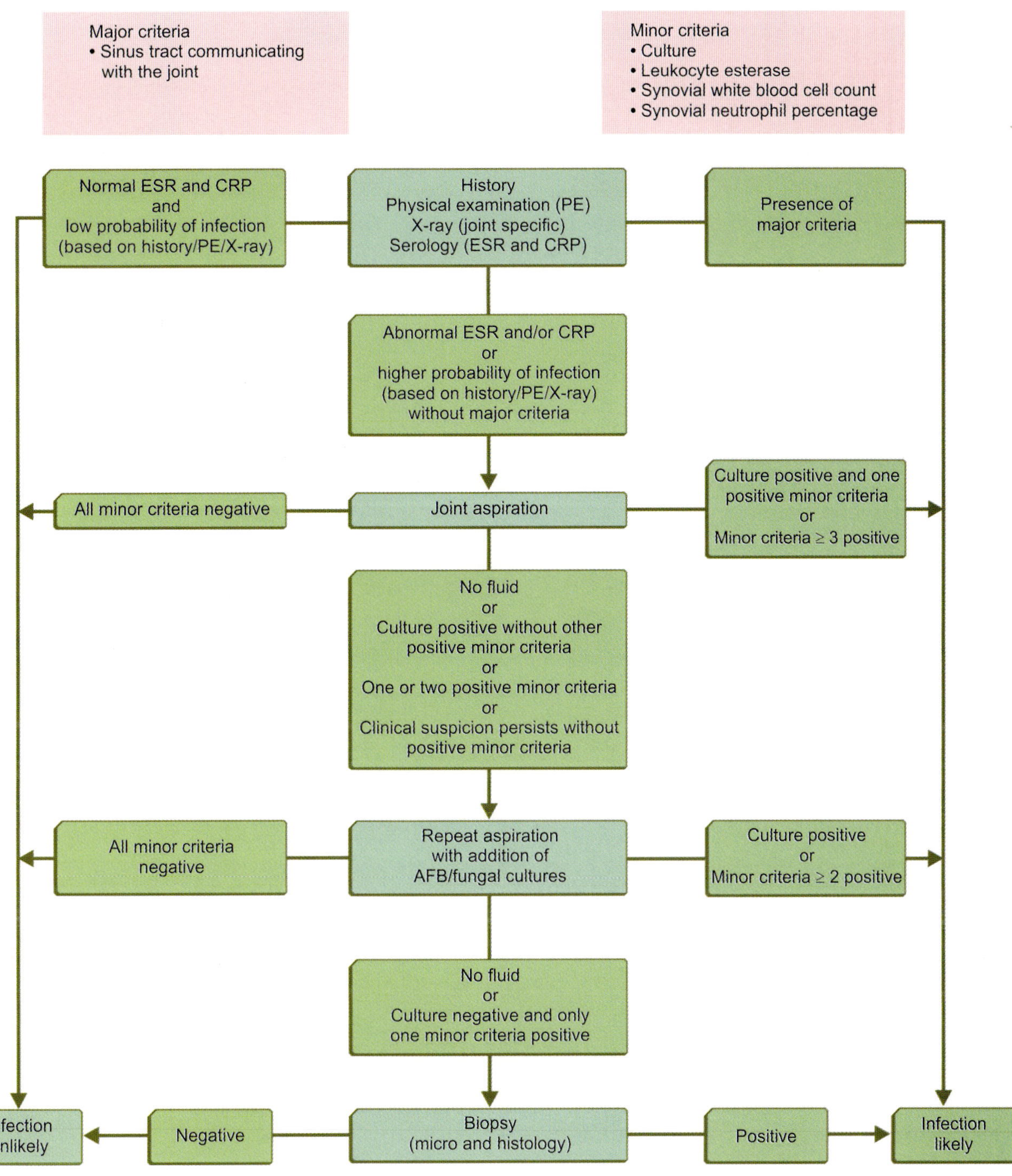

the infection,[54] but even then its specificity is low. The disadvantage is additional radiation to the patient and lack of cost-effectiveness. Gallium uptake also depends on inflammation, blood flow, and other factors. For example, ^{99m}Tc scintigraphy they can accumulate in areas of inflammation and heterotopic bone formation.

Indium-labeled or technetium-labeled WBC scintigraphy has also been used on the principle of

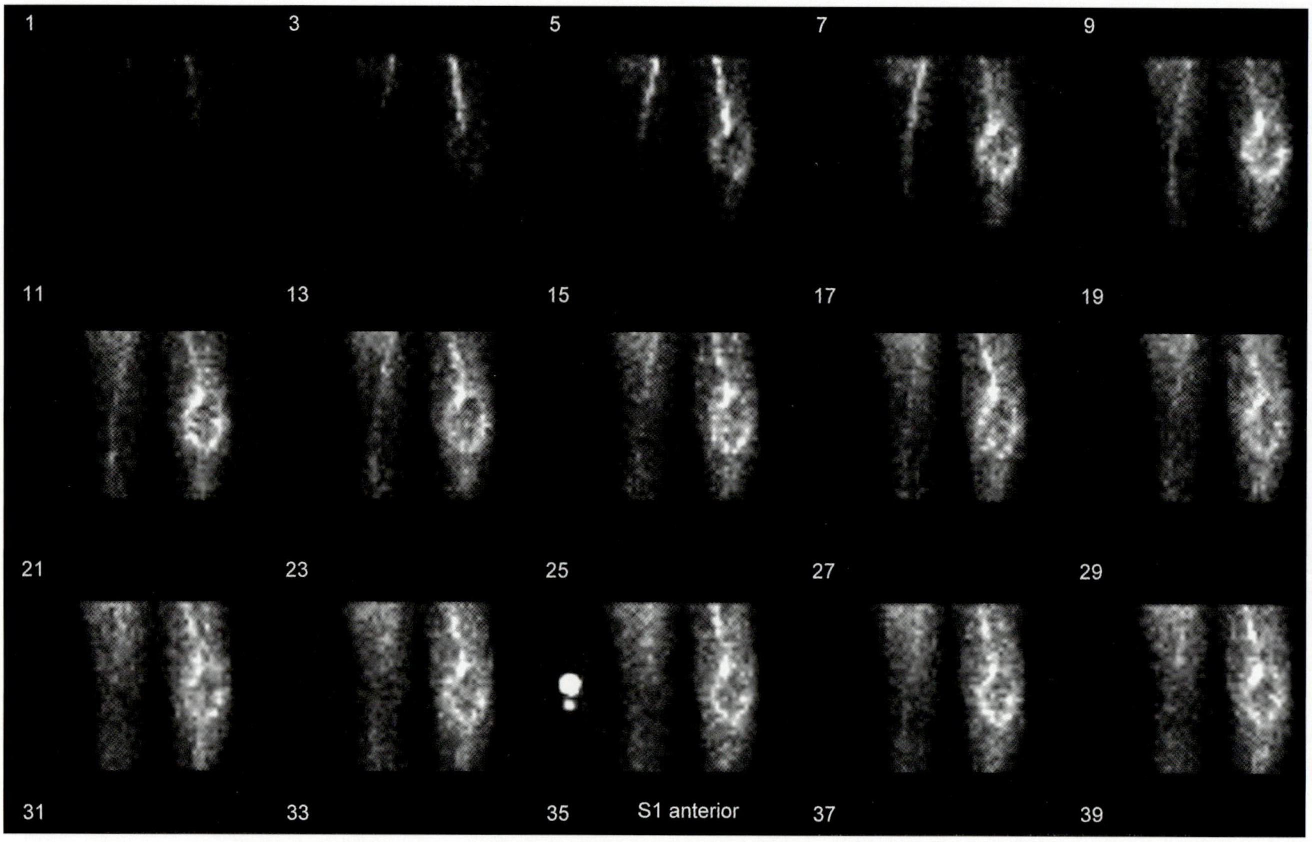

Figure 23.2 Hyperemia in left knee around femur and tibial component and joint in flow phase

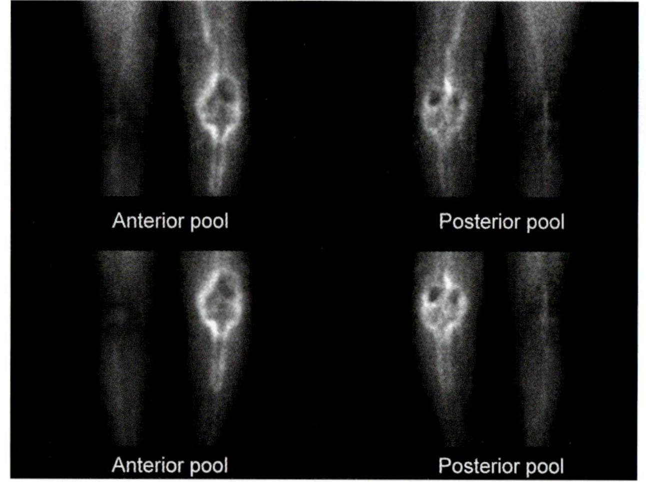

Figure 23.3 Hyperemia in left knee around femur and tibial component and joint during pool phase

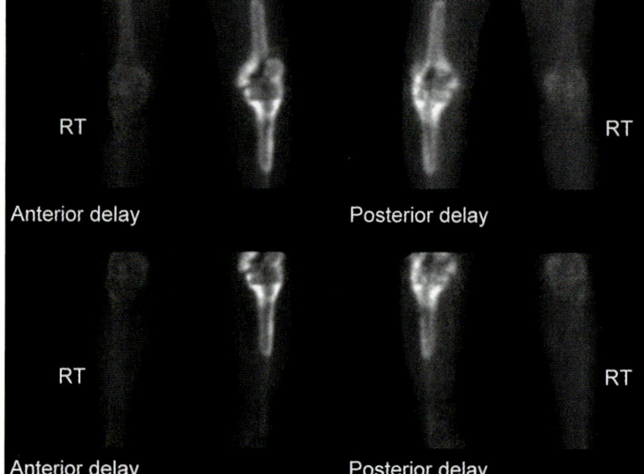

Figure 23.4 Increased uptake during delayed phase in left knee around femur and tibial component and joint. Increased uptake in all three phases is indicative of infection. Please note: in early postoperative period, there may be an increase in uptake even in joints without infection

leukocytes accumulating at the site of inflammation.[56] The commonly used tracers are ^{111}In-oxine and ^{99m}Tc-hexamethyl propylene amine oxime (HMPAO). It has the advantage of not accumulating in the area of bone remodeling or increased bone turnover in absence of infection. WBC scan is also negative in most of cases of aseptic loosening because most of aseptic infiltrate contains histiocytes, macrophages, lymphocytes, while most of labeled cells are neutrophils. The results of indium-labeled studies showed sensitivity between 77% and 100% and specificity between 73% and 100%.

WBC scan has the disadvantage of *in vitro* labeling of WBCs and requires specialized equipment and personnel. Finally, they may produce false positive results in early postoperative period and false negative when the patient is under the coverage of antibiotic because this test depends on migration of WBCs.

Leukocyte/bone marrow scintigraphy (combined ^{111}indium-labeled leukocyte/^{99m}Tc-sulfur colloid marrow) is gold standard among nuclear studies in detection of PJI with accuracy more than 90%.[51,53,54,57-59] But recent investigations suggest FDG-PET appears to be more accurate in detecting PJI. The investigation is based on the principle that both labeled leukocytes and sulfur colloids accumulate in marrow but only leukocytes accumulate in infection site. Although it is highly sensitive and specific, it puts patients through additional radiation. The disadvantages are *in vitro* labeling, handling of the blood products, and is expensive.[53,54]Instead of ^{111}indium-labeled leukocyte/^{99m}Tc-sulfur colloid, sulesomab and Tc-labeled nanocolloid can be used.[53] Late leukocyte scintigraphy, serial time leukocyte scintigraphy and *in vivo* leukocyte scintigraphy/anti-granulocyte scintigraphy are other type of studies available.

Antigranulocyte antibodies are increasingly being tried in diagnosis of PJI. The most commonly used monoclonal antibodies in the imaging of prosthesis infection are granulocyte-specific monoclonal antibody technetium-99m-BW-250/183 and sulesomab (also called as LeukoScan) that is obtained from mice [Fab fragment against the glycoprotein reactive antigen-90(NCA-90)].[60]

In their meta-analysis, Pakos et al. found that the use of Tc-labeled antigranulocyte antibodies in periprosthetic infection has sensitivity and specificity of 90% and 80%, respectively.[60]

When using combination of SPECT/CT with ^{99m}Tc-labeled antigranulocyte antibodies in the diagnosis of low grade PJI, SPECT not only increases the sensitivity due to its exact localization of tracer uptake but also its combination with CT increases the specificity by adding anatomic detail. Comparing with SPECT alone, the combination of SPECT and CT was able to differentiate between periprosthetic and corticomedullary uptake and was thus helpful in identifying low-grade infections. It also helps in knowing the extent of lesion, so it is useful in deciding extend of debridement during surgery or biopsy of the region.[52]

In recent years, FDG-PET[61] has gained popularity in diagnosis of periprosthetic infection. PET uses fluorine-18-flurodeoxyglucose as a tracer and its uptake is dependent on cellular glucose metabolism.

PET finding suggestive of infection is increased uptake at bone–prosthesis interface of femur or tibia, increased uptake at periprosthetic area, activity in periprosthetic area without corresponding activity on marrow image.[58] The location of the uptake is more important than the intensity of uptake. But there is lack of consensus regarding the criteria for diagnosing PJI using PET.

The pooled sensitivity and specificity of FDG-PET is around 84%.[54] It has been reported to have better results than triple phase bone scintigraphy[63] and indium-labeled leukocytes in hips.[64]The FDG-PET is more accurate for hips than knees.[54]

Advantages are that FDG-PET images are superior to images of other nuclear imaging techniques and less time consuming. It also has been suggested that FDG-PET improves the accuracy of sampling tissues in PJI[65] and is also useful in follow-up during treatment with antibiotics.[55] The disadvantage is it is not widely available, is expensive, and requires an experienced nuclear radiologist to interpret the results. False positives may also occur due to aseptic loosening due to accumulation of FDG by macrophages and giant cells present in those areas.[66] Although FDG-PET is not able to differentiate between septic and aseptic loosening, the negative scan rules out the need for revision.[62]

F-18 Fluoride PET has also been tried in the diagnosis of loosening in both septic and aseptic cases. Kobayashi et al. performed this test in THAs and found that F-18 Fluoride PET is useful in detecting loosening due to septic and aseptic case. It differs from FDG-PET by its specificity in identifying bone remodeling.[67]

MOLECULAR MARKERS

As there is no single test to identify PJI, the search for the perfect test continues. As a result of this many molecular methods have been tried and proposed as alternative or add-on to the existing tests. Some of these tests identify the organisms and while others are based on the response of the host. These tests are done on synovial fluid, sonication fluid, tissue culture, or blood. The molecular markers/tests that commonly proposed are PCR, interleukin (IL-1), IL-6, IL-8, IL-17, procalcitonin, α-2 macroglobulin, and vascular endothelial growth factor (VEGF).[33,68-75]

Polymerase Chain Reaction

PCR test is recommended currently for those cases in which there is a high suspicion of infection, but no organism has been identified by any other means. PCR is normally done on scraping of the implants or from the sonicated fluid of the explanted implants.[70,76-79] Bergin et al. showed sonication gives better results than scraping.[77] PCR on sonicated fluid of explanted implants offers better sensitivity compared with synovial fluid culture or tissue culture.[69,72,78-81] The type of PCR used varies among studies and include broad-based PCR, reverse transcriptase PCR, and/or multiplex PCR.

PCR is not only fast but results are available within a day;[69,79] it has the advantage of not being affected by previous antibiotic treatment.[70,71] Some of these tests have shown promise in identifying the antibiotic resistance genes (like *MecA* gene of MRSA).[78] One study suggested it will help in rapid implementation of first-line antibiotic therapy and reduce the use of broad-spectrum antibiotics,[78] where others even showed the ability to differentiate septic from aseptic failure.[70] But their routine clinical applicability is still questionable.

PCR has its own disadvantages like being a complex test to perform high false positive rate due to contamination[69,76] and difficulty in identifying the viability of bacteria in PCR positive cases especially those with negative culture results.[79] So the positive results in patients with no signs of infection should be interpreted carefully. Broad-based PCR techniques also require sequencing to identify the bacteria and they are of limited value in polymicrobial infections.[69] Multiplex PCR said to be more accurate and overcome these disadvantages.[70]

Interleukin-6

Interleukin-6 (IL-6) is an important cytokine in the immune system, which is secreted by activated monocytes/macrophages and has shown great promise in identifying the periprosthetic infection.[74,82] Different studies using different cutoff values reported sensitivity ranging from 60 to 100% and specificity from 50 to 100%.[73,74,82]

Normally serum IL-6 peaks 6–12 hours after surgery and returns to normal by 48–72 hours.[83,84] The normal level of serum IL-6 level is approximately 1 pg/mL, and it can increase to 30–430 pg/mL for as long as 3 days following total joint arthroplasty. Di Cesare et al. found that IL-6 levels of 10 pg/mL as a cutoff point for diagnosing PJI has enough sensitivity, specificity, PPV, and NPV.[74] Not only does it helps in identifying the infection, it also has the advantage of measuring patient response to infection after surgery because it returns to normal quickly after surgery.[74]

While Berbari et al. in their meta-analysis concluded that the serum IL-6 level has the highest accuracy for the diagnosis of prosthetic joint infection, followed by the CRP level, the ESR, and the WBC count;[19] another one study that evaluated the combination of CRP and serum IL-6 found that combination more useful for identifying PJI than IL-6 alone.[85]

The applicability of serum IL-6 levels in conditions like inflammatory arthropathies, prior antibiotic treatment before surgery, multiple sclerosis, Paget disease, immunodeficiency disorders,[74] and polyethylene wear[82]is limited because of elevated IL-6 in those conditions.

Synovial fluid IL-6 levels has also been evaluated as a marker for infection.[33,75,86]In trials their cutoff value varied between 1826 and 13350 pg/mL, and the sensitivity and specificity varied between 60–100% and 94–100%, respectively.[33,75,86] Because of its wide variation, further research is needed in using this marker in the diagnosis of periprosthetic infection.

IL-8, VEGF, and α-2 Macroglobulin

IL-8, VEGF, and α-2 macroglobulin have been evaluated as part of 46 proteins in synovial fluid by Jacovides et al.[33] Out of 46 markers, they found 5 proteins (IL-8, VEGF, α-2 macroglobulin, CRP, IL-6) have reasonable accuracy in diagnosing PJI. But they felt further investigations were needed to evaluate their routine clinical use.

Interleukin-1

Apart from IL-6, the interleukin that has shown promise in identifying the periprosthetic infection is IL-1. IL-1 is an inflammatory cytokine produced by macrophages, monocytes, and lymphocytes that form part of inflammatory response against infection. Out of 11 proteins of the interleukin family IL-1α and IL-1β levels were investigated by Deirmengian et al. in periprosthetic infections and he found synovial IL-1β (cutoff value 112 pg/mL) to have a high level of significance with 100% sensitivity, specificity, PPV, NPV.[75]

Procalcitonin

Procalcitonin is a hormone synthesized by C cells of thyroid. Levels increase 2–4 hours after sepsis and reach peak after 6 hours. The studies that evaluated the use of calcitonin in the diagnosis of PJI reported variable sensitivity and specificity between 30% and 100% and 30% and 98%, respectively.[73,82] The cutoff value also varied between studies.[73,82] Its use in diagnosis of PJI is limited because of lack of standard threshold and limited sensitivity.

Synovial TNF-α, IL-4, IFN-γ levels have also shown to be increased in PJI.[86] Gollwitzer et al. recommended combinations of synovial fluid IL-4, IL-6, LL-3, and HHD-3 to be good predictors of PJI.[86]

NONRECOMMENDED TESTS

The following tests are no longer recommended for the diagnosis of periprosthetic infection:

Role of Serum WBC Count

Because of their low sensitivity and specificity, WBC count and differential count have no role in diagnosis of prosthetic joint infection.[29,87,88] Elevations of WBC count occur only in small percentage of patients with deep infections. Apart from that the elevation of WBC with fever is normal in postoperative period of hip and knee arthroplasty.[89,90]

Role of Gram Stain and Swabs

Because of their ease of use and cost-effectiveness, swabs were used widely. But recommendation of international consensus meeting on periprosthetic infection was strongly against taking swabs. Swabs have increased the risk of contamination, decreased inoculum volume for growth of culture and inhibition of organisms and having no added advantage and less sensitivity than tissue culture.[91-93] Normally three to five samples are taken one each from tibia, femur, and capsule/synovial tissue. If two swabs are used, both aerobic and anaerobic culture can be done. Although the sensitivity of swab culture varies from 53% to 61%, its specificity is almost 98–99%.[22,27,93]

It is also important to note draining sinuses should not be cultured. They are prone to give false results about organisms and misguide antibiotic treatment. Tetreault et al. in their recent study found superficial cultures have concordance with deep cultures only in 47% of cases.[94]

Because of its low sensitivity (12–43%) and false positive results due to contamination, intraoperative Gram-stain has limited role in the diagnosis of periprosthetic infection. But most of the studies reported high specificity (92–100%).[95-101]

REFERENCES

1. Bozic KJ, Kurtz SM, Lau E, et al. The epidemiology of revision total knee arthroplasty in the United States. Clin Orthop Relat Res. 2010;468(1):45-51.
2. Sadoghi P, Liebensteiner M, Agreiter M, et al. Revision surgery after total joint arthroplasty: a complication-based analysis using worldwide arthroplasty registers. J Arthroplasty. 2013;28(8):1329-32.

3. Parvizi J, Pawasarat I, Azzam K, et al. Periprosthetic joint infection: the economic impact of methicillin-resistant infections. J Arthroplasty. 2010;25(6 Suppl):103-7.
4. Bhandari M, Smith J, Miller LE, Block JE. Clinical and economic burden of revision knee arthroplasty. Clin Med Insights Arthritis Musculoskelet Disord. 2012;5:89-94.
5. Hernández-Vaquero D, Fernández-Fairen M, Torres A, et al. Treatment of periprosthetic infections: an economic analysis. Scientific World Journal. 2013;2013: 821650.
6. Hellmann M, Mehta S, Bishai D, Mears S, JM. Z. The estimated magnitude and direct hospital costs of prosthetic joint infections in the United States, 1997 to 2004. J Arthroplasty. 2010;25(5):766-71.e1.
7. Pulido L, Ghanem E, Joshi A, Purtill JJ, Parvizi J. Periprosthetic joint infection: the incidence, timing, and predisposing factors. Clin Orthop Relat Res. 2008;466(7):1710-5.
8. Renaud A, Lavigne M, Vendittoli P-A. Periprosthetic joint infections at a teaching hospital in 1990-2007. Can J Surg. 2012;55(6):394-400.
9. Singh JA, Vessely MB, Harmsen WS, et al. A population-based study of trends in the use of total hip and total knee arthroplasty, 1969-2008. Mayo Clin Proc. 2010;85(10):898-904.
10. Singh JA. Epidemiology of knee and hip arthroplasty: a systematic review. Open Orthop J. 2011;5:80-5.
11. Kim SH, Gaiser S, Meehan JP. Epidemiology of primary hip and knee arthroplasties in Germany: 2004 to 2008. J Arthroplasty. 2012;27(10):1777-82.
12. Kurtz SM, Ong KL, Schmier J, et al. Future clinical and economic impact of revision total hip and knee arthroplasty. J Bone Jt Surg. 2007;89(suppl_3):144-51.
13. Bauer TW, Parvizi J, Kobayashi N, Krebs V. Diagnosis of periprosthetic infection. J Bone Joint Surg Am. 2006;88(4):869-82.
14. Rasouli MR, Harandi AA, Adeli B, Purtill JJ, Parvizi J. Revision total knee arthroplasty: infection should be ruled out in all cases. J Arthroplasty. 2012;27(6):1239-43.e1-2.
15. Bozic KJ, Lau E, Kurtz S, Ong K, Berry DJ. Patient-related risk factors for postoperative mortality and periprosthetic joint infection in Medicare patients undergoing TKA. Clin Orthop Relat Res. 2012;470(1):130-7.
16. Sendi P, Banderet F, Graber P, Zimmerli W. Clinical comparison between exogenous and haematogenous periprosthetic joint infections caused by *Staphylococcus aureus*. Clin Microbiol Infect. 2011;17(7):1098-1100.
17. Della Valle CJ, Sporer SM, Jacobs JJ, et al. Preoperative testing for sepsis before revision total knee arthroplasty. J Arthroplasty. 2007;22(6 Suppl 2):90-3.
18. Greidanus NV, Masri BA, Garbuz DS, et al. Use of erythrocyte sedimentation rate and C-reactive protein level to diagnose infection before revision total knee arthroplasty: a prospective evaluation. J Bone Joint Surg Am. 2007;89(7):1409-16.
19. Berbari E, Mabry T, Tsaras G, et al. Inflammatory blood laboratory levels as markers of prosthetic joint infection: a systematic review and meta-analysis. J Bone Joint Surg Am. 2010;92(11):2102-9.
20. Ghanem E, Parvizi J, Burnett RSJ, et al. Cell count and differential of aspirated fluid in the diagnosis of infection at the site of total knee arthroplasty. J Bone Joint Surg Am. 2008;90(8):1637-43.
21. Cipriano CA, Brown NM, Michael AM, et al. Serum and synovial fluid analysis for diagnosing inflammatory arthritis. J Bone Joint Surg Am. 2012;94:594-600.
22. Spangehl MJ, Masri BA, O'Connell JX, et al. Prospective analysis of preoperative and intraoperative investigations for the diagnosis of infection at the sites of two hundred and two revision total hip arthroplasties. J Bone Joint Surg Am. 1999;81(5):672-83.
23. Kusuma SK, Ward J, Jacofsky M, et al. What is the role of serological testing between stages of two-stage reconstruction of the infected prosthetic knee? Clin Orthop Relat Res. 2011;469(4):1002-8.
24. Jackson DW, Evans NA, Thomas BM. Accuracy of needle placement into the intra-articular space of the knee. J Bone Joint Surg Am. 2002;84-A(9):1522-7.
25. Della Valle C, Parvizi J, Bauer TW, et al. American Academy of Orthopaedic Surgeons clinical practice guideline on the diagnosis of periprosthetic joint infections of the hip and knee. J Bone Joint Surg Am. 2011;93(14):1355-7.
26. Ali F, Wilkinson JM, Cooper JR, et al. Accuracy of joint aspiration for the preoperative diagnosis of infection in total hip arthroplasty. J Arthroplasty. 2006;21(2):221-6.
27. Font-Vizcarra L, García S, Martínez-Pastor JC, Sierra JM, Soriano A. Blood culture flasks for culturing synovial fluid in prosthetic joint infections. Clin Orthop Relat Res. 2010;468(8):2238-43.

28. Ghanem E, Houssock C, Pulido L, et al. Determining "true" leukocytosis in bloody joint aspiration. J Arthroplasty. 2008;23(2):182-7.
29. Schinsky BMF, Valle CJ Della, Sporer SM, et al. Perioperative testing for joint infection in patients undergoing revision total hip arthroplasty. J Bone Joint Surg Am. 2008;90(9):1869-75.
30. Salinas M, Rosas J, Iborra J, Manero H, Pascual E. Comparison of manual and automated cell counts in EDTA preserved synovial fluids. Storage has little influence on the results. Ann Rheum Dis. 1997;56(10):622-6.
31. De Jonge R, Brouwer R, Smit M, et al. Automated counting of white blood cells in synovial fluid. Rheumatology (Oxford). 2004;43(9):1201; author reply 1201-2.
32. Parvizi J, Jacovides C, Adeli B, et al. Coventry Award: synovial C-reactive protein: a prospective evaluation of a molecular marker for periprosthetic knee joint infection. Clin Orthop Relat Res. 2012;470(1):54-60.
33. Jacovides CL, Parvizi J, Adeli B, Jung KA. Molecular markers for diagnosis of periprosthetic joint infection. J Arthroplasty. 2011;26(6 Suppl):99-103.e1.
34. Parvizi J, Jacovides C, Antoci V, Ghanem E. Diagnosis of periprosthetic joint infection: the utility of a simple yet unappreciated enzyme. J Bone Joint Surg Am. 2011;93-A(24):2242-8.
35. Aggarwal VKV, Tischler E, Ghanem E, Parvizi J, JP. Leukocyte esterase from synovial fluid aspirate: a technical note. J Arthroplasty. 2013;28(1):193-5.
36. Wetters NG, Berend KR, Lombardi AV, et al. Leukocyte esterase reagent strips for the rapid diagnosis of periprosthetic joint infection. J Arthroplasty. 2012;27(8 Suppl):8-11.
37. Schäfer P, Fink B, Sandow D, et al. Prolonged bacterial culture to identify late periprosthetic joint infection: a promising strategy. Clin Infect Dis. 2008;47(11): 1403-9.
38. Larsen LH, Lange J, Xu Y, Schønheyder HC. Optimizing culture methods for diagnosis of prosthetic joint infections: a summary of modifications and improvements reported since 1995. J Med Microbiol. 2012;61(Pt 3):309-16.
39. Butler-Wu SM, Burns EM, Pottinger PS, et al. Optimization of periprosthetic culture for diagnosis of *Propionibacterium acnes* prosthetic joint infection. J Clin Microbiol. 2011;49(7):2490-5.
40. Shuman EK, Urquhart A, Malani PN. Management and prevention of prosthetic joint infection. Infect Dis Clin North Am. 2012;26(1):29-39.
41. Tetreault MW, Wetters NG, Aggarwal V, et al. The Chitranjan Ranawat Award: should prophylactic antibiotics be withheld before revision surgery to obtain appropriate cultures? Clin Orthop Relat Res. 2014;472(1):52-6.
42. Burnett RSJ, Aggarwal A, Givens SA, et al. Prophylactic antibiotics do not affect cultures in the treatment of an infected TKA: a prospective trial. Clin Orthop Relat Res. 2010;468(1):127-34.
43. Trampuz A, Piper KE, Jacobson MJ, et al. Sonication of removed hip and knee prostheses for diagnosis of infection. N Engl J Med. 2007;357(7):654-63.
44. Janz V, Wassilew GI, Hasart O, Tohtz S, Perka C. Improvement in the detection rate of PJI in total hip arthroplasty through multiple sonicate fluid cultures. J Orthop Res. 2013;31(12):2021-4.
45. Bjerkan G, Witsø E, Bergh K. Sonication is superior to scraping for retrieval of bacteria in biofilm on titanium and steel surfaces *in vitro*. Acta Orthop 2009;80(2):245-50.
46. Monsen T, Lövgren E, Widerström M, Wallinder L. *In vitro* effect of ultrasound on bacteria and suggested protocol for sonication and diagnosis of prosthetic infections. J Clin Microbiol. 2009;47(8):2496-501.
47. Trampuz A, Piper KE, Hanssen AD, et al. Sonication of explanted prosthetic components in bags for diagnosis of prosthetic joint infection is associated with risk of contamination. J Clin Microbiol. 2006;44(2):628-31.
48. Borens O, Yusuf E, Steinrücken J, Trampuz A. Accurate and early diagnosis of orthopedic device-related infection by microbial heat production and sonication. J Orthop Res. 2013:1-4.
49. Tsaras G, Maduka-ezeh A, Inwards CY, et al. Utility of intraoperative frozen section. J Bone Joint Surg Am. 2012;94-A(18):1700-711.
50. Glithero P, Grigoris P, Harding L, Hesselwood S, Mcminn D. White cell scans and infected joint replacements. J Bone Jt Surgery(Br). 1993;75-B(3):371-4.
51. Love C, Marwin SE, Tomas MB, et al. Diagnosing infection in the failed joint replacement : a comparison of coincidence detection 18F-FDG and 111In-labelled leukocyte/99m Tc-sulfur colloid marrow imaging. J Nucl Med. 2004;45(11):1864-71.

52. Graute V, Feist M, Lehner S, et al. Detection of low-grade prosthetic joint infections using 99mTc-antigranulocyte SPECT/CT: initial clinical results. Eur J Nucl Med Mol Imaging. 2010;37(9):1751-9.
53. Sousa R, Massada M, Pereira A, et al. Diagnostic accuracy of combined 99mTc-sulesomab and 99mTc-nanocolloid bone marrow imaging in detecting prosthetic joint infection. Nucl Med Commun. 2011;32(9):834-9.
54. Gemmel F, Van den Wyngaert H, Love C, et al. Prosthetic joint infections: radionuclide state-of-the-art imaging. Eur J Nucl Med Mol Imaging. 2012;39(5):892-909.
55. Prandini N, Lazzeri E, Rossi B, et al. Nuclear medicine imaging of bone infections. Nucl Med Commun. 2006;27(8):633-44.
56. Scher DM, Pak K, Lonner JH, et al. The predictive value of indium-111 leukocyte scans in the diagnosis of infected total hip, knee, or resection arthroplasties. J Arthroplasty. 2000;15(3):295-300.
57. Joseph T, Mujtaba M, Chen A, et al. Efficacy of combined technitium-99m sulfur colloid/indium-111 leukocyte scans to detect infected total hip and knee arthroplasties. J Arthroplasty. 2001;16(6):753-8.
58. Van Acker F, Nuyts J, Maes A, et al. FDG-PET, 99mtc-HMPAO white blood cell SPET and bone scintigraphy in the evaluation of painful total knee arthroplasties. Eur J Nucl Med. 2001;28(10):1496-504.
59. Segura AB, Munoz A, Brulles RY, et al. What is the role of bone scintigraphy in the diagnosis of infected joint prostheses? Nucl Med Commun. 2003;25:527-32.
60. Pakos EE, Trikalinos TA, Fotopoulos AD, Ioannidis JPA. Prosthesis infection: diagnosis after total joint arthroplasty with antigranulocyte scintigraphy with 99mTc-labelled monoclonal antibodies: a meta-analysis. Radiology. 2007;242(1):101-8.
61. Chryssikos T, Parvizi J, Ghanem E, et al. FDG-PET imaging can diagnose periprosthetic infection of the hip. Clin Orthop Relat Res. 2008;466(6):1338-42.
62. Delank KS, Schmidt M, Michael JWP, et al. The implications of 18F-FDG PET for the diagnosis of endoprosthetic loosening and infection in hip and knee arthroplasty: results from a prospective, blinded study. BMC Musculoskelet Disord. 2006;7:20.
63. Reinartz P, Mumme T, Hermanns B, et al. Radionuclide imaging of the painful hip arthroplasty: positron-emission tomography versus triple-phase bone scanning. J Bone Joint Surg Br. 2005;87(4):465-70.
64. Pill S, Parvizi J, Tang P, et al. Comparison of fluorodeoxyglucose positron emission tomography and 111indium-white blood cell imaging in the diagnosis of periprosthetic infection of the hip. J Arthroplasty. 2006;21 sep(6 suppl 2):91-7.
65. Choe H, Inaba Y, Kobayashi N, et al. Use of 18F-fluoride PET to determine the appropriate tissue sampling region for improved sensitivity of tissue examinations in cases of suspected periprosthetic infection after total hip arthroplasty. Acta Orthop 2011;82(4):427-32.
66. Stumpe KD, Notzli HP, Zanetti M, et al. FDG PET for differentiation of infection and aseptic loosening in total hip replacements : comparison with conventional radiography and three-phase bone scintigraphy. Radiology. 2004;231(2):333-41.
67. Kobayashi N, Inaba Y, Choe H, et al. Use of F-18 fluoride PET to differentiate septic from aseptic loosening in total hip arthroplasty patients. Clin Nucl Med. 2011;36(11):e156-61.
68. Mariani BD, Martin DS, Levine MJ, Booth RE, Tuan RS. The Coventry Award. Polymerase chain reaction detection of bacterial infection in total knee arthroplasty. Clin Orthop Relat Res. 1996;(331):11-22.
69. Gomez E, Cazanave C, Cunningham SA, et al. Prosthetic joint infection diagnosis using broad-range PCR of biofilms dislodged from knee and hip arthroplasty surfaces using sonication. J Clin Microbiol. 2012;50(11):3501-8.
70. Portillo ME, Salvadó M, Sorli L, et al. Multiplex PCR of sonication fluid accurately differentiates between prosthetic joint infection and aseptic failure. J Infect. 2012;65(6):541-8.
71. Esteban J, Alonso-Rodriguez N, Del-Prado G, et al. PCR-hybridization after sonication improves diagnosis of implant-related infection. Acta Orthop. 2012;83(3): 299-304.
72. Cazanave C, Greenwood-Quaintance KE, Hanssen AD, et al. Rapid molecular microbiologic diagnosis of prosthetic joint infection. J Clin Microbiol. 2013;51(7):2280-7.
73. Glehr M, Friesenbichler J, Hofmann G, et al. Novel biomarkers to detect infection in revision hip and knee arthroplasties. Clin Orthop Relat Res. 2013;471(8):2621-8.
74. Di Cesare PE, Chang E, Preston CF, et al. Serum interleukin-6 as a marker of periprosthetic infection

following total hip and knee arthroplasty. J Bone Joint Surg Am. 2005;87-A(9):1921-7.

75. Deirmengian C, Hallab N, Tarabishy A, et al. Synovial fluid biomarkers for periprosthetic infection. Clin Orthop Relat Res. 2010;468(8):2017-23.
76. Suda AJ, Kommerell M, Geiss HK, et al. Prosthetic infection: improvement of diagnostic procedures using 16S ribosomal deoxyribonucleic acid polymerase chain reaction. Int Orthop. 2013;37(2):2515-21.
77. Bergin PF, Doppelt JD, Hamilton WG, et al. Detection of periprosthetic infections with use of ribosomal RNA-based polymerase chain reaction. J Bone Joint Surg. Am. 2010;92(3):654-63.
78. Titécat M, Loïez C, Senneville E, et al. Evaluation of rapid mecA gene detection versus standard culture in staphylococcal chronic prosthetic joint infections. Diagn Microbiol Infect Dis. 2012;73(4):318-21.
79. Kobayashi N, Inaba Y, Choe H, et al. Rapid and sensitive detection of methicillin-resistant *Staphylococcus* periprosthetic infections using real-time polymerase chain reaction. Diagn Microbiol Infect Dis. 2009;64(2): 172-6.
80. Tunney MM, Patrick S, Curran MD, et al. Detection of prosthetic hip infection at revision arthroplasty by immunofluorescence microscopy and PCR amplification of the bacterial 16S rRNA gene. J Clin Microbiol. 1999;37(10):3281-90.
81. Achermann Y, Vogt M, Leunig M, Wüst J, Trampuz A. Improved diagnosis of periprosthetic joint infection by multiplex PCR of sonication fluid from removed implants. J Clin Microbiol. 2010;48(4):1208-14.
82. Bottner F, Wegner A, Winkelmann W, et al. Interleukin-6, procalcitonin and TNF-alpha: markers of peri-prosthetic infection following total joint replacement. J Bone Joint Surg Br. 2007;89(1):94-9.
83. Kragsbjerg P, Holmberg H, Vikerfors T. Serum concentrations of interleukin-6, tumour necrosis factor-alpha, and C-reactive protein in patients undergoing major operations. Eur J Surg. 1995;161(1):17-22.
84. Baigrie R, Lamont P, Kwiatkowski D, Dallman M, Morris P. Systemic cytokine response after major surgery. Br J Surg. 1992;79(8):757-60.
85. Buttaro MA, Tanoira I, Comba F, Piccaluga F. Combining C-reactive protein and interleukin-6 may be useful to detect periprosthetic hip infection. Clin Orthop Relat Res. 2010;468(12):3263-7.
86. Gollwitzer H, Dombrowski Y, Prodinger PM, et al. Antimicrobial peptides and proinflammatory cytokines in periprosthetic joint infection. J Bone Joint Surg Am. 2013;95(7):644-51.
87. Williams JL, Norman P, Stockley I. The value of hip aspiration versus tissue biopsy in diagnosing infection before exchange hip arthroplasty surgery. J Arthroplasty. 2004;19(5):582-6.
88. Toossi N, Adeli B, Rasouli MR, Huang R, Parvizi J. Serum white blood cell count and differential do not have a role in the diagnosis of periprosthetic joint infection. J Arthroplasty. 2012;27(8 Suppl):51-4.e1.
89. Deirmengian GK, Zmistowski B, Jacovides C, O'Neil J, Parvizi J. Leukocytosis is common after total hip and knee arthroplasty. Clin Orthop Relat Res. 2011;469(11):3031-6.
90. Czaplicki AP, Borger JE, Politi JR, Chambers BT, Taylor BC. Evaluation of postoperative fever and leukocytosis in patients after total hip and knee arthroplasty. J Arthroplasty. 2011;26(8):1387-9.
91. Wilson ML, Winn W. Laboratory diagnosis of bone, joint, soft-tissue, and skin infections. Clin Infect Dis. 2008;46(3):453-7.
92. Perry JL, Ballou DR, Salyer JL. Inhibitory properties of a swab transport device. J Clin Microbiol. 1997;35(12):3367-8.
93. Aggarwal VK, Higuera C, Deirmengian G, Parvizi J, Austin MS. Swab cultures are not as effective as tissue cultures for diagnosis of periprosthetic joint infection. Clin Orthop Relat Res. 2013;471(10):3196-203.
94. Tetreault MW, Wetters NG, Aggarwal VK, et al. Should draining wounds and sinuses associated with hip and knee arthroplasties be cultured? J Arthroplasty. 2013;28(8 supplement):133-6.
95. Spangehl MJ, Masterson E, Masri BA, O'Connell JX, Duncan CP. The role of intraoperative gram stain in the diagnosis of infection during revision total hip arthroplasty. J Arthroplasty. 1999;14(8):952-6.
96. Morgan PM, Sharkey P, Ghanem E, et al. The value of intraoperative Gram stain in revision total knee arthroplasty. J Bone Joint Surg Am. 2009;91(9):2124-9.
97. Ghanem E, Ketonis C, Restrepo C, et al. Periprosthetic infection: where do we stand with regard to Gram stain? Acta Orthop 2009;80(1):37-40.

98. Parvizi J, Ghanem E, Menashe S, Barrack RL, Bauer TW. Periprosthetic infection: what are the diagnostic challenges? J Bone Joint Surg Am. 2006;88 Suppl 4:138-47.
99. Oethinger M, Warner DK, Schindler SA, Kobayashi H, Bauer TW. Diagnosing periprosthetic infection: false-positive intraoperative Gram stains. Clin Orthop Relat Res. 2011;469(4):954-60.
100. Della Valle CJ, Scher DM, Kim YH, et al. The role of intraoperative Gram stain in revision total joint arthroplasty. J Arthroplasty. 1999;14(4):500-4.
101. Banit D, Kaufer H, Hartford J. Intraoperative frozen section analysis in revision total joint arthroplasty. Clin Orthop Relat Res. 2002;401:230-8.

Chapter 24

Infected Total Knee Arthroplasty and its Management

W Klauser, D Kendoff, A Zahar

INTRODUCTION

Periprosthetic joint infection (PJI) is one of the most feared and challenging complications following knee replacement. Despite improved antibiotic prophylaxis and treatment, including systemic single-shot administration and local antibiotics in bone cement, infections occur in about 0.5–1.9% of primary cases; in revision total knee replacement, the rate of infection has been reported to be as high as 8–10%.[1-4] While the definitive diagnosis of PJI remains the key for success, a designated concept of preoperative planning and treatment is mandatory. Treatment options can include an early attempt of irrigation and debridement, up to the very last options including resection arthroplasty or fusion of the knee. As accepted worldwide, a two-stage exchange protocol has become the gold standard procedure, while a designated one-stage approach has only been advocated by a few specialized centers so far, with comparable outcomes.[5-11]

The therapeutic goal in either one- or two-stage revisions in PJI is defined by the complete eradication of the infection in combination with the maintenance of joint function. Both techniques should be available, depending on the status of the patient, the surgeon's expertise and the hospital set-up. Most often, an implant removal is followed by a 6- to 12-week course of systemic antibiotic treatment and delayed reimplantation of a new prosthesis, with an interval knee spacer applied. The introduction of mobile antibiotic-impregnated spacers seemed to improve the functional outcome of the two-stage approach and has gained increased popularity.[12-14]

Evaluating the current available literature and guidelines for the treatment of PJI, there is no clear evidence that a two- or more-stage procedure has a clearly higher success rate than a one-stage approach.[9,15-17] Although the two-stage technique is described in a large number of articles as the gold standard in infection eradication, the most mentioned recommendations, e.g. the duration of antibiotic treatment, static versus mobile spacer, interval of spacer retention, cemented versus uncemented implant fixation are based on level III-IV evidence studies or even expert opinions, rather than on prospective randomized or comparative data.[15,18,19]

To the best of our knowledge, the one-stage exchange offers some advantages, with a comparable success rate of infection control. Obvious advantages are mainly based on the need for only one operative procedure, reduced time on antibiotics, reduced hospitalization time and reduced relative overall costs.[20-24]

The following manuscript will give a detailed description of the clinical approach for PJI in total knee replacement, including diagnostics, preoperative planning, surgical treatment algorithm and postoperative set-up. Based on the experience of the authors' institution and strategies of a distinct one-stage approach in PJI, additional emphasis is given to all the detailed requirements that provide the basis for a high surgical and postoperative success rate for this technique as well as the more frequently used two-stage procedure. Alternative treatment options will only be briefly described.

CLASSIFICATION

Current guidelines of the American Academy of Orthopedic Surgeons (AAOS), the Infection Disease Society of America (IDSA) and the Liestal algorithm from Switzerland make a clear distinction between early and late prosthetic infections. An early infection is considered to occur within 3 weeks after the implantation of a prosthesis or, in case of a late hematogenous infection, within 3 weeks after the onset of acute symptoms.[18,19,24,25] After 3 weeks, the infection should be considered as a late infection, irrespective of the stability of the implant. Consequently, the term 'septic loosening' should never be considered, because in 60% of the cases, one or more components of the joint replacement is well-fixed, without any clinical or radiologic signs of loosening.[26] It is important to realize that periprosthetic infection does not only reflect an infection of the prosthetic interface, but also an infection of the surrounding bone and soft tissues.

Types of Classification

- Infections occurring within the first three postoperative weeks should be considered as *acute infections*
- Infections occurring after the third postoperative week are considered as *late infections.*

Consequently, we aggressively treat an acute infected total knee arthroplasty (TKA) (<3 weeks) with a local debridement, soft tissue revision and lavage and polyethylene liner exchange, including preservation of the initially implanted prosthesis. In this scenario, systemic antibiotics are adapted to the algorithm described by Zimmerli et al.[24] Any late infection (>3 weeks), however, should always be treated with a definite complete implant removal.

Due to the general advancements of diagnostic algorithms and further developments of systemic and local treatment options, we also adapted our infection classification system to the staging system described by McPherson et al.[27,28] This includes: the type and timing of infection, current systematic medical and immune status of the host patient and current local extremity grade based on all possible local compromising factors.

Related to the background of this strict distinction between early and late infections is the development of a biofilm on the surface of the implant. Bacteria like coagulase-negative staphylococci rapidly produce an active 'mucus-like' surface, which forms a biofilm that adheres to the surface of the implant.[29] This biofilm basically prevents the access of systemically administered antibiotics; thus, the bacteria cannot be approached without removing the implant, not even with local mechanical debridement of the prosthesis.[30] Consequently, we suggest removing all implanted material after 3 weeks, in case of a deep infection. It is, therefore, important to underline that any partial exchange of only one part of the components should not be considered a definitive treatment option, although it has been suggested in a few reports in the literature.

DIAGNOSTICS

Any painful knee following TKA should be considered to be infected until otherwise proven. Therefore, even without obvious signs of infection, such as redness or swelling, a low-grade infection should be ruled out in every single case. There is clear evidence that some general health conditions like diabetes mellitus, immunosuppression, urinary tract infections, or relevant obesity are more likely to develop PJI after joint replacement.[18,19] Especially in these patients, special attention needs to be given for a possible deep infection. The patient's history needs to be evaluated closely to find possible ways of bacterial contamination.

According to our experience, current evidence and recent clinical practice guidelines by the AAOS and[18] the international consensus group on PJI,[31] we defined the following mandatory preoperative testing for every single TKA patient with unclear pain:

- Laboratory monitoring of C-reactive protein (CRP) and erythrocyte sedimentation rate (ESR)[32-34]
- Aspiration of the affected joint with prolonged microbiologic culture time between 8 and 14 days; patients should be off antibiotics for a minimum of 14 days prior to aspiration[35]
- Synovial fluid analysis of white blood cell count and percentage of neutrophils[36-38]
- Repeat aspiration in cases of internal negative culture results in combination with either obvious signs of infection or pre-existing external positive culture results[33]
- Biopsy of the joint in cases of persistent negative aspiration results with obvious signs of infection.[5]

Procalcitonin has been shown to be a sensitive marker of septicemia, but not in cases of late PJI, where values can be within normal ranges.[24] The sensitivity of serum CRP is about 72.5%, while the specificity is 80.9% and a related positive predictive value of 59.2% and negative predictive value of 88.5%. A painful TKA with normal serum CRP levels, therefore, is most probably not infected. Painful TKAs with elevated serum CRP levels might be infected, however, and therefore require further diagnostic evaluation. In order to increase the accuracy of diagnostics with serum testing, a joint aspiration should be performed in every painful TKA.[34,38]

JOINT ASPIRATION

The most relevant and needed preoperative diagnostic test, especially in the case of a planned one-stage exchange, is based on joint aspiration with precise identification of the bacteria. The presence of a positive bacterial culture and the corresponding antibiograms are essential for a one-stage procedure. Specific antibiotic-loaded acrylic cement is based on this diagnostic tool, in order to achieve a high topical antibiotic elution directly at the surgical site for the one-stage procedure.[39]

This strict aspiration algorithm is the gold standard for every planned TKA revision in our hospital, including all late or early aseptic loosening cases. Furthermore, we expand this regime to all cases of unclear pain or malfunction after primary or revision TKA, based on our own aspiration study, which showed that between 4 and 7% of all our patients initially planned for an aseptic TKA revision had evidence of a subtle low-grade infection.[10]

Aspiration should always take place under strict sterile conditions, while the antibiotics administered before are withheld for 14 days prior to the procedure.[35] Otherwise, false negative cultures may result. We also do not recommend the use of local anesthetics; bacteriostatic characteristics might result in false negative cultures. It has been shown that a combination of serum CRP levels and joint aspiration including cultures result in a reported accuracy of 92.4%.[5] An increase of accuracy up to 98% can be reached by taking additional tissue samples (from arthroscopy or an open approach) with combined histological examination and cultures.

Furthermore, we recommend that bacteriologic cultures are performed for 10–14 days, because of slow growing germs or small colony variants.[35] It has been proven, for instance, that *propionibacteria* and *Peptostreptococcus* can be detected on traditional culture plates only after an incubation time of 10–12 days. Based upon the final microbiologic results and the susceptibility of the identified bacteria, the microbiologist can determine an adequate individualized antibiotic treatment plan for the patient, which is especially important for a one-stage protocol.

IRRIGATION AND DEBRIDEMENT

As described above, only in the phase of early infection (<3 weeks) might an adequate aggressive debridement in combination with irrigation and exchange of the polyethylene liner be successful.[25] Component retention in cases of chronic infections has shown high failure rates and poor outcome.[40,41]

A rather long-term combined antibiotic treatment for 4–6 weeks can be emphasized in these patients. However, a limited success rate of only 40% has been shown if this period is extended to 6 weeks after primary operation.[42] The surgical technique is comparable to the standard principles of primary implantation; however, it includes an aggressive debridement of all affected soft tissues and should include a complete synovectomy, at least at those anatomic sites that are accessible during surgery. In addition, an exchange of the poly liner needs to be performed. If the patella was initially resurfaced, removal of the component should be performed as well. Cultures should be taken, as described above, from various anatomic regions of the knee. Both components should be inspected for loosening; thus, the implant interfaces should be exposed.[43,44]

High-pressure jet lavage irrigation should include around 9 L, usually saline, while it remains unclear if antibacterial solutions improve the outcome.[45,46] Following irrigation, a second-look debridement can be done, while new instruments might be used to fulfill the poly liner exchange.

Concerning the duration of the intravenous (IV) antibiotic therapy after the surgical procedure, a time interval of 4–6 weeks has been widely accepted. Following IV antibiotic therapy, a continuous oral antibiotic therapy should be started, based on the bacteria and the patient's individual management, for a period of 3 months up to 1 year, in a curative set-up. In cases of suppression therapy, this oral intake might be extended to a lifelong suppression therapy.

TWO-STAGE EXCHANGE

In cases of late infection, a septic knee revision is indicated. This includes the removal of all foreign material as well as debridement of the soft tissues and bone at the time of first surgery. A spacer is usually placed in the knee and systemic antibiotics are administered for an interval of 4–6 weeks. Thereafter, a second revision is required to implant the new components if the knee is free of infection. However, if there is any suspicion that infection might persist, repeat debridement might be performed and a new spacer put in place.

Radical debridement and removal of all foreign material is essential for any revision for infection. Even solid implants have to be removed, sometimes even requiring extended osteotomies. While it is mandatory to remove all components of the implant, femoral or tibial stems, bone cement, cement restrictors, screws and wires in two-stage procedures, the general debridement does not have to be as aggressive as in one-stage exchange, since a planned second approach will be performed some weeks later for the reimplantation. During the resection, all septic membranes must be radically excised. Special care needs to be taken to properly debride the posterior capsule, since it might be the source of reinfection.

Removing cemented implants is sometimes even easier and less invasive than removing ingrown cementless components. In a few cases of well-fixed uncemented components, cortical windows are required to gain access to the interface. High-speed burrs and curved saw blades can aid removal; however, occasionally, significant destruction and related bone loss cannot be prevented.

A multiple osteotome (double bonk) technique should be used in the knee to drive cement from between the tibial base plate and the tibial platform. Narrow, straight osteotomes with symmetrically coned blades should be used to remove all accessible bone cement. This may be less destructive than aggressive extraction using the mallet and special extraction devices. Removal of the implant might necessitate special or universal extraction forceps, if available; otherwise, general punches are required. Curved chisels, long rongeurs, curetting instruments, long drills and cement taps are used to remove the cement. General debridement of bone and posterior soft tissues must be as radical as possible, including all areas of osteolysis and nonviable bone.

Multiple tissue samples for microbiologic examination from different surgical areas should be gained during surgery. We recommend taking at least 3–6 samples from the anterior capsule, the synovial, the femoral and tibial components' interface, the posterior capsule, and the patella. As recently shown, it is not necessary to hold the standardized prophylactic antibiotic infusion before taking the samples; thus, the infusion can be started within 1 hour prior to surgery.[31]

Generally, we recommend the use of pulsatile jet lavage throughout the procedure; however, after the removal of all foreign material and completed debridement, the intramedullary canals are packed with polymeric biguanide hydrochloride (polyhexanid)-soaked swabs.

THE SPACER

After complete debridement of all infected tissues and membranes, an antibiotic-loaded cement spacer is inserted.[47] The role of the spacer is to preserve the joint space and reduce soft tissue contracture, while effective topical antibiotic concentration is delivered by elution from the bone cement.[48,49] Ideally, it should also allow for an optimized exposure for second-stage reimplantation. The local bactericidal concentration of antibiotics eliminates the bacteria remaining after debridement at the local site of surgery, which is always combined with a systemic ongoing antibiotic therapy.[50,51]

In general, dynamic versus static spacers can be compared in the knee joint.[52] While a general improvement of function before second-stage reimplantation can mostly be achieved with an articulating spacer, there is current evidence that the overall range of motion at a mean follow-up time of 2 years after reimplantation does not significantly vary (<5°) between patients who received an articulating (dynamic) versus a nonarticulating (static) spacer in two-stage exchanges (ICM group 2013).[31] Furthermore, the use of articulating spacers does permit dislocation as a distinct complication. However, no clear contraindications have been described in the literature for either type of spacers, although many authors believe that a massive bone loss and the need for plastic reconstructive surgery are relative contraindications for the use of a articulating spacer (ICM).[31] There is no evidence that one technique does provide a better eradication of infection over the other after 2 years and there is no evidence that any industrial spacer shows bacteriologic superiority to any 'home made' type.[31]

In most scenarios, industrial manufactured versus hand-molded spacers made of PMMA bone cement are used. The advantages of industrial spacers are based on a smooth surface, the ease of use, congruent articulation and homogeneous dissemination of the antibiotics in the cement. They mostly contain aminoglycosides like gentamicin or tobramycin. Hand-molded spacers can be formed intraoperatively by hand according to the individual anatomical situation and the mixing of individual antibiotics can be done based upon the susceptibility of the germs (**Figures 24.1 to 24.3**).

Antibiotic-loaded bone cement spacers may contain water soluble, heat resistant antibiotics in crystalline form; the powder should be mixed together with the powder of

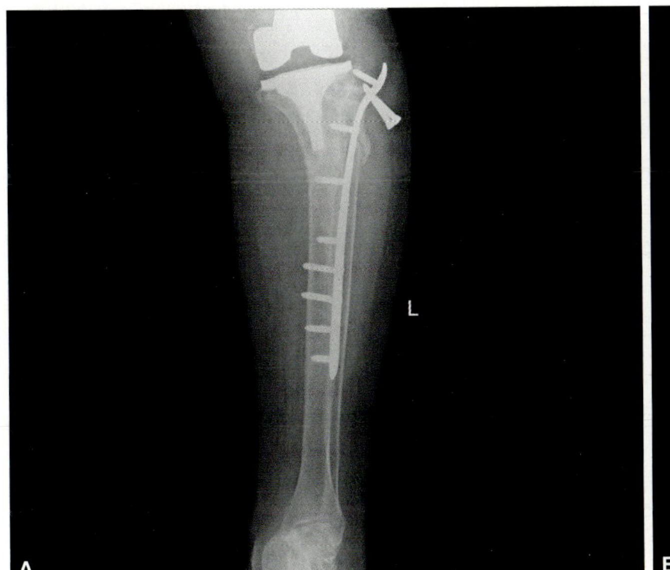

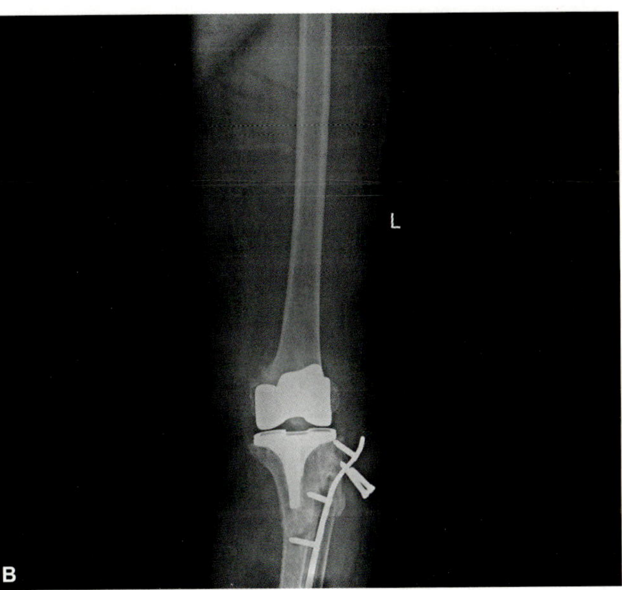

Figures 24.1A and B Patient with infected pseudarthrosis of tibia shaft after TKA implantation, 3 years after primary implantation and combined large anterior skin defect

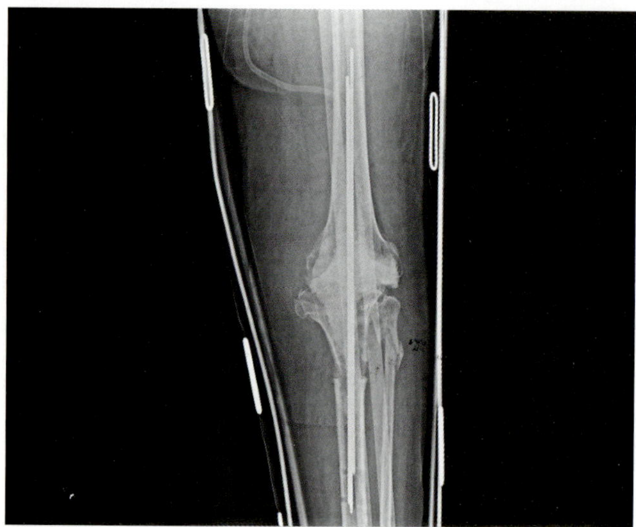

Figure 24.2 Nonarticulating spacer application, based on Kirschner-rods, for a period of 6 weeks before secondary reimplantation

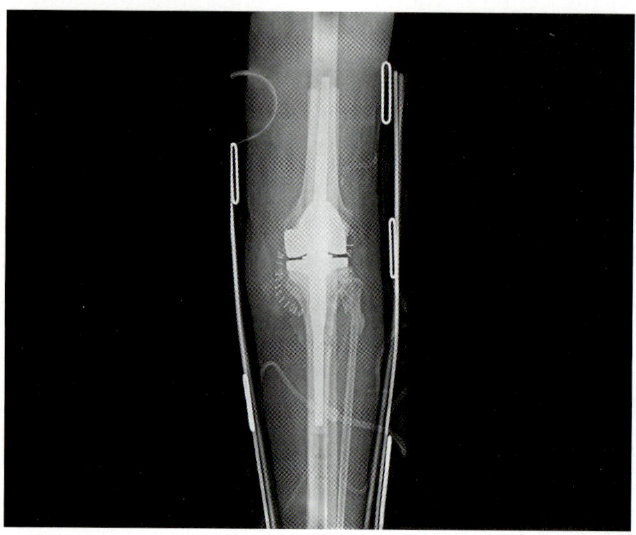

Figure 24.3 Two-staged reimplantation of long stemmed fully cemented rotating hinged implant with combined muscular gastroc-flap

the PMMA bone cement before liquid is added. With an antibiotic-loaded spacer, the total amount of antibiotics can be up to 20% of the total mass of the spacer, because the spacer has no definitive fixation function and is removed after several weeks. Care should be taken with the total amount of local antibiotics used.[53] Although rarely described, topical antibiotics may be nephrotoxic and can lead to renal failure. In comparison, when using the antibiotic-loaded cement for definitive fixation of a new implant during reimplantation, a maximum of 10% antibiotic should be added to the cement, to retain its biomechanical properties.[54,55]

In cases of recurrence or wound healing disturbances between the reimplantation stages, an exchange of the spacer may be indicated. Based upon the results of intraoperative microbiologic testing of the initial surgery, a new antibiotic combination may be considered for this subsequent spacer.[56,57]

ANTIBIOTIC THERAPY

Antibiotic treatment should be carried out based upon the results of bacterial cultures obtained before and during the surgery. A microbiologist recommends the antibiotic treatment according to the susceptibility of the germ, concomitant diseases of the patient and the laboratory tests, which should be carried out on a regular basis postoperatively.[53]

Antibiotic treatment is started during the first-stage surgery, and in the most frequent scenarios, it is continued until 4–6 weeks postoperatively. However, it can be extended individually, depending on the affected bacteria and the patient's progress. In the first 2 weeks, IV administration through a central venous line is recommended; subsequently, oral administration is carried out. Since oral administration is not always possible, especially in cases of multiresistant organisms, the whole treatment period might have to be administered IV.[58]

Two weeks prior to the reimplantation, the antibiotic treatment is terminated and the inflammatory markers of the patient are controlled. If the CRP levels dropped relevantly, the reimplantation can be planned. However CRP levels usually never normalize during that time period. Additionally, an aspiration of the knee joint should rule out infection persistence. Due to possible false negative culture results before reimplantation, the discontinuation of systemic antibiotics 2 weeks prior to aspiration is recommended.[32] In second-stage surgery, soft tissue samples should be obtained again, because the antibiotic treatment was withheld 2 weeks before surgery.

REIMPLANTATION

In most scenarios, reimplantation usually takes place between 2 and 3 months after the initial explantation and debridement. After spacer placement and confirmed negative aspiration results, a planned reimplantation can take place.[59] Evaluation of the use of ESR and CRP values before reimplantation has shown that they do show statistically significant reductions; however, they do not revert to normal values.[60,61] Therefore, no cutoff value to identify if the knee is persistently infected or not has been described yet.

During the procedure, antibiotics should not be administered if infection is no longer suspected.[62] Therefore, a conventional perioperative antibiotic prophylaxis can be given, if the organism was identified preoperatively.

Surgically, a full synovectomy should be performed. Some surgeons prefer to perform an anterior synovectomy, followed by the proximal tibia cut and then approach the posterior aspects of the knee, including a completed synovectomy of the posterior aspects. The femoral preparation is relatively specific to the implant system and the knee system used, i.e., semiconstrained versus full-constrained implants. There is still ongoing controversy on whether the stems should be fully cemented or partially, while a long cemented version allows for a broader delivery of local antibiotics throughout the infected field. On the other hand, diaphyseal engaging, uncemented stems might improve the alignment and the ease of removal in case of reinfection.

Generally, the second-stage procedure should be seen as another opportunity to complete debridement of the joint. Postoperative antibiotics are usually continued until intraoperative cultures are finalized and negative. The related wound control is obligatory, while movement restrictions are mainly based on the local skin conditions and wound healing procedure.

ONE-STAGE EXCHANGE

Indications

There are very few arguments against a one-stage revision in general; consequently, we have been able to fulfill around 85% of all our infected cases in the Endo-Klinik with this technique.[10,63] The mandatory infrastructural requirement is based on the clear evidence of bacteria preoperatively, in combination with the administration of patient-specific topical and systemic antibiotics.

Contraindications

The following criteria exist for deviating from a one-stage approach to a two-stage procedure:

- Failure of ≥ 2 previous one-stage procedures
- Infection spreading to the nerve-vessel bundle
- Unknown preoperative pathogen specification
- Nonavailability of appropriate antibiotics
- High antibiotic resistance.

Preoperative Preparation and Planning

It needs to be stressed again that the presence of a positive bacterial culture and antibiogram is absolutely mandatory for one-stage exchange. The proposed cemented fixation with specific antibiotics is considered to be the treatment of choice in order to achieve a high topical therapeutic level of antibiotic elution from the cement.[55] Although currently not commercially available, future-oriented approaches might include local antibiotic implant or silver coatings, which could be used in a one-stage approach as well.

Technical success does not only depend on the removal of all hardware material (including cement and restrictors) in combination with the topical antibiotics within the cement. Furthermore, a very extensive and complete debridement of any infected soft tissues and associated bone material is mandatory for this technique. It always includes a full synovectomy, even in the posterior aspects of the knee.

Operative Technique

Skin Incision and Debridement

Old scars in the line of the skin incision should be excised. The prior incision from the last operative approach should be used. In the presence of a sinus, it should be integrated into the skin incision and radically excised to the joint capsule. The tourniquet should be applied, but not inflated from the start of the operation. Surgery should be started without a tourniquet; consequently, the interfaces between infected tissue, scar and surrounding healthy bleeding soft tissue can be distinguished more clearly at debridement. All nonbleeding tissues and related bones need to be radically excised. After the completion of debridement and implant removal, the tourniquet can be helpful for the final intramedullary cement removal as well as for the process of recementation at the knee site. Biopsy material, preferably 5–6 samples, should be taken as a routine measure from all relevant areas of the operation site for combined microbiologic and histologic evaluation.[5,35] Prophylactic antibiotics should not be administered before these samples are taken.

Implant Removal and Completion of Debridement

As described above, in cases of long or partially cemented stems, curved chisels, long forceps, curretting instruments, long drills and cement taps are used to remove the cement. All cement and stoppers need to be removed radically. Generally, the debridement of bone and posterior soft tissues must be as radical as possible. It must include all areas of osteolysis and nonviable bone. Finalization of the aggressive debridement often exceeds the amount of resected materials in a two-stage approach. Thus, a resection of the collateral ligaments sometimes becomes necessary, which necessitates the use of fully cemented long stemmed revision implants and a higher level of constraint such as a rotating hinge, which is frequently used in our one-stage set-up (**Figures 24.4A and B**). We recommend the general use of pulsatile lavage throughout the procedure; however, after complete implant removal and debridement, the intramedullary canals are packed with polymeric biguanide hydrochloride (polyhexanid)-soaked swabs. The complete team now rescrubs, while new instruments are used for reimplantation. A second dose of antibiotic is given after 1.5 hours of the operating time or if blood loss at this point exceeds 1 L.

Reimplantation

In cases of inadequate bone stock, we do not recommend the use of allografts; however, there are few reports on the use of antibiotic-impregnated allografts in such cases

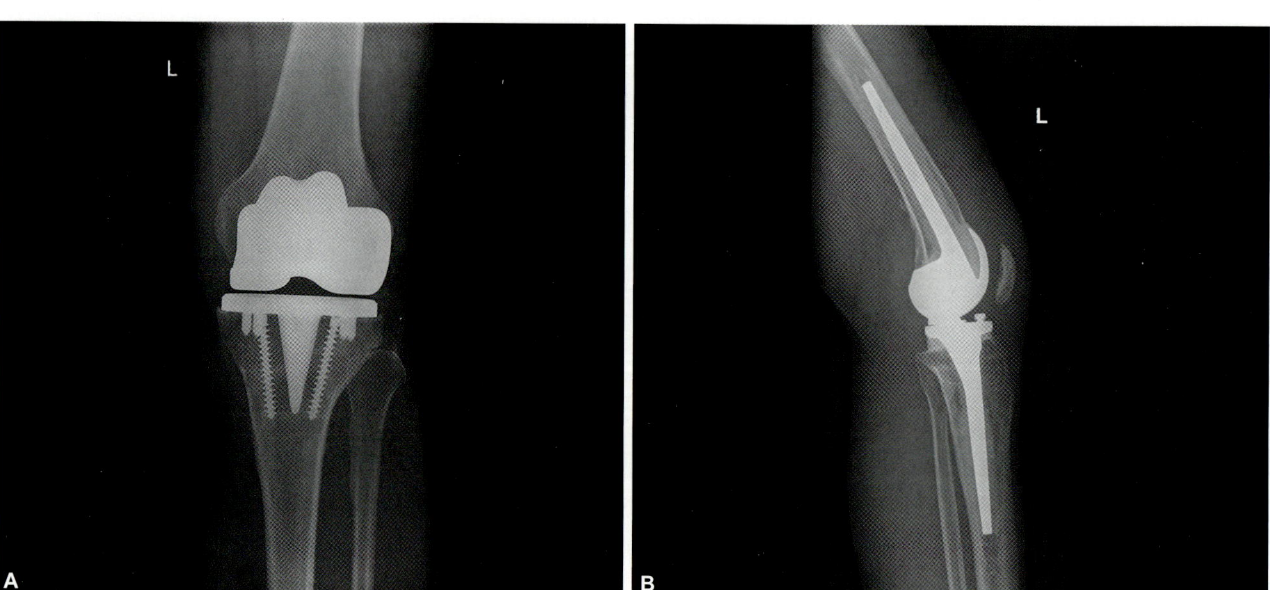

Figures 24.4A and B One-staged exchange due to *Staphylococcus epidermidis* infection of a conventional TKA, 4 years after implantation. Due to affected soft tissues around the collateral ligaments, a rotating hinge implant including patient specific antibiotics was used

(Winkler et al.).[64,65] We prefer to fill even small defects with bone cement. The use of trabecular metal cones in larger, contained bone defects of the distal femur or the proximal tibia has helped us to control more challenging situations **(Figures 24.5A and B)**. Variations in the depth and width of the metal cones allow for a proper reconstruction of the resulting bone loss, including an excellent biocompatibility and related stiffness and porous structure. Consequently, a combined fixation of the cement with the prosthesis and tantalum cones offers an excellent addendum to the treatment portfolio. In addition, it has been suggested that tantalum may additionally have some antibacterial properties, although this has not yet been proven clinically.[66]

Antibiotic-loaded cement is prepared in the meantime. It is mandatory that the following criteria are fulfilled:[31]

- Appropriate antibiotic (antibiogram, adequate elusion characteristics)
- Bactericidal (exception: clindamycin)
- Powder form (liquid antibiotic should not be used)
- Maximum addition of 10%/PMMA powder (for biomechanical stability).

Antibiotics (e.g. vancomycin) might change the polymerization behavior of the cement, causing the acceleration of cement curing. Generally, current principles of modern cementing techniques should be applied. In order to achieve an improved cement-bone interface, the tourniquet should be inflated prior to cementing in TKA cases.

Postoperative Antibiotics

In the one-stage approach, associated postoperative systemic antibiotic administration is usually for a period of 10–14 days (exception: streptococci).[10,53] While a prolonged administration of IV antibiotic for 6 weeks is common in the two-stage approach, the rationale for this extended period has not been completely clarified in studies. In contrast, there is evidence for possible relevant systemic and organ-specific complications after any prolonged antibiotic administration.[67]

Postoperative Care and Rehabilitation

A major advantage of the one-stage technique is based on the possible immediate physiotherapeutic approach and mobilization of all patients. The related postoperative hospitalization time ranges from 12 to 20 days (mean: 14) in our set-up. The physiotherapeutic approach at any one stage cannot be generalized. Due to the variety of soft tissue and bone damage and the extent of infection, in most cases, an individual plan is required. Postoperative rehabilitation in these patients aims to reduce associated

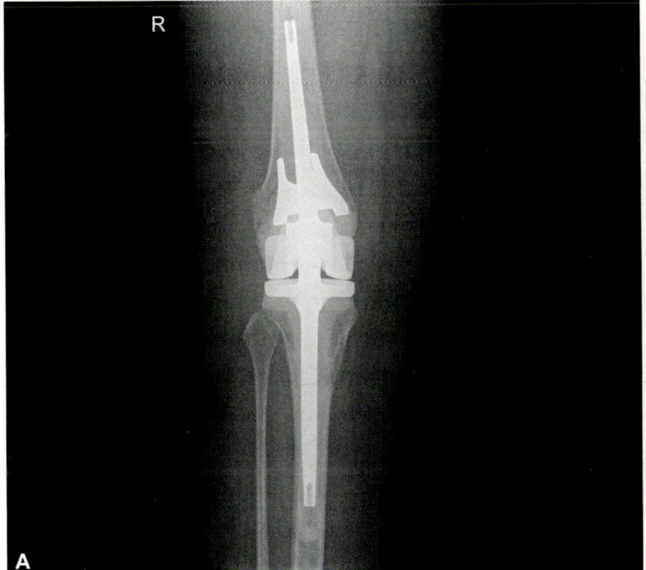

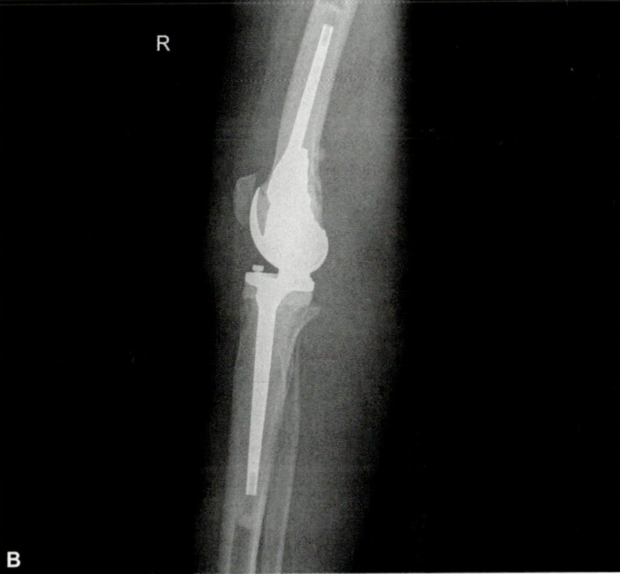

Figures 24.5A and B Example of one-staged exchange in combination of rotating hinge implant with tantalum cone

muscular movement restrictions, stiffness, or fibrosis of the affected knee joint. We generally recommend early mobilization within the first few postoperative days using walking aids. Weight-bearing should be adapted to the intraoperative findings and substance defects and might be increased to full weight-bearing within the first 2 weeks after surgery. In quite a large number of patients, the adequate bone stock and relative low soft tissue involvement allow an immediate mobilization under full weight-bearing.

Postoperative Complications

The persistence or recurrence of infection remains the most relevant complication in the one-stage technique. Failure rates with two-stage exchange have been described to range from 9 to 20% with nonresistant bacteria.[17,68,69] Our unpublished data as well as reports from other groups show comparable results in the short and mid-term follow-up, using the one-stage approach.[11,70] As a consequence, we advise our patients of a possible risk of recurrent or new infection of about 10–20%.

Although we are unable to present general comparative data evaluating the functional outcome between a two- and one-stage approach, we truly believe that neither any articulating spacer nor partial or complete immobilization of the knee joint will result in a better functional outcome.

We consider the risk of direct damage to the sciatic or peroneal nerve and main vessels to be relatively low with an experienced surgeon, even in such an extended aggressive debridement, and relatively comparable to a two-stage exchange. The general risk of intra- and postoperative fractures should also be comparable to the two- or more-stage exchange.

Outcome

As reported, the two-stage approach has become the most used technique worldwide, with a reported reinfection rate in the range of 9–20%.[68,71] Although advocated as the 'gold standard,' we established and have followed the above-described one-stage approach in our clinic for over 35 years in over 85% of all our infected TKA cases so far.[63]

Accordingly, far more studies have been published and emphasized the two-stage revision technique.[72] Very few studies or case series evaluating one-stage exchange are currently available. Although most reports are from or with our institution, some international experience exists, with comparable high success rates of 75–90%.[10,73,74]

Besides obvious surgical benefits, by eliminating a second major operative procedure, in our experience, a further advantage arises from the associated reduced duration of postoperative systemic antibiotics. This is rarely more than 14 days in our current set-up.

Alternative Treatment Options

There are additional surgical and nonsurgical options apart from the one- or two-stage revision in the treatment of PJI, which every surgeon should know about. These include chronic suppression of infections in the case of patients with concomitant diseases where surgery is not an option or where focal infections cannot be cured by surgery, excision arthroplasty, fusion or amputation. This chapter will mainly focus on these surgical options and give a brief overview over these different techniques.

Chronic Antibiotic Suppression

Generally, an antibiotic treatment will not eliminate infection. The goal is rather to keep function and stability of the prosthesis without sinus or pain not compromising the general health condition of the patient. Adequate counseling therefore is necessary.

In general, this type of therapy is considered, when it is not feasible to remove the prosthesis in patients with serious comorbidities where it might not be advisable to perform surgery. Additional criteria for this treatment include well-fixed components, low virulence of the pathogen, good susceptibility to oral antibiotic therapy and a low level of side effects of the antibiotic that will be administered. If these indications were carefully considered, a 86% success rate at 52, 6 months follow-up could be achieved, as published previously (**Figures 24.6A and B**).[75]

However, this therapy seems to depend highly on the selection criteria since other studies with larger amounts of patients only report good outcomes of 18–24%.[76,77]

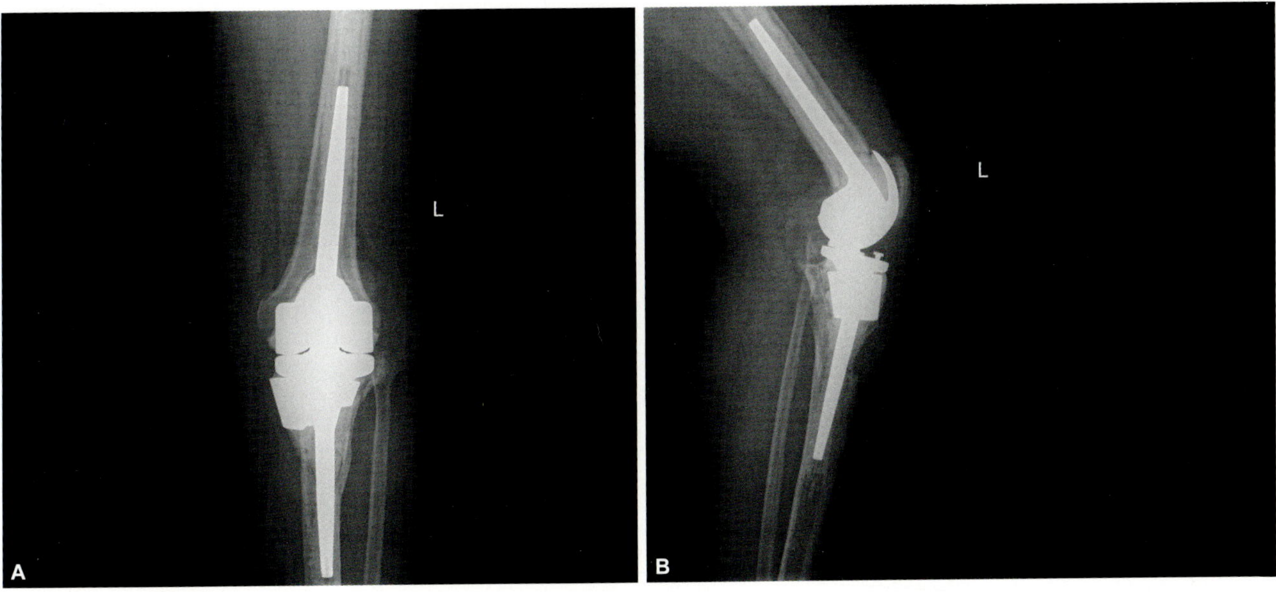

Figures 24.6A and B Status-post five-times reinfection of cemented rotating hinge in combination with tantalum cone and additional complete osseous destruction of the tibial tubercle and loss of function for 1.5 years

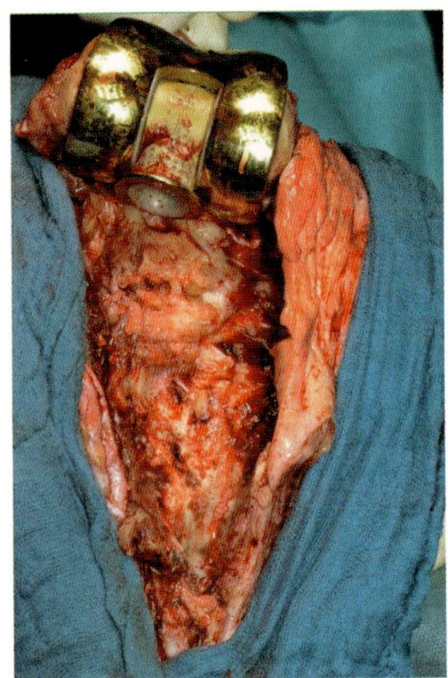

Figure 24.7 Intraoperative situs visualizes the destruction of the complete proximal tibia

Relative contraindications to this therapy include the presence of other implants that are not yet infected and presence of cardiac valvular prosthesis (**Figure 24.7**).

Excision Arthroplasty

Removal of all foreign material, along with soft tissue and bone debridement without reimplantation of new components or cement spacers defines resection arthroplasty. In our opinion, the indications for this surgical therapy are very limited and we have not performed this type of procedure over the past several years. Indications for this therapy might include a low demand, disabled patient that requires the capability of sitting which is more feasible than in a patient with a knee fusion. It is generally considered as a salvage procedure and results for eradication of infection range from 50 to 89%.[78,79]

Arthrodesis

Knee fusion has had a long tradition at our institution in the treatment of periprosthetic infections. Yet, the number of knee fusions has declined over the past decades with the good results of either one-stage or two-stage knee revision surgeries that could be achieved. In our institution, about only 1% of periprosthetic infections TKA are treated with knee arthrodesis annually.

Good candidates for knee arthrodesis are generally considered to be younger and more active and might also have a history of chronic drug abuse. Patients might present with loss of extensor mechanism, compromised bone stock and have a history of multiresistant pathogens

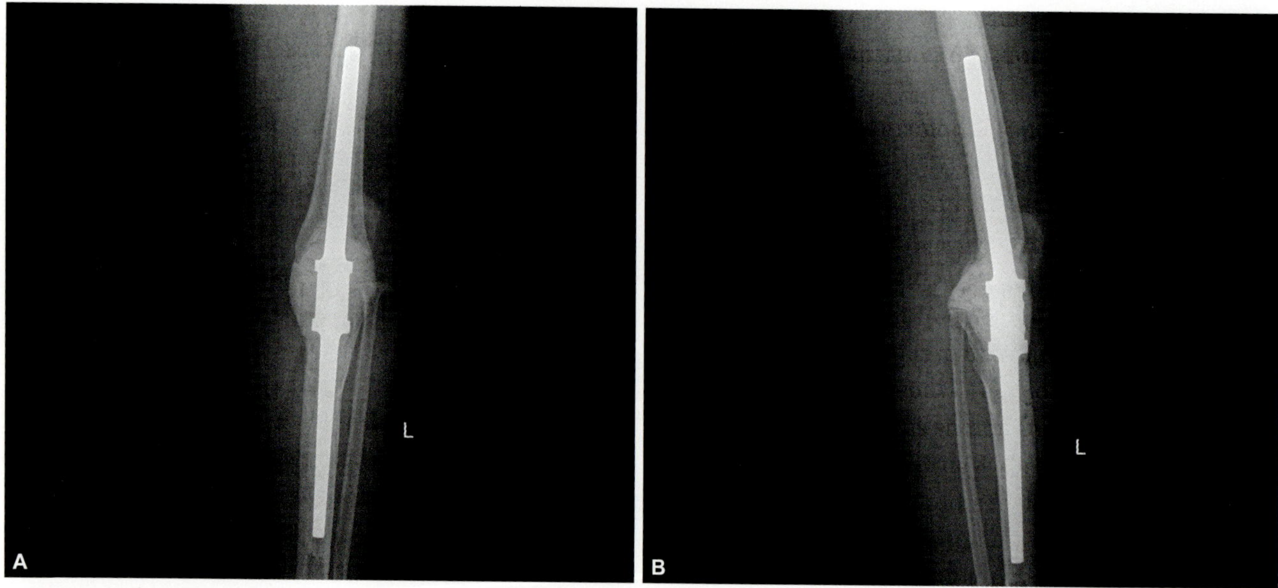

Figures 24.8A and B One-staged exchange to an arthrodesis rod, due to the severe destruction of tibial tubercle and long-term history of infection. As always including patient specific antibiotics

or multiple revision surgeries in their previous history. Different techniques have been described to achieve fusion and might include external fixation, double plating and intramedullary nailing which is the preferred treatment choice at our hospital. The nailing technique can also be performed in a one-staged technique (**Figures 24.8A and B**), while local antibiotics can be added. While the risks of fusion should not be neglected and include persistent pain and infection, functional limitations and limb length inequality as well as rotational malalignment problems, we consider this surgery as salvage therapy which allows for eradication of infection in severely compromised situations. In a recent report on two different techniques of fusion in patients with PJI of the knee, external fixation proved to be less susceptible to deep infection than intramedullary nailing techniques (4.9% vs 8.3%), however the rate of successful fusion was higher in the series of intramedullary nailing (95% vs 67%). However, it also needs to be noted that the rate of complications in this series was 40%.[80]

Amputation

Above-knee amputation is rarely indicated. It has been suggested that amputation might be the only treatment option in patients that present with a life threatening systemic sepsis. However in our experience, these situations are best handled in a manner, where open debridement is performed along with continuous lavage and suction drains applied.

We generally perform amputation rather in those situations where patients present after multiple previous revision surgeries due to persisting infections with general bone loss that might make fusion impossible.

In a described series, the prevalence of above-knee amputations directly related to infections of total knee replacement was 0.103% (19 of 18443 primary TKAs).[81]

Outcome of this surgical therapy is considered to be poor in the literature due to higher energy levels that are required to stay mobile. In one series, only 30% could ambulate regularly and 52% were confined to a wheelchair.[82]

REFERENCES

1. Bozic KJ, Kurtz SM, Lau E, et al. The epidemiology of revision total knee arthroplasty in the United States. Clin Orthop Relat Res. 2010;468(1):45-51.
2. Bozic KJ, Ries MD. The impact of infection after total hip arthroplasty on hospital and surgeon resource utilization. J Bone Joint Surg Am. 2005;87(8):1746-51.

3. Kurtz SM, Lau E, Schmier J, et al. Infection burden for hip and knee arthroplasty in the United States. J Arthroplasty. 2008;23(7):984-91.
4. Kurtz SM, Ong KL, Lau E, et al. Prosthetic joint infection risk after TKA in the medicare population. Clin Orthop Relat Res. 2010;468(1):52-6.
5. Fink B, Makowiak C, Fuerst M, et al. The value of synovial biopsy, joint aspiration and c-reactive protein in the diagnosis of late peri-prosthetic infection of total knee replacements. J Bone Joint Surg Br. 2008;90(7):874-8.
6. Siegel A, Frommelt L, Runde W. [Therapy of bacterial knee joint infection by radical synovectomy and implantation of a cemented stabilized knee joint endoprosthesis]. Chirurg. 2000;71(11):1385-91.
7. Steinbrink K, Frommelt L. Treatment of periprosthetic infection of the hip using one-stage exchange surgery. Orthopade. 1995;24(4):335-43.
8. Buchholz HW, Elson RA, Engelbrecht E, et al. Management of deep infection of total hip replacement. J Bone Joint Surg Br. 1981;63-B(3):342-53.
9. Wongworawat MD. Clinical faceoff: one- versus two-stage exchange arthroplasty for prosthetic joint infections. Clin Orthop Relat Res. 2013;471(6):1750-3.
10. Kordelle J, Frommelt L, Kluber D, Seemann K. Results of one-stage endoprosthesis revision in periprosthetic infection cause by methicillin-resistant *Staphylococcus aureus*. Z Orthop Ihre Grenzgeb. 2000;138(3):240-4.
11. Singer J, Merz A, Frommelt L, Fink B. High rate of infection control with one-stage revision of septic knee prostheses excluding MRSA and MRSE. Clin Orthop Relat Res. 2012;470(5):1461-71.
12. Fehring TK, Odum S, Calton TF, Mason JB. Articulating versus static spacers in revision total knee arthroplasty for sepsis. The Ranawat Award. Clin Orthop Relat Res. 2000;380:9-16.
13. Haddad FS, Masri BA, Campbell D, et al. The PROSTALAC functional spacer in two-stage revision for infected knee replacements. Prosthesis of antibiotic-loaded acrylic cement. J Bone Joint Surg Br. 2000;82(6):807-12.
14. Pietsch M, Wenisch C, Traussnig S, Trnoska R, Hofmann S. Temporary articulating spacer with antibiotic-impregnated cement for an infected knee endoprosthesis. Orthopade. 2003;32(6):490-7.
15. Engesæter LB, Dale H, Schrama JC, Hallan G, Lie SA. Surgical procedures in the treatment of 784 infected THAs reported to the Norwegian arthroplasty register. Acta Orthop. 2011;82(5):530-7.
16. Kurd MF, Ghanem E, Steinbrecher J, Parvizi J. Two-stage exchange knee arthroplasty: does resistance of the infecting organism influence the outcome? Clin Orthop Relat Res. 2010;468(8):2060-6.
17. Mortazavi SMJ, Vegari D, Ho A, Zmistowski B, Parvizi J. Two-stage exchange arthroplasty for infected total knee arthroplasty: predictors of failure. Clin Orthop Relat Res. 2011;469(11):3049-54.
18. Parvizi J, Adeli B, Zmistowski B, Restrepo C, Greenwald AS. Management of periprosthetic joint infection: the current knowledge: AAOS exhibit selection. J Bone Joint Surg Am. 2012;94(14):e104.
19. Osmon DR, Berbari EF, Berendt AR, et al. Executive summary: diagnosis and management of prosthetic joint infection: clinical practice guidelines by the infectious diseases society of America. Clin Infect Dis. 2013;56(1): 1-10.
20. Winkler H, Stoiber A, Kaudela K, Winter F, Menschik F. One stage uncemented revision of infected total hip replacement using cancellous allograft bone impregnated with antibiotics. J Bone Joint Surg Br. 2008;90(12):1580-4.
21. Buechel FF. The infected total knee arthroplasty: just when you thought it was over. J Arthroplasty. 2004;19:51-5.
22. Callaghan JJ, Katz RP, Johnston RC. One-stage revision surgery of the infected hip. A minimum 10-year follow-up study. Clin Orthop Relat Res. 1999;369:139-43.
23. Goksan SB, Freeman MA. One-stage reimplantation for infected total knee arthroplasty. J Bone Joint Surg Br. 1992;74(1):78-82.
24. Zimmerli W, Trampuz A, Ochsner PE. Prosthetic-joint infections. N Engl J Med. 2004;351(16):1645-54.
25. De Man FHR, Sendi P, Zimmerli W, et al. Infectiological, functional, and radiographic outcome after revision for prosthetic hip infection according to a strict algorithm. Acta Orthop. 2011;82(1):27-34.
26. Ince A, Rupp J, Frommelt L, Katzer A, Loehr JF. Is 'aseptic' loosening of the prosthetic cup after total hip replacement due to nonculturable bacterial pathogens in patients with low-grade infection? Clin Infect Dis. 2004;39:1599-1603.
27. McPherson EJ, Woodson C, Holtom P, et al. Periprosthetic total hip infection: outcomes using a staging system. Clin Orthop Relat Res. 2002;403:8-15.

28. Cierny G 3rd, DiPasquale D. Periprosthetic total joint infections: staging, treatment, and outcomes. Clin Orthop Relat Res. 2002;403:23-8.
29. Trampuz A, Osmon DR, Hanssen AD, Steckelberg JM, Patel R. Molecular and antibiofilm approaches to prosthetic joint infection. Clin Orthop Relat Res. 2003;414:69-88.
30. Ehrlich GD, Stoodley P, Kathju S, et al. Engineering approaches for the detection and control of orthopedic biofilm infections. Clin Orthop Relat Res. 2005;437:59-66.
31. ICG: International Consensus Group on Periprosthetic Infection. Consensus Statements. Thomas Jefferson University, Philadelphia, USA 01.08.2013.
32. Della Valle C, Parvizi J, Bauer TW, et al. Diagnosis of periprosthetic joint infections of the hip and knee. J Am Acad Orthop Surg. 2010;18(12):760-70.
33. Parvizi J GE, Menashe S, Barrack RL, Bauer TW. Periprosthetic infection: what are the diagnostic challenges? J Bone Joint Surg Am. 2006;88:137-47.
34. Schinsky MF, Della Valle CJ, Sporer SM, Paprosky WG. Perioperative testing for joint infection in patients undergoing revision total hip arthroplasty. J Bone Joint Surg Am. 2008;90(9):1869-75.
35. Schafer P, Fink B, Sandow D, Margull A, Berger I, Frommelt L. Prolonged bacterial culture to identify late periprosthetic joint infection: a promising strategy. Clin Infect Dis. 2008;47(11):1403-09.
36. Della Valle CJ, Sporer SM, Jacobs JJ, et al. Preoperative testing for sepsis before revision total knee arthroplasty. J Arthroplasty. 2007;22:90-3.
37. Ghanem E, Parvizi J, Burnett RS, et al. Cell count and differential of aspirated fluid in the diagnosis of infection at the site of total knee arthroplasty. J Bone Joint Surg Am. 2008;90(8):1637-43.
38. Trampuz A, Hanssen AD, Osmon DR, et al. Synovial fluid leukocyte count and differential for the diagnosis of prosthetic knee infection. Am J Med. 2004;117(8):556-62.
39. Hanssen AD, Spangehl MJ. Practical applications of antibiotic-loaded bone cement for treatment of infected joint replacements. Clin Orthop Relat Res. 2004;427:79-85.
40. Schoifet SD, Morrey BF. Treatment of infection after total knee arthroplasty by débridement with retention of the components. J Bone Joint Surg Am. 1990;72(9):1383-90.
41. Rasul AT Jr, Tsukayama D, Gustilo RB. Effect of time of onset and depth of infection on the outcome of total knee arthroplasty infections. Clin Orthop Relat Res. 1991;273:98-104.
42. Romanò CL, Manzi G, Logoluso N, Romanò D. Value of debridement and irrigation for the treatment of periprosthetic infections. A systematic review. Hip Int. 2012;22 (Suppl 8):S19-24.
43. Sherrell JC, Fehring TK, Odum S, et al. The Chitranjan Ranawat Award: fate of two-stage reimplantation after failed irrigation and debridement for periprosthetic knee infection. Clin Orthop Relat Res. 2011;469(1):18-25.
44. Koyonos L, Zmistowski B, Della Valle CJ, Parvizi J. Infection control rate of irrigation and débridement for periprosthetic joint infection. Clin Orthop Relat Res. 2011;469(11):3043-8.
45. Dirschl DR, Wilson FC. Topical antibiotic irrigation in the prophylaxis of operative wound infections in orthopedic surgery. Orthop Clin North Am. 1991;22(3):419-26.
46. Roth RM, Gleckman RA, Gantz NM, Kelly N. Antibiotic irrigations. A plea for controlled clinical trials. Pharmacotherapy. 1985;5(4):222-7.
47. Jamsen E, Sheng P, Halonen P, et al. Spacer prostheses in two-stage revision of infected knee arthroplasty. Int Orthop. 2006;30(4):257-61.
48. Springer BD, Lee G-C, Osmon D, et al. Systemic safety of high-dose antibiotic-loaded cement spacers after resection of an infected total knee arthroplasty. Clin Orthop Relat Res. 2004;427:47-51.
49. Cui Q, Mihalko WM, Shields JS, Ries M, Saleh KJ. Antibiotic-impregnated cement spacers for the treatment of infection associated with total hip or knee arthroplasty. J Bone Joint Surg Am. 2007;89(4):871-82.
50. Hanssen AD, Rand JA, Osmon DR. Treatment of the infected total knee arthroplasty with insertion of another prosthesis. The effect of antibiotic-impregnated bone cement. Clin Orthop Relat Res. 1994;309:44-55.
51. Westrich GH, Walcott-Sapp S, Bornstein LJ, et al. Modern treatment of infected total knee arthroplasty with a 2-stage reimplantation protocol. J Arthroplasty. 2010;25(7):1015-21.
52. Mabry TM, Hanssen AD. Articulating antibiotic spacers: a matter of personal preference. Orthopedics. 2007;30(9):783-5.
53. Frommelt L. Principles of systemic antimicrobial therapy in foreign material associated infection in bone tissue, with special focus on periprosthetic infection. Injury. 2006;37:S97-94.

54. Wahlig H, Dingeldein E, Buchholz HW, Buchholz M, Bachmann F. Pharmacokinetic study of gentamicin-loaded cement in total hip replacements. Comparative effects of varying dosage. J Bone Joint Surg Br. 1984;66(2):175-9.
55. Fink B, Vogt S, Reinsch M, Buchner H. Sufficient release of antibiotic by a spacer 6 weeks after implantation in two-stage revision of infected hip prostheses. Clin Orthop Relat Res. 2011;469(11):3141-7.
56. Kubista B, Hartzler RU, Wood CM, et al. Reinfection after two-stage revision for periprosthetic infection of total knee arthroplasty. Int Orthop. 2012;36(1):65-71.
57. Maheshwari AV, Gioe TJ, Kalore NV, Cheng EY. Reinfection after prior staged reimplantation for septic total knee arthroplasty: is salvage still possible? J Arthroplasty. 2010;25:92-7.
58. Kilgus DJ, Howe DJ, Strang A. Results of periprosthetic hip and knee infections caused by resistant bacteria. Clin Orthop Relat Res. 2002;404:116-24.
59. Insall JN, Thompson FM, Brause BD. Two-stage reimplantation for the salvage of infected total knee arthroplasty. J Bone Joint Surg Am. 1983;65(8):1087-98.
60. Kusuma SK, Ward J, Jacofsky M, Sporer SM, Della Valle CJ. What is the role of serological testing between stages of two-stage reconstruction of the infected prosthetic knee? Clin Orthop Relat Res. 2011;469(4):1002-8.
61. Ghanem E, Azzam K, Seeley M, Joshi A, Parvizi J. Staged revision for knee arthroplasty infection: what is the role of serologic tests before reimplantation? Clin Orthop Relat Res. 2009;467(7):1699-705.
62. Parvizi J, Della Valle CJ. AAOS Clinical Practice Guideline: diagnosis and treatment of periprosthetic joint infections of the hip and knee. J Am Acad Orthop Surg. 2010;18(12):771-2.
63. von Foerster G, Kluber D, Kabler U. Mid- to long-term results after treatment of 118 cases of periprosthetic infections after knee joint replacement using one-stage exchange surgery. Orthopade. 1991;20(3):244-52.
64. Winkler H, Kaudela K, Stoiber A, Menschik F. Bone grafts impregnated with antibiotics as a tool for treating infected implants in orthopedic surgery - one stage revision results. Cell Tissue Bank. 2006;7(4):319-23.
65. Winkler H, Janata O, Berger C, Wein W, Georgopoulos A. In vitro release of vancomycin and tobramycin from impregnated human and bovine bone grafts. J Antimicrob Chemother. 2000;46(3):423-8.
66. Schildhauer TA, Robie B, Muhr G, Köller M. Bacterial adherence to tantalum versus commonly used orthopedic metallic implant materials. J Orthop Trauma. 2006;20(7):476-84.
67. Hoad-Reddick DA, Evans CR, Norman P, Stockley I. Is there a role for extended antibiotic therapy in a two-stage revision of the infected knee arthroplasty? J Bone Joint Surg Br. 2005;87(2):171-4.
68. Azzam K, McHale K, Austin M, Purtill JJ, Parvizi J. Outcome of a second two-stage reimplantation for periprosthetic knee infection. Clin Orthop Relat Res. 2009;467(7):1706-14.
69. Bauer T, Piriou P, Lhotellier L, et al. Results of reimplantation for infected total knee arthroplasty: 107 cases. Rev Chir Orthop Reparatrice Appar Mot. 2006;92(7):692-700.
70. Jenny JY, Barbe B, Gaudias J, Boeri C, Argenson JN. High infection control rate and function after routine one-stage exchange for chronically infected TKA. Clin Orthop Relat Res. 2013;471(1):238-43.
71. Goldman RT, Scuderi GR, Insall JN. 2-stage reimplantation for infected total knee replacement. Clin Orthop Relat Res. 1996;331:118-24.
72. Haleem AA, Berry DJ, Hanssen AD. Mid-term to long-term follow up of two-stage reimplantation for infected total knee arthroplasty. Clin Orthop Relat Res. 2004;428:35-9.
73. Buechel FF, Femino FP, D'Alessio J. Primary exchange revision arthroplasty for infected total knee replacement: a long-term study. Am J Orthop (Belle Mead NJ). 2004;33(4):190-8.
74. Schmitz HC, Schwantes B, Kendoff D. One-stage revision of knee endoprosthesis due to periprosthetic infection and Klippel-Trenaunay syndrome. Orthopäde. 2011;40(7):624-6, 628-9.
75. Rao N, Crossett LS, Sinha RK, Le Frock JL. Long-term suppression of infection in total joint arthroplasty. Clin Orthop Relat Res. 2003;414:55-60.
76. Bengtson S, Knutson K. The infected knee arthroplasty. A 6-year follow-up of 357 cases. Acta Orthop Scand. 1991;62(4):301-1.
77. Hanssen AD, Rand JA. Evaluation and treatment of infection at the site of a total hip or knee arthroplasty. Instr Course Lect. 1999;48:111-22.
78. Falahee MH, Matthews LS, Kaufer H. Resection arthroplasty as a salvage procedure for a knee with infection after a total arthroplasty. J Bone Joint Surg Am. 1987;69(7):1013-21.

79. Wasielewski RC, Barden RM, Rosenberg AG. Results of different surgical procedures on total knee arthroplasty infections. J Arthroplasty. 1996;11(8):931-8.
80. Mabry TM, Jacofsky DJ, Haidukewych GJ, Hanssen AD. Comparison of intramedullary nailing and external fixation knee arthrodesis for the infected knee replacement. Clin Orthop Relat Res. 2007;464:11-5.
81. Sierra RJ, Trousdale RT, Pagnano MW. Above-the-knee amputation after a total knee replacement: prevalence, etiology, and functional outcome. J Bone Joint Surg Am. 2003;85-A(6):1000-4.
82. Pring DJ, Marks L, Angel JC. Mobility after amputation for failed knee replacement. J Bone Joint Surg Br. 1988;70(5):770-1.

Chapter 25

Salvage after Failed Total Knee Arthroplasty

Mojieb Manzary

INTRODUCTION

Total knee arthroplasty (TKA) has revolutionized humanity with the outstanding functional results that it imparts to those who receive it. It has been one of the most successful and gratifying surgeries in the field of orthopedics in terms of excellent resolution of the patient's symptoms.

It provides a pain free, well aligned, and durable knee joint for the prospective patient to perform his or her daily and/or recreational activities. In some unfortunate subset of patient population, a difficult decision has to be taken by the patient and the surgeon together for an alternate surgical option after all attempts to reconstruct a failed TKA to a successful revision arthroplasty have been unsuccessful. Those surgical alternatives, which will be discussed in this chapter, include arthrodesis of the knee, amputation above the knee, and resection arthroplasty of the knee.

KNEE ARTHRODESIS

In selected groups of TKA patients, in particular those who were unfortunate enough to develop refractory infection in their knees with TKA that did not have a satisfactory outcome even after a two-stage reimplantation, an alternative does exist to provide them with stable painless lower limb albeit with the sacrifice of motion at the knee.[1,2]

Compared to above knee amputation, which may not be acceptable to a number of patients due to concerns of loss of a body part or body image or due to social, cultural, and/or religious reasons, a knee arthrodesis has a better functional outcome with less energy expenditure.[1] Although, the most common indication for knee arthrodesis in contemporary orthopedic practice will be a refractory infection, other causes resulting in a nonreconstructable knee joint with either metaphyseal bone loss, or ligamentous imbalance that failed multiple revision procedures, insufficient or loss of extensor mechanism or its disruption.[1,2] In a nonarthroplasty set-up, knee arthrodesis could also be used in cases of tumor resection with intact soft tissue mechanism, Charcot arthropathy.[1] Historically, knee arthrodesis was used for the treatment of poliomyelitis as well as tuberculous or postseptic arthritis.[1] The decision to limit the number of revisions that a patient has to undergo for a resistant infection could turn out to be a difficult task to undertake.

Some authors believe in giving patients at least a second chance of two-stage reimplantation if the first attempt of two stage of the reimplantation failed with a recurrence of infection. The literature is very clear about the lower chances of success with increment numbers of revisions particularly for infections.[1,2] The success of arthrodesis is dependent on multiple factors, most important of which is absence or presence of active infection, presence of infection has been shown to lessen the chances of union as well as prolonging the time required to achieve bony union.[1-3] Other factors include, the degree of bone defect which is usually larger in cases of constrained total knee replacement (TKR) and in cases of revision TKR in comparison to primary TKR especially with those with less constraint used, and the ability to produce a rigid compression across the fusion site.[1-3]

Finally, the comorbidities of the patient, the etiology for which the TKR was originally done carries significance in whether a successful bony union will result or not. The main contraindication for arthrodesis is ipsilateral hip and ankle degenerative disease, contralateral hip or knee arthrodesis, and contralateral knee amputation extensive segmental bone defect. The most acceptable position for arthrodesis is 10–15° of knee flexion, and 5–7° of valgus with slight external rotation of the lower extremity.[1,2,4,5] This degree of flexion allows a better sitting position, it also improves the gait making it more efficient, in compared to the knees fused in full extension. There is usually some degree of shortening of the fused limb resulting in leg length discrepancy, which is directly proportional to the degree of flexion. 15° of flexion is usually associated with 2 cm of shortening.[1,2,4]

Technique

Various techniques have been described for successful knee arthrodesis. The most commonly used are the intramedullary techniques as well as those using double plating technique and use of the external fixator or its variants. Both can be used in infected TKR situations, after the removal of the prosthesis or the spacer, the surfaces could be opposed after freshening the edges of the condyles and two plates could be applied medially and anteriorly in compression mode.[1,6] The incision that was used for the removal of the prosthesis and/or the spacers could as well be used for insertion of the plates, or the nails that usually come in two parts. The femoral segment is inserted retrograde in the femur, and the tibial part is inserted antegrade in the tibia and coupled together in the knee.

Plates (Figures 25.1 to 25.3)

The proponents of using the plates cite advantages of using the same incision, avoidance of spreading the infection proximally and distally by an intramedullary nail, avoidance of pin tract infection, loosening of pins, and a relatively easier and earlier rehabilitation.[5,6] Nichols et al.,[6] reviewed 11 patients with failed TKR, who had arthrodesis with 100% union, with an average time to union of 5.6 months.[6] Pritchett et al.[5] described successful knee arthrodesis in 26 patients of various etiologies using tension band plate.[5]

However, only 10 of their patients, (10/26) 38% had a failed TKR, while the rests of their patients were having native diseased knees.[5] The original description of knee arthrodesis with the use of plates came from Lucas and Murray in 1961, with 17 out of their 18 patients achieving bony union.[7] They advocated the use of 1.3 cm wide plates applied anteriorly and medially, however with modification of their technique[6] using the more contemporary broad 4.5 dynamic compression plate (DCP) plates applied

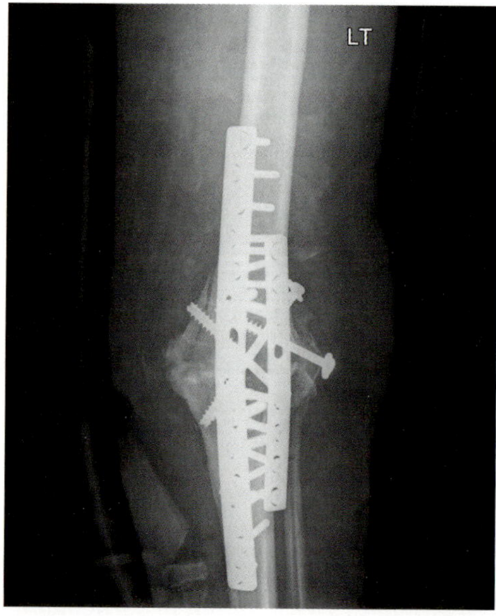

Figure 25.1 Arthrodesis with two dynamic compression plates—anteroposterior view

in staggered fashion allows more intimate bone to plate contact, and also allows compression to yield more rigid construction.[6] Applying the plate laterally and medially avoids the overstuffing of the anterior compartment that some authors have reported causing difficulty in skin closure.[6]

The patella could be osteotomized, to be used as a vascularized autogenous bone graft, and/or secured to the anterior and distal part of the construct, as a buttress, adding further rigidity.[6] Various cutting guides from the TKA instrumentations could be used to achieve the desired 7° of valgus in the femur as well as the 10° of flexion and desired external rotation of about 6–7°.[6] Cutting of the bone surfaces will also allow them to be freshened as well as be intimately opposed to achieve bony consolidation.[1,2]

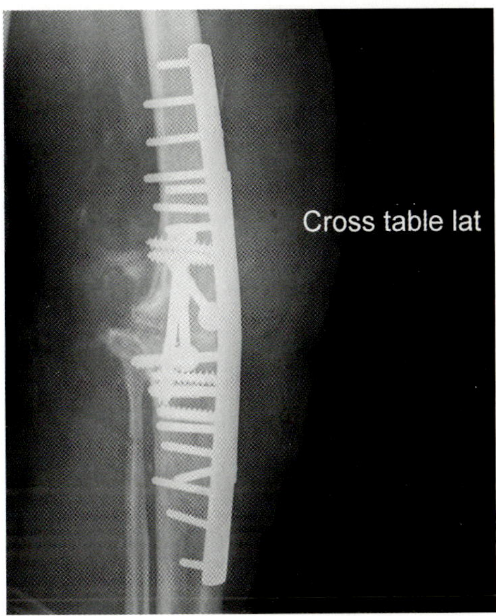

Figure 25.2 Arthrodesis with two dynamic compression plates—lateral view

Contouring of the plates allows the final desired position of the fusion to be obtained and maintained.[5,6] The two main problems reported in the literature are wound complications at the distal part of the wound, necessitating removal of the plate and debridement.[6] Stress fracture above the plate proximally (**Figures 25.4 and 25.5**) has been reported as well, treatment of which could be by an antegrade intramedullary nail. In these cases the length of the nail needs to be chosen carefully to bypass the fracture site while being overlapped by the plate (**Figures 25.6 and 25.7**) and, see figure, the proximal screws may need to be removed. Placement of plates in staggered fashion should minimize the chances of these types of fractures.[6]

Intramedullary Device

Multiple reports in the literature have advocated the use of intramedullary device/nails for arthrodesis.[1,2,8,9] The major attractive feature cited by its proponents are the mechanical advantage of a load sharing device, avoidance of pins and their complications, avoidance of

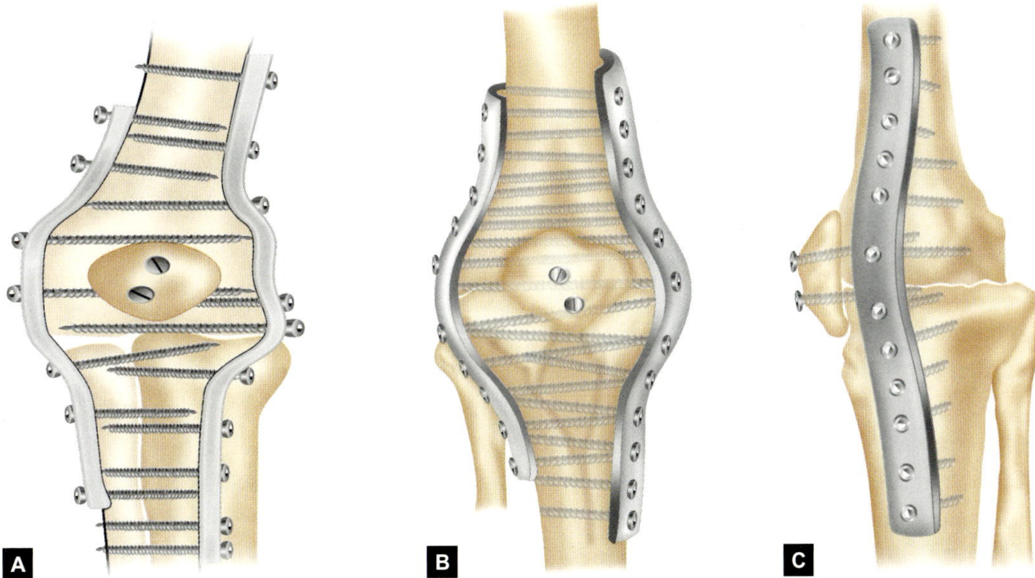

Figures 25.3A to C Diagrammatic representation of plating for arthrodesis

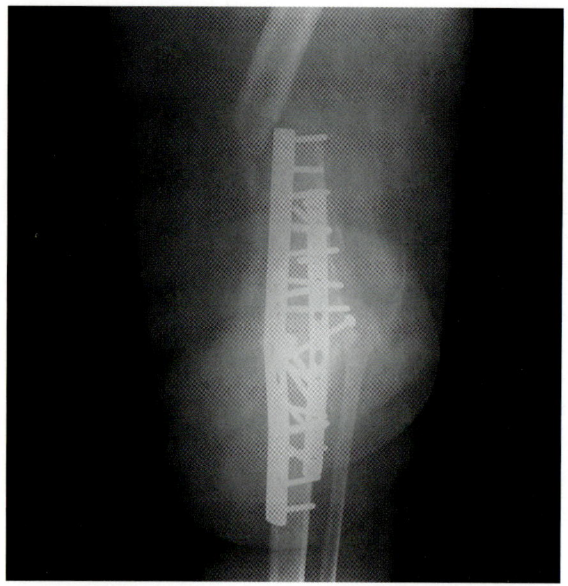

Figure 25.4 Stress fracture above the plate proximally—AP view

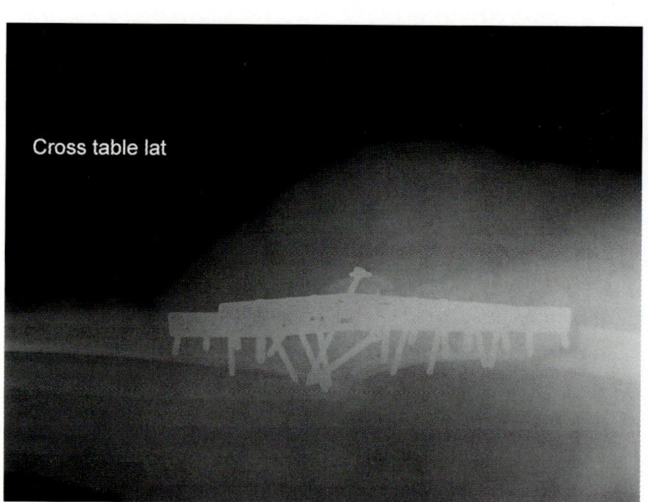

Figure 25.5 Stress fracture above the plate proximally—lateral view

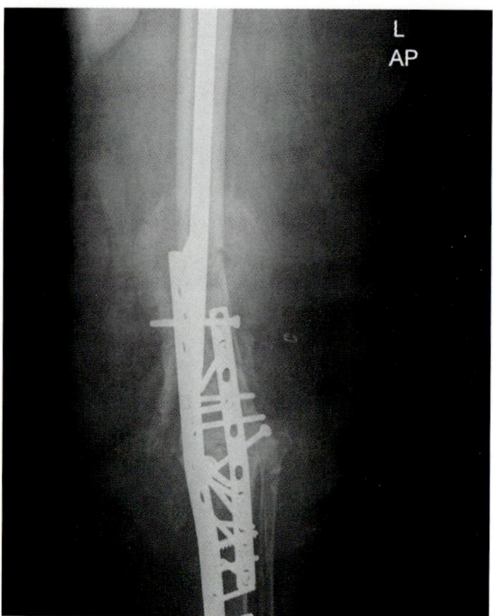

Figure 25.6 Stress fracture above the plate treatmented by an antegrade intramedullary nail

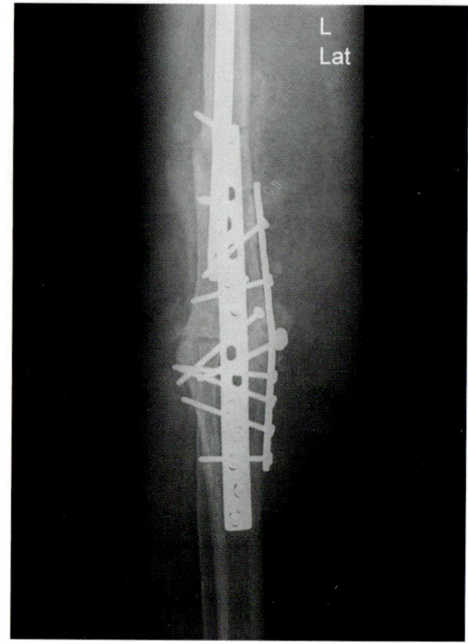

Figure 25.7 Fracture above the plate treatmented by an antegrade intramedullary nail

plate and its potential disadvantage of difficulty in wound closure or fracture above the plate (**Figures 25.8 and 25.9**).[1,8,10,11]

However, concerns remain about the possibility of the nail spreading the infection proximally and distally throughout the intramedullary canal, nail migration, lack of tibial rotational control, loss of femoral valgus alignment.[9] Bargiotas et al.[10] achieved clinical and radiographic union in ten out of their twelve patients with an infected TKR following two-stage arthrodesis using intramedullary nail.[10] In all of their cases they followed the two-stage protocol with a spacer and intravenous antibiotic for the interim period of 6–8 weeks in between the two stages. In only one of their twelve cases, infection persisted requiring an above knee amputation. Incavo et al. described their experience of using custom made intramedullary

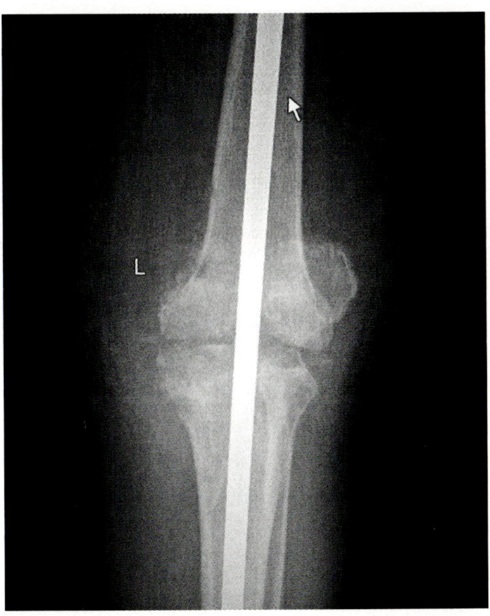

Figure 25.8 Use of intramedullary nails for arthrodesis—AP view

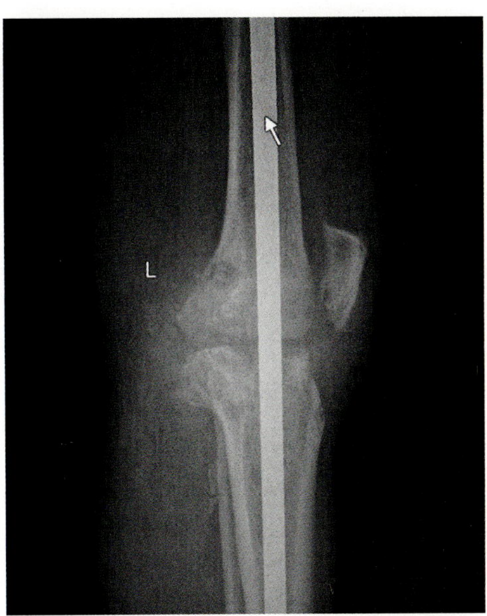

Figure 25.9 Use of intramedullary nails for arthrodesis—lateral view

nail for knee arthrodesis in 22 cases, 17 out of those cases were following infected primary or revision TKR.[12]

None of the infected cases in their series were treated in one-stage arthrodesis. The custom long nail was designed to have a gradual buildup of valgus and anterior bow to reach an apex at or around the tibiofemoral contact point. Other factors include the size of the bone defect at the site of the arthrodesis, rigid construct with compression along the fusion site, maximal contact of opposing bony surfaces, as well as the degree of infection control all serve as predictors affecting the union across the arthrodesis site. Recently the use of shorter modular titanium nail have been reported to show good results, however a major technical issue is the difficulty in removing those nails, if and when required for example in case of a recurrent infection or fracture.[9,11,12] In those circumstances, sectioning of the nail, or over reaming by a trephine or creating a window proximally or distally to push the nail out may be few technical hints for removal of those nails.

External Fixator

Use of external fixator or one of its variants, remain one of the most common mode of knee arthrodesis (**Figure 25.10**). Its main advantages are the short operating time and less blood loss. It also allows for surgical compression across the arthrodesis site with the appropriate alignment desired. Upon achieving solid union and removal of the pins no implants are leftover.[1,9,13] Its main disadvantages are pin tract infection and loosening, pin pullout and breakage, fracture through the pin sites, inability to early weight bear, the awkward feeling of discomfort by the patients having an apparatus of a wide field applied to their knee limiting their activity

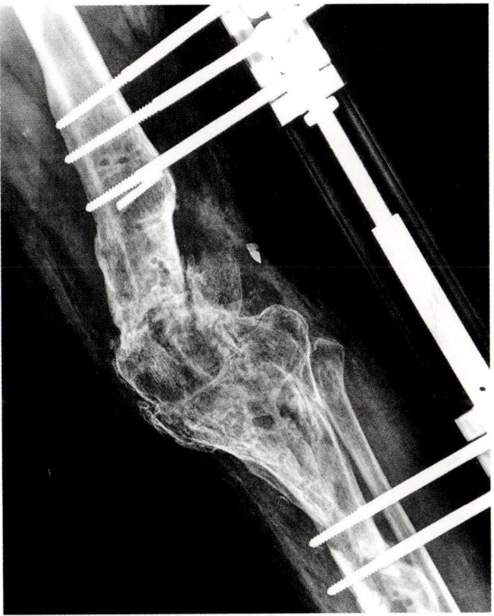

Figure 25.10 Knee arthrodesis using an external fixator

and mobility. There usually is a learning curve particularly with the use of more modern contemporary hybrid frames techniques. The fixation is usually nonrigid. Long healing times have usually been observed in comparison to the intramedullary (IM) nailing techniques.[9]

In comparison to the intramedullary technique, use of external fixator or rods were shown to give a more easier control of the opposed fragment with the ability to align the whole lower extremity at the knee in appropriate valgus and/or external rotation and flexion.[9,13] Use of biplane type of external fixator does not add any additional advantage in terms of achieving union, although it adds more stability.[1,2,9,13] The choice of external fixator may give the surgeon the option of attempting a one-stage arthrodesis following implant removal and extensive debridement, however the severity of the infection and its extent of involvement must be taken into consideration before deciding on one- or two-stage procedure.[1,2,9,13] The use of Ilizarov circular external fixator, frame has been reported as a method to obtain an arthrodesis by Spina et al.[13] they too used a two or even three-stage debridement for treatment of their severely infected knees prior to applying the final construct.[13] Their mean time to union was 9.3 months. A further advantage that the authors cited in their patients was the ability to early weight bear with the application of the Ilizarov frame. They also commented on use of simultaneous distraction osteogenesis technique to avoid leg length discrepancy.[13]

In a nonrandomized comparative study between intramedullary rods and external fixators for arthrodesis following infected TKR, Mabry et al.[9] showed better fusion rates in the IM rod group, but with longer operative times and more blood loss. They also showed a higher incidence of recurrent infection in the IM group in comparison to external fixator.[9] The average time for union in both groups was 5.4–5.7 months.

In conclusion, arthrodesis is a very good choice for the refractory case of failed TKR whether due to infectious or noninfectious etiology. The choice of the most appropriate surgical technique, available from the vast array of surgical options, is very much dependent on the severity of infection and the degree of bone defects, the experience of the surgeon and resources available. Two-stage arthrodesis should be carried out with use of intramedullary device and/or dual plates, single stage could be attempted with external fixator if the surgeon is pretty certain the debridement has been extensive enough to bring his infection under control.[1,2,6,9,10,13] The expectations as well as the functional outcome need to be clearly addressed with the patients, particularly the loss of motion at the knee that will be undergoing the fusion.[1,2]

ABOVE KNEE AMPUTATION

Total knee replacement has been such a rewarding procedure in terms of pain relief and functional improvement that the talk about knee amputation in the 21st century seems to be out of context. However, in a very small minority of patients, and after every attempt has been made to salvage the TKR, particularly after recurrent infection refractory to most aggressive medical and surgical therapy, the last resort remains to amputate the lower limb above the knee at the transfemoral level.[2,12,15] It could also be used in patients with medical comorbidities precluding them to be fit to undergo multiple surgical procedures.[2] Although the above knee amputation after TKR is commonly thought to be due to infection, other causes such as periprosthetic fractures, massive bone loss, and vascular etiologies, leading to ischemia, may also lead to above knee amputation.[15] Causes not related to TKR include diabetic neuropathy and malignant tumor around the knee (proximal tibia or distal femoral region).[15] The prevalence of the above knee amputation (AKA) has been reported to be between 0.14% and 0.18%.[15]

Isiklar et al. reported on nine above knee amputations in eight patients out of 5045 TKR done in their institutions.[12] The Mayo Clinic series of 18,443 TKRs showed that the minority of AKAs were secondary to complications directly related to the TKR itself, (25 out of 18,443) 0.14%, whereas (42 out of 18,443) 0.22% AKAs were performed for causes not related to TKR.[15] Of the group of the AKA following TKR, those related to the TKR complications were 37% whereas those not related were 63%. In the Mayo Clinic series, the great majority of those AKA related directly to complications after TKR were due to severe uncontrollable infections, which at times, were life threatening as well as associated with massive bone loss in some cases.

A significant proportion of these patients had a diagnosis (requiring primary TKR) of post-traumatic arthritis and rheumatic arthritis, both of which have been shown, by some authors, to have a higher incidence of infection. The biggest concern after AKA, is the functional results particularly the ability to ambulate independently or with minimal use of walking aids.[2,13-16] In the series of Pring et al. (7 out of 23), 30% patients were able to ambulate (with an above knee fitting prosthesis) with minimal or no use of wheelchair, those who did ambulate did so within 6–17 months post AKA surgery.[16] In terms of quantitative assessment of the amputees energy requirement, which have been described by Waters et al. the AKA individual (for vascular amputees) has 44% velocity of the normal individual compared to 59% of the normal individual for the patients with BKA and 66% for patients with Syme's amputation.[17] The figures are somewhat more impressive for the traumatic amputees, 63% for AKA compared to 87% for BKA.[17] In the series of Sierra et al.[15] from Mayo Clinic, only 9 out of 25 cases following AKA were fitted with prosthesis and only five of those nine patients ever used it for walking.

In summary, the knee amputation is probably the least favorable choice amongst surgeons and patients. It is usually reserved as a last resort in cases of severe life threatening septicemia or in cases of massive bone loss with infection. Often in those cases multiple salvage procedures have been attempted but yielded unsatisfactory results. The functional outcome following AKA is not very impressive with most series showing a non or minimal ambulatory status for majority of the patients, and a very small number of patients with AKA do actually maintain the ability to ambulate without much difficulty. It should also be noted that the clinical outcome in most earlier series had a large mortality prevalence, which comes as no surprise, since most of these patients are of old age by the time they have required the above knee amputation, in addition they also might have more comorbidities as well.

In more recent reviews, it appears that the functional outcome of this group of amputees is comparatively better, and their acceptance of the AKA prosthesis and to wear it for a longer part of the day performing more activities of daily living is also superior.[14] This change could be partly explained by the more improved options available in the prosthesis as well as relatively healthier and younger patient groups who might be getting the AKA who are potentially more active.[14]

RESECTION ARTHROPLASTY

This commonly known surgery in the domain of total hip arthroplasty, also known as a Girdlestone hip arthroplasty, is not that commonly practiced in the field of TKA. Its main use is in patients who're extremely low demand and flail, this procedure enables them to sit up in a chair comfortably without much discomfort in contrast to the knee arthrodesis.[2,18] The few reports in the literature describe this procedure as an option in low demand sedentary patients who could sit comfortably. Falahee et al.[18] reported resection arthroplasty in 26 cases and found only five out of those 26 patients were able to walk on their knees without external support. The mean arc of motion was about 36°.

The biggest concern in these patients is the extreme instability of the knee, which will affect the patient's ability to ambulate independently.[18] The patients with most disability before TKR do benefit the most, while those who have the least benefit, are better served by arthrodesis. Resection arthroplasty can potentially serve as an interim period after which patients could always get an arthrodesis if they elect to do so. Those groups of patients seem to be very well satisfied with the result of the arthrodesis.

CONCLUSION

Failure of TKA is a genuinely challenging as well as distressing problem to both the treating surgeon and the patient equally. The most refractory cases leading to a choice to be made for an alternative surgical option from the above-mentioned choices is refractory infection. The surgical solution chosen has to be made on individual basis, considering the patient's current level of activity, comorbidities, severity of infection and the severity of bone loss. The young and active patient could be well served by arthrodesis, while the elderly and less active could be served with resection arthroplasty with clear understanding of the limitation of postoperative activity and the requirement of wearing the brace. Amputation is usually reserved for the severely ill with life or limb threatening sepsis or who have failed all alternative surgical options.

REFERENCES

1. Conway JD, Mont MA, Bezwada HP. Arthrodesis of the knee. J Bone Joint Surg Am. 2004;86-A:835-48.
2. Jones RE, Russell RD, Huo MH. Alternative to revision total knee arthroplasty. J Bone Joint Surg Br. 2012;94:137-40.
3. Knutson K, Hovelius L, Lindstrand A, Lidgren L. Arthrodesis after failed knee arthroplasty. Clin Orthop Relat Res. 1984;191:202-11.
4. Siller TN, Hadjipavlou A. Knee arthrodesis: long term results. Can J Surg. 1976;19:217-9.
5. Pritchett JW, Mallin BA, Mathews AC. Knee arthrodesis with a tension-band plate. J Bone Joint Surg Am. 1988;70: 285-8.
6. Nichols SJ, Landon GC, Tullos HS. Arthrodesis with dual plates after failed total knee arthroplasty. J Bone Joint Surg Am. 1991;73(7):1020-4.
7. Lucas DB, Murray WR. Arthrodesis of the knee by double plating. J Bone Joint Surg Am. 1961;43:795-808.
8. Incavo SJ, Lilly JW, Bartlett CS, Churchill DL. Arthrodesis of the knee, experience with intramedullary nailing. J Arthroplasty. 2000;15(7):871-6.
9. Mabry TM, Jacofsky DJ, Haidukewych GJ, Hanssen AD. Comparison of intramedullary nailing and external fixation knee arthrodesis for the infected knee replacement. Clin Orthop Relat Res. 2007;464:11-5.
10. Bargiotas K, Wohlrab D, Sewecke JJ. Arthrodesis of the knee with a long intramedullary nail following the failure of a total knee arthroplasty as the result of infection. J Bone Joint Surg Am. 2006;88:553-8.
11. Christie MJ, DeBoer DK, McQueen DA, Cooke FW, Hahn DL. Salvage procedures for failed total knee arthroplasty. J Bone Joint Surg Am. 2003;85-A:58-62.
12. Isiklar ZU, Landon GC, Tullos HS. Amputation after failed total knee arthroplasty. Clin Orthop Relat Res. 1994;299:173-8.
13. Spina M, Gualdrini M, Fosco M, Giunti A. Knee arthrodesis with the Ilizarov external fixator as treatment for septic failure of knee arthroplasty. J Orthop Traumatol. 2010;11:81-8.
14. Fedorka CJ, Chen AF, McGarry WM, Parwizi J, Klatt BA. Functional ability after above the knee amputation for infected total knee arthroplasty. Clin Orthop Relat Res. 2011;469(4):1024-32.
15. Sierra RJ, Trousdale RT, Pagnano MW. Above-the-knee amputation after a total knee replacement, prevalence, etiology, and functional outcome. J Bone Joint Surg Am. 2003;85:1000-4.
16. Pring DJ, Marks L, Angel JC. Mobility after amputation for failed knee replacement. J Bone Joint Surg Br. 1988;70(5):770-1.
17. Waters RL, Perry J, Antonelli D, Hislop H. Energy cost of walking of amputees: the influence of level of amputation. J Bone Joint Surg Am. 1976;58(1):42-6.
18. Falahee MH, Matthews LS, Kaufer H. Resection arthroplasty as a salvage procedure for a knee with infection after a total arthroplasty. Journal Bone Joint Surg Am. 1987;69(7):1013-21.

Chapter 26

Revisions Following Aseptic Failures

Ashok Rajgopal, Attique Vasdev, Vivek Dahiya, Himanshu Gupta

Primary total knee arthroplasty (TKA) has shown good patient satisfaction and clinical results with survivorship ranging between 88% and 93% at 15–20 years. An increase in the number of primary TKAs, has led to a corresponding increase in revision TKA for both infection and aseptic failures. Aseptic failure is predominantly a mechanical failure and is often due to technical errors unrecognized at the time of primary surgery. Varying degrees of success (46–92%) has been reported following revisions for aseptic failure especially when compared to those of primary TKA. Friedman et al. reported improvement in function, instability, motion and pain after revision for aseptic loosening but found it to be significantly less than that after primary TKA. Bostrom and Hass in their series reported that aseptic revisions did quite well, if addressed with a proper surgical technique and appropriate choice of implant. Insall described similar results of primary TKA and revision TKA but with a higher incidence of extensor mechanism problems and less pain relief after revision. Wang et al. reported similar results of aseptic revision TKA to that of primary TKA at midterm follow-up. Patil et al. observed that patient selection and preoperative diagnosis had an effect on the outcome of aseptic revisions. Gofton et al. demonstrated a Kaplan-Meier survivorship of 93.5% at 8.6 years.

Rajgopal et al. retrospectively reviewed the results of 142 patients, revised for septic and aseptic failures. Their study revealed no statistical differences in the knee society scores and the Kaplan-Meier survivorships in both the groups.

Revision in aseptic failure of TKAs may be indicated in situations of component loosening, malrotation, osteolysis with polyethylene wear, ligamentous laxity in coronal or sagittal plane, periprosthetic fractures, patellofemoral complications, malalignment of components and a deficient extensor mechanism. Polywear may cause pain and instability either due to osteolysis and/or loosening.

Once aseptic failure is recognized it is important to operate early as delay may only lead to massive osteolysis and metallosis (**Figure 26.1**). Instability is an important cause of aseptic failure and may present, due to primary ligament imbalance or incompetence leading to subluxation or dislocation. Instability may be present in the coronal, sagittal or in both these planes. Instability

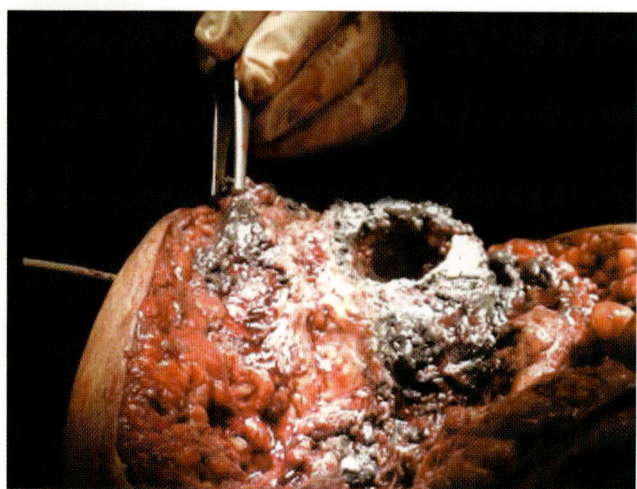

Figure 26.1 Metallosis

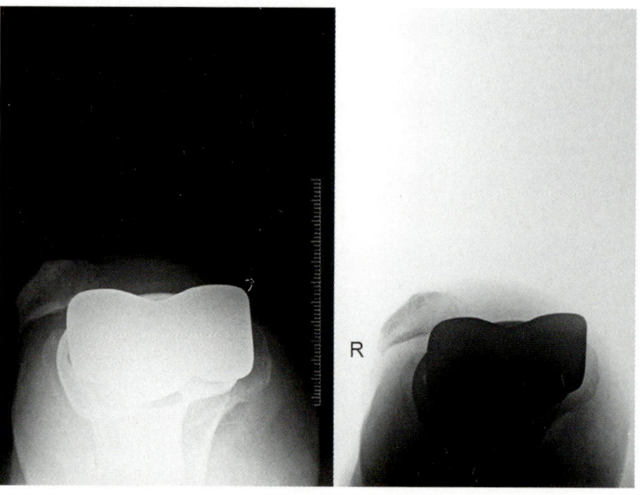

Figure 26.2 Patellar maltracking as on the skyline view

may present early as in cases of component malalignment, flexion-extension gap mismatch that may cause midflexion instability and the inability to restore the mechanical axis during primary surgery. Early instability may also occur due to unrecognized intraoperative damage to the medial collateral ligament or the posterior cruciate ligament (in cruciate retaining designs). Late instability is often due to polyethylene wear. Sagittal plane instability may occur due to wear or breaking of the post in posterior stabilized knees or the rupture or attenuation of the posterior cruciate ligament in cruciate retaining knees. Coronal plane instability is often due to asymmetrical polywear on the medial or lateral side leading to varus or valgus instability.

Another important and often missed cause of aseptic failures is osteolysis. It is often the main cause of delayed surgery as the extent is often missed in routine radiographs. Computed tomography (CT) scans and even magnetic resonance imaging (MRI) may be required in cases of suspicion. Whereas small lesions may only require observation and close follow-up, larger lesions usually require revision surgery with bone grafts or metal augments.

Maltracking patella (**Figure 26.2**) may lead to extensor mechanism failure that may be due to lack of understanding of a particular prosthetic design or a technical error such as femoral component malrotation during surgery. It may lead to either subluxation or dislocation of the patella (**Figure 26.2**), polywear in cases of patellar resurfacing, fractures or extensor mechanism ruptures.

PREOPERATIVE ASSESSMENT

History and physical examination form an important part of the preoperative assessment of a patient with aseptic failure. It often leads to the etiology of failure giving the surgeon an idea of what to expect during surgery. A history of constitutional symptoms like fever, chills, or persistent urinary tract infection may be suggestive of infection. A history of prolonged drainage or delayed wound healing may also point to infection. Pain present even during rest and from initial surgery itself may also suggest the presence of infection. History of pain while getting up or starting to walk may point to mechanical failure. Scars need be assessed for adequate healing and any evidence of sinuses should be noted. The knee itself should be examined for signs of instability, range of motion and patellar tracking. A thorough examination also rules out the referred pain from the spine of hip and establishes the knee as the primary cause of pain. Limb evaluation should include gait, hip abductor function and limb length. Scoliosis should be ruled out. The neurological and vascular status of the lower limbs should be assessed and recorded. Sudeck's osteodystrophy should particularly be ruled out.

Laboratory evaluation forms an important part of assessment of a patient suspected of aseptic failure. Complete blood counts, erythrocyte sedimentation rate and C-reactive protein (CRP) are basic requirements for the evaluation of infection. In case of any abnormality of these parameters or an effusion, aspiration of the joint should be done. The synovial fluid should be looked for signs of purulence and any polyethylene or metal debris. The aspirate should be then sent for cell count, cultures (aerobic, anaerobic and fungal) and for CRP of the aspirate itself.

Radiographic assessment includes anteroposterior standing, lateral and skyline views. These are evaluated for the component size, position and fixation. Any evidence of loosening, migration, polyethylene wear, osteolysis, and implant breakage can also be noted. The skyline or Merchant's view is useful in assessing the patellofemoral articulation and extensor mechanism tracking (**Figure 26.2**). If available, previous films can be compared to the recent ones to look for any migration, progressive osteolysis and progressive radiolucent lines. A full length hip to ankle X-ray or orthoscannogram allows a more accurate assessment of the affected limb and detects osseous tissues away from the joint such as stress fractures, malunions, previous unrelated joint or limb surgery with implant *in situ* that may interfere with the present surgery. Specialized views may include oblique X-rays to better visualize the periprosthetic bone to detect early osteolysis and stress X-rays to look for any ligamentous instability. Fluoroscopically positioned radiographs enhance visualization of the implant fixation interface and help in detecting early component loosening. Standing lateral views on the affected side alone are useful in quantifying flexion contracture and recurvatum.

CT scans are accurate in assessing the tibial and femoral rotation. These also quantify bone loss and osteolysis more accurately than plain radiographs. CT scans are also more accurate than plain radiographs in evaluating a stiff arthroplasty or extensor mechanism complications like patellofemoral pain, tilt, maltracking, subluxation or dislocations.

The role of MRI in evaluating the painful knee is not well established, though with modification in the pulse sequence parameters to reduce artifacts it may prove to be an important tool in assessing particle disease, osteolysis, synovitis and joint infection. MRI may also give useful information on the surrounding soft tissue envelope, including nerves, tendons and ligaments.

The role of radioisotope studies like the Tc-99m labeled bone scan, gallium scan, indium labeled white blood cell scan or the sulfur colloid bone marrow scan in aseptic failures is not well defined, though if normal in the painful knee with no obvious cause may suggest that surgery should be avoided.

Once infection is ruled out and the exact mode of failure of the prior arthroplasty is established, thought should be given to the prosthesis and the type of constraint required for revision. This is based upon the amount of bone loss and the osteolysis anticipated. Requirement of bone grafts, augments, wedges, metaphyseal sleeves and stems should be thought of in advance. Preoperative templating is especially useful in revisions with extra-articular deformities as these may require osteotomies to accommodate stems. Modularity of the revision system allows for the attachment of stems, augments and wedges. The soft tissue around should be assessed and if difficulty in closure is anticipated, a plastic surgery opinion should be considered.

SURGICAL TECHNIQUE

Prior to skin incision, a thorough examination of the knee under anesthesia should be done to look for the range of motion and stability. The previous skin incision or the lateral most incision is used to preserve the blood supply to the medial aspect of the lateral skin flap. Previous transverse incisions cannot be avoided should be crossed at 90°. To prevent subcutaneous ischemia, flaps should be kept as thick as possible. A medial parapatellar arthrotomy is then performed. Synovial fluid obtained should be sent for culture. In case of stiff knees, a quadriceps snip may need to be done early to prevent damage to the tibial tubercle and the extensor mechanism. This provides good exposure and the weight-bearing protocol need not be altered. Rarely to achieve additional exposure, a V-Y quadricepsplasty may be required. Though this provides excellent exposure, postoperatively immobilization in extension is required and may lead to an extensor lag. Occasionally in case of severe patella baja a tubercle osteotomy as described by Whiteside and Ohl may be necessary. This may also be useful in the removal of long cemented stems or stems with lot of bony ingrowth. The lateral soft tissue should be left attached to the bone and the osteotomy hinged open. This maintains fragment vascularity and makes closure easier. In situations with a good preoperative range of motion, a medial subperiosteal exposure allows the tibia to be externally rotated and subluxated anteriorly allowing adequate exposure. This release may be incorporated into final medial release required for balancing. Re-establishing the gutters is a critical part of the exposure especially in the stiff knee. A fixed varus deformity is corrected by subperiosteal release of the deep and superficial portions of the medial collateral ligament and the pes anserine insertion along the proximal medial aspect of the tibia. The distal insertion of the superficial medial collateral ligament can elevate subperiosteally in an incremental fashion. Once external rotation of the tibia is achieved, the semimembranosus and posterior capsules are released to allow full exposure of the proximal end of the tibia. In case of a fixed valgus deformity lateral 'pie crusting,' i.e. small, multiple horizontal incisions in the lateral structures (posterior capsule, lateral collateral ligament and iliotibial band), is often sufficient. More severe fixed valgus deformities may require a complete release of the lateral supporting structures from the femoral condyle like a subperiosteal femoral peel or lateral epicondylar osteotomy.

Exposure of the failed knee should be followed by thorough debridement of the suprapatellar and the parapatellar regions. A large amount of polyethylene and polymethylmethacrylate debris and bony fragments are produced in a failed knee and need to be removed meticulously. These often get incorporated in the synovium that gets inflamed and thickened due to metallosis and polyethylene debris. A complete synovectomy further facilitates exposure. Varus-valgus stability at this stage must be re-evaluated in full extension and in 30° flexion as the effects of posterior structures may be misleading in full extension.

EXPLANTATION

Implants are often not loose, as revision may be for reasons other than loosening. Porus coated implants or those with cemented stem are difficult to remove. Caution is required as one may end up losing good bone stock while removing the implant. It is advised to remove the polyethylene insert first. If the insert is all polyethylene then the polyethylene can be sawn off at the level of the tibia. This opens up the flexion-extension space. Special instruments such as the microsagittal or the reciprocating saw may be required to create a plane between the implant-cement interface. A Gigli saw may also be useful to create this interface. Thin or flexible osteotomes can then be passed around especially the posterior condyles where the saw blades cannot reach (**Figure 26.3**). A prosthesis specific extractor may be then used to extract the femoral component. Alternatively a blow on the proximal flange of the femur with a punch may also be used.

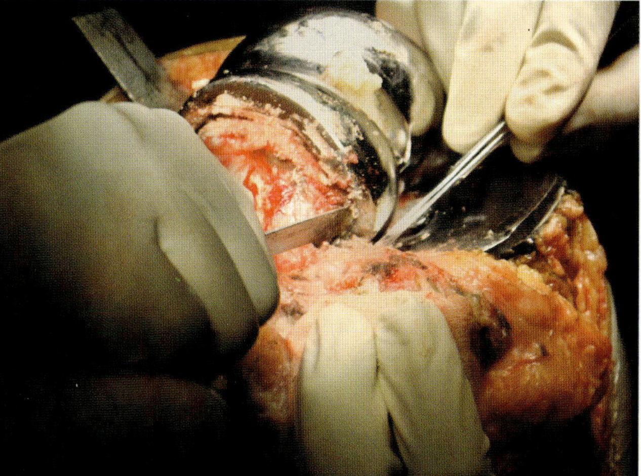

Figure 26.3 Thin osteotome used to create an interphase between the posterior femoral condyle and the femur implant

Once the femur is removed the tibia is addressed. Metal backed tibial components are removed similar to the femur. It is important to expose the tibia along its periphery in order to saw all around the tibial base plate. External rotation facilitates this process. The tibia can then be 'knocked' out using a punch. In the event of the presence of a stem, the tibial base plate may first be disengaged by removing the bolt that fixes the base plate to the stem. The bolt is then put back into the stem alone and the stem is then removed with the help of a slap hammer engaged to the bolt.

Once the components are removed (**Figures 26.4 and 26.5**), all granulation tissue, cement debris and soft tissues are meticulously removed off the bone surface. Cement is removed from the surfaces with the help of a narrow osteotome by cracking the surface without causing bone loss. A thorough wash with pulsatile lavage at this stage removes any residual debris.

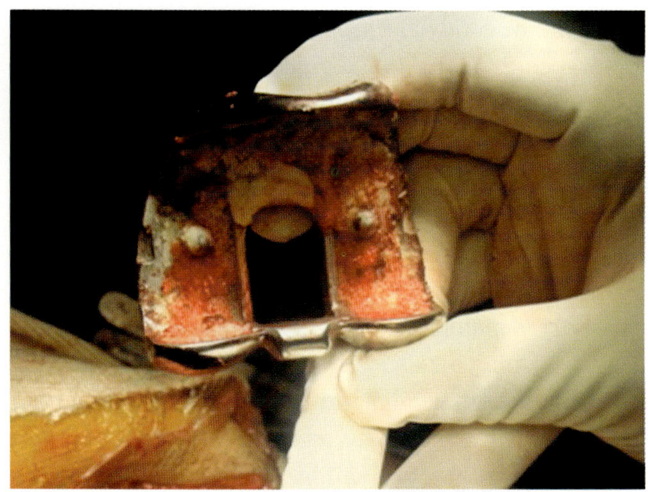

Figure 26.4 Explantation femur

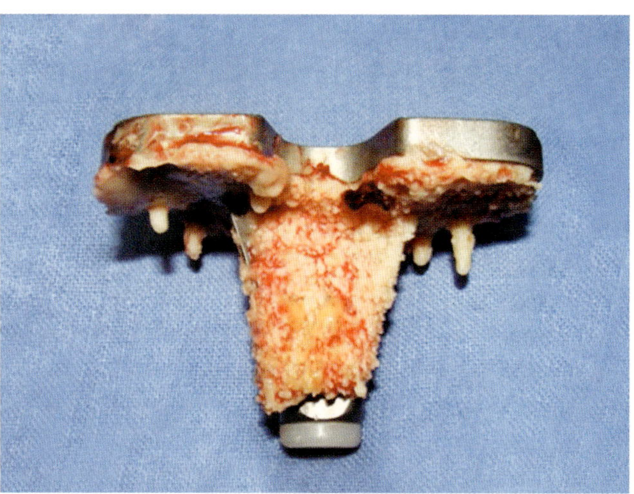

Figure 26.5 Explantation tibia

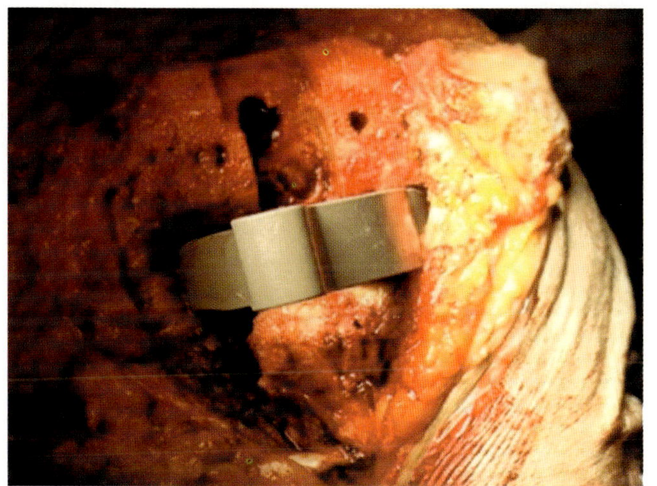

Figure 26.6 Flexion gap

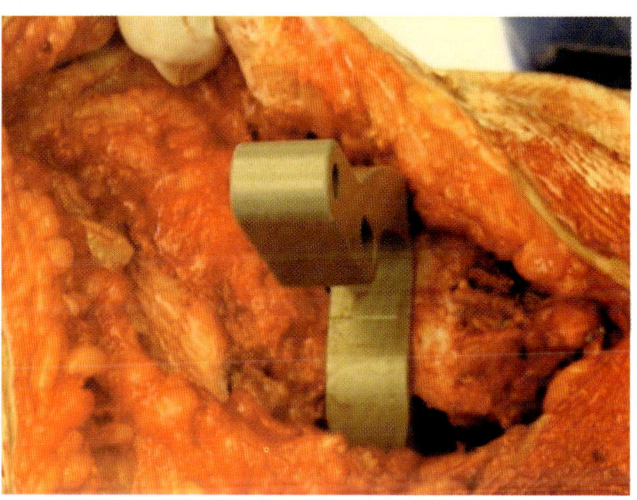

Figure 26.7 Extension gap

TRIALS

Once the implants have been removed it is important to establish the sequence to reimplantation. Though the aim is to achieve equal flexion and extension gaps (**Figures 26.6 and 26.7**), it is often not possible in revision situations and adjustments are often necessary. It is important to remember that any changes in the femur may affect the flexion gap whereas the tibia will affect both the flexion and the extension gap. Upsizing or downsizing the femur may increase or decrease the flexion gap to a limited extent whereas the extension gap can be increased or decreased to a much larger extent.

The reimplantation or revision may be divided into:

1. Re-establishing the tibial surface
2. Recreating the femur and re-establishing the flexion gap
3. Establishing a stable extension gap

Re-establishing the Tibial Surface

Re-establishing the tibial surface is the foundation of revision arthroplasty as it affects both the flexion and extension gaps. It is paramount to create a flat surface perpendicular to the mechanical axis. Bone cuts may be taken free hand or using the standard extramedullary jig. The intramedullary canal is an excellent guide to create a surface that is flat and also perpendicular to the mechanical axis. This can be achieved with the help of stems either straight or offset. As the center of the tibial diaphysis is on an average 4 mm medial to the center of the articular surface, using a press fit straight stem may lead to overhang on the medial side or lead to more valgus as the press fit stem lies in valgus. This is overcome by using a narrow fully cemented stem or a press fit offset stem extension. The tibial tubercle is used as a guide to position the tibial component in proper rotation. Modular augments such as wedges, blocks, trabecular metal cones, bone grafts are often required to recreate the proximal tibia to support a flat perpendicular tibial surface as close to the original tibial height as possible.

Recreating the Femur and Re-establishing the Flexion Gap

Recreating the femur and re-establishing the flexion gap (**Figure 26.8**) involves sizing the femur and placing the femoral component in correct femoral rotation. Establishing the joint line is also critical at this stage. Femoral component sizing has a bearing on the flexion space as it restores the anteroposterior dimensions and the posterior condylar offset. It is better to select a larger femoral component and augment the femoral condyles in order to restore the femoral condylar offset and the anteroposterior width as a small component will lead to flexion instability by failing to restore the femoral offset. The most reliable consistent landmark is the medullary canal. Stems, either press fit or fully cemented, help establish the component size and position. Augments are necessary to maintain this position. It is important to ream to get a position parallel to the bone and prevent reaming in the medial or lateral plane. At this stage it is important to remember the reason for revision. A stiff knee requires a larger flexion gap that can be achieved by downsizing the femur or decreasing the extension gap, whereas in a knee with midflexion instability the flexion gap needs to be reduced. This can be achieved by upsizing the femur.

Femoral rotation is important for patellar tracking and normal knee kinematics. Ideally, components should be placed parallel to the transepicondylar axis. Using the transepicondylar axis helps establish correct rotation (**Figure 26.9**). Often in revision situations the epicondyles are not palpable. In such situations the trochlear notch and posterior articular surfaces can be used to determine the rotation. The resected tibial platform can also be used as a guide to set the femoral rotation. It is essential to look for patellar tracking at this stage. If the patella does not track

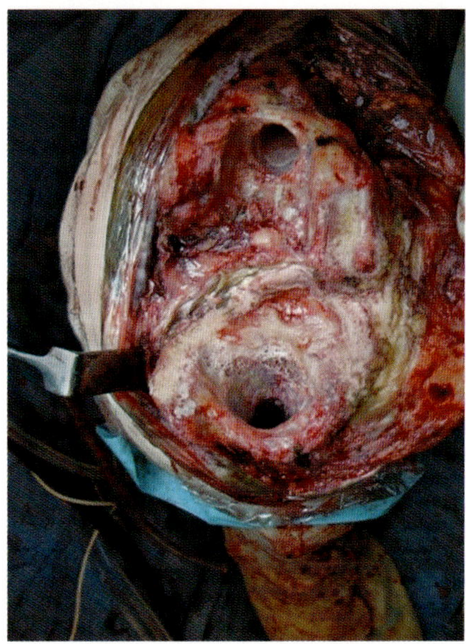

Figure 26.8 Building from flexion

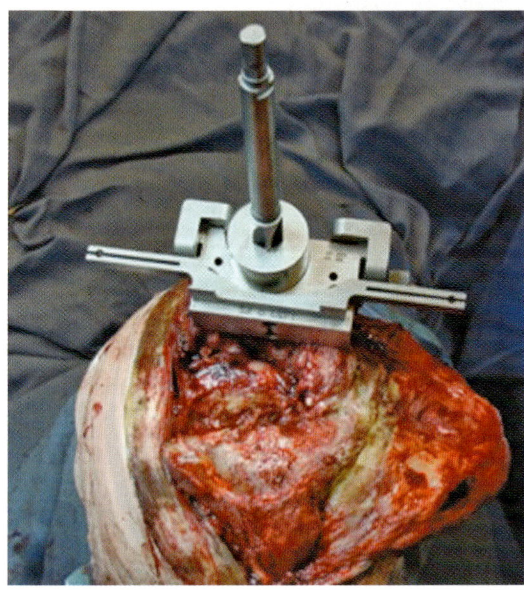

Figure 26.9 Femoral component rotation

centrally then revisiting external rotation of the femur and possibly the tibia may be required.

Establishing a Stable Extension Gap

Once the tibial platform is established and the provisional tibial and femoral components put into position, the largest tibial polyethylene that will fill the flexion gap and stabilize the knee in flexion is placed into the tibial tray. The knee is then extended. If the knee can be fully extended without a flexion attitude or recurvatum then it is a balanced knee and the polyethylene insert is of correct size. Often this is not the case. The gaps may be unequal at this stage and adjustments may be required. If the gaps are tight in both, flexion and extension, then reducing the height of the polyethylene insert may be sufficient. Similarly, if the gaps are loose both in extension and flexion, increasing the height of the insert may help. The problem arises when one of the gaps is asymmetrical.

If the knee is tight in flexion but loose in extension, the femur can be distalized using distal femoral augmentation till the gaps are equal. This is possible if the femur component is of the correct size. If the femur is oversized, the joint line is lowered. In such situations, the femur should be downsized and a thicker insert used. Often the femur may be of the correct size but placed posteriorly. Here, an offset stem extension directed posteriorly moves the component anteriorly opening the flexion space. This may occasionally lead to patellofemoral stuffing. Care should be taken to avoid this situation.

If the knee is tight in extension but stable in flexion additional distal femoral cuts may be required. This is often possible through slots in the trial prosthesis itself. Any distal femoral augments should be removed. One should be careful not to elevate the joint line. An offset stem extension directed anteriorly moves the component posteriorly decreasing the flexion space. An undersized femoral component may need to be upsized to increase the posterior offset reducing the flexion gap. A minor mismatch can often be managed by releasing the posterior capsule from the posterior femur especially when there is a flexion contracture preoperatively (**Flow chart 26.1**).

Flow chart 26.1 Algorithm for managing unequal flexion extension gaps

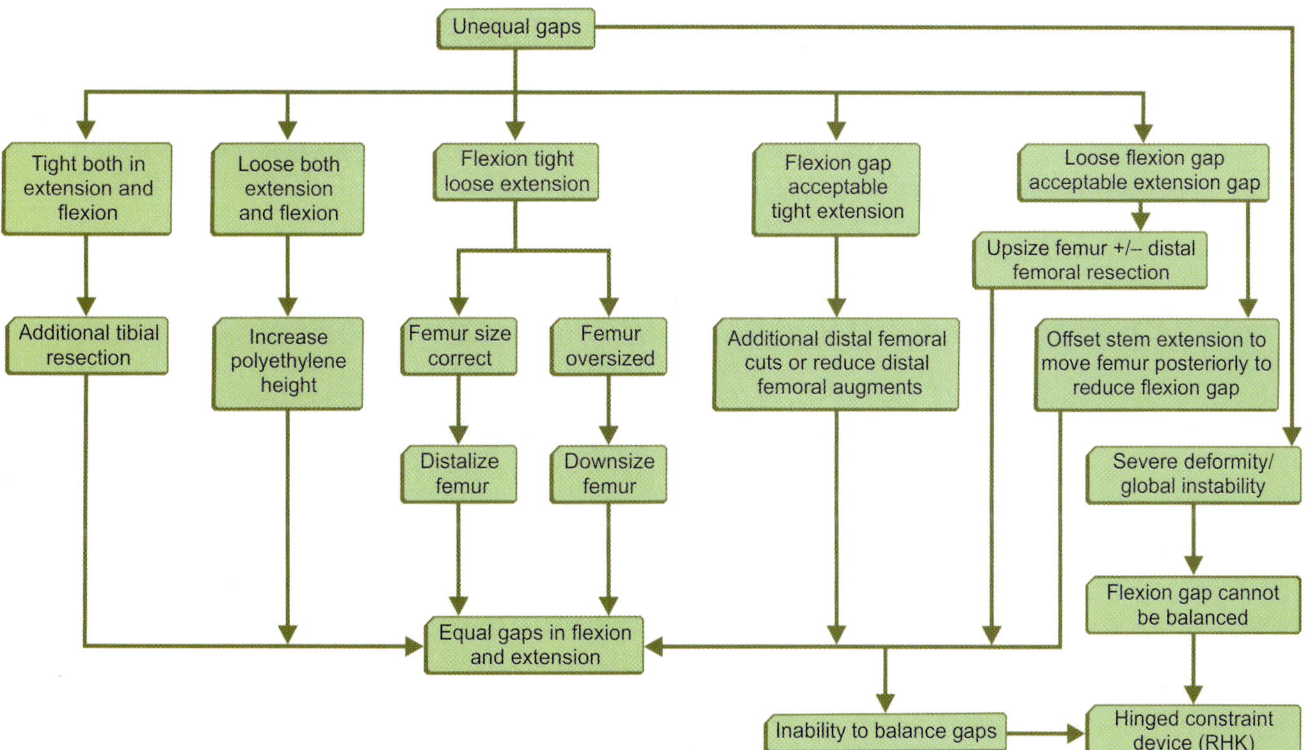

In cases where the flexion gap cannot be balanced in spite of using the largest possible insert or there is severe varus-valgus instability in extension and collateral damage especially the medial is present one should not hesitate to switch to a hinged constraint device line a Rotating Hinge Knee (RHK) or S-ROM Noiles Rotating Hinge (**Flow chart 26.1**).

REIMPLANTATION

The bone surfaces are thoroughly cleaned with pulsatile lavage. Any sclerotic bone is drilled. No attempt should be made to sacrifice the bone as this may further deplete bone stock. The surfaces are should be dried with sponges. The rotation of the tibia is made on the bone with a cautery. The position of the distal flange of the femur is also marked to prevent excessive impaction of the final implant. The implants are assembled before mixing the cement. We recommend the use of antibiotic impregnated cement in all revisions. The cement is coated on the implants. The tibial canal is filled with cement and the tibial surface coated with cement. The tibial component is first inserted and gently impacted into the canal taking care to maintain the rotation. The femur is then impacted into position. The polyethylene inserted is then fixed and the knee gently extended.

Once the cement is cured, the tourniquet may be released and hemostasis obtained and the wound closed over a drain. Most patients are allowed weight bearing and knee mobilization as per tolerance on the second postoperative day. Drains are removed after 24 hours. A quadriceps snip does not require any change in the postoperative protocol. A V-Y plasty requires needs immobilization in extension for 3–6 weeks to allow the quadricepsplasty to heal. Weight bearing may need to be delayed if extensive bone grafting or a tubercle osteotomy has been performed.

COMPLICATIONS

Complications include avulsion of the patellar tendon, fractures of the patella or tibia and femur

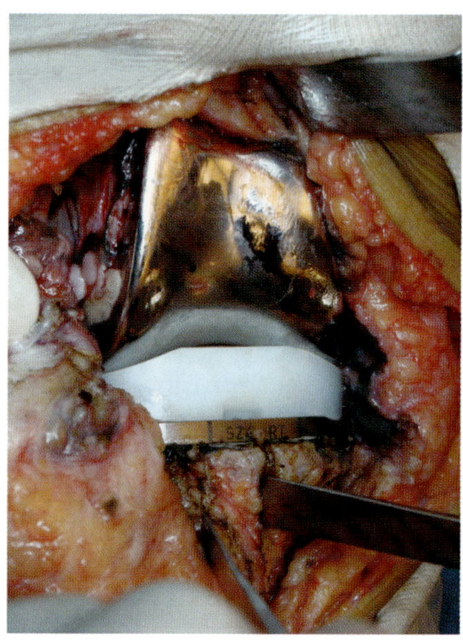

Figure 26.10 Tibial component malrotation

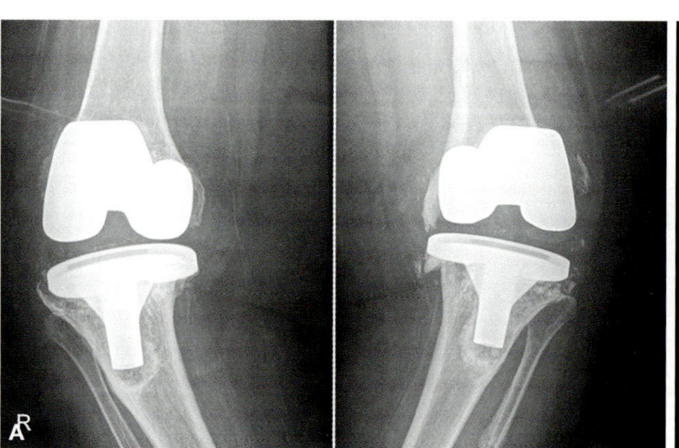

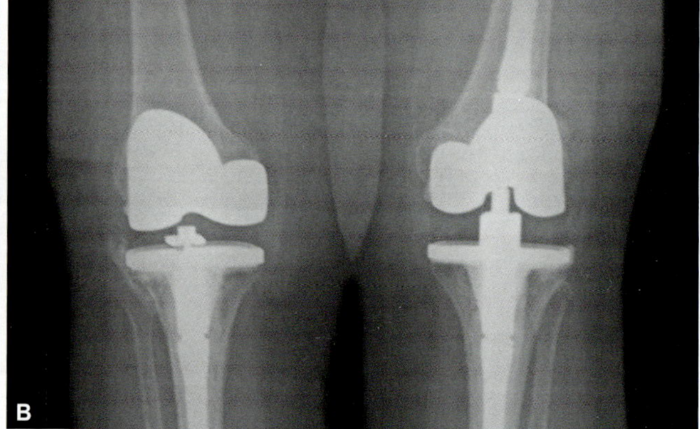

Figures 26.11A and B Radiographs of a patient with bilateral aseptic failure of total knee replacement. (A) Preoperative anteroposterior view; (B) Postoperative anteroposterior view

during implantation, collateral avulsion, component malposition (**Figure 26.10**), maltracking of the patella (**Figure 26.2**), stiffness, delayed wound healing, infection, and neurovascular injuries.

A systemic approach, identifying the reason for aseptic failure, ruling out infection, optimizing exposure, minimizing bone loss, managing bone defects, balancing and reconstructing bone gaps and getting well fixed implants are essential in obtaining a well aligned functional limb following revision for aseptic failures (**Figures 26.11A and B**).

BIBLIOGRAPHY

1. Baker P, Cowling P, Kurtz S, et al. Reason for revision influences early patient outcomes after aseptic knee revision. Clin Orthop Relat Res. 2012;470(8):2244-52.
2. Berger RA, Crossett LS, Jacobs JJ, Rubash HE. Malrotation causing patellofemoral complications after total knee arthroplasty. Clin Orthop Relat Res. 1998;356:144-53.
3. Bertin KC, Freeman MAR, Samuelson KM, Ratcliffe SS, Todd RC. Stemmed revision arthroplasty for aseptic loosening of total knee replacement. J Bone Joint Surg Br. 1985;67:242-8.
4. Bostrom MP, Hass SB. Revision total knee arthroplasty due to aseptic failure. Am J Knee Surg. 1996;9(2): 91-8.
5. Brand MG, Daley RJ, Ewald FC, Scott RD. Tibial tray augmentation with modular metal wedges for tibial bone stock deficiency. Clin Orthop. 1989;248:71-9.
6. Brooks PJ, Walker PS, Scott RD. Tibial component fixation in deficient tibial bone stock. Clin Orthop. 1984;184:302-8.
7. Friedman RJ, Hirst P, Poss R, Kelley K, Sledge CB. Results of revision total knee arthroplasty performed for aseptic loosening. Clin Orthop Relat Res. 1990;255:235-41.
8. Insall JN, Dethmers DA. Revision of total knee arthroplasty. Clin Orthop Relat Res. 1982;170:123-30.
9. Jiranek WA, Hanssen AD, Greenwald AS. Current concepts review antibiotic loaded bone cement for infection prophylaxis in total joint replacement. J Bone Joint Surg Am. 2006;88(11):2487-500.
10. Khaw FM, Kirk LM, Gregg PJ. Survival analysis of cemented press - fit condylar total knee arthroplasty. J Arthroplasty. 2001;16(2):161-7.
11. Kurtz S, Mowat F, Ong K, et al. Prevalence of primary and revision total hip and knee arthroplasty in the United States from 1900 through 2002. J Bone Joint Surg Am. 2005;87(7):1487-97.
12. Moreland JR. Mechanisms of failure in total knee arthroplasty. Clin Orthop. 1988;226:49-64.
13. Pun SY, Ries MD. Effect of gender and preoperative diagnosis on results of revision total knee arthroplasty. Clin Orthop Relat Res. 2008;466(11):2701-5.
14. Patil N, Lee K, Huddleston JI, Harris AH, Goodman SB. Aseptic versus septic revision total knee arthroplasty: patient satisfaction, outcome and quality of life improvement. Knee. 2010;17:200-3.
15. Ranawat CS, Flynn WF Jr, Saddler S, Hansraj KK, Maynard MJ. Long-term results of the total condylar knee arthroplasty. A 15-year survivorship study. Clin Orthop Relat Res. 1993;286: 94-102.
16. Rajgopal A, Vasdev A, Gupta H, et al. Revisions following aseptic and septic failures. J Orthop Surg (Hong Kong). 2013;21(3)285-9.
17. Rand JA, Bryan RS. Results of revision total knee arthroplasties using condylar prostheses. A review of fifty knees. J Bone Joint Surg Am. 1988;70(5):738-45.
18. Su DH, Chan CW, Seow KH. Results of revision total knee arthroplasty. Singapore Med J. 2000;41(1): 6-8.
19. Vince KG, Droll KP, Chivas D. Your next revision arthroplasty: why start in flexion? Orthopaedics. 2007;30:791-2.
20. Vince KG. Why knees fail. J Arthroplasty. 2003;18:39-44.
21. Vince KG. A step-wise approach to revision TKA. Orthopaedics. 2005;28:999-1001.
22. Wang CJ, Hsieh MC, Huang TW, et al. Clinical outcome and patient satisfaction in aseptic and septic revision total knee arthroplasty. Knee. 2004;11:45-9.
23. Whiteside LA, Ohl MD. Tibial tubercle osteotomy for exposure of the difficult total knee arthroplasty. Clin Orthop. 1990;260:6-9.
24. Windsor RE, Scuderi GR, Moran MC, Insall JN. Mechanisms of failure of the femoral and tibial components in total knee arthroplasty. Clin Orthop Relat Res. 1989;248 (15):15-9.

Chapter 27

Total Knee Arthroplasty in the Stiff Knee

Ashok Rajgopal, Attique Vasdev, Vivek Dahiya, Vipin Tyagi

Sitting with the knees flexed is a basic essence of living. It is extremely distressing and disabling for patients who have stiff knees. There is a social awkwardness in their gait and in their ability to sit with their knees bent or on the floor as in certain religious customs. Such patients often look toward the option of total knee arthroplasty (TKA) (**Figures 27.1A to D**).

A stiff knee by description is defined as a knee with less than 50° arc of motion.[1,2] Knees may be stiff in flexion or extension and it is important to identify the root cause of stiffness as it may have a profound effect on the end result. Knees stiff in extension are those where full extension is possible and a further arc of motion of 50° or less is present. Knees stiff in flexion are patients with a fixed flexion deformity with a further 50° arc of motion or less. Stiffness in flexion can be a result of contracture of posterior soft tissue structures, post high tibial osteotomy, mechanical bone block, or juxta-articular adhesions. Stiffness in extension may be due to quadriceps contracture, patella baja, heterotopic ossification, or intra-articular adhesions.[3] The contraindications for the take down of a stiff knee have become relatively limited because long-term results of this procedure have now been better defined as reported in various series.

Hsu et al.[4] in their study evaluated the outcome of total knee arthroplasty and analyzed the prognostic factors in patients with stiff knees and concluded that the most important factor related to the final arc of knee motion was the preoperative arc of knee motion. Fosco et al.[2] evaluated the results of total knee arthroplasty performed on 32 stiff knees to those with flexible knees with a mean follow-up of 4.5 years. They reported a 25% complication rate but had excellent or good results in 92% of the stiff group to 96% of the control group patients. Aglietti et al.[1] reported the results of total knee arthroplasty in a series of 20 stiff (range of motion, less than 50°) and six ankylosed knees, replaced with posterior stabilized condylar prosthesis. There was a significant improvement in the range of motion from 32° to 78° in their series. Rajgopal et al.[3] in their series of 84 knees in 53 patients with spontaneously ankylosed knees, having a preoperative range of motion between 0° and 20°(average 14°) showed a significant average gain of 61° in the arc of motion following total knee arthroplasty. Postoperatively, the average knee score was 75.2 (range 58–87) and an average functional score was 84.7(54–95), significantly more than the average preoperative knee score of 14.6 and the average preoperative functional score of 26.8. Montgomery et al.[5]

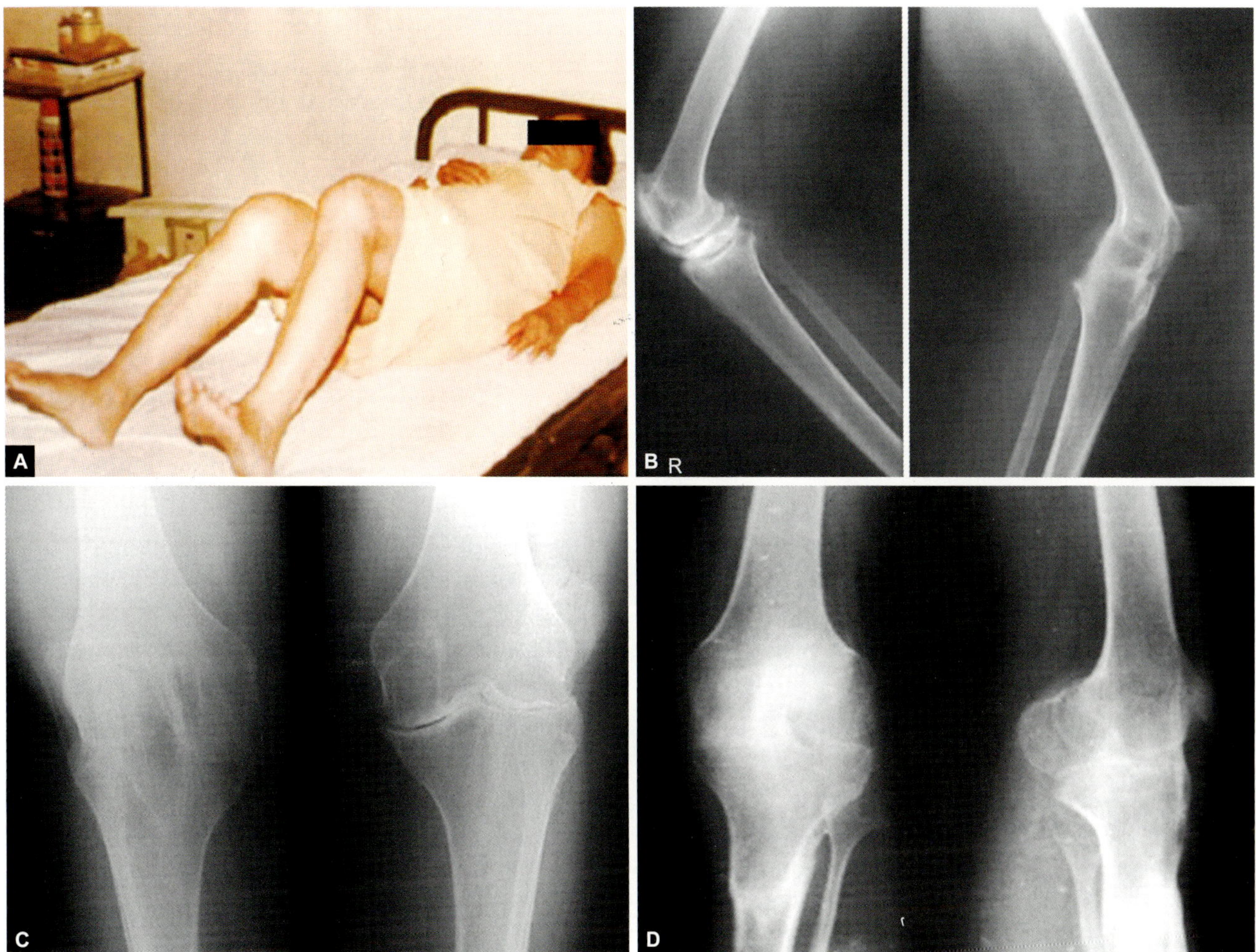

Figures 27.1A to D (A) Patient with bilateral stiff knees; (B to D) X-rays showing bony ankylosis

reviewed 71 patients (82 knees) who underwent total knee arthroplasty for an average range of motion of 36° (0°–50°). Following surgery, the average range of motion improved to 93° (range 35°–130°) and the knee score improved to 80 (range 0–98). They concluded that in stiff or ankylosed knees the total knee arthroplasty can produce good or excellent results and lead to significant improvement in range of motion. Kim and Kim[6] studied the outcome of 82 patients (99 knees) with ankylosed knees, who underwent total knee arthroplasty with a condylar constrained or a posterior stabilized prosthesis with a follow-up was 8.9 years. In their study there was a significant improvement of the Hospital for Special Surgery, knee society and the western Ontario and McMaster osteoarthritis index scores. Bhan et al.[7] retrospectively reviewed the results of 90 total knee arthroplasties in 52 patients with stiff or ankylosed knee with average follow-up of 6.5 years. The arc of flexion improved from 35°–69° preoperatively to 1°–94° postoperatively in the stiff knees and from 0° to 3°–77° in the ankylosed knees.

Growing experience in TKA with the advent of newer and better-constrained implants has made it technically possible to do a TKA in most patients with a stiff knee. It is wise to assess each patient individually with special focus on the functional ability of the extensor mechanism.[3,8,9] Complications, long-term results and the possibility of failure, revision and rearthrodesis should be explained to the patient in detail.[10-12] Evaluation of the desire of the patients and ability to comply with the postoperative therapy or protocols before offering a TKA to a patient with a stiff knee is absolutely important. Caution should be exercised in situations where stiffness is due to prolonged immobilization as in neurological conditions like stroke as TKA alone will not correct the underlying cause. Patients with severe pain leading to limited motion should not be subjected to surgery before ruling out reflex sympathetic dystrophy.

PREOPERATIVE EVALUATION

Preoperative planning should include a through history, a detailed clinical examination and a radiological evaluation. The condition of the overlying skin taking into account any previous surgical scars[9,13] should be noted. The power of the quadriceps, presence of any fibrosis of soft tissue around the knee, neurological status of the affected lower limb and the patellofemoral mobility should be assessed as all these may require attention at the time of surgery. The preoperative range of motion of the affected knee should also be meticulously recorded.

Radiographic examination evaluation should include a standard anteroposterior (AP) and lateral views to assess the limb alignment, bone loss and the quality of bone. Preoperatively a scanogram (full length standing X-rays) with emphasis laid on proper positioning of the limb during execution of the radiographs is helpful as external rotation may accentuate the varus deformity due to the anterior bowing of the femur. A scanogram is especially useful in assessing the alignment axis in presence of deformities with a stiff knee. CT scans should be done in patients with suspicion of bony ankylosis. This extent of defects in subchondral or metaphyseal region can be better assessed with CT scans and help in determining the need of grafts, wedges or stems.[3] The availability of a wide range of options in terms of constraint, stems and augments is helpful to overcome intraoperative challenges seen during surgery.

SURGICAL TECHNIQUE

The type of anesthesia, choice of prosthesis, incision, exposure, alignment, ligament stability, trial reduction and final implantation, all form an important part of the surgical planning for the stiff knee. Surgery is carried out under tourniquet and in laminar flow operating rooms. Epidural anesthesia for surgery may have an additional benefit of postoperative pain analgesia. Examination under anesthesia should be done for the patient's range of motion and ligamentous stability.

Surgical exposure is often one of the biggest challenges while attempting a TKA on a stiff knee.[2,3,6,10,11,14-16] The condition of the skin and the presence of any prior incisions are taken into account in deciding the incision as use of soft tissue expanders[17,18] may be required in tight or adherent skin from prior trauma or infection. An anterior midline[19,20] or medial parapatellar incision with medial parapatellar arthrotomy regardless of the associated deformity is sufficient in most cases. In cases where there are previous incisions the lateral most incision should be used. Care should be taken during exposure in the presence underlying disease conditions such as rheumatoid arthritis. Concomitant subchondral cysts may weaken the bone and affect soft tissue. These can jeopardize the integrity of extensor apparatus and collaterals making them susceptible to avulsion on attempting flexion.[3] Often the patellofemoral ankylosis is present and routine patellar eversion is difficult. Joint level may be difficult to identify and the normal patellar position is altered. Inadequate exposure may lead to component malpositioning, unbalanced flexion and extension gaps, patellar tendon ruptures, collateral ligament and tibial tuberosity avulsions. Enhancement of exposure can be done by using basic techniques like extending the quadriceps incision proximally, performing a lateral retinacular release, and externally rotating the tibia to enhance medial subperiosteal dissection along the proximal tibia.[3] If still adequate exposure and patellar eversion is not achieved, extensile exposure techniques like quadriceps snip, V-Y quadricepsplasty femoral peel, tibial tubercle osteotomy, or transepicondylar osteotomy with skeletonization can be used.[2,3,10-12,14-16,21-25]

Flexion is often limited due to adhesions below the quadriceps mechanism proximally. Any such residual adhesions should be looked for and excised from both the patellofemoral and suprapatellar areas. The tourniquet often restricts flexion and may have to be released temporarily and flexion reassessed. Osteotomy of the patellofemoral ankylosis is done in cases of bony ankylosis of the patellofemoral joint. The integrity of the collateral ligaments especially the medial collateral ligament should

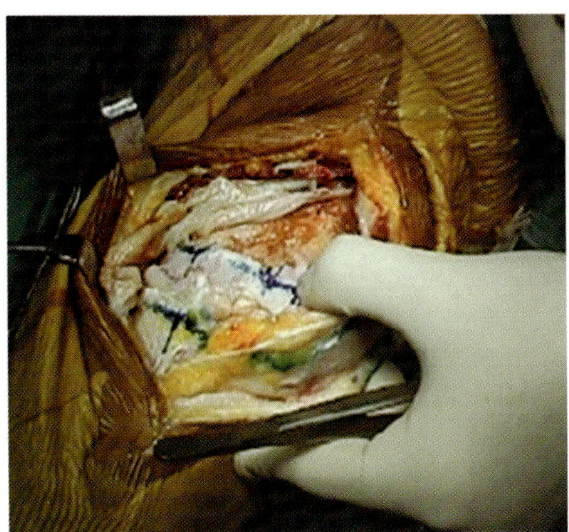

Figure 27.2 1 cm bone excised at the level of the joint in bony ankylosis

now be re-evaluated as it eventually determines the choice of implant. The above-mentioned methods usually are enough to displace the extensor mechanism laterally. A medial sleeve may similarly elevate from the distal femur, femoral condyle and the medial tibial plateau to enhance exposure. This allows good exposure of the anterior, medial and lateral aspects of the stiff knee. Minimal joint mobility should now be looked for to make identification of the joint line easier.[6,10] In case of bony ankylosis, 1 cm bone is excised at the level of the joint and the posterior cortex osteotomy (**Figure 27.2**) completed with osteoclasis. A vestigial anterior cruciate ligament is often seen even in bony ankylosis that further helps in identifying the joint level. Often an intact posterior cruciate ligament is also visualized. After the initial bony resection is done in position of ankylosis, the knee is slowly and carefully flexed and all subsequent femoral and tibial cuts done in flexion to avoid any inadvertent neurovascular damage. In patient with fibrous ankylosis, following an adequate soft tissue release, the knee can be carefully flexed and bony preparation completed. Standard alignment jigs such as intramedullary alignment guide for the femur and extra or intramedullary alignment guide for the tibia are adequate for taking cuts once flexion is achieved. Posterior cuts further improve mobility. Adequate posterior soft tissue release while preserving an envelope of soft tissue is important in postoperative stability. Care should be taken for correct placement of the femoral component in external rotation as preventing internal rotation is important to the success of surgery.[3] It is easy to malposition the femoral component in view of the distorted anatomy. Correct rotation of the femoral component is determined by using one of the described methods like the transepicondylar axis, the posterior condylar axis or the anteroposterior axis as described by Whiteside. We recommend taking the distal cut in 3° of valgus and this is adequate even in patients with severe valgus deformities. Once adequate flexion is obtained, soft tissue release as required for a varus or a valgus knee is done to obtain correction. All femur cuts are then taken using standard blocks. After completing the femur the final tibial cut is taken using the extramedullary jig. If required spacer blocks can be used to assess if a good rectangular gap has been achieved (**Figures 27.3A and B**). The ligaments should be reassessed at this stage to look for any collateral damage especially the medial collateral and if required a more constrained implant should considered. Trial reduction is attempted and near full extension and achievable flexion is strived for. Flexion may be limited at this stage and adhesions under the quadriceps looked for and excised. Stability and ligament imbalance at this stage determines the amount of constraint required. If the soft tissue dissection is carried out subperiosteally by keeping an intact soft tissue envelope throughout (**Figure 27.4**), the incidence of intraoperative instability requiring constrained implants may be reduced. Only in situations where the presence of medial collateral ligament is in doubt a more constrained prosthesis like the LCCK, rotating hinge (**Figures 27.5A and B**) or a TC3 is required. Patellar resurfacing depends on the surgeons' discretion. We routinely do not resurface the patella though we carefully excise all the osteophytes.

Care should be taken to note that the patellar tracking is good before final implantation. Documentation of flexion achieved on the operating table is made, as that is usually the index of the final range of flexion achieved.

The wound is closed over drains after carefully repairing the extensor mechanism using Vicryl sutures. Skin is closed with standard staples. Wound is dressed and a compression bandage applied before the torniquet is released. Some surgeons prefer releasing the tourniquet before closure and coagulate any bleeding vessels. The lateral genicular artery especially should be looked

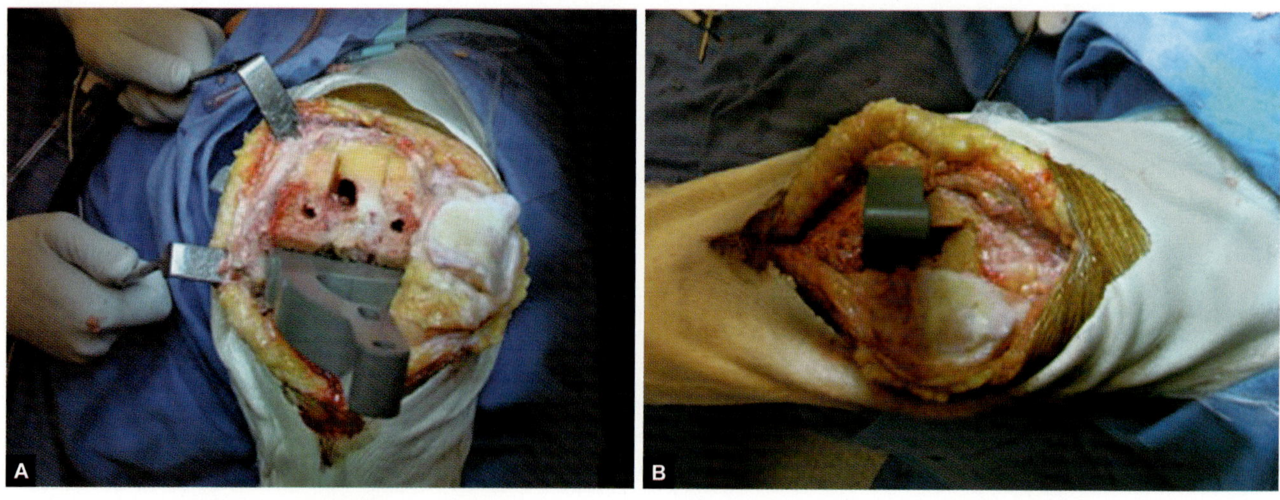

Figures 27.3A and B Spacer blocks used to assess if good rectangular gaps have been achieved

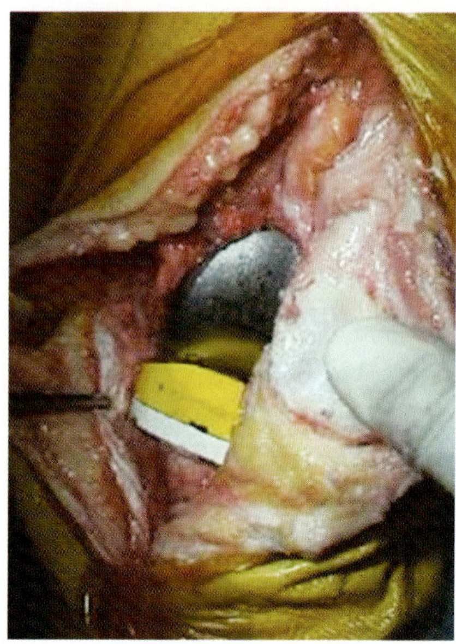

Figure 27.4 Soft tissue dissection carried out subperiosteally by keeping an intact soft tissue envelope

for where a lateral release has been done. The limb postoperatively is often left in 15° of flexion to reduce the risk of peroneal nerve palsy.

POSTOPERATIVE MANAGEMENT

Our goal in TKA in stiff knee is to achieve maximum range of motion in both flexion and extension. Static quadriceps exercises and ankle movements are started from the first postoperative day especially in patients with quadriceps snip or transepicondylar osteotomy. The drain is removed after 24 hours range of motion exercises are started soon after surgery and the patient made to ambulate with a walker. Patients are encouraged to perform knee flexion exercises and straight leg raises as per pain tolerance. Ambulation is increased on a daily basis and patients progressed to cane or crutches as tolerated. A removable night splint is used in patients where a residual flexion contracture remained after surgery. Range of motion exercises are carried out extensively for a minimum of 6 months after surgery. In patients where a V-Y quadricepsplasty is done a restricted range of assisted motion and delayed full weight bearing is advised using a hinged knee brace. Such patients are allowed active flexion and passive extension after 4–6 weeks. Manipulation under anesthesia is considered when extensive physiotherapy fails to increase flexion to more than 80° at the end of 6 weeks postoperatively. This usually helps in achieving a good range of flexion.[3]

COMPLICATIONS

Preoperative planning and adequate knowledge of extensile exposure techniques are important for avoiding potentially disastrous complications[2,6,9,11,21,26] both intra- and postoperatively. The take down of the stiff knee comes with the possibility of certain postoperative complications such as superficial and full thickness necrosis, an increase

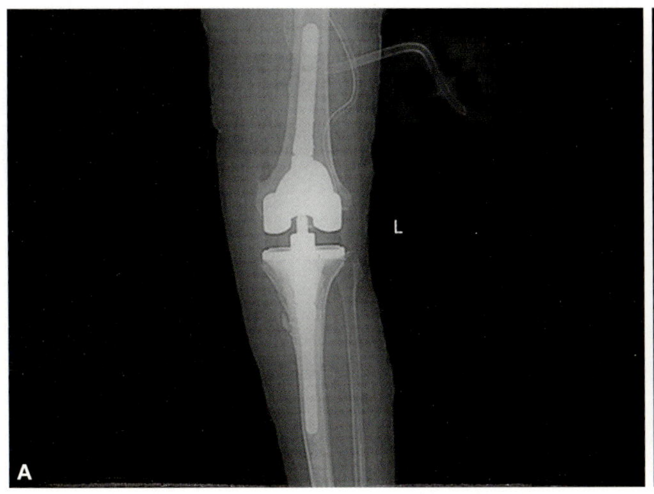

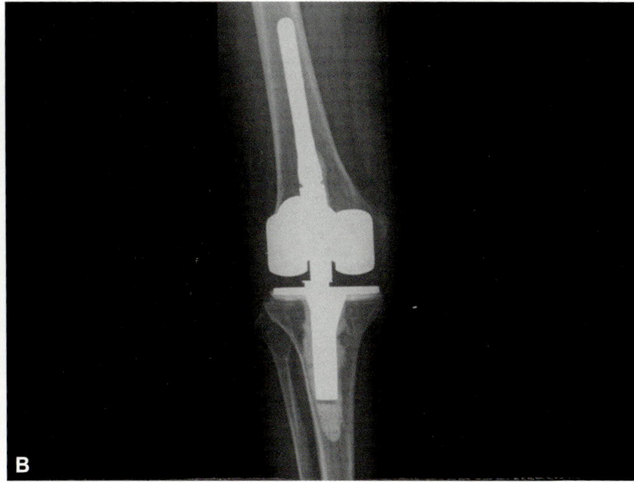

Figures 27.5A and B (A) A-LCCK; (B) B-RHK

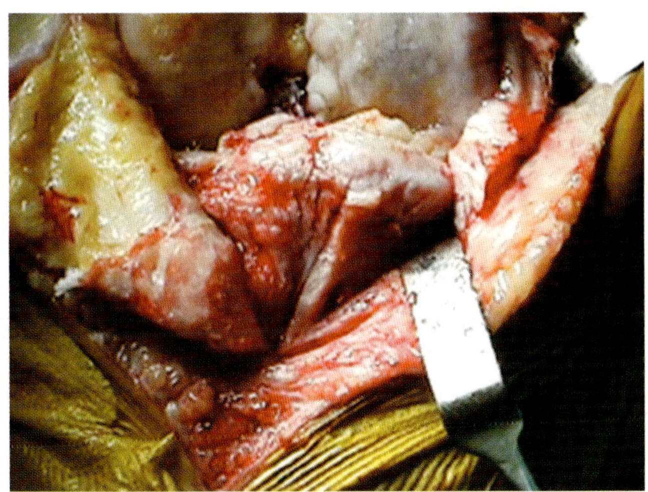

Figure 27.6 Patellar tendon avulsion

risk of postoperative infection which may require subsequent surgical intervention. Careful handling of the soft tissues and laminar airflows reduce such incidences. The integrity of the extensor mechanism should be preserved carefully. Patellar tendon avulsion (**Figure 27.6**) can be prevented with the help of fixation pins or clips on the medial side of patellar tendon insertion and external rotation of the tibia with avoidance of forceful flexion. Postoperatively the patient should be mobilized as early as possible to get optimal results as often there is a loss of range of motion despite what is achieved on the operating table. If adequate range of motion is not obtained one should not hesitate to manipulate under anesthesia.

Though TKA is reliable for achieving pain relief, increasing range of motion, maintaining stability and improving walking and sitting abilities in patients with stiff knees the expectations for outcome should be carefully reviewed with the patient. Even a small increase in the range of motion should be considered a success.

REFERENCES

1. Aglietti P, Windsor RE, Buzzi R, Insall JN. Arthroplasty for the stiff or ankylosed knee. J Arthroplasty. 1989;4(1):1-5.
2. Fosco M, Filanti M, Amendola L, Savarino LM, Tigani D. Total knee arthroplasty in stiff knee compared with flexible knees. Musculoskelet Surg. 2011;95(7):7-12.
3. Rajgopal A, Ahuja N, Dolai B. Total knee arthroplasty in stiff and ankylosed knee. J Arthroplasty. 2005;20:585-90.
4. Hsu CH, Chen WS, Lin PC, Wang JW. Total knee arthroplasty in patients with stiff knees. J Arthroplasty. 2012;27:286-92.
5. Montgomery WH 3rd, Insall JN, Haas SB, Becker MS, Windsor RE. Primary total knee arthroplasty in stiff and ankylosed knees. Am J Knee Surg. 1998;11:20-3.
6. Kim YH, Cho SH, Kim JS. Total knee arthroplasty in bony ankylosis in gross flexion. J Bone Joint Surg Br. 1999;81:296-300.
7. Bhan S, Malhotra R, Kiran EK. Comparison of total knee arthroplasty in stiff and ankylosed knees. Clin Orthop Relat Res. 2006;451:87-95.

8. Nayak N, Bourne RB, Rorabeck CH, Mulliken B, Robinson E. Techniques of exposure for the stiff total knee. Knee. 1995;2(4):189-94.
9. Della Valle CJ, Berger RA, Rosenberg AG. Surgical exposures in revision total knee arthroplasty. Clin Orthop Relat Res. 2006;446:59-68.
10. Bae DK, Yoon KH, Kim HS, Song SJ. Total knee arthroplasty in stiff knees after previous infection. J Bone Joint Surg Br. 2005;87:333-6.
11. Kim YH, Kim JS. Does TKA improve functional outcome and range of motion in patients with stiff knees? Clinical Orthop Relat Res. 2009;467:1348-54.
12. Kim YH, Kim JS. Total knee replacement for patients with ankylosed knees. J Bone Joint Surg Br. 2008;90:1311-6.
13. Scott RD, Siliski JM. The use of a modified V-Y quadricepsplasty during total knee replacement to gain exposure and improve flexion in the ankylosed knee. Orthopedics. 1985;8:45-8.
14. Camanho GL. Total arthroplasty in ankylosed knees: a case series. Clinics. 2009;64:183-7.
15. Kim YH, Kim JS, Cho SH. Total knee arthroplasty after spontaneous osseous ankylosis and takedown of formal knee fusion. J Arthroplasty. 2000;15:453-60.
16. Schurman 2nd JR, Wilde AH. Total knee replacement after spontaneous osseous ankylosis: a report of three cases. J Bone Joint Surg Am. 1990;72:455-9.
17. Mahomed N, McKee N, Solomon P, Lahoda L, Gross AE. Soft tissue expansion before total knee arthroplasty in arthrodesed knee. A report of two cases. J Bone Joint Surg Br. 1994;76:88-90.
18. Manifold SG, Cushner FD, Craig-Scott S, Scott WN. Long term results of total knee arthroplasty after the use of soft tissue expanders. Clin Orthop. 2000;380:133-9.
19. Insall JN. A midline approach to the knee. J Bone Joint Surg Am. 1971;53:1584-6.
20. Barrack RL, Smith P, Munn B, Engh G, Rorabeck C. The Ranawat Award. Comparison of surgical approaches in total knee arthroplasty. Clin Orthop Relat Res. 1998;356:16-21.
21. Naranja RJ Jr, Lotke PA, Pagnano MW, Hanssen AD. Total knee arthroplasty in previously ankylosed or arthrodesed knee. Clin Orthop Relat Res. 1996;331:234-7.
22. Lu H, Mao CS, Lin J. Total knee arthroplasty in presence of severe flexion contracture: a report of 37 cases. J Arthroplasty. 1999;14:775-80.
23. Garvin KL, Scuderi G, Insall JN. Evolution of the quadriceps snip. Clin Orthop. 1995;321:131-7.
24. Whiteside LA. Exposure in difficult total knee arthroplasty using tibial tubercle osteotomy. Clin Orthop. 1995;321:32-5.
25. Arsht SJ, Scuderi GR. The quadriceps snip for exposing the stiff knee. J Knee Surg. 2003;16(1):55-7.
26. McAuley JP, Harrer MF, Ammeen D, Engh GA. Outcome of knee arthroplasty in patients with poor preoperative range of motion. Clin Orthop Relat Res. 2002(404):203-7.

Chapter 28

Hinged Knee Prosthesis

Ashok Rajgopal, Attique Vasdev, Himanshu Gupta, Vipin Tyagi

Primary total knee replacement (TKR) has proved to be very successful with survivorship rates as high as 95% in 15 years.[1] However, with an increase in primary TKR there is an expected corresponding increase in revision surgeries[2-4] with 5–13% of primary TKRs requiring revision.[3] These patients often present with massive bone loss, soft tissue deficiencies, and global instability. In such situations, the role of semiconstrained or posterior stabilized implants is limited and requires hinged devices to restore function and stability.

Walldius[5] in 1951 developed a hinged prosthesis initially made of acrylic and later with metal. Shiers[6] in 1954 reported on a similar device with better biomechanical characteristics. These devices looked promising as these were self-aligning and stabilizing to the presence of intramedullary rods, and the extent of damage to the knee did not matter. Extreme deformities could be corrected with these prostheses by resecting extra bone and soft tissues. Both these were uncemented devices. Once methacrylate cement was available newer prosthesis such as the Guepar, which could be used with bone cement, became available. The problem with these designs was the amount of rigid constraint provided by these implants. The rigid hinges allowed movement in only one plane and were truly fixed hinges. Movement was possible only in flexion and extension with no rotational ability. This inability of the prosthesis to accommodate gait related rotational stresses led to torsional stresses being transferred to the bone cement interfaces directly from the metal hinged articulation. This led to a large production of metal debris that caused early failure because of aseptic loosening, implant breakage, or both.[7-14] Freeman in 1973[15] reported a survival rate of 88% using the Wallidus prosthesis in primary osteoarthritis. Jones et al. in 1979[16] had a survival rate of 89% at a maximum of 3 years with the Guepar prosthesis, though 29% had poor results. Bargar et al.[10] in 1980 also reported a survivorship of 87% for a 2–4 years follow-up. Grimer et al.[11] Insall,[16] and Oglesby and Wilson[17] reported a survivorship of 80%, 96% and 90% using the Stanmore, Guepar, and Walldius prosthesis, respectively for primary knee replacement. Bargar et al.[10] and Karpinski and Grimer[18] in their series of revision surgery had a survivorship rate of 76% and 90%, respectively at 4 years.

Knutson et al.[14] in 1986 in a nationwide multicenter investigation of 8000 cases reported a cumulative survivorship of 65% at 6 years with rigid hinged knees in primary osteoarthritis patients. They attributed poor results of these early rigid hinged knees to metal on metal-bearing surfaces and small stems leading to poor medullary fill and significant bone removal to accommodate large implants.

With the availability of Endo-Model rotating hinge, the Kinematic rotating hinge and the St George rotating knee rotation around the vertical axis were made available. Better results were achieved both due to a metal on polyethylene-bearing surface and the axial rotation component.

Survivorship as high as 96% with the Endo-Model prosthesis by Petrou et al. 2004[19] at 7–15 years was reported for primary knee replacement. Barrack et al.[20] Westrich et al.[21] both in 2000, and Jones et al. in 2001[22] all reported survivorship rates of 100% with the S-ROM, Finn, and S-ROM components, respectively, over a 2–6 years follow-up for revision situations.

The major drawback of these designs was the lack of modularity, though some of these designs are still available today. Shindell et al. in 1986[23] in their series reported a 56% failure rate with the Noiles rotating hinge over a 32-month follow-up with failures predominantly in patients over 90 kg in revision situations. Rand et al. in 1987[8] in their series of 38 Kinematic rotating hinge knees (RHKs) at an average 55-month follow-up reported a high incidence of patellar instability (22%), infection (16%), and component breakage (6%). They reported a survivorship of only 57%.

In Europe especially in Germany with the addition of some anteroposterior translation between the tibial metal post and the femoral polyethylene cam led to the wide use and popularity of the GSB prosthesis.[24] However, the midterm results of this prosthesis were poor as both the polyethylene in the femoral cam and the tibial polyethylene inserts were nonmodular, leading to extensive wear that required for the whole prosthesis to be exchanged.

With the availability of modularity with newer prosthesis like the NexGen RHK, S-ROM Noiles modular knee, and the Stryker MRH, better knee kinematics with rotation ability throughout the flexion extension could be achieved. The linkage of these designs was different from the previous designs. Here the hinge was secured to the femoral component and inserted into the tibial component freely with a hinge-post extension. This mechanism along with a rotating articulation surface stresses on the cement interfaces that are not only reduced but transferred to the soft tissues reducing wear and debris generation. Compared with previous hinged designs, the amount of bone resection required in present day designs is reduced. The availability of modular fluted canal filling stems with variable offsets for a more reliable alignment, and press fit fixation, metaphyseal sleeves, trabecular metal cones, and modular wedges to fill large bone defects encountered in difficult revision situations have all helped reduce failure rates. These modern day rotating hinge devices have a more conforming articulation allowing for the femoral condyles to interact with the tibial surface as the main articulating surface. These highly conforming articular surfaces increase stability by means of condylar contact and not by the constraint mechanism alone greatly reducing shear stress on the hinge.[25] There is only partial transfer of varus–valgus, mediolateral, and anteroposterior loads from the hinge post extension to the tibial stem. Improvement in the design of the patellar groove providing for better patellar tracking, screw home phenomenon in extension by rotation around the vertical axis, and a rollback mechanism of the femur during flexion that may decrease the pressures at the patellofemoral joint during flexion have all helped reduce failure rates further.

The importance of joint line position and flexion extension gaps was emphasized by Joshi and Navarro-Quilis[26] while implanting a RHK. Any imbalance in the flexion extension gaps could lead to instability in the arc of motion, though the knee may be stable in extension and 90° flexion. They reported four cases of instability and three cases of dislocation in their series. This mechanism was best described by Wang and Wang[27] who suggested that an excessive flexion gap led to instability in flexion, and posterior dislocating forces on the prosthesis could cause mechanical failure.

Rajgopal et al.[28] in 2012 reported their midterm results using exclusively the NexGen RHK. They followed up 44 patients for average of 62 months. They advocated judicious use of the hinged knee and limiting it to patients with severe global deformities, severe bone loss extensor mechanism disruption, or severely comminuted fractures around the knee in both primary and revision situations. They also attributed their better results to use of the same prosthetic design over the years.

In spite of all improvements in current day designs of the RHK, the bone cement interfaces and the hinge mechanisms remain areas of concern. Though loads are significantly reduced in present day rotating hinge designs, some sheer and torsional stresses are still transferred to the bone cement interfaces; thus the need for well-fixed long intramedullary stems. A posteriorly located articulating hinge mechanism bears most of the weight throughout the range of motion (ROM), leading to high stresses on the hinge increasing polywear resulting in early failure. In designs where the femoral condyles articulate with a highly conforming rotating polyethylene surface and those which have a hinge-post extension (e.g. NexGen RHK) fare better as here the most of the loads are transferred not from the hinge mechanism but rather from the condyles. Maximizing contact area distributes the stresses in the polyethylene across a larger surface area. Also with the use of the hinge post extension inserted freely into the tibial component not only are the varus-valgus, anteroposterior, and mediolateral movements achieved, but also their loads are partially transferred to the tibial stem via the long hinge post extension. Any reduction in the stresses should have an impact on reducing the mechanical failure rates.

Implant dislocation is another thing to be taken into account while using the RHK. Flexion laxity especially if exceeds the jump height of the hinge mechanism may lead to separation of the post from the tibial mechanism (**Figures 28.1A and B**).[29] This is possible as the rotating hinge is commonly used where the ligaments and the collaterals are either insufficient or absent (**Figures 28.2A and B, 28.3A and B, and**

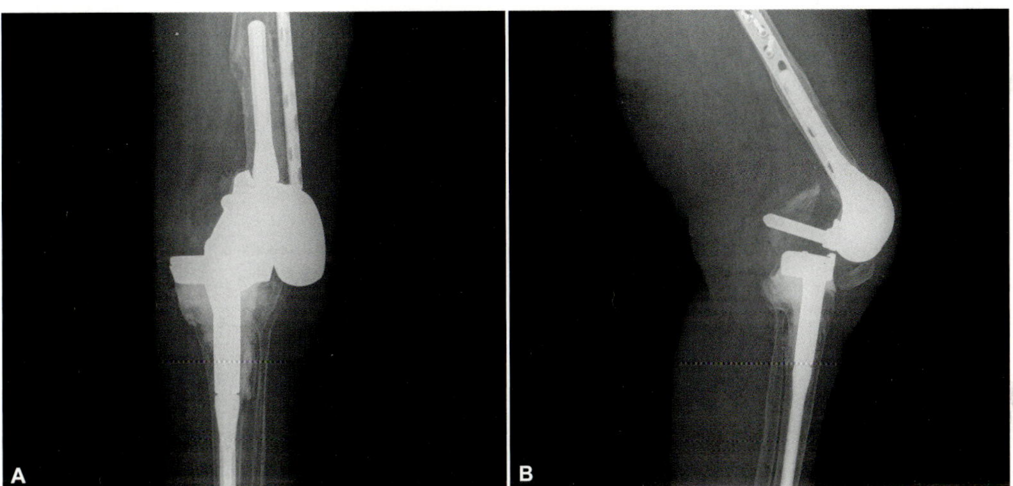

Figures 28.1A and B (A) Dislocated rotating hinge knee (RHK)—anteroposterior view; (B) Dislocated RHK—lateral view

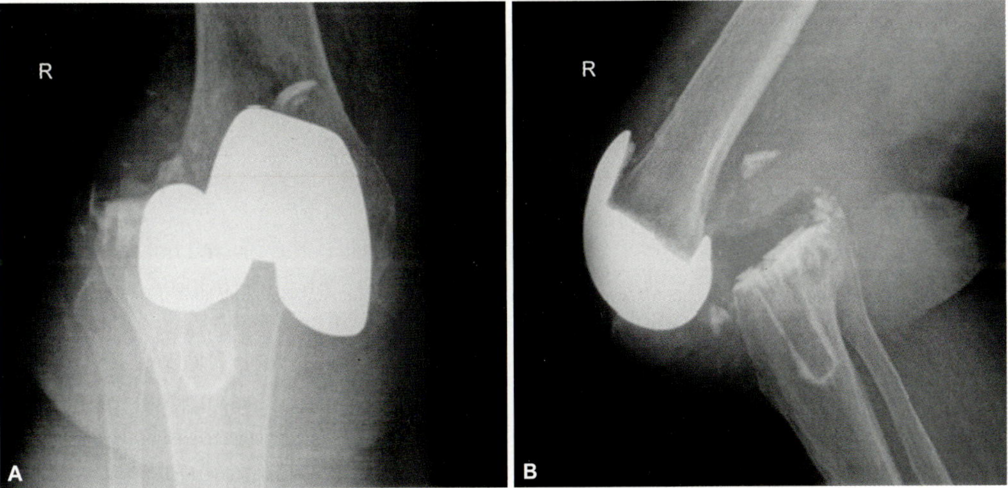

Figures 28.2A and B Gross instability

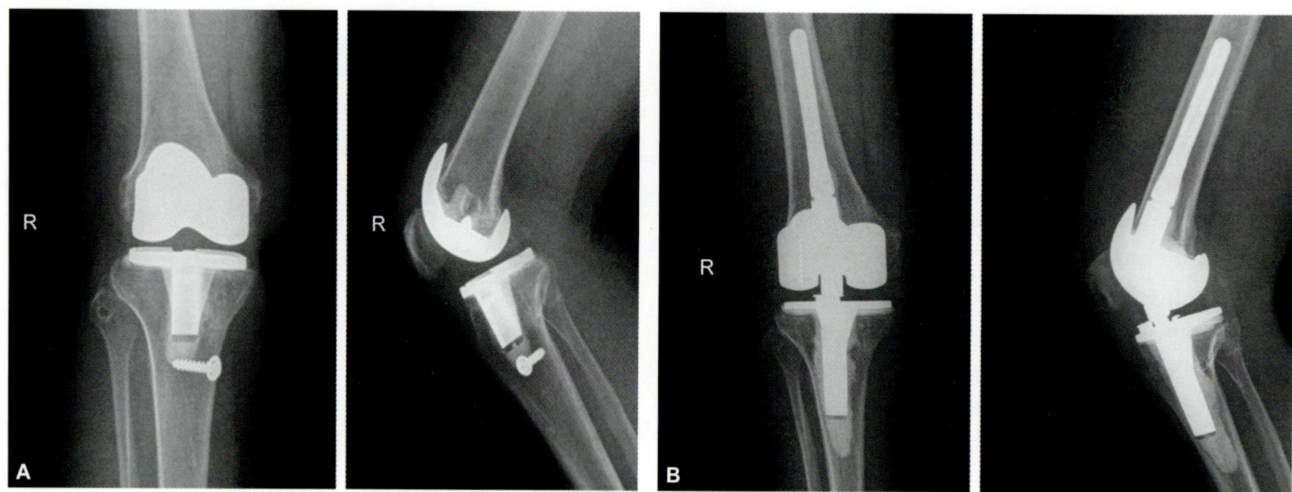

Figures 28.3A and B (A) Failed medial collateral ligament (MCL) reconstruction following total knee replacement; (B) Rotating hinge knee following failed MCL reconstruction

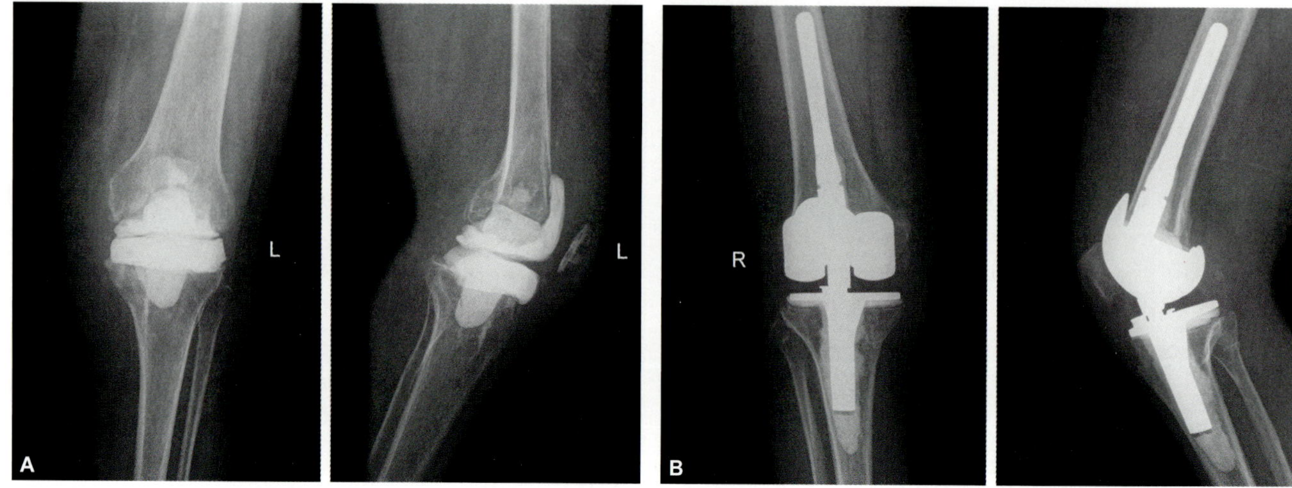

Figures 28.4A and B (A) Stage one following Infected TKA; (B) RHK as stage two procedure

28.4A and B). Adult cadaveric studies show that in the absence of ligaments it is possible to distract the knee joint by 20–32 mm.[30] Ward et al. in 2003[31] measured the stem lengths and taper lengths of the rotating hinges made by various manufactures. In their study the Howmedica, Techmedica, Intermedics/Sulzer Medica, and Wright Medical Technology/Dow Corning Wright designs required a minimal distraction of 39 mm before dislocating. The Biomet knee prosthesis required 33 or 44 mm of distraction to dislocate, depending on the polyethylene thickness, whereas the S-ROM knee required only 26 mm of distraction to dislocate. The hinge-post extension of the NexGen RHK is designed to provide a minimum jump height of 40 mm.

PERSONAL EXPERIENCE

We evaluated our midterm results and survivorship using the NexGen RHK.[31] From a cohort of 47 patients, we retrospectively analyzed the results of 44 patients (46 knees) who underwent the NexGen RHK. Clinical outcomes were measured using the Knee Society Scores (KSS), the ROM, and serial radiography. The mean follow-up was 62 months (36–96 months). There was an improvement in the KSS from 47 preoperatively to 81 postoperatively. Functional score improved from 17 to 67.5 at follow-up. The ROM improved from 65°–96° at follow-up. Radiological analysis showed nonprogressive radiolucent lines in 7 knees (5 femurs, 2 tibiae). These were less than 2 mm with no evidence of loosening or subsidence. The mean postoperative alignment was in 5.5° valgus (range: 4°–7°). Two patients had an intraoperative fracture of the medial tibial condyle due to osteopenia. Both were treated with cancellous screw fixation. Two patients had subluxation of the patella at 90° flexion. One patient developed superficial infection that was treated with oral antibiotics. Our data suggest that the midterm results with the NexGen RHK in our patients were better than other series where different implants were used due to the use of a single type of modern rotating hinged implant (NexGen rotating hinge) due to better understanding and experience gained over years. The outcome reported in our series is encouraging for indications such as severe bone loss (**Figures 28.5A and B**), instability (**Figures 28.2, 28.3A and B, and 28.4A and B**), periprosthetic fractures (**Figures 28.6A to D**), tumors (**Figures 28.7A to C and 28.8A and B**), and extensor apparatus disruption. We also advocate the use of the rotating hinge in selected neglected primary situations (**Figures 28.9A to C and 28.10A to C**) where regular or even semiconstrained options would not give a well-balanced aligned knee.

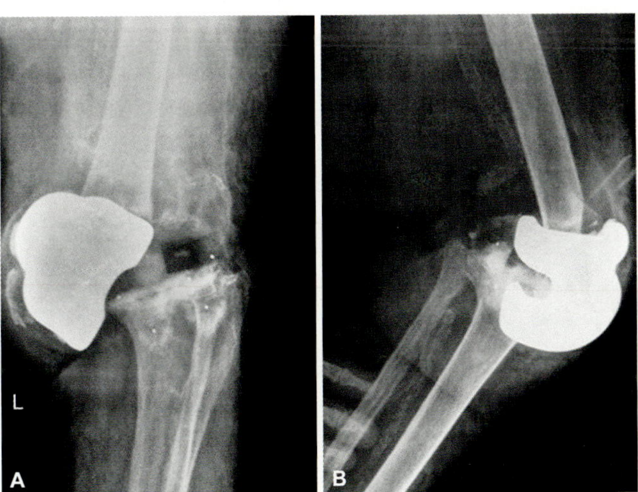

Figures 28.5A and B Severe bone loss

WHY WE CHOSE TO USE THE NEXGEN RHK?

In the NexGen RHK, 95% (as shown in laboratory studies) of the load is carried by the tibial condyles due to its modular hinge mechanism that is similar to the loading pattern of a primary implant design. The patellofemoral contact area is maximized due to the trochlear groove, allowing the patella to track deeply as in the case of primary implant designs. This allows smooth translation from flexion to extension and also resists lateral subluxation. Normal patellar tracking is also facilitated by the central position of the hinge axis that prevents the patella from shifting posteriorly during flexion. Being a modular design that allows the use of augments, the basic bone cuts of the NexGen RHK are the same as that of the primary NexGen system, thus minimizing bone loss. The locking hinge mechanism has a 'jump height' of 40 mm thus resisting subluxation. The NexGen RHK allows 25° of internal and external rotation. This helps in displacing torsional loads from cement interfaces to soft tissues. The highly dished articular tibial surface and the femoral condyles have virtually a conformity ratio of 1:1 that maximizes contact area distributing stresses in the polyethylene to a large surface area. Another important feature is the simplicity of putting the hinge-post extension pin and the tibial articular surface after cementing the NexGen RHK femoral and tibial components without any excessive distraction.

The indications for a hinged knee in our experience are limited and should be used judiciously. These are most often used in revision situations. Present day indications for the use of the modular hinged knees include severe bone loss, global instability, complex periprosthetic fractures, inability to balance flexion extension gaps, tumors around the knee, and extensor apparatus disruption. The hinged knee is also a good option in selected cases of primary neglected degenerative arthritis in patients presenting very late where less constrained options like the CCK or the TC3 fail to give a well-aligned and balanced knee. The RHK is best used as a salvage procedure should other options for revision fail.

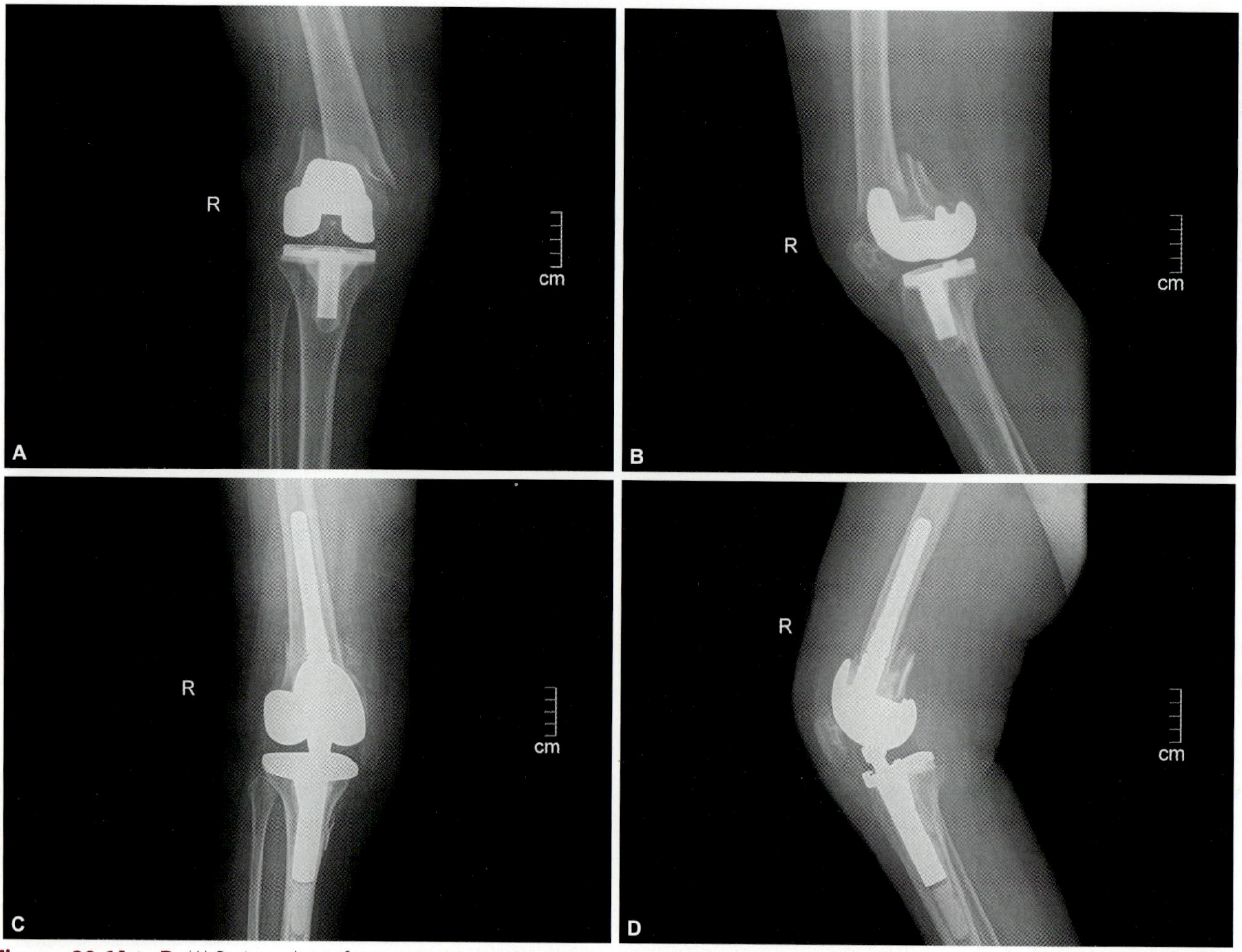

Figures 28.6A to D (A) Periprosthetic fracture—anteroposterior view; (B) Periprosthetic fracture—lateral view; (C) Periprosthetic fracture—postoperative anteroposterior view; (D) Periprosthetic fracture—postoperative lateral view

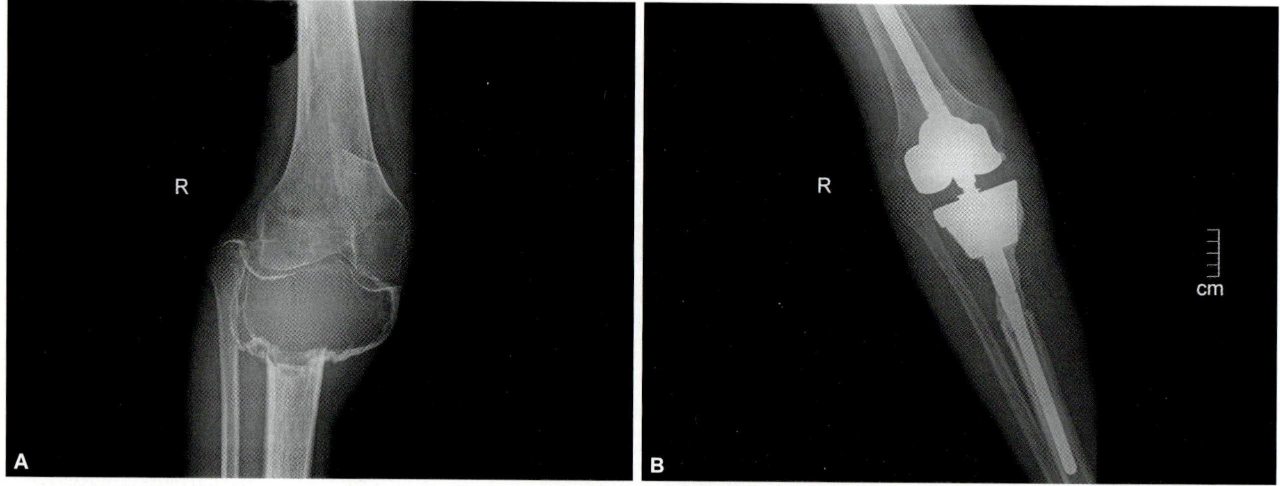

Figures 28.7A and B

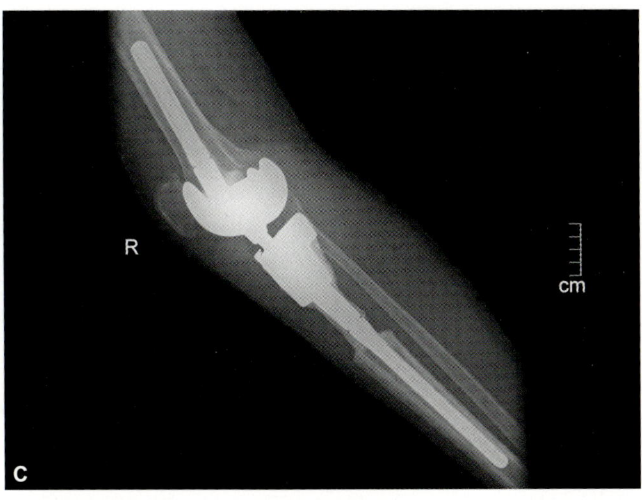

Figure 28.7C

Figures 28.7A to C (A) Giant cell tumor (GCT) proximal tibia; (B) GCT rotating hinge knee (RHK) and trabecular metal (TM) cone—anteroposterior view; (C) GCT—RHK and TM cone—lateral view

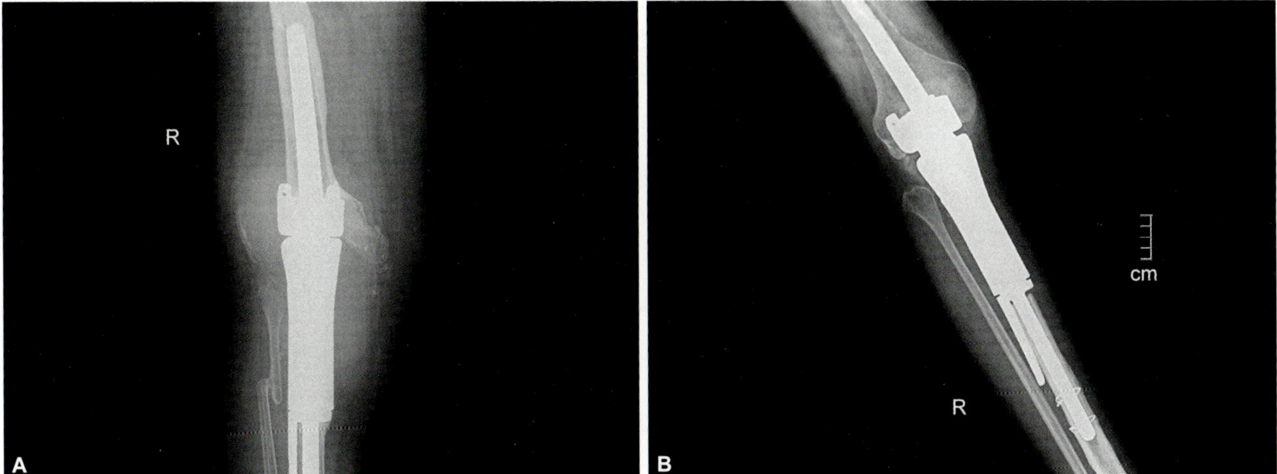

Figures 28.8A and B (A) Hinged tumor prosthesis; (B) Hinged tumor prosthesis

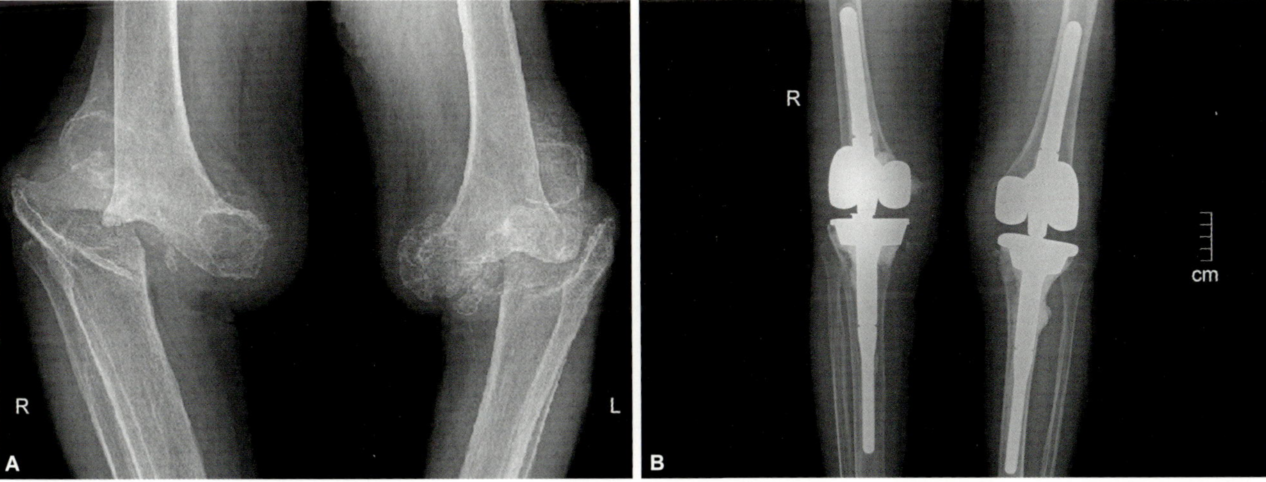

Figures 28.9A and B

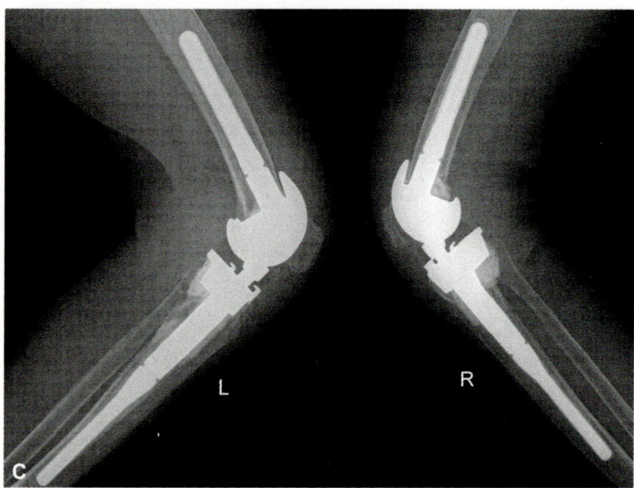

Figure 28.9C

Figures 28.9A to C (A) Complex neglected primary OA preoperative radiograph; (B) Complex neglected primary OA—postoperative anteroposterior view; (C) Complex neglected primary OA—postoperative lateral view

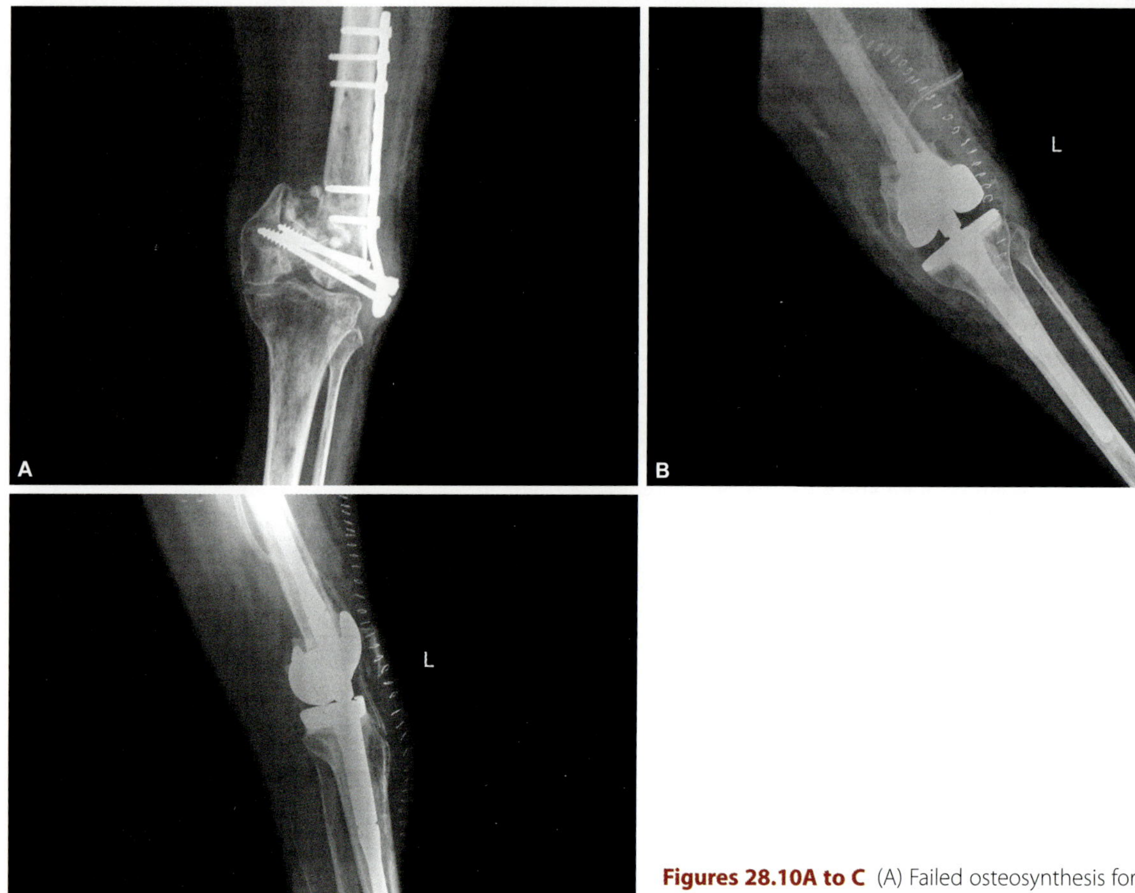

Figures 28.10A to C (A) Failed osteosynthesis for distal end femur; (B) Primary rotating hinge knee (RHK) for failed osteosynthesis distal end femur—anteroposterior view; (C) Primary RHK for failed osteosynthesis distal end femur—lateral view

REFERENCES

1. Ranawat CS, Flynn WF Jr, Deshmukh RG. Impact of modern technique on long term results of total condylar knee arthroplasty. Clin Orthop Relat Res. 1994;309:131-5.
2. Barrack RL. Evolution of the rotating hinge for complex total knee arthroplasty. Clin Orthop Relat Res. 2001;392:292-9.
3. Kurtz S, Mowat F, Ong K, et al. Prevalence of primary and revision total hip and knee arthroplasty in the United States from 1990 through 2002. J Bone Joint Surg. 2005;87-A:1487-97.
4. Springer BD, Sim FH, Hanssen AD, Lewallen DG. The modular segmental kinematic RH for nonneoplastic limb salvage. Clin Orthop Relat Res. 2004;421:181-7.
5. Walldius B. Arthroplasty of the knee joint using endoprosthesis. Acta Orthop Scand Suppl. 1957;24:19.
6. Shiers LGP. Arthroplasty of the knee: preliminary report of a new method. J Bone Joint Surg Br. 1954;36:553.
7. Jones RE, Skedros JG, Chan AJ, Beauchamp DH, Harkins PC. Total knee arthroplasty using the S-ROM mobile bearing hinge prosthesis. J Arthroplasty. 2001;16:279-87.
8. Rand JA, Chao EY, Stauffer RN. Kinematic rotating hinge total knee arthroplasty. J Bone Joint Surg. 1987;69-A:489-97.
9. Walker PS, Emerson R, Potter T, et al. The kinematic rotating hinge: biomechanics and clinical application. Orthop Clin North Am. 1982;13:187-99.
10. Bargar WL, Cracchiolo A, Amstutz HC. Results with the constrained total knee prosthesis in treating severely disabled patients and patients with failed total knee replacements. J Bone Joint Surg Am. 1980;62:504-12.
11. Grimer RJ, Karpinski MRK, Edwards AN. The long-term results of Stanmore total knee replacements. J Bone Joint Surg Br. 1984;66:55-62.
12. Inglis AE, Walker PS. Revision of failed knee replacements using fixed-axis hinges. J Bone Joint Surg Br. 1991;73:757-61.
13. Jones RE, Barrack RL, Skedros J. Modular, mobile-bearing hinge total knee arthroplasty. Clin Orthop. 2001;392:306-14
14. Knutson K, Lindstrand A, Lidgren L. Survival of knee arthroplasties: a nation-wide multicentre investigation of 8000 cases. J Bone Joint Surg Br. 1986;68:795-803.
15. Freeman PA. Walldius arthroplasty: a review of 80 cases. Clin Orthop. 1973;94:85-91.
16. Insall JN. Total Knee Replacement. In: Insall JN (Ed). Surgery of the Knee. New York: Churchill Livingstone; 1984. pp. 587-695.
17. Oglesby JW, Wilson FC. The evolution of knee arthroplasty. Clin Orthop. 1984;186:96-103.
18. Karpinski MRK, Grimer RJ. Hinged knee replacement in revision arthroplasty. Clin Orthop. 1987;220:185-91.
19. Petrou G, Petrou H, Tilkeridis C, et al. Medium-term results with a primary cemented rotating hinge total knee replacement: a 7- to 15-year follow-up. J Bone Joint Surg Br. 2004;86:813-7.
20. Barrack RL, Lyons TR, Ingraham RQ, Johnson JC. The use of a modular rotating hinge component in salvage revision total knee arthroplasty. J Arthroplasty. 2000;15:858-66.
21. Westrich GH, Mollano AV, Sculco TP, et al. Rotating hinge total knee arthroplasty in severely affected knees. Clin Orthop. 2000;379:195-208.
22. Jones RE, Barrack RL, Skedros J. Modular, mobile-bearing hinge total knee arthroplasty. Clin Orthop. 2001;392:306-14.
23. Shindell R, Neumann R, Connolly JF, Jardon OM. Evaluation of the Noiles hinged knee prosthesis: a five-year study of seventeen knees. J Bone Joint Surg Am. 1986;68:579-85.
24. Sprenger TR, Doerzbacher JF. Long-term follow-up of the GSB II total knee used in primary total knee arthroplasty. J Arthroplasty. 2002;17:176-83.
25. Hernandez-Vaquero D, Sandoval-Garcia MA. Hinged total knee arthroplasty in the presence of ligamentous deficiency. Clin Orthop Relat Res. 2010;468:1248-53.
26. Joshi N, Navarro-Quilis A. Is there a place for rotating hinge arthroplasty in knee revision surgery for aseptic loosening? J Arthroplasty. 2008;23:1204-11.
27. Wang CJ, Wang HE. Early catastrophic failure of rotating hinge total knee prosthesis. Case report. J Arthroplasty. 2000;15:387-91.
28. Rajgopal A, Vasdev A, Chidgupkar AS, Dahiya V, Tyagi VC. Mid-term results of rotating hinge knee prostheses. Acta Orthop Belg. 2012;78:61-7.
29. Gustke KA. Preoperative planning for revision total knee arthroplasty: avoiding chaos. J Arthroplasty. 2005;20(Suppl 2):37-40.
30. Krackow KA, Mihalko WM. The effect of severe femoral bone loss on the flexion-extension joint space in revision total knee arthroplasty: a cadaveric analysis and clinical consequences. Orthopedics. 2001;24:121-6.
31. Ward WG, Haight D, Ritchie P, Gordon S, Eckardt JJ. Dislocation of rotating hinge total knee prosthesis: a biomechanical analysis. J Bone Joint Surg Am. 2003;85:448-53.

Chapter 29

Anesthesia and Pain Management of Total Knee Arthroplasty

Yatin Mehta, Bijaya Kumar Shadangi

INTRODUCTION

Technological development related to the total knee arthroplasty is one of the finest advancements in orthopedic surgery. Worldwide knee arthroplasty is a leading surgical procedure but causes significant perioperative morbidity. During the perioperative period of knee arthroplasty, the pain at times may be variable but can be severe particularly in the postoperative period. As an anesthesiologist and perioperative physician one may play a significant role in influencing the perioperative morbidity, while encountering a multitude of challenges in providing anesthesia and postoperative pain management.[1] Most of the patients who required total knee arthroplasty are almost always associated with comorbidities like osteoarthritis, rheumatoid arthritis, obesity, diabetes mellitus, and other significant diseases. Adequate pain control enables early ambulation and initiation of knee physiotherapy that not only speeds up recovery but also reduces the length of the stay in the hospital along with decreasing the hospital acquired infection and thromboembolic disease.[1-3] Better anesthetics and surgical techniques along with better implants have resulted in a good perioperative course of the patients.[4]

PREDICTORS INFLUENCING THE OUTCOME OF KNEE ARTHROPLASTY

Patients undergoing bilateral knee replacement have a higher rate of postoperative complications like cardiopulmonary events, need of blood transfusions and related complications, especially if associated with pre-existing coronary artery diseases. With appropriate and adequate hemodynamic monitoring and adequate analgesia, the outcome is excellent, not only during intraoperative period but also during the first 48 hours of the postoperative period. Bilateral knee arthroplasty, on a male more than 75 years old, with other comorbid illnesses is an independent risk factor for morbidity. Relative contraindications for simultaneous bilateral total knee arthroplasty include the following: ASA grade III and above, decreased cardiopulmonary reserve, liver dysfunction, neurological disorder and renal dysfunction.

Preoperative Evaluation

Most of the patients posted for knee arthroplasty are usually elderly with obesity and multiple comorbidities. A thorough but complete preoperative assessment and maximum medical optimization with an appropriate planning is essential for a possible positive outcome. Not only does it help in identifying the risk factors and prognostication but it also ensures the patients have a smoother perioperative course following this major surgery.

A multidisciplinary care team approach is required so that, preoperative, intraoperative and postoperative pain management can be smoothly integrated. Adopting this will help in developing a comprehensive perioperative care for the elderly, especially for prevention of common postoperative complications like atelectasis, delirium, pneumonia and various stages of respiratory failure.

ASSESSMENT AND OPTIMIZATION OF COMORBIDITIES

Degenerative Diseases

Most common degenerative diseases like osteoarthritis, rheumatoid arthritis usually affect the various joints including the knee, besides involving various other organs in this disease process, as explained in **Table 29.1.**

TABLE 29.1 Organs involved and their manifestations in degenerative diseases

Systems involved	*Systemic manifestation*
• Pulmonary system	Pleural effusion, interstitial pulmonary fibrosis
• Cardiovascular	Conduction defects, pericarditis, pericardial effusion, valvular involvement and related problem
• Endocrine system	Defective immune system, steroid use related to adrenal insufficiency
• Hematological issues	Anemia, thrombocytopenia and platelets dysfunction, susceptibility to infection.

Cardiovascular Diseases

Assessments of exercise tolerance of the patients are unreliable because of limited mobility and debilitation and usually mask the underlying pulmonary as well as cardiac dysfunction. Dobutamine stress echocardiography is helpful in evaluating the functional ability of cardiopulmonary system. In the absence of any clinical predictors, one may not perform the stress echocardiography. A normal 2D-echocardiography may be advised for LV function, wall movement and valvular abnormality, if the history of symptoms warrants it. With the help of radiological images of the spine and other joints, adequate preparation and careful positioning is accomplished for smooth intubation and to secure the airway. Neck stabilization and fibro-optic intubation at times may be essential in order to avoid protrusion of the odontoid process either compressing the spinal cord or compromising the vertebral blood flow to brain by excessive neck extension particularly in cases of bamboo spine of ankylosing spondylitis.

MULTIDIMENSIONAL MODEL OF PERIOPERATIVE RISK STRATIFICATION

In order to achieve effective perioperative assessment and sharing of patient-related information with other colleagues of the department, *Holt and Silverman* postulated a multidimensional model of perioperative risk stratification. Following are the factors that are incorporated in the *Holt and Silverman* postulation.

ASA Physical Status Scoring for Physical Condition of the Patient

Pulmonary Diseases

These patients are associated with multifold increase in risk factors for postoperative pulmonary complications. Preoperative spirometry is helpful, and if COPD is severe, it may necessitate a thorough investigation and ABG analysis. Optimization of lung functions may be advised, if required, with the help of respiratory physicians. Cessation of cigarette smoking at least 4–6 weeks in advance will be helpful in a great way to tide over the acute crisis.

Renal Dysfunction

This may be due to the chronic and excessive use of NSAIDs (analgesics: particularly diclofenac sodium), secondary to progressive diabetes or hypertension.

Diabetes Mellitus

Adequate blood sugar control is of paramount importance for achieving the maximal benefit of surgery and reducing chances of infection. It is also essential to study the possible associated complications including cardiovascular disease, autonomic neuropathy and nephropathy.

Concurrent medications that the patient might be receiving to control the pain (analgesics like aspirin), to limit the progression of the disease process (steroids), to suppress active inflammation like NSAID (aspirin) and disease modifying antirheumatoid drugs like methotrexate and their undesired side effects after prolonged use also need to be taken into consideration.

PREOPERATIVE MEDICATIONS

Most of the medications (except a few like: hypoglycemic agents, angiotensinogen converting enzyme inhibitors and diuretics) should be continued till the morning of the surgery.

- *Acid prophylaxis:* Either by H_2-blockers/proton pump inhibitors (e.g. pantoprazole)
- Antihypertensive medications should be continued.
- *Antiplatelet drugs:* Clopidogrel should be discontinued at least 5–7 days before surgery
- Thromboprophylaxis
- Because of high-risk of venous thromboembolism in these groups of patients, thromboprophylaxis should be considered and with adequate pain control early ambulation should be instituted.
  - Physiological thromboprophylaxis, can be achieved by precautionary advice and education and leads to decreased risk. Adequate hydration during NPO status through existing intravenous line, and early mobilization with the help of physiotherapist should be considered.
  - *Mechanical thromboprophylaxis:* Most widely used methods include the following.
    - Antiembolism stockings during and after surgery in postoperative period.
    - Intermittent pneumatic compression devices.
    - Foot impulse devices.
  - Pharmacological thromboprophylaxis
- Pharmacological agents/medications can also be tried through the intravenous, subcutaneous or oral route during knee arthroplasty. The following are the common medications used for these purpose.
  - Indirect thrombin/factor x inhibitors, heparin, low molecular weight heparin (LMWH).
  - Direct thrombin inhibitors (lepirudin, argatroban, dabigatran).
  - Direct factor Xa inhibitors (rivaroxaban, apixa).
  - Vitamin K antagonist (warfarin, acenocoumarol).
  - Antiplatelet agents (clopidogrel).
  - *Regional anesthesia:* It can decrease the reflex stress hormone release, resulting in attenuation of pain, activation of local fibrinolysis and to some extent, inhibition of platelets activation and the local anesthetic itself inhibit platelet aggregation.
- *Steroids:* Patients with preoperative steroids intake should continue these till the morning of the surgery.
- *β_2-agonist*: If the patient is on regular bronchodilators, these should be taken till the morning of the surgery.

ANESTHETIC MANAGEMENT

The anesthetic technique may vary from patient to patient depending upon the existing medical conditions of the patient, complexity of the procedure followed and expected intraoperative complications.

Anesthesia/analgesic techniques for knee arthroplasty should target to have a good intraoperative environment and maximal analgesia, rapid patient recovery, with least possible side effects like sedation, postoperative respiratory, depression, nausea and vomiting, hypotension and motor blockade and finally, allowing for effective joint rehabilitation.

The most commonly followed anesthetic techniques for knee arthroplasty are as follows:

- Central neuroaxial blockade.
  - Intrathecal/spinal.
  - Epidural with indwelling catheters.
  - Combined spinal and epidural with indwelling catheters.
- General endotracheal anesthesia.
- Peripheral nerve blocks (with/without USG and catheters).
- Combination of the above procedures.

Sometimes the length of surgery, patient factors and other medical issues of the patient and patient preference affect the choice of anesthesia.[5] But typically most specialized centers use spinal and/or epidural with indwelling catheters with/without general anesthesia for knee arthroplasty.

CENTRAL NEUROAXIAL BLOCKADE

This method of administering anesthesia has several important implications not only for stable intraoperative period but also the postoperative outcome like rapid patient recovery with better postoperative pain management.[6]

Advantages of Central Neuroaxial Blockade

Most specialized centers for knee arthroplasty use either an epidural anesthetic technique alone or combined spinal epidural, barring a few that use spinal anesthesia alone. If correctly carried out, it will have following benefits:

- Regional anesthesia provides good surgical conditions and analgesia extending into postoperative period
- Airway manipulation is avoided
- Common complications of general anesthesia, like deep vein thrombosis, pulmonary embolism, pneumonia, respiratory depression
- Communication between the patient and operating room personnel including surgeons should not be lost throughout the procedure
- Epidural analgesia to manage/improve the immediate postoperative pain—the greatest advantage (addition of opioids/catheters can extend the analgesic period)
- Overall reduction in morbidity and mortality
- Less intra- and postoperative blood loss due to decreased blood pressure and peripheral vasodilation
- Attenuation of property of prothrombotic effect of stress response
- Motor blockade achieved by spinal anesthesia is more profound than general anesthesia
- Regional anesthesia may be associated with a lower incidence of postoperative confusion and cognitive dysfunction as compared to GA.

The local anesthetic agent used in regional anesthesia usually blocks nociceptive transmission in the peripheral nervous system and central nervous system depending upon the site, where they are used.[6] At times, to enhance the quality and duration of the anesthesia and analgesia adjuvants like opioids (morphine/fentanyl), anesthesia and analgesia adjuvants like opioids (morphine/fentanyl), nervous.

Placement of an epidural catheter definitely has certain extra-advantages over single shot epidural/spinal anesthesia, like extension of the anesthesia period when the intraoperative surgical time is increased than the expected/anticipated besides the above benefits.[7] Decreased incidence of deep vein thrombosis is seen, in patients receiving continuous epidural infusion for postoperative pain management. Sometimes regional anesthesia is supplemented with sedation since the duration of surgery is long and the patients often are uncomfortable while lying in a particular position. Sedation with intermittent bolus doses of midazolam and fentanyl or infusion of propofol (target controlled infusion) or dexmedetomidine infusion, with the supplementation of oxygen, are often used. If the patient still needs deep asleep during the procedure after regional anesthesia, then general endotracheal anesthesia can be supplemented with or without spontaneous breathing using laryngeal mask airway (LMA).

Complications of Neuroaxial Anesthetics

The most common complication experienced after neuroaxial anesthetics with the patients is short-term backache. But the postdural puncture headache, at the present time is almost nonexistent with even 25G and above sizes spinal needles in TKR group. Nerve injury due to needle trauma is also very rare. But there have been reports of paresthesias by patients during the needle placement, so it is important to decrease the level of sedation to as low as possible before the neuroaxial block. It should be prudent to maintain some degree of verbal contact during the procedure to allow reporting of paresthesias or pain during needle injection or during injection of local anesthetics. In extreme cases, damage to spinal cord/conus medullaris by needle trauma is although very rare, but is a dreaded complication during central neuroaxial blockade while performing above the L_2 space.

Serious complications following neuroaxial blockade like cardiac arrest, neurological injury and cauda equine syndrome are extremely rare and reported to be less than 0.1%.[8] Other extremely rare complications like infection and anterior spinal artery syndrome are avoided by appropriate technique.

REGIONAL ANESTHESIA AND ANTICOAGULATION

The American Society for Regional Anesthesia recommends for delaying the placement of epidural or spinal 10 to 12 hours after the last dose of the commonly used LMWH. For thromboprophylaxis treatment in the postoperative period, it recommends the first dose to be administered not earlier than 24 hours postoperatively, the indwelling epidural catheter be removed before initiating the therapy and at the same time, the LMWH administered no sooner than 2 hours after catheter removal.

In order to reduce the risk of bleeding or the formation of hematoma 'warfarin' should be discontinued at least 5 days and clopidogrel at least 7 days before surgery and fondaparinux may be administered at least 6 hours after the surgery and 12 hours after removal of catheters.

General Anesthesia

The use of opioids mostly during general anesthesia is associated with side effects such as nausea, vomiting, pruritus, sedation, respiratory depression and urinary retention. The above side effects can have negative effects on the patient comfort and safety as well as delaying the start of physiotherapy that will negatively impact functional rehabilitation.

General endotracheal tube anesthesia or general anesthesia with spontaneous respiration using LMA is an option. It can also apply to those patients, in whom regional anesthesia is contraindicated like in patients with severe aortic and mitral stenosis. In most musculoskeletal disorder where regional anesthesia will be technically difficult, general anesthesia may be administered. To reduce intraoperative blood loss tranexamic acid may be used during the procedure, provided those patients are not at increased risk of thromboembolic episode, at a dose of 20–25 mg/kg although the blood loss generally is not much with neuroaxial block and application of tourniquet.

Tourniquet Release Response (Intraoperative Period)

During the tourniquet release, there will be a variable response on hemodynamics. Generally, the blood pressure falls appreciably after the tourniquet release and should be corrected promptly. It has been seen that approximately 20% reduction in mean arterial pressure usually occurs within a minute of tourniquet release. There will be a compensatory rise in heart rate but this physiological response may be variable depending upon autonomic dysfunction in diabetics or patients on β-blockers. About 4% of patients had a heart rate decrease greater than 10 beats per minute as observed in a study conducted by Kahn RL et al.[9] With adequate fluid management or changing the position or by administrating short-acting vasoactive drugs like ephedrine during the procedure the hypotension and bradycardia can be corrected.

Peripheral Nerve Blocks

Peripheral nerve blocks may be considered as the sole anesthetic technique and also for postoperative pain management in many centers during knee arthroplasty. Peripheral nerve blocks are also useful in patients who cannot be considered for regional (spinal/epidural) or general endotracheal tube anesthesia because of various reasons. It provides some stable hemodynamics and is devoid of postoperative complications including hypotension, respiratory depression, nausea, vomiting, and urinary retention as commonly seen in other techniques of anesthesia.

Peripheral nerve blocks can be achieved either with single injection of local anesthetic of various concentrations or with the use of indwelling catheter for intermittent boluses doses or continuous infusion of local anesthetic. But the limitations of the use of indwelling catheter include more cost with additional time consumption and finally well-trained skilled personnel that are required for placement and management of catheter. It also includes the increase in incidence of risk of infections and nerve injury. It mandates the use of either syringe pump or infusion pump for continuous infusion.

Nerve blocks can also be used as a supplement to general endotracheal anesthesia either for postoperative analgesia or during intraoperative period. The following are the nerves that innervate the knee from lumbosacral plexus. The obturator and femoral nerves are responsible for the pain originating from the anterior aspect of the knee and the sciatic nerve innervates the posterior part of knee.[10]

INTRAOPERATIVE COMPLICATION

- *Blood loss:* As most surgeons apply tourniquet during the intraoperative period, the blood loss becomes more apparent during the postoperative period (average 500–1000 mL per knee) and even slightly more if it is a revision arthroplasty. So regular hemoglobin and hematocrit estimation will guide the estimating and treating the blood loss.
- *Hypothermia:* A more frequent complication, so measures need to be taken to maintain normothermia, particularly, in the elderly as in the orthopedic theater the room temperature usually kept low. The normothermia can be maintained by water mattress, convective air blankets, e.g. Bair Hugger and warming the IV fluids (fluid warmers).
- *Bone cement implantation syndrome:* During or after the application of bone cement (prepolymerized polymethyl methacrylate or PMMA), there may be a possibility of severe fall in blood pressure and oxygen saturation. A decrease in consciousness and fat embolism syndrome, which though rare, can also occur during this event. It may be the result of release of microembolism of air, bone marrow, fat globules or platelet aggregation plug into the circulation by the high intramedullary pressure during cement or prosthesis insertion. Microemboli phenomenon may at times reach the lungs and the consequences of pulmonary embolism may follow. Surgeons try to reduce this by drilling multiple holes in the bone.
- Pre-emptive administration of intravenous hydrocortisone before cementing is sometimes helpful.
- *Thromboembolism:* venous thromboembolism is also a known complication in the form of DVT or pulmonary thromboembolism. But acute arterial thrombus in the operated limb is also documented after knee arthroplasty. Early identification of the problem and prompt treatment will ensure a positive outcome. Adequate prophylaxis either by pharmacological or mechanical and chemical prophylaxis should be followed.
- Tourniquet release complications.
- *Postoperative delirium:* More common after general anesthesia, but also seen with patients who opted for regional anesthesia. Use of haloperidol during preoperative period and if required postoperatively, has shown to have reduced the incidence and severity of delirium.

POSTOPERATIVE PAIN MANAGEMENT

Patients after total knee arthroplasty usually experience severe pain in the immediate postoperative period. The primary aim of postoperative analgesic use includes maximum pain relief with minimum side effects and[11] to allow aggressive but 'continuous passive movement' (CPM: physiotherapy) of the operated leg. The maximum[12] achievements in the rehabilitation milestones/benchmarks are only possible with the aggressive management of postoperative analgesia, without loss of motor tone in the limbs.

The patients need early mobilization of joints in the immediate postoperative period and poorly controlled pain may prevent this early mobilization of the knee joint and subsequently results in adhesions, capsular contracture and to some extent muscular atrophy.[13] So the final functional outcome of the surgery either will be delayed or badly affected.

Postoperative pain can also present with severe reflex spasms of the quadriceps muscle causing further pain and inhibit the proper muscle function required for physiotherapy. This spasm will be more pronounced as soon as the patient starts to ambulate. These afferent nociceptive inputs are usually blocked by epidural infusions so that these reflex responses do not occur.

MULTIMODAL APPROACH TO PAIN MANAGEMENT

Actual advantages of controlling postoperative pain after knee arthroplasty are generally maximized when a multimodal strategy is implemented to facilitate the patient's convalescences. The principle of multimodal surgery includes control of postoperative pain of the patient to allow early mobilization, early enteral nutrition, education and attenuation of the postoperative stress response with the help of regional anesthetic techniques and use of combination of analgesic agents (multimodal analgesia) and peripheral nerve blocks. This approach usually decreases perioperative morbidity, decreases length of hospital stay and improves patient satisfaction without compromising patient safety.

Epidural Anesthesia and Analgesia

Continuous epidural infusion/patient controlled epidural analgesia (PCEA) with infusion pump/PCA pump, is one of the most favored method for postoperative analgesia after knee arthroplasty. Depending upon the patient tolerance and response this epidural infusion may be supplemented with patient controlled (through PCA pump) devices with boluses of 3–5 mL at regular intervals. **Table 29.2** shows different doses of opioids for pain relief.

Local anesthetics can also be used in epidural infusion with various strengths. The choice of local anesthetic for continuous epidural infusion varies. Bupivacaine, ropivacaine, or levobupivacaine are widely used local anesthetics because of differential and preferential clinical sensory blockade with minimal impairment of the motor function. The concentrations used for postoperative epidural analgesia are <0.125% bupivacaine or levobupivacaine or <0.2% ropivacaine.

PATIENT CONTROLLED EPIDURAL ANALGESIA (PCEA)

It has been seen that PCEA allows for individualization of postoperative analgesic requirement and has several advantages over continuous epidural analgesia like lesser amount of drug use, greater patient satisfaction and above all superior analgesia with a higher degree of patient satisfaction. Besides the demand dose, the provision of either continuous or background infusion is more popular than with intravenous PCA in definitely providing superior analgesia, compared to the use of demand dose alone. According to several studies, addition of an opioid to the local anesthetics can provide analgesia that is superior to either agent alone especially in continuous epidural infusions. **Table 29.3** shows various possible combinations of opioids for PCEA.

TABLE 29.2 Epidural doses of opioids

Drugs	*Epidural single dose*	*Epidural continuous infusion*	
Fentanyl	50–100 µg	25–100 µg/h	Commonly used drugs
Morphine	1–5 mg	0.1–1 mg/h	
Sufentanil	10–50 µg	10–20 µg/h	Not commonly used
Alfentanil	0.5–1 mg	0.2 mg/h	

TABLE 29.3 Patient controlled epidural analgesia (PCEA) regimen

Local anesthetic and opioids	*Continuous rate (back ground) mL/h*	*Demand dose (mL)*	*Lockout interval (min)*
0.0625–0.125% bupivacaine and 5 µg/mL fentanyl	4–6	3–7	10–15
0.125% levobupivacaine and 4µg/mL fentanyl	4	2	10
0.2% ropivacaine and 4 µg/mL fentanyl	4	3	10

Intravenous PCA Pump

Intravenous PCA use may provide advantages, such as patient satisfaction and this may be the result of superior analgesia and of perceived control over analgesic medication and decreased postoperative pulmonary complications. Intravenous PCA optimizes delivery of analgesic opioids and minimizes other side effects. These PCA devices may be adjusted for multiple variables including the demand (bolus) dose, lockout interval and background infusion. The optimal demand dose for morphine is 1 mg and that for fentanyl is 20 µg.

TRANSDERMAL PCA

Without venous access transdermal PCA may be used to deliver opioids for postoperative pain relief. Recently, fentanyl iontophoretic transdermal system (fentanyl ITS) has been introduced in medical practice for postoperative pain relief. This is a preprogrammed system applied to the patients' upper outer arm or chest for 24 hours.

Peripheral Nerve Blocks

Recent literature supports the use of single shot or continuous peripheral nerve blocks to provide postoperative analgesia with minimal motor blockade and improved rehabilitation. Ultimately, it facilitates early and more effective joint mobilization and physiotherapy without any muscle spasm. Additional benefits include, avoidance of systemic side effects of opioids and epidural analgesia (hypotension, urinary retention). To minimize the motor blockade in postoperative period low concentration of local anesthetic solutions should be used. The rate of infusion of local anesthetic solution may vary between 5 mL/h and 10 mL/h after total knee arthroplasty and may be continued for 48–72 hours. Using electronic infusion pumps or elastomeric devices. Rare but some serious complication can also be encountered during continuous peripheral nerve block like infection, hematoma, systemic toxicity, catheter knotting, dislodging, and shearing. Most centers nowadays use USG-guided blocks or peripheral nerve stimulators for total knee arthroplasty.

Femoral Nerve Block

Single shot femoral nerve block provides analgesia to the anterior aspects of the knee for up to 24 hours.[14-16,18] Continuous femoral nerve block has low incidence of side effects but the analgesic efficacy of this technique is comparable to both continuous epidural analgesia and continuous lumbar plexus block following total knee arthroplasty. However, as part of the posterior aspect of the knee is innervated by the sciatic nerve, a femoral block alone does not cover this area and supplementary drugs may be required.

Sciatic Nerve Block

Single shot sciatic nerve block either with USG-guided or peripheral nerve stimulator combined with the femoral nerve provide very good postoperative analgesia for up to 24 hours, with a highest success rate. Single sciatic nerve block with continuous femoral nerve block combination is the best-suited postoperative analgesic after total knee arthroplasty.

Lumbar Plexus Block

It includes the blockade of[17] femoral, obturator and lateral femoral cutaneous nerves. It has been seen that these improve analgesia and facilitate earlier mobilization following total knee arthroplasty.

Obturator Nerve Block[18]

Addition of single shot obturator nerve block to single shot sciatic and femoral nerve blocks may improve analgesia, as femoral nerve block alone in isolation has been shown to spare to the obturator nerve.

STEP-DOWN ANALGESIA

The concept of concomitant and step-down analgesia is becoming common in clinical practice. Most clinicians are of the opinion that regular oral acetaminophen should be given to all patients undergoing total knee arthroplasty unless contraindicated. The routine use of nonsteroidal anti-inflammatory drugs (NSAIDs) can also be considered provided the risk of bleeding events, pre-existing renal dysfunction and gastrointestinal ulceration in these group of patients in the preoperative period has been ruled out.

Intravenous Acetaminophen (Paracetamol)

Its opioid sparing effect made it an integral part of multimodal analgesia in acute postoperative pain along with other NSAIDs.[19] Acetaminophen has no associated postoperative bleeding unlike other NSAIDs and is a cost-effective analgesic. It has been demonstrated that it has great efficacy in patients undergoing total joint arthroplasty.

Intra-articular Analgesia

Local peripheral administration of opioids along with local anesthetics after knee arthroplasty may even provide analgesia for up to 24 hours after surgery and provide better rehabilitation. Higher doses of opioids with local anesthetic solutions into intra-articular spaces result in superior analgesia.

Parvataneni et al.[20] demonstrated a better pain relief and patient satisfaction levels with intra-articular infiltration of bupivacaine, morphine, and epinephrine and a femoral block than a femoral block alone. Similar results were presented by Toftdhal et al.[21] Their data suggested that local infiltration analgesia with ropivacaine, ketorolac, and epinephrine resulted in faster postoperative mobilization. Ropivacaine, though pharmacologically similar to bupivacaine, has less cardiac and neurotoxicity allowing patients to tolerate larger doses.[22] Epinephrine reduces the toxicity of the local anesthetic by reducing the rate of drug release into circulation by vasoconstriction via its α-adrenergic effects. We routinely use periarticular infiltration with 150 mL ropivacaine (0.2%), ketorolac (30 mg/mL), epinephrine (0.5 mg/mL), and 0.5 mL clonidine (150 mg/mL) divided into three syringes of 50 mL each. 100 mL is injected before final cemented of implants into the posterior capsule and the intercondylar area and the remaining 50 mL into the anterior capsule after final cementing of implants into position. Clonidine exerts its effect via its α_2-adrenergic actions. It results in potentiation of the actions of local anesthetic agents and local opioids via synergistic effects.[23,24]

Gabapentin and Pregabalin

Besides the common NSAIDs and COX-2 inhibitors anti-neuropathic drugs like gabapentin and pregabalin can inhibit central neuronal sensitization. Even preoperative administration of gabapentin leads to reduction in postoperative pain and morphine consumption. Gabapentin administered one hour before surgery in patients undergoing knee surgery had significantly improved postoperative analgesia with better range of knee motion postoperatively. Combination of gabapentin and pregabalin, rather than a drug in isolation is known to improve the final outcome of knee arthroplasty.

Finally, the anesthetic and analgesic management of the patient during and after total knee arthroplasty always has a considerable influence on medical and surgical outcomes. It is equally important for an anesthesiologist to periodically upgrade and improve anesthetic and analgesic techniques in order to achieve maximum medical and surgical outcome with minimal side effects and complications. Majority of anesthesiologists are of the opinion that central neuroaxial blockade supplemented by additional analgesic nerve and lumbar plexus blockade have definite advantages over general anesthesia. Local infiltration of the surgical site has offered a new dimension to the issue of pain management.

REFERENCES

1. Calum RK Grant, Matthew R Checketts. Analgesia for primary hip and knee arthroplasty: the role of regional anaesthesia. CEACCP. 2008;8(2):56-61.
2. William-Russo P, Sharrock RE, Haas SB, et al. Randomized trial of epidural versus general anesthesia: outcomes after primary total knee replacement. Clin Orthop. 1996;331:199-208.
3. Mohaney OM, Noble PC, Davidson J, Tullos HS. The effect of continuous epidural analgesia on postoperative pain, rehabilitation and duration of hospitalization in total knee arthroplasty. Clin Orthop Rel Res. 1990;260:30-7.

4. Capdevila X, Barthelet Y, Biboulet P, et al. Effects of perioperative analgesic technique on the surgical outcome and duration of rehabilitation after major knee surgery. Anesthesiology. 1999;91:8-15.
5. Rodgers A, Walker N, Schug S, et al. Reduction of postoperative mortality and morbidity with epidural and spinal anesthesia: results from overview of randomized trails. BMJ. 2000;321:1493.
6. Gandhi K, Viscusi E. Multimodal pain management techniques in hip and knee arthroplasty. J New York Sch Reg Anesth. 2009;13.
7. Sharrock NE, Hass SB, Hargett MJ. Effects of epidural anesthesia on the incidence of deep vein thrombosis after knee arthroplasty. J Bone Joint Surg Am. 1991;73:502-6.
8. Auroy, Narachi P, Messiach A, et al. Serious complications related to regional anesthesia: result of a post-operative surgery in France. Anesthesiology. 1997;87;479-86.
9. Kahn RL, Marinol V, Urquhart B, Sharrock ME. Hemodynamic changes associated with tourniquet use under epidural anesthesia for total knee arthroplasty. Reg Anesth. 1992;17:228-32.
10. Paul JE, Arya A, Hurlburt L, et al. Femoral nerve block improves analgesia outcomes after total knee arthroplasty. Anesthesiology. 2010;113:1144-62.
11. Apfelbaum JL, Chen C, Mehta SS, Gan TJ. Postoperative pain experience: results from a national survey suggest postoperative pain continues to be undermanaged. Anesth Analg. 2003,97:534-40.
12. Kehlet H, Dahl JB. The value of multimodal or balanced analgesia in postoperative pain treatment. Anesth Analg. 1993;77:1048-56.
13. Seet E, Leong WL, Yeo AS, Fook-Choog S. Effectiveness of 3-in-1 continuous femoral block of differing concentration compared to patient controlled intravenous morphine for post-total knee arthroplasty analgesia and knee rehabilitation. Anaesth Intensive Care. 2006;34:25-30.
14. Duarte VM, Fallis WM, Solonowsky D, Kwarteng K, Yeung CK. Effectiveness of femoral nerve blockade for pain control after total knee arthroplasty. J Perianesth Nurs. 2006;21:311-6.
15. Davies AF, Segar EP, Murdoch J, Wright DE, Wilson IH. Epidural infusion or combined femoral and sciatic nerve blocks as peri-operative analgesia for knee arthroplasty. Br J Anesth. 2004;93:368-74.
16. Kandasami M, Kinnionmonth AW, Sarungi M, Bains J, Scott NB. Femoral nerve block for total knee replacement: a word of caution. Knee. 2009;166:98-100.
17. Allen HW, Liu SS, Ware PD, Nairn CS, Owens BD. Peripheral nerve blocks improve analgesia after total knee replacement surgery. Anesth Anal. 1998;87:93-7.
18. Barrington MJ, Olive D, Low K, et al. Continuous femoral nerve block or epidural analgesia after total knee replacement: a prospective randomized controlled trial. Anesth Analg. 2005;101:1824-9.
19. Sinatra Rs, Jahr JS, Reynolds LW, et al. Efficacy and safety of single and repeated administration of 1 gm intravenous acetaminophen injection (Paracetamol) for pain management after major orthopedic surgery. Anesthesiology. 2005;102:822-31.
20. Parvataneni HK, Shah VP, Howard H, et al. Controlling pain after total hip and knee arthroplasty using a multimodal protocol with local periarticular injections: a prospective randomized study. J Arthroplasty. 2007;22(6):33-8.
21. Toftdahl K, Nikolajsen L, Haraldsted V, et al. Comparison of peri- and Intra-articular analgesia with femoral nerve block after total knee arthroplasty: a randomized clinical trial. Acta Orthop. 2007;78(2):172-9.
22. Mather LE, Copeland SE, Ladd LA. Acute toxicity of local anesthetics: underlying pharmacokinetic and pharmacodynamic concepts. Reg Anesth Pain Med. 2005;30(6): 553-66.
23. Joshi W, Reuben SS, Kilaru PR, Sklar J, Maciolek H. Postoperative analgesia for outpatient arthroscopic knee surgery with intra-articular clonidine and/or morphine. Anesth Analg. 2000;90: 1102-6.
24. Paech MJ, Pavy TJ, Orlikowski CE, Lim W, Evans S. Postoperative epidural infusion: a randomized double-blind dose finding trial of clonidine in combination with bupivacaine and fentanyl. Anesth Analg. 1997;84: 1323-8.

Chapter 30

Rehabilitation in Total Knee Arthroplasty and Ligament Injuries

Kalpana Aggarwal, Shivani Jain, Alok Mohan

THE STRUCTURE AND COMPONENTS OF KNEE JOINT

The knee joint is a ginglymus type of joint. Its primary function is weight-bearing and it also provides stability that helps to maintain an erect posture.[1] It is called a modified hinged joint because other than the primary movements of flexion and extension, it also provides rotation and some translation. Because of its location between the hip and the ankle, it works as a part of open and closed kinematic chain, while sitting, standing, walking, and exercising.

The static stability of the joint is provided by the ligaments, while the musculoskeletal units provide dynamic stability to the knee joint.

The knee has three major and four accessory components. Its major components are as follows:

1. Posterior capsulofibrous complex
2. Medial collateral ligament
3. Lateral collateral ligament.

The accessory components are comprised of the fibrotendinous sheaths of varying strengths:

1. The anteromedial sheath
2. The anterolateral sheath
3. The posteromedial sheath
4. The posterolateral sheath.

Of all the muscles, quadriceps is the most important one that provides stability and power to the knee joint.[1] However, this muscle is also the first to atrophy in any eventuality. Unfortunately, its recovery is very slow. Thus, a good therapist takes all important steps to prevent the atrophy of quadriceps and rehabilitates it appropriately without losing time.

The knee joint primarily has two degrees of freedom.[2,3] The first degree of freedom is in the transverse axis along with the movement of flexion and extension in the sagittal plane. The second degree of freedom is in the longitudinal axis of the tibia (leg) in the form of rotation. However, this occurs only when the knee is in flexion. No rotation is possible in extension owing to the taut collateral and cruciate ligaments in this position. In high sitting when the knee is flexed to 90° (this prevents hip rotation) with the toes pointing slightly outward (neutral position), the medial rotation is performed with toes pointing inward completely. It is around 30° (fick angle).[17] The lateral rotation occurs when the toes point outward maximally. It ranges around 40° (fick angle*).[1] These angles vary with

*The angle between the line corresponding to the 2nd metatarsal in neutral position and maximum intoeing and out toeing.

the change in the angle of knee flexion. Lateral rotation is an important component of foot abduction, whereas medial rotation plays an important role in foot adduction.

To measure the passive angle of rotation, the therapist makes the patient lie prone with the knee flexed to 90° and will turn the foot inward (medial rotation) and outward (lateral rotation). The passive angle is of course more than the active range of motion. The longitudinal axis of the femoral shaft does not coincide with the long axis of the tibial shaft (leg), hence forming an obtuse angle of 170°–175°, opening outward. This angle is known as physiological valgus of the knee. Physiological valgus is more in females owing to a wider pelvis. This angle also determines pathological variations like genu valgum and genu varum.

Major movements of the joint are flexion and extension. Active flexion with a flexed hip is 140°, and with extended hip is 120°. The passive flexion is around 160°, allowing the heel to touch the buttock. The flexion deficit can be calculated by two ways:

1. The difference between the degree of flexion achieved and the maximum expected angle (160°)
2. The distance between the heel and the buttock.

There is no absolute extension of the knee, since in the position of reference the limb is maximally extended. Thus, the knee extension deficit is a negative angle. For example, if the leg is flexed to 120°, the extension deficit will be said to be –120°.

INJURIES OF KNEE JOINT

As it is located between two long lever arms (tibia and femur), the knee joint is subjected to extreme load-stress and strain.[2] Owing to the bony incongruence and the stability factors, this complex synovial joint is susceptible to various injuries. These injuries may be the result of the direct or indirect force. Indirect forces such as valgus strain, varus injury, hyperextension thrust, twisting injury, or a combination of these may cause various injuries and trauma in and around the knee joint. These injuries then require surgeries like ligament reconstruction or repairs.

Such knee joint injuries form a major section of sport injuries. Degenerative conditions or prolonged abuse of the knee in the form of obesity, faulty postures, etc. are the other common causes of knee joint injuries and may eventually need surgeries like total or unicompartmental knee arthroplasties.

Whatever the cause of injury may be, once the damage has been corrected surgically, our target as physical therapists should be to rehabilitate the patients to their normal level of activity, whether it is in the sports field or for normal day-to-day activities. Once the patient has undergone surgery, there are several different treatment protocols that may be followed depending upon the nature of injury, the corrective surgery, and the surgeon's expectations of the outcome of the aforesaid surgery (**Tables 30.1 to 30.5**).

In order to understand the nature of a rehab program that may be appropriate for any condition pertaining to the knee joint, it is first important to understand the kind of exercises that can be done and their effect on the biomechanics. It may then be easier to customize an exercise program to suit the needs of the patient.

TYPES OF EXERCISE

There are two basic types of exercise that are inherent to any rehabilitation protocol:[4,5]

1. Isometric exercises
2. Isotonic exercises.

Isometric exercises are a type of strength training in which the joint angle and muscle length do not change during contraction. Isometrics are done in static positions, rather than being dynamic through a range of motion.

Isometric exercises involve a pushing or pulling motion that result in a tightening or contraction of a large muscle group without moving the joint. Normally, exercises involve joint movement that can be painful in the postoperative phase or immediately after an injury. However, the lack of joint movement during isometric exercises is a bonus, because it maintains muscle tone and strength without causing any discomfort.

Some of the common examples of isometric exercises are the following:

- Quadriceps setting exercises
- Hamstring setting exercises.

TABLE 30.1 Rehabilitation protocol after total knee arthroplasty[21,23,27]

Postoperative phase	*Weight-bearing status*	*Braces*	*Exercises*	*Activities*	*Restrictions*
Phase 1 (Day 0–6)	• Walker aided weight-bearing • Gait training with a walker	No brace	• Ankle toe movements • Isometric quads, hams and gulteals • Active SLR and short arcs • Dynamic quads in sitting • CPM if required	• Assisted toilet activities • Chair sitting for meals	• Unassisted walking • Forced knee flexion
Phase 2 (Day 7–21)	Elbow crutch/ single-stick-aided full weight-bearing (FWB)	No brace	• Short arcs • SLR • Active abduction • Dynamic quads • Heel slides • Balance training	• Supervised toilet activities • Chair sitting • Gait training • Stair climbing	Same as above
Phase 3 (Day 21–week 6)	Stick aided FWB	No brace	Active exercises as above gradually increasing difficulty levels	Independent functional and social recreational activities	Lotus position, kneeling and squatting
Phase 4 (Week 6 onward) Long term	Independent walking	No brace	• Stationary cycling • Exercises as above to continue	• Normal activities of daily living • Car driving • Swimming • Low-impact sports like golf to start after 3 months	Unaccustomed activities without appropriate training/practice

In an isotonic contraction, the muscle tension remains unchanged, while the muscle length changes. Lifting an object or moving a joint is an example of an isotonic contraction.[6-8,10]

There are two types of isotonic exercises:

1. Concentric exercises
2. Eccentric exercises.

Concentric Exercises

In a concentric contraction, the muscle tension rises to meet the resistance and then remains the same as the muscle shortens. This type is typical of most exercises. The external force on the muscle is less than the force that the muscle is generating. In other words, it is a muscle contraction in which muscle shortening occurs.

Eccentric Exercises[22]

In eccentric exercises, the muscle lengthens due to the resistance being greater than the force the muscle is producing. Eccentric training is the lowering phase of an exercise.

Some examples of isotonic exercises are as follows:

- Straight leg raises
- Heel slides
- Short arcs.

Exercises can also be classified as open kinetic chain and closed kinetic chain exercises.[11-14]

Open kinetic chain or open chain exercises are exercises in which the distal segment is free, for example, SLR, in which the distal segment of the leg (foot) is free and not in contact with any surface. In these exercises, the force applied by the body is sufficient to overcome the resistance. These exercises involve a single-joint and a single-muscle group. These are effective for strengthening and rehabilitation objectives. Open chain exercises often involve isolation movements that promote more shearing forces. Open chain exercises are postulated to be advantageous in rehabilitation settings because they can be easily manipulated to selectively target-specific

TABLE 30.2 Rehabilitation after anterior cruciate ligament reconstruction[25]

Postoperative phase	*Goals*	*Exercises*	*Activities/weight bearing*	*Restrictions/ precautions*	*Criteria for progression to next phase*
Phase 1 (Day 0–14)	• Protect graft function • Minimize effects of immobilization • Control inflammation	• Cryotherapy • Limb elevation • Ankle foot pumps • Isometric quads, hams and gluteals • Active abduction and SLR exercise	• Toilet activities • Bed to chair transfer • Partial weight-bearing (PWB) walking with a walker/2 elbow crutches • Independence in activities of daily living (ADLs)	Restricted flexion as per surgery—knee to be immobilized in a knee brace	• Good quads power 3+/5 • SLR without extension lag • Complete knee extension
Phase 2A (Day 15–21)	• Restore normal gait • Attempt to regain full ROM • Protect graft fixation • Improve strength, endurance and proprioception to prepare for functional activity	• Exercises as above to continue • Remove knee brace • Short arcs • Dynamic quadriceps in high sitting • Proprioceptive and balance training	• Stick-aided full weight-bearing (FWB) walking • Stair climbing	Restrict full squats	• Good quads control • AROM 0–90° • Independent normal gait
Phase 2B (Day 21–42)	• Restore normal gait • Restore full ROM • Protect graft fixation • Improve strength, endurance and proprioception to prepare for functional activity	• Theraband resisted strengthening exercises • Weight-bearing closed chain exercises • Exercise cycling • Treadmill walking • Leg press • Leg curls • Swimming	Normal ADLs and gymnasium exercises as advised for operated leg only	Restrict sporting activities	• Normal gait • Full ROM • Sufficient strength and proprioception as compare to contralateral limb • Stable graft on Lachman and KT-1000 **(Figure 30.6)** testing at 6 weeks
Phase 3 (Week 6–12)	• Improve confidence in the knee • Avoid overstressing graft fixation • Progress strength, power and proprioception to prepare for normal functional activities	• Increased resistance in all the above exercises • Advanced proprioception and balancing exercises	Normal ADLs and gymnasium exercises as above	Restrict sports	• Sufficient strength and proprioception to initiate functional activities • Stable graft on Lachman and KT-1000 testing • Physicians clearance to initiate advance CKC exercise and functional progression
Phase 4 (3–6 months)	Return to unrestricted activity	• Initiate plyometric training • Agility exercises • Gradually increase resistance training	• Continue proprioception and aerobic conditioning	Restrict sports	• No patellofemoral joint or soft tissue complain • All criteria met for return to sports • Physician clearance to resume full activity • Stable graft on Lachman and KT-1000 testing
Phase 5 6–9 months	• Maintenance of strength, endurance and proprioception • Patient education concerning any possible limitation	• Advance proprioception and balance training • Plyometric and agility training	• Isokinetic training • Start low level running • Progress to full speed at the end of 9 months	Start low impact sports	Same as phase 4 criteria
Phase 6 9 months onward	Safe return to athletics	Continue strengthening and flexibility programs	• Advance plyometric exercises • Isokinetic training	Gradually return to sports	

TABLE 30.3 Rehabilitation after medial patellofemoral ligament repair[25]

Postoperative phase	*Weight-bearing status*	*Bracing*	*Exercises*	*Activities*	*Restrictions*
Phase 1 (Day 0–Week 2)	Walker/B/L elbow crutch aided partial weight-bearing (PWB) walking	Knee brace locked in extension	• Cryotherapy • Active ankle toe movements • Isometrics for quads hams and gluteals	Toilet activities	• No knee flexion • Only partial weight-bearing as tolerated
Phase 2 (Week 3–6)	Same as in phase 1 gradually weaning off support	Knee brace locked in extension for walking	• Phase 1 exercises to continue • Side leg raises—start knee flexion in supine (Remove knee brace for exercises only)	Functional ADLs	• No straight leg raises • No antigravity knee extensions • No forced knee flexion, cross leg sitting and kneeling
Phase 3 (Week 7–12)	Independent unaided walking	Remove knee brace—wear a knee support with patellar cut-out	• Full ROM • Active stretching of all muscle groups • PRE and strength training • Stationary cycling	• Gym activities • Swimming	No forced knee flexion
Phase 4 (Week 13 onward)	Independent	Functional knee support for sports training	• Exercises as above to continue • Sports-specific exercises and isokinetic training to start at 16 weeks postoperative • Advanced plyometrics and agility training between 16 and 20 weeks	Gradual return to sports by the end of 24 weeks from surgery	• No unaccustomed activity without appropriate training • Knee support during contact sports

muscles, or specific heads of certain muscles, at different phases of contraction.

Some examples of open chain lower body exercises are:

- Leg extension
- Leg curl
- SLR
- Bench press.

Closed kinetic chain (CKC) or closed chain exercises are those exercises in which the distal segment is fixed in space and cannot move. In these exercises, the force applied is not sufficient to overcome the resistance. The extremity remains in constant contact with the immobile surface. These exercises usually involve multiple joints and muscle groups, making them more utilitarian and oriented toward athletic activities. Closed chain exercises are considered safer and more 'functional' compared to open chain exercises. In the lower extremity, they concentrate on a cocontraction of the quadriceps, hamstrings, hip flexors, gastrocnemius, and the soleus muscles.

Some examples of closed chain lower body exercises are:

- Squats
- Lunges
- Cycling
- Step-ups and step-downs.

Isometric Exercises

Quadriceps Setting Exercise[15]

Quads sets are common isometric exercises that help to strengthen the quadriceps muscles, which are the key protectors of the knee. Begin by sitting/lying on any firm

TABLE 30.4 Rehabilitation after poly ligament repair[26]

Postoperative phase	*Weight-bearing status*	*Bracing*	*Exercises*	*Activities*	*Restrictions*
Phase 1 (Day 0–Week 6)	Walker-aided non-weight-bearing (NWB) with knee brace locked in extension	Static knee brace with knee in extension	• Active ankle toe movements • Isometric quads, hams and gluteals	NWB independent toilet activities and other ADLs	• No weight-bearing • No knee flexion
Phase 2 (Week 6–12)	Stick aided FWB with dial Loc brace **(Figure 30.7)**	Dial Loc knee brace (0–45°) increasing ROM by 15° a week	• Exercises as in phase 1 to continue • SLR • AROM within dial Loc brace	• FWB walking • Independence in all ADLs	No forced movements/floor sitting
Phase 3 (3–6 months)	Independent unaided walking	Discontinue dial Loc brace	• Full knee ROM exercises • Theraband resisted PRE • CKC • Proprioception and balance training	Gradually get back to normal functional activities	Same as in phase 2
Phase 4 (6–9 months)	Normal		• Initiate plyometric training • Agility exercises • Isokinetic training	At the end of this phase the patient starts with low level sports activities	No contact sports
Phase 5 (9 months onward)	Normal	Functional knee support during contact sports	• Sports-specific training • Advanced plyometrics	Continue flexibility and strengthening exercises with an aim to gradually return to sports with functional knee support	

surface with legs outstretched in front. Contract or tighten the quadriceps muscle. The kneecap will move slightly. Hold for 5 seconds and then relax. Repeat 8–12 times.

Hamstring Tightening Exercise[15]

During this exercise, sit on a firm surface with the legs stretched out in front. Contract the muscles at the back of the knee simultaneously digging the heel into the ground as if trying to bend the knee. However, do not let the knee bend. Hold for 5 seconds and then relax. Repeat 8–12 times.

Open Chain Isotonic Exercises[13,15]

Straight Leg Raise

Lie down on a firm surface with both the knees stretched out. Gently lift one leg up toward the ceiling to around 45° and hold for 8–10 seconds. Repeat 10 times. Perform the same with the other leg. To increase the difficulty level, lower down the angle of hip flexion or use weights.

Short Arc Exercises

Lie down on a firm surface with both the knees stretched out. Place a bolster under one knee such that it is bent to around 45°. Lift up the leg toward the ceiling pulling the toes toward yourself and hold for 8–10 seconds. Repeat 10 times. Perform the same with the other leg. Increase the difficulty level by using weights.

Prone Knee Bending

Lie down in prone lying on a firm surface and bend one knee such that heel approximates the buttock. Hold for 8–10 seconds. Repeat 10 times. Perform the same

TABLE 30.5 Rehabilitation after posterior cruciate ligament repair[26]

Postoperative phase	*Weight-bearing status*	*Bracing*	*Exercises*	*Activities*	*Restrictions*
Phase 1 (Day 0–Week 6)	Walker-aided PWB with knee brace	Static knee brace with posterior tibial thrust	• Active ankle toe movements • Isometric quads, hams and gluteals	PWB independent toilet activities and other ADLs	• Only partial weight-bearing • No knee flexion
Phase 2 (Week 7–12)	Stick aided FWB with dial Loc brace	Dial Loc knee brace (0-45°) increasing ROM by 15° a week	• Exercises as in phase 1 to continue • SLR • AROM within dial Loc brace	• FWB walking • Independence in all ADLs	No forced movements/floor sitting
Phase 3 (4–6 months)	Independent unaided walking	Discontinue dial Loc brace	• Full knee ROM exercises • Theraband resisted PRE • CKC • Proprioception and balance training	Gradually get back to normal functional activities	Same as in phase 2
Phase 4 (7–9 months)	Normal		• Initiate plyometric training • Agility exercises • Isokinetic training	At the end of this phase the patient starts with low level sports activities	No contact sports
Phase 5 (9 months onward)	Normal	Functional knee support during contact sports	• Sports-specific training • Advanced plyometrics	Continue flexibility and strengthening exercises with an aim to gradually return to sports with functional knee support	

with the other leg. Increase the difficulty level by using weights.

Dynamic Quadriceps Exercises

In high sitting, extend the knees pulling up the toes toward the head. Hold for 8–10 seconds. Repeat 10 times. Perform the same with the other leg. Increase the difficulty level by using weights (**Figure 30.1**).

Closed Chain Isotonic Exercises[13,15]

Heel Slides

Lie down on a firm surface with both the knees stretched out. Slide one heel on the surface bringing the heel toward the buttock. Hold for 8–10 seconds. Repeat 10 times. Perform the same with the other leg. Increase the difficulty level by using weights.

Calf Raises

Stand against the wall and lift up the body toward the ceiling by raising the heels up and standing on the toes. Hold for 8–10 seconds and repeat for 10 times. Increase the difficulty level by using weights or increasing the hold time.

Wall Squats

Stand up with the back against a wall and feet about 24 inches away from the wall. Place a small exercise ball

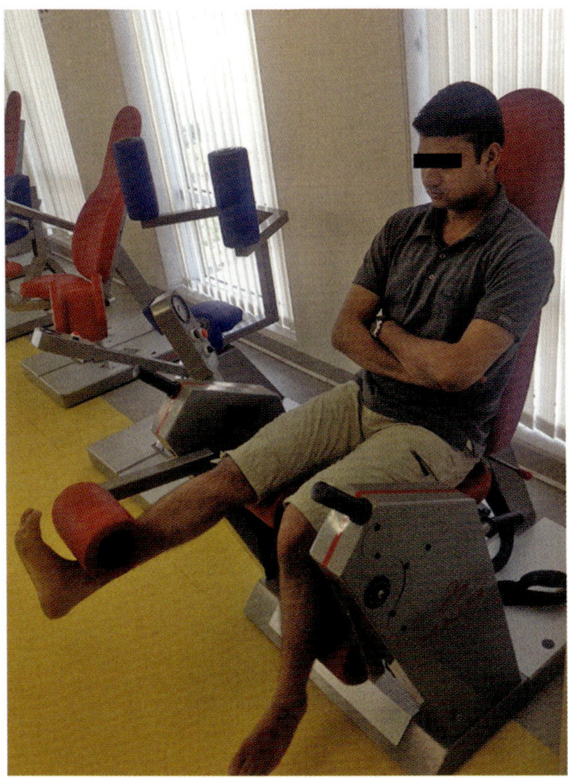

Figure 30.1 Leg extension

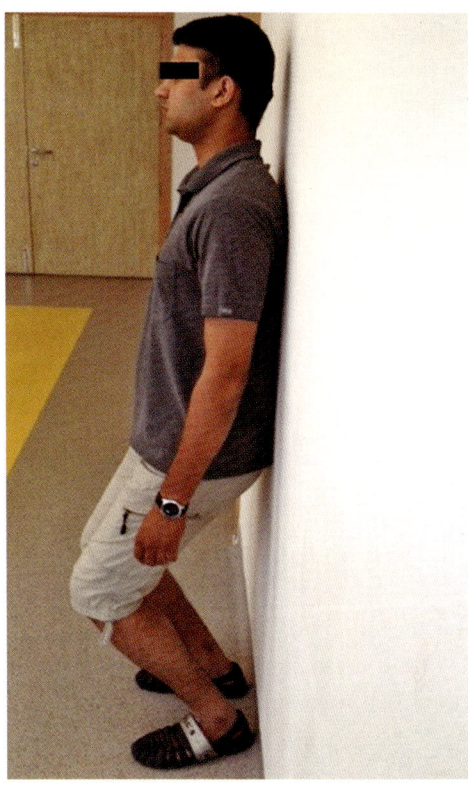

Figure 30.2 Wall squats

between both the knees to keep them stable. Push the heels down into the floor and lower down into a squat.

Mini squat: Knees should be flexed at about an angle of about 30° when in the squat position, do not let them cross the sagittal axis of your ankles.

Half squat: Knees should be bent to an angle of 90°.

Hold for 10–20 seconds and then return to a standing position. Relax for a minute and then repeat. Increase the hold time as the knees and heels become stronger (**Figure 30.2**).

Step-ups

With a stool of 4–6 inch height in front of you, place one leg on the step and then bearing the weight on the top leg, pull yourself up. Avoid pushing up with the other leg (the leg on the ground). Repeat 8–10 times.

Step-down

To perform the step-down exercise, start by standing on top of a step. From there, slowly step-down with one leg until the knee is bent at a 90° angle. Then take the other leg and place it on the ground, keeping the first leg bent. Once feet are on the ground, lift the first leg up off the ground without straightening it. Once completed, return to the step and repeat the exercise.

Cross-overs

Perform step-up and step-down in one go.

Lateral Step-ups

Stand on the side of a stool. Climb up the stool with the leg closer to it and then pull up the body, bearing the weight on the top leg. Do not push with the other leg. Repeat the same with the other leg.

Stretching Exercises[16]

Hamstring Stretching Exercise

During this exercise sit on a chair or on the bed with the back fully supported and legs stretched out in front of you (If you are sitting on a chair then rest your heels on a similar chair or on a stool of the same height.) Allow the knee to stretch out completely while pushing down with the patella. Repeat the same 8–12 times.

Quadriceps Stretches

While standing, bend one knee such that the heel approximates the buttock. Keeping the body straight, try to touch the heel to the buttock till a comfortable stretch is felt on the anterior thigh. Hold for 30–40 seconds. Repeat the same with the other leg.

Calf Stretches

Stand facing the wall with the toes of one foot fixed on the wall. Keep the other leg at a comfortable distance keeping the knee straight and foot fixed on the ground. Now, gently move the whole body forward keeping the back leg straight, till a gentle stretch is felt in the calf of the behind leg.

Knee Proprioception Exercises[5,18,19]

Balance Board

Stand on the balance board and shift the body weight front and back and side-to-side maintaining the body balance. To begin, start without weights using just the body weight. Progress to the exercise with medicine ball wherein the therapist throws the medicine ball toward the patient in different directions (up, down, left, and right) and the patient tries to catch it maintain the balance on the board. Gradually progress to the heavier medicine ball (**Figure 30.3**).

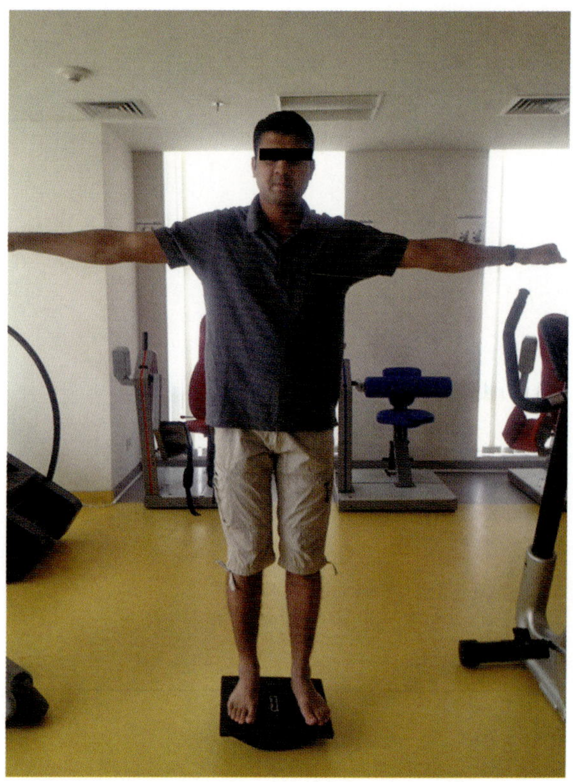

Figure 30.3 Double stance balancing

Tandem Walking

Make the patient walk on a straight line first with open eyes and then with closed eyes in a protected environment. Progress to walking with weights.

One-leg Balance

Stand straight on one-leg with the knee slightly bent. Bend the other knee to keep the foot off the ground. Make sure that hips remain in level, and hold the balance for 1 minute; then switch sides. To increase the difficulty of the exercise, close your eyes or stand on an uneven surface. Wobble board and trampoline balancing further increase the difficulty levels of this exercise (**Figure 30.4**).

One-leg Heel Raises

Stand on one leg and hold onto something for a better balance. Bend the other knee to keep the leg off the ground.

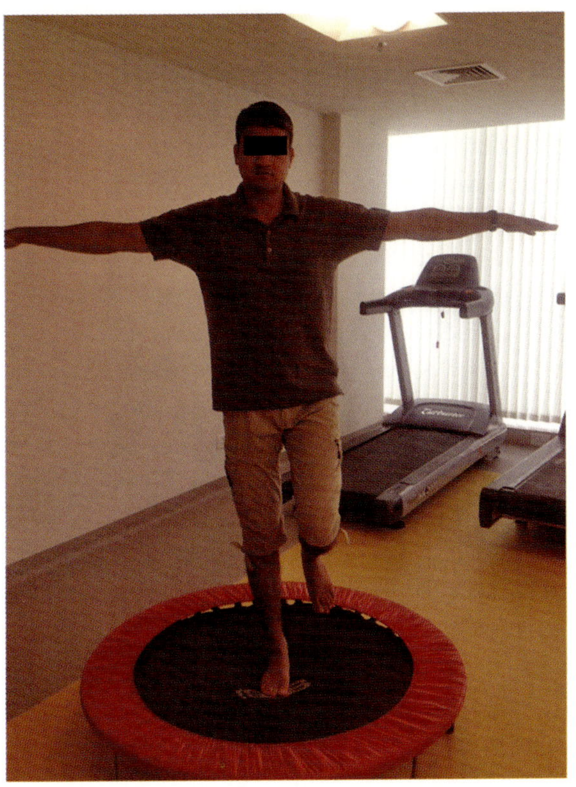

Figure 30.4 Single leg balancing—trampoline

Raise the body up as high on the fixed toes as possible, and then slowly sink back to the starting position. Immediately progress to another repetition. Perform 20 repetitions and then switch sides. To increase difficulty, do not hold onto anything, hold weights or close the eyes.

Progressive Resisted Exercises[5,19,20,23]

This is a strength training method in which the overload is constantly increased to facilitate adaptation. Progressive resistance is essential for building muscle and reaching goals. The body adapts to exercise and needs to be constantly challenged in order to continue to grow and change. There are many ways to achieve progressive resistance:

- Increase the weights. Do the same number of repetitions and sets each week, but increase the weights
- Increase the number of repetitions. Use the same weight for each workout, but increase the repetitions each week
- Increase the number of sets each time one works out

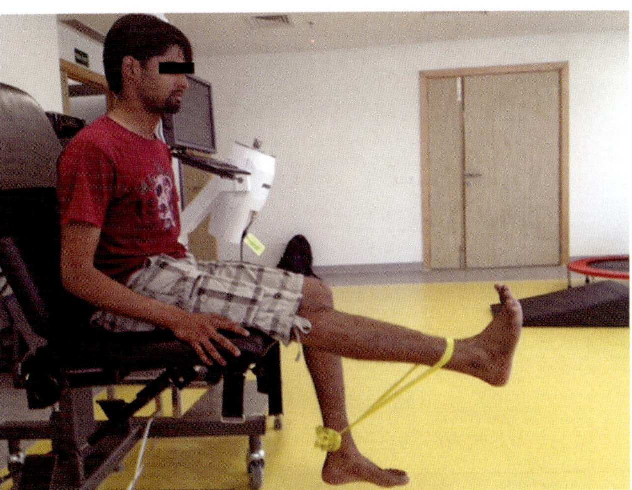

Figure 30.5 TheraBand-resisted leg extensions

- Lengthen the time under tension—or how long your muscle fibers are under stress. Use the same weight and repetitions, but slow down the exercise. For example, 1 count to lift the weight, 3 counts to lower the weight.

The health benefits associated with a progressive resisted exercise (PRE) make it a useful intervention in physical therapy. A reduced ability of muscles to generate force, due to injury, pathology, or disuse, is a common impairment in patients seen by physical therapists. If a lack of force generation by muscles is an impairment contributing to an inability to perform everyday activities, then this provides a rationale for physical therapists to apply the principles of PRE when designing treatment programs.

TheraBand Exercises[19]

TheraBands are useful tools that can be used as a part of any strengthening exercise program. They offer graded resistance when used in conjunction with normal open and closed chain isotonic exercises (**Figure 30.5**).

Agility Exercises[2,16]

Agility exercises are normally prescribed for high demand patients like sportsmen and athletes. Normally after any sports injury, to get back to competitive sports the athlete

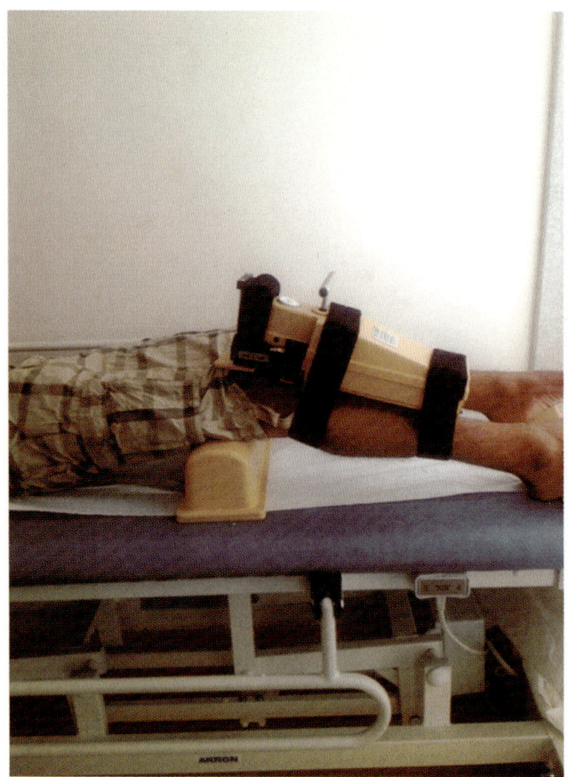

Figure 30.6 KT 1000

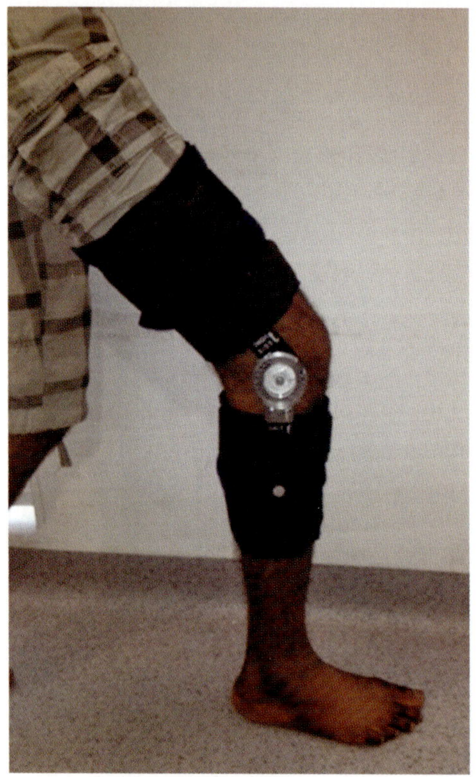

Figure 30.7 ROM knee brace

goes through an intensive rehabilitation program that starts at the basic level of isometric exercises and over a period of time advances to intense sports training by way of agility or plyometric exercises. They help to build dynamic power, co-ordination and balance thus becoming very useful in the eventual return of the individual to active sports. These exercises should only be performed after a thorough warm up.

Some examples of plyometric exercises are:

- *Lateral plyometric jumps*—the athlete has to jump sideways over hurdles
- *Shuttle runs*—these are short repeated sprints through two markers set about 25 m apart. They can be performed as side to side runs, forward-backward runs and forward-touch-return runs
- *Dot drills*—use a dot drill mat or place small 'X' marks with tape on the ground in the pattern of five on a dice. Begin with a warm up and jump from dot to dot with both feet at a time. Progress to one foot hopping and follow a specific jump pattern
- *Forward-backward sprints*—set-up two markers about 10 yards apart. After a good warm up, sprint forward from the first cone to the far cone. Stop at the far cone and run or jog backward to the start. Stop and quickly accelerate in a sprint back to the far cone
- *Stair running*—while not technically an agility drill, running stairs is a great way to develop quickness and foot speed while getting an excellent interval workout. Running stairs provides a cardiovascular benefit similar to that of running and is a great way to build sprint power. Many athletes are trained at a stadium of a local outdoor stair way with about a hundred steps.

Gym Exercises

- Stationary cycling progressing from free cycling to uphill training
- Treadmill walking progressing to running
- Quadriceps table
- Leg curl
- Leg press.

Practical Guidelines for Resistance Training[9,19,21,24]

- Warm up
- Adjust equipment
- Exercise large muscle groups first
- Legs or large muscles in the upper body
- Begin any resistive training program slowly and with lower intensities
- Ultimately, you must overload
- Strengthen weak side
- Working arms and legs independently
- Isolate the muscle group
- Protect the back
- Total body workout
- Should be done no more than 2–3 times per week
- May alternate days
- May alternate equipment to save time.

REFERENCES

1. Kapandji IA. The physiology of the joints. Vol. 2. 5th edn. Churchill Livingstone, Edinburgh, London, Melbourne, New York; 1987.
2. Maria Zuluaga, et al. Sports Physiotherapy Applied Sciences and Practice, 1st edn, Churchill Livingstone, Edinburgh, London, Melbourne, New York; 1992.
3. David J Magee. Orthopaedic Physical Assetment, 5th edn, Saunders Elsevier, New Delhi; 2008.
4. S Brent Brotzman, Kelvin E Wilk. Clinical Orthopaedic Rehabilitation. 2nd edn, Mosby, Philadelphia; 2003.
5. American College of Sports Medicine. Progression models in resistance training for healthy adults. Med Sci Sports Exerc. 2002;34:364-80.
6. Bubbico, Aaron, Kravitz, Len. Eccentric Training. Idea Fitness. 2010;7:10.
7. Lindstedt SL, LaStayo PC, Reich TE. When active muscles lengthen: properties and consequences of eccentric contractions. New Physiol Sci. 2001;16:256-61.
8. LaStayo PC, Woolf JM, Lewek MD, et al. Eccentric muscle contractions: their contribution to injury, prevention, rehabilitation, and sport. J Orthop Sports Phys Ther. 2003;33(10):557-71.
9. Mayhew TP, Rothstein JM. Measurement of muscle performance with instruments. In: Rothstein JM (Ed.), Measurement in Physical Therapy. New York, NY: Churchill Livingstone Inc.; 1985:ch 3.
10. Bahr R, Fossan B, Loken S, Engebretsen L. Surgical treatment compared with eccentric training for patellar tendinopathy (jumpers knee) a randomized controlled trial. J Bone Joint Surg. 2006;88(8):1689-98.
11. Fitzgerald GK. Open versus closed kinetic chain exercise: issues in rehabilitation after anterior cruciate ligament reconstructive surgery. Phys Ther. 1997;77(12):1747-54.
12. Graham VL, Gehlsen GM, Edwards JA. Electromyographic evaluation of closed and open kinetic chain knee rehabilitation exercises. J Athl Train. 1993;28(1):23-30.
13. Blackburn JR, Morrissey MC. The relationship between open and closed kinetic chain strength of the lower limb and jumping performance. J Orthop Sports Phys Ther. 1998;27(6):430-5.
14. Prokopy MP, Ingersoll CD, Nordenschild E, et al. Closed-kinetic chain upper-body training improves throwing performance of NCAA Division I softball players. J Strength Cond Res. 2008;22(6):1790-8.
15. Robert A Donatelli, Michael J Wooden. Orthopaedic Physical Therapy, 3rd edn, Churchill Livingstone, A Harcourt Health Science Company, New York, Edinburgh, London, Philadelphia; 2001.
16. M Dena Gardiner, Principles of Exercise Therapy, 4th edn, CBS Publishers & Distributors, New Delhi, Bengaluru, Chennai, Kochi, Pune; 2007.
17. Seto JL, Brewster CE. Treatment approaches following foot and ankle injury. Clin Sports Med. 1994;13(4):695-718.
18. Winnett RA, Carpinelli RN. Potential health-related benefits of resistance training. Prev Med. 2001;33:503-13.
19. Kraemer WJ, Ratamess NA, French DN. Resistance training for health and performance. Curr Sports Med Rep. 2002;1:165-71.
20. Srinivas M, Srikanth BV, Raviendra KB, Jalaja P. A comparative study of proprioceptive exercises versus conventional training program on osteoarthritis of knee. Res J Recent Sci. 2012;1(12):31-35.
21. Smith TO, King JJ, Hing CB. The effectiveness of proprioceptive-based exercise for osteoarthritis of the

knee: a systematic review and meta-analysis. Rheumatol Int. 2012;32(11):3339-51.

22. Todd E, George D. Closed kinetic chain exercise: a comprehensive guide to multiple joint exercises. J Chiropr Med. 2001;2(2):78.
23. Miller JP, Croce RV. Analysis of isokinetic and closed chain movements for hamstring reciprocal coactivation. J Sport Rehabil. 2007;16:319-25.
24. Jette AM, Delitto A. Physical therapy treatment choices for musculoskeletal impairments. Phys Ther. 1997;77:145-54.
25. Romeyn RL, Jennings J, Davies GJ. Surgical treatment and rehabilitation of combined complex ligament injuries. North Am J Sports Phys Ther. 2008;3(4):212-25.
26. OSU sports medicine, Multiple ligament knee injuries combined ACL and PCL repair rehabilitation guidelines.
27. Myer GD, Paterno MV, Ford KR, Quatman CE, Hewett TE. Progression through the return-to-sport-phase. J Orthop Sports Phys Ther. 2006;36(2):385-402.

SECTION 2

Arthroscopy and Sports Injuries of the Knee

Chapter 31

Knee Anatomy

Vivek Pandey, Saumitra Goyal, P Sripathi Rao

The femoral condyles and the tibial plateaus are not inherently stable in their relationship. The knee joint depends on the static and dynamic soft tissue forces to enhance its stability. Owing to the various axes of movement in the joint, the knee is susceptible to complex stresses. Injuries to the knee are more often combined ligament–meniscus disruptions than isolated events. For the interpretation of common problems around the knee, the physician needs to have a reasonable knowledge of anatomy. Diagnosis and management of such injuries and other pathologies demand a thorough knowledge of the anatomy of the joint and its surroundings. The aim of this chapter is to provide readers with comprehensive details of anatomy of the knee with pertinent surgically important details with sufficient illustrations.

BONY ARCHITECTURE

Patella

It is the largest sesamoid bone of the body developed in the quadriceps muscle. It articulates against the anterior articular surface of the distal femur forming the patellofemoral articulation. Asymmetrically oval in shape with a distal apex, its superior border provides insertion to the tendinous fibers of rectus femoris and vastus intermedius, whereas the medial and lateral borders provide attachment to vastus medialis and vastus lateralis. The medial and lateral borders converge distally and form distal pole that provides attachment to the patellar tendon. Posteriorly, it is covered with 6.5 mm thick hyaline cartilage that is the thickest in the body. The anterior surface is slightly convex in all directions. The anterior surface has three parts: the rough superior third receives the insertion of the quadriceps tendon. The superficial portion of this tendon continues over the anterior surface and is densely adhered to the bone. The middle third reveals numerous vascular orifices and is crossed by numerous vertical striations giving a bristled appearance as seen on the axial radiograph. The inferior third ends in a V-shaped point, which provides attachment to the patellar tendon. The posterior part of the patella is divided into seven facets (**Figures 31.1A and B**). Grossly, a vertical (median) ridge divides it into the medial and lateral facets. The lateral facet is two-thirds, and the medial one is one-third of the patella. The medial facet is slightly convex, whereas

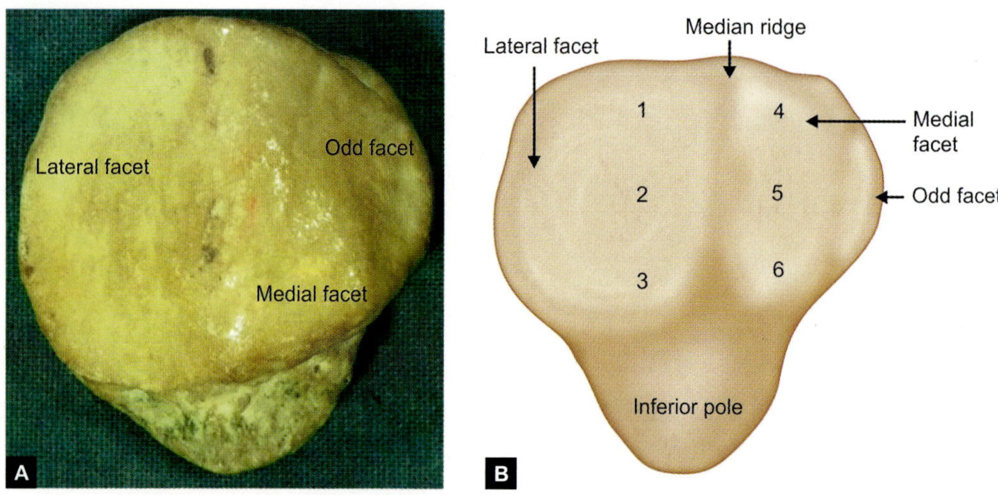

Figures 31.1A and B Articular surface of the left patella (A) divided into facets. Diagrammatic description of facets on the articular side (B)

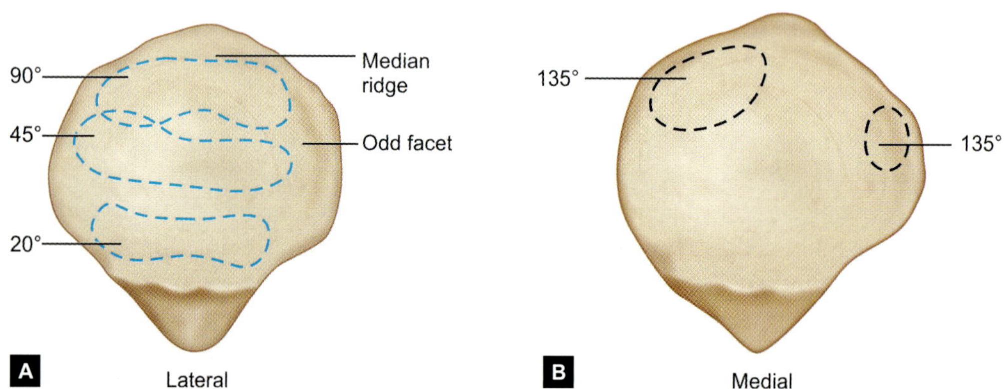

Figures 31.2A and B Patellofemoral contact area at different degrees of flexion

the lateral one possesses sagittal convexity and coronal concavity. Vertically, both medial and lateral facets are roughly divided into equal thirds. The medial-most part of the medial facet is known as the odd facet.

Posterior part of the patella articulates with femoral trochlea that is separated from the medial and lateral femoral condyle by two ridges, medial and lateral. The medial ridge is less distinct than lateral. The patella glides within the trochlear groove in various degrees of knee flexion. The area of contact between the patella and trochlea has been investigated using casting and dye techniques. It varies in various degrees of flexion but never more than one-third of the patellar surface area[1] (**Figures 31.2A and B**). It moves proximally with increasing flexion.[1]

The main function of patella is to increase the lever arm of the quadriceps mechanism. As the knee flexion increases, it increases the load across the patellofemoral joint. However, the area of contact also increases with increasing flexion dissipating the forces over larger area.[2]

Femur

The distal end of the femur is formed by two condyles, medial and lateral. These condyles are asymmetrical and provide attachment to various tendons and ligaments. All surfaces of the condyles are articular except the sides. The medial condyle is bigger and has a more symmetrical curvature. The lateral femoral condyle has an increasing radius of curvature posteriorly. The lateral femoral condyle projects more anteriorly whereas the medial femoral condyle projects more distally. The inferior and posterior surfaces of both condyles articulate with the tibial plateau, whereas the anterior and trochlea surfaces articulate with the patella. Anteriorly, two condyles are separated by a trochlear groove. This complex anatomy should be restored in the distal femoral fractures.

The intercondylar notch is situated between two condyles inferiorly that is home for cruciate ligament. The medial wall of the lateral femoral condyle provides an attachment to the anterior cruciate ligament (ACL), whereas the lateral wall of the medial femoral condyle houses the posterior cruciate ligament (PCL). The mean width of the notch is widest proximally and narrows distally (1.8–2.3 cm). The height of the notch is maximum in the middle (2.4 cm), whereas it decreases proximally (1.3 cm) and distally (1.8 cm).[3] The dimensions of the notch is an area of interest for all knee surgeons as the risk of ACL tear is high in people with narrow notch. It may be due to impingement by the narrow notch over the ACL.[4,5] Notch is especially narrow in the chronic ACL tear where the surgeon might have to perform notchplasty before the ACL reconstruction.

The medial wall of the lateral femoral condyle has two distinct ridges, the lateral intercondylar ridge (LIR) and bifurcate ridge[6] (**Figure 31.3**). The LIR that is also known as resident's ridge marks the anterior end of ACL insertion. It runs proximal to distal. The bifurcate ridge runs anteroposteriorly and marks the division of ACL bundles. The posterolateral (PL) bundle is in front of the bifurcate ridge whereas the anteromedial (AM) bundle of the ACL is behind the bifurcate ridge. The lateral aspect of the lateral condyle has a lateral epicondyle that provides attachment to the lateral collateral ligament (LCL). Just below and anterior to the lateral epicondyle is a shallow groove in which the popliteus tendon is attached. On the medial surface of the medial femoral condyle, the medial epicondyle is a C-shaped ridge with a central depression. The medial collateral ligament originates from the sulcus. Adductor tubercle is superior and posterior to the medial epicondyle and provides attachment to the adductor magnus tendon. The line joining the two epicondyles (most prominent part of lateral epicondyle and sulcus region of

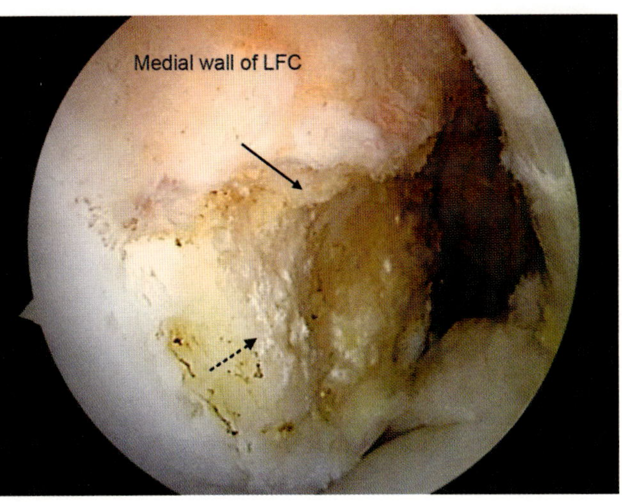

Figure 31.3 Arthroscopic image of the medial wall of the lateral femoral condyle (LFC) (right knee in 90° flexion) showing lateral intercondylar ridge (black arrow-continuous) and bifurcate ridge (black arrow-interrupted)

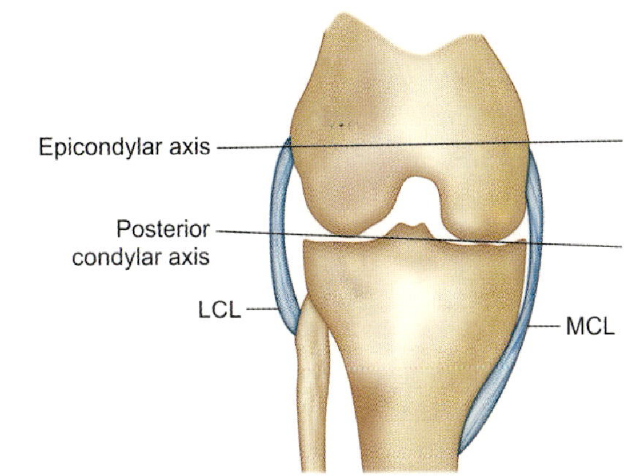

Figure 31.4 Diagrammatic representation of the knee showing epicondylar and posterior condylar axis
Abbreviations: LCL, lateral collateral ligament; MCL, medial collateral lilgament

medial epicondyle) is referred to as the epicondylar axis. This axis is rotated externally with reference to the posterior condylar axis (**Figure 31.4**). It is an important referencing axis for total knee replacement. In relation to the posterior condylar axis, the epicondylar axis is 3.5° and 1° externally rotated in males and females respectively.[7] It can be as high as 10° in patients with valgus knee and osteoarthritis.[8] The lateral surface of medial femoral condyle houses the PCL and meniscofemoral ligaments (MFLs).

There is definite difference in the morphology of the condyles in males and females of different racial groups. The mediolateral width of condyles for any given anteroposterior width (aspect ratio) is less in females with respect to males in both Asian and Caucasian races.[9-11] This racial and sexual dimorphism is now being taken into consideration while developing newer prosthesis for total knee replacement (gender specific components). However, it is still unclear whether the universal prosthesis can adversely affect the outcome when used in different races or sex.

Tibia

The upper end of the tibia flares out into two distinct condyles, medial and lateral. The upper surface of condyle is known as plateau that is covered by thick hyaline cartilage. The tibia plateau slopes posteriorly, generally varying from 5° to 10° from the intramedullary canal (**Figure 31.5**). The medial tibial plateau is nearly flat or slightly concave with a squared-off posterior edge. The lateral tibial plateau is slightly convex with posterior edge having 10° posterior inclination with respect to the shaft of tibia. The gender and race do affect the morphology of proximal tibia too.[11,12] Rims of these plateaus are in contact with menisci but central portions receive condyles of femur. The median portion of the tibia between the two plateaus is known as intercondylar eminence with medial and lateral tibial spines (**Figure 31.6**). Contrary to the popular belief, tibial spines do not provide attachment to the ACL or menisci but may act as side-to-side stabilizers for femoral condyles. The area in front of the spines is slightly depressed and houses the anterior horn of medial meniscus, ACL and anterior horn of lateral meniscus, anterior to posterior. Behind the spines, posterior intercondylar groove separates the two plateaus. It provides attachment to the posterior horn of lateral meniscus and medial meniscus, anterior to posterior. PCL originates from posterior intercondylar area 1 cm below the joint line and about 8-9 mm lateral to medial tibial spine.[13] Anteriorly, two condyles merge into a vascular triangular area that leads onto the tibial tuberosity. Tibial tuberosity provides attachment to the patellar tendon. The anterolateral aspect of the lateral tibial condyle has a prominence known as Gerdy's tubercle that provides attachment to Iliotibial band (ITB). On the posteroinferior aspect of the lateral condyle, there is a small circular facet that provides articulation with the head of fibula. The medial surface of medial condyle gives attachment to medial collateral ligament. The posterior surface of medial condyle has a small groove that gives attachment to insertion of semimembranosus muscle.

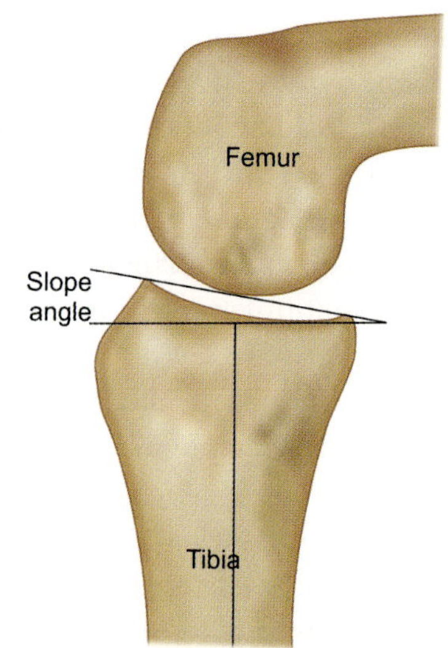

Figure 31.5 Diagrammatic illustration of posterior slope of tibia

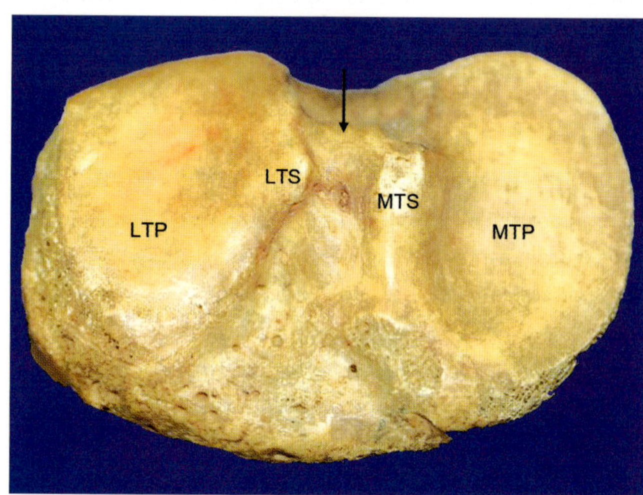

Figure 31.6 Upper surface of the tibia showing two tibial condylar surfaces (plateau) with tibial spines in between the plateau. Black arrow pointing toward the retrocondylar ridge (McGuire's ridge)
Abbreviations: MTP, medial tibial plateau; LTP, lateral tibial plateau; LTS, lateral tibial spine; MTS, medial tibial spine

Tibiofibular Joint

During the fetal development, both tibia and fibula are in contact with the femur. However the growth of tibia is faster than fibula, so fibula forms a separate tibiofibular joint but retains the original capsule. The capsule is further strengthened by accessory anterior and posterior ligaments. The articular surface of fibula is directed superolaterally to articulate with posteroinferior facet of tibia on lateral condyle. The superior tibiofibular joint (STF) is a plane synovial joint (inferior is a syndesmosis) with slight movement. The styloid process projects superiorly from the PL aspect of the fibular head. It is an attachment site for the LCL, biceps femoris tendon, arcuate ligament and fabellofibular ligament.

The anterior aspect of the STF joint gives rise to tibialis anterior, extensor hallucis and extensor digitorum muscles whereas the posterior aspect gives rise to soleus. There is a small opening in the interosseous membrane, two fingerbreadth below the STF joint, through which the anterior tibial artery enters the anterior compartment of the leg. It is endangered during any procedures around the STF joint or proximal metaphysiodiaphyseal fractures.

HYALINE CARTILAGE

It is a complex connective tissue that can withstand tremendous force over several cycles. It is composed of hydrated proteoglycans interspersed within collagen fibrils. Proteoglycans are complex glycoproteins with a central protein core to which glycosaminoglycan are attached. It is divided into several zones. The deepest layer closest to the subchondral bone is the layer of calcified cartilage followed by tidemark or zone of calcification (**Figure 31.7**). Beyond this region, the chondrocytes are in abundance but their density decreases toward the superficial surface of cartilage. Being avascular, superficial chondrocytes derive their nutrition synovial fluid and deeper ones from subchondral bone. Hyaline cartilage is prone to damage termed as chondromalacia. Outerbridge[14] classified changes in the cartilage appearance based upon arthroscopic findings: grade 0 is normal, white and firm; grade I is softening in consistency while external appearance is normal; grade II represents fissures/fibrillation in an area < 1/2 inch; grade III marks fissures/fibrillation > 1/2 inch; and grade IV represents loss of cartilage up to subchondral bone. Chondromalacia in early stages is difficult to diagnose with the help of magnetic resonance imaging. Hyaline cartilage also suffers damage due to pathological changes occurring in the subchondral bone where in it can result in osteonecrosis or osteochondritis dissecans.

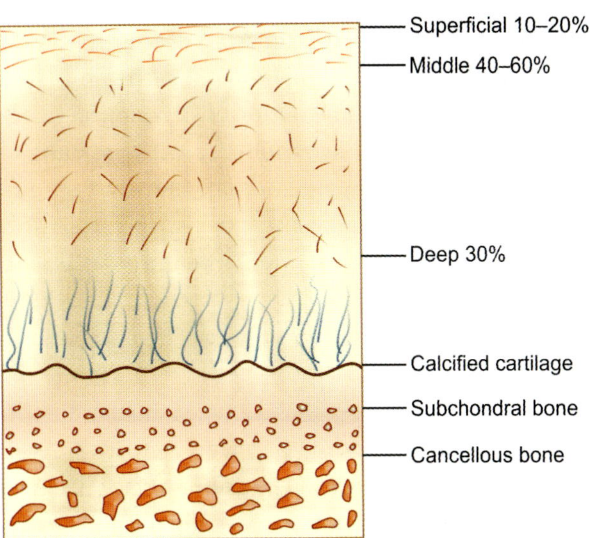

Figure 31.7 Diagrammatic representation of the histological appearance of normal hyaline cartilage

CRUCIATE LIGAMENTS

These are originally referred to as crucial ligaments because of the cruciate or crossed arrangement of both the ligaments in the knee. Cruciate ligaments are intra-articular but extrasynovial ligaments. They are named anterior and posterior based on their relationship to the intercondylar eminence of the tibia. Cruciate ligaments provide anteroposterior stability to the knee. Numerous sensory fibers are present in the cruciate ligament providing proprioceptive function. Neural innervation to cruciate ligaments comes from the posterior articular branch of the tibial nerve.[15] These nerves penetrate posterior capsule and run along periligamentous vessels. A small number of fibers with mechanoreceptor function (slowly adapting Ruffini type and fast adapting Pacinian corpuscles) is also observed in the substance of cruciates.[16,17] Both the ACL and PCL have slow conducting pain fibers.[18] The vascularity to the cruciate ligament does not arrive from subchondral bone.[19] It is mostly derived from the middle genicular artery and minor contribution comes from lateral inferior genicular arteries.[20,21] The presence of ample vascularity in the ACL and proprioceptive fibers in the ACL has prompted surgeons to retain the tibial stump or a remnant bundle while ACL reconstruction so that this may help in quick vascularization of the ACL graft and may help in better proprioception through remnant bundle.[22-24]

Ultrastructure

It mostly consists of type I collagen fibers (90%) and remainder is type III (10%). It is inserted into the bone via a fibrocartilaginous enthesis. This is divided into four zones. Zone 1 represents the end of the ACL fibers, zone 2 represents the ACL intermeshing with fibrocartilage, and zone 3 shows progressive mineralization of fibrocartilage that ends up merging with bone of zone 4.

Anterior Cruciate Ligament

It originates from a rough, nonarticular area in front of the intercondylar eminence, lateral to the medial tibial spine extending a little below the transverse meniscal ligament and fanning a slip to anterior horn of the lateral meniscus. It extends upwards and laterally to be inserted onto the medial surface of the lateral femoral condyle. In extension, attachment on the lateral femoral condyle takes an oval shape or segment of a circle. The anterior margin of attachment is straight whereas the posterior side is convex. The tibial attachment is stronger than femoral. The average length and width of the ACL is 38 mm (range: 22–41 mm) and 11 mm (range: 7–12 mm) respectively.[16,25] The maximal tensile strength of the ACL is 1725 ± 270 N, which is less than the peak force occurring in the athletic activities.

In the last two decades, there has been tremendous research in the area of ACL anatomy and function. From gross appearance of a single cord like structure, many authors have confirmed that it is composed of two or three or more distinct bundles with a specific function of each. However, it is now widely accepted that the ACL has two functional bundles: the AM and PL bundle.[15,16,26-28] These two bundles are defined by their insertion on tibia. However, controversy still exists about the anatomical division of bundles. On histological examination by Odensten et al., there was no evidence of separate bundles.[29]

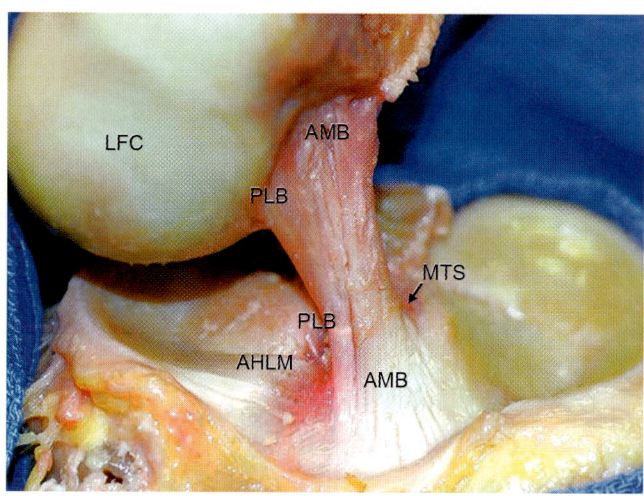

Figure 31.8 Anatomic image of the right knee showing the orientation of anterior cruciate ligament

Abbreviations: LFC, lateral femoral condyle; AMB, anteromedial bundle; PLB, posterolateral bundle; AHLM, anterior horn of Lateral Meniscus; MTS, medial tibial spine

a. *Femoral insertion:* The two bundles of the ACL originate posterior to the lateral intercondylar ridge (resident's ridge). In an extended knee, this ridge runs from proximosuperior to distal-inferior direction along the ACL fibers (**Figure 31.3**). This landmark, resident's ridge, which was described by William Clancy Jr is of surgical importance as none of the ACL fibers are attached anterior to it. The AM bundle originates from proximal part of the lateral femoral condyle and inserted upon the AM part of tibial insertion. The PL bundle originates distally and inserts in the PL aspect of tibial insertion (**Figure 31.8**). The shape of the femoral attachment is described as either oval [29] or as a segment of a circle.[27] The location of the two bundles on femoral condyle changes with flexion and extension of the knee. Posterolateral bundle (PLB) is posterior (deep) and inferior in extension whereas it is more shallow (anterior) and inferior in flexion.

   Area of ACL attachment at femoral site: Various authors report a varying area of attachment due to different dissection techniques of synovium preservation or excision. With synovium covering preserved, Odensten and Harner reported area of the ACL attachment as 155 mm^2 and 113 ± 27 mm^2 respectively.[29,30] After complete removal of synovium, Mochizuki and Seibold reported 65 mm^2 and 83 ± 19 mm^2 respectively.[31,32]

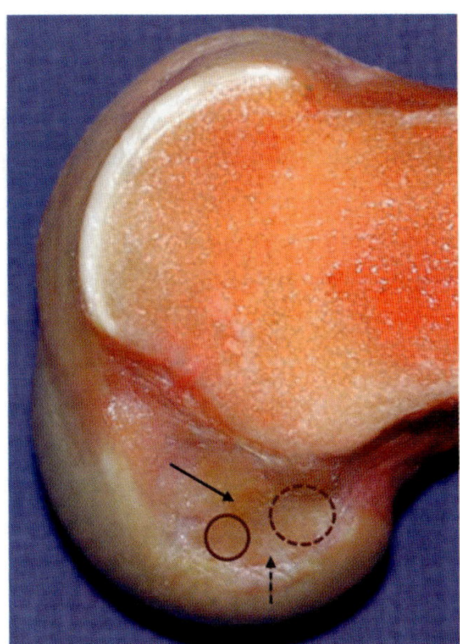

Figure 31.9 Anatomic image of cadaveric dissected right knee showing the attachment areas of anteromedial bundle (interrupted circle) and posterolateral bundle (continuous circle) of ACL over the medial wall of lateral femoral condyle. The two black arrows point toward lateral intercondylar (continuous arrow) and bifurcate (interrupted arrow) ridges. Note: the area represented by the circle is not the true footprint area of the bundles

Osseous landmark of two bundles: The two bundles lie posterior to the LIR. The area posterior and inferior to this ridge houses the two bundles of ACL. The area below the LIR is further divided by a vertical ridge that runs inferior toward the cartilage known as the bifurcate ridge.[6] The PLB is anterior to the bifurcate ridge whereas the anterolateral bundle (ALB) is posterior to the bifurcate ridge. Harner and Seibold confirmed that the two bundles share equal area, front and behind of the bifurcate ridge whereas Mokizuki could not confirm it.[31-33] He observed that AMB has 1.5 times larger area than PLB (**Figure 31.9**).

b. *Tibial insertion:* Contrary to the popular belief, the ACL does not attach onto the tibial spines.[34] It attaches anterolateral to the medial tibial spine in the anterior intercondylar fossa. Anteriorly, certain fibers passing beneath the transverse meniscal ligament and laterally certain fibers merge with the anterior horn of lateral meniscus. The tibial insertion site is 120% larger than the femoral footprint and is triangular or oval in shape.[30] It has a diameter of approximately 11 mm (range: 9–13 mm) in the frontal plane and 17 mm (range: 14–20 mm) in the sagittal plane.[20,29,30,35] The AMB occupies a slightly larger area than the PLB. Distance between the two centers of AMB and PLB is about 8 mm. The area of tibial insertion may vary from 114 ± 36 to 136 ± 33 mm^2.[32,33] AMB and PLB are named according to their attachment onto the tibia. AMB is anterior and medial whereas PLB is slightly posterior and lateral to AMB.

Identification of the center of ACL and center of two bundles is vital in single and double bundle anatomic ACL reconstruction. Currently, single bundle anatomic ACL reconstruction is the most popular technique. Kato et al. concluded on a porcine model that mid-mid reconstruction most closely restores knee kinematics and provides the most stable joint among all single bundle reconstruction.[36] It means that the tibial and femoral tunnels are placed at the center of tibial and femoral footprints incorporating the footprints of both AM and PL bundle, albeit partially. Various authors have used different landmarks to identify the center of the ACL on tibia and femur.

Techniques to identify anatomic center of ACL on tibial footprint: Accurate placement of femoral footprint can be established using several methods.

- 7 mm anterior to the PCL
- The posterior border of anterior horn of lateral meniscus
- Just lateral to medial tibial spine.

McGuire's 'over the back ridge' Morgan et al. suggested that the center of ACL is 7 mm anterior to PCL whereas Zantop et al. contradicted it.[37,38] According to Zantop, 7 mm anterior to PCL belongs to the center of PLB. Colombet et al. also suggested that if PCL is used as landmark, we may end up placing the tibial tunnel too far posteriorly.[39] Zantop also suggested that the posterior border of anterior horn of lateral meniscus corroborates with the center of AMB.[38] Medial tibial spine is another landmark that is helpful in establishing the center of ACL. Edwards et al. stated that the center of PLB and AMB is 4 ± 1 and 5 ± 1 mm lateral to medial tibial spine respectively.[35] McGuire described presence of 'over the back ridge' (OTB) behind the two spines at the end of posterior tibial slope that can be taken as reference point.[40] The same ridge was mentioned as 'Retroeminence ridge' by Colombet et al.[39] This ridge is quite consistent. The center of AMB and PLB is approximately 17 ± 2 mm and 10 ± 1 mm anteriorly respectively from the OTB ridge. However, identification of this ridge arthroscopically may not be easy. Use of fluoroscopy is quite accurate in identifying the center of the footprint of ACL on tibia that is at 43% of the 'Amis-Jacob line.'

Currently, the center of tibial attachment is taken just lateral to medial tibial spine in the line of the posterior border of the anterior horn of lateral meniscus.

Techniques to identify anatomic center of ACL on femoral footprint: Accurate placement of the femoral footprint can be established using several methods.

- Ruler method
- Bernard-Hertel quadrant method
- Ridge method
- Fluoroscopic method.

In the ruler method that is popularized by Charley Brown and Tim Spalding, the midpoint of the anteroposterior (shallow-deep in 90° flexion of knee) length of the femoral wall that is measured below the intercondylar ridge is considered as close to the femoral ACL center of footprint.[41,42] The high-low position of the ACL center is selected at the midpoint of the bifurcate ridge. Bernard et al. devised a quadrant method using fluoroscopy to identify the center of the footprint of ACL on the femur.[43] Fluoroscopy is considered as most accurate method to identify the center of ACL footprint in both femur and tibia.[44,45] Another way to place ACL femoral tunnel accurately is by identifying the LIR and bifurcate ridge. However, they may not be present in all cases, especially the bifurcate ridge.

Spatial orientation of two bundles: In an extended knee, both bundles remain parallel to each other with PLB tight and AMB moderately lax. In flexion, the femoral attachment site becomes horizontal with the AMB becoming tight and PLB lax. During the movement of the knee, the behavior of the ACL remains nonisometric with varying tension in both bundles.

Function of ACL

The ACL is a primary restraint to anterior translation of tibia over femur. The AMB remains primary anterior restraint in 90° flexion, whereas the PLB remains restraint in extension exhibiting reciprocal relationship.[25] Sakane also confirmed using robotic studies that the PLB carries more load in extension and AMB carries more load beyond a 45° flexion.[46] Consequently, an isolated rupture of AMB will have more effect on the anterior drawer (performed at 90° flexion), and failure of PLB will have more effect on the Lachman test (performed at 15°–20° flexion). The PLB also plays role in resisting internal and external rotation. The current technique of single bundle anatomic ACL reconstruction emphasizes on placement of the femoral tunnel more horizontally in order to replicate the PLB to control rotations more effectively. The single bundle transtibial ACL reconstruction technique is under heavy criticism as it places femoral tunnel too vertical, consequently only reconstructing the AMB. This can control anterior translation effectively but has lesser impact on rotational stability. Also, better understanding of anatomy, biology and function of individual bundles has led to the development of the concept of 'Augmentation' of ACL. In this, isolated bundles (AMB/PLB), which are ruptured, are reconstructed, whereas the normal bundle is spared.

Posterior Cruciate Ligament

The PCL is the primary restraint to the posterior drawer contributing approximately 90% of the resistance along the flexion arc.[47] It is a very strong ligament with tensile loads reported in range of 739–1627 N.[48,49] Its strength is derived from a broad cross-sectional area and broad footprint over femur and tibia. It is a 32–38 mm long ligament whose diameter is 1.5 times more than the ACL and footprint 3 times larger than that of diameter.[27,33,50] To mimic this anatomic dumbbell shape of ligament is difficult and this makes the PCL reconstruction difficult.

The PCL is functionally divided into AL and PM bundles based upon femoral and tibial insertion.[27] AL bundle tightens in flexion whereas the PM bundle tightens in extension. Harner et al. demonstrated that the AL bundle possesses superior structural properties than the PM bundle.[50] The AL bundle is 2.1 times stiffer than the PM bundle and possesses 2.7 times ultimate strength as compared with PM bundle. Hence, the current surgical recommendation for single bundle PCL reconstruction is to reconstruct the AL bundle. Also, the AL bundle tightens in knee flexion that is more important for PCL function. But this bundle description of PCL is oversimplification. Makris et al. dissected 24 pairs of knee and proposed that the PCL region is divided into four anatomic and functional fiber regions (anterior, central, posterior-longitudinal and posterior-oblique) whose tensioning and relaxing patterns are different in varying position of the knee.[51] In a study on 12 cadaveric knees, Hatshushika et al. found an interesting topographical correlation between the tibial and femoral attachments.[52] Femoral fibers followed high and low configuration but tibial footprint followed a parabolic or transverse type of attachment. This complex anatomy of the PCL renders PCL reconstruction difficult with current techniques by merely placing tubular/flat graft with circular tunnels.

The tibial footprint of PCL is located between the posterior horns of two menisci about 1–1.5 cm below posterior tibial margin in the 'PCL facet'. The ALB arises from the superior part of facet above the shelf and posteromedial bundle (PMB) arises below the shelf. The lowermost fibers of the PLB merge with tibial periosteum and posterior tibial capsule. The ALB and PLB fibers further extend upwards and medially to be attached onto the medial femoral condyle. The ALB is attached mostly to the roof of the intercondylar notch and PLB to the medial side of the wall (**Figures 31.10A to D**). This division of fibers is based upon the tensioning pattern in flexion-extension

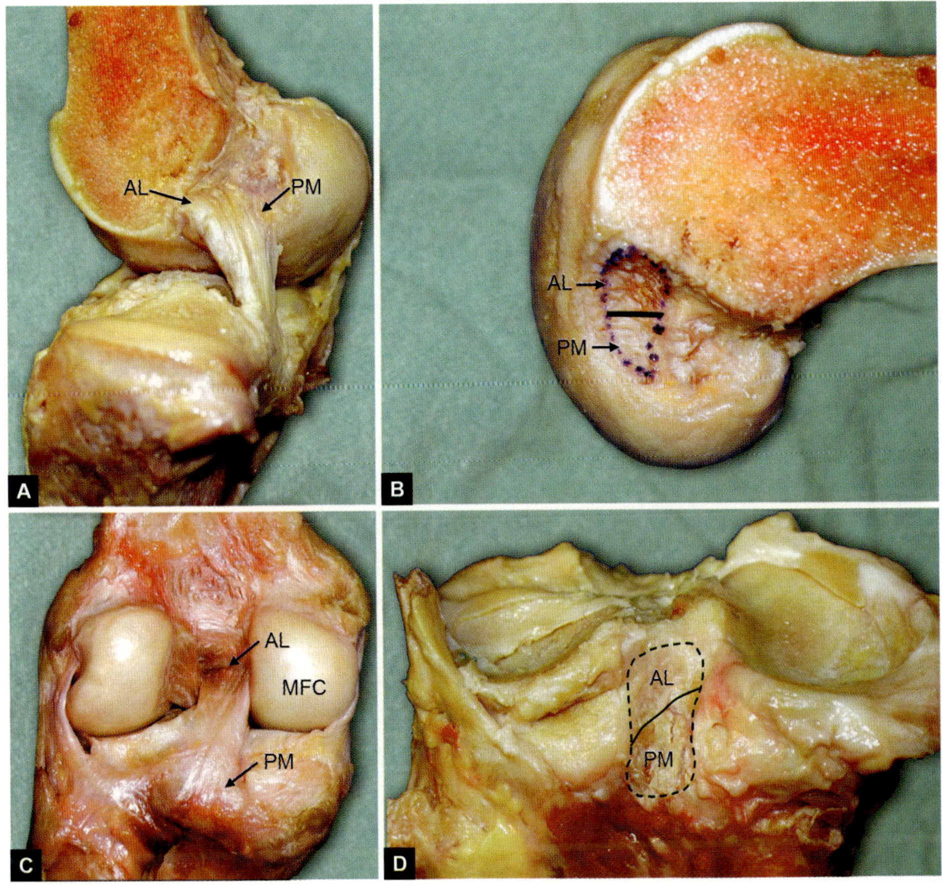

Figures 31.10A to D Anatomic images of cadaveric dissected right knee show attachment of the PCL fibers; the AL bundle and the PM bundle over the tibia and femur. (A) Image shows both AL bundle and PM bundle attachment over MFC with knee in extension; (B) Image reveals the area occupied by both bundles over MFC when seen in knee flexed where in AL bundle occupies near the roof or high position and PM bundle occupies low position near articular cartilage; (C) Image shows the attachment and orientation of the PCL fibers from the back of knee; (D) Image shows the origin of PCL fibers over the back of tibia

Abbreviations: AL, anterolateral; PM, posteromedial; MFC, medial femoral condyle

and is based upon dissection rather than true anatomic division.[27,53] The ALB has a larger cross-sectional area and is much stronger than PLB. Recently, another interesting observation was made by Hoof et al. on embalmed nine cadaveric knees using CT scan.[54] They replaced PCL by best fitting cylinder on a CT model and suggested that average tibial and femoral footprint of PCL was 189.1 mm^2 and 293.3 mm^2. The mean diameter of best-fit cylinder was 10.5 mm and mean coverage on the tibial and femoral footprint was 76.5% and 46.5%, respectively. The central axis of this cylinder was central on tibial footprint and anterolateral on femoral footprint of the PCL. The practical implication of this study is profound, indicating that with the existing techniques of PCL reconstruction it is difficult to restore the anatomical footprint of PCL over tibia and femur.

The PCL is also flanked by MFL, anteriorly (ligament of Humphrey) and posteriorly (ligament of Wrisberg).[55] Both anterior and posterior MFL arise from the posterior horn of lateral meniscus and are attached onto the medial femoral condyle anterior and posterior to the PCL respectively (**Figure 31.11**). Their presence is quite variable. A review of 16 anatomic studies (1022 cadaveric knees) done by Gupte et al. revealed that 91.1% knee have at least one MFL.[56] Posterior MFL was more frequent than anterior (70.4% versus 48.2%) MFL offers a significant biomechanical advantage to the knee due to its size, stiffness and strength.[55] Recent biomechanical analysis revealed that aMFL and pMFL stiffness is almost equal to the PM bundle of PCL (265N, 443N).[57] MFL also guides the movement of lateral meniscus. Unpublished study of Demeo and Bergfeld (2004) proved that they offer 30–60% resistance for posterior drawer in 90° knee flexion. Due to their varied but definite functional role in the knee, they should be preserved during the PCL reconstruction.

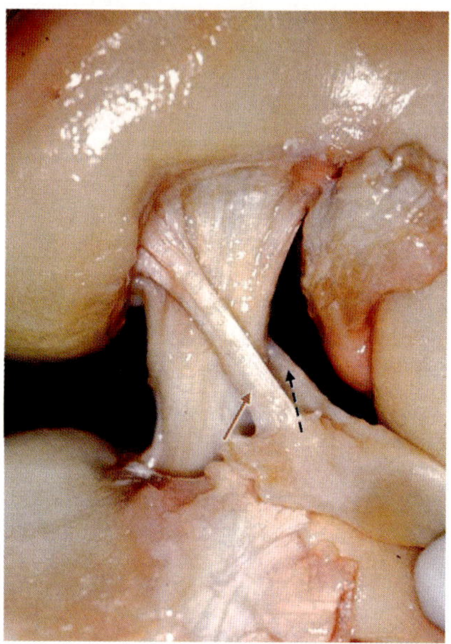

Figure 31.11 Anatomic image of the knee shows anterior (continuous brown arrow) and posterior (interrupted brown arrow) meniscofemoral ligaments that are anterior and posterior to the PCL

Function of PCL complex: Its primary function is to restrain posterior tibial translation as the knee moves from extension to flexion especially from 30° to 90° flexion.[47,53] Posteromedial and PL capsules, collaterals provide posterior restraint between 0° and 30° flexion. It is also secondary restraint to varus, valgus and external rotation at high flexion angles. Covey et al. demonstrated that posterior translation of tibia increases by twofold (7.23 ± 0.65 mm) at 90° flexion, as compared with 20° flexion (3.41 ± 0.77 mm) at 74 N posteriorly directed force over tibia after selective sectioning of the PCL. Greater than 12 mm posterior drawer is not PCL injury alone indicating damage to posterior capsule.[58]

MENISCUS

The two menisci (lateral and medial) are C-shaped fibrocartilage interposed between the femur and tibia covering approximately two-third of the tibial plateau (**Figure 31.12**). Arising from the tibia, they serve to deepen the articular surface of the tibia improving the articulation between the femur and tibia. The peripheral border of meniscus is thick, convex and attached to the joint capsule; the inside opposite border tapers to a thin free edge. The proximal surface of menisci is concave and in contact with femoral condyles. The distal surface is flat and rests over the tibial plateau. Each meniscus has two horns, anterior and posterior. The posterior horn of the medial meniscus is larger than the anterior horn whereas the two horns of the lateral meniscus are equal in size. Both menisci assume their typical shape early in the prenatal developmental stage.[59] The blood supply to meniscus originates from superior and inferior, medial and lateral genicular vessels. The vessels are present throughout the meniscal substance in fetus but in adults, only outer one-third is vascular.[59,60]

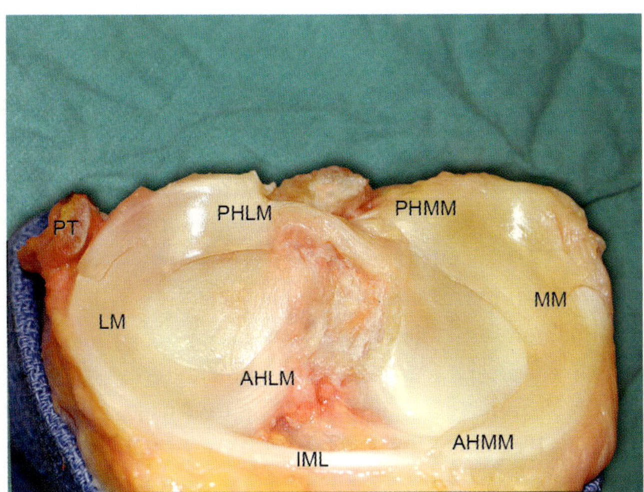

Figure 31.12 Anatomic image of the right knee shows both the meniscus and its parts

Abbreviations: MM, medial meniscus; AHMM, anterior horn of medial meniscus; PHMM, posterior horn of medial meniscus; LM, lateral meniscus; AHLM, anterior horn of lateral meniscus; PHLM, posterior horn of lateral meniscus; PT, popliteus tendon; IML, intermeniscal ligament

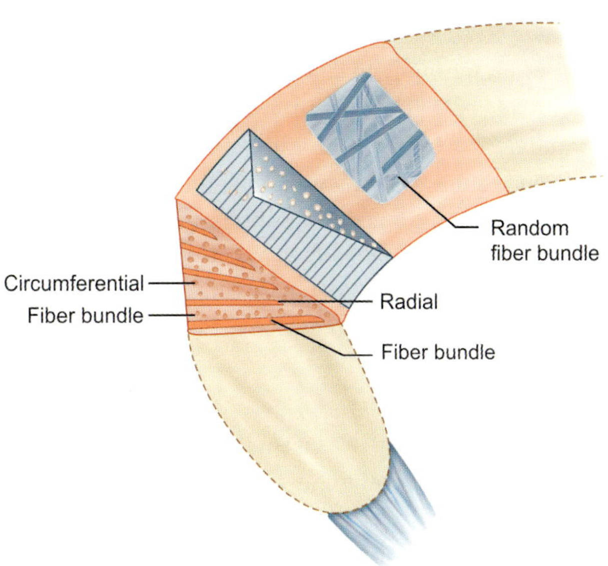

Figure 31.13 Diagrammatic illustration of meniscal ultrastructure reveals intricate arrangement of circumferential and radial fibers within meniscus

Menisci are mostly composed of collagen (75%). All four types of collagen are present but mostly type 1 collagen predominates (90%). Histologic examination reveals fibroblasts and fibrocartilaginous cells dispersed in an organized matrix of eosinophilic collagen fibers. A network of collagen fiber is oriented in circumferential direction forming the dominant pattern. This circumferential pattern is optimal for compressive loads. Radial fibers are present at the surface and midsubstance and may function as to restrain motion between the circumferential fibers and resisting longitudinal split (**Figure 31.13**). The presence of 0.6% elastin fiber ensures the meniscal recoil into the original shape after deformation. In the degenerative menisci, metaplasia of the cell population occurs toward chondroid cell appearance. The substance of menisci is prone to degenerative and traumatic tears. It can also undergo calcification known as chondrocalcinosis, a disease that is associated with calcium pyrophosphate dihydrate deposition.

- *Medial meniscus*: It is a C-shaped structure approximately 3.5 cm in length. It occupies approximately 50% of the medial tibial plateau. Its posterior horn or meniscal root is attached in posterior part of intercondylar fossa just anterior to the PCL attachment. The meniscal root is an important part in the stability of meniscus. If the root is avulsed from its attachment, it is akin to total meniscectomy jeopardizing the function of meniscus and it can accelerate the arthritic changes in the knee. Hence, it establishes the importance of root re-attachment if avulsed.[61-63] The anterior horn is attached 7 mm anterior to the ACL attachment in the line of medial tibial spine. The body is attached to the capsule of the knee. In the middle, the medial meniscus periphery is attached to the femur via deep MCL. The meniscus is attached to the tibial margin by coronary ligament. The two anterior horns of medial and lateral meniscus are connected by intermeniscal ligament.
- *Lateral meniscus*: It is almost circular, more uniform in shape and covers 70% of the tibial articular surface. The anterior horn is attached in front of the intercondylar eminence behind the ACL with which it blends over the margins. The posterior horn is attached behind the intercondylar eminence in front of the posterior horn of medial meniscus. The posterior horn is connected to medial femoral condyle by MFL of Humphrey and ligament of Wrisberg that run anterior and posterior to the PCL, respectively. On periphery, it is loosely attached to capsule but not to the LCL. The capsular attachment is briefly interrupted by popliteal hiatus.

Posteriorly, it is attached to popliteus tendon. By virtue of its attachment to popliteus and medial femoral condyle via MFLs, its motion is coupled with femoral condyle during flexion and rotation. This coupled motion renders lateral meniscus more mobile, almost by 1 cm. Hence, it is prevented from getting entrapped between the femur and tibia and lesser prone for injury as compared with medial meniscus.[64]

Function of Meniscus

The menisci are responsible for several important functions including: (1) tibiofemoral load transmission; (2) shock absorption; (3) lubrication; (4) prevention of synovial impingement; (5) contribution to the joint stability by increasing conformity; (6) distribution of synovial fluid; (7) assistance in gliding motion.

The most pivotal role of meniscus is load transmission both in extension and flexion of the knee. At least 50% of the compressive loads are transmitted in extension and 85% in 90° flexion of the knee.[65] In a meniscectomized knee where the area of contact reduces by 50–75%, the contact pressure per unit area increases between the tibia and femur by 235% and this accelerates the degeneration of hyaline cartilage.[65,66] Fairbank first observed such changes in a meniscectomized knee with the presence of osteophytes at the site of meniscectomy, flat femoral condyle and narrowing of joint space.[67] In biomechanical studies by Ahmed et al. and Ihn et al. showed that there is a linear correlation between contact pressures on the joint surface and the volume of meniscal tissue removed.[65,68]

Another important function of menisci is to act as shock absorbers. Normal knee has 20% more shock absorbing capacity than meniscectomized knee.[69] Inability of the knee joint to absorb the shock may translate into more injury to the cartilage resulting into cartilage damage. Medial meniscectomy in association with ACL tear leads to increased anterior translation significantly. Peripheral concavity of meniscus leads to an increased congruity of the knee joint and hence serves to increase joint stability. The presence of type 1 and 2 nerve fibers in horns of meniscus perhaps provides proprioceptive mechanism. So, it would always be prudent to save as much as meniscus as possible and resect as much as necessary.

MEDIAL ASPECT OF THE KNEE

According to Warren and Marshall, the supporting structures of knee on medial side can be divided into three principal layers.[70]

Layer I: Deep fascial layer that invests the sartorius muscle.
Layer II: Superficial medial collateral ligament (SMCL) and other variable structures.
Layer III: Joint capsule.

Layer I: It is a layer deep to the subcutaneous tissue. It invests sartorius muscle medially and medial gastrocnemius posteriorly. It can be separated from SMCL by sharp dissection. Anteriorly, layer I and layer II fuse to form medial patellar retinaculum. Anterosuperiorly, layer 1 is continuous with fascia of vastus medialis. Anteroinferiorly, layer I invests into the sartorius muscle that finally inserts into the tibial periosteum. Semitendinosus and gracilis muscles are between the layers I and II. These two tendons fuse together into the sartorius fascia approximately 3 cm prior to their attachment onto the tibia.

Layer II: Superficial MCL is the largest and main content of this layer. According to Brantigan and Voshell, SMCL consists of parallel and oblique portions.[71] It has one femoral and two tibial attachments. The femoral attachment of superficial MCL (parallel fibers) arises from a depression that is an average 3.2 mm (range: 1.6–5.2 mm) proximal and 4.8 mm (range: 2.5–6.3 mm) posterior to medial epicondyle (**Figure 31.14**).

The distal end of parallel fibers of SMCL is attached onto the proximal tibia 4.6 cm inferior to the tibial articular surface immediately posterior to the insertion of the pes anserinus. The broad insertion continues distally, up to 7.5 cm, and blends with periosteum (**Figures 31.15A and B**). The oblique portion of the superficial MCL that courses posteriorly is known as a posterior oblique ligament (POL). It begins mid medially and blends with the capsule, medial meniscus and semimembranosus tendon and inserts just below the tibial articular surface. POL is anatomically and functionally distinct from MCL.[72,73]

POL originates just anterior and inferior to the medial head of gastrocnemius. It courses inferiorly and displays three arms: superficial, central, and capsular. The superficial arm remains parallel to the superficial MCL. The central arm is the main component and attaches to semimembranosus tendon, deep MCL, posterior capsule and medial meniscus. The capsular arm of distal part of semimembranosus tendon attaches to the medial head of gastrocnemius.[73,74]

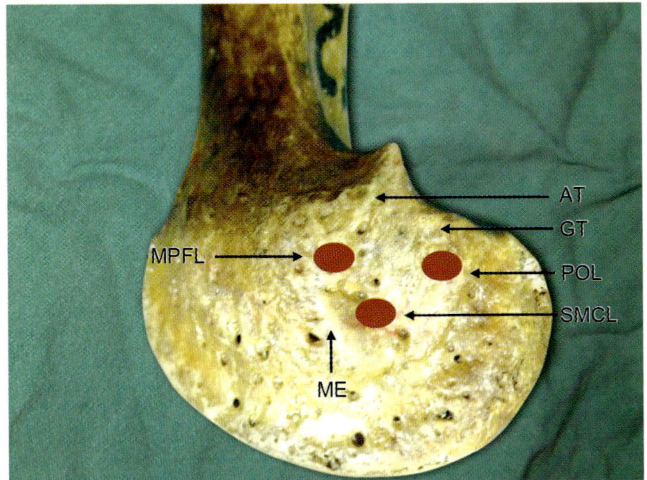

Figure 31.14 Medial surface of the medial femoral condyle revealing the attachment of various ligaments and their inter-relationship with various tubercle

Abbreviations: MPFL, medial patellofemoral ligament; ME, medial epicondyle; SMCL, superficial medial collateral ligament; POL, posterior oblique ligament; GT, gastrocnemius tubercle; AT, adductor tubercle

Practically, the MCL complex includes parallel fibers of MCL, POL and deep MCL. Latter is a part of layer III. MCL complex receives dynamic reinforcement from pes anserinus, vastus medialis and semimembranosus during flexion and extension. Pes anserinus and vastus medialis support during extension and semimembranosus during flexion.[75,76] This may explain that certain individuals who have good muscular support continue to remain asymptomatic despite injury to medial side of the knee.

Superiorly, fibers of layer II form medial patellofemoral ligament, parapatellar retinaculum and inferiorly forming medial meniscopatellar ligament that is attached to anterior horn of medial meniscus.

Medial patellofemoral ligament (MPFL): This ligament needs a special mention due to recent increase in focus on its role in patellar stability. It is a distinct ligament in layer 2 of the medial side of the knee (**Figures 31.15A and B**). Medially, it has a broad base attachment over the medial border of the patella. Its midpoint lies roughly at 41.4% of the distance between the proximal and distal pole.[77] The femoral attachment can be variable as described by various authors.[78-80] It courses medially to be attached between the attachment of adductor magnus tendon

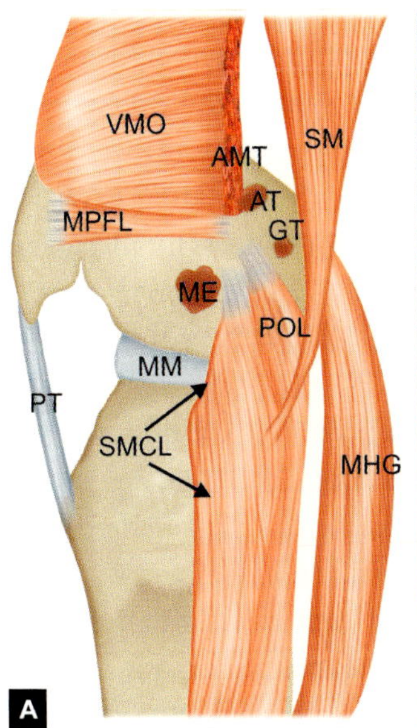

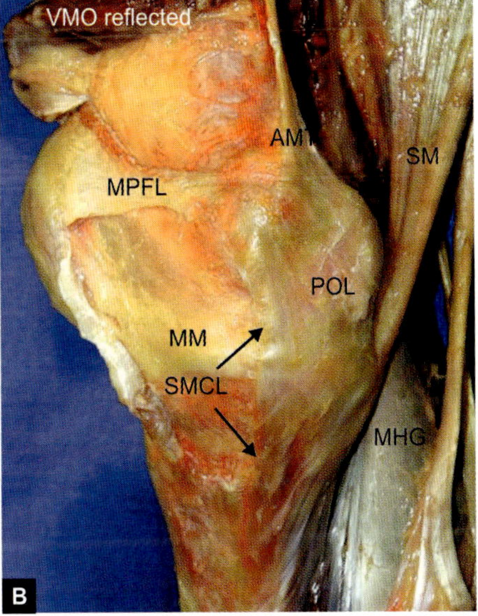

Figures 31.15A and B Diagrammatic representation (A) and anatomic image (B) of second layer of the medial side of the knee

Abbreviations: MPFL, medial patellofemoral ligament; ME, medial epicondyle; SMCL, superficial medial collateral ligament; POL, posterior oblique ligament; GT, gastrocnemius tubercle; AT, adductor tubercle; PT, patellar tendon; VMO, vastus medialis obliquus; AMT, adductor magnus tendon; MM, medial meniscus; SM, semimembranosus; MHG, medial head of gastrocnemius

and superficial MCL. MPFL attachment on femur is 10.6 mm (range: 8.0–13.4 mm) proximal and 8.8 mm (range: 6.1–10.3 mm) posterior to the medial epicondyle. Also, it is 1.9 mm (range: 1.3–3.2 mm) anterior and 3.8 mm (range: 2.1–6.3 mm) distal to adductor tubercle.[74]

The term posteromedial corner (PMC) refers to the structures posterior to parallel fibers of the MCL. It comprises of POL, posteromedial capsule, semimembranosus tendon, oblique popliteal ligament (OPL) and posterior horn of medial meniscus. The differentiation between MCL complex and PMC injury is vital as former can be managed conservatively whereas the latter is usually a part of extensive multiligament injury that needs operative intervention. Otherwise, it can render knee severely unstable in valgus and will lead to the failure of reconstructed ACL or PCL due to undue strain.

Layer III: Capsule of the knee joint form layer 3. It can be separated from layer 2 except near patella, where it is too thin. Beneath the SMCL, layer 3 thickening forms deep MCL that is vertically oriented short fibers. It is attached below the medial epicondyle and then to the margins of tibia and meniscus (**Figure 31.16**).

Anteriorly, deep MCL can be well separated from SMCL whereas posteriorly, it blends with SMCL in the cephalad direction. Caudally, the meniscotibial component of deep MCL can be separated from SMCL and is referred as coronary ligament.

Posteromedially, layer 2 and 3 merge and their structure is strengthened by various arms of semimembranosus that has five insertions: (1) direct arm on posteromedial corner of tibia; (2) second arm insertion deep to SMCL; (3) third arm blends with oblique fibers of SMCL; (4) fourth arm over medial meniscus; (5) fifth arm running proximally and laterally across posterior capsule and form OPL.

Semimembranosus acts as dynamic stabilizer of the knee on the medial side especially by dynamic function to the posteromedial corner.[72,73] It prevents impingement of posteromedial meniscus posteriorly in deep flexion by pulling it posteriorly through its attachment onto the meniscus.

Function of MCL: It is the 'prime static stabilizer of the medial side of the knee against valgus forces'[70] and primary restraint against valgus stress in flexion, especially at 25° flexion. A study by Haimes et al. proved that selective

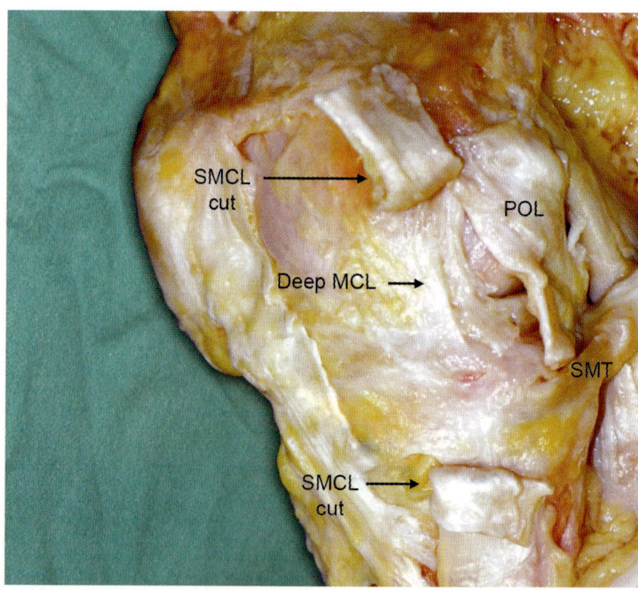

Figure 31.16 Anatomic image of right knee showing deep MCL as a part of third layer of the knee

Abbreviations: POL, posterior oblique ligament; SMT, semimembranosus tendon

sectioning of MCL causes increased valgus instability at 15°, 30°, 60° and 90° but not at full extension.[81] Deep MCL fibers have minimal role in providing valgus stability. Superficial MCL is also an important static stabilizer against external rotational forces.[82] Though MCL is not an important sagittal stabilizer in the presence of intact ACL and PCL, but in their absence MCL acts as a secondary stabilizer for anterior-posterior stability.[81,83]

Function of Deep MCL: By its attachment to the medial meniscus, the deep meniscus is supposed to stabilize the medial meniscus.[71,84]

Function of PMC: Posteromedial (PM) capsule and POL provides valgus stability in an extended knee: the load bearing position of the knee during gait.[72] It accounts for approximately 30% of valgus stability in extension. With flexion, the PM capsule becomes lax and superficial MCL becomes the primary restraint against valgus forces. Also, the PM capsule and POL restrain internal rotation at all flexion angles but do not appear to have any restraint over controlling external rotation.[82] They also prevent posterior translation and valgus abduction even with intact PCL.[81] In biomechanical studies where MCL has already been divided, serial sectioning of POL and PM capsule further increases valgus and rotational instability. Hence, after an isolated injury to the MCL, POL and PM capsule become important restrains against valgus and rotation forces.[81,85]

LATERAL SIDE OF THE KNEE

The structures on the lateral side of the knee also consist of three layers that were described by Seebacher.[86]

Layer I: (a) Fascia lata; (b) ITB; (c) biceps femoris.

Layer II: Anteriorly-quadriceps retinaculum; posteriorly-patellofemoral ligament.

Layer III: Lateral capsule.

Layer I: It is composed of ITB and its anterior expansion and biceps femoris and its posterior expansion (**Figure 31.17**). These structures are interconnected by fascia. Eventually, layer I merges with prepatellar bursa anteriorly and posteriorly with deep fascia of popliteal fossa. ITB that is formed by fascia investing tensor fascia lata continues distally, remains attached to linea aspera through lateral intermuscular septum, passes over the lateral femoral epicondyle and ends at Gerdy's tubercle at the anterolateral aspect of the tibia. Posteriorly, the fascia lata merges into the biceps fascia. The biceps femoris muscle that is formed by union of two heads, long and short, ends in a common tendon. It further divides into three layers: superficial, middle, and deep. Superficial layer inserts upon proximal tibia as wide expansion. Middle layer envelops LCL and is separated from LCL by a bursa. The deep layer bifurcates and inserts upon fibular styloid process and on Gerdy's tubercle. The biceps femoris acts as weak knee flexor and external rotator of the knee. It is an important static and dynamic stabilizer of the knee especially beyond 30° of flexion.[87] The ITB is essentially a passive fibrous structure that remains anterior to the axis of the knee in extension and posterior in flexion.[88,89] It is an important static lateral stabilizer of the knee. Its contracture is seen in chronic valgus deformity of the knee that needs release during total knee replacement as a part of balancing. Also, ITB's connection to biceps femoris and vastus lateralis through lateral intermuscular septum forms a sling behind lateral femoral condyle assisting the ACL in preventing posterior displacement of femur when tibia is fixed and the knee joint is in near extension.

Layer II: This layer was described by Fulkerson and Gossling.[90] This layer is made up of lateral knee retinaculum

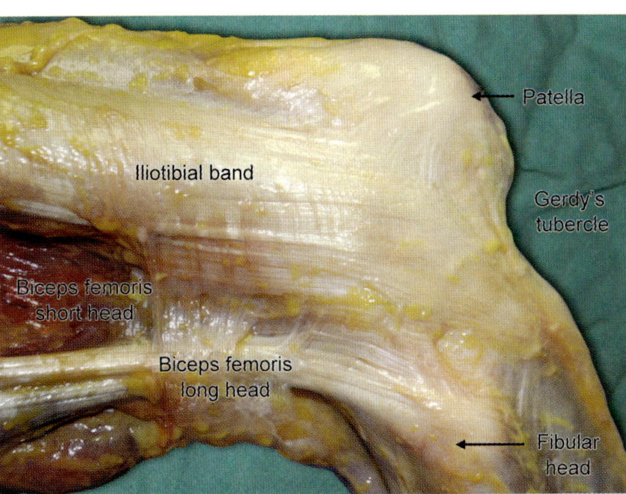

Figure 31.17 Anatomic image of right knee showing structures present in the first layer of lateral side of the knee

that is composed of two major parts: superficial oblique retinaculum and deep transverse retinaculum. Superficial layers runs obliquely from the ITB to patella. The deep layer has epicondylopatellar band (transverse patellofemoral ligament), transverse retinaculum and patellotibial band. The epicondylopatellar band provides superolateral support to patella. Transverse retinaculum that runs from ITB to the lateral border of patella is the main lateral support to the patella. The patellotibial band runs inferiorly between the patella and tibia (**Figures 31.18A and B**).

Layer III: The layer III or the deepest layer has several distinct structures as lateral capsule, LCL, fabellofibular ligament, arcuate ligament, popliteus and popliteofibular ligament (PFL).

The lateral capsule is a loose thin structure on the lateral side attached proximally to the edge of the femur and distally onto the tibia. It attaches the inferior margin of the lateral meniscus to the lateral tibial margin as coronary ligament.[86,91] The tendon of popliteus passes through a hiatus in coronary ligament. The LCL is attached proximally onto the lateral epicondyle of the femur, runs beneath the lateral retinaculum and inserts into the head of fibula (**Figure 31.19**). The fabellofibular ligament lies between the LCL and arcuate ligament. Proximally, it is attached to the fabella and distally into the styloid process of fibula.[92] The arcuate ligament is a Y-shaped ligament whose vertical limb is attached to the fibular styloid process. The upper lateral limb, which is dense and strong, is attached to the lateral femoral condyle and popliteus whereas the

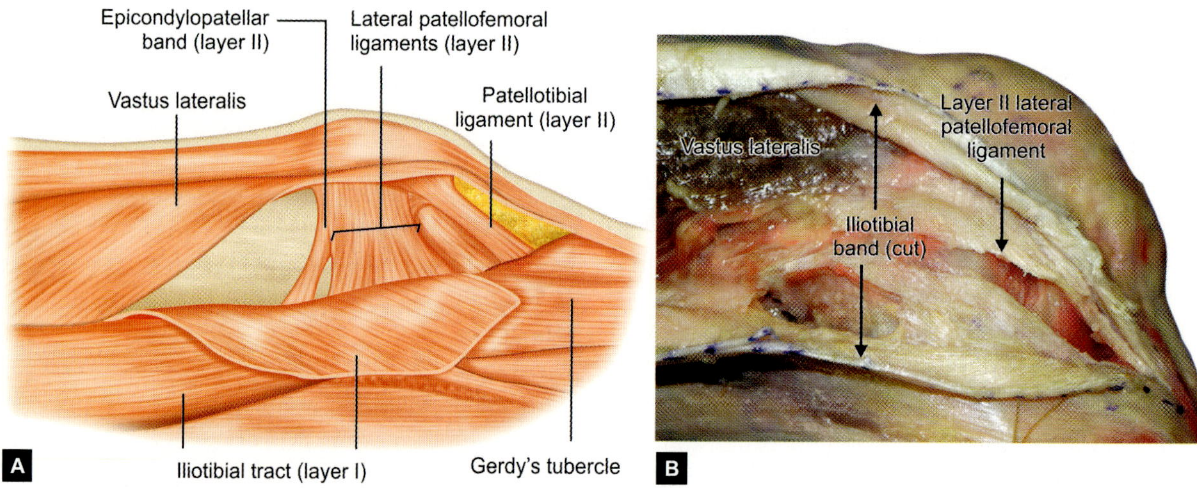

Figures 31.18A and B Diagrammatic representation of structures present in the second layer lateral side of knee (A), and anatomic image of the right knee showing structures present in the second layer of the lateral side of the knee (B)

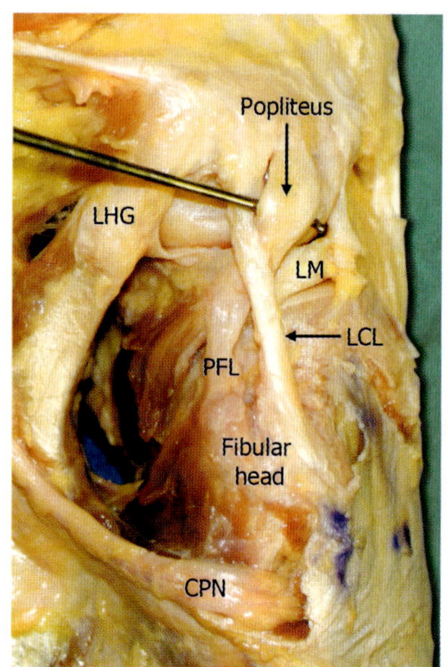

Figure 31.19 Anatomic image showing the structure present in the third layer of the knee (lateral side) with probe under the popliteus tendon

Abbreviations: LCL, lateral collateral ligament; PFL, popliteofibular ligament; LM, lateral meniscus; LHG, lateral head of gastrocnemius; CPN, common peroneal nerve

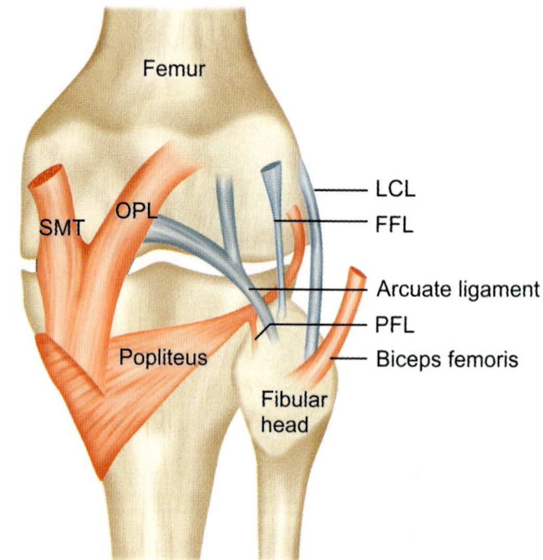

Figure 31.20 Diagrammatic illustration of the third layer of the knee on the lateral side showing arcuate complex and other structures

Abbreviations: LCL, lateral collateral ligament; PFL, popliteofibular ligament; FFL, fabellofibular ligament; OPL, oblique popliteal ligament; SMT, semimembranosus tendon

weaker medial limb curves upwards over popliteus muscle and merges with OPL[64] (**Figure 31.20**). Below the arch of medial crescentic limb, emerges the tendon of popliteus to get inserted onto the tibia. Both fabellofibular and arcuate ligament is present only in 67% of the knees. In case the fabellofibular ligament is dominant with large fabella, the arcuate ligament may be absent. In the absence of fabella, only the arcuate ligament may be present.[86] Popliteus arises from a depression anterior and inferior to the lateral epicondyle of femur. It courses inferolaterally, passes below the medial limb of the arcuate ligament and flares as thin, flat popliteus muscle to be inserted upon a triangular area on upper medial aspect of tibia above the soleal line. It gives a direct attachment to the fibular head known as

PFL.[93] PFL lies deep to the arcuate ligament and attaches on the most posterior and proximal points of the fibular head. The popliteal tendon is also attached to the arcuate ligament and lateral meniscus through popliteomeniscal fascicle.[94,64] The primary role of the popliteus muscle is to unlock the knee to allow flexion by producing external rotation of the femur in tibia fixed position.[64,95,96] It also appears to control the motion of meniscus when the knee is in motion. The PCL, LCL, and popliteus-arcuate ligament complex are very important in stabilizing the knee against varus stress, external rotation, and posterior drawer. Damage to one or more of these structure leads to PL instability of the knee.[97,98]

ANTERIOR ASPECT OF THE KNEE

Along with the patella, the distal quadriceps muscles and the associated tendinous structures are collectively referred to as the extensor mechanism of the knee. The quadriceps complex is formed by the central rectus femoris muscle, flanked by the vastus medialis and the vastus lateralis on either side. The fourth component, the vastus intermedius, lies deep to the rectus femoris (**Figure 31.21**). The quadriceps tendon was thought to be a trilamellar organization with common attachments of rectus femoris superficially, vastus medialis and lateralis in the middle and vastus intermedius; deep but actually consists of an intricate blending of all four-tendon fibers. Rieder and associates noted the rectus tendon to be a fan shaped structure, extending 5–8 cm proximally from the superior pole of the patella, 3–5 cm wide at the attachment.[99] Some of the rectus fibers insert at the superior pole, however the majority continue over the anterior aspect of patella to form the infrapatellar tendon.

The vastus medialis muscle is formed by two distinctly arranged fibers groups innervated by separate branches of the femoral nerve. The prominence of the vastus medialis muscle is formed by oblique (VMO) fibers whose direction tends much more toward the transverse (55°–70°) than the majority of the vastus medialis muscle fibers[99] (**Figure 31.22**). The VMO is tendinous only few millimeters proximal to the patella inserting on superomedial border, majority continuing to form the medial retinaculum.

The vastus lateral is muscle belly usually terminates about 2–3 cm proximal to the patella converging at an

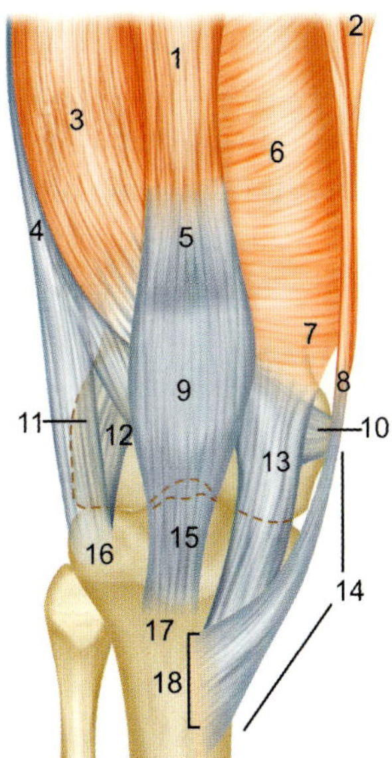

Figure 31.21 Knee joint; anterior aspect
Abbreviations: 1, rectus femoris muscle; 2, gracilis muscle; 3, vastus lateralis muscle; 4, Iliotibial band; 5, quadriceps tendon; 6, vastus medialis muscle; 7, vastus medialis obliquus; 8, sartorius; 9, patella; 10, medial patellofemoral ligament; 11, lateral femoral condyle; 12, lateral longitudinal patellar retinaculum; 13, medial longitudinal patellar retinaculum; 14, medial collateral ligament; 15, patellar ligament; 16, Gerdy's tubercle; 17, tibial tuberosity; 18, pes anserinus

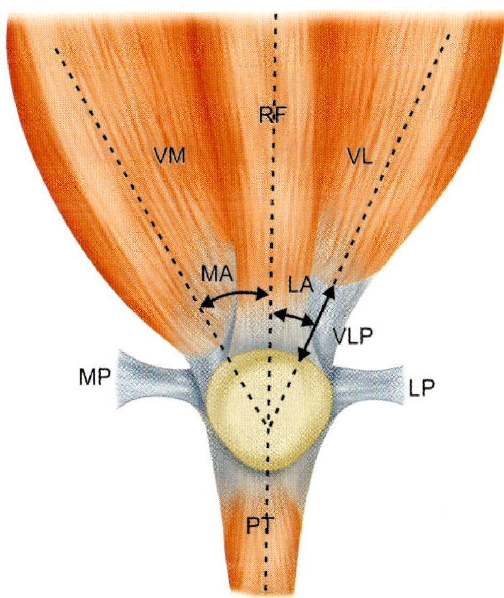

Figure 31.22 Quadriceps parameters
Abbreviations: RF, rectus femoris; VM, vastus medialis; VL, vastus lateralis; PT, patellar tendon; MP, MPFL; LP, LPFL (part of lateral retinaculum); MA, angle between VM and RF (55°–70°); LA, angle between VL and RF (22°–45°); VLP, distance between distal fibers of VL and the superolateral corner of the patella
Note: VM and MP width is more than lateral counterparts

angle of 22°–45° to the patella.[99] The lateralis like the medialis is also distinctly divided into vastus lateralis longus and obliquus with the medial most fibers inserting on the superolateral border and continuing distally to form the lateral retinaculum. The most lateral fibers merge with the fibers of ITB with very few crossing distally to form the patellar tendon.

The intermedius tendon lies deep to the rectus and inserts directly to the proximal pole of the patella. The tendon blends with fibers of lateralis and medialis on either side forming a more complex arrangement than the traditional trilamellar concept of quadriceps tendon.

Deep to the quadriceps complex lies a flat highly variable muscle called the articularis genu.[99] It arises from the anterior aspect of supracondylar portion of the femur inserting in the joint capsule and its function is still obscure.

Patellar Tendon and Infrapatellar Fat Pad

Distal to the patella is the patellar tendon or patellar ligament, broad flat band made up predominantly of rectus fibers that connect the inferior pole of the patella to the tibia. The patellar tendon inserts on the tibial tubercle, or tibial tuberosity measuring about 46 mm in length, with a range of 35 to 55 mm[2,100].

The infrapatellar fat pad, or Hoffa's fat pad, is an intracapsular but extrasynovial structure. It has a thick central body extending from the inferior pole of patella and the patella tendon anteriorly to the anterior horns of medial and lateral meniscus to which it is attached with thinner extensions on either side. It helps in reducing joint friction but also may be a site for loose bodies to hide. Inflammation causes anterior knee pain and is called Hoffa's disease with hypertrophied fat pad getting impinged between anterior structures and femoral condyles. Excessive resection of the fat pad may also lead to loss of blood supply to the patella or the tendon.

FASCIAL STRUCTURES

The medial and lateral retinacular structures complement the extensor mechanism, inserting onto the proximal tibia allowing active knee extension in isolated transverse patella fracture.

The fascia lata stretches across the anterior surface of the knee investing the quadriceps complex and forms the retinacula with aponeurotic contributions from vastus medialis and lateralis. Superficial fascia of vastus lateralis and biceps femoris, termed as arciform fibers traverse the anterior aspect of the patella and blends in midline with the superficial fascia of the sartorius and vastus medialis from medial aspect.

Dye and coworkers described in detail the fascial layers anterior to patella.[100] The deepest prepatellar fascial structure is composed of the deep fibers of the rectus femoris that extend to continue as the fibers of the patella tendon. Intermediate layer receives contributions from medialis and lateralis fibers running obliquely. The most superficial layer being formed by an extremely thin expansion of fascia lata with transverse fiber orientation, Dye et al. also noted prepatellar bursa complex of three distinct bursae in between the layers.[100]

POSTERIOR ASPECT OF THE KNEE AND POPLITEAL FOSSA

The diamond shaped popliteal fossa lies behind the knee. It is actually a narrow interval between the diverging hamstring tendons superiorly and converging fleshy heads of gastrocnemius inferiorly. The popliteal surface of the femur, posterior capsule of the knee joint and popliteus muscle with its fascia form the anterior wall while deep fascia pierced by small saphenous vein and posterior femoral cutaneous nerve forms the posterior wall of the fossa. Popliteal vessels along with branches of sciatic nerve and few lymph nodes are contained within the fat in the fossa.

Posterior to the ITB, the biceps tendon can be palpated laterally in a flexed knee that forms the proximal lateral boundary. The semitendinosus and semimembranosus taking origin from the ischial tuberosity form the proximal and medial boundaries of popliteal fossa with their distal attachment on the posteromedial aspect of tibia. The gracilis muscle tendon lies medial to the tendon of the semitendinosus while the sartorius muscle arising from the anterior superior iliac spine runs distally and medially across the front of the thigh. Together, the tendons of the sartorius, gracilis, and semitendinosus form the pes anserinus that attaches onto the proximal medial surface of tibia overlying superficial MCL.

The two heads of the gastrocnemius muscle arise from the popliteal surface of the corresponding femoral condyles with the lateral head having largely fleshy origin whereas the portion of the medial head arising close to the MCL being tendinous. The two heads merge to form a common tendon with the soleus, which narrows distally and inserts into the tendocalcaneus. There is a small plantaris muscle posteriorly that arises from the lateral supracondylar line of femur deep to the lateral head of gastrocnemius. It is absent in about 7% population.

Within the popliteal fossa, the common peroneal nerve can be found sloping downwards across the lateral boundary medial to the biceps tendon. It overlies the plantaris, lateral head of gastrocnemius and posterior capsule of joint before disappearing into the peroneus longus around the neck of fibula and dividing into deep and superficial peroneal nerves. In its course it gives off the following branches: peroneal communicating nerve, lateral cutaneous nerve, superior and inferior genicular nerves, and the recurrent genicular nerve. The first two pierce the roof of fossa with the former joining the sural nerve while the latter supplying the skin over the upper parts of peroneal and extensor compartments of the leg. The genicular nerves accompany the arteries by same names and supply the lateral part of joint capsule, while the superior part is supplied by the recurrent genicular nerve.

The tibial nerve runs vertically down the middle of the fossa along with the popliteal vessels and disappears by passing deep between the heads of gastrocnemius beneath the fibrous soleal arch. It gives motor branches to all muscles in the popliteal fossa and only one cutaneous branch, sural nerve.

Throughout the fossa, the popliteal artery is the deepest of the large neurovascular structures. It begins at the tendinous opening in the adductor magnus continuing from the femoral artery and ends below the lower border of the popliteus dividing into anterior and posterior tibial arteries. At all times it runs medial to the nerve with the popliteal vein lying between the nerve and artery. It overlies the little fat posterior to the popliteal surface of the femur and the popliteal ligament to which it is firmly fixed by fibrous tissue and middle genicular artery.

The popliteal artery gives off muscular branches to the muscles in the popliteal fossa and sural arteries, which are end arteries and if severed can lead to ischemic necrosis of the heads of gastrocnemius. The genicular arteries are five in number, upper and lower, lateral and medial, and middle genicular arteries. Their course is discussed with the arterial anastomoses around the knee. The middle genicular artery pierces the posterior ligament of knee joint to supply the cruciate ligaments along with posterior division of the obturator nerve. The popliteal vein formed by the union of two venae comitantes of the anterior and posterior tibial arteries also receives tributaries from the accompanying popliteal artery branches and from the short saphenous vein.

The posterior capsule of the knee consists of vertical fibers reinforced by the OPL proximally and medially and the arcuate ligament laterally. The OPL is a broad, flat expansion of the semimembranosus that is attached proximally to the margin of the intercondylar fossa and posterior surface of the femur close to the articular margins of the condyles. It has openings for the passage of the popliteal vessels and nerves. The OPL forms part of the floor of the popliteal fossa, and the popliteal artery rests on it. At the site of the popliteal hiatus, the capsule is displaced inferiorly toward the fibula head, forming the arcuate ligament between the lateral meniscus and the fibular styloid.

The popliteus muscle slopes upward and laterally at the back of the knee, taking origin from the popliteal surface of tibia above the soleal line and inserting on the lateral surface of the lateral femoral condyle just below the epicondyle. The cord like tendon of this muscle enters the joint beneath the arcuate popliteal ligament giving few superficial attachments to it, while almost half of the muscle is attached to the posterior convexity of the lateral meniscus. The popliteus 'unlocks' the knee also controls excursion of lateral meniscus to avoid being caught between the two bones.

CAPSULE

The articular capsule encapsulates the joint from all around and is discreetly thickened in certain areas that act as ligaments. Anteriorly, the capsule is thin and merges with the patellar tendon. Proximally, it is attached three to four fingerbreadth above the patella. Posteriorly, the capsule is attached just above the femoral condyles and over the roof of the intercondylar fossa. In this area, the capsular fibers are reinforced by OPL (flat, broad band) that is an extension of semimembranosus tendon. OPL extends superolaterally and attached over intercondylar fossa margins and over lateral femoral condyle. Large foramina for vessels and nerves perforate the OPL and the popliteal artery rests against it. Inferiorly, the capsule is circumferentially attached to tibial margin all around except where the popliteus tendon passes posterolaterally. Arcuate popliteal ligament is located on the lower lateral side of the knee below the popliteal hiatus and helps in strengthening the capsule. It extends inferiorly toward the back of the fibular head and superiorly over the posterior surface of the joint.

Bursae of the Knee: The knee joint vicinity has plenty of bursae as most of the tendons crossing the joint are parallel to the bones and pull lengthwise to the joint.

Anteriorly, there are three bursae; prepatellar bursa (between patella and skin), subcutaneous infrapatellar bursa (between skin and patellar tendon) and deep infrapatellar bursa (between patellar ligament and tibial tuberosity). Prepatellar and subcutaneous bursae prevent friction while flexion-extension and kneeling.

Anteromedially, pes anserine bursa lies between the tendons of sartorius, gracilis and semitendinosus and tibia. Its inflammation can be misinterpreted as osteoarthritis of knee.

Laterally, there are bursae between LCL and biceps femoris, popliteus and lateral tibial plateau and popliteus and LCL. Posteriorly, there is a subtendinous bursa of lateral and the medial head of gastrocnemius that separates them from capsule. Bursa associated with lateral head of gastrocnemius may occasionally communicate with the knee joint cavity.

BLOOD SUPPLY TO THE KNEE AND ANASTOMOSIS AROUND KNEE

The arterial anastomosis is contributed by eight separate arteries that provide nourishment to the patella and fascioligamentous structures of the knee (**Figure 31.23**): two medial and two lateral genicular arteries from the popliteal artery, descending genicular artery from the femoral artery, a genicular branch from the lateral circumflex artery, and anterior and posterior tibial recurrent arteries.

The supreme or descending genicular artery is given off at the Hunter's canal from the superficial femoral artery, while the four geniculate arteries take origin from the popliteal artery and course around the heads of gastrocnemius and pass anteriorly. The recurrent tibial

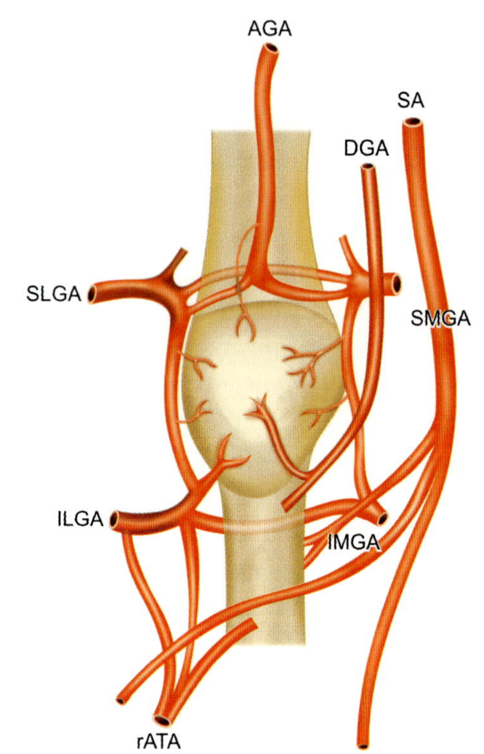

Figure 31.23 Popliteal fossa

Abbreviations: AGA, anterior genicular artery; DGA, descending genicular artery; SA, saphenous artery; SMGA, IMGA, superior and inferior medial genicular arteries; SLGA, ILGA, superior and inferior lateral genicular arteries; rATA, recurrent branch of anterior tibial artery

artery arising 1 cm below the proximal tibiofibular joint is a branch of the anterior tibial artery. The patella has extensive supply via the extraosseous and intraosseous plexus, while the tendon is supplied by the deep vessels in the fat pad and superficial retinacular vessels.

NERVES AROUND THE KNEE JOINT

The knee joint and the structures around it are mainly supplied by the tibial and the peroneal nerve branches (**Figure 31.24**). Superficial branches on the AM and anterolateral aspect can sometimes get injured during surgery and may lead to painful neuroma or paresthetic conditions. Articular nerves arise from two distinct groups of anterior afferent and posterior afferent.[101]

The posterior afferent group consists of posterior articular nerve and the obturator nerve. The anterior group comprises of branches from the femoral, common peroneal and saphenous nerves.

The tibial nerve, which is a branch of the sciatic nerve, runs through the popliteal fossa. It supplies both heads of gastrocnemius, plantaris, popliteus and soleus muscles. It gives a sural cutaneous branch. It gives an articular branch known as the posterior articular nerve. The posterior articular nerve is the largest and most consistent nerve supplying the knee.[101] It winds around popliteal vessels and forms a plexus over OPL. Then those plexus fibers perforate the OPL and supply the fibrous capsule and external part of the menisci with few fibers also coursing through the synovial membrane of cruciate ligaments and reach infrapatellar fat pad. The terminal portion of the posterior branch of the obturator nerve accompanies the middle genicular artery to pierce the posterior capsule of the knee joint.

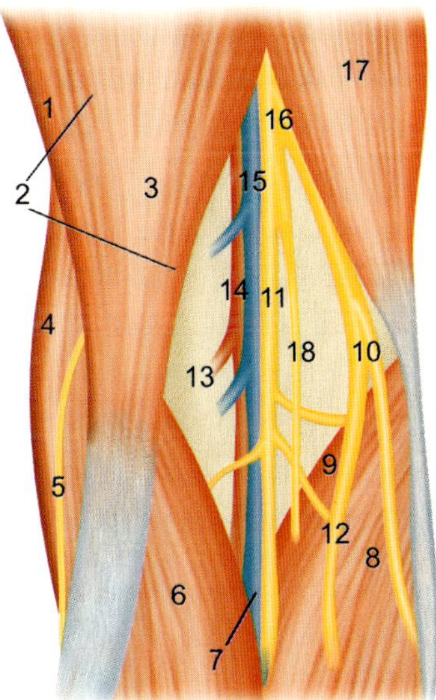

Figure 31.24 Nerve supply to the knee joint (anterior aspect)
Abbreviations: 1, gracilis; 2, semimembranosus; 3, semitendinosus; 4, sartorius; 5, saphenous nerve; 6, medial head of gastrocnemius; 7, short saphenous vein; 8, lateral head of gastrocnemius; 9, plantaris muscle; 10, common peroneal nerve; 11, tibial nerve; 12, peroneal communicating nerve; 13, sural artery; 14, popliteal artery; 15, popliteal vein; 16, sciatic nerve; 17, biceps femoris; 18, sural communicating nerve

The predominant supply of the anterolateral and the AM capsule and associated ligaments is the anterior group of afferents. Articular branches from the terminal portion of femoral nerve supplying the quadriceps muscle form the plexus on the anterior aspect of knee, along with branches from the saphenous and common peroneal nerve. The nerve to vastus medialis is the largest branch that bifurcates underneath the medial retinaculum and supplies a major portion of the AM capsule and nerve to vastus lateralis forming its lateral counterpart (**Figures 31.25A and B**). Deep to the quadriceps motor branches to vastus intermedius give off articular afferent to the suprapatellar pouch. Located on the medial side is mainly the saphenous nerve with infrapatellar and sartorial branch. The infrapatellar branch traverses the sartorius muscle and joins patellar plexus (formed by medial, intermediate and lateral cutaneous nerve of thigh); it innervates the AM capsule, patellar tendon and the AM skin. The sartorial branch accompanies the saphenous nerve and supplies medial aspect of the leg. These can be easily injured during the medial dissection of the knee.

The common peroneal nerve runs medial to the biceps tendon in popliteal fossa on the lateral side. It then runs behind the fibula and winds around the neck of the fibula. It then enters the anterolateral compartment of the knee supplying anterior and lateral compartment of the leg. It also gives rise to sural communicating nerve and nerve to supply the upper lateral aspect of the leg. It gives rise to two articular branches: a lateral articular nerve near the posterior joint supplying the lateral capsule and the LCL and a recurrent peroneal nerve that enters the joint anteriorly. Close to the lateral epicondyle lies the lateral

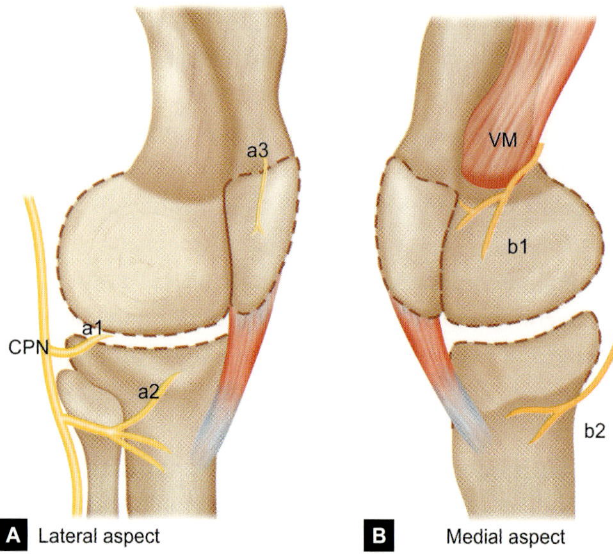

Figures 31.25A and B Arterial anastomoses around knee
Abbreviations: CPN, common peroneal nerve; a1, lateral articular nerve; a2, recurrent peroneal nerve; a3, articular branch of the nerve to vastus intermedius; VM, vastus medialis; b1, articular branch of the nerve to VM (femoral nerve); b2, saphenous nerve

retinacular nerve, within a bursa that is commonly implicated in pain associated with the runner's knee.

The complex innervations of the capsule are associated with the presence of certain mechano and proprioreceptors responsible for sensory input and stabilizing feedback to the knee. Neural elements are located within the ACL and PCL in their richly vascularized synovial coverings but unlike PCL, specialized Golgi-like tendon receptors are not found in the ACL attachments. Controversy exists in meniscal nerve supply with Wilson et al. suggesting up to middle third of the body of meniscus being innervated but Kennedy and coworkers did not find any such fibers in their dissection of 15 knees. They also found that axons, free nerve endings and Golgi-type receptors were limited to perimeniscal capsular tissues.

ACKNOWLEDGMENT

We profusely thank Dr Charles Brown for providing high quality images of knee dissection and consent to use them in the chapter on knee anatomy. Several of those images have been extensively used in this chapter for illustration.

REFERENCES

1. Goodfellow J, Hungerford DS, Zindel M. Patello-femoral joint mechanics and pathology. Functional anatomy of the patello-femoral joint. J Bone Joint Surg Br. 1976;58:287-90.
2. Kaufer H. Mechanical function of the patella. J Bone Joint Surg Am. 1971;53:1551-60.
3. Koukoubis TD, Glisson RR, Bolognesi M, Vail TP. Dimensions of the intercondylar notch of the knee. Am J Knee Surg. 1997;10:83-7.
4. LaPrade RF, Burnett QM 2nd. Femoral intercondylar notch stenosis and correlation to anterior cruciate ligament injuries. A prospective study. Am J Sports Med. 1994;22:198-202.
5. Good L, Odensten M, Gillquist J. Intercondylar notch measurements with special reference to anterior cruciate ligament surgery. Clin Orthop Relat Res. 1991;185-9.
6. Ferretti M, Ekdahl M, Shen W, Fu FH. Osseous landmarks of the femoral attachment of the anterior cruciate ligament: an anatomic study. Arthroscopy. 2007;23:1218-25.
7. Berger RA, Rubash HE, Seel MJ, Thompson WH, Crossett LS. Determining the rotational alignment of the femoral component in total knee arthroplasty using the epicondylar axis. Clin Orthop Relat Res. 1993;40-7.
8. Griffin FM, Insall JN, Scuderi GR. The posterior condylar angle in osteoarthritic knees. J Arthroplasty. 1998;13:812-5.
9. Booth RE, Jr. Sex and the total knee: gender-sensitive designs. Orthopedics. 2006;29:836-8.
10. Cheng FB, Ji XF, Lai Y, et al. Three dimensional morphometry of the knee to design the total knee arthroplasty for Chinese population. Knee. 2009;16:341-7.
11. Hitt K, Shurman JR 2nd, Greene K, et al. Anthropometric measurements of the human knee: correlation to the sizing of current knee arthroplasty systems. J Bone Joint Surg Am. 2003;85-A:115-22.
12. Kwak DS, Surendran S, Pengatteeri YH, et al. Morphometry of the proximal tibia to design the tibial component of total knee arthroplasty for the Korean population. Knee. 2007;14:295-300.
13. Johannsen AM, Anderson CJ, Wijdicks CA, Engebretsen L, LaPrade RF. Radiographic landmarks for tunnel positioning in posterior cruciate ligament reconstructions. Am J Sports Med. 2013;41:35-42.

14. Outerbridge RE. The etiology of chondromalacia patellae. J Bone Joint Surg Br. 1961;43-B:752-7.
15. Arnoczky SP. Anatomy of the anterior cruciate ligament. Clin Orthop Relat Res. 1983;19-25.
16. Duthon VB, Barea C, Abrassart S, et al. Anatomy of the anterior cruciate ligament. Knee Surg Sports Traumatol Arthrosc. 2006;14:204-13.
17. Schultz RA, Miller DC, Kerr CS, Micheli L. Mechanoreceptors in human cruciate ligaments. A histological study. J Bone Joint Surg Am. 1984;66:1072-6.
18. Ikeuchi M, Wang Q, Izumi M, Tani T. Nociceptive sensory innervation of the posterior cruciate ligament in osteoarthritic knees. Arch Orthop Trauma Surg. 2012;132:891-5.
19. Ellison AE, Berg EE. Embryology, anatomy, and function of the anterior cruciate ligament. Orthop Clin North Am. 1985;16:3-14.
20. Petersen W, Tillmann B. Structure and vascularization of the cruciate ligaments of the human knee joint. Anat Embryol (Berl). 1999;200:325-34.
21. Scapinelli R. Vascular anatomy of the human cruciate ligaments and surrounding structures. Clin Anat. 1997;10:151-62.
22. Kazusa H, Nakamae A, Ochi M. Augmentation technique for anterior cruciate ligament injury. Clin Sports Med. 2013;32:127-40.
23. Mifune Y, Ota S, Takayama K, et al. Therapeutic advantage in selective ligament augmentation for partial tears of the anterior cruciate ligament: results in an animal model. Am J Sports Med. 2013;41:365-73.
24. Papalia R, Franceschi F, Vasta S, et al. Sparing the anterior cruciate ligament remnant: is it worth the hassle? Br Med Bull. 2012;104:91-111.
25. Amis AA, Dawkins GP. Functional anatomy of the anterior cruciate ligament. Fibre bundle actions related to ligament replacements and injuries. J Bone Joint Surg Br. 1991;73:260-7.
26. Chhabra A, Starman JS, Ferretti M, et al. Anatomic, radiographic, biomechanical, and kinematic evaluation of the anterior cruciate ligament and its two functional bundles. J Bone Joint Surg Am. 2006;88(Suppl. 4):2-10.
27. Girgis FG, Marshall JL, Monajem A. The cruciate ligaments of the knee joint. Anatomical, functional and experimental analysis. Clin Orthop Relat Res. 1975;106:216-31.
28. Petersen W, Zantop T. Anatomy of the anterior cruciate ligament with regard to its two bundles. Clin Orthop Relat Res. 2007;454:35-47.
29. Odensten M, Gillquist J. Functional anatomy of the anterior cruciate ligament and a rationale for reconstruction. J Bone Joint Surg Am. 1985;67:257-62.
30. Harner CD, Baek GH, Vogrin TM, et al. Quantitative analysis of human cruciate ligament insertions. Arthroscopy. 1999;15:741-9.
31. Mochizuki T, Muneta T, Nagase T, et al. Cadaveric knee observation study for describing anatomic femoral tunnel placement for two-bundle anterior cruciate ligament reconstruction. Arthroscopy. 2006;22:356-61.
32. Siebold R, Ellert T, Metz S, Metz J. Femoral insertions of the anteromedial and posterolateral bundles of the anterior cruciate ligament: morphometry and arthroscopic orientation models for double-bundle bone tunnel placement–a cadaver study. Arthroscopy. 2008;24:585-92.
33. Harner CD, Livesay GA, Kashiwaguchi S, et al. Comparative study of the size and shape of human anterior and posterior cruciate ligaments. J Orthop Res. 1995;13:429-34.
34. Bicer EK, Lustig S, Servien E, Selmi TA, Neyret P. Current knowledge in the anatomy of the human anterior cruciate ligament. Knee Surg Sports Traumatol Arthrosc. 2010;18:1075-84.
35. Edwards A, Bull AM, Amis AA. The attachments of the anteromedial and posterolateral fibre bundles of the anterior cruciate ligament: Part 1: tibial attachment. Knee Surg Sports Traumatol Arthrosc. 2007;15:1414-21.
36. Kato Y, Ingham SJ, Kramer S, et al. Effect of tunnel position for anatomic single-bundle ACL reconstruction on knee biomechanics in a porcine model. Knee Surg Sports Traumatol Arthrosc. 2010;18:2-10.
37. Morgan CD, Kalman VR, Grawl DM. Definitive landmarks for reproducible tibial tunnel placement in anterior cruciate ligament reconstruction. Arthroscopy. 1995;11:275-88.
38. Zantop T, Petersen W, Sekiya JK, Musahl V, Fu FH. Anterior cruciate ligament anatomy and function relating to anatomical reconstruction. Knee Surg Sports Traumatol Arthrosc. 2006;14:982-92.
39. Colombet P, Robinson J, Christel P, et al. Morphology of anterior cruciate ligament attachments for anatomic reconstruction: a cadaveric dissection and radiographic study. Arthroscopy. 2006;22:984-92.

40. McGuire DA, Hendricks SD, Sanders HM. The relationship between anterior cruciate ligament reconstruction tibial tunnel location and the anterior aspect of the posterior cruciate ligament insertion. Arthroscopy. 1997;13:465-73.
41. Brown CH Jr, Spalding T, Robb C. Medial portal technique for single-bundle anatomical anterior cruciate ligament (ACL) reconstruction. Int Orthop. 2013;37:253-69.
42. Getgood A, Spalding T. The evolution of anatomic anterior cruciate ligament reconstruction. Open Orthop J. 2012;6:287-94.
43. Bernard M, Hertel P, Hornung H, Cierpinski T. Femoral insertion of the ACL. Radiographic quadrant method. Am J Knee Surg. 1997;10:14-21; discussion-2.
44. Lobenhoffer PBM, Agneskirchner J. Quality assurance in cruciate ligament surgery. Arthroscopy. 2003;16:202–8.
45. Passler HH, Hoher J. Intraoperative quality control of the placement of bone tunnels for the anterior cruciate ligament. Unfallchirurg. 2004;107:263-72.
46. Sakane M, Fox RJ, Woo SL, et al. In situ forces in the anterior cruciate ligament and its bundles in response to anterior tibial loads. J Orthop Res. 1997;15:285-93.
47. Butler DL, Noyes FR, Grood ES. Ligamentous restraints to anterior-posterior drawer in the human knee. A biomechanical study. J Bone Joint Surg Am. 1980;62:259-70.
48. Kennedy JC, Hawkins RJ, Willis RB, Danylchuck KD. Tension studies of human knee ligaments. Yield point, ultimate failure, and disruption of the cruciate and tibial collateral ligaments. J Bone Joint Surg Am. 1976;58:350-5.
49. Marinozzi G, Pappalardo S, Steindler R. Human knee ligaments: mechanical tests and ultrastructural observations. Ital J Orthop Traumatol. 1983;9:231-40.
50. Harner CD, Xerogeanes JW, Livesay GA, et al. The human posterior cruciate ligament complex: an interdisciplinary study. Ligament morphology and biomechanical evaluation. Am J Sports Med. 1995;23:736-45.
51. Makris CA, Georgoulis AD, Papageorgiou CD, Moebius UG, Soucacos PN. Posterior cruciate ligament architecture: evaluation under microsurgical dissection. Arthroscopy. 2000;16:627-32.
52. Hatsushika D, Nimura A, Mochizuki T, et al. Attachments of separate small bundles of human posterior cruciate ligament: an anatomic study. Knee Surg Sports Traumatol Arthrosc. 2013;21:998-1004.
53. Race A, Amis AA. PCL reconstruction. In vitro biomechanical comparison of 'isometric' versus single and double-bundled 'anatomic' grafts. J Bone Joint Surg Br. 1998;80:173-9.
54. Van Hoof T, Cromheecke M, Tampere T, et al. The posterior cruciate ligament: a study on its bony and soft tissue anatomy using novel 3D CT technology. Knee Surg Sports Traumatol Arthrosc. 2013;21:1005-10.
55. Kusayama T, Harner CD, Carlin GJ, Xerogeanes JW, Smith BA. Anatomical and biomechanical characteristics of human meniscofemoral ligaments. Knee Surg Sports Traumatol Arthrosc. 1994;2:234-7.
56. Gupte CM, Smith A, Jamieson N, et al. Meniscofemoral ligaments–structural and material properties. J Biomech. 2002;35:1623-9.
57. Gupte CM, Bull AM, Thomas RD, Amis AA. A review of the function and biomechanics of the meniscofemoral ligaments. Arthroscopy. 2003;19:161-71.
58. Grood ES, Stowers SF, Noyes FR. Limits of movement in the human knee. Effect of sectioning the posterior cruciate ligament and posterolateral structures. J Bone Joint Surg Am. 1988;70:88-97.
59. Clark CR, Ogden JA. Development of the menisci of the human knee joint. Morphological changes and their potential role in childhood meniscal injury. J Bone Joint Surg Am. 1983;65:538-47.
60. Arnoczky SP, Warren RF. Microvasculature of the human meniscus. Am J Sports Med. 1982;10:90-5.
61. Allaire R, Muriuki M, Gilbertson L, Harner CD. Biomechanical consequences of a tear of the posterior root of the medial meniscus. Similar to total meniscectomy. J Bone Joint Surg Am. 2008;90:1922-31.
62. Harner CD, Mauro CS, Lesniak BP, Romanowski JR. Biomechanical consequences of a tear of the posterior root of the medial meniscus. Surgical technique. J Bone Joint Surg Am. 2009;91(Suppl. 2):257-70.
63. Marzo JM, Gurske-DePerio J. Effects of medial meniscus posterior horn avulsion and repair on tibiofemoral contact area and peak contact pressure with clinical implications. Am J Sports Med. 2009;37:124-9.
64. RJ L. The popliteus muscle and the lateral meniscus. J Bone Joint Surg Br. 1950;32:93.

65. Ahmed AM, Burke DL. In-vitro measurement of static pressure distribution in synovial joints—Part I: tibial surface of the knee. J Biomech Eng. 1983;105:216-25.
66. Baratz ME, Fu FH, Mengato R. Meniscal tears: the effect of meniscectomy and of repair on intraarticular contact areas and stress in the human knee. A preliminary report. Am J Sports Med. 1986;14:270-5.
67. Fairbank TJ. Knee joint changes after meniscectomy. J Bone Joint Surg Br. 1948;30B:664-70.
68. Ihn JC, Kim SJ, Park IH. In vitro study of contact area and pressure distribution in the human knee after partial and total meniscectomy. Int Orthop. 1993;17:214-8.
69. Voloshin AS, Wosk J. Shock absorption of meniscectomized and painful knees: a comparative in vivo study. J Biomed Eng. 1983;5:157-61.
70. Warren LF, Marshall JL. The supporting structures and layers on the medial side of the knee: an anatomical analysis. J Bone Joint Surg Am. 1979;61:56-62.
71. Brantigan OC VA. The tibial collateral ligament: its function, its bursae, and its relation to the medial meniscus. J Bone Joint Surg Am. 1943;25:121-31.
72. Robinson JR, Bull AM, Thomas RR, Amis AA. The role of the medial collateral ligament and posteromedial capsule in controlling knee laxity. Am J Sports Med. 2006;34:1815-23.
73. Sims WF, Jacobson KE. The posteromedial corner of the knee: medial-sided injury patterns revisited. Am J Sports Med. 2004;32:337-45.
74. LaPrade RF, Engebretsen AH, Ly TV, et al. The anatomy of the medial part of the knee. J Bone Joint Surg Am. 2007;89:2000-10.
75. Brantigan OC VA. The mechanics of the ligaments and menisci of the knee joint. J Bone Joint Surg Am. 1941;23:44-66.
76. Ml W. The Knee: Form, Function, and Ligament Reconstruction. New York, NY: Springer-Verlag; 1985.
77. Steensen RN, Dopirak RM, McDonald WG 3rd. The anatomy and isometry of the medial patellofemoral ligament: implications for reconstruction. Am J Sports Med. 2004;32:1509-13.
78. Amis AA, Firer P, Mountney J, Senavongse W, Thomas NP. Anatomy and biomechanics of the medial patellofemoral ligament. Knee. 2003;10:215-20.
79. Feller JA, Feagin JA Jr, Garrett WE Jr. The medial patellofemoral ligament revisited: an anatomical study. Knee Surg Sports Traumatol Arthrosc. 1993;1:184-6.
80. Tuxoe JI, Teir M, Winge S, Nielsen PL. The medial patellofemoral ligament: a dissection study. Knee Surg Sports Traumatol Arthrosc. 2002;10:138-40.
81. Haimes JL, Wroble RR, Grood ES, Noyes FR. Role of the medial structures in the intact and anterior cruciate ligament-deficient knee. Limits of motion in the human knee. Am J Sports Med. 1994;22:402-9.
82. Griffith CJ, LaPrade RF, Johansen S, et al. Medial knee injury: Part 1. Static function of the individual components of the main medial knee structures. Am J Sports Med. 2009;37:1762-70.
83. Ritchie JR, Bergfeld JA, Kambic H, Manning T. Isolated sectioning of the medial and posteromedial capsular ligaments in the posterior cruciate ligament-deficient knee. Influence on posterior tibial translation. Am J Sports Med. 1998;26:389-94.
84. Ml W. The Knee: Form, Function, and Ligament Reconstruction. New York, NY: Springer-Verlag; 1985.
85. Wijdicks CA, Griffith CJ, LaPrade RF, et al. Medial knee injury: Part 2. Load sharing between the posterior oblique ligament and superficial medial collateral ligament. Am J Sports Med. 2009;37:1771-6.
86. Seebacher JR, Inglis AE, Marshall JL, Warren RF. The structure of the posterolateral aspect of the knee. J Bone Joint Surg Am. 1982;64:536-41.
87. Terry GC, LaPrade RF. The biceps femoris muscle complex at the knee. Its anatomy and injury patterns associated with acute anterolateral-anteromedial rotatory instability. Am J Sports Med. 1996;24:2-8.
88. Kaplan EB. The iliotibial tract; clinical and morphological significance. J Bone Joint Surg Am. 1958;40-A:817-32.
89. Kaplan EB. Some aspects of functional anatomy of the human knee joint. Clin Orthop. 1962;23:18-29.
90. Fulkerson JP, Gossling HR. Anatomy of the knee joint lateral retinaculum. Clin Orthop Relat Res. 1980;183-8.
91. Last RJ. Anatomy: Regional and Applied, 8th edition. Churchill Livingstone, London;1990.
92. Kaplan EB. The fabellofibular and short lateral ligaments of the knee joint. J Bone Joint Surg Am. 1961;43-A:169-79.

93. Maynard MJ, Deng X, Wickiewicz TL, Warren RF. The popliteofibular ligament. Rediscovery of a key element in posterolateral stability. Am J Sports Med. 1996;24:311-6.
94. Staubli HU, Birrer S. The popliteus tendon and its fascicles at the popliteal hiatus: gross anatomy and functional arthroscopic evaluation with and without anterior cruciate ligament deficiency. Arthroscopy. 1990;6:209-20.
95. Basmajian JV, Lovejoy JF Jr. Functions of the popliteus muscle in man. A multifactorial electromyographic study. J Bone Joint Surg Am. 1971;53:557-62.
96. Mann RA, Hagy JL. The popliteus muscle. J Bone Joint Surg Am. 1977;59:924-7.
97. Baker CL Jr, Norwood LA, Hughston JC. Acute posterolateral rotatory instability of the knee. J Bone Joint Surg Am. 1983;65:614-8.
98. Hughston JC, Andrews JR, Cross MJ, Moschi A. Classification of knee ligament instabilities. Part II. The lateral compartment. J Bone Joint Surg Am. 1976; 58:173-9.
99. Reider B, Marshall JL, Koslin B, Ring B, Girgis FG. The anterior aspect of the knee joint. J Bone Joint Surg Am. 1981;63:351-6.
100. Dye SF, Campagna-Pinto D, Dye CC, Shifflett S, Eiman T. Soft-tissue anatomy anterior to the human patella. J Bone Joint Surg Am. 2003;85-A:1012-7.
101. Kennedy JC, Alexander IJ, Hayes KC. Nerve supply of the human knee and its functional importance. Am J Sports Med. 1982;10:329-35.

Chapter 32

History of Arthroscopy

P Sripathi Rao

The desire to know about and peep into body cavities has always been an obsession with humankind. By all accounts, the earliest evidence for this has been the discovery of primitive proctoscopes in the ruins of Pompeii. Hebrew literature does refer to the vaginal speculum. Open cavities like the rectum and vagina were definitely more accessible than closed cavities since illumination was not necessary.

The urinary bladder with its plethora of secrets was the first closed visceral structure to be visualized through an endoscopic device. In 1806, Botzini, a German surgeon (1773–1809), presented his 'Lichtleiter' to the Joseph Academy of Medical Surgery in Vienna. This device consisted of two tubes. The first tube conducted candlelight into the bladder and the second tube served as the viewing channel.[1] This attempt was not received with the attention that it deserved.

Pierce Segalas presented a Bozzini like instrument to the Academic des Sciences in 1826. His use of glow-worms (lampyrids) as a source of light was challenged by Herteloupe who labeled it as an act of plagiarism.[2]

In 1853, Desormaux laboriously constructed an endoscope that he called the 'gasogene cystoscope'. This device utilized the light emitted by the combustion of gasoline and turpentine as a source of illumination. Light was conducted into the bladder by a set of mirrors. As cumbersome and hazardous it was, the gasogene cystoscope is considered to be the harbinger of endoscopy.[3]

FR Cruise of Dublin (1865) improved on the illumination of the gasogene cystoscope by using a mixture of petrol and camphor for combustion. He added a mahogany case to protect the surgeon's hands from the heat of the lamp.[4]

The first modern cystoscope as developed by Max Nitze in 1876. A platinum loop heated by electricity provided the light. A water-cooled goose quill served for the safe passage of the platinum loop into the bladder.

The year 1880 was a watershed year for endoscopy, as Edison developed the incandescent light bulb. It was but a logical step to utilize the light bulb for endoscopic illumination. The first cystoscope of this description was developed by Leiter and Nitze in Germany in 1886. They took photographs of the interior of the bladder in 1890. In the year 1910, Hans Christian Jacobeus used an endoscope with an incandescent light bulb for the diagnosis of abdominal conditions. Its use was extended to the thorax in the treatment of pleural adhesions caused by tuberculosis. The instrument came to be called the 'laparothoracoscope'.[3]

Dr Nordentoft, a Danish surgeon presented his work on suprapubic cystoscopy, laparoscopy, and knee arthroscopy at the 41st Congress of the German Society of Surgeons in Berlin in the year 1912. He used a 5 mm endoscope, similar to the Jacobeus laparothoracoscope in design and construction. Though Nordentoft's paper received scant notice, he was the first surgeon to use an endoscope to look at the interiors of the knee joint.[5]

The three significant contributors to the development of arthroscopy after the 1st World War were Professor Kenji Takagi from Tokyo; Eugene Bircher, a Swiss physician and Michael Burman of the Hospital for Joint Disease in New York.

PROFESSOR KENJI TAKAGI (1888–1963)

Tuberculosis of the knee joint was a significant cause of morbidity in Japan. In an effort at early diagnosis of this malady, Takagi developed arthroscopes to view the interior of the knee joint. His first arthroscope was 7.3 mm in diameter and unwieldy for practical use. Takagi persisted in his endeavor to design narrower scopes and presented a 3.5 mm diameter arthroscope in 1931. A constant striver in the improvement of design and optics, Takagi can be credited to be the first innovator in arthroscopy. He also discussed distension of the knee joint with saline for better visualization.[3,6]

EUGENE BIRCHER (1882–1956)

In 1921, Eugene Bircher, a Swiss surgeon and politician published his experience with the arthroendoscope in the diagnosis of meniscal pathology in the knee joint.[3] Following the diagnostic arthroendoscopy, Bircher managed the meniscal pathology through an arthrotomy. His endoscope suffered from a limited field of vision and poor illumination. Perhaps disillusioned, Bircher abandoned arthroscopy in later years and concentrated on developing air-arthrography to diagnose meniscal pathology.

MICHAEL BURMAN (1883–1943)

As a resident at the Hospital for Joint Disease, New York, Burman began using the arthroscope (made by a Mr R Wappler) on cadaver knee joints. Burman later worked with Professor George Schmorl, professor of pathology in Dresden, Germany on a project to study the effects of dyes injected into the knee, on degenerative joint cartilage. He continued a clinical trait of arthroscopy on live patients and published the results of his research in a paper 'arthroscopy or direct visualization of joints'. Though his initial findings were published in art form from Dresden, his later pictures remained unpublished for want of an interested publisher.

The Second World War impeded the publication of further developments and experience in the field of arthroscopy. It took more than 15 years for serious work to resume.

MASAKI WATANABE (1911–1994)

A young intelligence officer in the Japanese army, Masaki Watanabe, rejoined the University of Tokyo after the end of the World War. Having seen the 12 scopes designed by Takagi, his mentor, Watanabe decided to pursue on further research on the arthroscope. He was helped by the Japanese electronic and optic industry in the production of the 13th and 14th arthroscopes. In order to document his arthroscopic findings, Watanabe added an additional light source introduced through an accessory portal. Armed with a video of arthroscopy, he traveled extensively in the USA, to show his film to the orthopedic fraternity. He made few converts to the field and returned to Japan.

The Number 21 Arthroscope

Watanabe concentrated on producing a better arthroscope than the number 14, in which the light guide could be housed in the sheath itself. His designs from numbers 15-19 proved to be impractical. His constant efforts produced the number 21 arthroscope in 1958. Thought the outer diameter of the arthroscope was 6 mm, it had an outstanding, carefully hand-grounded lens. The number 21 arthroscope had a field of vision of 101° (almost equivalent to the human eye) and a depth of focus from zero to infinity. With its special features, the number 21 arthroscope hit the publication line and sold modestly around the world. The last arthroscope to utilize the incandescent light bulb, the number 21 arthroscope eventually suffered a foreseeable fate–breakage of the offset tungsten bulb inside the joint. Despite its drawbacks, Watanabe number 21 was the first arthroscope to be used by many arthroscopists around the world.

After the Number 21 Arthroscope

The incandescent light bulb gave way to the incorporated fiber light in 1967 the number 22 arthroscope. The first ultrathin fiberoptic endoscope with a diameter of 2 mm was named the number 25 arthroscope. This arthroscope formed the basis of the dyonic needle scope.

ARTHROSCOPIC SURGERY AND THE CONCEPT OF TRIANGULATION

The transition of the arthroscope from a mere diagnostic tool to an operative modality was carefully guided by Watanabe. He successfully excised a xanthomatous tumor from the superior recesses of the knee in 1955 and went on to perform the first loose body removal in 1961 and partial meniscectomy in 1962.

Arthroscopic surgery of the knee was facilitated by the concept of 'triangulation'. Simply put, triangulation is the technique by which instruments are brought from different portals to operate on the lesion under vision. The arthroscope, the lesion and the surgeon form the three sides of the triangle. Watanabe contributed extensively to the improvement in arthroscopic design, enhancement of illumination and widening the field of vision. As his innovations empowered arthroscopists to operate on a wider spectrum of knee joint pathology, Watanabe is credited with the development of the concept of triangulation.

In 1951, the first atlas of arthroscopy was published by Watanabe, with Takeda and Ikenchi as [1]coauthors. The atlas was revised in 1969 with photographs of joint disease replacing illustrations.

ARTHROSCOPY IN THE UNITED STATES

Dr Robert Jackson of Toronto went to Tokyo University in 1964 with the objective of learning tissue culture techniques. He returned committed to the technique of arthroscopic surgery and its advancement in the Western World. In addition to practicing arthroscopic surgery, Jackson exhibited great zeal in spreading its knowledge, technique and skills through teaching sessions, lecture, learning laboratories and audiovisual presentations. Richard O'Connor joined him in the instructional courses. A free-thinking maverick, Dr Connor refined the technique of partial meniscectomy and developed better cutting instruments.

Dr John Joyce III and S Ward Casscells took leading roles in the teaching of arthroscopy in North America. Robert Metcalf was the first to establish an independent surgical center for arthroscopy that was a successful financial model.

John B McGinty's significant contribution to the spread of arthroscopy was in from the book which he edited 'Operative Arthroscopy'. Lanny Johnson extended arthroscopy to other diarthrodial joints. The credit for developing the motorized shaver belongs to Lanny Johnson. He also introduced 'abrasive arthroplasty' in degenerative joint disease. Richard Caspari started exclusively using the television monitor for visualization and contributed significantly to the development of shoulder arthroscopy.[3]

ARTHROSCOPY IN EUROPE

Harold Eikelaar was the first person to receive a PhD in arthroscopy from the University of Groningen in the Netherlands in 1975. The Storz company in Germany helped him to develop the 30° forward oblique arthroscope which enlarged the field of vision when rotated inside the joint.

The teaching of arthroscopy in Europe was taken forward by Eriksson and Gillquist. Gillquist also promoted the central portal to the knee, through the patellar tendon. David Dandy, in addition to promoting arthroscopy in England, coauthored the first textbook on arthroscopy.

REFERENCES

1. Bush RB, Leonhardt H, Bush IV, Landes RR. Dr. Bozzini's Lichtleiter. A translation of his original article (1806). Urology. 1974;3(1):119-23.
2. Herteloupe CLS. Lettre a I' Academie des Sciences; 1827.
3. Jackson RW. A history of arthroscopy. Arthroscopy. 2010;26(1):91-103.
4. Murphy LJT. History of Urology. Springfield, IL: Charles C Thomas; 1972.
5. Keiser CW, Jackson RW. Severin Nordentoft: the first arthroscopist. Arthroscopy. 2001;17(5):532-5.
6. Takagi K. Practical experience using Takagi's arthroscope. J Jpn Orthop Assoc. 1933;8:132.

Chapter 33

Portals in Knee Arthroscopy

Nicholas A Antao, Nirav N Antao

The word portal comes from 'porte' that means door. However, the entry to the knee is through a keyhole incision and not a door, and the terminology used is portal and not porthole. The patient for arthroscopic surgery lies in a supine position after general, regional, or local anesthesia.[1] The procedure is mostly performed with a well-padded tourniquet applied at least 8 fingerbreadths above the top of the patella. The knee should be free to bend to 90° or more, with or without a leg holder, either on a straight table or a table bent to allow the knee to hang (**Figure 33.1**). The leg holder allows you to apply valgus/varus forces to the knee and the freedom to put the knee in a figure of four position to see the lateral compartment (**Figures 33.2 and 33.3**). It is also vital that the 11 no. blade is perfectly fitted into the knife handle because it has the potential to get stuck in the fat pad if not attached properly to it. Surface marking of the patella, ligamentum patellae, tibial tubercle, medial and lateral joint line, and the posterior contours of the medial and lateral femoral condyle should be done at the beginning stage of arthroscopy (**Figure 33.4**). The cardinal keys to a successful arthroscopy are the presence of adequate light, distension of the joint, precise location of the portals for good visualization, and smooth instrumentation. It is very important to make sure that the arthroscopy equipment like camera, light source, light cable, television monitor, shaver system, and arthroscopy instrumentation are in perfect workable condition before induction of anesthesia.

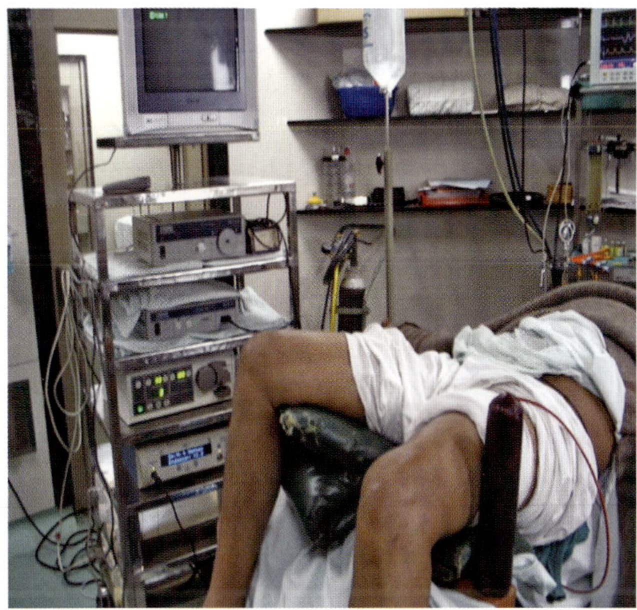

Figure 33.1 Position of the knee for arthroscopy

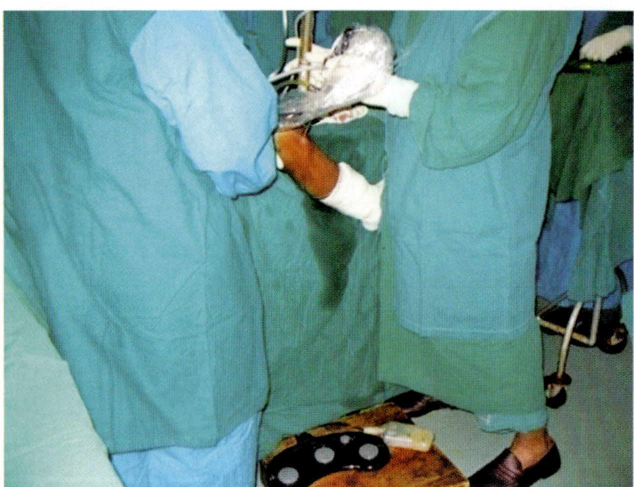

Figure 33.2 Valgus position of the knee to see medial compartment

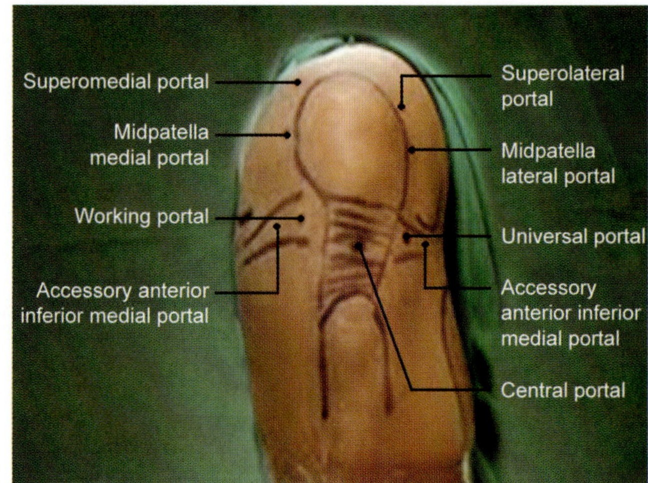

Figure 33.4 Surface marking of the knee with various portals

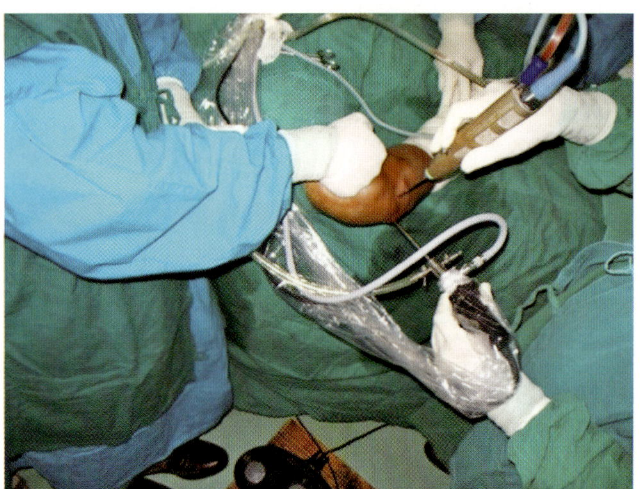

Figure 33.3 Figure of four position of the knee to see lateral compartment

The inflow cannula may or may not be used as most arthroscopes sheaths have irrigation through the sheath. Always drain the blood from the joint either through aspiration or irrigation, so that the returning fluid from the sheath is as clear as the inflow fluid. It is therefore absolutely necessary to thoroughly lavage the joint clear of blood or fat globules.

PORTALS

The portals are divided into anterior, posterior, and accessory. Anterior and posterior portals can be further subdivided into primary and secondary portals. Primary portals are more frequently used. The primary anterior portals are inferior lateral also known as universal and inferomedial (working portal). The secondary anterior portals are midlateral, midmedial, central, superomedial or superolateral and accessory inferomedial, and inferolateral. The posterior primary ones are the posteromedial and posterolateral, and the posterior secondary ones are the high superior or low inferior ones to the posteromedial or posterolateral portal.[2,3] The trans-septal portal is also an accessory posterior portal.[2]

UNIVERSAL (INFEROLATERAL) PORTAL

This is the first portal that is made blind, while the rest of the portals are made under vision of the camera. Therefore, it is important to make sure that this portal is made properly and accurately to avoid portal problems. It is also called the anterolateral portal. This portal is very vital because the scalpel blade could accidentally slice a bit of cartilage of the lateral condyle, the menisci, or cruciate ligaments if not done properly. If this first portal is poorly placed, then the whole arthroscopy could become incredibly difficult. This portal is most widely used by almost all arthroscopy surgeons and hence called universal portal.[4-7]

The universal portal is ideally taken at the soft spot on the outer side of the inferior pole of the patella at the intersection of the transverse perpendicular line drawn at the inferior pole of the patella and vertical line from the outer border of the tibial tubercle. This point corresponds to a point just about a centimeter lateral to the outer border of ligamentum patellae below the inferior pole of the patella and above the lateral joint line. It is important to palpate the spot just above the infrapatellar fat pad. If the portal is too superior, then the chances of hitting the lateral femoral condyle articular cartilage increase and the posterior horns of the menisci are not properly visualized. However, if the portal is far too inferior, one can get lost in the fat pad, or damage the anterior horn of the lateral meniscus. If it is too medial, then the damage to the ligamentum patellae and articular cartilage of the patella is likely to occur. A far too lateral portal can increase the chances of being lost in the fat pad or can make entry into the knee joint particularly difficult due to less joint space being available.[4-7] This portal has limitations of not adequately visualizing the PCL, anterior horn of lateral menisci, and posterior horn of menisci in tight knees.

INCISION

It is important to infiltrate the portal spot with lidocaine containing adrenaline to avoid bleeding and reduce pain. Alternatively, the incision can also be taken without infiltration before introducing the arthroscope sheath with blunt trocar. The incision is made with an 11 no. blade with the knee straight angling the scalpel toward the intercondylar notch and the sharp end of the blade facing laterally to avoid accidental damage to the ligamentum patellae. It should be about 4 mm either vertical or transverse in line with the crease or Langer lines (**Figure 33.5**). The benefit of taking a vertical incision is that the scope can be moved up and down easily. However, a drawback of this approach is that the chances of damaging the transverse branches of the infrapatellar branch of the medial saphenous nerve (**Figure 33.6**) increase giving rise to painful neuroma.[3] The transverse incision is preferred, as it avoids injury to the nerve[8] and gives the freedom of greater side to side mobility to the scope making the incision with the knee straight, in which position the knee cap is up and out of the way. The surgeon should use the index finger as a stop on the scalpel blade to prevent deeper penetration. The scalpel is removed and

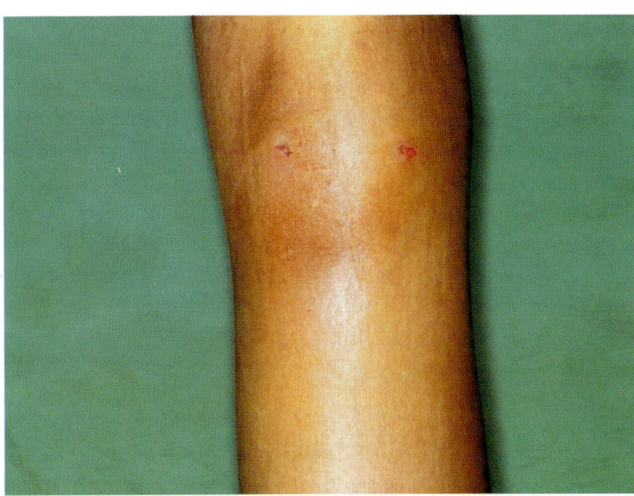

Figure 33.5 Transverse incision for portal

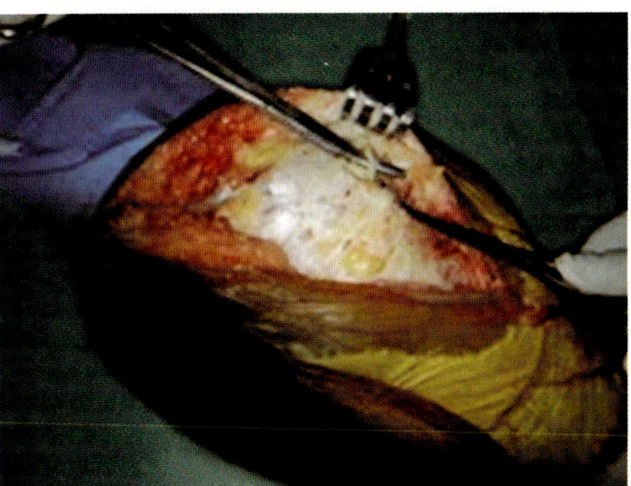

Figure 33.6 Infrapatellar transverse branches of the medial saphenous nerve crossing the knee dissected and isolated with a mosquito

the sheath of the arthroscope, containing a blunt trocar, is inserted in the same direction into the knee flexed at 30°. It is directed toward the intercondylar notch after which the knee is extended to 0° to guide the sheath with trocar into the suprapatellar pouch. The blunt trocar is then removed and the telescope is inserted into the sheath.[6]

INFEROMEDIAL PORTAL (ANTEROMEDIAL PORTAL/WORKING PORTAL/INSTRUMENT PORTAL)

This portal is made under direct vision, with the help of an 18 no. spinal needle to locate the ideal point of entry for the operating instrument. This enables access to the pathology without much difficulty, without stressing the operating instrument and without scuffing the articular cartilage of the medial femoral condyle. Once the point of entry is selected, sometimes after multiple attempts with the needle, the final selected point is infiltrated with lidocaine containing adrenaline. It is normally 1 cm below the universal portal, 1 cm above the medial joint line, 1 cm medial to the ligamentum patellae and 1 cm below the inferior pole of the patella.[4-7] The point of entry is then incised to make a 4 mm incision with the 11 no. blade facing away from ligamentum patellae after which the entry point is dilated with a mosquito. It is helpful to view the whole of the lateral compartment, to palpate the medial meniscus and posterior horn of the medial meniscus and the anterior horn of the lateral meniscus with the probe. The entry point should not be too medial to avoid troublesome entry into a pad of fat that obscures the operating view and makes instrument entry difficult, or too inferior to avoid damage to the meniscus and the condyles.

ACCESSORY ANTERIOR INFERIOR MEDIAL PORTAL

It is a portal that is placed just 5–8 mm medial to the inferior medial portal under vision to make sure that there is no damage to the menisci and articular cartilage while using the 18 no. needle. It came into prominence with the advent of double bundle anatomical anterior cruciate ligament (ACL) reconstruction. The portal helps to give a better view of the anatomic footprint of the ACL on the medial wall of the lateral femoral condyle. Similarly, an accessory anterior inferior lateral portal can be made lateral to the universal portal.

SUPEROLATERAL PORTAL

This portal is located above the superior pole of the patella 2.5 cm lateral to the superolateral part of the outer border of the patella lateral to the quadriceps tendon. It is useful to view the tracking and dynamics of the patellofemoral articulation. It can act also as the drainage portal for entry and outflow, to resect the plicae, to remove loose bodies, for synovectomy and for the release of the lateral retinaculum.[4,5,7]

SUPEROMEDIAL PORTAL

This portal is located 2.5 cm medial to the superomedial border of the patella, medial to quadriceps tendon, and is often used as an inflow portal. It also used to remove plicae, loose bodies, placation of the medial retinaculum and synovectomy.[4,5,7]

MIDPATELLAR LATERAL/MEDIAL PORTAL

This portal was described by Dr Dinesh Patel to avoid crowding of instruments while operating and to facilitate arthroscopy surgery by better viewing of the anterior compartment structures and the popliteal tunnel. It is taken at the midpoint of the patella in straight position, just 8–10 mm lateral to the outer border of patella on the lateral side. The arthroscope is introduced from this portal in the midlateral/midmedial position looking from the top and the inferior lateral and inferior medial portals are free to use operating instruments. It is difficult to view the posterior horns with this portal. A proper selection of the portal is necessary; a site far off the medial and lateral edges can jeopardize the view of the joint. The portal at times is used during the procedure for arthroscopic fixation of the avulsed tibial spine with the ACL attached with a cannulated screw.[9]

CENTRAL PORTAL

This portal was described by Dr Guilquist (**Figure 33.7**). It is also known as the Swedish portal. It is made through the tendon of the ligamentum patellae 1 cm below the inferior pole of the patella. The knee is flexed to 90°, and the skin and the subcutaneous tissue are incised. The tendon is split with mosquito or trocar. This portal allows the inferomedial and lateral portals to be made available for bimanual manipulation in the anterior joint. This portal allows good view of the posterior compartment in the intercondylar notch. This portal can damage the patellar tendon, and can be very difficult in situations where there is thickening and hypertrophy of infrapatellar pad of

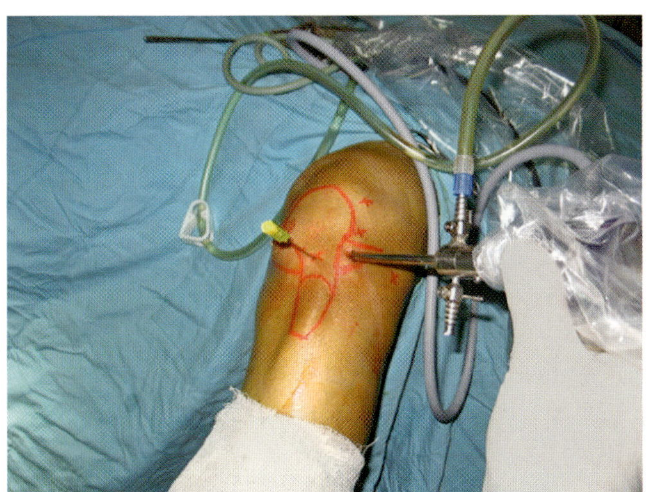

Figure 33.7 Central portal (Guilquist portal) being depicted by a spinal needle

fat. This portal can be also used for viewing the femoral footprint of the ACL and anatomical reconstruction.[10]

POSTERIOR PORTALS (POSTEROMEDIAL)

This portal is located in a small triangular soft spot formed by the posteromedial edge of the femoral condyle and posteromedial edge of the tibia. The posteromedial compartment is small, but any arthroscope can be inserted into it with due care and delicate technique (**Figures 33.8A and B**).

PREREQUISITES BEFORE DOING THIS PORTAL

The knee has to be maximally distended with saline so that the soft spots bulge and it becomes easier to identify especially in the obese and muscular patients. The bony landmarks need to be marked before distension.[11] The knee should be flexed to 90° to allow the neurovascular structures to fall back posteriorly.[12]

SURFACE MARKING

Anatomically, the entry point of the portal is 1 cm above the joint line 2.5 cm superior to the medial femoral condyle, anterior to the medial head of gastrocnemius, posterior to the medial collateral ligament and medial femoral epicondyle and superior to pes anserinus.[11,13] It is necessary to take care to avoid injury to the infrapatellar branch of medial saphenous nerve 1 cm above the joint line that runs into the fat above the sartorius.

An 18 no. spinal needle is used 2.5 cm superior to the medial femoral condyle to make the entry point and is directed to puncture the capsule to enter the joint. The accepted point is then infiltrated with lidocaine with adrenaline. An 11 no. scalpel blade is used to make the point of entry with a stab incision that is then widened with a mosquito to dissect the sartorial fascia and the capsule

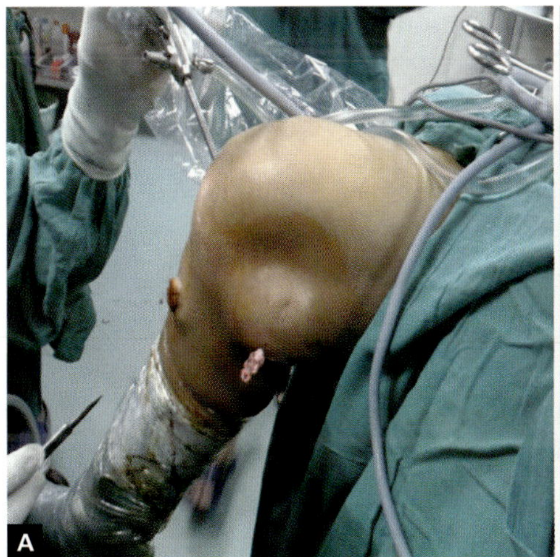

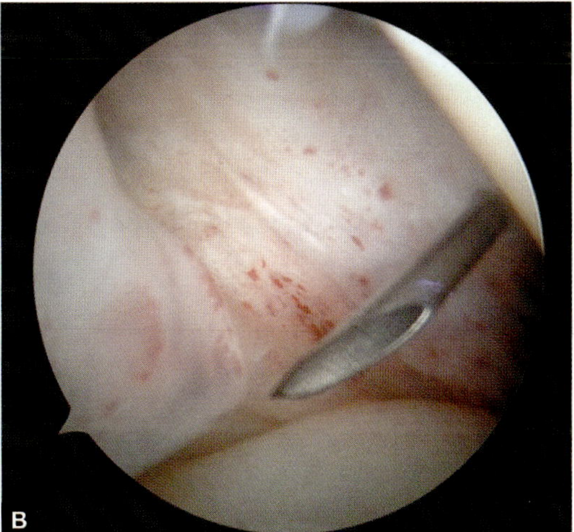

Figures 33.8A and B Spinal needle showing posterior medial portal from the outside and inside

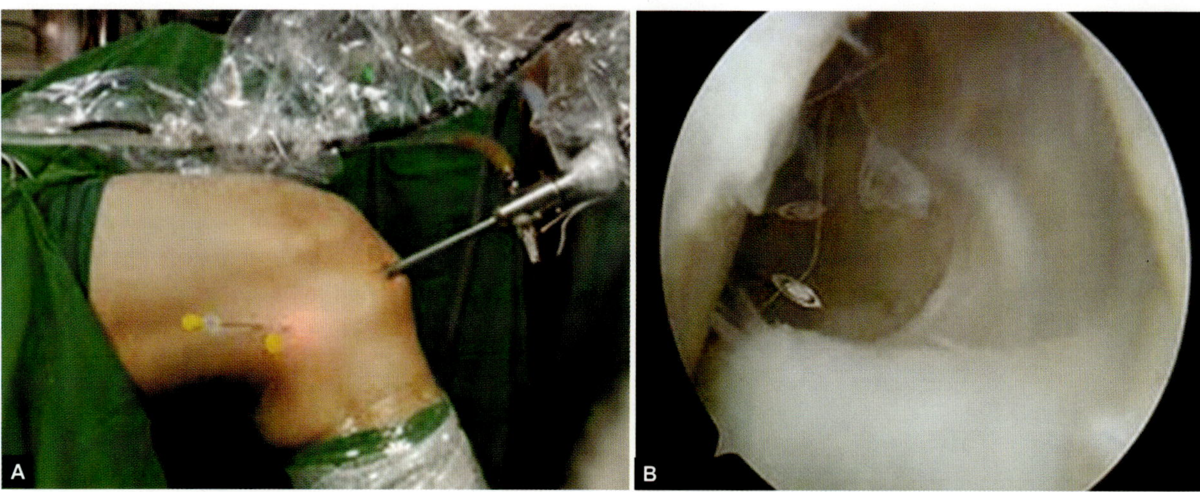

Figures 33.9A and B Spinal needle showing posterolateral lateral portal from the outside and inside

to protect the saphenous nerve.[12] A Wissinger rod is then passed through the entry point and the cannula/sheath of the scope is then driven over the rod.

Uses of this Portal

This portal is very helpful to visualize the posterior horn of the meniscus and for the repair or resection of the avulsed root and torn posterior part of the meniscus. It is also useful in the resection of meniscal cysts, the removal of loose bodies and cysts located in the posterior compartment, in synovectomy of the posterior compartment, in the facilitation of the trans-septal portal and most frequently for surgery of the PCL either during reconstruction or fixation of the avulsed PCL with bony stump.[11-14]

Risks

This portal runs the risk of injury to the saphenous nerve.

POSTEROLATERAL PORTAL

It is essential to flex the knee to 90° with maximal distension using saline to facilitate the entry point to this portal.[12]

Anatomical Landmarks

This portal is situated 2 cm above the lateral joint line at the point of intersection of the posterior margin of the femoral cortex and the posterior aspects of the fibula, behind the posterior edge of the iliotibial band. [11,12,15] An 18 no. spinal needle is used to localize this point. The accepted point is then infiltrated with lidocaine with adrenaline and then incised with 11 no. scalpel blade, dilated later with a mosquito penetrating the capsule. The Wissinger rod is then used to enter the joint and a cannula/sheath is driven over it to the joint **(Figures 33.9A and B)**.

Uses of the Portal

Portal is used to visualize the posterior compartment, remove the loose bodies in the posterior compartment, make the trans-septal portal, and for synovectomy of the posterior compartment.

Risks

This portal has to be made carefully to avoid damage to the articular cartilage. It can also damage the peroneal nerve and the tendon of biceps femoris.

POSTERO ACCESSORY SECONDARY PORTALS

Posteromedial/posterolateral accessory portals are either slightly inferior or superior to the main portal. They are used to make additional portals to facilitate the use of operating instruments during surgery in the posterior compartment.[12-15]

TRANS-SEPTAL PORTAL

This portal was first described by Ahn. It is made by using a combination of posteromedial and posterolateral portals. The procedure involves removal of the septum with a shaver blade behind the PCL to get a good view of the posterior part of the knee. [2,16]

Uses of the Portal

To do surgery in the posterior compartment like synovectomy, adhesiolysis, removal of loose bodies, fixation of the avulsed bone fragment with PCL and cysts in the posterior compartment.[2,13-16]

MANAGEMENT OF ARTHROSCOPY PORTALS

After the procedure, it is important to empty the joint. The portals can either be kept open or sutured or closed with a tape. The evidence-based medicine suggests that there is no difference in the final outcome with either technique.[3] I like to keep the portals open in order to avoid hemarthrosis and pain due to the distension. I always use a Jones compression bandage after the procedure. The bulky dressing is removed after 3–5 days. The patient is encouraged to do quadriceps exercises and crutch walking depending upon the type of operative procedure.

COMPLICATIONS OF ARTHROSCOPY

Arthroscopy of the knee is considered a safe and successful procedure. As with any operative procedure, there are associated complications. While the complication rate is very low, it is important to be aware of the types of complications and their management. Knee pain, swelling, bruising and discomfort around the portal site are commonly seen post-surgery and typically resolve with time. They are not considered complications.

IATROGENIC ARTICULAR CARTILAGE DAMAGE

This kind of damage is the most common complication often encountered during the learning phase of arthroscopy. It may occur if the sheath with trocar is introduced too forcibly or during instrumentation if the portals are not well angulated to the lesion/pathology. It is seen more often in tight knees, stiff knees and due to the use of sharp trocar. It is therefore essential to avoid using the sharp trocar and only use blunt trocar. The cartilage scuffing normally heals well with time but in deeper and broader lesions with a loose flap of articular cartilage, it needs to excised. Postoperatively one might encounter residual synovitis till the cartilage lesion is healed.

HEMARTHROSIS

Hemarthrosis is more common after operative procedures like ligament reconstruction and lateral release.[17-19] A small amount of hemarthrosis subsides with ice therapy, compression bandage and quadriceps exercises. A tense hematoma needs to be aspirated and lavaged. The patient should be advised crutch walking and non-weight-bearing mobilization till the pain disappears.

THROMBOEMBOLISM

Thromboembolism has the tendency to occur postoperatively in middle-aged groups, especially those who have significant risk factors or previous history of thrombosis or embolism.[17] It is rarely seen in younger patients and those who participate/engage in sports. One must always be aware of this entity and take proper precautions. Small reported the incidence of thromboembolism in 0.17% of patients postarthroscopy.[19]

Infection at the Portal Site

This is normally a result of prolonged surgery more frequently seen with the medial portal than the lateral portal. It is important to take the precaution of sending the fluid for culture and sensitivity and to use appropriate antibiotics when the wound ends are inflamed. Sometimes, the portal takes a little longer time than usual to heal.

Synovial Fistula

In this rare complication, the portal takes an unusually long time to heal, with discharge of synovial fluid from the joint through the portal. When this situation arises, the fluid needs to be sent for culture and sensitivity and the patient's knee should be immobilized in a plaster cast for 2–3 weeks with the patient ambulating on crutches without bearing weight. DeLee's retrospective study of 118,590 arthroscopic surgeries reported 30 cases of synovial fistulae, 70% of which successfully responded to conservative treatment involving immobilization in cast.[20]

Nerve Injury

Neurological injury can occur during arthroscopy as a result of: (1) direct trauma to a nerve, (2) as a result of pressure in compartment syndrome due to extravasation of fluid, (3) prolonged use of tourniquet, (4) and rarely due to autonomic system disturbances as in reflex sympathetic dystrophy.[21]

The incidence of nerve injury is often from incorrect placement of the portals and sharp trocars. It therefore can be reduced by correctly placing the portal and using the blunt trocar. A nerve that is frequently damaged is the infrapatellar branch of the medial saphenous nerve at the anterior inferomedial portal with a vertical incision and the saphenous nerve usually from the posteromedial portal during inside out meniscal repair. Damage to the infrapatellar branch can sometimes be unavoidable due to the wide variability in its path.[8,17] The common peroneal nerve can be prone to injury during a posterolateral portal especially in lateral meniscus inside out repair. This can be avoided by proper flexion of the knee, direct dissection and identification and use of adequate retraction. The other cause is neuropraxia due to improper tensioning and padding of tourniquet and longer duration of tourniquet use.[21]

COMPLEX REGIONAL PAIN SYNDROME (CRPS)

Formerly referred to as reflex sympathetic dystrophy, this is a rare complication characterized by pain that is out of proportion.[17] Studies have reported that patients with patellofemoral injury, disease or surgery or damage to cutaneous nerves or the saphenous nerve and its branches are potentially vulnerable to CRPS.[17] The rehabilitation and treatment period can be very long.

COMPARTMENT SYNDROME

This occurs as a result of prolonged surgery, due to extravasation of fluid used for distention of the joint and also unidentified capsular injuries before surgery. Such an entity is an emergency procedure and has to be immediately decompressed after diagnosis to prevent disabling sequelae of compartment syndrome.

REFERENCES

1. Jackson RW. Current concepts review: arthroscopic surgery. J Bone Joint Surg. 1983; 65-A:416-20.
2. Ahn JH, Ha CW. Posterior trans-septal portal for arthroscopic surgery of the knee. Arthroscopy. 2000;16:774-9.
3. Hussein R, Southgate GW. Management of knee arthroscopy portals. Knee. 2001:8(4):329-31.
4. Dandy DJ. Arthroscopy of the knee. Br J Hosp Med. 1982;27(4):360, 362, 365.
5. Johnson LL. Arthroscopic Surgery: Principles and Practice, 3rd edition. The CV Mosby Company, United States; 1986.
6. McGinty JB, Freedmann PA. Arthroscopy of the knee. Clin Orthop. 1976;121:173-80.
7. Shahriaree H. O'Connor Textbook of Arthroscopic Surgery. JB Lippincott Company, United States; 1984.
8. Ebraheim NA, Mekhail AO. The infrapatellar branch of the saphenous nerve: an anatomic study. J Orthop Trauma. 1997;11:195-9.
9. Patel D. Proximal approaches to arthroscopic surgery of the knee. Am J Sports Med. 1981;9(5):296-303.
10. Guilquist J, Hagberg G. A new modification of the technique of arthroscopy of the knee joint. Acta Chir Scand. 1976;142:123-30.
11. Pace JL, Wahl CJ. Posterior portals for arthroscopic surgery of the knee. Arthroscopy. 1994;10(6):608-13.
12. Ahn JH, Lee SH, Jung HJ, Koo KH, Kim SH. Arthroscopy of the posterior knee compartments: neurovascular anatomic relationships during arthroscopic transverse capsulotomy. Arthroscopy. 2010;26(5):637-42.
13. McGinnis MD 4th, Gonzalez R, Nyland J, Caborn DN. The posteromedial knee arthroscopy portal: a cadaveric study

defining a safety zone for portal placement. Arthroscopy. 2011;27(8):1090-5.

14. Ogilvie-Harris DJ, Biggs DJ, Mackay M, Weisleder L. Posterior trans-septal portal for arthroscopic surgery of the knee joint. Arthroscopy. 2000;16(7):774-9.
15. Kim SJ, Kim HJ. High portal: practical philosophy for positioning portals in knee arthroscopy. Arthroscopy. 2001;17(3):333-7.
16. Ahn JH, Chung YS, Oh I. Arthroscopic posterior ligament reconstruction using the posterior trans-septal portal. Arthroscopy. 2003;19:101-7.
17. Allum R. Complications of arthroscopy of the knee. J Bone Joint Surg Br. 2002;84-B:937-45.
18. DeLee JC. Complications of arthroscopy and arthroscopic surgery: results of a national survey. J Arthroscopic Rel Surg. 1985;1:214-20.
19. Small NC. Complications in arthroscopy: the knee and other joints. Arthroscopy. 1986;2:253-8.
20. Rodeo SA, Forster RA, Weiland AJ. Neurological complications due to arthroscopy. J Bone Joint Surg Am. 1993;75(6):917-26.
21. Hamula M. Arthroscopic trans-septal portal to treat extension deficits from arthrofibrosis. Knee. 2004;11(6):501-2.

Chapter 34

Clinical Examination and Diagnostic Arthroscopy of the Knee Joint

P Sripathi Rao, Vivek Pandey

A detailed clinical examination is mandatory before embarking upon the management of ligament injuries of the knee joint. The contralateral knee should also be tested as it serves as a comparative standard. This chapter does not deal with the routine steps of knee examination, namely limb alignment, points of tenderness, range of motion, and the neurovascular status. These steps are valuable in arriving at a clinical diagnosis. Attention must also be paid to ascertain the mechanism of injury and symptoms narrated by the patient.

ANTERIOR INSTABILITY

The anterior cruciate ligament (ACL) is the primary restraint to the abnormal anterior translation of the tibia on the femur. The diagnosis of the ACL tear is made by the demonstration of abnormal anterior translation of tibia. The mechanism of injury to the ACL typically involves rapid deceleration, hyperextension, or pivoting on a fixed spot.[1] When the foot is planted on the ground, a blow to the lateral aspect of knee joint can rupture the ACL along with medial structures. Feeling or hearing a pop in the joint and acute hemarthrosis is associated feature.

Lachman Test

First described by Torg, this test was originally performed with the knee joint in 15° of flexion.[2] It is now performed with the knee in 30° of flexion and neutral rotation.[3] The Lachman test is highly sensitive and highly specific (near 95%).[4]

With the patient placed supine and the knee in 30° of flexion, the examiner stabilizes the distal femur with one hand (**Figure 34.1**). Sustained anterior pressure is applied on the proximal tibia with the other hand. The abnormal anterior translation of the tibia (in comparison with the opposite knee) with a soft end point indicates a positive test. Anterior translation of 1–5 mm is defined as grade I, 6–10 mm as grade II, and more than 10 mm as grade III.[5] A variation in the Lachman test has been described for testing of patients with muscular thighs, where the patient's leg is cradled in the examiners axilla.[5]

Anterior Drawer Test

This test has low sensitivity (22–95%) in the unanesthetized patient.[6] The thick posterior horns of the menisci,

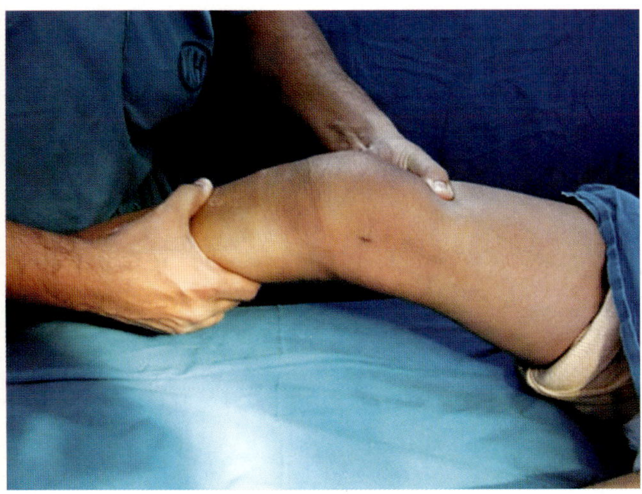

Figure 34.1 The knee is kept in 30° flexion to elicit Lachman test

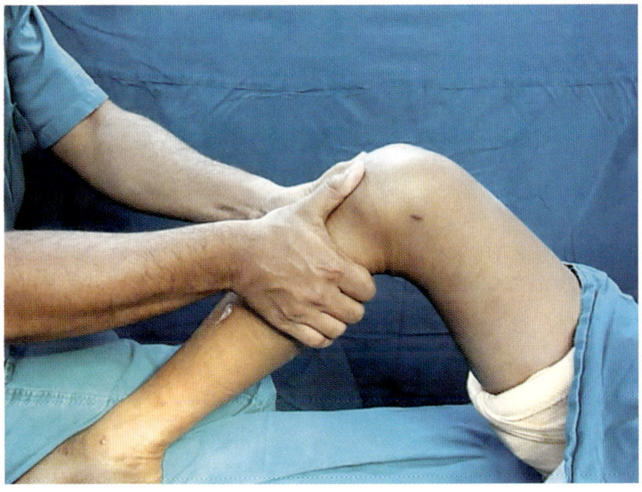

Figure 34.2 With the knee in 90° flexion and examiner stabilizing the foot, the thumb stays over the joint line to assess the grade of anterior drawer

hamstring spasm, the bony contours of the joint and the inability to flex the acutely injured knee to 90° serve as limitations to this test.[7] With the patient supine and knee flexed to 90°, the joint should be observed from the side to confirm the absence of the posterior sag. The hamstrings are then relaxed by instruction and gentle palpation. The examiner grasps the proximal tibia with his hands, with the thumbs placed on the anterior joint line (**Figure 34.2**). The increased anterior translation of the tibia with a soft end point indicates a positive result.

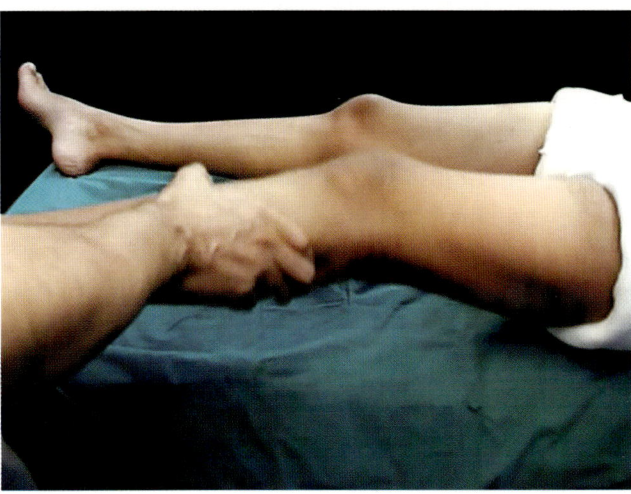

Figure 34.3 The hip is kept slightly abducted and the knee in valgus and the leg in internal rotation. The pivot shift can be observed with the knee moving from extension to early flexion

Pivot Shift Test

The term pivot shift was first coined by Galway and Macintosh.[8] The test demonstrates the reduction in the lateral tibial condyle from a state of anterior subluxation.[9] A positive test suggests that the laxity is clinically significant indicating that the patient would need the ACL reconstruction.[10]

The knee is held in extension and internal rotation with the application of valgus stress on the distal thigh (**Figure 34.3**). As the knee is flexed from this position, the lateral tibial plateau relocates posteriorly with a clunk at 30°–40° of flexion.[11] This relocation of the lateral tibial plateau is caused by the Iliotibial band, which becomes a flexor of the knee beyond 30° of flexion. Ligament laxity and stretching of the Iliotibial band, medial collateral injury, and a bucket handle tear of the meniscus may interfere with the performance of the test.[12]

POSTERIOR INSTABILITY

The posterior cruciate ligament (PCL) assisted by the collateral ligaments and the posterolateral corner (PLC) provides restraint to the posterior translation of the tibia on the femur. Injuries of the PCL may occur in sports and dashboard injuries. Hyperextension injuries to the PCL may be associated with damage to the other structures and or dislocation of the knee joint.[13-15] Instability is only occasionally noted in PCL deficiency with patients usually complaining of pain, stiffness and knee swelling. Isolated PCL injuries are not as common as those with PLC involvement.[14] PCL deficiency is diagnosed by the posterior drawer, Lachman, posterior sag, and quadriceps active tests.

Posterior Drawer Test

This test has been reported to be the most specific and sensitive test for the diagnosis of the isolated PCL tear.[13] False negative results may be obtained if the knee is held in internal rotation during the testing, because of the intact meniscofemoral ligaments.[13]

The patient is placed supine with the knee in 90° of flexion and neutral rotation. In this position, the tibial plateau is 1 cm anterior to the medial femoral condyle. The examiner places both his hands on the proximal tibia, with his thumbs over the anterior joint line. The posterior translation is noted on exerting backward pressure and graded as I (0–5 mm), II (6–10 mm) and III (more than 10 mm). The quality of the end point (firm, soft, absent) is indicative of the state of the PCL.[16]

Posterior Lachman Test

This test is of the value in the acutely injured knee that cannot be flexed to 90° for the posterior drawer test.[17] The patient's knee is held in 30° of flexion by the examiner. A posteriorly directed force is then applied in neutral rotation and the excessive posterior translation is graded.

Posterior Sag Test

This is a static test and is found to be 100% specific and 79% sensitive for PCL deficiency.[18] The patient is placed supine with the knees flexed to 90° and the feet planted flat on the table. Both the knees are then viewed from the side (**Figure 34.4**). If the proximal tibia is found to sag posterior to the anterior portion of the femoral condyles, the test is considered positive.[19]

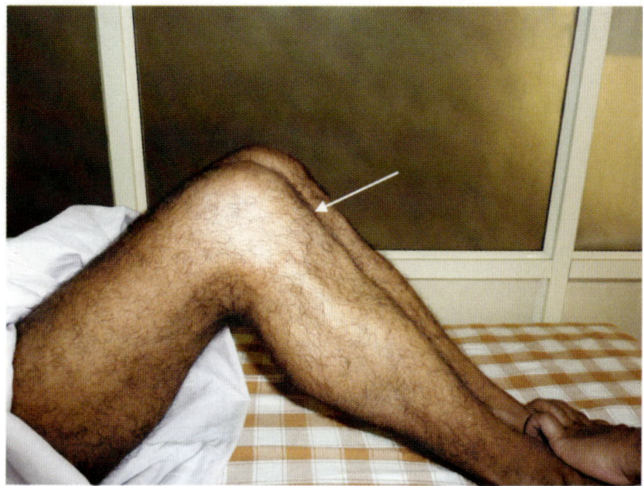

Figure 34.4 With the knee in 90° flexion, the right knee can be seen sagging posteriorly (white arrow) due to the deficient PCL

Quadriceps Active Test

Originally described by Daniel et al.[20] this test uses the patient's quadriceps contraction as the displacing force. Its reliability in testing PCL deficiency has been questioned. With the patient placed supine and the knee flexed to 90°, the patient is asked to slide his fixed foot anteriorly. This induces a quadriceps contraction and the posteriorly displaced tibia is observed to relocate anteriorly. This dynamic reduction in tibia is considered a positive test if the tibia shifts by a minimum of 2 mm.[20]

VARUS INSTABILITY

The lateral collateral ligament is the primary restraint to varus instability with support from the PLC.

Varus Stress Test at 0° and 30°

With the patient placed supine, the knee is held in 30° flexion and slight internal rotation. The examiner holds the distal medial thigh with one hand and the proximal tibia with the other hand. A varus force is exerted in this position and the test is repeated with the knee in extension (**Figures 34.5A and B**). The test is deemed positive if the knee opens more than on the contralateral joint. A grading

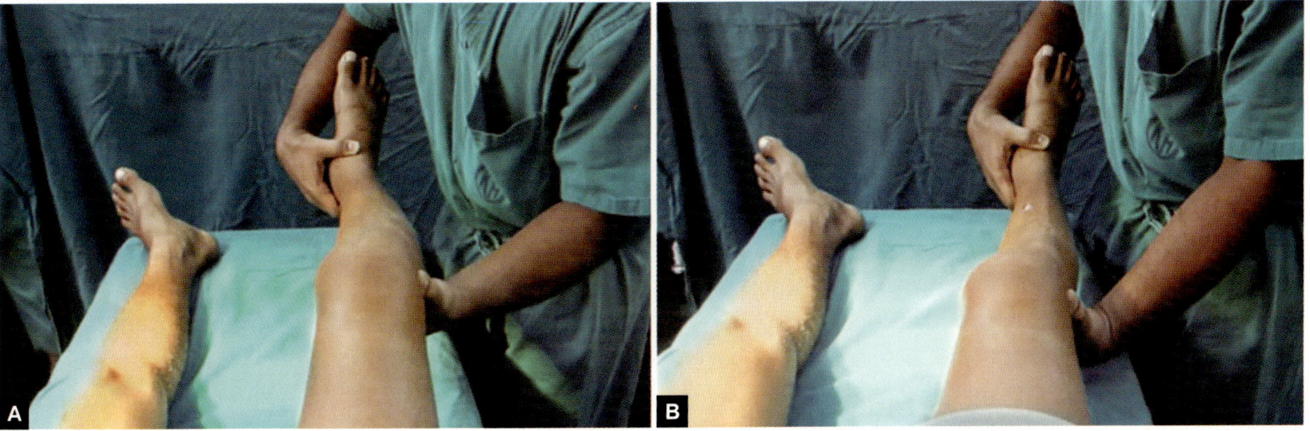

Figures 34.5A and B The varus test is being performed in 30° flexion (A) and full extension (B) with the thumb at the joint line to assess the degree of joint opening

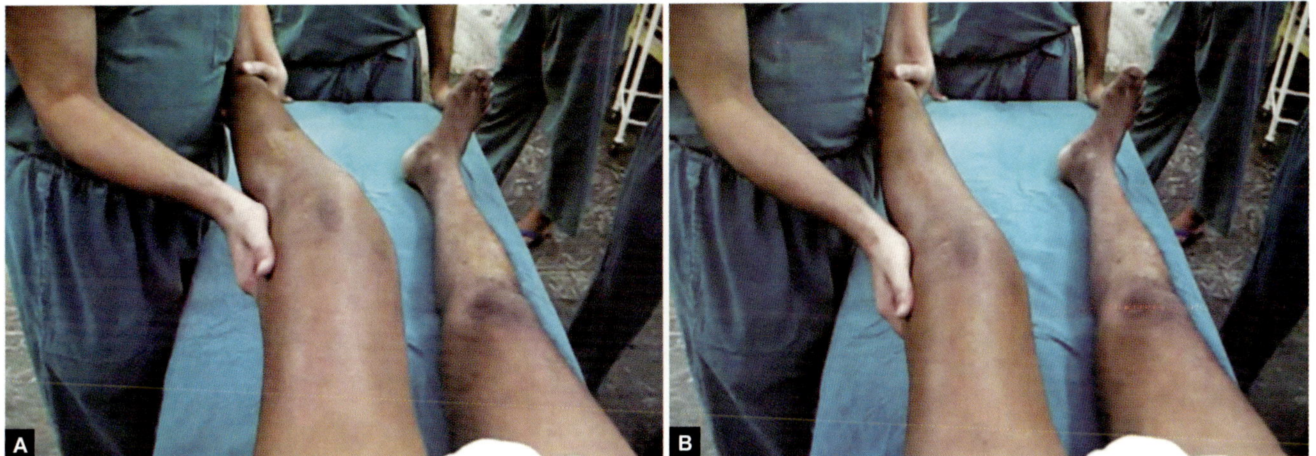

Figures 34.6A and B The valgus test is being performed in 30° flexion (A) and full extension (B) to assess the degree of joint opening

system (grade I to III) similar to that used in other knee ligament tests can be employed.

Pathologic opening predominantly noticed in 30° flexion indicates injury to the lateral collateral ligament and posterolateral ligament. When there is significant opening at 0°, a combination injury to the LCL, PLC, PCL and perhaps the ACL is suspected.[21]

VALGUS INSTABILITY

The superficial fibers of the medial collateral ligament are the primary restraint to valgus stress at 30° flexion.[22,23] Secondary stabilizers like the deep portion of the medial collateral ligament, posterior oblique ligament and ACL come into play only in extension.

Valgus Stress Test in 30° and 0°

The patient is placed supine with the hip slightly abducted and the knee flexed 30° over the side of the table. The examiner stabilizes the lateral aspect of the thigh with one hand and applies valgus stress by holding at the ankle with the other hand. The test is repeated with the knee in extension (**Figures 34.6A and B**).

Maximum instability at 30° flexion with relative stability at extension signifies isolated MCL injury. A positive test in extension suggests additional injury to the PMC, POL and cruciate ligaments.[24]

ROTATORY INSTABILITIES

Rotatory instabilities do not affect knee function when the knee is extension but do so with the knee in flexion.[25] Isolated rotatory instabilities may manifest during cutting, pivoting or rapid deceleration activity.[25]

Anteromedial Rotatory Instability (AMRI)

Excessive valgus movement of the knee coupled with external rotation has been described to be AMRI.[26] The PM corners has been shown to be a restraint to AMRI. Perhaps the most common form of knee instability, AMRI may also be the most frequent cause of ACL disruption. When AMRI is combined with ALRI, the functional disability can be severe.[9]

Slocum Test

The anterior drawer test is first performed in the standard manner. The test is then repeated with the knee in 15° of external rotation, thus tightening the PMC and reducing the anterior tibial translation. If in external rotation, anterior tibial translation remains unchanged, the test is considered to be positive.[26]

Anterolateral Rotatory Instability (ALRI)

Injury to the middle third of the lateral capsular ligament is considered to be the cause of ALRI.[27] Tests like the pivot shift and the anterior drawer with the tibia in neutral rotation indicate the presence of ALRI. If ALRI is suspected and not demonstrated by these two tests, the following additional tests are suggested.

Jerk Test of Houghston

Considered to be the opposite of the pivot shift test, this test has been described to be the most specific test for ALRI.[27]

The patient is placed supine with the knee in 90° flexion and moderate internal rotation. The joint is slowly extended while applying valgus stress. In a positive test, result the tibia displaces anteriorly and internally at 30° flexion and the examiner feels a 'jerk.'

Losee Test

Concerned that the internal rotation employed in the pivot shift test could create impingement between the lateral femoral condyle and the tibial plateau (resulting in pain and hamstring spasm), Losee[11] suggested that the tibia be held in external rotation. The starting position of the knee is 45° of flexion and external rotation. Valgus stress is applied as the knee is extended. A positive test is the observation of anterior shifting of the lateral tibial plateau at about 20° flexion.

Flexion Rotation Drawer Test

This test was first described by Noyes et al.[28] when the examiner holds the knee in 15° of flexion; the femur drops posteriorly and rotates externally in an ACL deficient knee. As the examiner flexes the knee tibial reduction and external rotation of the femur are observed at 40° of flexion.

Posteromedial Rotatory Instability (PMRI)

When the medial capsular ligament, MCL, POL and ACL are torn the proximal medial tibia could displace posteriorly. If the PCL is also torn, the whole of the tibia sags posteriorly. Clinically PMRI is diagnosed when the medial tibial plateau displaces posteromedial on application of a valgus stress.[25]

Posterolateral Rotatory Instability (PLRI)

The PLC consists of dynamic and static structures. The dynamic structures include the ITB, the biceps tendon and the popliteus muscle tendon complex. The static structures are the LCL, the arcuate ligament complex, the patellofemoral ligament and the PLC.[25,27] Injury to the PLC results in PLRI that is often associated with ACL deficiency.[29]

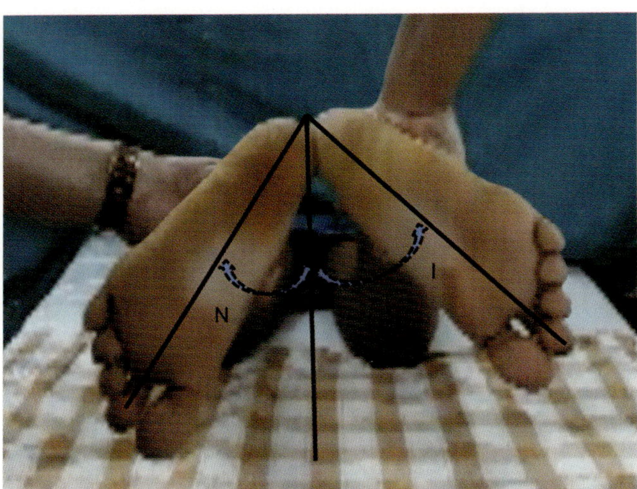

Figure 34.7 With the patient in prone position, the dial test is being performed in 30° flexion of the knee. The right side (I-index knee) is seen to have increased external rotation as compared to the left side (N-normal knee)

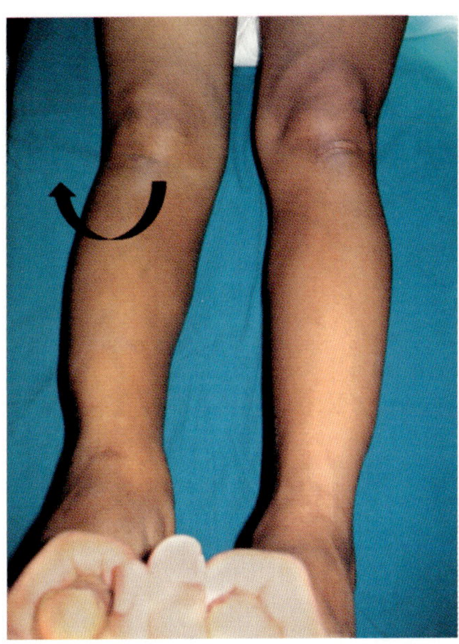

Figure 34.8 The right leg is demonstrating increased recurvatum and external rotation with varus when lifted by great toe

Dial Test at 30° and 90°

This test assesses abnormal external tibial rotation and also helps to differentiate between isolated PCL tear and PCL tear with PLC injury.

The test can be performed with the patient supine or prone. The examiner holds the patients feet with the knee in 30° of flexion and exerts maximum external rotation force (**Figure 34.7**). The thigh foot angle is measured on both sides. The test is then repeated with the knees in 90° flexion. A difference in the thigh foot angle of more than 10° between the two sides is considered significant. If the test is positive at 30° of knee flexion and negative at 90°, it is considered to be indicative of isolated PCL injury. If the test is positive in 30° and 90°, a combination of PCL and PLC injury is diagnosed.[30,31]

External Rotation Recurvatum Test

The patient is placed supine on the table with his or her legs together. The examiner lifts the limbs off table while holding the great toes on both sides. If the knee falls into varus, hyperextension, and external rotation (**Figure 34.8**), it is considered to be a positive test for PLRI.[32,33]

DIAGNOSTIC ARTHROSCOPY OF THE KNEE

The arthroscope has emerged as a useful tool in the diagnosis and management of intra-articular pathology of the knee joint. A thorough knowledge of the superficial and deep anatomy of the knee joint, arthroscopic instrumentation and theatre setup are of fundamental importance before embarking on arthroscopic surgery. Though postoperative sepsis is uncommon with this technique, arthroscopy demands the same amount of preoperative preparation and theatre asepsis as any open orthopedic procedure.[34]

Patient Positioning for Arthroscopic Surgery

Straight Leg Position

The patient is placed supine and the surgeon stands on the side of the table. A side post may be mounted against the upper lateral thigh. This position permits valgus-varus stresses to be applied with ease.[34]

Flexed Knee Position

The patient's knee is flexed at 90° and the leg is suspended over the distal end of the table. The surgeon stands at the foot end of the table. A leg holder may be required to stabilize the knee joint.[34]

PORTALS

Since the anterior aspect of the knee is relatively free of neurovascular structures, standard portals are established at AL and AM sites. Most arthroscopic work is possible through these standard portals. Accessory portals may be created for better visualization, accesses or joint distension. It is advisable to mark the borders of the patella, quadriceps tendon, patellar tendon, femoral and tibial condyles and the joint line before marking the first portal. Precisely placed portals are the key to successful arthroscopy, as they provide for adequate accesses and complete viewing.

Standard Portals

Anterolateral Portal (Arthroscopy or Viewing Portal)

Made adjacent to the patellar tendon at the level of the inferior pole of patella (**Figure 34.9A**). A thumb placed over the lateral tibial articular surface prevents iatrogenic trauma to the lateral meniscus (LM). The portal is made with a # 10 knife blade with the sharp edge directed superiorly (**Figure 34.9B**). The knee is flexed to 90° while creating the portal. The standard AL portal enables visualization of the entire knee. If the portal is too high, the movement of the scope is hindered by the lateral femoral condyle. If the portal is placed too medial, the infrapatellar fat pad may interfere with visualization.

Anteromedial Portal (Instrument or Operative Portal)

Usually made at a little higher location. Its exact location is dictated by the location of the intra-articular pathology. A spinal needle placed through the proposed site is manipulated in the joint to reach the lesion and confirm the site (**Figure 34.9C**). Most locations in the knee can be reached through this portal except the posterior third of the LM.

Accessory Portals

Superolateral and Superomedial Portals

Made about 2 cm superior to the patella (**Figure 34.9D**). The superolateral (SL) portal is ideal for viewing the patellofemoral joint, the infrapatellar fat pad, for retrieval

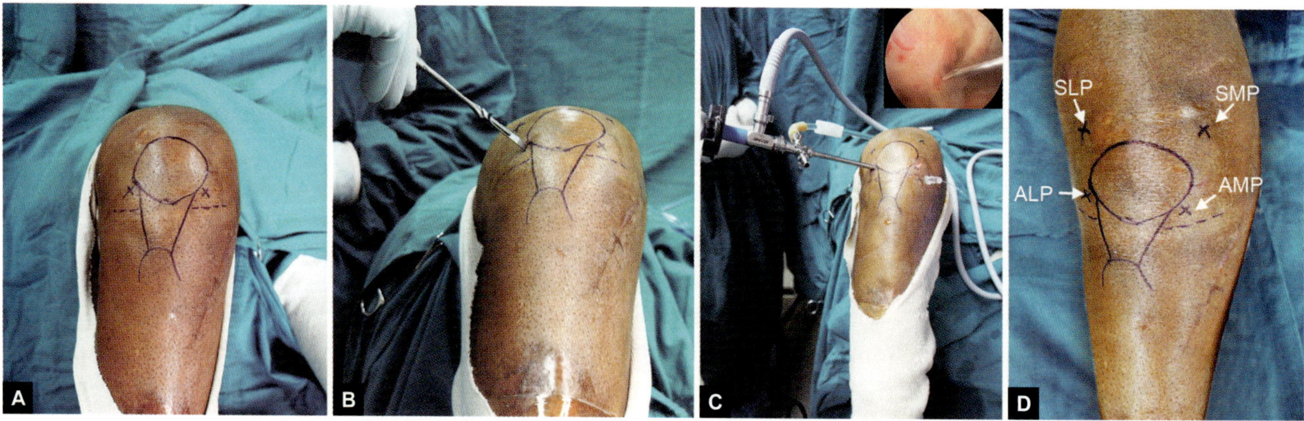

Figures 34.9A to D Composite image revealing portals and its placement. Image (A) shows the position of AL and AM portals in 90° flexion of the right knee. The hashed line indicates the level of the joint line. Image (B) shows the placement of the AL portal with the knife facing upward. Image (C) shows the placement of the AM portal with the help of a needle that is seen in the arthroscopic image (inset). Image (D) indicates all the portals.

Abbreviations: ALP, anterolateral portal; AMP, anteromedial portal; SLP, superolateral portal; SMP, superomedial portal

of loose bodies from the lateral gutter, for synovectomy of the suprapatellar fossa and excision of a pathological medial plica. The superomedial portal can be used as an additional inflow portal. However, this portal can interfere with quadriceps function.

Posteromedial Portal

Made 1 cm above the PM joint line and 1 cm posterior to the PM margin of the medial femoral condyle. The portal is best made with while viewing the posteromedial compartment (PMC) through the AL portal, with the knee in 90° of flexion. Light emanating from the arthroscope can be seen at the portal site (**Figure 34.10A**). A spinal needle confirms the accuracy of portal placement (**Figure 34.10B**). The saphenous nerve is at risk while making the portal. The portal is of use during the PCL reconstruction, synovectomy, removal of loose bodies, and retrieval of last meniscal fragments.

Posterolateral Portal

Created in similar fashion after transillumination with the arthroscope. Rarely used this portal is situated at the intersection of the posterior margin of the femur with extension of the posterior margin of the fibula. Typically this is approximately 2 cm superior to the PL joint line at the posterior edge of the Iliotibial band and the anterior edge of the biceps tendon.

Central (Transpatellar Tendon or Gillquist) Portal

Made vertically through the fibers of the patellar tendon in its proximal third. Though it can be used to view the intercondylar notch; it is less often used now because of the possible scarring of the patellar tendon.

Midpatellar Portal

Described by Patel to provide access to the anterior, lateral and medial structures as well as the popliteus tunnel, located on either side of the patella at its widest part, the portals are designed to provide a bird's eye view of the joint. The PCL and the posterior horns of the meniscus are difficult to view through these portals.

Arthroscopic Anatomy and Diagnostic Viewing

The knee joint should be systematically viewed before embarking on operative work on an identified lesion.

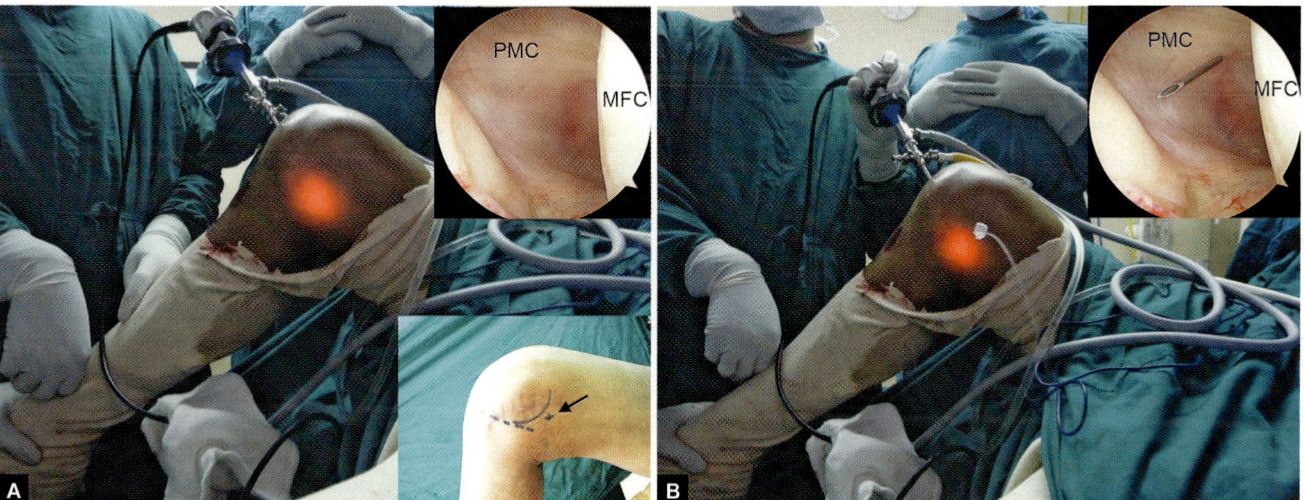

Figures 34.10A and B The composite image shows the technique of the placement of the PM portal. Image (A) shows light emanating at the site of the PM portal in the knee that is kept at 90° flexion. The black arrow shows the surface marking for the PM portal. The arthroscopic image (inset) shows the PMC. Image (B) shows the accurate placement of the needle in the PMC that is confirmed in the arthroscopic image (inset).
Abbreviations: PMC, posteromedial compartment; MFC, medial femoral condyle

Such systematic viewing reduces the incidence of missed lesions.

The conical or blunt obturator is locked with the arthroscope sleeve and the assembly is carefully introduced into the joint in the direction of the intercondylar notch, with the knee in flexion. After the capsule is pierced, the sleeve is directed towards the suprapatellar fossa, while simultaneously extending the knee. The obturator is then exchanged for the arthroscope and the joint is distended with irrigation fluid.

Systematic viewing of the knee joint:

Suprapatellar Fossa

The ideal location to begin the diagnostic arthroscopy of the knee joint (**Figure 34.11**). Rotation of the arthroscope facilitates the viewing of the roof (quadriceps tendon and capsule) the floor (synovial membrane) and the medial and lateral capsule. The suprapatellar plica is a normally occurring fold of synovium. A large plica may harbor loose bodies. The plica forms a complete membrane in 4–20% of adults and can subdivide the suprapatellar fossa into the superior and inferior portion.[35]

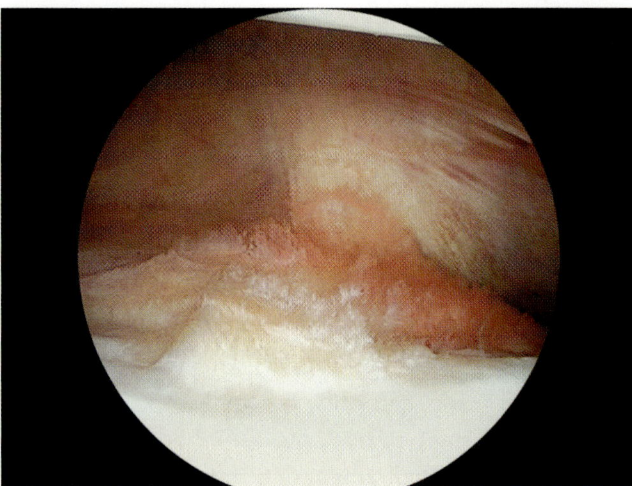

Figure 34.11 The arthroscopic image of the suprapatellar pouch

Patellofemoral Articulation

Withdrawal of the scope from the suprapatellar fossa enables visualization of the patellofemoral articulation (**Figure 34.12**). By rotational and side-to-side movements of the arthroscope, the patellar facets, trochlear notch of the femur, and the infrapatellar fat pad are visualized. Thumb pressure on the patella helps in better visualization of the facets. The facets of the patella seat themselves on the trochlea within 40° of the flexion. Patellofemoral tracking is better appreciated through the SL portal.

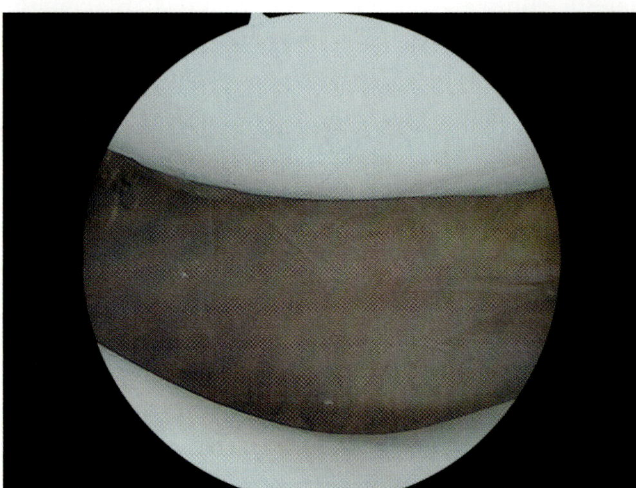

Figure 34.12 The arthroscopic image of the patellofemoral joint showing a patella on top with a trochlear notch below

Medial Gutter

Bounded by the medial capsule and the edge of the medial femoral condyle (**Figure 34.13**), the medial gutter can house loose bodies. The medial plica is a redundant fold of synovial membrane stretching from the medial capsule to the infrapatellar fat pad (**Figure 34.14**). If fibrosed and contracted, the medial plica can become symptomatic and may need to be resected.[36]

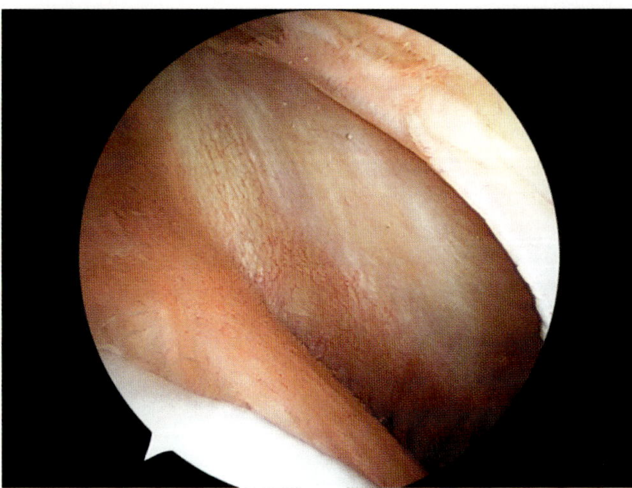

Figure 34.13 The arthroscopic image of the medial gutter of the right knee

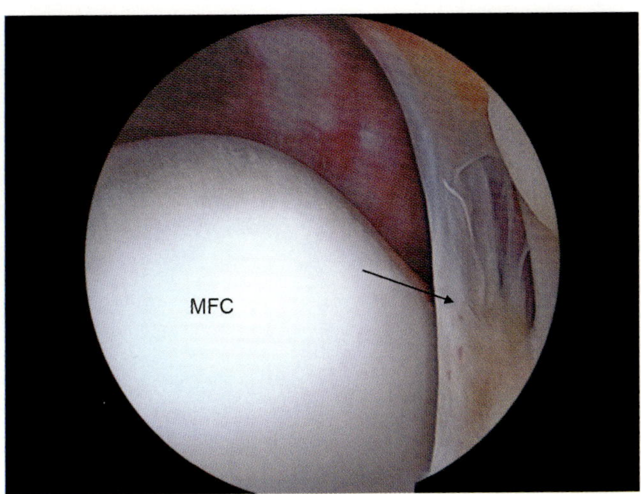

Figure 34.14 The arthroscopic image of the medial plica (black arrow)
Abbreviation: MFC, medial femoral condyle

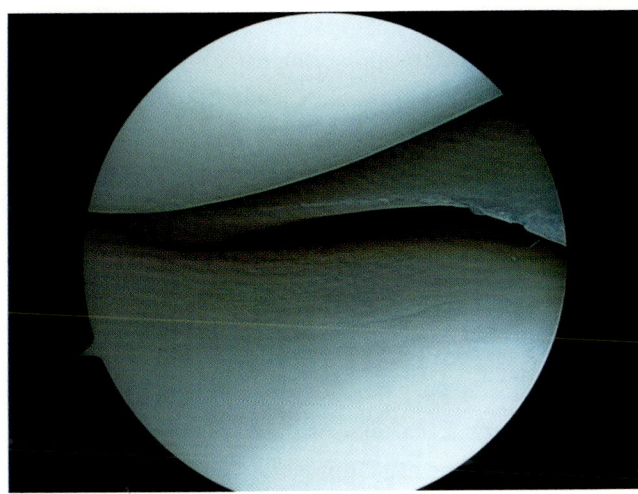

Figure 34.15 The arthroscopic image of the medial compartment of the right knee showing the medial meniscus between the medial femoral condyle and the medial tibial plateau

Medial Compartment

This compartment is entered by moving the arthroscope over the edge of the medial femoral condyle and pass the meniscosynovial junction while simultaneously flexing the knee. The entire medial meniscus can be viewed by the moving and rotating the arthroscope (**Figure 34.15**). External rotation, valgus and extension enable better visualization of the posterior third of the medial meniscus. The meniscus should be probed and gently pulled to ascertain its integrity. The probe should be used to palpate the superior and inferior surface of the meniscus. The state of the hyaline cartilage over the medial femoral condyle and tibial plateau should be documented. Normal dimpling of the cartilage under the probe should not be misconstrued for cartilage softening.

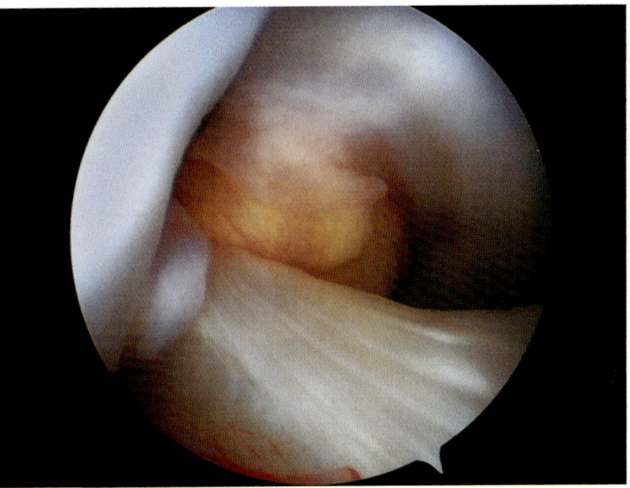

Figure 34.16 The arthroscopic image of the intercondylar notch showing the presence of the ACL

Intercondylar Notch

The ACL can be visualized from its tibial attachment to its femoral attachment at the back of the lateral condyle of the femur (**Figure 34.16**). The probe is used to assess the tension of this ligament. The proximal attachment of the PCL to the medial femoral condyle is now visualized. The inferior plica is a thin film of synovial membrane stretching from the infrapatellar fat pad to the roof of the intercondylar notch, anterior to the ACL. If thick, the plica can hamper visualization of the ACL or the passage of instruments and may have to be bypassed or excised.[36]

Lateral Compartment

This compartment is accessed by placing the arthroscope in the triangle bounded by the ACL, the anterior horn of the LM and the lateral femoral condyle, the knee is then moved to the figure of 4 position in order to view the LM (**Figure 34.17**). Being smaller in radius than the medial meniscus, the LM can be viewed in its entirely in one field of vision. The popliteus tendon, placed obliquely behind

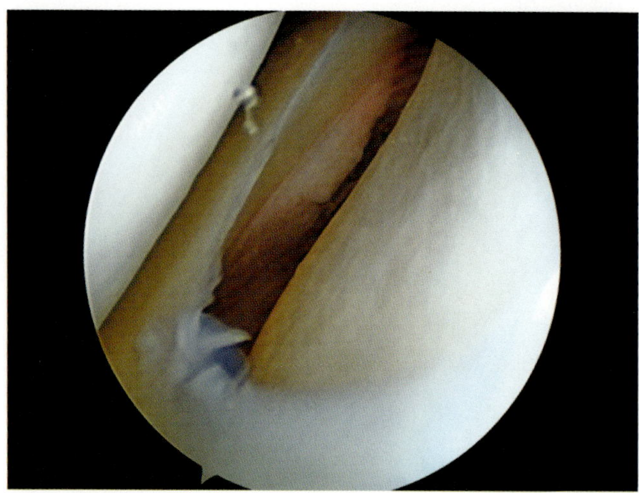

Figure 34.17 The arthroscopic image of the lateral compartment showing the presence of the LM

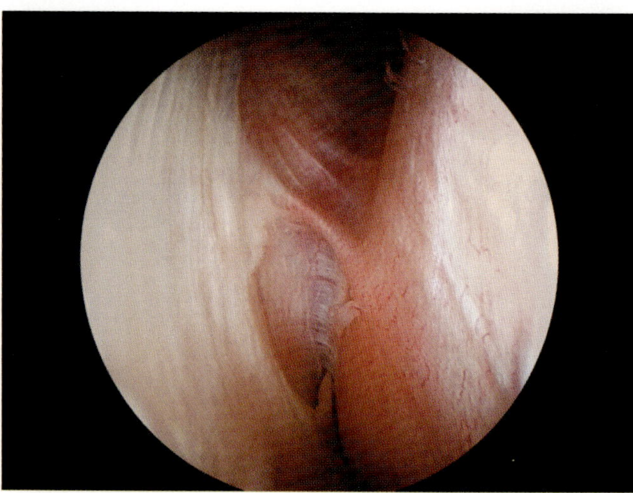

Figure 34.19 The arthroscopic image of the lateral gutter characterized by the presence of synovial folds

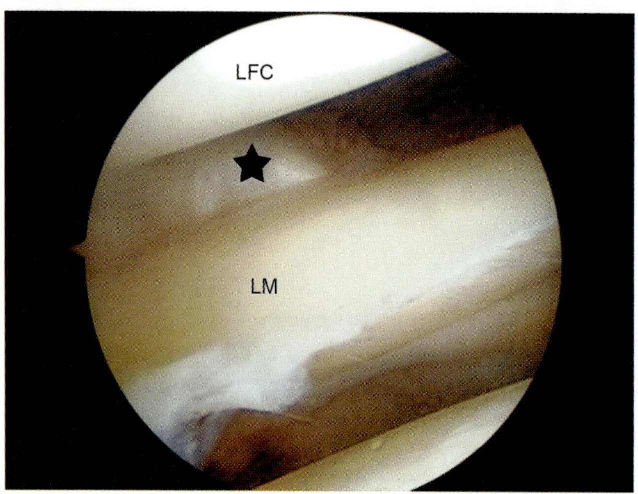

Figure 34.18 The arthroscopic image of the popliteus (black star) behind the LM
Abbreviations: LM, lateral meniscus; LFC, lateral femoral condyle

the posterior third of the LM, is palpated at this juncture (**Figure 34.18**). Loose bodies may be harbored in the popliteus hiatus.

Posteromedial and Posterolateral Compartments

The PMC can be viewed by gently advancing the arthroscope posteriorly, between the ACL and the medial femoral condyle, with the knee in 80° of flexion. This may not be possible in patients with tight knees or degenerative knee joints with osteophytosis.[36] The posterior horn of the medial meniscus, the posterior capsule and the distal extension of the PCL are viewed in the PMC.

The PL compartment may be entered from the space between the ACL and the lateral femoral condyle with application of gentle varus stress. The posterior aspect of the LM and the PL capsule can be inspected in the PL compartment.

Lateral Gutter

The lateral gutter is bounded by the lateral femoral condyle and the lateral capsule (**Figure 34.19**). Though the lateral gutter can be viewed through the AL portal, operative procedures are easier through the SL portal. The popliteus tendon in its hiatus can be seen at the inferior limit of the lateral gutter. A consistent synovial fold runs transversely between the lateral femoral condyle and the lateral capsule at the bottom of the lateral gutter.[35]

REFERENCES

1. Noyes FR, Grood ES, Butler DL, Malek M. Clinical laxity tests and functional stability of the knee: biomechanical concepts. Clin Orthop Relat Res. 1980;146:84-9.
2. Torg JS, Conrad W, Kalen V. Clinical diagnosis of anterior cruciate ligament instability in the athlete. Am J Sports Med. 1976;4:84-93.

3. Markolf KL, Burchfield DM, Shapiro MM, et al. Biomechanical consequences of replacement of the anterior cruciate ligament with a patellar ligament allograft. Part I: insertion of the graft and anterior-posterior testing. J Bone Joint Surg Am. 1996;78:1720-7.
4. Katz JW, Fingeroth RJ. The diagnostic accuracy of ruptures of the anterior cruciate ligament comparing the Lachman test, the anterior drawer sign, and the pivot shift test in acute and chronic knee injuries. Am J Sports Med. 1986;14(1):88-91.
5. Lubowitz JH, Bernardini BJ, Reid JB 3rd. Current concepts review: comprehensive physical examination for instability of the knee. Am J Sports Med. 2008;36:577-94.
6. Donaldson WF 3rd, Warren RF, Wickiewicz T. A comparison of acute anterior cruciate ligament examinations. Initial versus examination under anesthesia. Am J Sports Med. 1985;13:5-10.
7. Shoemaker SC, Markolf KL. Effects of joint load on the stiffness and laxity of ligament-deficient knees. An *in vitro* study of the anterior cruciate and medial collateral ligaments. J Bone Joint Surg Am. 1985;67:136-46.
8. Galway HR, MacIntosh DL. The lateral pivot shift: a symptom and sign of anterior cruciate ligament insufficiency. Clin Orthop Relat Res. 1980;147:45-50.
9. Ellison AE. The pathogenesis and treatment of anterolateral rotatory instability. Clin Orthop Relat Res. 1980;147:51-5.
10. Kocher MS, Tucker R, Briggs KK. Relationship between subjective and objective assessment of outcomes after anterior cruciate ligament reconstruction. J Knee Surg. 2005;18:73-81.
11. Losee RE, Johnson TR, Southwick WO. Anterior subluxation of the lateral tibial plateau. A diagnostic test and operative repair. J Bone Joint Surg Am. 1978;60:1015-30.
12. Losee RE. Concepts of the pivot shift. Clin Orthop Relat Res. 1983;172:45-51.
13. Clancy WG, Jr, Shelbourne KD, Zoellner GB, et al. Treatment of knee joint instability secondary to rupture of the posterior cruciate ligament. Report of a new procedure. J Bone Joint Surg Am. 1983;65:310-22.
14. Fanelli GC, Edson CJ. Posterior cruciate ligament injuries in trauma patients: Part II. Arthroscopy. 1995;11:526-9.
15. Gollehon DL, Torzilli PA, Warren RF. The role of the posterolateral and cruciate ligaments in the stability of the human knee. A biomechanical study. J Bone Joint Surg Am. 1987;69:233-42.
16. Shelbourne KD, Davis TJ, Patel DV. The natural history of acute, isolated, nonoperatively treated posterior cruciate ligament injuries. A prospective study. Am J Sports Med. 1999;27:276-83.
17. AJ T. Diagnosis of knee ligament injuries. Scott WN Ligaments and Extensor Mechanism. St Louis: CV Mosby; 1991.
18. Rubinstein RA Jr, Shelbourne KD, McCarroll JR, VanMeter CD, Rettig AC. The accuracy of the clinical examination in the setting of posterior cruciate ligament injuries. Am J Sports Med. 1994;22:550-7.
19. Barton TM, Torg JS, Das M. Posterior cruciate ligament insufficiency. A review of the literature. Sports Med. 1984;1:419-30.
20. Daniel DM, Stone ML, Barnett P, Sachs R. Use of the quadriceps active test to diagnose posterior cruciate-ligament disruption and measure posterior laxity of the knee. J Bone Joint Surg Am. 1988;70:386-91.
21. LaPrade RF, Terry GC. Injuries to the posterolateral aspect of the knee. Association of anatomic injury patterns with clinical instability. Am J Sports Med. 1997;25:433-8.
22. Grood ES, Noyes FR, Butler DL, Suntay WJ. Ligamentous and capsular restraints preventing straight medial and lateral laxity in intact human cadaver knees. J Bone Joint Surg Am. 1981;63:1257-69.
23. Warren LF, Marshall JL. The supporting structures and layers on the medial side of the knee: an anatomical analysis. J Bone Joint Surg Am. 1979;61:56-62.
24. Marshall JL, Baugher WH. Stability examination of the knee: a simple anatomic approach. Clin Orthop Relat Res. 1980;146:78-83.
25. Larson RL. Physical examination in the diagnosis of rotatory instability. Clin Orthop Relat Res. 1983;172:38-44.
26. Slocum DB, Larson RL, James SL. Late reconstruction of ligamentous injuries of the medial compartment of the knee. Clin Orthop Relat Res. 1974;100:23-55.
27. Hughston JC, Andrews JR, Cross MJ, Moschi A. Classification of knee ligament instabilities. Part II. The lateral compartment. J Bone Joint Surg Am. 1976;58:173-9.
28. Noyes FR, Bassett RW, Grood ES, Butler DL. Arthroscopy in acute traumatic hemarthrosis of the knee. Incidence of

anterior cruciate tears and other injuries. J Bone Joint Surg Am. 1980;62:687-95.

29. O'Brien SJ, Warren RF, Pavlov H, Panariello R, Wickiewicz TL. Reconstruction of the chronically insufficient anterior cruciate ligament with the central third of the patellar ligament. J Bone Joint Surg Am. 1991;73:278-86.
30. Cooper DE. Tests for posterolateral instability of the knee in normal subjects. Results of examination under anesthesia. J Bone Joint Surg Am. 1991;73:30-6.
31. Grood ES, Stowers SF, Noyes FR. Limits of movement in the human knee. Effect of sectioning the posterior cruciate ligament and posterolateral structures. J Bone Joint Surg Am. 1988;70:88-97.
32. Hughston JC, Andrews JR, Cross MJ, Moschi A. Classification of knee ligament instabilities. Part I. The medial compartment and cruciate ligaments. J Bone Joint Surg Am. 1976;58:159-72.
33. Hughston JC, Norwood LA Jr. The posterolateral drawer test and external rotational recurvatum test for posterolateral rotatory instability of the knee. Clin Orthop Relat Res 1980;147:82-7.
34. Rao PS, Acharya KKV. Diagnostic Knee Arthroscopy. In: Kulkarni GS (Ed.). Textbook of Orthopaedics and Trauma. Jaypee Brothers Medical Publishers, New Delhi, India; 2008.
35. Tingstad E. The Knee. McGinty JB Operative Arthroscopy. Lippincott Williams and Wilkins, United States; 2003.
36. Howard WW RJ. Arthroscopy of the Knee: Basic Setup and Technique. Lippincott Williams and Wilkins, United States; 2003.

Chapter 35

The Menisci: Menisectomy and Meniscal Repair

Vivek Dahiya, Attique Vasdev, Himanshu Gupta, Ashok Rajgopal

Menisci (medial and lateral) are C-shaped triangular structures that occupy the space between the femoral condyles and the tibial plateau. They enhance the stability of the knee joint by deepening and hence increasing the contact area between the femoral condyles and the tibial plateau. They help in dissipating the contact hoop forces evenly across the articular surface. By virtue of the nerve endings in their anterior and posterior thirds, they contribute to the proprioception in the knee joint. The menisci also aid in lubrication in the knee joint.[1,2]

Menisci are made up of thick collagen (90% type 1 collagen) fibers arranged in a circumferential pattern augmented by some radially oriented fibers. This arrangement gives them good tensile strength and aids in evenly distributing forces across the articular surface.[2] The circumferential fibers absorb the compressive forces, whereas the radial fibers help prevent longitudinal splitting.[3]The disruption of the meniscal integrity leads to uneven loading of the joint cartilage leading to early osteoarthritis.[4] Each meniscus is divided into three segments: anterior third, middle third (body), and the posterior third. It is the outer 20–30% that is vascular (red zone) and is supplied by the medial and lateral geniculate arteries, respectively. The inner two-thirds of the menisci are relatively avascular (white zone). This distribution of blood supply determines the treatment of meniscal tears.[5]

The medial meniscus is the larger of the two and covers about 50% of the medial tibial plateau (**Figure 35.1**). The anterior third is attached to the medial tibial spine just (7 mm) anterior to the anterior cruciate ligament (ACL) insertion. The posterior third attaches the anterior to

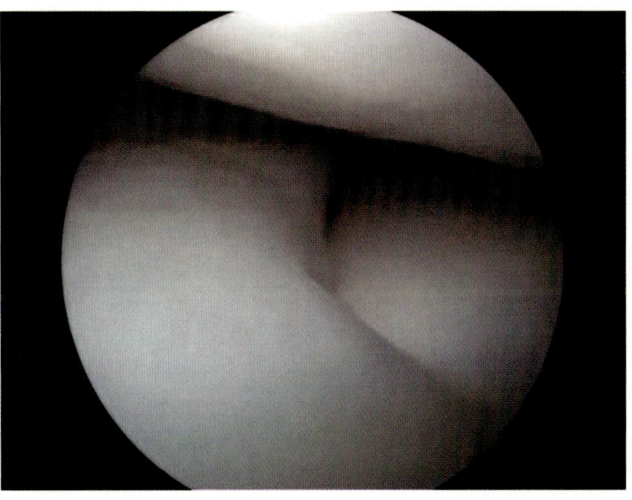

Figure 35.1 Normal meniscus

the posterior cruciate ligament. Medially, it is attached to the femoral condyle and tibial plateau by means of the coronary ligaments that form the deep portion of the medial collateral ligament.[6] The peripheral capsular attachment of the medial meniscus is continuous. This relative immobility of the medial meniscus renders it at a higher risk of injury when compared with the lateral meniscus.[7,8]

The lateral meniscus, which is the smaller of the two menisci, covers about 70% of the lateral tibial plateau. The anterior third attaches anterior to the tibial spine sharing some fibers with the ACL. The posterior third is attached just posterior to the tibial spine.[6] The peripheral capsular attachment is interrupted by the popliteus hiatus through which the popliteus tendon passes. The meniscofemoral ligaments attach the posterior third of the lateral meniscus to the lateral margin of the posterior medial femoral condyle. The anterior part is called the ligament of Humphrey, and the posterior one is called the ligament of Wrisberg. It is more mobile than the medial meniscus and may displace up to 1 cm. This may explain why meniscal injuries occur less frequently on the lateral side.[7,8]

The discoid meniscus is a developmental anomaly in which the meniscus is thickened and is disk-shaped. Discoid medial menisci are very rare with a reported incidence of 0.06–0.3%[9,10] of the general population. Discoid lateral menisci are more common with a reported incidence of 1.4–15.5%.[11] Korean and Japanese have a higher incidence (16%) than the Caucasians (5%).[12] They are of three types: partial, complete and the Wrisberg.[13] Partial and complete variants are determined by the amount of coverage of the tibial plateau. They have normal tibial attachments and are stable. The Wrisberg type has no posterior capsular and tibial attachment. The only attachment is the meniscofemoral ligament of Wrisberg. These are highly mobile and unstable.

The incidence of meniscal tears is about 61/100, 000 persons per year in the United States[14] and 60–70/100,000 persons in Europe.[15] This is a highly estimated figure as many tears are asymptomatic and a similar high number is seen in degenerative knees. Meniscal tears are more common in males (male: female = 2.5:1 to 4:1). ACL injuries are associated with almost a third of meniscal tears, more commonly the lateral meniscus.[16,17]

Meniscal tears can occur from both acute events and chronic degeneration. Sports activities, in which sudden stopping and turning movements occur, lead to a majority of tears. Thirty-two percent of meniscal tears occur during a sports injury, 39% during activities of daily living such as squatting and 29% do not have any identifiable cause/event.[16] These twisting injuries are accompanied by a sudden onset of pain in the involved knee followed by a delayed onset of swelling. The knee feels tender especially over the involved compartment (medial joint line tenderness for a medial meniscus tear and lateral joint line tenderness for a lateral meniscus tear). Mechanical symptoms such as locking, catching and giving way are frequently seen. Joint effusion is present and pain is felt on deep flexion or on squatting. Special tests include joint line tenderness, McMurray and Apley grinding tests. Joint line tenderness is the most sensitive test with a sensitivity of 74%. A positive McMurray test with a palpable clunk is very specific for a meniscal tear (98% specificity), but has a sensitivity of only 15%. A positive Apley grinding test has a specificity of 70% and sensitivity of 60%.[18-20] Symptoms of associated ligament injuries may also manifest. Chronic degenerative tears are present with episodes of mechanical symptoms. On top of the underlying pain of the degenerative process in the knee, the patient may complain of locking and/or catching of the knee. An injury or twisting episode is not necessary to produce these symptoms. Magnetic resonance imaging is the investigation of choice to detect meniscal tears. X-rays are often performed to rule out any osseous injury.

Meniscal tears are classified on the basis of tear location, tear pattern or blood supply. On the basis of tear location, they are anterior horn tears, tears of the body, posterior horn tears and root avulsions. Tears classified on the basis of pattern of tear (**Figures 35.2 to 35.6**) are flap tears, radial tears, complex/degenerative tears, longitudinal tears, bucket handle tears, parrot beak tears and horizontal tears.[21] Cooper et al. described a circumferential zone classification based on the blood supply of the meniscus. Zone 0 is the meniscosynovial junction, zone 1 is the outer third of the meniscus, zone 2 includes the middle third and zone 3 is the central third of the meniscus.[22]

Treatment of meniscal tears has evolved from conservative to surgical, from an open to arthroscopic

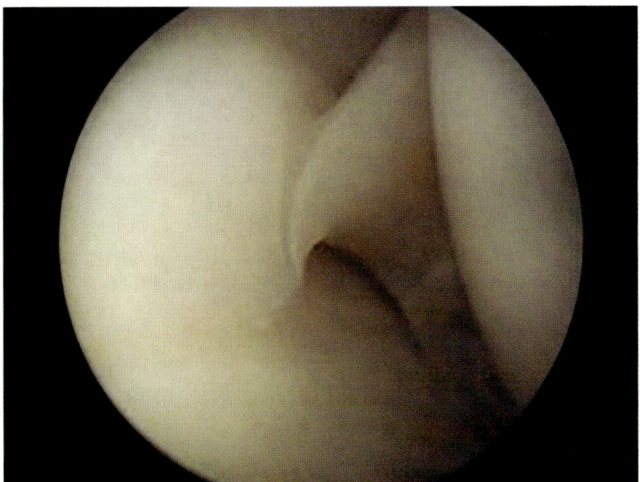

Figure 35.2 Parrot beak tear of medial meniscus

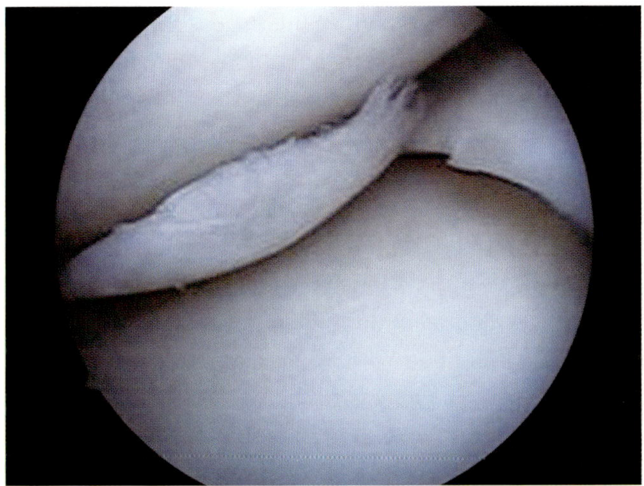

Figure 35.3 Flap tear of medial meniscus

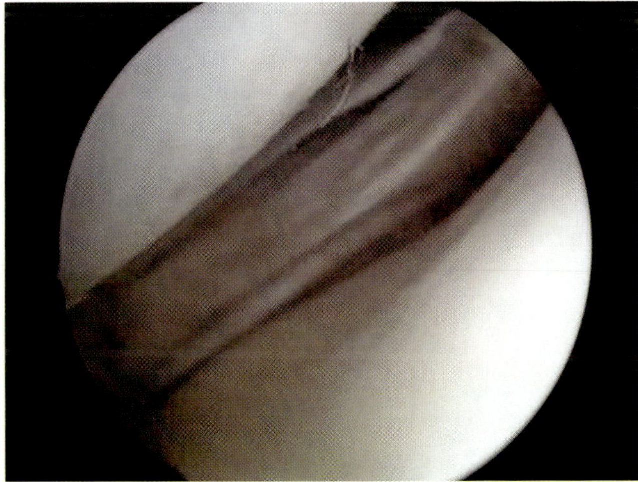

Figure 35.4 Undisplaced bucket handle tear of medial meniscus

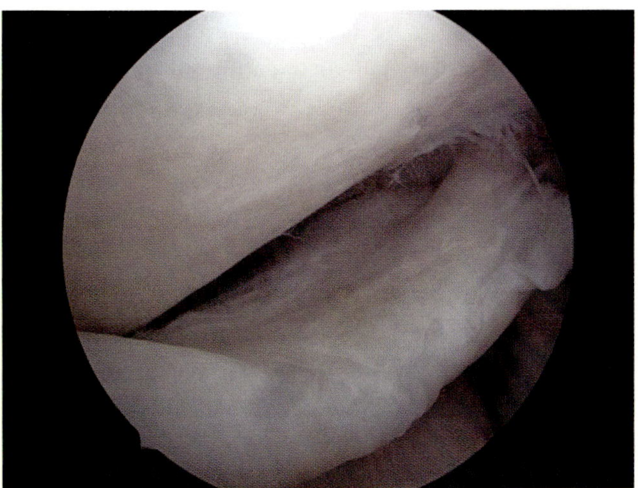

Figure 35.5 Displaced bucket handle tear of medial meniscus

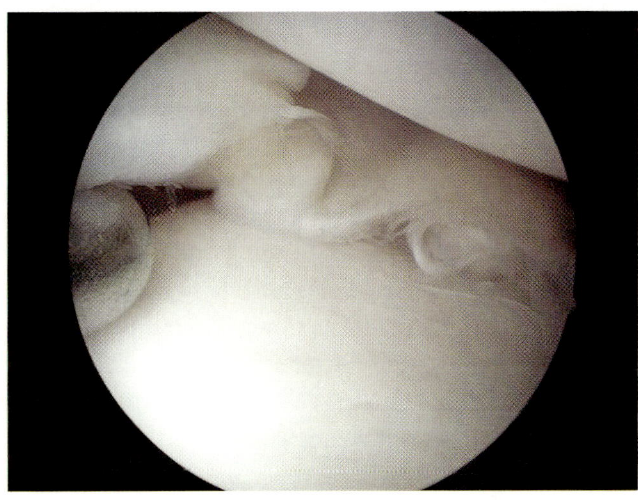

Figure 35.6 Complex tear medial meniscus

technique and from total meniscectomy to partial meniscectomy and meniscal repair. Meniscal allograft transplant is a salvage procedure to replicate the meniscal function.

Nonoperative treatment consists of activity modification, physical therapy, local ice packs, and anti-inflammatory medication. Once the acute pain subsides, the patients are prescribed with the range of motion (ROM) exercises and after attaining full ROM any muscle imbalance is corrected.[23]

Historically, the surgical treatment of an injured meniscus was open complete excision. Bland Suttons in 1897 had described menisci as functionless remnants of intra-articular leg muscles. McMurray[24] advocated a total meniscectomy for any meniscal tear and had gone to the extent of stating that 'a far too common error is shown in the incomplete removal of the injured meniscus.' This philosophy was shown to be detrimental to the articular cartilage as described by Fairbanks in 1948, who described the changes in the knee joint following a meniscectomy which included ridge formation, narrowing of the joint space and flattening of the femoral condyle.[25] Further studies delineated the importance of preserving the meniscus as demonstrated by decreased contact areas and increased peak contact stress after a partial and/or total meniscectomy.[26,27] Post-meniscectomy 74% of knees had at least one Fairbank change and 39.4% had degenerative arthritis as compared with 6% of the contralateral normal knee.[27] Results of lateral meniscectomy are worse than that of medial meniscectomy, and resection of both menisci produced worse results than the excision of a single meniscus. With the evolution of arthroscopic techniques, in the present day almost all procedures related to the meniscus are done using arthroscopically.

Meniscal tears in young patients and those associated with ACL tears should be repaired. If the meniscus is not repairable, then a partial meniscectomy should be done. During a partial meniscectomy, unstable fragments should be removed to create a smooth transition, thus maintaining a functional meniscus. The short-term results of partial meniscectomy are excellent.[28,29] Every attempt must be made to preserve as much meniscus as possible.

The decision to repair a meniscus is dictated by the location of the tear.[30,31] The indications for a meniscal repair are: acute symptomatic tears, longitudinal orientation, peripheral red-red and red-white tears, > 7–10 mm in length, concomitant ACL reconstruction and patients who prefer the procedure. Chronic tears, degenerative tears, tears in the avascular zone and those associated with infection/rheumatoid arthritis are contraindications for a meniscal repair. Meniscal repair includes inside-out techniques, outside-in techniques and all-inside meniscal repair techniques.

The inside-out technique of meniscal repair is the gold standard and has given the best results to date (**Figure 35.7**). This technique is indicated for the tears of the body and posterior horn. A 73–91% rate of success has been reported.[32,33] Relook arthroscopies have demonstrated a 65–83% rate of meniscal healing.[34,35] Concomitant ACL reconstruction improves meniscal healing rates.[36] Meticulous adherence to the surgical detail is a must to avoid neurological complications. The outside-in technique is more indicated for anterior horn tears.

All-inside meniscal repair devices are increasingly being used because of shorter operating times, smaller incisions and ability to be used in areas of the meniscus that are difficult to reach via an open procedure. They include the meniscus Arrow, T-Fix, SD Sorb staple, Biostinger, Fastener, Clearfix screw, Dart, FasT-Fix, Rapidloc, Maxfire, Cinch, and the Sequent. The newer devices are suture based and allow for compression across the meniscal tear. The success rate is around 85% based on the published reports. As the follow-up increases, the failure rates increase too (0–43%). Further studies are required to be able to formulate evidence-based guidelines for the use of all-inside devices for meniscal repair.[37,38]

Meniscal root tears are being increasingly identified, as their significance in the meniscal function is understood and recognized. Lateral meniscal root tears occur commonly with ACL tears. Medial meniscal root tears occur in a bimodal pattern. In the < 40 age group, they are seen in conjunction with other ligament tears secondary to sports injury, whereas in the >40 age group seemingly trivial trauma (getting up from a chair) leads to these tears. Indication for repair is a young patient with an ACL tear who is desirous of going back to sports.[39,40]

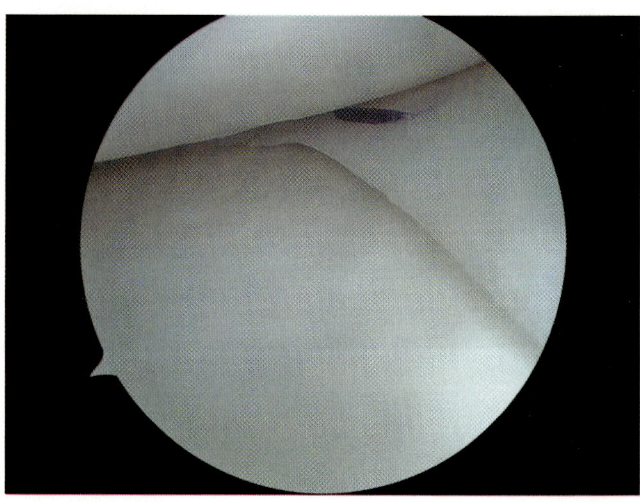

Figure 35.7 Inside out meniscal repair

Rehabilitation after a meniscal surgery is tailored around the procedure performed. In the case of a meniscal root tear, debridement or a partial meniscectomy focuses on achieving full ROM, strengthening of muscles and early return to full activity. Weight-bearing as tolerated is started immediately after surgery. In the event of a meniscal repair, weight-bearing is restricted for 4 weeks. The knee is immobilized in a knee brace for 2 weeks, and then passive movements from 10° to 100° are started. Full weight-bearing in a protective ROM brace is started and the brace continued for 6 weeks. The protocol for a patient undergoing a meniscal surgery with an ACL reconstruction is highly surgeon dependent and varies from accelerated exercise regimens to the more traditional protocols.

REFERENCES

1. Bessette GC. The meniscus. Orthopedics. 1992;15(1):35-42.
2. Fithian DC, Kelly MA, Mow VC. Material properties and structure function relationships in the menisci. Clin Orthop Relat Res. 1990;252:19-31.
3. Renstrom P, Johnson RJ. Anatomy and biomechanics of the menisci. Clin Sports Med. 1990;9:523-38.
4. Rath E, Richmond JC. The menisci: basic science and advances in treatment. Br J Sports Med. 2000;34(4):252-7.
5. Arnoczky SP, Warren RF. Microvasculature of the human meniscus. Am J Sports Med. 1982;10(2):90-5.
6. JohnsonDL, Swenson TM, Livesay MS, et al. Insertion site anatomy of the human menisci: gross, arthroscopic and topographical anatomy as a basis for meniscal transplantation. Arthroscopy. 1995;11:386-94.
7. Last RJ. Some anatomical details of the knee joint. J Bone Joint Surg Br. 1948;30B:683-8.
8. Last RJ. The popliteus muscle and the lateral meniscus. J Bone Joint Surg Br. 1950;32:93.
9. Dickason JM, Del Pizzo W, Blazina ME, et al. A series of 10 discoid medial menisci. Clin Orthop. 1992;168:75-9.
10. Schonholtz GJ, Koenig TM, Prince A. Bilateral discoid medial menisci: a case report and literature review. Arthroscopy. 1993;9:315-7.
11. Dickhaut SC, DeLee JC. The discoid lateral meniscus syndrome. J Bone Joint Surg Am. 1982,64:1068-73.
12. Ikeuchi H. Arthroscopic treatment of the discoid lateral meniscus: Technique and long-term results. Clin Orthop. 1982;167:19-28.
13. Washington ER 3rd, Root L, Liener UC. Discoid lateral meniscus in children: long-term follow-up after excision. J Bone Joint Surg Am. 1995;77:1357-61.
14. Nielse AB, Yde J. Epidemiology of acute knee injuries: a prospective hospital investigation. J Trauma. 1991;31: 1644-8.
15. Hede A, Jensen DB, Blyme P, Sonne-Holm S. Epidemiology of meniscal lesions in the knee: 1215 open operations in Copenhagen 1982-84. Acta Orthop Scand. 1990;61:435-7.
16. Drosos GI, Pozo JL. The causes and mechanisms of meniscal injuries in the sporting and nonsporting environment in an unselected population. Knee. 2004;11:143-9.
17. Poehling GG, Ruch DS, Chabon SJ. The landscape of meniscal injuries. Clin Sports Med. 1990;9:539-49.
18. Hegedus EJ, Cook C, Hasselblad V. Physical examination tests assessing a torn meniscus in the knee: a systematic review with meta-analysis. J Orthop Sports Phys Ther. 2007;37:541-50.
19. Meserve BB, Cleland JA, Boucher TR. A meta-analysis examining clinical test utilities of assessing meniscal injury. Clin Rehabil. 2008;22:143-61.
20. Terry GC, Tagert BE, Young MJ. Reliability of the clinical assessment in predicting the cause of internal derangements of the knee. Arthroscopy. 1995;11:568-76.
21. Freddie F. Master Techniques in Knee Surgery; Sports Medicine, 3rd edn. USA Lippincott William & Wilkins; 2010.
22. Cooper DE, Arnoczky SP, Warren RF. Meniscal repair. Clin Sports Med. 1991;10(3):529-48.
23. Insall S, Scott NM. Surgery of the Knee, 4th edn. Churchill Livingstone, USA, 2006.
24. McMurray TP. The semilunar cartilages. Br J Surj. 1942;29:407-14.
25. Fairbanks TJ. Knee joint changes after meniscectomy. J Bone Joint Surg Br. 1948;30:664-70.
26. Tapper EM, Hoover NW. Late results after meniscectomy. J Bone Joint Surg Am. 1969;51:517-26
27. Johnson RJ, Kettelkamp DB, Clark W, Leaverton P. Factors affecting late results after meniscectomy. J Bone Joint Surg Am. 1974;56:719-29.

28. Jareguito JW, Elliot JS, Leitner T, Dixon LB, Reider B. The effects of partial lateral meniscectomy in an otherwise normal knee: a retrospective review of functional, clinical and radiographic results. Arthroscopy. 1995;11:29-36.
29. Burks RT, Metcalf MH, Metcalf RW. Fifteen-year follow-up of arthroscopic partial meniscectomy. Arthroscopy. 1997;13:673-9.
30. Dehaven KE. Decision-making factors in the treatment of meniscus lesions. Clin Orthop. 1990;252:49-54.
31. Newman AP, Daniels AU, Burks RT. Principles and decision making in meniscal surgery. Arthroscopy. 1993;9:33-51.
32. Barber FA. Meniscus repair: results of an arthroscopic technique. Arthroscopy. 1987;3:25-30.
33. Jorgensen U, Sonne-Holm S, Lauridsen F, Rosenklint A. Long-term follow-up of meniscectomy in athletes. A prospective longitudinal study. J Bone Joint Surg Br. 1987;69(1):80-3.
34. Horibe S, Shino K, Nakata K, et al. Second look arthroscopy after meniscal repair: a review of 132 menisci repaired by an arthroscopic inside out technique. J Bone Joint Surg Br. 1995;77:245-9.
35. Rubman MH, Noyes FR, Barber-Westin SD. Arthroscopic repair of meniscal tears that extend into the avascular zone. A review of 198 single and complex tears. Am J Sports Med. 1999;26:87-95.
36. Ranalletta M, Rossi W, Paterno M, et al. An arthroscopic study in anterior cruciate ligament deficient knees. Arthroscopy. 2007;23(3):275-7.
37. Gill SS, Diduch DR. Outcomes after meniscal repair using the meniscus arrow in knees undergoing concurrent anterior cruciate ligament reconstruction. Arthroscopy. 2002;18:569-77.
38. Lozano J, Ma C, Cannon W. All inside meniscal repair: a systematic review. Clin Orthop Relat Res. 2006;455:134-41.
39. Beasley L, Armfield RD, West RV, et al. Medial meniscus root tears: an unsolved problem—demographic, radiographic and arthroscopic findings. Pittsburgh Orthop J. 2005;16:155.
40. Habata T, Uematsu K, Hattori K, Takakura Y, Fujisawa Y. Clinical features of the posterior horn tear in the medial meniscus. Arch Orthop Trauma Surg. 2004;124:642-5.

Chapter 36

Meniscal Allograft Transplantation

Dinshaw Pardiwala, Sujit Kadrekar, Waseem Siddiqui

INTRODUCTION

The meniscus has several roles that are essential to the normal knee function, including load transmission, shock absorption, joint stability, lubrication, and nutrition.[1] There is a severe compromise in these indispensable functions with meniscectomy, and this may predispose the knee to early degenerative joint disease.[2,3] With this increased awareness, efforts are now aimed at meniscal preservation. Meniscal repair is the treatment of choice whenever possible, but this procedure is not possible for many complex meniscal tears. Moreover, patients with a previous meniscectomy have symptomatic knee pain with functional disabilities caused by meniscal deficiency, which if unaddressed, leads to severe arthritis warranting either unicompartmental or total knee arthroplasty.

Keeping post-meniscectomy joint deterioration in mind, meniscus surgery in the past 75 years has seen a dramatic evolution in techniques from total meniscectomy to meniscus transplantation. Milachowski et al. performed the first meniscal transplantation on 24 November 1984 at Munich University Hospital.[4] Although the procedure was conceived almost 30 years back, it has gained credibility and popularity only now. Meniscal allografts have been found to be a feasible option for meniscal transplant in young patients with irreparable meniscal tears and previously meniscectomized knees.[5] Menisci are 'immune privileged,' and basic science studies have found little evidence of rejection.[6] The grafts readily heal at the repair site, and biomechanical testing has found that the grafts reduced joint forces compared to meniscectomy.[7]

Prosthetic meniscal replacements have been largely unsuccessful because of the inability to replicate the complex biomechanical properties of the normal meniscus.[8] However, with the increased awareness that even partial meniscectomy causes a compromise in meniscal functions, and may predispose the knee to early arthritis, the use of absorbable meniscal implants for partial meniscal defects is under intense research. Methods such as tissue engineering to replace or regenerate the meniscus also show promise, although they are as yet experimental.

BIOMECHANICS

The primary function of the meniscus is to distribute loads by increasing the contact area through which the load is transmitted across the knee.[9] Biomechanical studies have shown that the lateral meniscus bears up to 75% of the load on the lateral side.[10,11] Total lateral meniscectomy causes a 45–50% decrease in the joint contact area and a 200–300% rise in contact stresses. Similarly, after a total medial meniscectomy, the contact area in the medial compartment is reduced 50–70%, and the contact stress is increased 100%.[12,13]

Menisci also act as spacers, allowing the initial tibiofemoral contact through the more compliant menisci, with the direct articular cartilage contact occurring at higher loads.[14] An intact meniscus decreases joint stiffness and diminishes the magnitude of vertical impulse loads.[15,16] The increase in the articular peak stress and impulse loading secondary to meniscectomy may be responsible for the increased articular wear and premature degeneration that is seen in these cases.

Menisci are also secondary anterior-posterior stabilizers of the knee and a medial meniscectomy in an ACL deficient knee can increase the anterior-posterior translation at 90° by 58%.[17]

INDICATIONS

The optimal indications for meniscal allograft transplantation still need to be defined. These procedures have been performed in a large spectrum of patients and have resulted in conflicting outcomes: from prophylactic transplants in young athletic individuals who have undergone complete meniscectomy before the onset of symptoms,[18] to patients with mild unicompartmental degenerative changes.[19] Early experience has shown that patients with significant knee arthritis had the most symptomatic improvement, but most grafts failed within 2 years. As a result, patients with grade IV chondromalacia or radiographic evidence of joint incongruity are not candidates for the procedure. Joint stability and alignment are other variables that have a direct effect on success.

Currently, meniscal transplantation is indicated in young patients with a prior meniscectomy, persistent pain in the involved compartment with or without recurrent effusions, intact articular cartilage, normal alignment and a stable joint.[5] Meniscal allograft transplantation can be considered in the presence of focal grade IV chondral changes, ligament instability or limb malalignment, provided these can be corrected prior to, or during the surgery.

Although controversial, it is generally believed that a patient should be symptomatic before replacing the meniscus. Prophylactic meniscal transplantation may be beneficial in the lateral compartment where there is a more rapid progression to degeneration after meniscectomy compared with the medial compartment because of the greater role in the stress protection of the lateral meniscus.[20,21] Prophylactic medial meniscus transplants may also be considered during the ACL reconstruction in patients who have had prior medial meniscectomy, so as to afford the increased stability by a functional medial meniscus.[22]

Contraindications to the meniscus allograft transplantation include morbid obesity with a BMI more than 30, femoral flattening, advanced arthrosis, uncorrectable malalignment or instability, and skeletal immaturity. Although an age limit has not been defined, typically patients are younger than 50 years of age and have knee demands that exceed the limitations of knee arthroplasty. Inflammatory and infective arthropathy, and synovial diseases like pigmented villonodular synovitis are also contraindications to the procedure.

ALLOGRAFT SELECTION AND BIOLOGY

Types of Allograft

Four types of allografts have been described: fresh, fresh-frozen, cryopreserved and lyophilized (freeze-dried). Each has its inherent advantages:

1. Viable donor cells in the transplanted meniscus are preserved only in fresh grafts and to a lesser extent in cryopreserved grafts. Viable meniscus cells in the graft may enhance the maintenance of the extracellular matrix and, thus, the allograft's mechanical integrity following transplantation.[6,23]
2. Sterilization to reduce the risk of disease transmission generally destroys viable cells and is not performed on fresh or cryopreserved grafts.

3. Deep freezing may denature histocompatibility antigens,[24] and make a graft less immunogenic, although its clinical significance is uncertain.
4. The material properties of a graft may be altered by processing. Lyophilized grafts are prone to reduced tensile strength, graft shrinkage, poor rehydration, and synovitis,[25] and are therefore best avoided in the clinical setting.

Allograft Risks

The use of allografts holds inherent risks, and these include a potential for immune reactions and the risk of disease transmission. Although meniscus allografts are considered 'immune-privileged,' they have been demonstrated to express class I and class II histocompatibility antigens, which confer a potential for host immune response.[26] However, there has been only one report of frank immunologic rejection of a cryopreserved, nontissue antigen-matched meniscal allograft in humans, based on histologic and clinical evidence.[27] Bone grafts are well known to be immunogenic, so the presence of bone plugs attached to the meniscal graft may increase the risk of immune reaction.[28,29]

Disease transmission like HIV is also theoretically possible given the pitfalls associated with graft-processing techniques. Stringent donor selection and screening is an essential first step in the procurement of the healthy allograft tissue[30] (**Figure 36.1**).

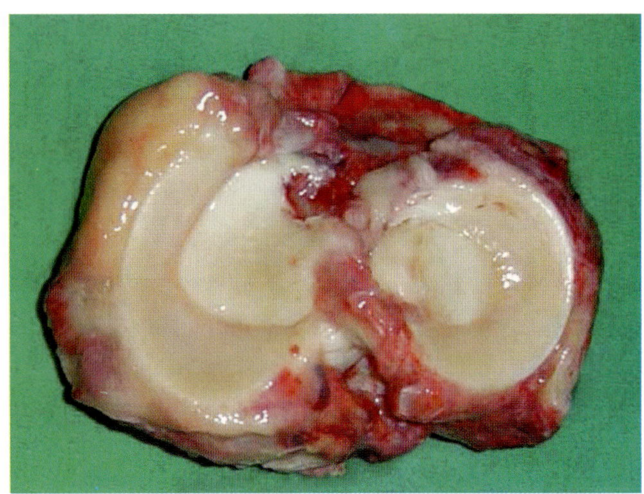

Figure 36.1 Allograft harvesting from a multiorgan donor (under 45 years of age) is performed under sterile conditions in an operating room. Both menisci are harvested, checked for macroscopic quality, and sized, prior to separation with its osseous support

Allograft Biology

The available information regarding graft biology has been generated from animal studies and what has been suggested is as follows:

- Allografts become repopulated with cells that appear to be derived from the host synovial membrane,[31] and the graft incorporates from the periphery toward the center.[32] Deep-frozen grafts have been shown to repopulate least completely, with the central region of the graft tending to remain hypocellular or acellular.[33]
- New capillaries from the capsular and synovial attachments revascularize the graft gradually and incompletely.[34]
- Graft revascularization and cellular repopulation are intrinsically associated with remodeling of the matrix structure.

Allograft Failure

Allografts fail due to either biological factors and/or biomechanical factors.[35] Hoop stress transmission and functional load transmission across the knee depend upon correct position and fixation of the anterior and posterior horn attachment sites.[35] The most common region of allograft failure due to tearing and degeneration is adjacent to the posterior horn of the medial meniscus. When the allograft's posterior horn attachment is fixed in an excessively posterior position, proper load sharing will not be re-established.[36] On the other hand, an excessively anterior position of a medial meniscal transplant may result in excessive compressive forces and meniscal damage.[37] Sizing of the allograft also plays a role in the ultimate success or failure of the implant. Undersized grafts result in poor congruity with the femoral condyle and may experience excessive loads.[35] Oversized grafts may be predisposed to extrude from the compartment, resulting in inadequate transmission of compressive loads across the knee.[35]

Allograft Sizing

Meniscal allografts are specific to compartment and side. Correct size of the allograft is important for successful healing, functionality and to maximize the graft's potential capacity to be chondroprotective.[38] Knee joint tolerance for size mismatch is minimal and graft size should be within 5% of the original meniscus.[39]

Different techniques have been employed in an attempt to match meniscal allografts with host size requirements. Currently, plain radiographs appear to serve as the gold standard of preoperative graft sizing. As per the method developed by Pollard:[40]

- Correct for magnification.
- In the coronal plane, calculate the width of the meniscus on the AP radiograph by measuring from the medial or lateral tibial metaphyseal margin, disregarding marginal osteophytes, to the peak of the respective tibial eminence.
- Calculate the length of the lateral meniscus as 70% of the tibial plateau sagittal length on the lateral radiograph (the sagittal length of the tibial plateau is defined as the distance measured at the joint line between a line running parallel to the tibia's anterior and posterior margins).
- Calculate the length of the medial meniscus as 80% of the tibial plateau sagittal length on the lateral radiograph MRI of the contralateral meniscus for sizing, remains controversial in view of numerous cases of demonstrated anatomic variability and asymmetry between left and right knees.[41,42]

Surgical Technique

For meniscal transplant to be successful the relationship of the meniscal allograft transplant with intra-articular bone and soft tissue must be anatomic.[43] The transplant is immediately expected to withstand strain along the circumferentially oriented collagen fibers at the periphery of the meniscus. The strain rate in these fibers is very low, which prevents excessive point loading of the articular cartilage.[43] This functional requirement for an effective low rate of strain, however, can only be accomplished by a technically challenging surgical technique that follows the following three requirements:

1. Attachment of the anterior and posterior horns of the transplant to the anatomically correct site of the tibial host.
2. Secure attachment of the peripheral edge of the transplant to the host capsule. Exact cephalad or caudal attachment of the transplant to the host capsule is essential to prevent premature peripheral capsular separation and for recruitment of peripheral host soft tissue structures that will then restrain improper rotational and anterior translation.
3. ***Proper sizing of the meniscus:***

There are different methods for meniscus allo-transplantation, and include both open and arthroscopic techniques, with or without the use of a bone block for lateral meniscus and bone plugs for medial meniscus. Arthroscopic techniques afford reduced surgical morbidity, avoid collateral ligament disruption, and allow earlier rehabilitation. Biomechanical cadaver studies have shown superiority of a bony fixation over soft tissue fixation technique at the attachments of the meniscal horns.[44-46] However, with bone plugs/block, the implantation technique including allograft sizing is more exacting and has an increased immunological potential due to the presence of allogeneic bone.

LATERAL MENISCUS ALLOGRAFT TRANSPLANT

Allograft Preparation

The meniscus allograft is prepared immediately prior to the surgical procedure, and involves sharp removal of all nonmeniscal soft tissue from the specimen, and fashioning of a single rectangular bone block that rigidly joins the anterior and posterior horns together in an anatomic relationship (**Figures 36.2A and B**). The bone block is precisely debrided of excess bone until it fit within the 9 mm slot on a sizing block. A template is trimmed until it exactly matches the finished bone block. Two high-strength 2-0 sutures are preinserted into the meniscal edge, whereas two high-strength coated polyester (no. 2)

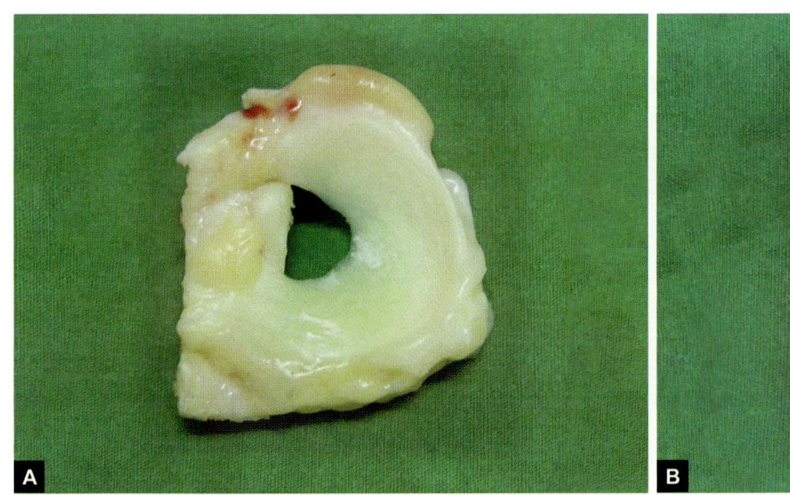

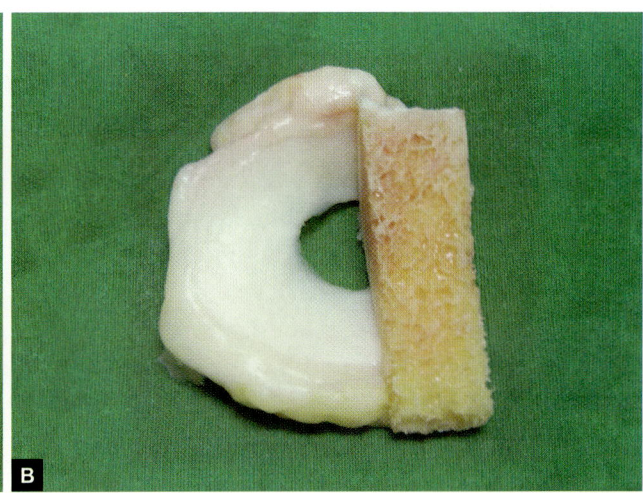

Figures 36.2A and B Lateral meniscus allograft with a single rectangular bone block rigidly joining the anterior and posterior horns together in an anatomic relationship

sutures are inserted 10 mm apart through the common bone block.

Diagnostic Arthroscopy

Under tourniquet control a diagnostic arthroscopy is performed through routine anterolateral and anteromedial portals. The lateral compartment should reveal no macroscopic chondral wear.

Removal of Remnant Meniscus

The meniscal remnants at the anterior and posterior horns are excised. The meniscocapsular junction is debrided until bleeding edges can be identified. The exact cephalad-caudal level of the peripheral meniscal rim is identified and the anatomic host site for the donor allograft is marked using knotted sutures. The presence of these markers placed 2 cm apart would subsequently prevent incorrect positioning of the transplant at the periphery when the implant would obscure an otherwise obvious view of the intended recipient edge.

Preparation of Meniscal Trough

Visualizing from the medial portal, a 9 mm meniscal gouge is inserted into the lateral portal and the recipient meniscal trough is created. The bone is removed from anterior to posterior, remaining in close proximity to the lateral border of the ACL. The trough is fashioned from 1 cm posterior to the anterior edge of the lateral tibial plateau and care is taken not to exit the bone posteriorly. With the use of a power burr, hand gouge and meniscal trough rasp, the trough is extended so as to exactly match the template of the finished allograft bone block. A 1 cm incision is made medial to the tibial tuberosity. Using an ACL tibial jig, two transosseous holes are placed 10 mm apart, into the middle of the trough, exiting the tibia adjacent to the tibial tuberosity.

Insertion and Fixation of the Meniscal Allograft

A miniarthrotomy is performed by enlarging the anterolateral portal to 3 cm length (**Figure 36.3**). After each of the sutures inserted in the graft bone block are inserted through its respective transosseous hole in the bottom of the bone trough, the allograft meniscus is introduced into the lateral compartment and recipient bony trough via the miniarthrotomy. A varus stress on the knee while flexing to 30° is required at this stage. The knee joint is taken through multiple range of motion movements to ensure that the meniscal allograft seats itself anatomically within the lateral compartment. The coincidental slopes of the host/donor lateral tibial eminence are matched, and the bone block is punched into its trough. The two bone trough sutures are tied together at the medial edge of the tibial tuberosity. Thereafter, a posterolateral incision and approach to expose the posterolateral capsule, similar to that used for lateral meniscus repairs, must be used to protect the peroneal nerve and assist in suture passage. Using a combination of zone specific meniscus suturing techniques (all-inside for posterior, inside-out for body, and outside-in for anterior), the periphery of the meniscal graft is sutured to the marked meniscocapsular junction of the host from posterior to anterior (**Figures 36.6A and B**). The stability, sizing, and anatomical position and of the graft is confirmed, and both incisions are sutured to terminate the procedure.

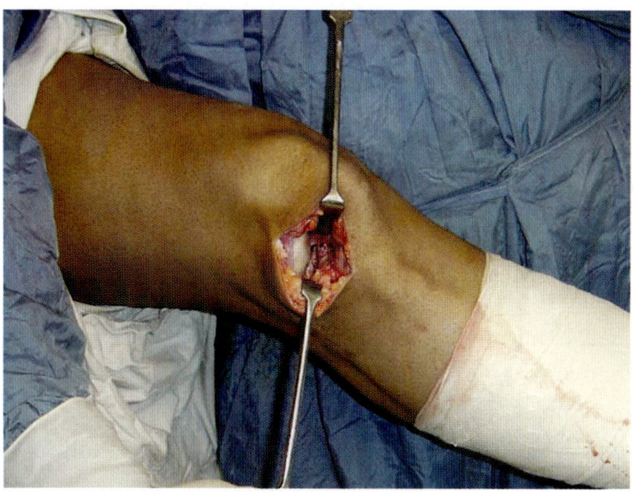

Figure 36.3 The miniarthrotomy for lateral meniscus allograft transplantation is performed by enlarging the anterolateral portal to 3 cm length

MEDIAL MENISCUS ALLOGRAFT TRANSPLANT

Diagnostic Arthroscopy

Under tourniquet control a diagnostic arthroscopy is performed through routine anterolateral and anteromedial portals. The medial compartment should reveal no macroscopic chondral wear.

Removal of Remnant Meniscus

The medial tibial eminence is excised with an osteotome to facilitate easy visualization and access to the posterior horn of the medial meniscus. The meniscal remnants at the anterior and posterior horns are excised. The meniscus rim is debrided until bleeding edges can be identified. This rim should not be completely excised since it is an important envelope limiting extrusion of the graft, and provides an excellent bed for meniscal fixation. The exact cephalad-caudal level of the peripheral meniscal rim is identified and the anatomic host site for the donor allograft is marked using knotted sutures.

Allograft Preparation

The transplant is prepared simultaneously on the back table and consists of removal of excessive peripheral soft tissue, preparation of 10 mm bone plugs (**Figure 36.4A**) at

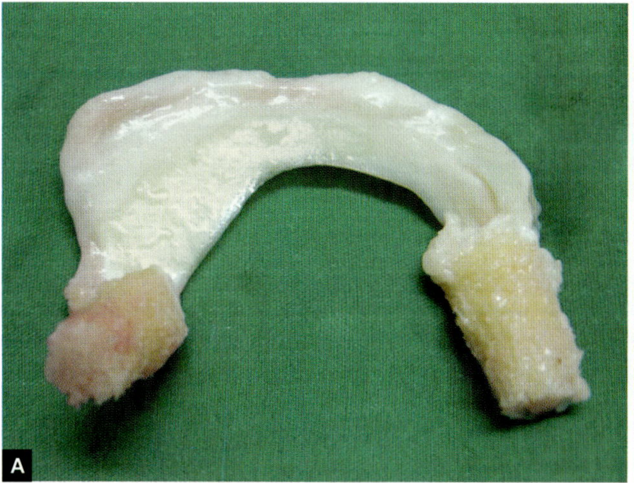

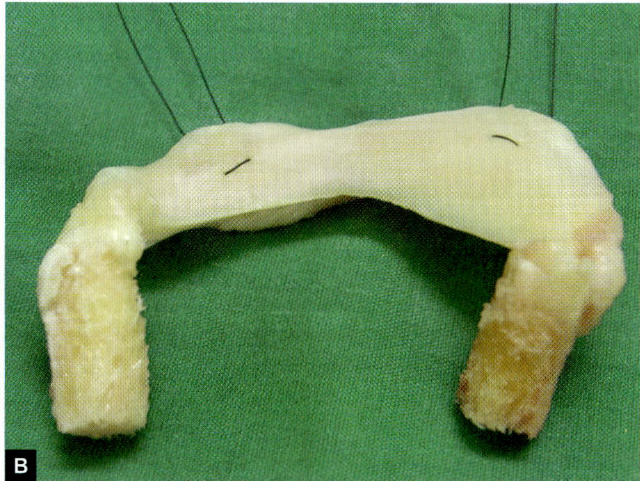

Figures 36.4A and B Medial meniscus allograft with bone plugs at the anterior and posterior horns for bony fixation

the anterior and posterior horns of the medial meniscus allograft, insertion of a high-strength coated polyester (no. 2) suture through a 1 mm hole in each bone plug, and insertion of two traction high-strength 1-0 sutures into the meniscal edge at the posteromedial and anteromedial junction (**Figure 36.4B**).

Preparation of Anterior and Posterior Horn Bone Tunnels

With the aid of an ACL tibial guide, two separate tunnels of 8 mm diameter are drilled from the medial tibial shin to the anatomic anterior and posterior meniscal horns. The intra-articular opening of each tunnel is expanded to 10 mm diameter using a small curette.

Insertion and Fixation of the Meniscal Allograft

The medial portal is extended distally to the level of the tibial plateau, and via this miniarthrotomy the allograft is inserted into the knee. Pull-through sutures in each bone plug are used to seat the plugs in their respective tunnels. Using a finger in the joint via the miniarthrotomy, the allograft is unfolded and anatomically seated in the position. This is aided by traction on the posteromedial and anteromedial sutures attached to the allograft periphery that are passed through the corresponding capsule using a suture-shuttle device. The horn sutures are tied together across the bone bridge between the transosseous tunnels. The extended medial portal is closed. Using a combination of zone specific meniscus suturing techniques (all-inside for posterior, inside-out for body, and outside-in for anterior), the periphery of the meniscal graft is sutured to the marked meniscocapsular junction of the host from posterior to anterior (**Figures 36.5A to D**).

CONCOMITANT PROCEDURES

The common concomitant procedures performed with meniscus transplantation are the ACL reconstruction and osteochondral transplantation. In such situations, the sequence of steps should be adapted to protect the graft from the ACL instrumentation, and maximize the efficiency of the operation. When a high tibial osteotomy is required in the same knee, we recommend that this be performed 4–6 months prior to the meniscus transplantation.

COMPLICATIONS

In addition to the usual potential complications of surgery and allograft usage, complications after this procedure are infrequent and include arthrofibrosis, loss of bony fixation, detachment of the allograft from the bone block, allograft tears, and failure to heal. There have been instances of progressive unexplained pain, infection, or persistent synovitis that have warranted allograft removal.[4,5,47-51]

POSTOPERATIVE REHABILITATION

The knee is immobilized in an extension brace. Our protocol incorporates gradual return of the knee range (restricted to 90° for the first 3 weeks) and restricted weight-bearing (toe-touch to partial weight-bearing) over the first 6 weeks postsurgery. The knee range is started on the second postoperative day, and full range of knee movements is achieved by 6 weeks. Full weight-bearing without crutches is started at 6 weeks, and the brace is continued during ambulation up to 8 weeks. Strenuous knee activity, and high impact are restricted for 6–8 months. A return to light sports is allowed after 1 year. To maximize allograft longevity, we recommend long-term activity modification.

RESULTS AND OUTCOMES

Clinical studies with short- to medium-term follow-up have shown that meniscal allografts do successfully revascularize and heal to the periphery. They undergo cellular repopulation and remodeling, can be of subjective benefit. Results are encouraging in terms of reducing knee pain and increasing function.[5] However, of the 39 clinical studies evaluating meniscal transplantation, most series have been small and there is a lack of uniformity between patient selection, type of allograft preservation, surgical technique, concomitant procedures, and follow-up. Despite the high success seen on second-look arthroscopy and clinical evaluation, the ultimate success of a meniscal

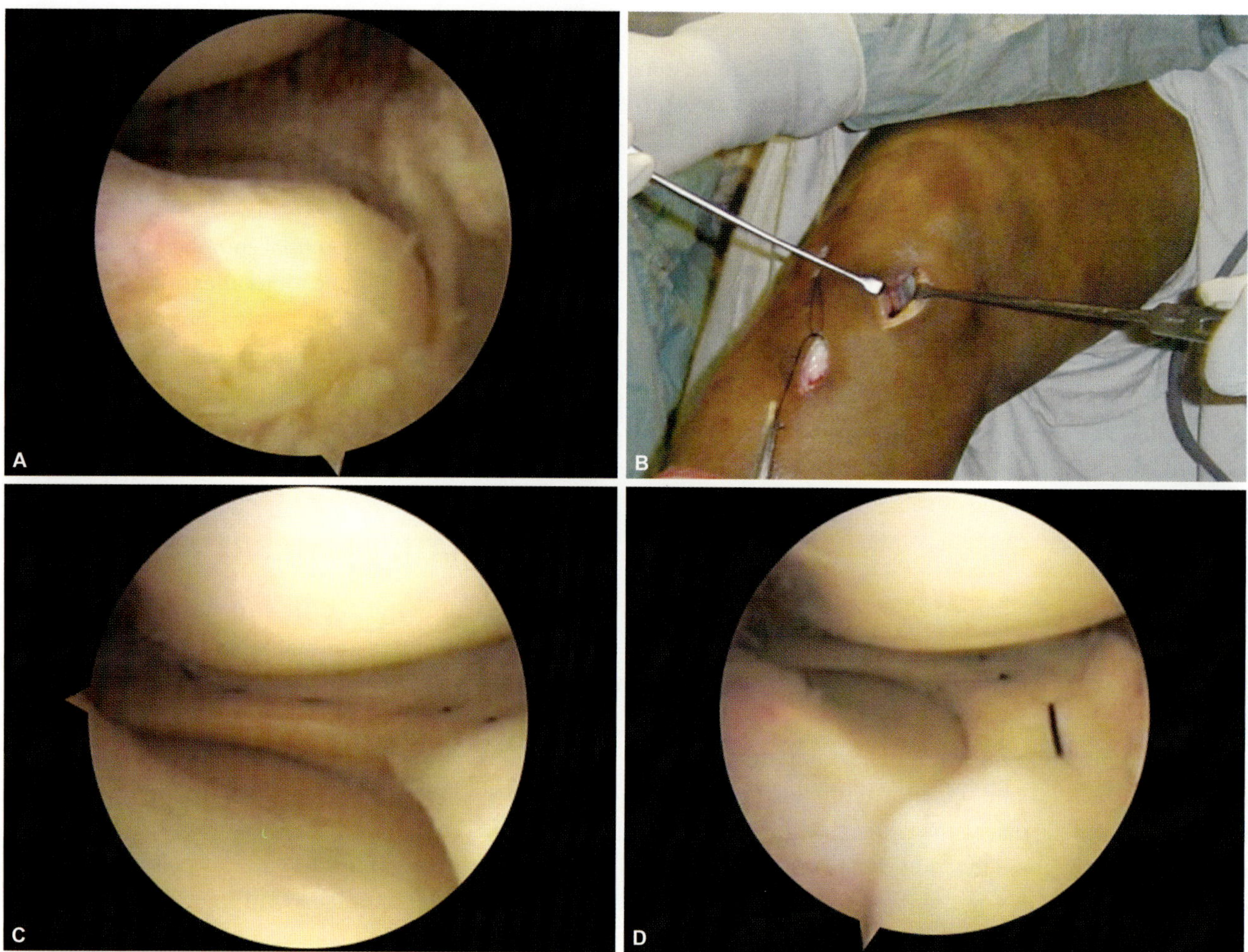

Figures 36.5A to D Medial meniscus allograft transplantation. (A) Arthroscopic image of medial meniscus deficient compartment; (B) The medial miniarthrotomy for graft insertion in the knee; (C and D) Arthroscopic images after zone-specific repair of the medial meniscus allograft

transplant can only be measured by its ability to prevent arthrosis. The durability of the allograft and its long-term ability to deter arthritis remains to be established.

Clinical and Functional Outcomes

All studies show significant improvement in subjective pain scales and functional activity scores with 75–90% patients reporting fair to excellent results.[52] Almost all studies report improved physical examination findings at follow-up with regard to pain, range of motion, effusion, stability, function tests, and IKDC score. There does not seem to be any difference between isolated meniscus transplants and combined procedures. No statistically significant difference has been noted in meta-analyses between allograft preservation techniques or fixation methods.

Radiological Outcome

Meniscus allograft transplantation has a chondroprotective effect in 30–40% of patients.[52] Although a significant number of patients showed no signs of progressive joint space narrowing, this has been observed in many patients in most series and tends to increase with longer follow-ups. It is unknown whether allograft transplantation delays the natural course of osteoarthritis after meniscectomy.

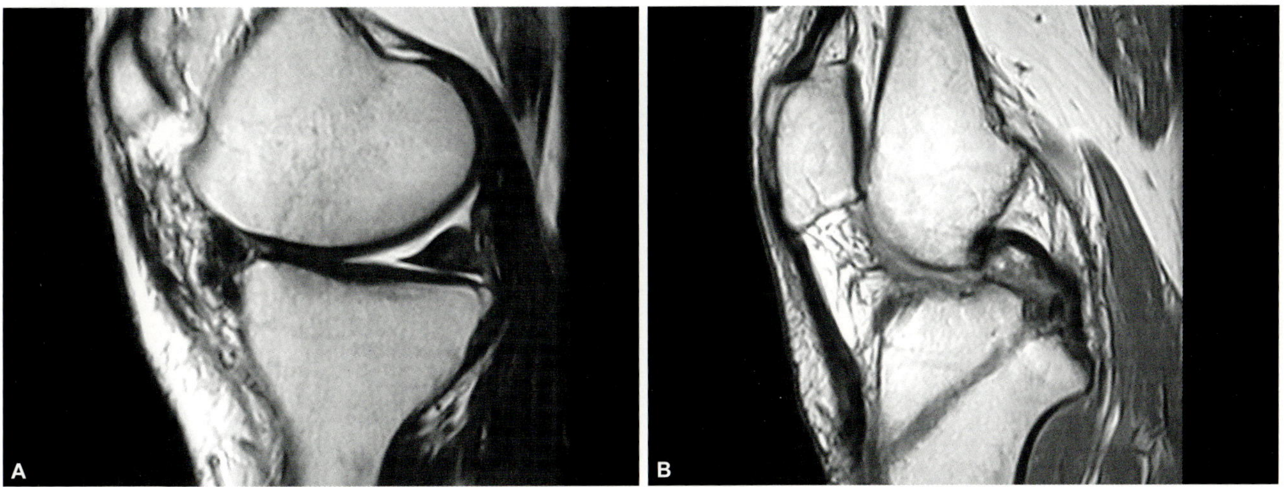

Figures 36.6A and B Postoperative MRI of medial meniscus allograft transplant showing healing of graft periphery to the capsular rim, and position of tunnel for bony fixation of the posterior horn

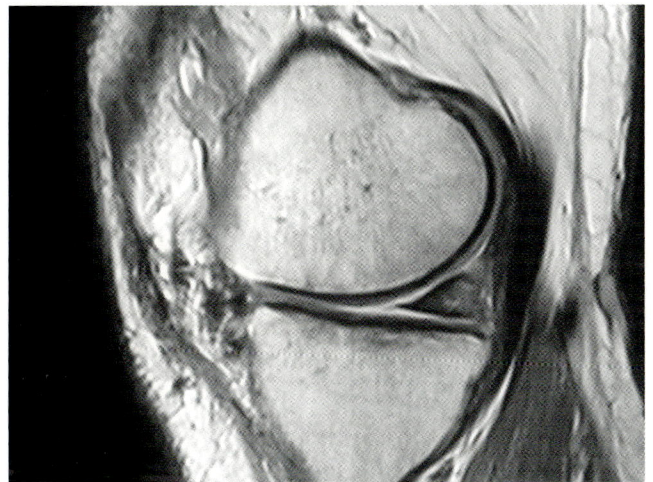

Figure 36.7 Postoperative MRI 2 years following medial meniscus allograft transplantation. The allograft reveals abnormal signals that reflect biological remodeling of the extracellular matrix of the allograft

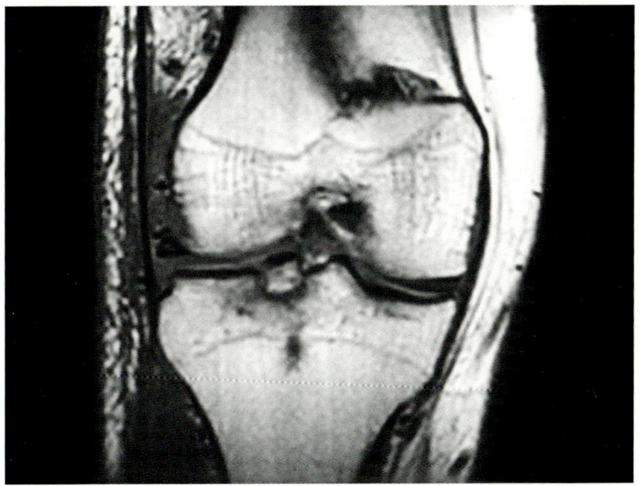

Figure 36.8 Meniscus extrusion noted in a postoperative weight-bearing MRI done 6 months after lateral meniscus allograft transplantation. Note appropriate seating of the allograft bone block within its recipient channel

MRI Analysis

In one recent long-term study, progression of cartilage degeneration according to MRI and radiological criteria was halted in 35% of patients, indicating a potential chondroprotective effect.[53] On MRI, healing of the allograft to the rim is observed in the vast majority of patients (**Figures 36.6A and B**). The allograft also often reveals abnormal signals that reflect biological remodeling of the extracellular matrix of the allograft (**Figure 36.7**). MRI can also reveal allograft extrusion (**Figure 36.8**), and this has been reported independent of surgical fixation technique. All allograft types reveal some extent of shrinkage, whether the etiology of shrinkage is a mechanical or biological process is unknown.

Survival Analysis

Based on available survivorship data, a clinical survivorship of 70% at 10 years can be anticipated for both medial and lateral allografts[52] (**Figures 36.9A and B**). Ligament

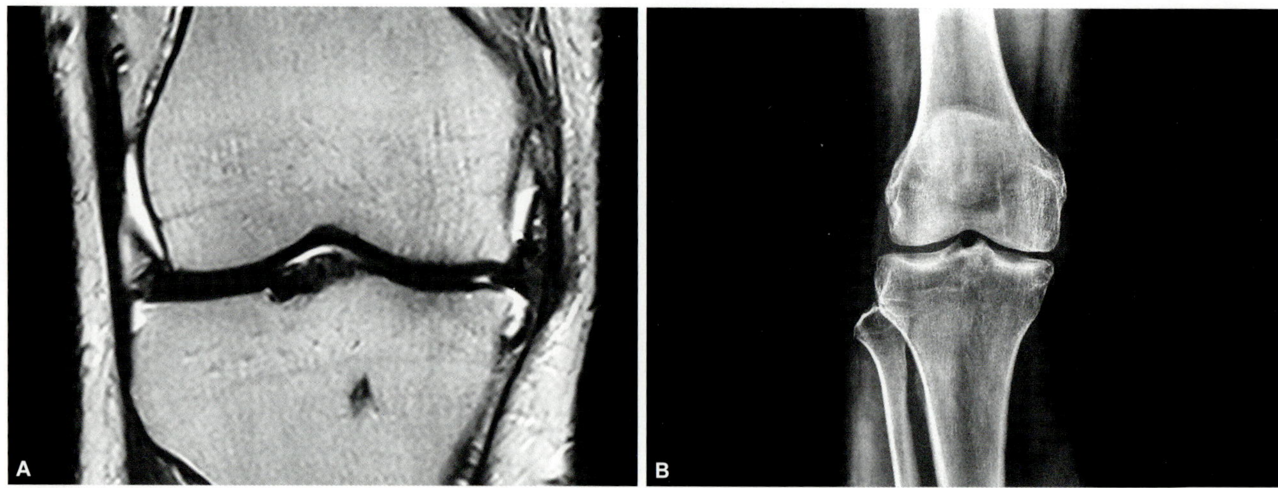

Figures 36.9A and B MRI and weight-bearing AP radiograph of a 10-year follow-up of medial meniscus allograft transplantation

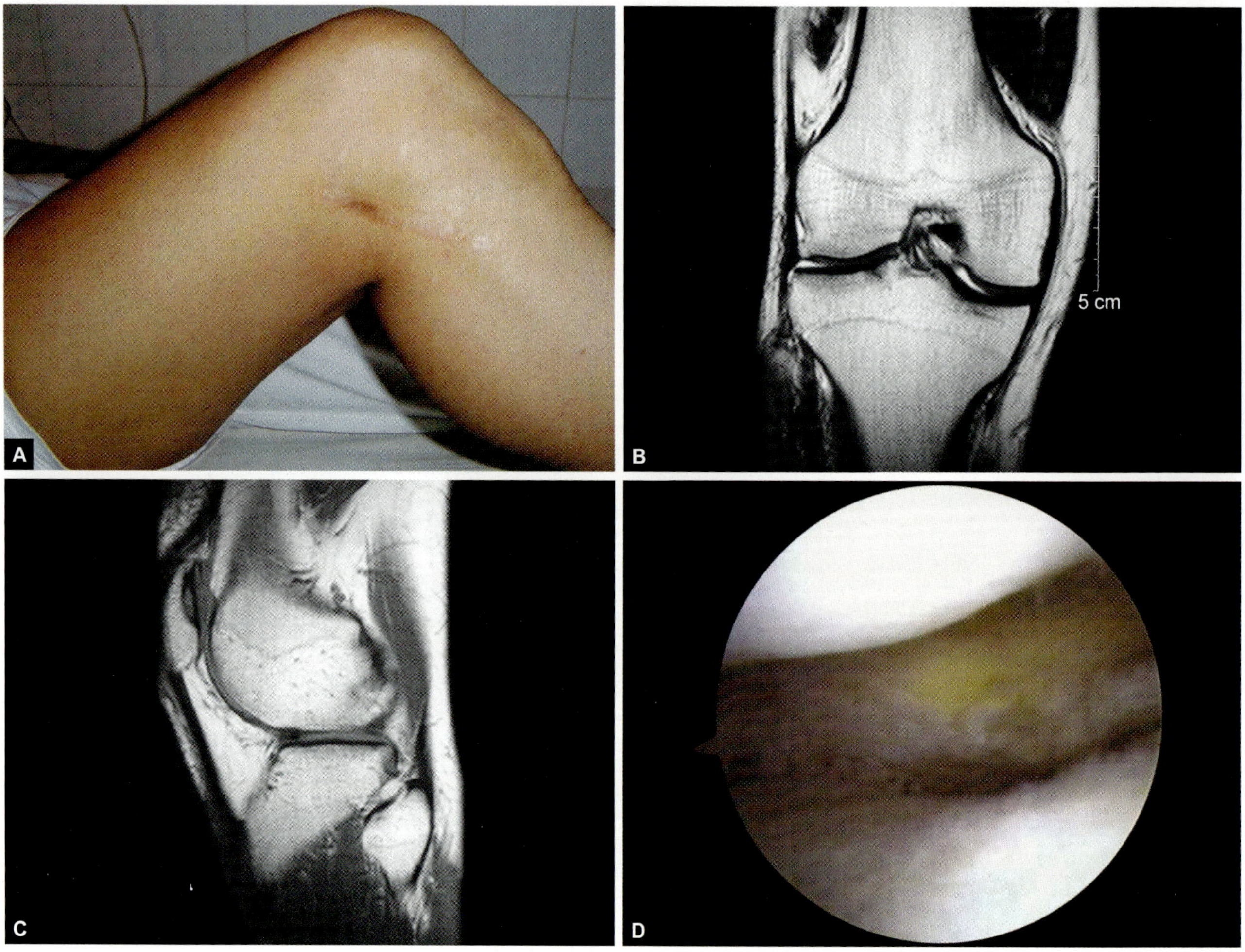

A
B
5 cm
C
D

Figures 36.10A to D

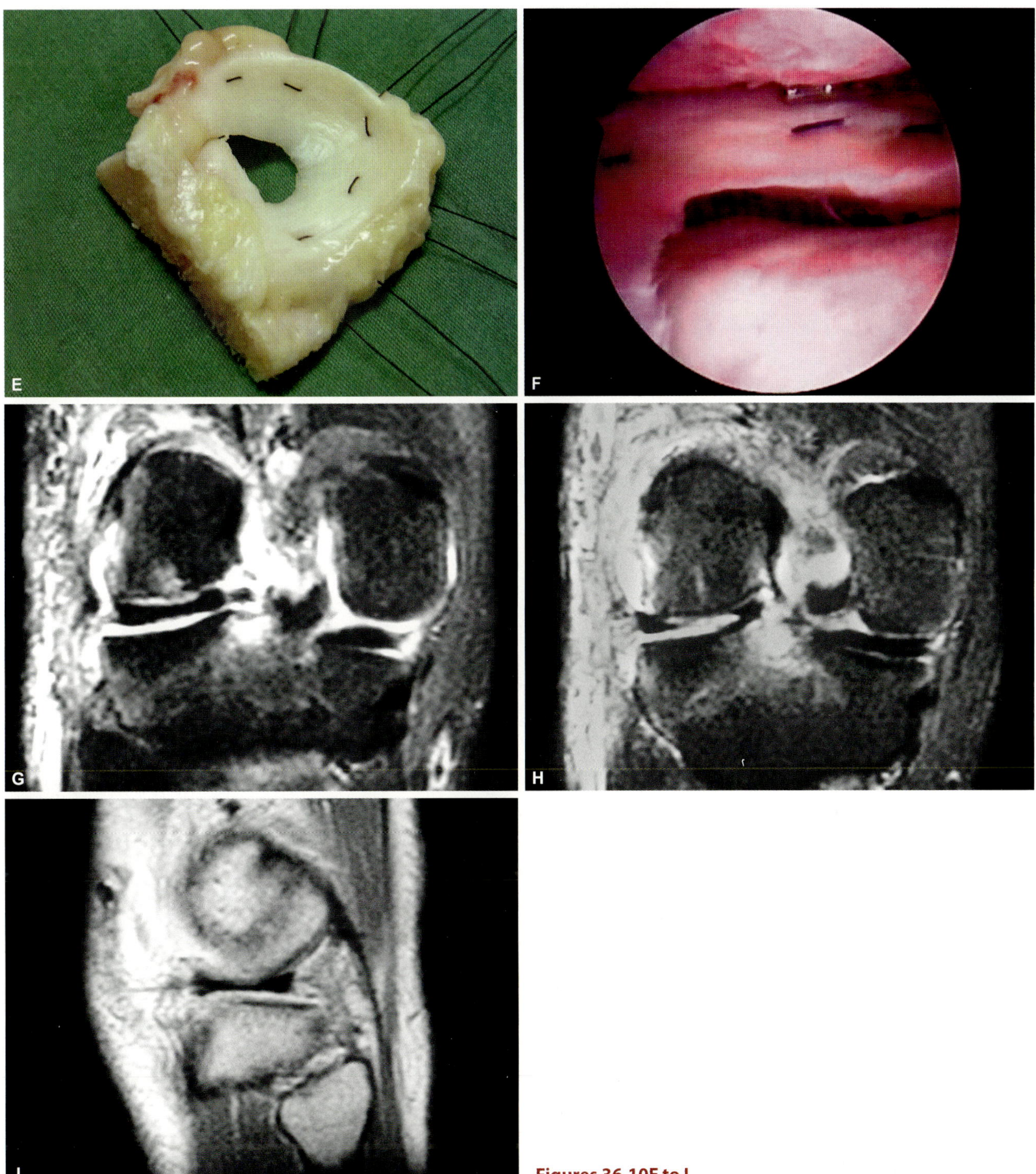

Figures 36.10E to I

Figures 36.10A to I Lateral meniscus allograft transplantation. (A) Preoperative clinical photograph showing presence of scar of open total meniscectomy; (B and C) Preoperative MRI showing lateral meniscus deficient knee; (D) Arthroscopic image of lateral meniscus deficient compartment; (E) Prepared lateral meniscus allograft with bone block connecting anterior and posterior horns; (F) Arthroscopic image after lateral meniscus allograft transplantation; (G to I) Postoperative MRI at 1 year showing healing of the meniscal periphery. There is no size mismatch, no extrusion, and no shrinkage of the transplant. Articular cartilage thickness and signal intensity is normal

instability, axial malalignment and cartilage degeneration are associated with a higher failure rate and inferior results.

REFERENCES

1. Arnoczky A, Adams M, DeHaven K, et al. Meniscus. In: Woo SL, Buckwalter JA (Eds). Injury and Repair of the Musculoskeletal Soft Tissues. Chicago, IL: American Academy of Orthopaedic Surgeons; 1987. p. 487.
2. Ferkel RD, Davis JR, Friedman MJ, et al. Arthroscopic partial medial meniscectomy: an analysis of unsatisfactory results. Arthroscopy. 1985;1:44-8.
3. Aglietti P, Buzzi R, Bassi PB. Arthroscopic partial meniscectomy in the anterior cruciate ligament deficient patient. Am J Sports Med. 1988;16:597-602.
4. Milachowski KA, Weismeier K, Wirth CJ. Homologous meniscal transplantation. Experimental and clinical results. Int Orthop. 1989;13:1-9.
5. Rijk PC. Meniscal allograft transplantation - Part I: background, results, graft selection and preservation, and surgical considerations. Arthroscopy. 2004;20:728-43.
6. Siegel MG, Robert CS. Meniscal allografts. Clin Sports Med. 1993;12:59-80.
7. Bylski-Austrow DI, Meade T, Malumed J, et al. Irradiated meniscal allografts: mechanical and histological studies in the goat. Trans Orthop Res Soc. 1992;38:175-83.
8. Sommerlath K, Gillquist J. The effect of a meniscal prosthesis on knee biomechanics and cartilage: an experimental study in rabbits. Am J Sports Med. 1992;20:73-6.
9. Teurlings L. Meniscal injuries. In: Arendt EA (Ed), Orthopedic Knowledge Update: Sports Medicine, 2nd edn. Rosemont, IL: AAOS; 1999. pp. 349-54.
10. Seedhom BB. Transmission of the load in the knee joint with special reference to the role of the menisci: II, experimental results, discussion and conclusions. Eng Med. 1979;8:220-8.
11. Walker PS, Erkman MJ. The role of menisci in force transmission across the knee. Clin Orthop. 1975;109:184-92.
12. Kettelkamp DB, Jacobs AW. Tibiofemoral contact area - determination and implication. J Bone Joint Surg Am. 1972;54:349-56.
13. Fukubayashi T, Kurosawa H. The contact area and pressure distribution pattern of the knee. Acta Orthop Scand. 1980;51:871-9.
14. Baratz ME, Fu FH, Mengato R. Meniscal tears: the effect of meniscectomy and of repair on intra-articular contact areas and stress in the human knee. Am J Sports Med. 1986;14:270-5.
15. Newman AP, Daniels AU, Burks RT. Principles and decision making in meniscal surgery. Arthroscopy. 1993;9:33-51.
16. Kurosawa H, Fukubayashi T, Nakajima H. Load bearing mode of the knee joint: physical behaviour of the knee joint with or without menisci. Clin Orthop. 1980;149:283-90.
17. Greis P, Bardana DD, Holmstrom MC, Burks RT. Meniscal injury: I. Basic science and evaluation. J Am Acad Orthop Surg. 2002;10:168-76.
18. Johnson BL, Bealle D. Meniscal allograft transplantation. Clin Sports Med. 1999;18:93-108.
19. Garrett JC. Meniscal transplantation: a review of 43 cases with 2 to 7 years follow-up. Sports Med Arthrosc Rev. 1993;1:164-7.
20. Allen PR, Denham RA, Swan AV. Late degenerative changes after meniscectomy. J Bone Joint Surg Br. 1984;66:666-71.
21. Jorgensen U, Sonne-Holm S, Lauridsen F, Rosenklint A. Long term follow-up of meniscectomy in athletes. A prospective longitudinal study. J Bone Joint Surg Br. 1987;69:80-3.
22. Barber FA. Accelerated rehabilitation for meniscus repairs. Arthroscopy. 1994;10:206-10.
23. Arnoczky SP, Milachowski KA. Meniscal allografts: where do we stand? In: Ewing JW (Ed), Articular Cartilage and Knee Joint Function: Basic Science and Arthroscopy. New York: Raven; 1990. pp. 129-36.
24. Brown KL, Cruess RL. Bone and cartilage transplantation in orthopedic surgery. A review. J Bone Joint Surg Am. 1982;64:270-9.
25. Jackson DW, Windler GE, Simon TM. Intra-articular reaction associated with the use of freeze-dried, ethylene oxide-sterilized bone-patella tendon-bone allografts in the reconstruction of the anterior cruciate ligament. Am J Sports Med. 1990;18:1-11.
26. Khoury MA, Goldberg VM, Stevenson S. Demonstration of HLA and ABH antigens in fresh and frozen human menisci by immunohistochemistry. J Orthop Res. 1994;12:751-7.
27. Hamlet W, Liu SH, Yang R. Destruction of a cryopreserved meniscal allograft: a case for acute rejection. Arthroscopy. 1997;13:517-21.

28. Bos GD, Goldberg VM, Zika JM, Heiple KG, Powell AE. Immune responses of rats to frozen bone allografts. J Bone Joint Surg Am. 1983;65:239-46.
29. Stevenson S. The immune response to osteochondral allografts in dogs. J Bone Joint Surg Am. 1987;69:573-82.
30. American Association of Tissue Banking. Standards for Tissue Banking McLean, VA: American Association of Tissue Banking; 1993.
31. Rodeo SA, Seneviratne A, Suzuki K, et al. Histological analysis of human meniscal allografts: a preliminary report. J Bone Joint Surg Am. 2000;82:1071-82.
32. Rijk PC. Meniscal allograft transplantation—part II: alternative treatments, effects on articular cartilage, and future directions. Arthroscopy. 2004;20:851-9.
33. Arnoczky SP, DiCarlo EF, O'Brien SJ, Warren RF. Cellular repopulation of deep-frozen meniscal autografts: an experimental study in the dog. Arthroscopy. 1992;8:428-36.
34. Jackson DW, McDevitt CA, Simon TM, et al. Meniscal transplantation using fresh and cryopreserved allografts: an experimental study in goats. Am J Sports Med. 1992;20:644-56.
35. Rodeo SA. Meniscal allografts—where do we stand? Am J Sports Med. 2001;29:246-61.
36. Alhalki MM, Hull ML, Howell SM. Contact mechanics of the medial tibial plateau after implantation of a medial meniscal allograft. A human cadaveric study. Am J Sports Med. 2000;28:370-6.
37. Noyes FR, Barber-Westin SD, Rankin M. Meniscal transplantation in symptomatic patients less than fifty-years old. J Bone Joint Surg Am. 2005;87:149-65.
38. Verdonk R, Kohn D. Harvest and conservation of meniscal allografts. Scand J Med Sci Sports. 1999;9:158-9.
39. Wilcox TR, Goble EM, Doucette SA. Goble technique of meniscus transplantation. Am J Knee Surg. 1996;9:37-42.
40. Pollard ME, Kang Q, Berg EE. Radiographic sizing for meniscal transplantation. Arthroscopy. 1995;11:684-7.
41. Wilcox TR, Goble EM, Doucette SA. Goble technique of meniscus transplantation. Am J Knee Surg. 1996;9:37-42.
42. Johnson DL, Swenson TM, Livesay GA, et al. Insertion-site anatomy of the human menisci: gross, arthroscopic, and topographical anatomy as a basis for meniscal transplantation. Arthroscopy. 1995;11:386-94.
43. Goble M. Meniscal allograft technique. Oper Tech Orthop. 2000;10:220-6.
44. Chen MI, Branch TP, Hutton WC. Is it important to secure the horns during lateral meniscal transplantation? A cadaveric study. Arthroscopy. 1996;12:174-81.
45. Paletta GA Jr, Manning T, Snell E, Parker R, Bergfeld J. The effect of allograft meniscal replacement on intra-articular contact area and pressures in the human knee: a biomechanical study. Am J Sports Med. 1997;25:692-8.
46. Alhalki MM, Howell SM, Hull ML. How three methods for fixing a medial meniscal autograft affect tibial contact mechanics. Am J Sports Med. 1999;27:320-8.
47. Zukor DJ, Cameron JC, Brooks PJ, et al. The fate of human meniscal allografts. In: Ewing JW (Ed). Articular Cartilage and Knee Joint Function. New York: Raven; 1990. pp.147-52.
48. Goble EM, Kohn D, Verdonk R, Kane SM. Meniscal substitutes-human experience. Scand J Med Sci Sports. 1999;9:146-57.
49. Cameron JC, Saha S. Meniscal allograft transplantation for unicompartmental arthritis of the knee. Clin Orthop. 1997;337:164-71.
50. Rath E, Richmond JC, Yassir W, Albright JD, Gundogan F. Meniscal allograft transplantation. Two to eight years results. Am J Sports Med. 2001;29:410-4.
51. Shelton WR, Dukes AD. Meniscus replacement with bone anchors: a surgical technique. Arthroscopy. 1994;10:324-7.
52. Verdonk P, Verdonk R. Results and Indication. In: Verdonk R, et al. (Eds). Meniscal Transplantation. ISAKOS: 2013.
53. Verdonk PC, Demurie A, Aimqvist KF, et al. Transplantation of viable meniscal allograft. J Bone Joint Surg Am. 2006;88:109-18.

Chapter 37

Cartilage Defects: Mosaicplasty/Microfracture/ Autologous Chondrocyte

David V Rajan, K Santosh Sahanand

INTRODUCTION

'Once articular cartilage is damaged it is not reversible, we can only delay or halt the progression of damage'. This was a common quote used in our clinical practice. This does not hold true today, as various advancements in our field have led to new procedures that help restore the damaged cartilage. In this chapter, we will be dealing with focal cartilage defects and not degenerated diffuse cartilage lesions.

BASIC SCIENCE

Hyaline cartilage is a viscoelastic substance that does the complex function of reducing the friction during joint movements and absorbing the shock during loading. Structurally, cartilage is composed of chondrocytes and extracellular matrix. In the past, cartilage was described as a tissue with sparse cells and homogenous amorphous extracellular matrix. Over the past 40 years we have understood more about their simple but unique structure. It has only one cell type namely chondrocytes, no vessels, no nerves but an array of fibrillar and nonfibrillar proteins in the extracellular matrix.[1]

The extracellular matrix constitutes 95% of the tissue volume that includes collagen, proteoglycans, and other glycoproteins.[2] These substances maintain sufficient amount of water within the matrix. A proportion of the water moves in and out of the extracellular matrix contributing to its material property, joint lubrication, and nutrition of chondrocytes by diffusion. Articular cartilage is divided into four zones: 1, superficial; 2, middle or transitional; 3, deep or radial; 4, layer of calcified cartilage[2] (**Figure 37.1**).

Type II collagen is the predominant type. Its arrangement varies with depth. The superficial layer has thin fibrils arranged parallel to the joint surface contributing resistance for joint shear stress. The middle layer has larger fibrils obliquely arranged and suitable for transmission of forces between superficial and deep layers and absorbing compressive load. Deep layer fibrils are arranged vertical to the joint surface and parallel to each other and resist compressive load. The fibrils cross into the calcified cartilage layer providing mechanical transition from the cartilage to bone.[3]

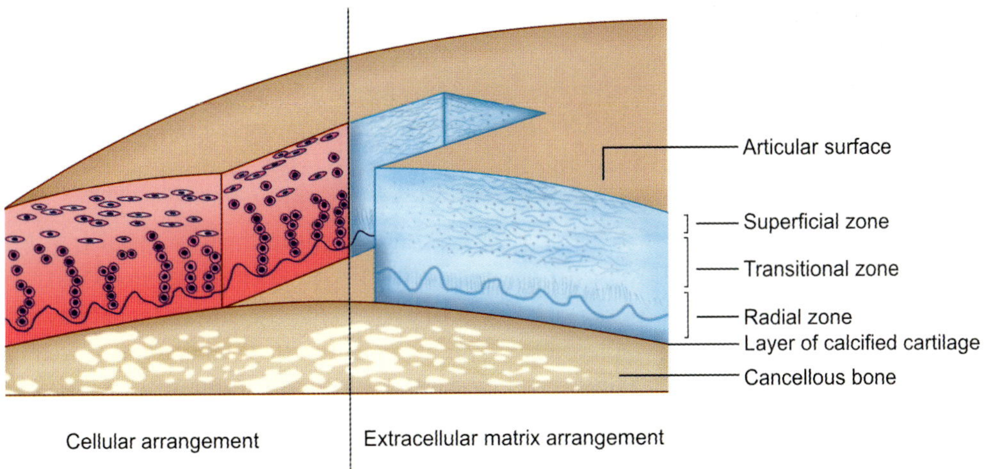

Figure 37.1 Schematic diagram of the cartilage anatomy

Proteoglycans consists of glycosaminoglycans arranged around the central protein core. Glycosaminoglycans are highly negatively charged so they have high affinity for water molecules. The negative charges between the closely arranged fibrils repel each other and keep the molecule in a relatively rigid state. Because of the relative rigidity of the intermingling fibrils, the capacity to swell up by absorbing water is decreased. So the tissue is in a semihydrated state.[4] If the same proteoglycans were uncontained as in a solution, they would occupy a much larger volume as compared to the cartilage.

Chondrocytes are derived from the mesenchymal stem cells (MSCs). They constitute only 2% of the tissue volume but they are responsible for the synthesis of the extracellular matrix.[5] The superficial zone has inactive flattened cells and deeper layers have spherical cells arranged in columns. The ability of chondrocytes to self-proliferate and synthesize extracellular matrix decreases with age.[6] After skeletal maturity, chondrocytes rarely replicate under normal conditions.[5]

The biomechanical property of the cartilage can be explained by the fluid phase—solid phase model: fluid phase being water and electrolytes, solid phase being collagen, proteoglycans, and other glycoproteins. On compressive loading of the cartilage, fluid is squeezed out of the solid phase that holds on to the fluid due to its affinity to water. But the deformation of the solid phase is prevented as they are in relatively rigid state due to their high negative charge and repulsion between fibrils. As the cartilage surface is less permeable water cannot be quickly squeezed out of the solid medium. So on high impact rapid loading situation, the fluid phase protects the solid phase from shock. On prolonged continuous loading the fluid is slowly squeezed out of the solid phase and the entire load is supported by the solid phase.[7]

Healing of the injured cartilage is limited as it is avascular and the only cellular component, namely chondrocyte, is trapped in the extracellular matrix. But if the subchondral bone is damaged, then access to the mediators of injury healing is established and healing response does take place. So healing of partial thickness and full thickness cartilage injury is different.

Partial thickness injury shows brief cellular response and no significant healing. Full thickness injury heals with fibrocartilage formation that degenerates over time.

EVALUATION

Clinical evaluation has less role in diagnosing a cartilage lesion but essential in diagnosing associated ligament insufficiency, malalignment and meniscal pathology. Plain X-rays can pick up joint space reduction in chronic cases. Full length X-rays are needed for malalignment quantification. CT arthrogram can be used to evaluate cartilage surface.

Magnetic resonance imaging (MRI) scans of 1.5 or 3.0 T field strength are useful for cartilage evaluation. Standard 2D and advanced isotropic 3D sequences provide a detailed morphological evaluation. T1 sequences are used for viewing cartilage and subchondral bone anatomy. T2 sequence shows clear demarcation between the synovial fluid and cartilage surface. Newer techniques like T1rho, T2 mapping, delayed gadolinium enhanced MRI of cartilage are useful in evaluating the collagen and proteoglycan.[8] With these advances an MRI is currently considered the gold standard in structural evaluation of cartilage defect and repair.[9] Arthroscopy concludes the evaluation in assessing the superficial cartilage morphology, stability of the lesion and wall of the lesion.

PRINCIPLES OF TREATMENT

Various factors are involved in decision making while treating cartilage injury. These can be categorized as patient factors, joint factors and cartilage factors.

Patient factors	*Joint factors*	*Cartilage factors*
• Age • Activity level • BMI • Disability relevance • Comorbidity • Smoking • Functional demand • Affordability	• Ligament insufficiency • Malalignment • Loss of meniscus • Inflammatory pathology	• Location • Grade • Size • Edge

The ability of chondrocytes to proliferate decreases with age. So cartilage repair procedures are less successful with increasing age. Postsurgery demand and expected load on the healing cartilage must be taken into consideration. Comorbidities like diabetes and smoking may hamper cartilage healing. Insurance coverage and economy of the patient are also factors that cannot be ignored.

Coexisting joint pathologies for example knee ACL insufficiency or varus malalignment or patellar instability must be addressed with stabilization or corrective osteotomy or patellar stabilization respectively along with cartilage repair procedures.

The most important factors are the cartilage factors. Location: whether the defect is in the weight-bearing area? Is it protected by meniscus from bone to bone contact (tibiofemoral or patellofemoral)? At what degree of flexion do the lesions come into contact will decide if the lesion would be symptomatic or not.

Grading commonly followed is ICRS (International Cartilage Repair Society) (**Figure 37.2**).

Defect size influences the congruity of the joint surface, large defect results in uncontained lesions whereas small lesions are contained (**Figures 37.3A and B**). The size and shape of the entire joint surface is a factor as the defect size increases. The arbitrary size of 2 cm^2 (16 mm diameter) was considered the upper limit, above which rim contact stress increases. A recent study has shown that rim stress becomes a factor for defect 0.76 cm^2 (10 mm diameter).[10] Symptomatic cartilage lesions ICRS grade 2 to 4, arbitrarily more than 1 cm^2 require treatment.

TREATMENT OPTIONS

International Cartilage Repair Society (ICRS) grade 1 cartilage defect is generally asymptomatic and does not warrant any intervention. ICRS grade 2 cartilage defect needs debridement of the unstable fragments and smoothening out the edges of the defect leaving the base intact to reduce edge loading.[11] This procedure is called chondroplasty.

International Cartilage Repair Society (ICRS) grade 3–4 defects require cellular reinforcement to stimulate healing. This can be achieved by either recruiting cells from the marrow from the base of the lesion or transplanting chondrocytes. Bone marrow-based techniques are microfracture, chondroneogenesis (microfracture covered with collagen), scaffold based (microfracture covered with scaffolds), and stem cell based (bone marrow mesenchymal stem cell transplantation). Chondrocytes based techniques are autologous osteochondral grafts [mosaicplasty/ osteochondral autograft transfer system (OATS)], cultured chondrocytes [autologous chondrocyte implantation (ACI)], osteochondral allograft.

The commonly followed techniques in clinical practice are discussed below.

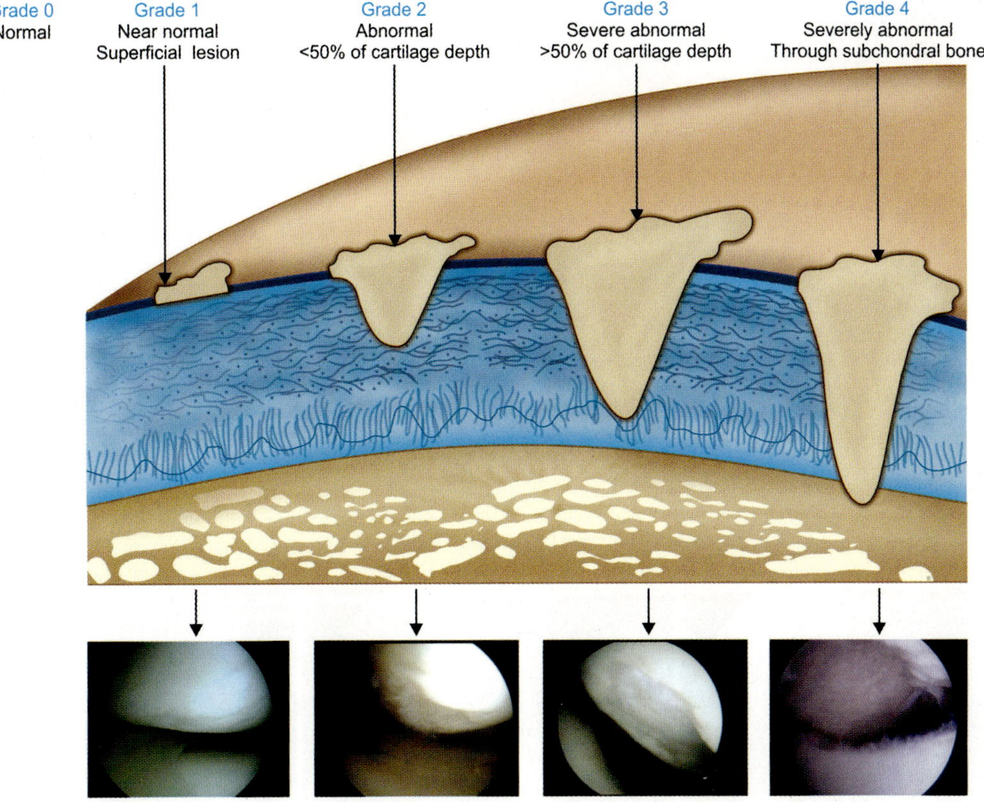

Figure 37.2 ICRS grading of cartilage defect with schematic and arthroscopic examples

CHONDROPLASTY

Chondroplasty is an effective treatment for pain associated with partial thickness cartilage defect. Mechanical debridement using arthroscopic shaver has its downside, so radio frequency (RF) chondroplasty is gaining popularity.

RF energy produces oscillation of electrolytes in intra- and extracellular fluid, and the resultant molecular friction produces localized heat. Three effects of RF on cartilage are neo surface formation, ablation and annealing. At temperatures 40–70°C collagen, triple helix uncoils, reforms when heat is removed, the fibrils are arranged parallel to the surface compared with before. This neo surface may reduce the shear stress compared to mechanical debridement. At > 100°C, the collagen is completely destroyed, so the irregular superficial tissue closer to the RF probe exposed to higher temperatures is ablated. Annealing effect reduces the permeability to water, so the stiffness of cartilage is retained[12] (**Figure 37.4**).

Chondroplasty for large flaps can start with mechanical debridement so that heating effect of RF on neighboring tissues can be reduced. By keeping the RF probe moving helps reduce point heating and localized damage.[12]

MICROFRACTURE

Marrow stimulation techniques include drilling, abrasion chondroplasty and microfracture. Microfracture is the most common cartilage procedure performed currently. Microfracture is preferred to other marrow

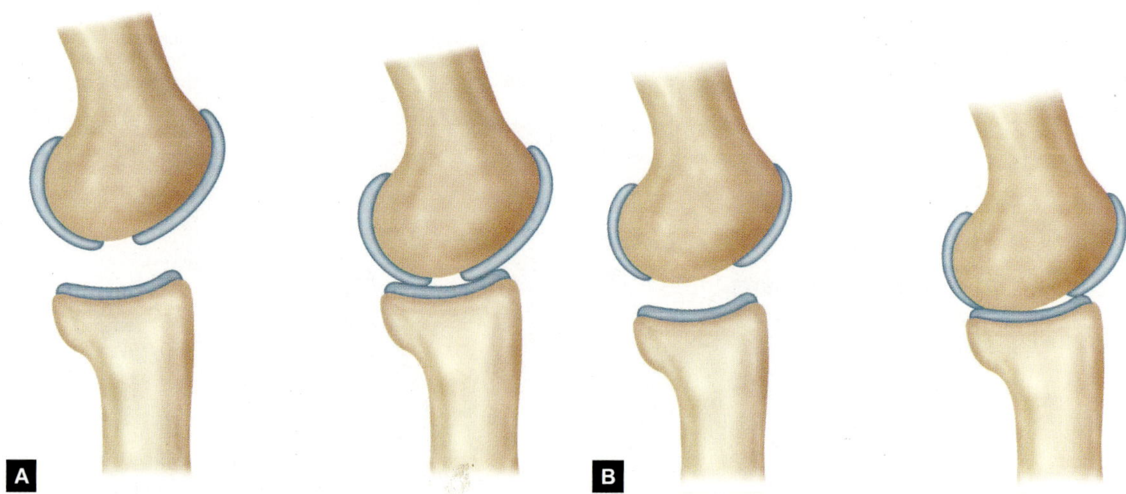

Figures 37.3A and B Schematic view showing how size, location of defect and size of condyle influence containment. (A) Contained defect; (B) Uncontained defect

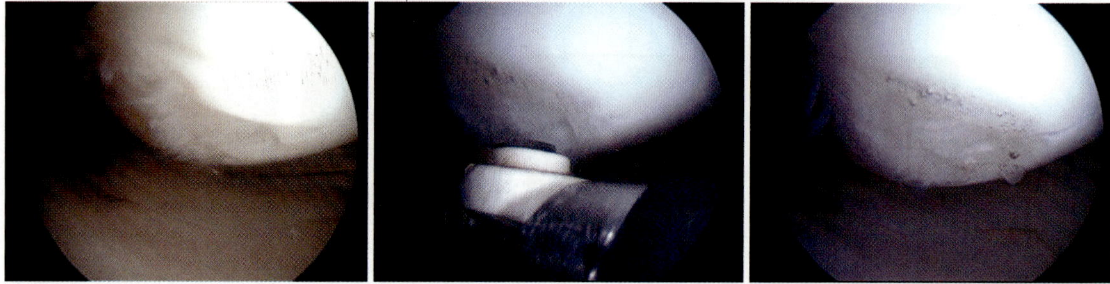

Figure 37.4 Radiofrequency chondroplasty. First picture showing arthroscopic view of ICRS grade 2 cartilage defect. Second showing radiofrequency chondroplasty using radiofrequency probe. Last picture postchondroplasty showing neo surface

stimulation techniques as the subchondral bone damage is less.

Microfracture involves perforation of the subchondral bone to gain access to the cells rich boned marrow. The resultant clot contains mesenchymal stem cells, platelets and various growth factors to aid fibrocartilage formation.[13]

Procedure

- Debridement of the base of the cartilage defect to remove debris
- Removal of the calcific cartilage layer using curette to enhance healing response[13]
- Debridement of the borders of the defect to create a vertical stable wall; a well shouldered lesion will reduce mechanical load on the lesion[14]
- Multiple perforation of the subchondral bone with awl of various angles (**Figure 37.5A**)
- Direction of perforation as perpendicular to surface as possible (**Figure 37.5B**)
- Use various angled awls and switch portals to achieve desired angle (**Figure 37.5C**)
- Perforation to the approximate depth of 2–4 mm is indicated by release of fat droplets[15]
- Start from periphery towards the center
- Leave 3–4 mm bone bridge between each perforation to avoid fracture
- Release the tourniquet or reduce pump pressure to check for bleeding from the perforation (**Figure 37.5C**).

Rehabilitation

This depends on the location of the defect. Defect in the weight-bearing area requires nonweight bearing for 6 weeks, followed by partial weight bearing for 2 weeks. ROM exercise is started early. Defect in patellofemoral

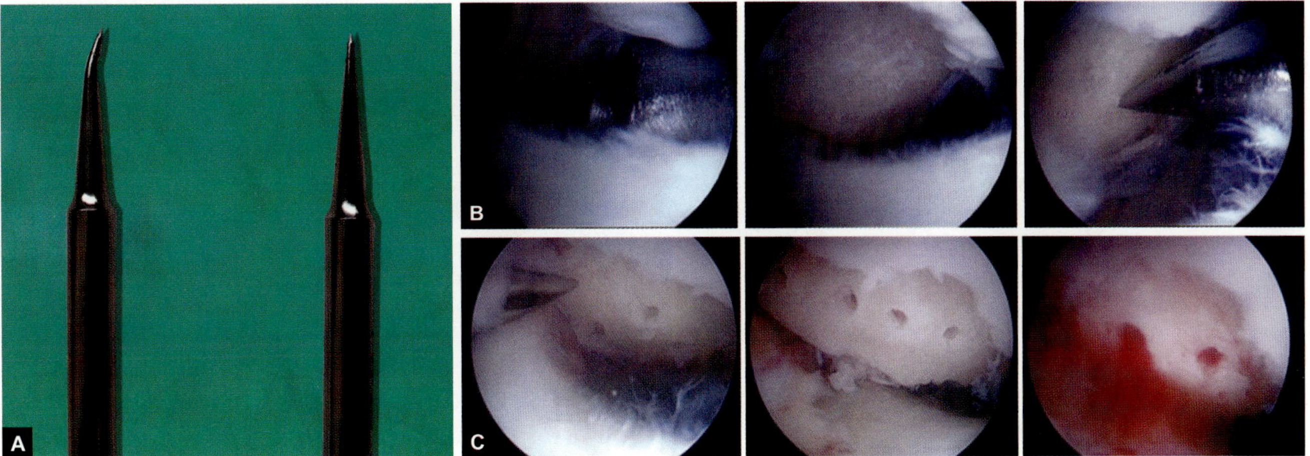

Figures 37.5A to C (A) Chondropic awl. Angled and straight awl; (B) Arthroscopic view of ICRS grade 4 defect debrided and calcified cartilage layer removed with scoop. Postdebridement view of the defect seen from anterolateral portal. Angled awl introduced from anteromedial portal and perforated perpendicular to the surface of subchondral bone; (C) Arthroscopic view switching the portals, viewing from anteromedial portal and awl through the anterolateral portal. Postmicrofracture view with 3 mm gap between the holes. View after releasing the tourniquet, marrow blood flowing out

area require restriction of ROM depending on region of patella and trochlea engagement that varies with flexion. Patella engages on trochlea from superior to inferior as knee flexion increases from 30° to 90°.

Advantages

- Arthroscopic procedure
- Single-staged procedure
- Simple instrumentation
- Cost-effective.

Disadvantages

- Chance of subchondral fracture
- Heals with fibrocartilage formation
- Chance of intralesional osteophyte formation
- Results of secondary procedures postmicrofracture are inferior.

MOSAICPLASTY

Osteochondral graft transfer procedure has evolved over 60 years from transfer of osteochondral blocks to cylindrical plugs using standardized tubular instruments. Mosaicplasty also called as OATS involves harvesting cylindrical osteochondral plugs from lesser weight-bearing areas of the joint into drill holes made in the defect area matching the contour of the cartilage surface.[16] This procedure can be done arthroscopically, it is better to start with miniarthrotomy before attempting full arthroscopic technique.

Procedure

Preparation of the defect by debridement (**Figure 37.6A**) and planning the size and number of osteochondral plugs is required. The various sizes are 2.7, 3.5, 6.5 and 8.5 mm diameter. Smaller grafts fill irregular defects but are fragile, have lower pull out strength and are difficult to handle. So larger grafts are preferred to minimize the number of plugs. But sizes more than 8.5 mm result in donor site morbidity.

Donor site for graft harvest is from the medial and lateral margins of the trochlea superior to the sulcus terminalis, and margin around notch area. But topographic analysis has shown that the medial and lateral parts of the trochlea match the weight-bearing areas of medial and lateral femoral condyles better.[17] Graft harvester is advanced to 15 mm depth and rotated 90° clockwise and

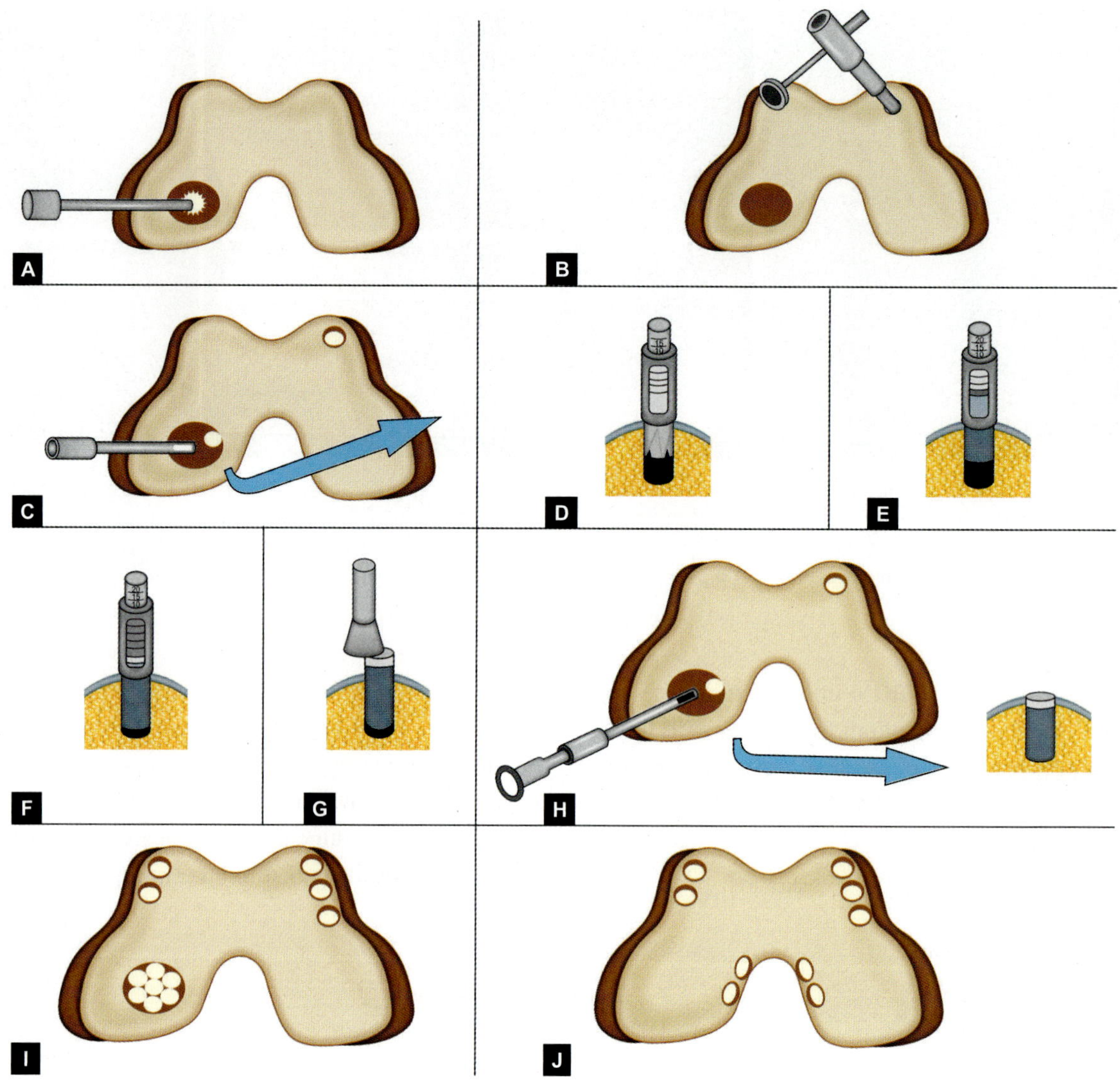

Figures 37.6A to J Mosaicplasty procedure: (A) Defect in the femoral condyle debrided and planning done for size and number of grafts required; (B) Graft harvest from the edge of trochlea using harvester introduced, twisted and removed; (C) Defect area drilled with corresponding size; (D) Closer view of the drilling; (E) Without removing the guide the graft introduced; (F) Graft gently tapped in till 2 mm remained outside; (G) Tamp used at the edge to tap it flush to avoid sinking in of graft; (H) Graft flush with surface; (I) Same procedure repeated till filling the defect; (J) Representation of donor sites for graft harvest in knee

counterclockwise to remove the cylindrical plug (**Figure 37.6B**). At least 3 mm bone bride must be present between the donor defects to maintain stability of donor site.

Drill guide is placed over the defect area and the drill hole made to the depth 2 mm short of the plug length (**Figure 37.6C**). The drill guide is kept in the same position and the graft is placed into the guide checking the orientation of the graft contour to match with the donor site contour (**Figure 37.6D**). The graft plug is gently tapped in to 2 mm short of the desired articular surface level (**Figures 37.6E and 37.6F**). A tamp is used to pass the graft further to place it flush to the normal surface by placing the tamp at the edge of the graft and remaining on the normal area so as to avoid inadvertent deeper placement of the graft (**Figure 37.6G**). The next drill hole is made as planned and the same sequence is followed to achieve sufficient coverage of the defect (**Figure 37.6H and I**).

Rehabilitation

ROM exercises are started immediately in the postoperative period: nonweight bearing for 3 weeks to prevent graft subsidence; partial weight bearing for 3–6 weeks; high demand sports activities after 6 months.

Advantages

- Single-staged procedure
- Restores hyaline cartilage
- Cost-effective.

Disadvantages

- Donor site morbidity
- In large defects acceptable contour cannot be restored
- Technically demanding.

AUTOLOGOUS CHONDROCYTE IMPLANTATION

It is a two-staged procedure that involves initial harvest of autologous chondrocytes for chondrocyte culture, followed by the second stage of implanting the expanded cell population in the defect. This was first clinically introduced by Brittberg in 1987.[18] Follow-up studies have shown autologous chondrocyte implantation (ACI) to have a better outcome especially in defects larger than 4 cm^2.[19] The classical method of first generation ACI involved suturing the defect with a periosteal patch and injecting the cultured chondrocytes. This method showed good symptomatic improvement but reported incidence of graft hypertrophy due to the periosteum. So the second generation ACI came up where collagen membrane was tried instead of periosteum. Third generation ACI involves loading cultured cells in various biomaterial scaffolds like collagen, hyaluronic/polylactide meshes or fibrin gel. Fourth generation ACI involves use of growth factor and gene manipulation in the culturing process.

Procedure

- Stage 1 involves graft harvest from lesser weight bearing area as shown in (**Figure 37.6J**). The graft is transported in a sterile medium to the lab
- In the laboratory, the cartilage is enzymatically digested and expanded in culture. After achieving sufficient quantity of cells depending on the defect size, target concentration should be around 30 million cells mL^{-1}
- The culturing process changes with the third generation, the cultured cells are loaded in scaffolds in the form of collagen, hyaluronic, PLA, PGA sponges or meshes as in MACI (matrix associated ACI)[1] or in gel form as in Gel MACI[20]
- After about 4–6 weeks of sufficient expansion of cells, culture is tested for cell concentration, viability and contamination and transported back for the second stage of implantation without breaking the sterility chain (**Figure 37.7**)
- In Stage 2, miniarthrotomy is performed based on the location of the lesion, but with newer generation ACI techniques arthroscopic technique is possible
- Defect area is cleared of debris, stable vertical walls are created (**Figure 37.8**) The floor of the defect is dried and diluted adrenaline soaked Neuro Patties can be used
- Classical method involves harvesting periosteum from proximal tibia and suturing over the defect with the cambium layer facing the defect using 6.0 Vicryl. Water tight compartment is checked with saline infusion into the lesion. Then cells are injected under the periosteum and then margins are sealed with fibrin glue

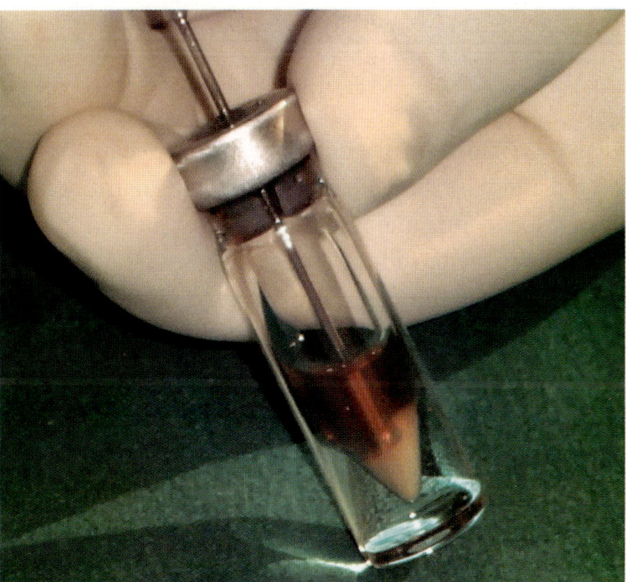

Figure 37.7 Cultured chondrocytes transported in sterile vials. Cells being aspirated for implantation

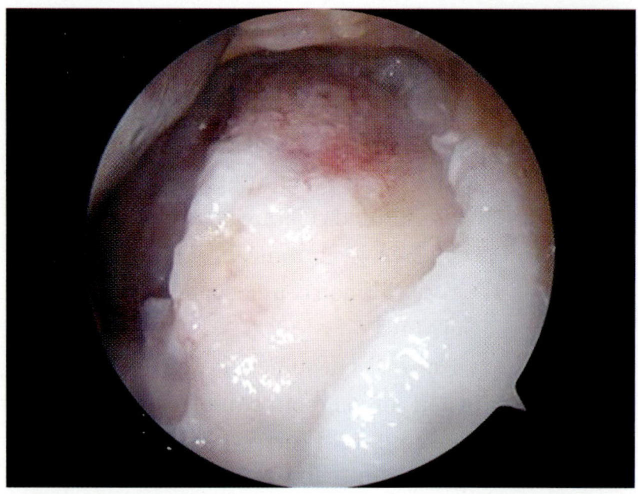

Figure 37.8 Grade 4 defect floor and margins debrided till stable vertical walls

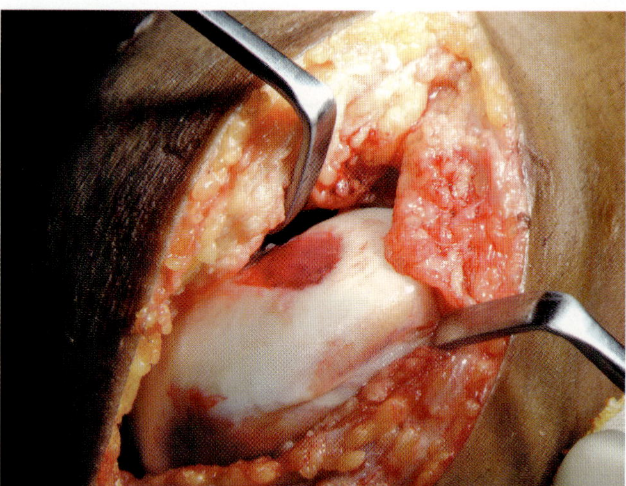

Figure 37.9 Gel ACI. Arthrotomy and gel ACI implantation in the medial femoral condyle

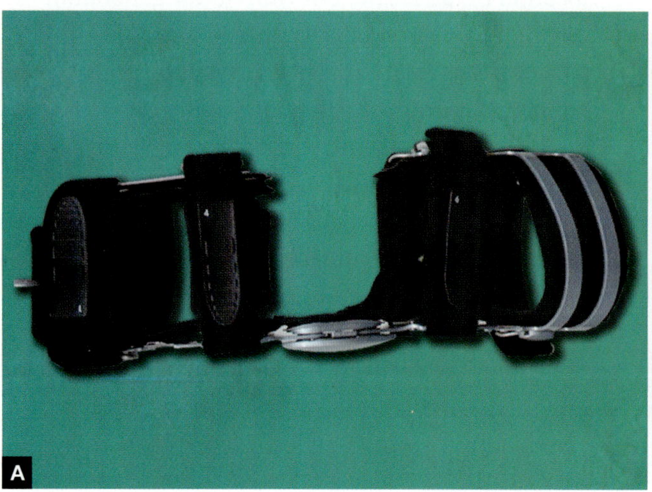

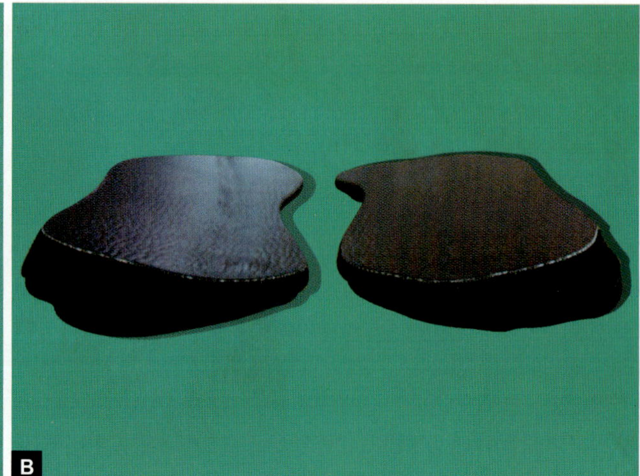

Figures 37.10A and B (A) Unloading brace; (B) Lateral wedge insoles used to medial joint unloading

- In MACI method, the defect area is templated first with foil and the exact shape and size of the matrix scaffold is cut and implanted in the defect and sutured
- Newer gel based ACI does not involve suturing the defect, the cell gel mixture sets in 8 minutes (**Figure 37.9**).

Rehabilitation

Rehabilitation is based on the phases of maturation of the graft.[21] The initial proliferative phase where cells multiply is followed by the matrix production phase where the extracellular matrix is synthesized and orients itself. During these phases, loading of the defect is avoided so patient is kept nonweight bearing for 6 weeks and ROM is started early to prevent adhesions and help cellular orientation. During the maturation phase the graft gains its stiffness, so the stimulus is gradually given from 6 weeks to 3 months with progressive partial weight bearing. Excess loading of the defect can be reduced by the use of unloading orthotics according to the compartment that needs to be unloaded such as the varus/valgus unloading knee brace (**Figure 37.10A**), lateral/medial wedge footwear (**Figure 37.10B**). Full weight bearing is started after 3 months with unloading orthotics. High impact sports activities can be started after 6 months.

Advantages

- Restores hyaline like cartilage
- Indicated for large size defects.

Disadvantages

- Two-staged procedure
- Costly
- Chances of graft hypertrophy, delamination and extrusion.

FUTURE TRENDS

One of the most promising fields in medical research is regenerative medicine and nanotechnology; this field holds immense potential to revolutionize medical treatment modalities. This contribution to cartilage repair is already in clinical practice like the ACI and many more promising newer techniques are awaited.

Delivering and maintaining the cells in the defect area has been a major obstacle in ACI. Various cell-targeting methods have been investigated, which improve the delivery and retention of the injected cells in the desired injured site. Nanoparticles have been developed with different antibodies, ligands that have the capacity to link to MSCs and cartilage matrix proteins. So when the MSCs with these nanoparticles are in contact with the injured cartilage they bind to them. Further nanoparticles are used in drug delivery, so slow release of differentiation mediator aid in cell differentiation in the desired lineage.[22] Dennis et al. reported studies with prochondrocytes directly coated with antibodies and ligands that can bind with cartilage extracellular matrix.[23]

Another novel technology being investigated for improved cell homing onto the lesion is the magnetic cell delivery system.[24] Magnetically labeled MSCs are guided by the magnetic field for delivery into the desired site. These stem cells not only were delivered but also retained with good regenerative potential.[25]

Medical research has opened innumerable new options, and several exciting new prospects are awaited. Currently techniques are available for restoring focal cartilage defects. There would be a time not far from now when we can restore diffuse cartilage degeneration probably with just an injection of autologous stem cells with 'magic' nanoparticles, capable of repairing diffuse early osteoarthritis. From the days when we used to say for osteoarthritis 'We can only halt or delay the progression of cartilage damage,' we are now saying 'We can replace the damaged cartilage,' but the days when we shall say 'We can restore your damaged cartilage' are probably not far.

REFERENCES

1. Mow VC, Ateshian GA, Ratcliffe A. Anatomic form and biomechanical properties of articular cartilage of the knee joint. In: Finerman GAM, Noyes FR (Eds). Biology and Biomechanics of the Traumatized Synovial Joint: The Knee as a Model. Rosemont, IL: AAOS; 1992. pp. 55-81.
2. Buckwalter JA. Articular cartilage. Instr Course Lect. 1983;32:349-70.
3. Newman AP. Articular cartilage repair. Am J Sports Med. 1998;26:309-24.
4. Buckwalter JA, Hunziker E, Rosenberg L, et al. Articular cartilage: composition and structure, In: Woo SL-Y, Buckwalter JA (Eds). Injury and Repair of the Musculoskeletal Soft Tissues. Park Ridge, IL: AAOS; 1988. pp. 405-25.
5. Alford W, Cole BJ. Cartilage restoration, part 1: basic science, historical perspective, patient evaluation, and treatment options. Am J Sports Med. 2005;33(2):295-306.
6. Chesterman PJ, Smith AU. Homotransplantation of articular cartilage and isolated chondrocytes. An experimental study in rabbits. J Bone Joint Surg. 1968;50(1):184-97.
7. Buckwalter JA, Mankin HJ. Articular cartilage. Part I: tissue design and chondrocyte-matrix interaction. J Bone Joint Surg. 1997;79A:600-11.
8. Welsh GH, Brittberg M, Vonk LA, et al. Is magnetic resonance imaging reliable in predicting clinical outcome after articular cartilage repair of the knee? A systematic review and meta-analysis. Am J Sports Med. 2013;41(7):1695-702.
9. Crema MD, Roemer FW, Marra MD, et al. Articular cartilage in the knee: current MR imaging techniques and applications in clinical practice and research. Radiographics. 2011;31(1):37-61.
10. Guettler JH, Demetropoulos CK, Yang KH, Jurist KA. Osteochondral defects in human knee: influence of defect

size on cartilage rim stress and load redistribution to surrounding cartilage. Am J Sports Med. 2004;32:1451-8.
11. Brittberg M, Winalski CS. Evaluation of cartilage injury and repair. J Bone Joint Surg Am. 2003;85-A:58-69.
12. Kosy JD, Schranz PJ, Toms AD, Eyres KS, Mandalia VI. The use of radiofrequency energy for arthroscopic chondroplasty in the knee. Arthroscopy. 2011;27(5):695-703.
13. Frisbie DD, Trotter GW, Steadman JR. Arthroscopic subchondral bone plate microfracture technique augments healing of large chondral defects in the radial carpal bone and medial femoral condyle of horses. Vet Surg. 1999;28:242-55.
14. Alford W, Cole BJ. Cartilage restoration, part 2: techniques, outcomes and future directions. Am J Sports Med. 2005;33:443-60.
15. Steadman JR, Rodkey WG, Rodrigo JJ. Microfracture: surgical technique and rehabilitation to treat chondral defects. Clin Orthop. 2001;391:S362-9.
16. Hangody L, Dobos J, Panics G, et al. Clinical experiences with autologous osteochondral mosaicplasty in an athletic population: a 17-year prospective multicenter study. Am J Sports Med. 2010;38:1125-33.
17. Bartz RL, Kamaric E, Noble PC, Lintner D, Bocell J. Topographic matching of selected donor and recipient sites for osteochondral autografting of the articular surface of the femoral condyles. Am J Sports Med. 2001;29:207-12.
18. Brittberg M, Lindahl A, Nilsson A, et al. Treatment of deep cartilage defects in the knee with autologous chondrocyte transplantation. N Engl J Med. 1994;331(14):889-95.
19. Harris JD, Siston RA, Pan X, Flanigan DC. Autologous chondrocyte Implantation: a systematic review. J Bone Joint Surg Am. 2010;92(12):2220-33.
20. Wysocka A, Mann K, Bursig H, Dec J, Gazdzik TS. Chondrocyte suspension in fibrin glue. Cell Tisse Bank. 2010;11(2):209-15.
21. Hirschmuller A, Baur H, Braun S, et al. Rehabilitation after autologous chondrocyte implantation for isolated cartilage defects of the knee. Am J Sports Med. 2011;39:2686-96.
22. Ansboro S, Greiser U, Barry F, Murphy M. Strategies for improved targeting of therapeutic cells: implications for tissue repair. Eur Cell Mater. 2012;23:310-9.
23. Dennis JE, Cohen N, Goldberg VM, Caplan AI. Targeted delivery of progenitor cells for cartilage repair. J Orthop Res. 2004;22:735-41.
24. Ochi M. Mesenchymal stromal cell transplantation in the regeneration of articular cartilage and bone using a magnetic cell delivery system. J Am Acad Orthop Surg. 2013;21:61,62.
25. Kamei G, Kobayashi T, Ohkawa S, et al. Articular cartilage repair with magnetic mesenchymal stem cells. Am J Sports Med. 2013;41(6):1255-64.

Chapter 38

Classification of Knee Ligament Injuries (Including Dislocations)

Raju Easwaran

INTRODUCTION

The importance of classifying anything in clinical science stems from the desire for standardizing communication among colleagues, to assist research and thereby improve patient care. Knee ligament injuries are very common these days due to increased participation in sports, extreme events, and road traffic accidents.[1] A good classification system helps streamline treatment protocols and serves as a yardstick for prognosticating the patient.

BASICS

Way back in 1968, the Committee of Medical Aspects of Sports, American Medical Association,[2] classified musculoskeletal injuries to two broad categories:

- *Sprain:* Injury limited to a ligament
- *Strain:* Injury to a muscle or its tendinous attachment to bone.

Sprain was further subclassified as given in **Table 38.1.**

The instability caused by the third-degree sprains was further subclassified by the same committee as follows:

TABLE 38.1 Classification of ligament sprains

Type of sprain	*Number of fibers torn*	*Tenderness*	*Instability*
First degree (mild)	Minimum	Localized	No
Second degree (moderate)	More	Generalized	No
Third degree (severe)	Complete disruption	Generally little to no tenderness	Yes

- *Mild (1+) instability:* Separation of joint surfaces < 5 mm
- *Moderate (2+) instability:* 5–10 mm of separation of joint surfaces
- *Severe (3+) instability:* > 10 mm of separation of joint surfaces.

EVOLUTION OF KNEE INSTABILITY CLASSIFICATION

Initial attempts at classifying knee ligament injuries were based on identifying the direction of displacement/

dislocation of tibia on the femur. Later it was realized that knee dislocations and multiple ligament injuries do not result from a unidirectional force, but rather a smorgasbord of forces in multiple directions.[3] A simple directional classification does not simulate clinical scenario in such injuries and fails to provide useful guidelines from the management perspective. Modern classification systems like that of Schenck[3] et al. have evolved into an anatomical system, identifying the ligaments involved, disregarding the direction of displacement, and are more useful from a management and prognosis perspective. Other authors[4,5] have attempted to classify these injuries based on the force sustained during injury as high-velocity and low-velocity injuries. On the basis of time duration, these injuries can be classified as acute or chronic,[6] with 3 weeks being the cutoff point.

DIRECTIONAL/POSITION CLASSIFICATION SYSTEM

Hughston[7,8] et al. in 1976 classified knee instability in a series of two papers into two broad types: straight and rotatory. Rotatory instability is one in which the tibial condyle rotates around the femur. This requires an intact posterior cruciate ligament (PCL) to act as a pivot, around which the tibia can rotate. They are further subdivided as simple and combined rotatory instability.

Depending on the direction of rotation, simple rotatory instabilities are subclassified as anteromedial, posterolateral, and anterolateral. Here, the first half of the word denotes the direction in which the rotation is taking place and the next half of the word denotes the affected tibial condyle. To give an example, posterolateral instability means that the lateral tibial condyle is rotating posteriorly. Depending on the injury combination, combined rotatory instabilities are subclassified as anteromedial + anterolateral, and anteromedial + posterolateral. In their cadaveric study, where they did selective sectioning of the ligaments, they did not encounter posteromedial instability with an intact PCL (**Figures 38.1 to 38.4**).

Straight instability of the knee is one in which the tibial condyles undergo pure linear translation on stress testing (**Figures 38.5 to 38.8**). Depending on the direction of displacement, straight instability is further subclassified as anterior, posterior, medial, and lateral. In straight anterior and posterior instability, careful attention has to be given to the clinical examination. It must be noted that the lateral and medial tibial condyles have an equal amount of anterior/posterior excursion. If one condyle moves more than the other, then an element of rotational instability is also involved.

This classification is very similar to an earlier published Kennedy[9] classification of knee dislocations. The only difference is the addition of the posteromedial rotatory dislocation in the Kennedy classification, which was not found in the above classification. The Kennedy classification is also based on cadaveric sectioning studies.

The advantage of this type of positional classification is its simplicity and guidance on how to carry out a closed reduction. If the surgeon is able to identify posterolateral dislocation using this system, then he can be alerted to the

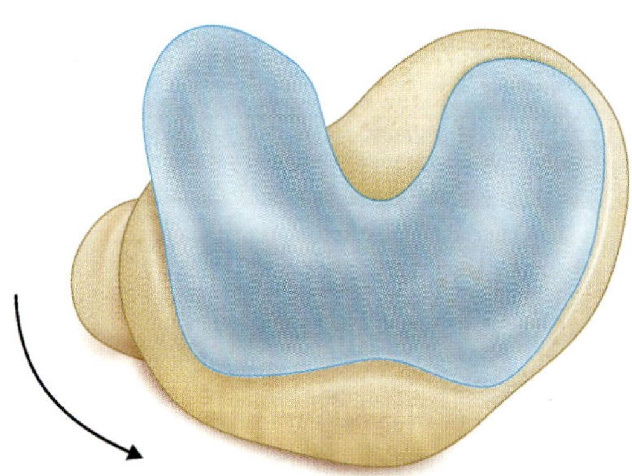

Figure 38.1 Anterolateral

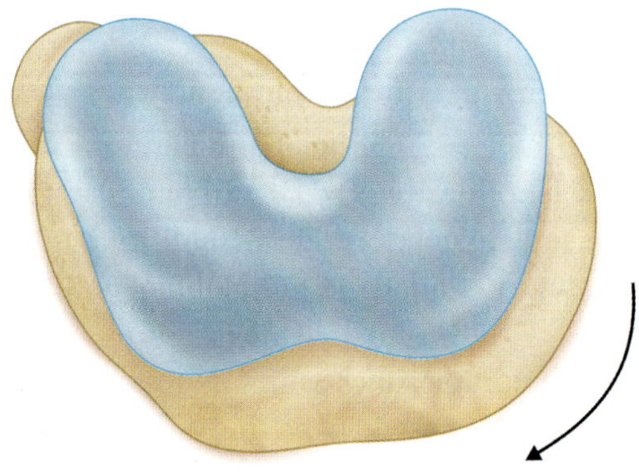

Figure 38.2 Anteromedial

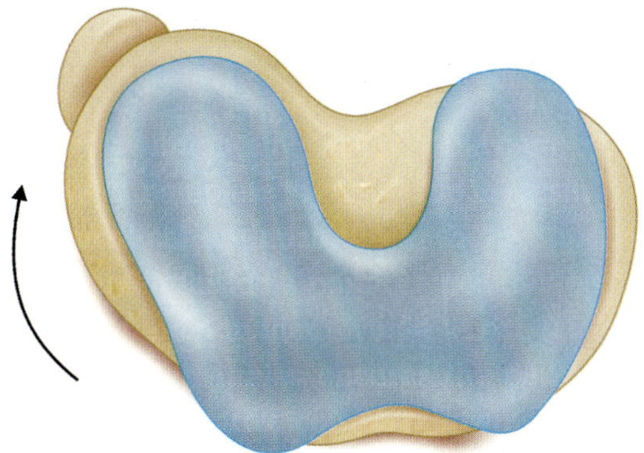

Figure 38.3 Posterolateral

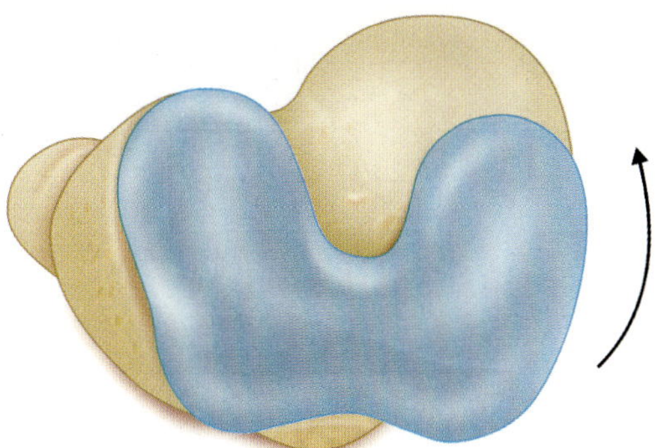

Figure 38.4 Posteromedial

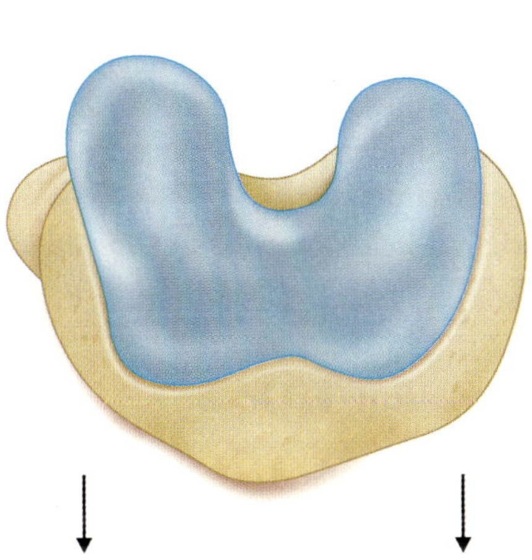

Figure 38.5 Straight anterior

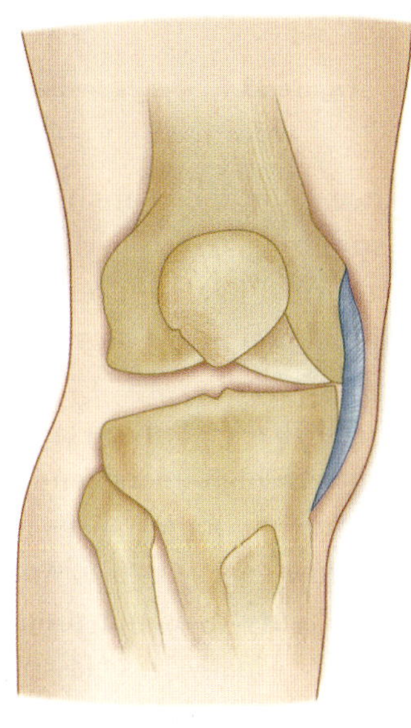

Figure 38.6 Straight lateral

very high percentage of irreducibility with closed methods and peroneal nerve injury that are associated with this dislocation.[10] There are two potential drawbacks:

1. In most clinical scenarios the dislocation has reduced by the time the patient has reached the hospital and hence the injury remains unclassifiable. Wascher[11] et al. found that up to 50% of knee dislocations reduce spontaneously by the time the patient reaches the caregiver.
2. It does not indicate which ligament is injured and hence, fails to guide treatment protocols.

ENERGY OF INJURY CLASSIFICATION SYSTEM

Dislocations are categorized as high-energy and low energy based on the mechanism of injury. Motor vehicle accidents, falls from great height and industrial accidents are classified as high energy. Sporting activities, minor falls, and minor injury in the obese patient are classified as low energy.[4,5]

The one advantage of this classification is that it can guide treatment protocol to a certain extent.

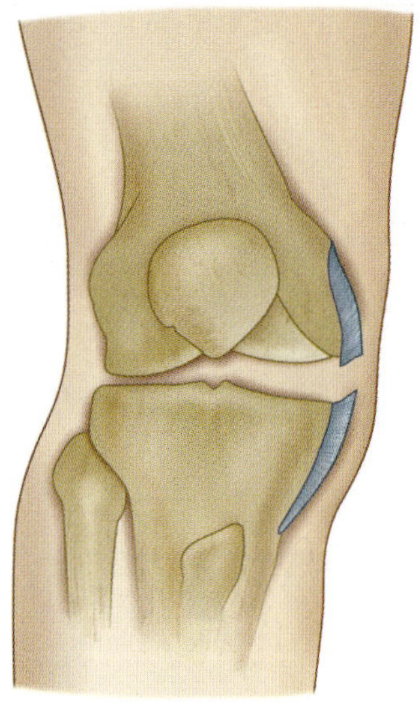

Figure 38.7 Straight medial

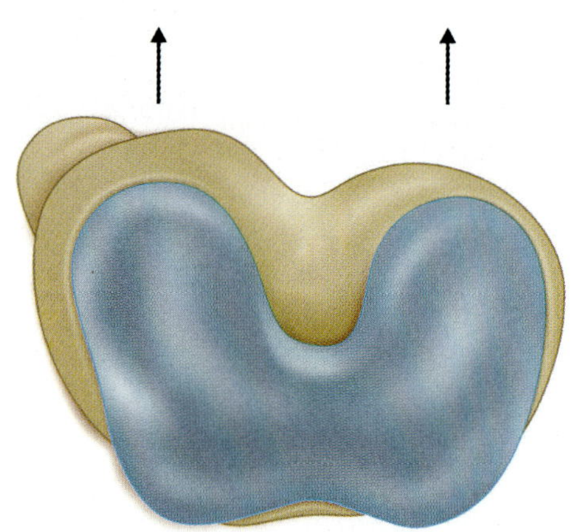

Figure 38.8 Straight posterior

High-energy knee dislocations are best treated initially with a joint spanning fixation till the patient has stabilized for a formal ligament reconstruction. Low-energy knee dislocation might be suitable for an early ligament reconstruction.[12]

The major drawback of this classification is the arbitrary line between high-energy and low-energy. The same sport in different circumstances might produce a high-energy or a low-energy injury. Another drawback is that energy of injury does not predict ligament or neurovascular injury. Finally, this classification does not allow uniform communication between clinicians for patient management and research purposes.

ANATOMICAL CLASSIFICATION

The anatomical classification system was developed by Schenck[3] et al. and was later modified by Wascher[11] et al. This system identifies the torn ligaments, instead of the direction of displacement and is thus able to provide useful guidelines for management and planning operative incisions. Associated fractures, neurologic, and vascular injuries are also included and hence this forms a good tool to prognosticate the patient. This system is also known as the KD system and generally higher the KD grade, worse the injury, and the prognosis.

This system relies on X-ray (for fracture dislocations) and functional examination of the patient. The examination could be done in the emergency room or more commonly in the operation theater, under anesthesia. MRI can also be used as an adjunct, but it is considered less reliable than a clinical examination.

The original Schenck classification is as given in **Table 38.2**.

Knee Dislocation (KD I)

It is a single cruciate intact knee dislocation in which the collaterals are torn. The most common type is the PCL intact dislocation, with the posterolateral corner and anterior cruciate ligament (ACL) torn. Since the PCL is intact, the risk of arterial injury and peroneal nerve palsy is low.

Knee Dislocation (KD II)

It is a rare injury in which both the cruciates are torn, but the collaterals are intact. The MRI may show edema to

TABLE 38.2 Anatomical classification of knee dislocations

KD I	One cruciate intact
KD II	Both cruciates torn, collaterals intact
KD III	Both cruciates and one collateral torn Subset KD IIIM and KD IIIL
KD IV	All four ligaments torn
KD V	Periarticular fracture or dislocation
C = Arterial injury N = Neurologic injury	

one or both the collaterals, but on examination, they are functionally intact.

Knee Dislocation (KD III)

This is the most common type of knee dislocation, in which in addition to a bicruciate (ACL + PCL) injury, one of the collaterals is torn. It is further subclassified as KD IIIM and KD IIIL depending on which side is torn. The KD IIIL injury has a high percentage of damage to the peroneal nerve. It corresponds to the posterolateral dislocation of the positional classification.

Knee Dislocation (KD IV)

This is a high-energy injury in which all the four ligaments of the knee are torn.

Knee Dislocation (V)

This is a fracture dislocation. The fracture can involve either the femoral or the tibial condyle. Dan Wascher[11] added this subcategory. This has now been further subclassified by Moore[13] into four types, depending on the number of ligaments involved. KD V1 is a single cruciate injury, KD V2 is a bicruciate injury, in KD V3 both cruciates and one collateral are involved, and finally in KD V4 all the ligaments of the knee are functionally torn. Small avulsion fractures are not classified as KD V injuries but as ligament disruptions (KD I or II).

For example, a knee dislocation with injury to the ACL, PCL, and MCL with popliteal artery injury shall be classified as KD IIIMC as per this classification.

CONCLUSION

Knee dislocations and multiligament injuries should be considered as two different facets of the same injury. They are difficult injuries to treat and recover from. It is essential that they are identified early and classified accurately for standardizing patient care. As a broad guideline all the torn ligaments need to be repaired or reconstructed in a single or staged manner. A good classification system should thus be able to guide the clinician regarding the severity of injury and help him or her plan the surgery. With the available literature, the anatomical classification is able to fulfill most of the above criteria, and hence, this system is the currently favored system for classification of these injuries.

REFERENCES

1. Engebretsen L, Risberg MA, Robertson B, Ludvigsen TC, Johansen S. Outcome after knee dislocations: a 2–9 years follow-up of 85 consecutive patients. Knee Surg Sports Traumatol Arthrosc. 2009;17(9):1013-26.
2. Committee on the Medical Aspects of Sports. American Medical Association: Standard Nomenclature of Athletic Injuries; 1968. pp. 99,101. American Medical Association.
3. Robert Schenck Jr. Classification of knee dislocations. Oper Tech Sports Med. 2003;11(3):193-8.
4. Shelbourne KD, Klootwyk TE. Low velocity knee dislocation with sports injuries. Treatment principles. Clin Sports Med. 2000;19(3):443-56.
5. Wascher DC. High-velocity knee dislocation with vascular injury. Treatment principles. Clin Sports Med. 2000;19(3):457-77.
6. McCoy GF, Hannon DG, Barr RJ, Templeton J. Vascular injury associated with low-velocity dislocations of the knee. J Bone Joint Surg Br. 1987;69(2):285-7.
7. Hughston JC, Andrews JR, Cross MJ, Moschi A. Classification of knee ligament instabilities. Part I. The medial compartment and cruciate ligaments. J Bone Joint Surg Am. 1976;58(2):159-72.
8. Hughston JC, Andrews JR, Cross MJ, Moschi A. Classification of knee ligament instabilities. Part II. The lateral compartment. J Bone Joint Surg Am. 1976;58(2):173-9.
9. Kennedy JC. Complete dislocation of the knee joint. J Bone Joint Surg Am. 1963;45:889-904.
10. Huang FS, Simonian PT, Chansky HA. Irreducible posterolateral dislocation of the knee. Arthroscopy. 2000;16(3):323-7.
11. Wascher DC, Dvirnak PC, DeCoster TA. Knee dislocation: initial assessment and implications for treatment. J Orthop Trauma. 1997;11(7):525-9.
12. Hobby BD, Wascher DC, Schenck RC Jr. Classification of knee dislocations and the surgical implications. In: Fanelli GC (Ed.). The Multiple Ligament Injured Knee: A Practical Guide to Management. New York: Springer; 2013. pp. 63-9.
13. Moore TM. Fracture-dislocation of the knee. Clin Orthop Relat Res. 1981;156:128-40.

Chapter 39

Anterior Cruciate Ligament Reconstruction

Ashok Rajgopal, Attique Vasdev, Vivek Dahiya, Himanshu Gupta

Tears of the anterior cruciate ligament (ACL) are one of the common ligamentous injuries in the knee. The ACL has been a subject of much deliberation and the treatment protocols have changed considerably over the past years. It has gone from stages of nonrecognition in the 60s with no treatment to emergency repairs in the 70s and 80s and then to repair and augmentation with autograft or synthetic material in the early 90s. At the same time in the late 80s and early 90s with the onslaught of arthroscopy, more and more reconstructions were coming into vogue using both synthetic material and central third of the patellar tendon using the semi-open technique. Injury to the ACL is very common among athletes as a result of hyperextension injury in combination with valgus angulation and internal rotation of the knee. ACL injury predisposes the knee to further injury, leading to early degenerative changes in the knee. These changes are primarily attributable to the loss of the essential function of the ACL namely to prevent anterior displacement of the tibia relative to the femur, as well as to restrain internal rotation and valgus angulation. However, the ACL is not merely a mechanical stabilizer of the knee. It also has important proprioceptive properties. It contains different sets of mechanoreceptors that provide the central nervous system with afferent information about the position of the joint by way of the tibial nerve. Following ACL rupture, recurring episodes of joint instability are associated with meniscus injury and damage to the joint cartilage.[1] Currently, surgical reconstruction is the preferred option to restore knee stability, be it the single-bundle or the double-bundle technique. Present day reconstructive techniques have reported long-term success rates between 70% and 90% in terms of functional stability and relief of symptoms with return to activity.[2-6] However, this leaves a substantial group of patients with unsatisfactory results in patients with continued pain, loss of motion secondary to operative intervention, and, in some cases, continued or recurrent instability. The surgical treatment of a torn ACL hence needs to be individualized to the needs of the person. Important factors include age, occupation, associated intra-articular injuries like meniscal tears, concomitant ligament injuries, and level of sports involvement. The willingness of the patient to participate in the postoperative rehabilitation program is another important parameter before suggesting surgery to the patient. Results of surgery performed anytime between 6 weeks and 1 year following injury are similar.

Though the contraindications for ACL reconstruction have considerably reduced over years, not all ACL tears need surgery. Indications for surgery should be patient specific and patients with advanced osteoarthritic changes should be treated conservatively with rehabilitation and bracing.

PREOPERATIVE EVALUATION

Assessment following acute injury may be difficult due to pain and swelling due to hemarthrosis. However, symptoms often lead to a working diagnosis. Patients often complain of hearing a 'pop' at the time of injury. They complain of inability to continue their activity following the injury. An effusion develops soon after injury. There may not be a history of any contact injury but there may be a history of a rotational trauma with sudden change of direction. The injury may be a combination of flexion-valgus-external rotation or flexion-varus-internal rotation, forced external rotation or hyperextension.

In cases of older ruptures a through clinical examination establishes a diagnosis.

Many tests are described namely:

- Anterior drawer test
- Lachman test
- Quadriceps active test
- Pivot shift test
- Losee test
- Flexion rotation drawer test.

The Lachman test is the most sensitive test for an ACL injury. It is not affected much by hamarthrosis and can be performed even in acute injuries without causing much pain. Clinical examination should tests for other associated injuries like meniscal or collateral ligament injury. Objective measurement of knee laxity can also be obtained with the help of a KT 1000 arthrometer.

The Lachman test is performed in 30° of flexion with an anterior force applied in the proximal end of the tibia and anterior translation of the tibial looked for. This is not affected by hemarthrosis and can be performed in acute injuries without much pain. This is more sensitive than the anterior drawers performed in 90° of flexion as it allows more anterior translation in isolated ACL tears.

The anterior drawer is performed with the knee flexed in 90° with the hip flexed at 45°. With the hand of the examiner around the proximal part of the patient's tibia, the hamstrings are palpated and the proximal tibia pulled and pushed forward and backward and translation of the proximal tibia looked for. The test is performed in neutral, internal, and external rotation of the foot.

The pivot shift is performed beginning with the knee in full extension with internal rotation and valgus stress applied to demonstrate anterolateral subluxation on flexion due to a torn ACL. Assessment is incomplete without plain radiographs (standard anteroposterior and lateral views) to look for associated fractures like Segond fracture, fibular head fractures or any bony ligament avulsions. Specialized views like the Frick tunnel view or a posteroanterior Rosenberg views are occasionally required to assess the intercondylar notch.

MRI other than to confirm the ACL tear, is done to assess associated intra- and extra-articular injuries like associated meniscal tears, patellar tendon avulsions, acute patellar dislocations that may have relocated, posterolateral complex injuries or bone bruising that may require modification of the postoperative protocol.

SURGERY

Timing of surgery is under considerable debate following ACL injuries. It is worthwhile waiting for the acute inflammatory phase to subside before surgery is undertaken. The patient should have attained 120° range of motion without much pain. This often takes up to 3 weeks following injury. A locked knee secondary to a bucket handle tear with considerable pain and a reasonable range of motion of the knee and no signs of acute inflammatory phase may be an indication for considering early surgery. Studies by Shelbourne et al.[7] showed a higher incidence of arthrofibrosis for patients operated within 1 week of injury compared to patients treated after 3 weeks. They also stated that patients recovered muscle strength earlier in spite the delay.

GRAFT SELECTION

Common sources of autograft for reconstruction of the ACL include:

- Autografts
  - The hamstring tendons [semitendinosus (ST) alone or both the ST and gracilis]
  - The patellar tendon
  - The quadriceps tendon
  - The Achilles tendon
  - The iliotibial band
  - Plantaris
- Allografts
- Synthetic (Gore-tex, Trevira, Stryker, Leeds-keio, Proflex, Kennedy LAD, LARS, and Lafil ligaments).

Autografts

Hamstring Tendons

Advantages: These can be harvested through a small incision that is cosmetically better. It does not compromise the extensor mechanism like in the patellar tendon graft. It has an elastic modulus similar to that of the native ACL. Scar formation is considerably less during graft remodeling, thus the possibility of a cyclops reduces.

Disadvantages: Graft harvesting has a learning curve due to anatomic variations. Internal rotation and terminal flexion is often compromised following hamstring reconstruction. There is also a possibility of hematoma following hamstring harvesting. Bungee effect, windshield wiper effects are known to occur following ACL reconstruction with hamstrings.

Patellar Tendon

This was considered the gold standard for ACL reconstructions till the increase in popularity of the hamstring tendons. The graft includes bone plugs from the patella and the tibial tuberosity along with the middle third of the patellar tendon.

Advantages: Easy to harvest with availability of variable width. Bone plugs provide strong primary fixation with bone-to-bone healing preventing 'bunge effect'. There is no loss of internal rotation after bone-patellar tendon-bone ACL reconstruction. Though the quadriceps is weakened after harvesting, this may be considered beneficial as normally it is a strong antagonist to the ACL.

Disadvantages: Mainly related to donor site morbidity. These include anterior knee pain, difficulty in kneeling following surgery, weakening of the extensor mechanism, possibility of patellar tendon rupture, and the risk of patella fracture. As the volume of graft increases during remodeling there is a higher possibility of cyclops formation that leads to a mechanical block to extension.

Quadriceps tendon: The quadriceps tendon is finding increasing use in ACL reconstructions especially in revision situations. It has the advantage of less donor site morbidity and bony fixation on one side with the patellar bone block. Due to its large cross section, the graft can be split for use in double-bundle ACL reconstructions. Quadriceps atrophy is a common complication following quadriceps tendon harvesting.

Allografts

Allografts have the advantage of no donor site morbidity, but are not easily available and are costly. They run the risk of disease transmission and are known to cause severe synovitis and recurrent effusion.

Synthetic Graft

Synthetic grafts have a high incidence of rupture with poor biocompatibility. There are reports of have very high incidence of postoperative synovitis after synthetic graft ACL reconstruction. These were extensively used in the past as augmentation to the ACL reconstruction. The proposed advantages were early weight bearing, faster rehabilitation, protection of graft, and increase stability. Later studies however did not show any advantages.

Graft selection is often based on the tensile strength of the graft material. As the middle third of the patellar tendon has a tensile strength similar to that of the intact ACL it was the graft of choice. The nonavailability of good fixation techniques to attach soft tissue to bone earlier added to the bone patellar tendon's popularity. The two stranded ST alone has less tensile strength than the normal ACL. However, the four-stranded ST alone or the two stranded ST along with the two stranded gracilis has twice the tensile strength of the normal ACL and has gained popularity especially now with the availability of much better fixation techniques of soft tissue to bone.

SURGICAL TECHNIQUE

A stepwise approach makes it easier to perform the surgery. The steps include:

- Examination under anesthesia
- Diagnostic arthroscopy
- Graft harvesting and preparation
- Notchplasty (if required)
- Preparing the femoral and tibial tunnels
- Graft passage
- Graft fixation in tunnels.

Examination Under Anesthesia

Before starting the surgery itself an examination under anesthesia must be performed. A positive Lachman and pivot shift test are clinical evidences of ACL injury. These should be done on the normal limb also to look for any laxity. The limb is then prepared and draped after applying a tourniquet.

Diagnostic Arthroscopy

Once the tourniquet is inflated the arthroscopy is performed using the standard portals and the structures visualized. The torn ACL is often adherent to the anterior surface of the posterior cruciate ligament and may be mistaken for an intact ACL. It is advisable to visualize the ACL at this stage in a figure of four positions. This enables accurate assessment of the proximal attachment and demonstrates detachment of the ACL from the femur (**Figure 39.1**).

Meniscal tears can either be repaired or excised at this stage through additional working portals. All the remnants of the ACL are also removed at this stage especially at the femoral attachment. It is advised to retain the tibial stump for its alleged role in providing proprioception and blood supply to the graft.

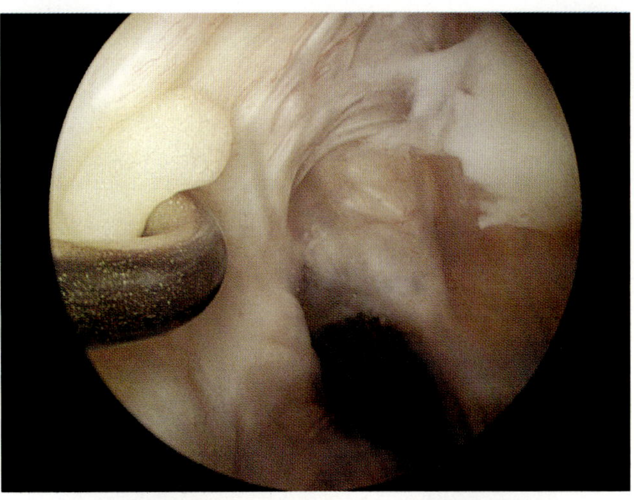

Figure 39.1 Torn anterior cruciate ligament

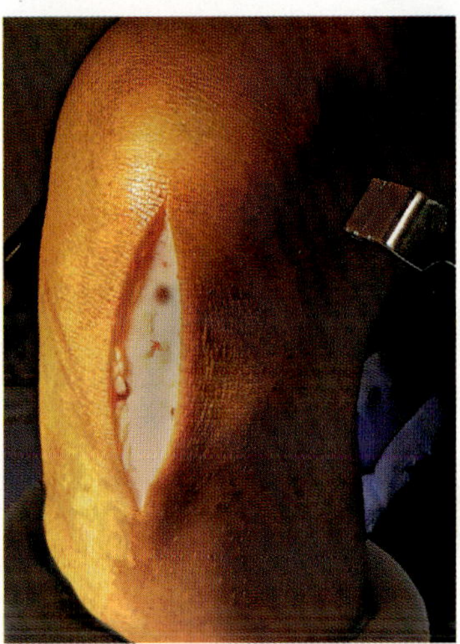

Figure 39.2 Incision anterior cruciate ligament BPTB graft harvest

Graft Harvesting and Preparation

Bone Patellar Tendon (Figures 39.2 to 39.7)

The patella and tibial tubercle landmarks are drawn on the skin, and a vertical incision is made from the inferior pole of the patella to 1 cm below the tibial tubercle. Skin flaps are developed to identify the full width of the tendon, and the paratenon is incised in line with the skin incision and reflected. Parallel incision is made in the tendon from the patella to the tibial tubercle. The middle third of the patellar tendon is used. The incision is carried proximally over the patella for a distance of 20–25 mm from the tendon

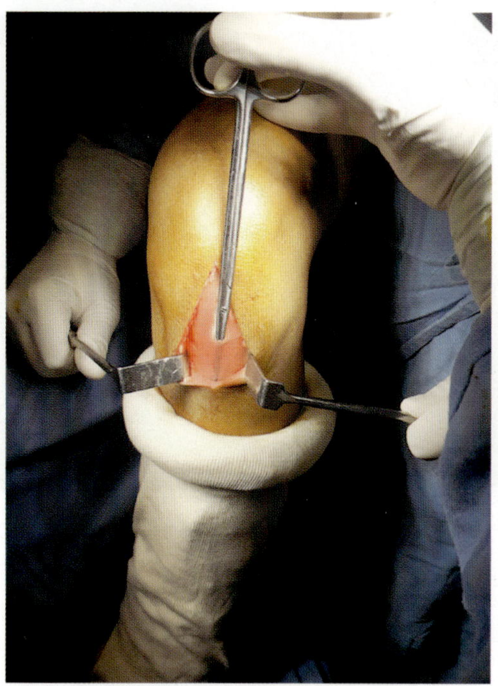

Figure 39.3 Opening the peritendon—anterior cruciate ligament BPTB graft harvest

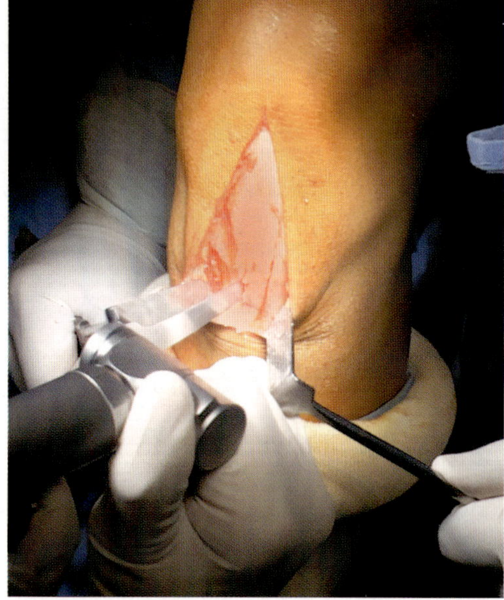

Figure 39.4 Anterior cruciate ligament BPTB graft harvest

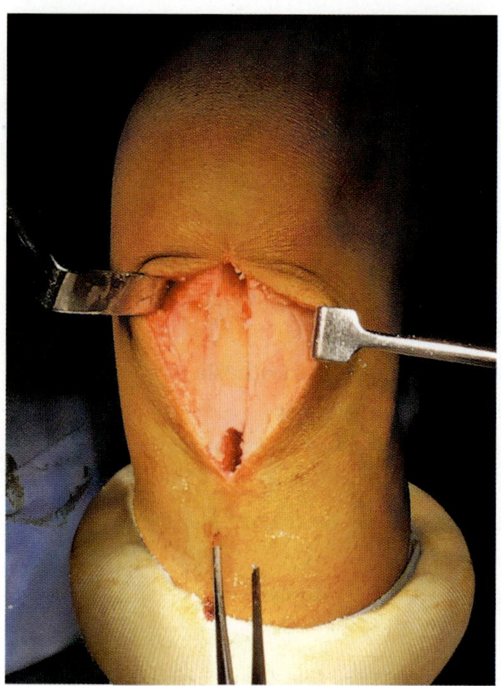

Figure 39.5 Post-anterior cruciate ligament BPTB graft harvest

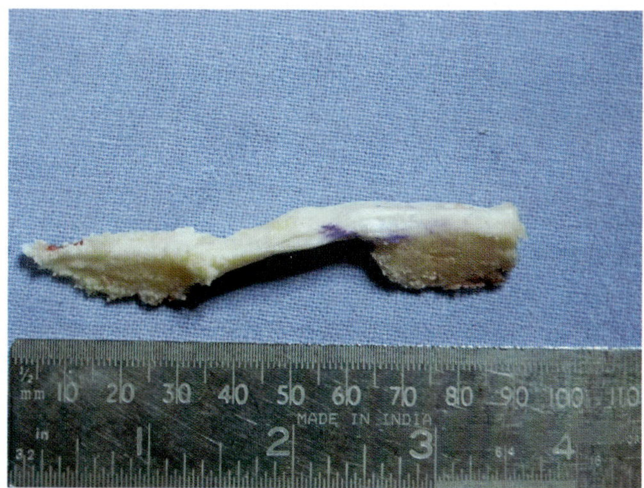

Figure 39.6 BPTB graft

insertion, as well as distally over the tibial tubercle, also 20–25 mm from the attachment site of the tendon. A narrow oscillating saw is used to cut bone plugs in a rectangular shape at the tibial tubercle and a triangular shape at the patella to a depth of approximately 8–10 mm and a length of 20–25 mm, which are then carefully removed with a narrow curved osteotome.

All excess soft tissue is removed from the graft, and the diameter of the bone plugs trimmed to the required width (8 or 10 mm) to facilitate an easy passage into the bone

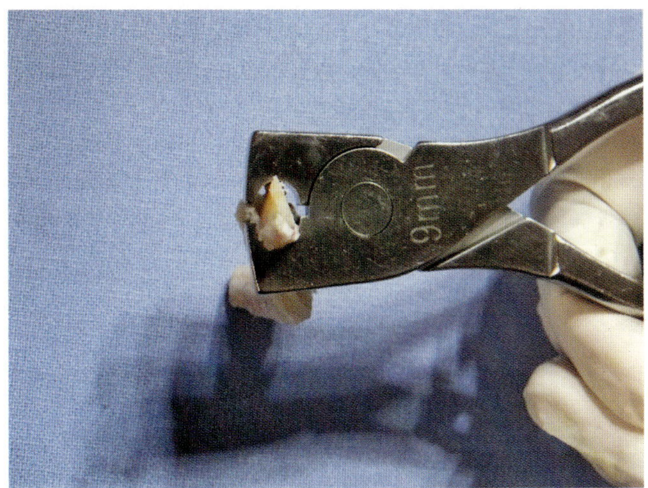

Figure 39.7 Sizing the BPTB graft

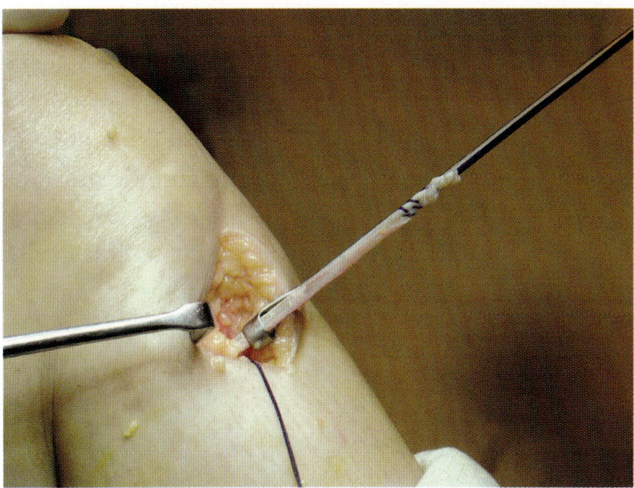

Figure 39.8 Harvesting semitendinosus

tunnels. The tibial tubercle plug is prepared for placement in the femoral tunnel. The edges of the bone plugs are smoothened for easy passage of the graft. Diameters of the bone plugs should be checked by passing the graft through the graft master or template for correct size. The tendon bone junctions are marked with a marking pen. Drill holes are then made in the patellar bone plug and in the tibial tubercle bone plug, for passage of strong (number five) nonabsorbable suture through these holes. These sutures facilitate passage and tensioning of the graft. Graft is measured to adjust the tunnel length to fill the tunnels with the bone plug totally.

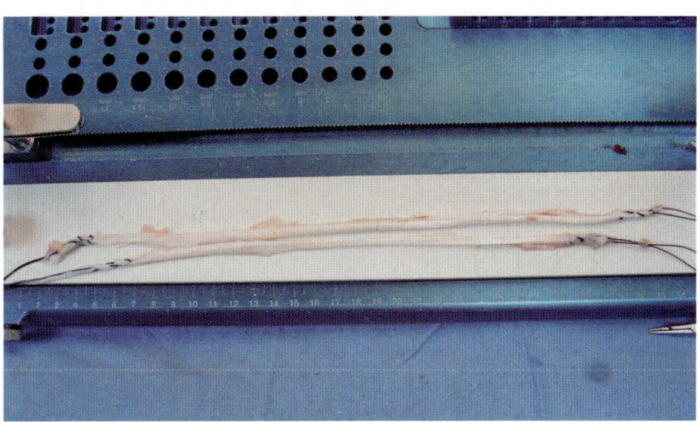

Figure 39.9 Hamstring graft

Hamstring Tendons (Figures 39.8 to 39.10)

The ST and gracilis tendons are harvested through a 3–4 cm incision overlying the pes anserinus centered approximately 2 cm medial to the tibial tubercle. The sartorius fascia is then incised parallel and distal to the palpable ST tendon exposing the ST and gracilis tendons that are then released from their tibial attachment. The tendons are separated, and each tendon is whipstitched with nonabsorbable suture. Using blunt dissection with the index finger, the tendons are freed from surrounding adventitia.

The extratendinous bands should be excised to completely free up the tendons to their respective sheaths. It is important to incise these fascial bands to

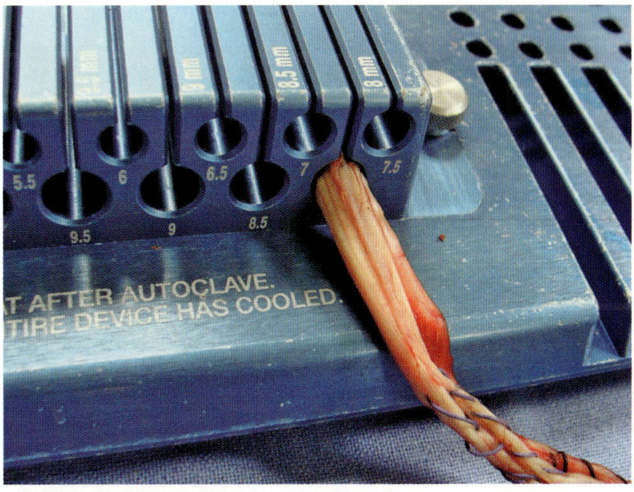

Figure 39.10 Sizing the hamstring graft

prevent premature amputation of the tendon while using a tendon stripper. The tendons are then harvested with a blunt-ended tendon stripper. The attached muscle tissue is removed from the fascia and the tendons cut to give an overall length of 24–26 cm, and the free ends are whipstitched. The tendons are looped to give a four-stranded graft either with ST alone or with the gracilis. The graft is then sized in the graft master in preparation for tunnel drilling.

Notchplasty

Notchplasty may be required to prevent impingement of the graft especially when the tibial tunnel is anterior. This leads to 'Cyclops' (**Figure 39.11**) formation preventing full extension. This was more common in the transtibial technique. The amount of bone to be removed remains controversial and intraoperative clinical judgment of the surgeon is required.

Various studies have attempted to establish guidelines for assessing the adequacy of the notchplasty. The relationship between the placement of the tibial tunnel and the required size of the notchplasty was described by Howell et al.[8] More anteriorly placed tibial tunnels in their study required up to 6 mm of bone removal from the intercondylar roof as compared with only minimal removal of bone for tunnels placed 2–3 mm posterior to the ACL tibial insertion site. Berg defined an adequate notchplasty on the basis of the notch width index that is the ratio of the intercondylar width to the total femoral condylar width at the level of the popliteal groove that should be at least 0.250 to prevent impingement of the graft.

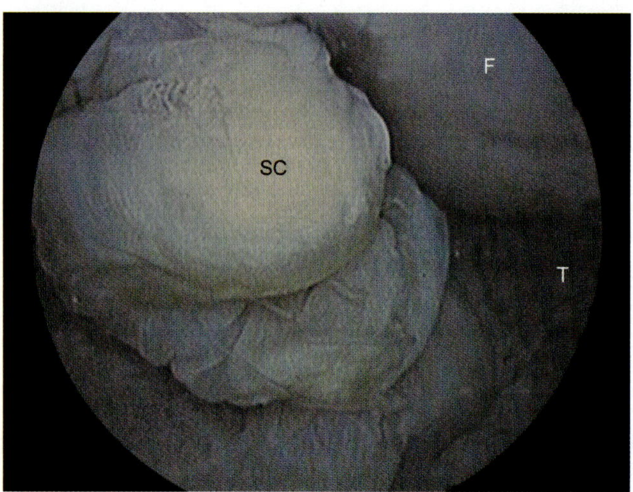

Figure 39.11 Cyclops
Abbreviations: SC–Cyclops; T–Tibial; F–Femur

The disadvantage of notchplasty lies in the removal of the osseous landmarks of the femoral ACL insertion.[9] This can compromise correct anatomic tunnel placement. It can lead to abnormal graft forces, graft failure,[10] and possible regrowth, and overgrowth of the notch.[11]

Preparing the Femoral and Tibial Tunnels

The placement of the femoral and tibial tunnels has a direct effect on the outcome of ACL reconstruction. While there is no debate about the tibial tunnel, the femoral tunnel has been a reason for significant controversy. The placement of the femoral tunnel has evolved from the over the top position to 'anatomic' placement of the tunnel in the ACL footprint. Biomechanical studies have shown improved knee kinematics and rotational stability with restoration of the native ligament orientation, origin, and insertion.[12-27] Transtibial ACL reconstruction techniques result in vertical graft orientation because of technical limitations in reaming an anatomic femoral tunnel. A nonanatomically positioned femoral tunnel is one of the most common causes of failure after ACL reconstruction.[13,28-36] To address the concern regarding nonanatomic graft placement with conventional transtibial ACL reconstruction, double-bundle ACL reconstruction has been advocated to more accurately restore rotational and translational knee stability by recreating the individual anteromedial (AM) and posterolateral bundles of the ACL. The procedure is, however, complex and technically difficult, with a number of complications associated with the preparation of four tunnels. Preparation of separate femoral tunnels for each bundle, particularly in the setting of a small femoral footprint, can result in nonanatomic tunnel position. Preparing two divergent femoral tunnels with a bony bridge in between can result in errant distal and anterior positioning of the posterolateral bundle tunnel.[37] This results in abnormal knee kinematics, impingement, and even over constraint of the knee, particularly in extension. Studies by Adachi et al.[38] and Hamada et al.[39] prospectively compared double and single-bundle reconstructions. They found no differences in stability, proprioception, or subjective functional outcomes. To overcome the technical difficulty associated with the double-bundle technique, ACL reconstruction with single-bundle anatomically positioned femoral and tibial tunnels centered in the footprints of the native ligament are fast becoming the technique of choice of surgeons.

Drilling of the femoral tunnel through a medial arthroscopic portal to reliably achieve an anatomic position with a low-risk of complications has been advocated by Bottoni [40] and Harner et al.[41] (**Figures 39.12 and 39.13**).

In the transtibial technique, a transtibial offset (**Figures 39.14 and 39.15**) is used to direct the guide pin in the required location. The offset is passed through the tibial tunnel and locked in over the top position by flexing the knee in 90° of flexion. The guide pin is positioned at 11 o'clock position in the right knee and 1 o'clock position in the left knee. The femoral canal is then drilled to 35–40 mm with the appropriate sized reamer. A possibility of a posterior wall blow out must be kept in mind while doing this technique.

The AM reaming technique evolved in an effort to increase graft obliquity, because the relatively vertical graft prepared with TTs limited anterior translation but not the rotatory instability seen in ACL insufficiency. Reconstructions performed with AM portal reaming yield more accurate femoral position, tibial position, and graft obliquity. In both cadaveric[42,43] and *in vivo*[44-46] studies,

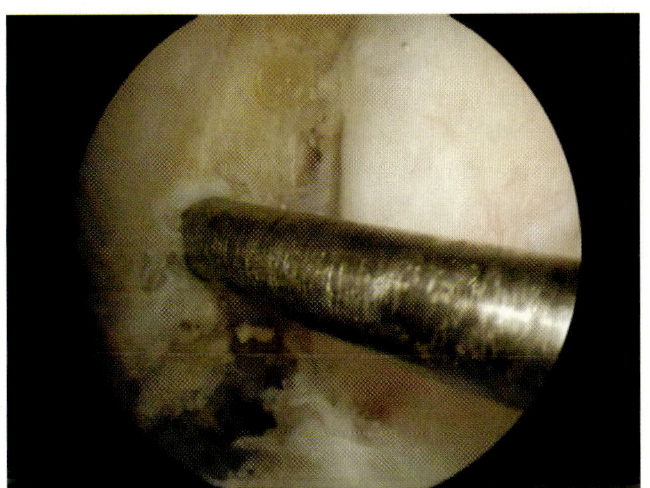

Figure 39.12 Anteromedial guidewire

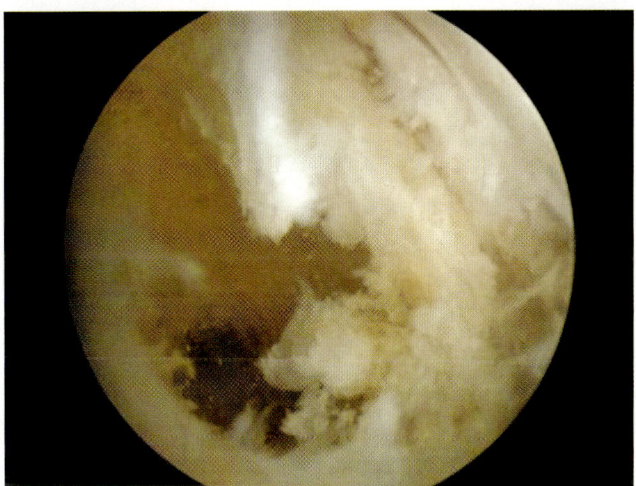

Figure 39.13 Anteromedial femoral tunnel

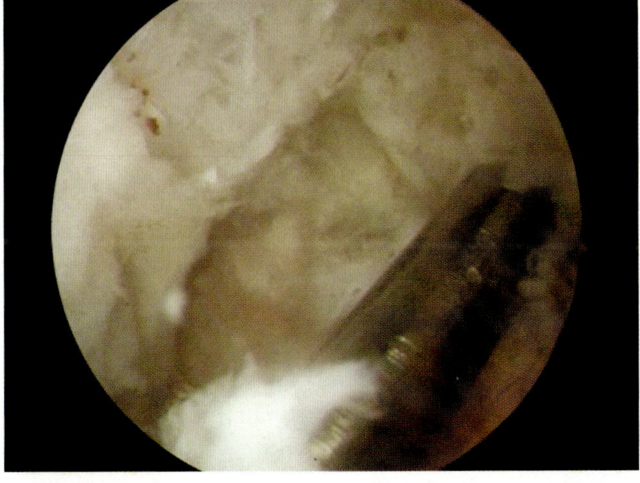

Figure 39.14 Transtibial anterior cruciate ligament guidewire

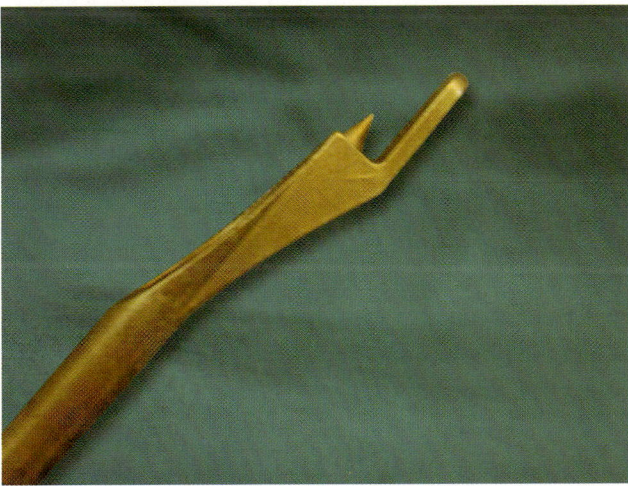

Figure 39.15 Transtibial femoral offset

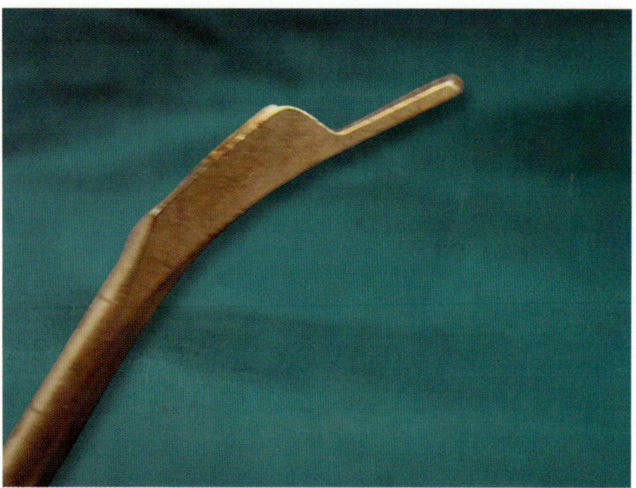

Figure 39.16 Anteromedial femoral offset

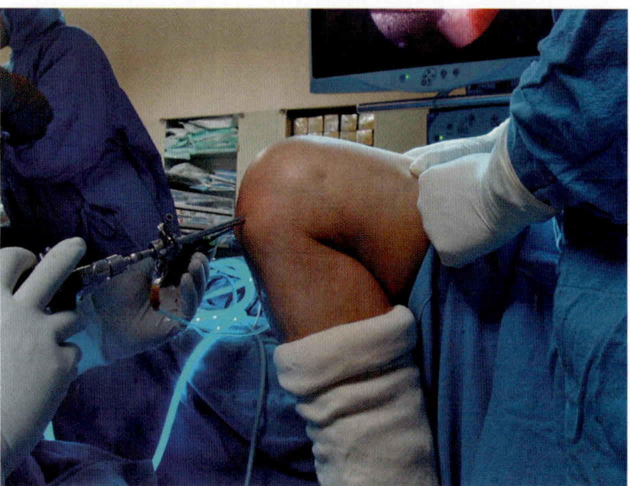

Figure 39.17 110° flexion for anteromedial femoral tunnel through anteromedial portal

femoral tunnels position and graft obliquity have been shown to be more closely replicated with AM compared with TTs.[47] A 6 or 7 mm angled offset guide (**Figure 39.16**) placed over the back of the posterior surface of the lateral femoral condyle keeping the knee in flexion of at least 110° (**Figure 39.17**) helps direct the guide pin in the desired location. A tunnel of 20–25 mm is then made in the lateral femoral condyle.

Despite the potential advantages of AM portal technique it has its problems. The learning curve is steep when transitioning from conventional transtibial ACL reconstruction techniques. Lubowitz[48] has reported a number of technical difficulties associated with AM portal reaming, which include short sockets (less than 20 mm) with insufficient tendon-bone interface for healing, posterior or lateral tunnel wall blowout, inferior exit of the guidewire from the lateral thigh that may injure critical neurovascular structures, iatrogenic injury to the medial femoral condyle with reamer passage, difficulty with visualization and instrumentation in the requisite hyperflexed position (**Figure 39.17**), bending of a rigid guidewire in the hyperflexed position, and difficulty with graft passage and fixation. The current trend today is to create the femoral tunnel through the AM portal that we also recommend.

The tibial tunnel is made by passing a tibial guide pin through the ACL footprint, approximately 5–7 mm anterior to the anterior border of the posterior cruciate ligament with the help of a tibial drill guide kept at 45°–55°. Other landmarks useful for tibial tunnel positioning include the posterior border of the anterior horn of the lateral meniscus and the interspinous region of the tibial plateau. With the knee in 90° of flexion the tibial tunnel is then made with the appropriate reamer corresponding to the size of the graft itself for the hamstrings option and 1 mm larger than the size of the bony plugs in the bone patellar tendon graft. Though all attempts should be made to produce the correct tibial tunnel length to prevent graft extrusion with tunnels that are too short, and prevent difficult distal fixation and femoral tunnel placement with tunnels that are too long, this is often not possible when reconstructing the ACL with the patellar tendon. In these situations adjustments in the tunnel lengths especially that of the tibia may be required. A longer or shorter tibial tunnel can be achieved by increasing or decreasing the angle of the tibial drill guide.

Graft Passage

Prior to graft passage all debris should be remove from the joint and the tunnels cleared of all soft tissue. This prevents a possibility of arthrofibrosis and also allows smooth passage of the graft. The graft may be passed into the tunnels by using a Beath pin passed through the femoral and the tibial tunnels and out of the anterolateral aspect of the thigh with the sutures of the graft threaded into the eye of the Beath pin. The Beath pin is then pulled out from the anterolateral surface allowing the graft to be pulled into

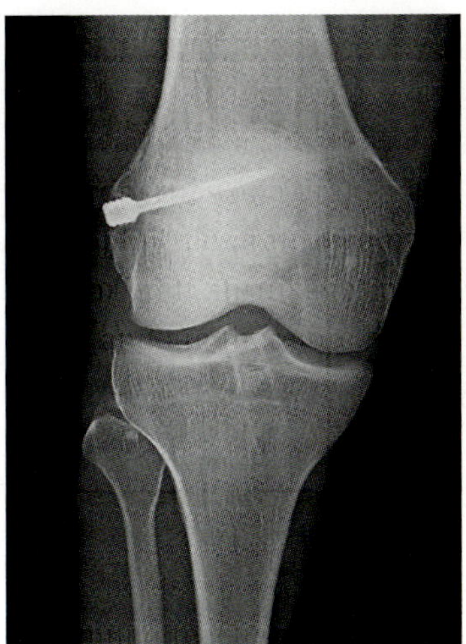

Figure 39.18 Transfix

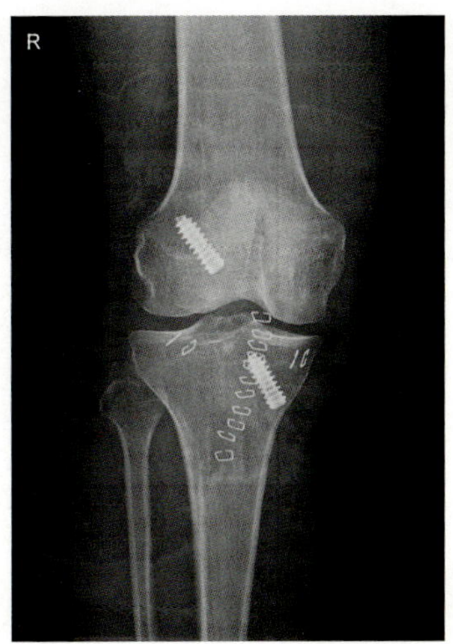

Figure 39.19 Intereference screws

the joint and the tunnels. In case of hamstrings the graft may also be looped over a Netlon wire that is then pulled on either side pulling the graft with it into the tunnel as in the case of certain suspensory systems like the Transfix (**Figure 39.18**).

Graft Fixation

The choice of graft fixation depends upon the type of graft and what the surgeon is familiar with. There are two basic types of fixation namely, bone to bone fixation that is achieved by bony ingrowth of the bone block as in the case of bone patellar tendon bone graft and bone to tendon fixation where tendon has to heal to the bone to achieve bony integration of the graft.

Bone to bone fixation is best achieved with interference screw placement into the gap between the bone block and the tunnel wall. This ensures high fixation strength and good bony integration of the graft. Tendon to bone fixation may be achieved by screws (headed or headless, titanium (**Figure 39.19**) or biodegradable), or transfixation systems (e.g. Transfix, Crosspins, and Rigidfix) or fixation buttons (e.g. Endobutton and Retrobutton).

Whatever the method of choice the femoral end is fixed first. The knee is then taken through several cycles of motion before tibial fixation especially when using tendon grafts to pretension the graft. This can be done with the help of a tensioner applying 25 lbs of longitudinal tension following which the graft is fixed into the tibial tunnel with the proximal tibia pushed posteriorly and the knee in 15° of flexion. Additional fixation may be used, if required (**Figures 39.20 to 39.22**). A compression bandage is then applied and the tourniquet released. We recommend using a knee brace in 10° of flexion for 10 days following surgery.

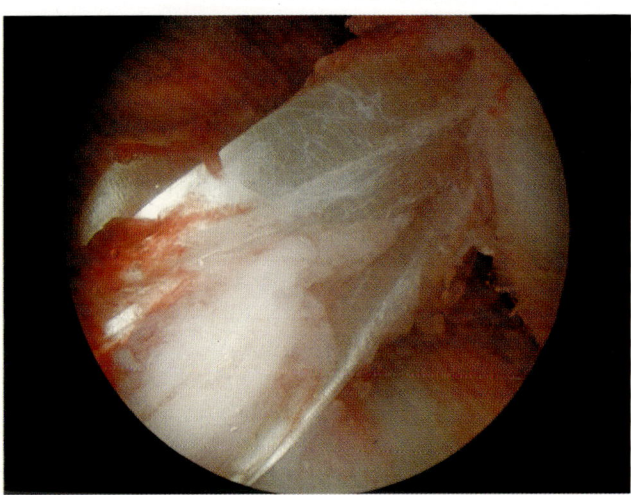

Figure 39.20 Reconstructed anterior cruciate ligament—hamstring

We recommend partial weight bearing with crutches and a brace, passive knee mobilization, patellar mobilization, straight leg raising, and static quadriceps exercises for the first 2 weeks following surgery. The brace is removed, full weight bearing with a stick and active knee quadriceps, hamstring, hip abductor, and adductor

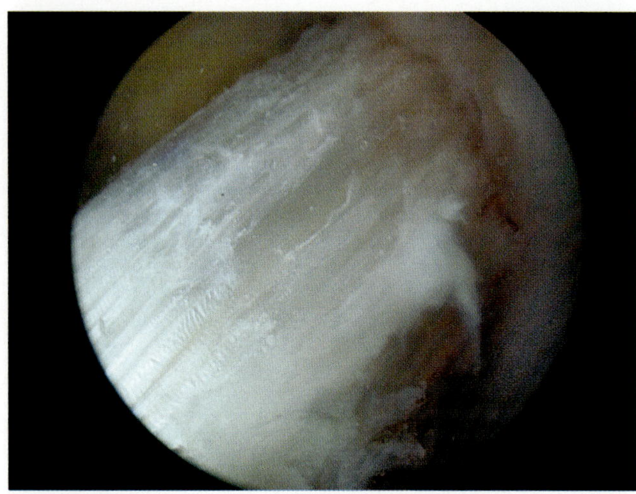

Figure 39.21 Reconstructed bone patella tendon graft as an anterior cruciate ligament

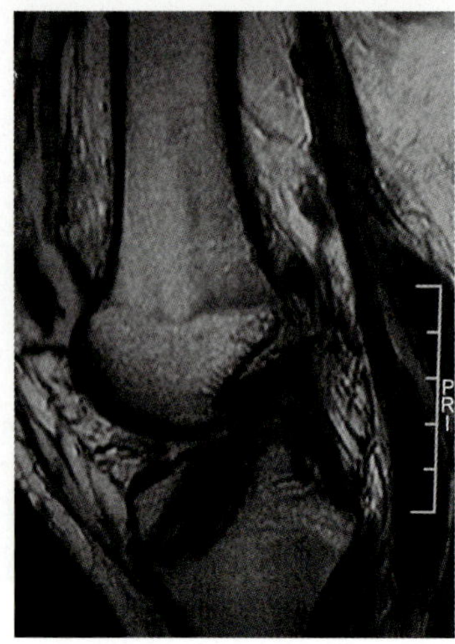

Figure 39.22 Two years postoperative MRI

exercises are encouraged from the third week following surgery. Stationary cycling is allowed as is stair climbing 4 weeks following surgery. Weight training not exceeding 2–3 kg is permitted after 6 weeks of surgery. More aggressive strengthening with weights and resistance bands, closed kinetic exercises and single leg balance training is initiated after 3 months of surgery that continued to 6 months postoperatively. Our preferred option is to delay return to contact sports by up to 9 months following surgery.

REFERENCES

1. Samuelsson K, Andersson D, Karlsson J. Arthroscopy. 2009;25:1139-74.
2. Harter RA, Ostering LR, Singer KM, et al. Long-term evaluation of knee stability and function following surgical reconstruction for the anterior cruciate ligament insufficiency. Am J Sports Med. 1988;16:434-43.
3. Holmes PF, James SL, Larson RL, Singer KM, Jones DL. Retrospective direct comparison of three intra-articular anterior cruciate ligament reconstructions. Am J Sports Med. 1991;19:596-600.
4. Howe JG, Johnson RJ, Kaplan MJ, Fleming B, Jarvinen M. Anterior cruciate ligament reconstruction using quadriceps patellar tendon graft: part I. Long-term follow up. Am J Sports Med. 1991;19:447-57.
5. Kaplan MJ, Howe JG, Fleming B, Johnson RJ, Jarvinen M. Anterior cruciate ligament reconstruction using quadriceps patellar tendon graft: II. A specific sport review. Am J Sports Med. 1991;19:458-62.
6. Komblatt I, Warren RF, Wickiewicz TL. Long-term follow up of anterior cruciate ligament reconstruction using quadriceps substitute for chronic anterior cruciate ligament insufficiency. Am J Sports Med. 1988;16:444-8.
7. Shelbourne KD, Wilckens JH, Mollabashy A, De Carlo M. Arthrofibrosis in acute anterior cruciate ligament reconstruction. The effects of timing of reconstruction and revolution. Am J Sports Med. 1991;19:332-6.
8. Howell SM, Barad SJ. Knee extension and its relationship to the slope of the intercondylar roof: Implications for positioning the tibial tunnel in anterior cruciate ligament reconstructions. Abstract, ACL study group. 19.3.1994 Ischgl (Austria).
9. van Eck CF, Morse KR, Fu FH. The anteromedial portal for anterior cruciate ligament reconstruction. Arthroscopy. 2009;25:1062-4.
10. Markolf KL, Hame SL, Hunter DM, Oakes D, Gause P. Biomechanical effects of femoral notchplasty in anterior cruciate ligament reconstruction. Am J Sports Med. 2002;30:83-9.
11. May DA, Snearly WN, Bents R, Jones R. MR imaging findings in anterior cruciate ligament reconstruction: evaluation of notchplasty. AJR Am J Roentgenol. 1997;169:217-22.

12. Arnold MP, Verdonschot N, van Kampen A. ACL graft can replicate the normal ligament's tension curve. Knee Surg Sports Traumatol Arthrosc. 2005;13:625-31.
13. Brophy RH, Voos JE, Shannon FJ, et al. Changes in the length of virtual anterior cruciate ligament fibers during stability testing: a comparison of conventional single-bundle reconstruction and native anterior cruciate ligament. Am J Sports Med. 2008;36:2196-203.
14. Cha PS, Brucker PU, West RV, et al. Arthroscopic double-bundle anterior cruciate ligament reconstruction: an anatomic approach. Arthroscopy. 2005;21:1275.
15. Järvelä T, Moisala AS, Sihvonen R, et al. Double-bundle anterior cruciate ligament reconstruction using hamstring autografts and bioabsorbable interference screw fixation: prospective, randomized, clinical study with 2-year results. Am J Sports Med. 2008;36:290-7.
16. Lee MC, Seong SC, Lee S, et al. Vertical femoral tunnel placement results in rotational knee laxity after anterior cruciate ligament reconstruction. Arthroscopy. 2007;23:771-8.
17. Loh JC, Fukuda Y, Tsuda E, et al. Knee stability and graft function following anterior cruciate ligament reconstruction: comparison between 11 o'clock and 10 o'clock femoral tunnel placement. Arthroscopy. 2003;19:297-304.
18. Musahl V, Plakseychuk A, VanScyoc A, et al. Varying femoral tunnels between the anatomical footprint and isometric positions: effect on kinematics of the anterior cruciate ligament-reconstructed knee. Am J Sports Med. 2005;33:712-8.
19. Pearle AD, Shannon FJ, Granchi C, Wickiewicz TL, Warren RF. Comparison of 3-dimensional obliquity and anisometric characteristics of anterior cruciate ligament graft positions using surgical navigation. Am J Sports Med. 2008;36:1534-41.
20. Petersen W, Tretow H, Weimann A, et al. Biomechanical evaluation of two techniques for double-bundle anterior cruciate ligament reconstruction: one tibial tunnel versus two tibial tunnels. Am J Sports Med. 2007;35:228-34.
21. Petersen W, Lenschow S, Weimann A, et al. Importance of femoral tunnel placement in double-bundle posterior cruciate ligament reconstruction: biomechanical analysis using a robotic/universal force-moment sensor testing system. Am J Sports Med. 2006;34:456-63.
22. Scopp JM, Jasper LE, Belkoff SM, Moorman CT 3rd. The effect of oblique femoral tunnel placement on rotational constraint of the knee reconstructed using patellar tendon autografts. Arthroscopy. 2004;20:294-9.
23. Yamamoto Y, Hsu WH, Woo SL, et al. Knee stability and graft function after anterior cruciate ligament reconstruction: a comparison of a lateral and an anatomical femoral tunnel placement. Am J Sports Med. 2004;32:1825-32.
24. Yasuda K, Kondo E, Ichiyama H, et al. Anatomic reconstruction of the anteromedial and posterolateral bundles of the anterior cruciate ligament using hamstring tendon grafts. Arthroscopy. 2004;20:1015-25.
25. Yasuda K, Ichiyama H, Kondo E, et al. An *in vivo* biomechanical study on the tension-versus-knee flexion angle curves of 2 grafts in anatomic double-bundle anterior cruciate ligament reconstruction: effects of initial tension and internal tibial rotation. Arthroscopy. 2008;24:276-84.
26. Yasuda K, Kondo E, Ichiyama H, Tanabe Y, Tohyama H. Clinical evaluation of anatomic double-bundle anterior cruciate ligament reconstruction procedure using hamstring tendon grafts: comparisons among 3 different procedures. Arthroscopy. 2006;22:240-51.
27. Zantop T, Diermann N, Schumacher T, et al. Anatomical and nonanatomical double-bundle anterior cruciate ligament reconstruction: importance of femoral tunnel location on knee kinematics. Am J Sports Med. 2008;36:678-85.
28. Pearle AD, Shannon FJ, Granchi C, Wickiewicz TL, Warren RF. Comparison of 3-dimensional obliquity and anisometric characteristics of anterior cruciate ligament graft positions using surgical navigation. Am J Sports Med. 2008;36:1534-41.
29. Heming JF, Rand J, Steiner ME. Anatomical limitations of transtibial drilling in anterior cruciate ligament reconstruction. Am J Sports Med. 2007;35:1708-15.
30. Rue JP, Ghodadra N, Bach BR Jr. Femoral tunnel placement in single-bundle anterior cruciate ligament reconstruction: a cadaveric study relating transtibial lateralized femoral tunnel position to the anteromedial and posterolateral bundle femoral origins of the anterior cruciate ligament. Am J Sports Med. 2008;36:73-9.
31. Rue JP, Ghodadra N, Lewis PB, Bach BR Jr. Femoral and tibial tunnel position using a transtibial drilled anterior cruciate ligament reconstruction technique. J Knee Surg. 2008;21:246-9.

32. Simmons R, Howell SM, Hull ML. Effect of the angle of the femoral and tibial tunnels in the coronal plane and incremental excision of the posterior cruciate ligament on tension of an anterior cruciate ligament graft: an *in vitro* study. J Bone Joint Surg Am. 2003;85:1018-29.
33. Anderson AF, Snyder RB, Lipscomb AB Jr. Anterior cruciate ligament reconstruction. A prospective randomized study of three surgical methods. Am J Sports Med. 2001;29:272-9.
34. Aune AK, Holm I, Risberg MA, Jensen HK, Steen H. Four-strand hamstring tendon autograft compared with patellar tendon-bone autograft for anterior cruciate ligament reconstruction. A randomized study with two-year follow-up. Am J Sports Med. 2001;29:722-8.
35. Barrett GR, Noojin FK, Hartzog CW, Nash CR. Reconstruction of the anterior cruciate ligament in females: a comparison of hamstring versus patellar tendon autograft. Arthroscopy. 2002;18:46-54.
36. Freedman KB, D'Amato MJ, Nedeff DD, Kaz A, Bach BR Jr. Arthroscopic anterior cruciate ligament reconstruction: a meta-analysis comparing patellar tendon and hamstring tendon autografts. Am J Sports Med. 2003;31:2-11.
37. Asagumo H, Kimura M, Kobayashi Y, Taki M, Takagishi K. Anatomic reconstruction of the anterior cruciate ligament using double-bundle hamstring tendons: surgical techniques, clinical outcomes, and complications. Arthroscopy. 2007;23:602-9.
38. Adachi N, Ochi M, Uchio Y, et al. Reconstruction of the anterior cruciate ligament. Single-versus double-bundle multistranded hamstring tendons. J Bone Joint Surg Br. 2004;86:515-20.
39. Hamada M, Shino K, Horibe S, et al. Single- versus bi-socket anterior cruciate ligament reconstruction using autogenous multiple-stranded hamstring tendons with endobutton femoral fixation: a prospective study. Arthroscopy. 2001;17:801-7.
40. Bottoni CR. Anterior cruciate ligament femoral tunnel creation by use of anteromedial portal. Arthroscopy. 2008;24:1319.
41. Harner CD, Honkamp NJ, Ranawat AS. Anteromedial portal technique for creating the anterior cruciate ligament femoral tunnel. Arthroscopy. 2008;24:113-5.
42. Steiner ME, Battaglia TC, Heming JF, et al. Independent drilling outperforms conventional transtibial drilling in anterior cruciate ligament reconstruction. Am J Sports Med. 2009;37:1912-9.
43. Gavriilidis I, Motsis EK, Pakos EE, et al. Transtibial versus anteromedial portal of the femoral tunnel in ACL reconstruction: a cadaveric study. Knee. 2008;15:364-7.
44. Dargel J, Schmidt-Wiethoff R, Fischer S, et al. Femoral bone tunnel placement using the transtibial tunnel or the anteromedial portal in ACL reconstruction: a radiographic evaluation. Knee Surg Sports Traumatol Arthrosc. 2009;17:220-7.
45. Hantes ME, Zachos VC, Liantsis A, et al. Differences in graft orientation using the transtibial and anteromedial portal technique in anterior cruciate ligament reconstruction: a magnetic resonance imaging study. Knee Surg Sports Traumatol Arthrosc. 2009;17:880-6.
46. Bedi A, Altchek DW. The 'footprint' anterior cruciate ligament technique: an anatomic approach to anterior cruciate ligament reconstruction. Arthroscopy. 2009;25:1128-38.
47. Bowers AL, Bedi A, Lipman JD, et al. Comparison of anterior cruciate ligament tunnel position and graft obliquity with transtibial and anteromedial portal femoral tunnel reaming techniques using high-resolution magnetic resonance imaging. Arthroscopy. 2011;27:1511-22.
48. Lubowitz JH. Anteromedial portal technique for the anterior cruciate ligament femoral socket: pitfalls and solutions. Arthroscopy. 2009;25:95-101.

Chapter 40

Double-bundle ACL Reconstruction: Principles and Surgical Technique

J Clement Joseph

The recent focus on restoring the anatomy and function of reconstructed anterior cruciate ligament (ACL) as close to the native ACL has resulted in the evolution of double bundle reconstruction. The potential benefits hypothesized are better rotational stability, lesser failure rates and less chances of osteoarthritis. This technique is a culmination of the principles of ACL reconstruction, which are to:

- Restore the bundle anatomy
- Restore the insertional anatomy
- Restore tensioning pattern
- Individualize surgery according to patients.

The anatomy of ACL has been well studied and is shown to have two bundles, anteromedial and posterolateral bundles with distinct functions at different ranges of flexion. The separation can be identified even in fetal development.[1]

The anteromedial bundle is relatively stronger and maintains a constant level of tension, with some increase when knee is flexed 60° and contributes to anteroposterior stability throughout knee motion. The posterolateral bundle tightens near extension and becomes lax beyond 30° of flexion and being more horizontally oriented, it is thought to contribute more to the rotational stability and AP stability near extension.[2-5] The anteromedial (AM) bundle is slightly larger, 28 to 38 mm in length and posterolateral (PL)being around 17 mm in length.

As a concept, double bundle reconstruction is a major advancement in ACL surgery, as it tries to reproduce the bundle anatomy, behavior, footprint coverage and possibility of restoring greater rotational stability. *In vitro* biomechanical studies have shown superior stability, especially rotational stability with double reconstructed knees.[6,7] Some clinical studies have shown better results and most other show comparable outcomes.[8-11] The studies describing double bundle reconstructions also vary in surgical techniques, graft choices, fixation methods, and rehabilitation protocols.[12] The presence of comorbid factors like meniscus tears and cartilage defects can also result in variable outcomes.

Double bundle reconstruction cannot be advised for all knees as a 'one size fits all' approach, especially when the footprint of ACL is small and notch is narrow. DB-ACL reconstruction also requires a certain level of proficiency in surgical skills, well-trained team members, instrumentation, and a variety of implant choices to suit the situation.[13] It has to be remembered, the first chance to reconstruct the ACL is the best one and a badly done, failed DB-ACL is very difficult to revise. It is very important to counsel the patient that a DB-ACL will be carried out only if the footprint is large enough and dimensions of notch are ideal. The patient should also be counseled about the requirements for rehabilitation and return to sports.

SURGICAL TECHNIQUE

The surgical technique described here has been done by one of the authors for the past 4 years and uses supine positioning, and transportal technique of making both the femoral tunnels, hamstring grafts and uses cortical (suspensory) fixation at both ends. A button fixation like Endobutton CL (Smith & Nephew) or tightrope RT (Arthrex) is used on the femoral side and suture discs are used on the tibial side. This fixation technique allows us to use a short length of graft (7 cm).

Usually a graft diameter of 7 mm is preferred for the AM bundle and a 6 or 7 mm graft for the PL bundle. Use of an interference screw requires a longer graft length (minimum 90 mm length) and makes it necessary to routinely harvest gracilis graft and also if the wall between the tunnels is thin, interference fixation can result in tunnel coalescence and thereby resulting in poor fixation strength. A doubled gracilis graft alone may be insufficient to perform the role of PL bundle and could be reason for ruptured PL bundles in many studies.

The procedure is carried out under spinal or epidural analgesia. The patient is positioned supine with a foot roll under the foot, when the knee is flexed to 90° and a lateral thigh support is positioned at the level of tourniquet so that the leg can maintain its position in 90° and vertical without any external support (**Figure 40.1**). The opposite leg can be left lying on the table. A Mayo's table can be attached above the pelvis and should not obstruct the hyperflexion of knee.

A diagnostic arthroscopy is performed first, addressing the meniscal and chondral lesions. The notch is cleared of soft tissue with a scoop and shaver. In acute cases the femoral footprint can be identified by the ACL remnant. In chronic cases with bone overgrowth, bony notchplasty may be necessary. The orientation and description of

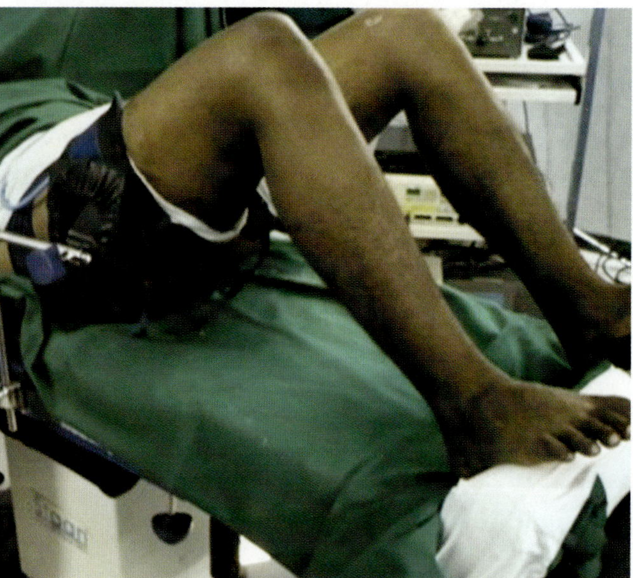

Figure 40.1 Positioning for anatomical DB-ACL reconstruction

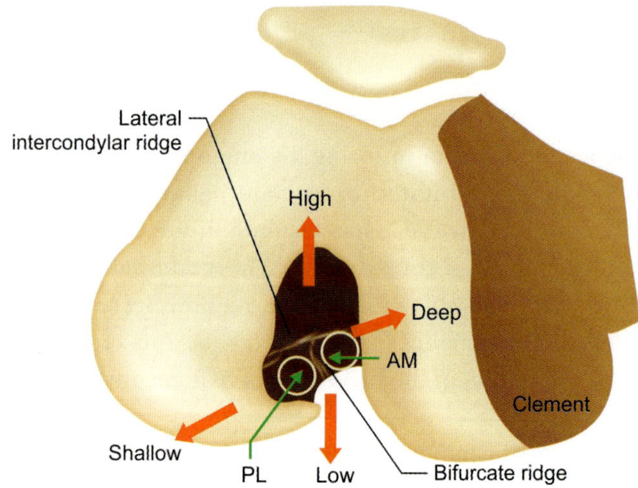

Figure 40.2 Notch anatomy and orientation

notch anatomy has also undergone changes recently. The clockface reference of the notchplasty is no longer used as the reference points of the clockface change with different angles of flexion. Any reference point in the lateral notch position towards the surgeon is referred as shallow and a point away from the surgeon is referred as deep. A point towards the ceiling is referred as high and a point towards the floor is referred as low (**Figure 40.2**).

The lateral intercondylar ridge is an osseous ridge on the lateral wall of intercondylar notch, that runs proximal to distal in an extended knee and the entire ACL footprint is behind (posterior) this ridge, the AM bundle occupying a posterior and proximal position and PL bundle located just distal to it, the bundles lying parallel to each other. But in a flexed knee, which is the position in which arthroscopy is done, the lateral intercondylar ridge becomes horizontal and the entire ACL footprint becomes horizontal and lies below the ridge, the AM lying at the back (deep and low) and PL lying toward the surgeon (shallow and low) (**Figure 40.2**). The bundles now adopt a crossing pattern. In the supine position, when the knee is flexed 90°, the femur is flexed 45° at the hip and the orientation of footprints also changes accordingly.

A tibial footprint of 14 mm is a contraindication for DB-ACL. A tibial footprint more than 16 mm can be considered for a DB-ACL. A femoral footprint of more than 16 mm is ideal for a DB-ACLR reconstruction. After confirming the footprint dimensions, a decision is made to perform a double bundle reconstruction.

Graft harvest is carried out using an oblique incision starting from a point 1 cm medial to the midline at the level of lower margin of tibial tuberosity, proceeding medially and distally for about 3 cm. The oblique incision allows a good exposure for harvesting the tendons and allows good retraction for the placement of tibial tunnels mediolaterally and the low position ensures that the tunnels and implants are not directly under the scar (**Figure 40.3**).

The semitendinosus tendon is harvested and prepared. Since cortical (suspensory) fixation is used in both the ends, a graft construct length of 7 cm is enough. A semitendinosus (ST) tendon length of 28 cm is required

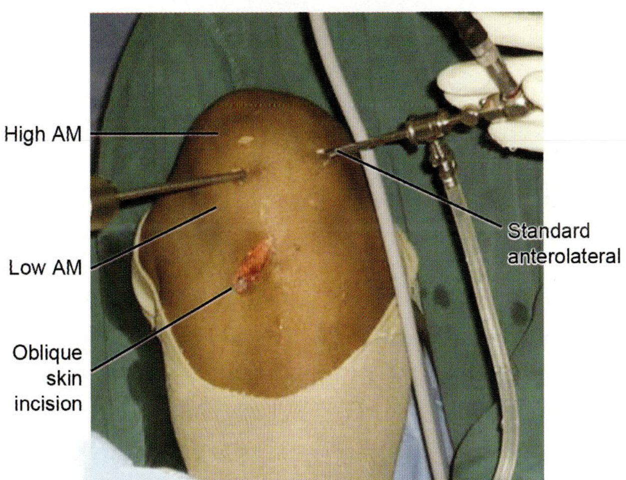

Figure 40.3 Portal anatomy and incision for graft harvest

for preparing two double stranded grafts (ST2 + ST2), thus conserving the gracilis. The tendon is divided at 14 cm; whipstitches are applied at the ends using either FiberWire or number 5 Ethibond sutures. So, when each half is folded on itself, the ensuring length will be 7 cm. It is very important to carefully apply the whipstitches so as to maintain a low profile so as not to increase the size of tibial tunnels. The grafts are sized and a diameter of 6 mm or 7 mm is acceptable. If the ST is thin, or the footprint is large enough, a doubled gracilis graft of same length can be added to one of the double strands, usually the AM bundle.

The accessory AM portal is made 1 cm below the standard AM portal, just lateral to the patellar tendon and entering the knee just above the medial meniscus. Horizontal incision ensures that the anterior horn of medial meniscus will not be damaged inadvertently (**Figure 40.3**). It is also important to shave a portion of fat pad, especially the portion under the scope, as the fat pad will rise up and obstruct the vision when the knee is flexed to 120°.

Femoral AM and femoral PL tunnels are made first followed by tibial PL and tibial AM tunnels. The AM tunnel is made with knee flexed in 120° and PL tunnel is made with knee flexed in 90°. Making tunnels in the same flexion angle will create parallel tunnels and it may preclude using suspensory fixation or interference fixation. The varying angles will ensure divergent tunnels.

The drilling procedure for AM tunnel starts with the knee flexed 90°, the starting point for AM tunnel is marked by an impression with a 45° Chondropick, which will prevent the Beath pin skiving off (**Figures 40.4A and B**). The Beath pin drill tip is kept in this impression and drilled slowly for few turns to get a then the knee is flexed to 120° and then the Beath pin is advanced out of the cortex. Keeping the Beath pin parallel to the floor can ensure a good tunnel length and the low accessory AM portal is very helpful for this positioning (**Figures 40.5 and 40.6**). The Beath pin is overdrilled with a 4.5 mm cannulated drill for the button passage and the tunnel is measured with a depth gauge. Then it is sequentially over-reamed with acorn drills to a desired diameter and depth.

The depth of final reaming depends on the type of fixation. Ideally 20 mm of graft should be accommodated inside the tunnel. In case of fixed loop devices like

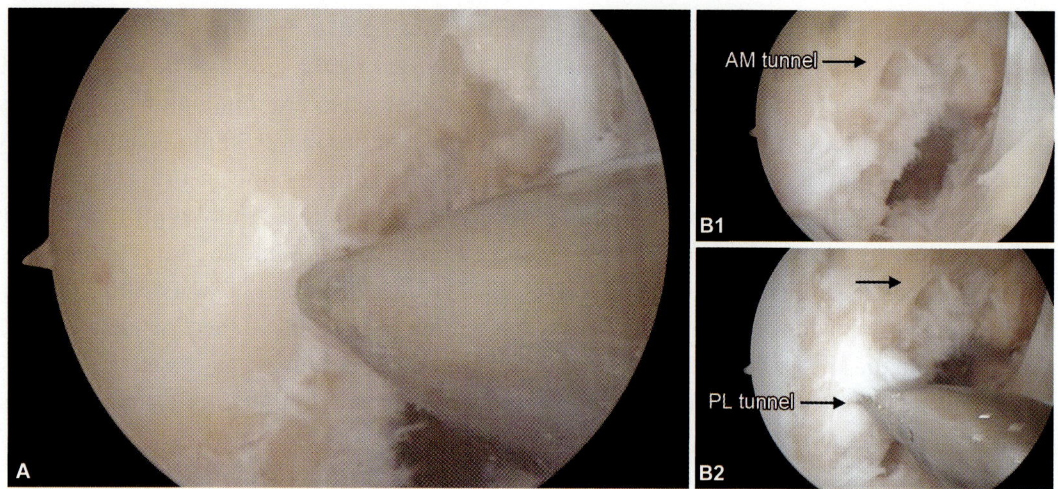

Figures 40.4A and B The starting point is marked with a 45° Chondropick (awl) is used to make a mark for drilling with Beath pin without skiving off

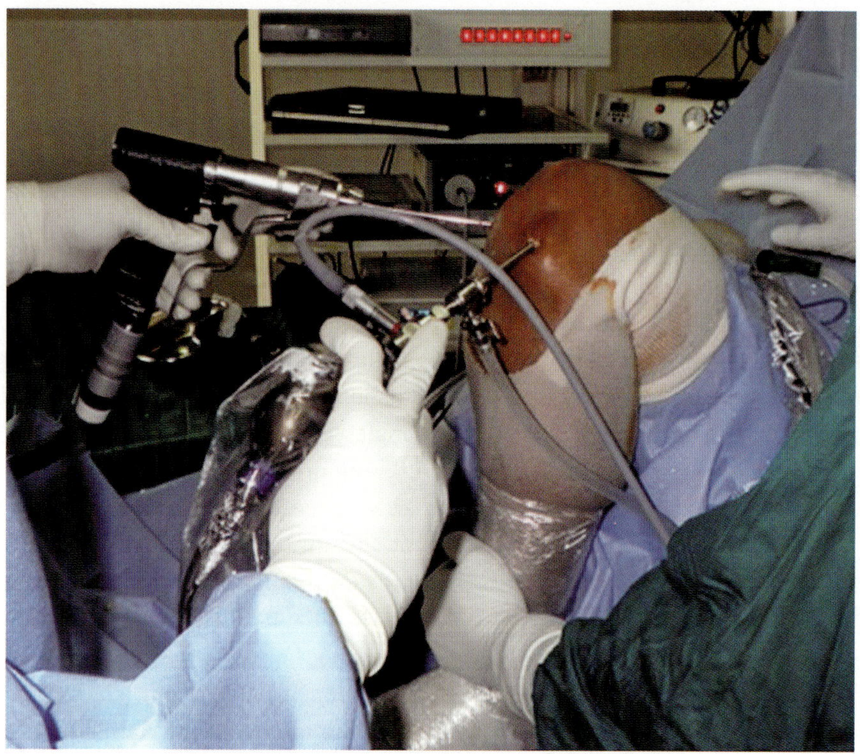

Figure 40.5 Anteromedial tunnel is made with knee flexed to 120°

Endobutton, the socket should be reamed 6 mm more (flipping distance), so as the button can come out, flip and seat over the cortex. For example, if the 4.5 mm tunnel length is 40 mm and if 20 mm of graft is planned to be accommodated inside the tunnel, a 6 mm of flipping distance is added and a socket of 26 mm is made with the acorn drill. The size of the Endobutton loop can be calculated by subtracting the length of graft to be accommodated from the total tunnel length (e.g. 40–20 = 20 mm loop). The length of the graft to be accommodated inside the tunnel is marked with a skin marker or a Vicryl suture. In short tunnels, 15 mm of graft can be accommodated as

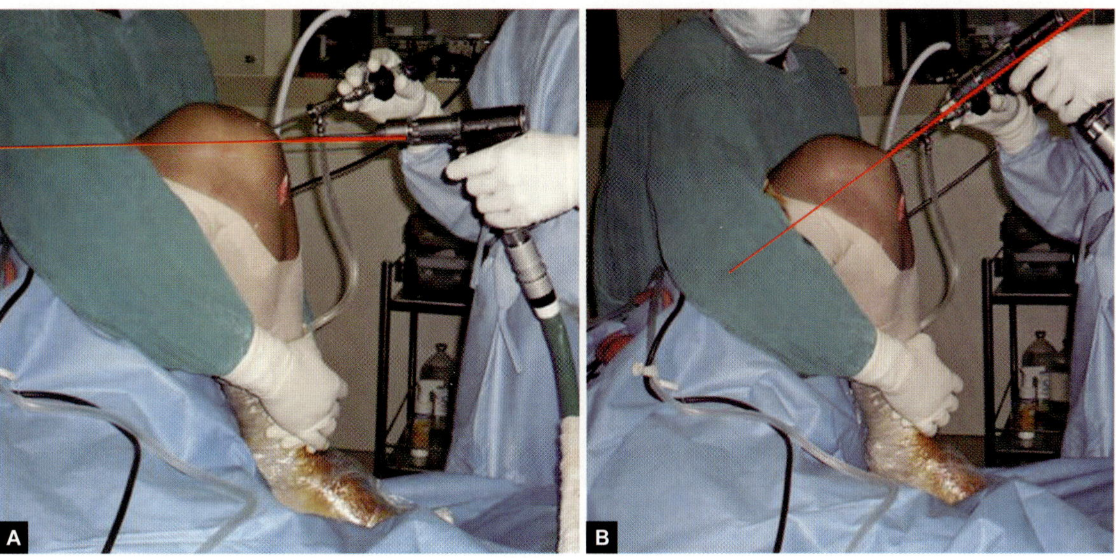

Figures 40.6A and B Keeping the Beath pin parallel to the floor ensures a good tunnel length. The accessory anteromedial portal is helpful in this regard

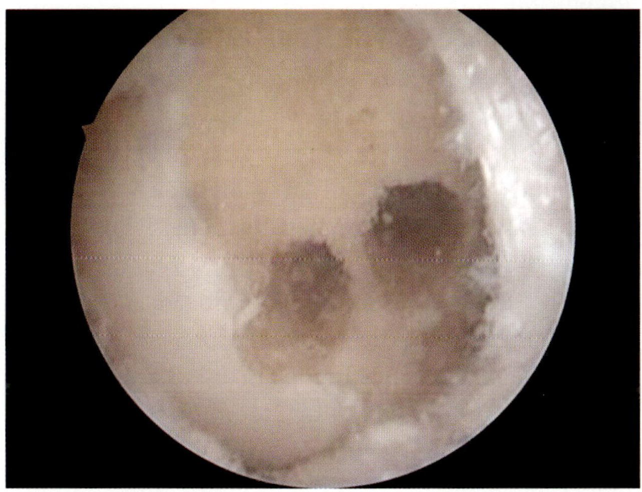

Figure 40.7 Postion of femoral tunnels

well. Adjustable loop suspensory devices (Tightrope RT) do not require the reaming of additional flipping distance and can be helpful in short PL femoral tunnels.

At this stage, the space for placement of PL tunnel is verified again. If there is no space, still the procedure can be converted into a single bundle procedure (**Figure 40.7**). Hence it is advantageous to drill the tunnels in this sequence. The PL femoral tunnel is made with knee flexed 90°. Once again the starting point is marked with a Chondropick, a Beath pin is passed from accessory anteromedial portal so as to exit from the lateral aspect of thigh. Any exit posterior to the biceps femoris tendon is not acceptable and should be revised. In a similar way, the Beath pin is over-reamed with 4.5 drill, through and through for the passage of the button and subsequent reaming done with the final diameter acorn drill for accommodating the graft.

Care should be exercised while reaming the femoral tunnels via portals, as the reamers can damage the cartilage or meniscus. The drill should always be introduced with the hand over the guide pin, close to the midline so as not to scratch the femoral condyles, with reverse rotatory movements and once the drill is in contact with lateral wall of the notch, the direction is fixed and power is used.

In the tibia, considerable amount of tibial ACL stump can be left for biological healing and proprioception, but early in early learning curve, necessary shaving can be performed to get an idea of placement of tunnels. In the tibia, the posterolateral tunnel is reamed first and then AM tunnel (**Figure 40.8**). The PL guidewire is passed with the aiming guide set at 50° angle, starting from a point 3 cm from the midline on the anteromedial surface of tibia [just anterior to medial collateral ligament (MCL) and avoiding injuring the MCL] and entering the joint 3–4 mm in front of the posterior horn of lateral meniscus. The guidewire is left in place.

The AM guidewire is passed with the aiming guide set at 55°, starting from a point 1 cm from the midline on the anteromedial surface of tibia (avoiding injury to the patellar tendon insertion) and entering in the center

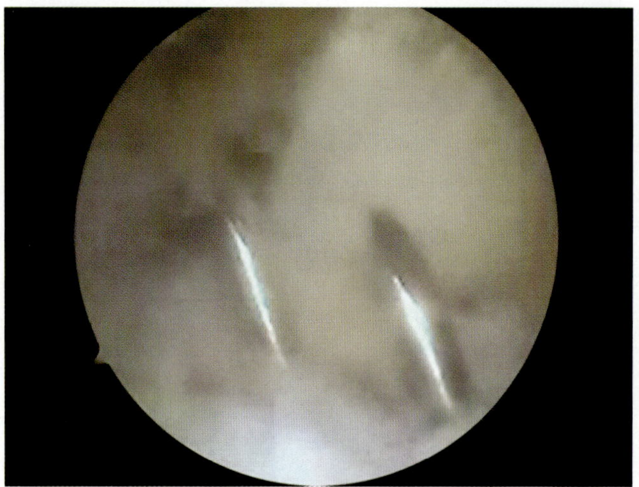

Figure 40.8 Guidewires for tibial tunnels

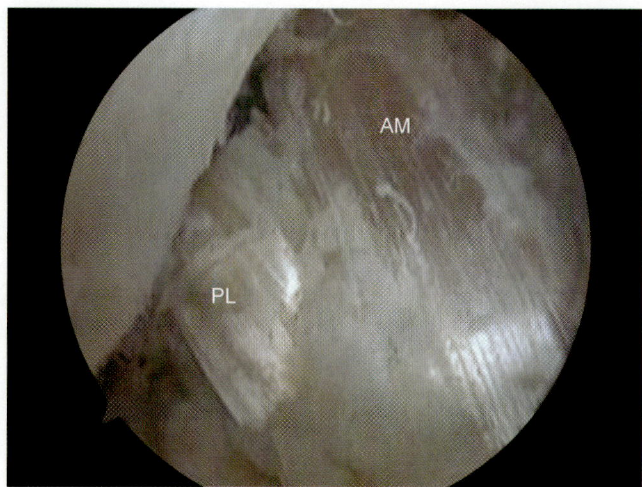

Figure 40.10 Double-bundle reconstruction

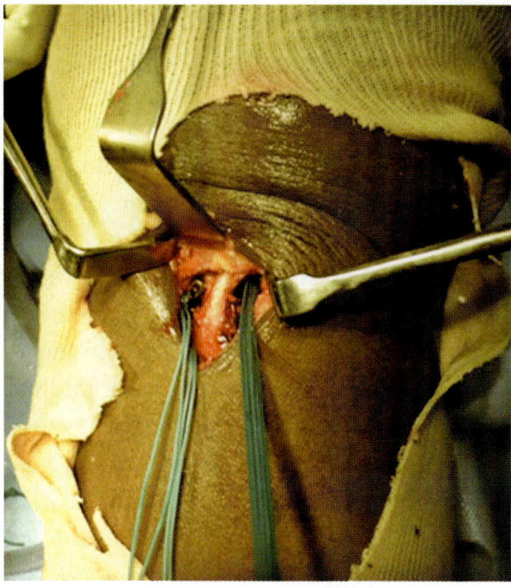

Figure 40.9 Position of tibial tunnels

of the anterior half of tibial footprint (**Figure 40.9**). The guidewires are left in place projecting 3–4 mm. Now as the knee is extended, the AM guidewire should pass inside the notch. If not, the position is considered too anterior and is revised. Similarly, the distance between the tunnels can also be judged at this stage. Sequential reaming of PL tunnel is done first and later AM tunnel, carefully avoiding violating the intervening wall.

At this stage, thorough joint lavage is given to remove the debris. A Beath pin loaded with number 2 Ethibond loop is passed through the PCL femoral tunnel from the accessory AM portal, the free ends exiting out of lateral thigh and loop being pulled inside the joint. A hook or probe is passed into the tibial PL tunnel and the loop is brought out through the tibial PL tunnel. The leading sutures and flipping sutures of the button are passed into the loop, pulled and are brought out of the lateral thigh. The graft is pulled into the socket and as the 20 mm mark enters few millimeters into the tunnel, the Endobutton is flipped and after the flip, the graft slides down, so that the mark is in line with the mouth of the tunnel.

The knee is hyperflexed to 120°, a Beath pin with number 2 Ethibond loop passed into the AM femoral tunnel and then with knee at 90°, the loop is retrieved out of joint through AM tibial tunnel. In a similar fashion, the graft is passed and the button is flipped. The grafts are checked for impingement by moving through ROM and then cyclic loading is performed (**Figure 40.10**). On the tibial side, the PL bundle is fixed first in full extension and then the AM bundle is fixed at 30° of flexion. The sutures are secured using six half hitches; first two in the same direction, the third in reverse direction and subsequent three are made reversing the direction as well as changing the posts.

REHABILITATION

DB-ACL reconstructions are rehabilitated using the same protocol as that of single bundle-anterior cruciate ligament (SB-ACL). It has been the personal observation of the author that the double bundle-anterior cruciate ligament (DB-ACL) reconstructed knees regain the range quite quickly and comfortably, probably due to exact anatomical placement and behavioral reproduction. Grafts need time to heal and more so with double bundles, and hence return to sports is allowed only after 9 months.

DISCUSSION

The concept of double-bundle reconstruction makes sense as to restoring the knee kinematics closer to the normal, but clear superiority in terms of outcomes and prevention of OA has yet to be proved. In addition, considerations like, implant costs, increased operating time, demands of the patients, and skill levels, are also important. One should also be aware of complications like tunnel coalescence, cortical blowout, inadvertent through and through drilling. Authors like Freddie Fu, have postulated that anatomically placed grafts may be at more risk of failure, as they face higher *in situ* forces due to their anatomical placement. However, in nonanatomical placements, the forces are absorbed by other structures like meniscus, condyles, etc. Hence, rehabilitation of any anatomical ACL reconstruction should be very gradual and careful, more so with DB-ACL reconstructions. DB-ACL grafts are theoretically weaker in the early phase, as they take time to heal and act synergistically. Moreover, each bundle sustains the entire load individually at respective flexion angles and thereby increasing the chance of failures.[13]

DB-ACL reconstruction as a technique restores knee kinematics especially in selected patients with greater rotatory instability, large footprints. Careful attention to technique, patient selection, and rehabilitation will ensure good results. DB-ACL reconstruction as a concept has even improved our SB-ACL reconstructions by focusing on the anatomical placement of grafts and using thicker grafts ensuring good amount of collagen is used to fill the footprint. Well-designed studies with standardized technique will decide the status and indications of this procedure in the future.

REFERENCES

1. Ferretti M, Levicoff EA, Machpherson TA, et al. The fetal anterior cruciate ligament: an anatomic and histology study. Arthroscopy. 2007;23:278-83.
2. Buoncristiani AM, Tjoumakaris FP, Starman JS. Anatomic double-bundle ACL reconstruction. Arthroscopy. 2006;22(9):1000-6.
3. Gabriel MT, Wong EK, Woo SL, Yagi M, Debski RE. Distribution of *in situ* forces in the anterior cruciate ligament in response to rotator loads. J Orthop Res. 2004;22:85-9.
4. Sakane M, Fox RJ, Woo SL, et al. *In situ* forces in the anterior cruciate ligament and its bundles in response to anterior tibial loads. J Ortho Res. 1997;15:285-93.
5. Zantop T, Herbort M, Raschke MJ, Fu FH, Petersen W. The role of the anteromedial and posterolateral bundles of the anterior cruciate ligament in anterior tibial translation and internal rotation. Am J Sports Med. 2007;35:223-7.
6. Yagi M, Kuroda R, Nagamune K, Yoshiya S, Kurosaka M. Double bundle ACL can improve rotational stability. Clin Orthop Relat Res. 2007;454:100-7.
7. Yagi M, Wong EK, Kanamori A, et al. Biomechanical analysis of an anatomic anterior cruciate ligament reconstruction. Am J Sports Med. 2002;30:660-6.
8. Muneta T, Koga H, Mochizuki T, et al. A prospective randomized study of 4-strand semitendinosus tendon anterior cruciate ligament reconstruction comparing single-bundle and double-bundle techniques. Arthroscopy. 2007;23(6):618-28.
9. van Eck CF, Kopf S, Irrgang JJ, et al. Single-bundle versus double-bundle reconstruction for anterior cruciate ligament rupture: a meta-analysis—does anatomy matter? Arthroscopy. 2012;28:405-24.
10. Hussein M, van Eck CF, Cretnik A, Dinevski D, Fu FH. Individualized anterior cruciate ligament surgery: a prospective study comparing anatomic single and double bundle reconstruction. Am J Sports Med. 2012;40:1781-8.
11. Hussein M, van Eck CF, Cretnik A, Dinevski D, Fu FH. Prospective randomized clinical evaluation of conventional single bundle, anatomic single bundle, and anatomic double bundle anterior cruciate ligament reconstruction: 281 cases with 3- to 5-year follow-up. Am J Sports Med. 2012;40:512-20.
12. van Eck CF, Schreiber VM, Mejia HA, et al. 'Anatomic' anterior cruciate ligament reconstruction: a systematic review of surgical techniques and reporting of surgical data. Arthroscopy. 2010;26(9):S2-12.
13. Marx RG. Single- versus double-bundle anterior cruciate ligament reconstruction. Clin Orthop Relat Res. 2013;471(2):363-7.

Chapter 41

Posterior Cruciate Ligament Reconstruction

Vivek Pandey, Charles H Brown, Sachin Tapaswi

Ideal and successful treatment of posterior cruciate ligament (PCL) injuries remains elusive due to its complex anatomy and biomechanics. Historically, the outcome of PCL reconstruction has been inferior as compared with anterior cruciate ligament (ACL) reconstruction. The results of reconstruction by various surgical techniques continue to vary in different studies. However, in the last two decades, continuous research on PCL anatomy, biomechanics, and function has provided newer insights into the treatment options and techniques including inlay or tunnel technique, graft and fixation options, single or double bundle, and rehabilitation methods. With the help of recent literature review, this chapter would focus on the basics of anatomy and biomechanics of PCL, their influence on the treatment option; natural history of tear and alteration in biomechanics; diagnostic modalities and their usefulness in various scenarios; various treatment options (single and double bundle), fixation methods, and rehabilitation.

ANATOMY

Posterior cruciate ligament (PCL) is the primary restraint to the posterior drawer contributing approximately 90% of the resistance along the flexion arc.[1] It is a very strong ligament with tensile loads reported in the range of 739–1627 N.[2,3] Its strength is derived from a broad cross-sectional area and broad footprint over femur and tibia. It is a 32–38 mm long ligament whose diameter is 1.5 times more than the ACL and footprint three times larger than that of diameter.[4-6] To recreate this dumbbell, shape of ligament is difficult and this makes the PCL reconstruction difficult. PCL is functionally divided into the anterolateral (AL) and PM bundles based on femoral and tibial insertion.[4] The AL bundle tightens in flexion whereas the PM bundle tightens in extension. Harner et al. demonstrated that the AL bundle possesses superior structural properties than the PM bundle. The AL bundle is 2.1 times stiffer than the PM bundle and possesses 2.7 times ultimate strength as compared with the PM bundle.[6] Hence, the current surgical recommendation for single bundle PCL reconstruction is to reconstruct the AL bundle. Also, the AL bundle tightens in knee flexion that is more important for the PCL function. But this bundle description of PCL is oversimplification. Makris et al. dissected 24 pairs of knee and proposed that the PCL region is divided into four anatomic and functional fiber regions (anterior, central, posterior-longitudinal and posterior-oblique) whose tensioning and relaxing patterns are different in varying positions of the knee.[7] In a study on 12 cadaveric knees, Hatshushika et al. found an interesting topographical correlation between tibial and femoral attachments.[8] Femoral fibers followed high and low configuration but tibial footprint followed a parabolic or transverse type of attachment. This complex anatomy of the PCL renders PCL reconstruction difficult with current techniques by merely placing tubular/flat graft within circular tunnels.

The tibial footprint of the PCL is located between the posterior horns of two menisci about 1–1.5 cm below the posterior tibial margin in the 'PCL facet.' The anterolateral bundle (ALB) arises from superior part of the facet above the shelf and posteromedial bundle (PMB) arises below the shelf. Lowermost fibers of PLB merge with tibial periosteum and posterior tibial capsule. ALB and PLB fibers further extend upward and medially to be attached onto the medial femoral condyle (MFC). ALB is attached mostly to the roof of the intercondylar notch and PLB to the medial side of the wall (**Figures 41.1A to D**). This division of fibers is based upon the tensioning pattern in flexion-extension and is based upon dissection rather than true anatomic division.[4,9] ALB has a larger cross-sectional area and is much stronger than PLB. Recently,

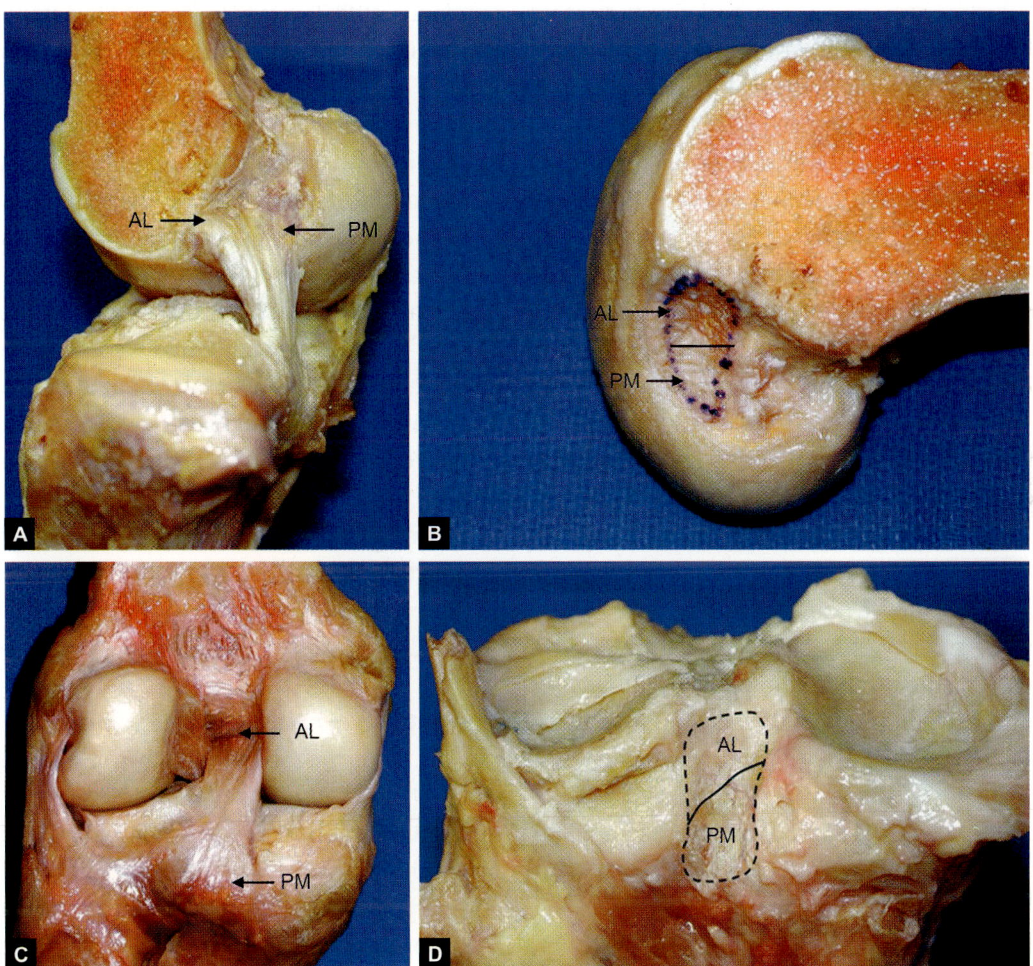

Figures 41.1A to D Images of cadaveric dissected 'right knee' shows attachment of posterior cruciate ligament (PCL) fibers; the AL bundle and PM bundle over tibia and femur. Image (A) shows both the AL bundle and PM bundle attachment over MFC with knee in extension. Image (B) reveals the area occupied by both bundles over the MFC when seen in knee flexed where in the AL bundle occupies near the roof or high position and the PM bundle occupies low position near articular cartilage. Image (C) shows the attachment and orientation of PCL fibers from the back of the knee. Image (D) shows the origin of PCL fibers over the back of the tibia. *Abbreviations:* AL, anterolateral; PM, posteromedial; MFC, medial femoral condyle

another interesting observation was made by Hoof et al. on embalmed nine cadaveric knees using CTscan.[10] They replaced the PCL by a best fitting cylinder on a CT model and suggested that average tibial and femoral footprint of the PCL was 189.1 mm^2 and 293.3 mm^2. The mean diameter of the best-fit cylinder was 10.5 mm and mean coverage on tibial and femoral footprint was 76.5% and 46.5%, respectively. The central axis of this cylinder was central on the tibial footprint and AL on the femoral footprint of the PCL. The practical implication of this study is profound indicating that with the existing techniques of PCL reconstruction; it is difficult to restore the anatomical footprint of the PCL over tibia and femur. Double-bundle PCL (DB PCL) reconstruction could be more logical as it covers more footprints. The experimental evidence is encouraging.[9,11,12] However, clinical evidence is not supportive.[13]

The PCL is also flanked by the meniscofemoral ligament (MFL), anteriorly (ligament of Humphrey) and posteriorly (ligament of Wrisberg).[14] Both anterior and posterior MFL arise from the posterior horn of lateral meniscus and are attached onto the MFC anterior and posterior to PCL, respectively. Their presence is quite variable. A review of 16 anatomic studies (1022 cadaveric knees) done by Gupte et al. revealed that 91.1% knee have at least one MFL.[15] Posterior MFL was more frequent than anterior (70.4% versus 48.2%). The MFL offers a significant biomechanical advantage to the knee due to its size, stiffness and strength.[14] Recent biomechanical analysis revealed that aMFL and pMFL stiffness is almost equal to the PM bundle of PCL.[16] The MFL also guides the movement of lateral meniscus rendering it less vulnerable for injuries due to more mobility. Unpublished study of Demeo and Bergfeld (2004) proved that they offer 30–60% resistance for posterior drawer in 90° knee flexion. Due to their varied functional role in the knee, they should be preserved during PCL reconstruction.

Function of PCL Complex

The primary function is to restrain posterior tibial translation as the knee moves from extension to flexion especially from 30°–90° flexion.[1,9] Posteromedial and posterolateral capsule, collaterals provide posterior restraint between 0° and 30° flexion. It is also secondary restraint to varus, valgus and external rotation at high flexion angles. Covey et al. demonstrated that posterior translation of tibia increases by two fold (7.23 ± 0.65 mm) at 90° flexion as compared with 20° flexion (3.41 ± 0.77 mm) at 74 N posteriorly directed force over tibia after selective sectioning of the PCL.[17] Greater than 12 mm posterior drawer is not PCL injury alone indicating damage to posterior capsule.[18]

Epidemiology and Mechanism of Injury

PCL injuries are not as common as ACL injuries. Overall incidence of PCL injury is 1% to 44%.[19] But the incidence can be as high as 95% in combined high velocity ligament injuries due to road traffic accidents. The PCL is injured in contact sports or during road traffic accidents.[20]

1. Hyperflexion of the knee with plantar flexed foot is most commonly observed mechanism in sports injuries.[21]
2. Hyperextension is the other mechanism of injury which can rupture posterior capsule too.
3. Isolated PCL tears are also observed during fall from two wheelers over the road with the knee flexed and posteriorly directed force (pretibial trauma).
4. Dashboard injury to the knee where passenger sustains posteriorly directed force over tibia also results in PCL tear with associated fractures and PCL injury. PCL injuries are quite frequent with periarticular fractures, in which it is missed over 60% of time.[22]

Altered Biomechanics of Knee after PCL Tear

Martin et al. demonstrated that chronic isolated tear of the PCL alters the medial compartment kinematics during weight bearing.[23] PCL tear causes persistent subluxation of medial tibia posteriorly so that MFC rides anteriorly over tibial upslope. This deranges the kinematics of medial compartment. The lateral compartment is not affected. Also, posteriorly subluxated tibia brings the patella closer to femoral trochlea causing increased contact pressure in the patellofemoral compartment. In 10 patients with grade 2 PCL tear, Cristian et al. demonstrated that their knees had decreased maximum valgus moment during stance phase and increased vertical ground reaction force during midstance phase of gait.[24] Skyhar et al. concluded after a cadaveric study that isolated sectioning of the PCL leads to increased pressure in the medial compartment of the knee and the patellofemoral joint.[25] This may explain the increased rates of osteoarthritis in the medial and patellofemoral compartment of the knee. For long, it was thought that an isolated PCL tear can be managed conservatively and is a more benign injury. However, Strobel et al. in 2003 concluded after knee arthroscopy of 181 patients with isolated PCL tear and revealed that 80% had MFC articular cartilage damage and 50% had patellar cartilage damage after 5 years.[26]

Effect of Posterolateral Corner (PLC) Injury, Hamstring and Gravity Over PCL

Injury to PLC causes increase in stress over the PCL and PCL replacement graft by 30%.[27] This effect is quantitatively maximum at low flexion angles.[28] Hamstring activity too increases forces over the PCL especially at 90° flexion of the knee. Gravity too increases the force over the PCL and graft especially in supine position by causing posterior sag.

Clinical Evaluation

Detailed history is helpful in eliciting the mechanism of injury and possible ligaments involved. Clinical features vary in acute and chronic setting of the PCL tear.

In acute PCL tear, there might be an abrasion over the knee or tibia indicating direct injury over the tibia. There might be effusion in the knee and tenderness in the popliteal fossa. If PLC is injured, there might be ecchymosis over the lateral aspect of the knee and upper end of the leg indicating posterolateral capsular tear. Assessment of neurovascular structures cannot be underestimated. Posteriorly directed force can disrupt popliteal artery resulting in vascular deficit. Involvement of common peroneal nerve is not uncommon especially in multiligament injury. Serial examination of pulse is of extreme importance in acute injuries. Absent/ feeble pulse or if ankle brachial index is less than 0.9 as compared with uninvolved knee, arteriogram is indicated in such situation which can be performed while doing CT or MR scan of the knee.

Chronic tears of the PCL result in instability and pain both. The patient may complain of instability while climbing stairs, walking up or down inclines (ramps) or while lifting heavy loads with the knee flexed. They might complain of knee pain suggesting involvement of the medial compartment of knee and patellofemoral joint causing arthrosis. On examination, the tibia sags posteriorly with knee flexion. The most accurate test is posterior drawer at 90° flexion with sensitivity of 90% and specificity of 99%.[29,30] The posterior drawer is graded from 1 to 3. Normally, the tibial plateau is 1 cm ahead of femoral condyle in 90° flexion. Grade 1 posterior drawer means that tibia can be pushed 3–5 mm posteriorly but step-off is still present. In grade 2, the tibial plateau is flush with femoral condyle where posterior drawer is between 5–10 mm. In grade 3, the tibial plateau is no more flush but is felt behind the femoral condyle where posterior drawer is more than 10 mm. Associated injuries of posterolateral corner (PLC), posteromedial corner or ACL should be confirmed by appropriate tests. Test for meniscus should be performed to rule out meniscal tears. Medial joint line tenderness may indicate developing arthrosis in medial compartment. Patellofemoral crepitus and facet tenderness indicate involvement of the patellofemoral joint.

Radiological Evaluation

Plain X-ray of the knee comprising A-P, lateral and Merchant's view is done to evaluate the knee. Narrowing of the medial compartment, avulsion fracture of PCL, involvement of the patellofemoral compartment, posterior sag, tibial slope and medial Segond fracture can be easily recognized. Medial Segond fracture indicates medial meniscus tear. The lower limb alignment is assessed by hip to ankle scanogram while standing. Varus malalignment are quite frequent with chronic PCL injuries.

Stress radiographs (Telos, Marburg, Germany) are the most essential part of radiographic evaluation. It is a simple method of objective evaluation of sagittal translation of the tibia over femur. It helps in differentiating partial from complete tears of PCL and the amount of sagittal translation posteriorly. It also objectively informs about

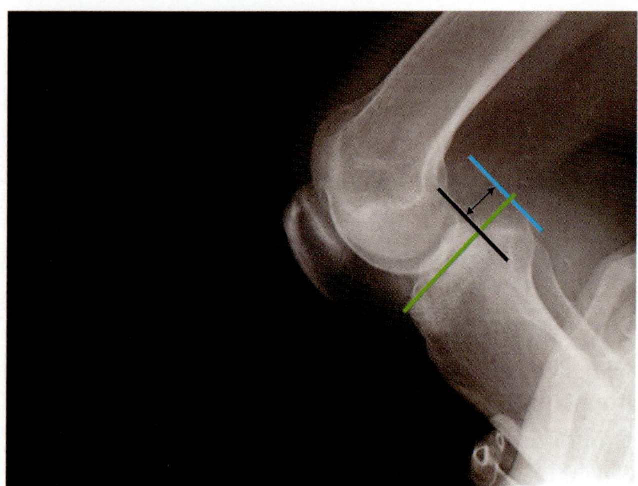

Figure 41.2 Plain radiograph of the left knee showing manual posterior drawer stress X-ray to assess insufficiency of the posterior cruciate ligament. The green line represents the tibial plateau. Black line represents the back of femoral condyle and blue line represents the end of tibial plateau. The arrow between blue and black represents the measure of posterior translation

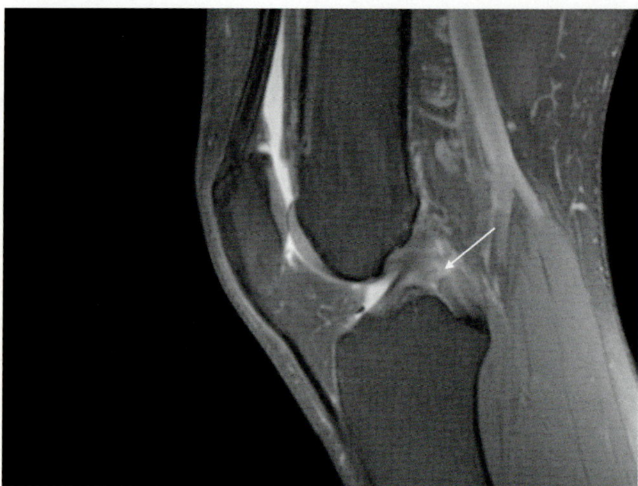

Figure 41.3 Proton density fat saturated sagittal T2 MR image reveals complete posterior cruciate ligament tear (white arrow)

the functional status of the PCL that appears healed on MRI but may remain functionally defunct. However, the availability of such instruments is a rarity in most centers of developing nations. In such scenario, a simple forced posterior drawer in 90° can help in approximate grading of posterior drawer (**Figure 41.2**).

Further evaluation is performed by MRI. MRI has accuracy of 96–100% in predicting PCL tears.[31] MRI is more sensitive (100%) in an acute tear setting rather than chronic.[29] MRI determines the location of the PCL injury, meniscal and cartilage pathologies and associated collateral ligament status. Grade 1 and 2 tears of the PCL on MRI may look normal. In such situation, clinical examination and stress radiographs are helpful to differentiate between functional or nonfunctional PCL (**Figure 41.3**).

Bone scan may be performed in chronic PCL tear to diagnose early medial compartment arthritis which may not be detected by X-ray or MRI.

Natural History of PCL Tear

Natural history of ligament tear comprises of 'what its absence does to the joint and what happens to itself.' In the absence of functional PCL, the biomechanics of knee joint is altered leading to arthritic changes in the medial compartment and the patellofemoral joint. The rate of articular cartilage involvement varies from 12% to 52% and rates of meniscal tear vary from 16% to 28%.[32-34] Radial tears in the middle and posterior part and longitudinal tear in the anterior horn of the lateral meniscus have been reported.[34] As far as the functional outcome is concerned, conservatively managed PCL tear may have a benign outcome in short term but gradually the joint function deteriorates. Parolie et al. concluded that 80% (20 out of 25) athletes report satisfactory outcome after a mean of 6.2 years.[35] Torg et al. followed 43 patients out of which 14 patients had isolated PCL tear and others had combined instability.[36] At a mean of 6.3 years (1–37 years), 5 (36%) patients with isolated PCL tear reported excellent outcome, 7 (50%) reported good outcome, whereas patients with combined instability fared poorly. One-hundred thirty-three patients of grade 1 and 2 isolated PCL tear followed by Shelbourne et al. for a mean period of 5.4 years with 68 were followed up on long-term.[19] There was no change between initial and final laxity. Radiographic changes in the knee and the subjective outcome of the patient had no correlation with grade of laxity. Regardless of laxity, 50% of the patients could return to same sport at same or higher level and 30% of them could return to the same sport at lower level. There are many reports about spontaneous healing of PCL after tear. The PCL has better chance of healing as compared with the ACL due to robust blood supply. After studying 18 patients over 1 year with stress radiographs and MRI, Mariani et al. reported that partial PCL tears heal well and complete PCL tears greater than 12 mm or PCL tear associated with other ligament injuries are less likely to heal.[37] Jung et al. too demonstrated that out of 46 cases of complete PCL tear, more than 72% heal (on MRI) after 2 months.[38] Tears associated with combined instability are less likely to heal. Shelbourne et al. followed 40 patients with isolated PCL tear and combined injuries for 3.2 ± 1.3 years and classified them into high (22), mid (14) and low grade (4) PCL injuries.[39] All low- and mid-grade injuries healed whereas 19 out of 22 high grade too healed. Even patients with combined instability showed signs of PCL healing. So, this concludes that isolated partial or complete tears of PCL stand a chance of healing and should be managed conservatively. The question arises at the end that whether PCL reconstruction would prevent arthritis of the knee or not? The answer remains elusive as no study has proven the theory that PCL reconstruction would prevent knee arthritis.[40]

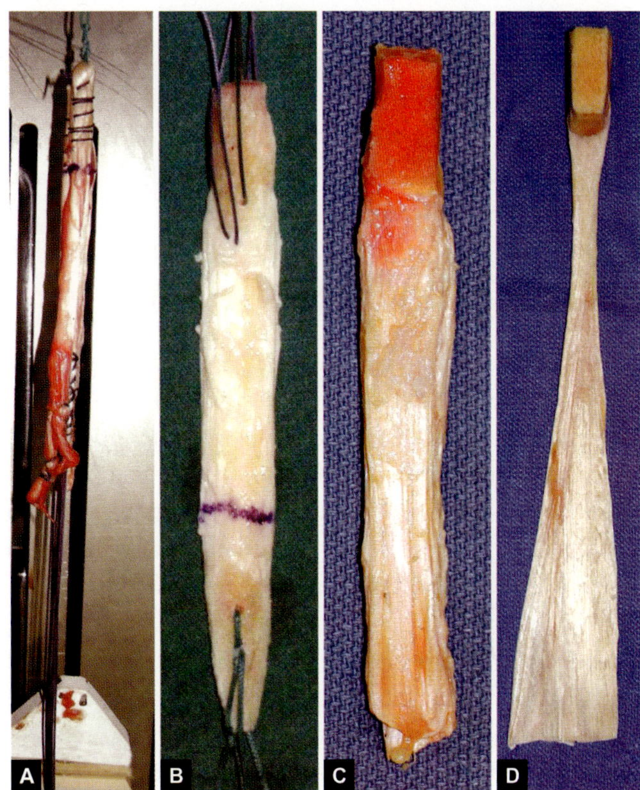

Figures 41.4A to D Image showing various graft options: (A) Quadrupled hamstring graft; (B) Bone-PT-bone graft; (C) Quadriceps tendon-bone graft; (D) Tendoachilles-bone graft

Nonoperative Treatment

Indications

1. Grade 1 and 2 isolated tears of PCL with secondary restrains (PLC and posteromedial corner) normal.
2. Undisplaced avulsion fracture of PCL. The decision is supported by appropriate clinical and radiological evaluation.

Principles of Conservative Management of PCL Tear

Phase 1: 0–6 Weeks

1. Rest, ice, compression and elevation for a few days and nonweight bearing gait training.
2. Knee immobilization in extension preferably in posterior tibial support PCL brace (**Figures 41.4A to D**) or cylindrical cast 3-4 weeks. It is important to eliminate posterior sag of the proximal tibia with the use of appropriate padding in the brace/cast. In the modified PCL brace, the femoral side straps of brace are tied firmly to push femur posteriorly whereas the tibial side straps are tied loosely to prevent further push to tibia posteriorly.
3. Quadriceps strengthening is the mainstay of rehabilitation which counteracts force of gravity and hamstrings which displace the tibia posteriorly.
4. Active straight leg-raising in knee brace, hamstring and gastrocnemius stretching.

Phase 2: 6–12 Weeks

Patient is permitted to mobilize the knee through the full range. Quads are continued to be strengthened further as they are PCL synergists. Proprioception training can be started. PCL braces can be given for 3-4 months especially while walking.

Phase 3: 13–18 Weeks

Initiation of running and sports specific training is started. Return to sports is by 4–5 months after clinical and radiological assessment of healing of the ligament and complete return of strength of the knee.

Role of PCL Braces in Rehabilitation

Varieties of commercial braces (PCL-Jack brace, Ossur CTi brace, DonJoy PCL brace) are available in the market. The purpose of a PCL brace is to prevent tibia from subluxating posteriorly under the influence of gravity and simultaneously push the femur down. This action can help healing of PCL in optimal length without getting elongated and prevents PCL graft from abrasive forces acting at killer turn of tibia.

An ideal PCL brace would be the one that can continue exerting such static effect during the complete range of knee movement and also let the length tension relation of PCL be maintained during the movement of the knee. Recently, Jansson et al. concluded that the currently available braces do not provide adequate support to PCL 'in motion' as they exert same forces throughout the range of movement whereas in the normal PCL, the tension varies throughout the flexion.[41] However, a static PCL brace which can support tibia from subluxation posteriorly, especially during healing phase, could be useful in early days of immobilization.

OPERATIVE TREATMENT

Indications

1. Grade 3 symptomatic PCL tear.
2. Combined instabilities.
3. Posterior drawer more than 10–12 mm on Telos stress radiography.
4. Displaced PCL bony avulsion (PCL appears buckled on MRI with displaced fragment).

Factors for PCL Reconstruction

1. Timing.
2. PCL remnant preservation or excision.
3. Graft selection.
4. Single or double bundle.
5. Tibial tunnel or inlay technique.
6. Fixation.

Timing

Acute Grade 3 PCL Tear

PCL reconstruction is usually done as an elective procedure after 3–6 weeks of initial injury. In the waiting period, other extra-articular instability, if significant, is dealt with. Also, the posterior capsule tends to heal which is not only important for posterior stability but also for all arthroscopic PCL reconstruction to prevent fluid extravasation. Delaying PCL reconstruction for long can lead to capsular scarring and persistent posterior subluxation especially in multiligament injuries. In such a situation even if PCL is reconstructed, the outcome is usually poor in the wake of persistent subluxation.

Chronic PCL Tear

If the knee is clinically unstable, stress X-rays reveal grade 3 posterior drawer or bone scan shows early arthritic changes in medial compartment, it would be prudent to go ahead with the PCL reconstruction. Further delay can lead to arthritic changes in the knee. If PCL reconstruction is performed in arthritic knee, the knee would be stable after reconstruction, but it may remain painful and the outcome would be poor.

PCL Remnant Preservation or Excision

The PCL has better healing potential as compared with the ACL due to robust blood supply. Also, the presence of mechanoreceptors in the residual remnant aids in better proprioception from the knee.[42] Hence, some authors believe that preserving the elongated PCL remnant aids in mechanical support to the knee, protects new graft from killer turn at tibia and it heals together with newly reconstructed PCL giving better support to the knee.[43] Kim et al. did a retrospective study on PCL/PLC reconstruction with and without remnant preservation and opined that though the two groups did equally same on objective scale but subjective scores of remnant preservation were better.[44] However, strong objective evidence in favor of stump preservation is still lacking. When single bundle PCL is reconstructed while preserving the PCL remnant, the graft should be brought underneath the remnant otherwise the reconstructed part will be twisted. However, a recent cadaveric biomechanical study performed by Jung et al. suggested that a curved path over the remnant PCL will give more intra-articular length to reconstructed PCL and better isometry than under the PCL remnant.[45] So, based on their observation, they recommend passage of graft over the remnant. In conclusion, if one chooses to preserve the stump, it is preferable to pass the graft posterior and superior to the stump to preserve isometry of graft.

Graft Selection

The intra-articular length for PCL graft required is 4 cm and average length of the PCL graft should be 8–12 cm depending upon the technique used. The diameter of the graft selected should be a minimum of 9 mm as it has to counteract gravitational, abrasive (at killer angle), and elongation forces. Though the graft choice (auto/allograft) varies between quadruple hamstrings; bone-patellar tendon-bone; bone-quadriceps, tendoachilles-bone; tibialis anterior and posterior, there is no ideal graft for PCL as none of them can closely resemble its complex anatomy which can be replicated during reconstruction (**Figures 41.5A and B**). Availability of allograft is scarce especially in developing nations.

Quadruple Hamstring Graft (QHG) (Both Semitendinosus and Gracilis)

It can be used for single bundle (SB) or double bundle (DB) reconstruction. It heals by tissue to bone healing and is associated with less morbidity. Since, it is used as graft in tunnel technique; it is prone for failure at the killer turn. If diameter of QHG of index side of knee is less than 8 mm, the semitendinosus tendon of the other side must be harvested in order to increase the diameter of graft to prevent failure of graft during rehabilitation. This should be explained to the patient preoperatively and appropriate consent should be obtained preoperatively.

Bone-Patellar Tendon-Bone (B-PT-B)

It allows bone to bone healing and can be used both as inlay or tunnel technique. The morbidity and complications associated with this graft are well described.

Quadriceps Tendon-Bone Graft (Quad-B) and Tendoachilles

Bone also allows bone-to-bone healing at tibial end and soft tissue-bone at the femoral end. They have large

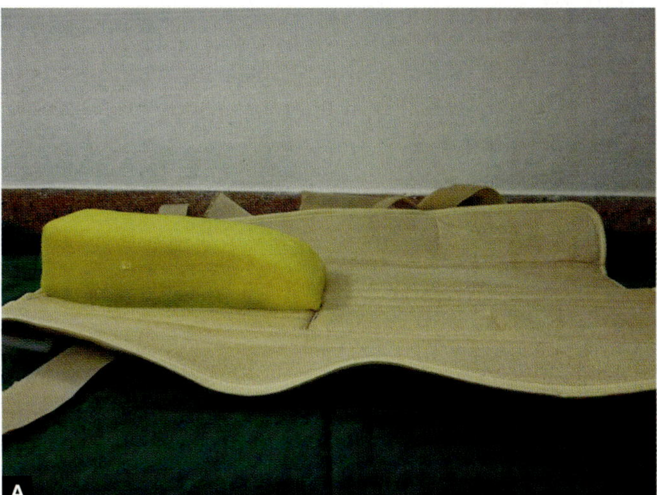

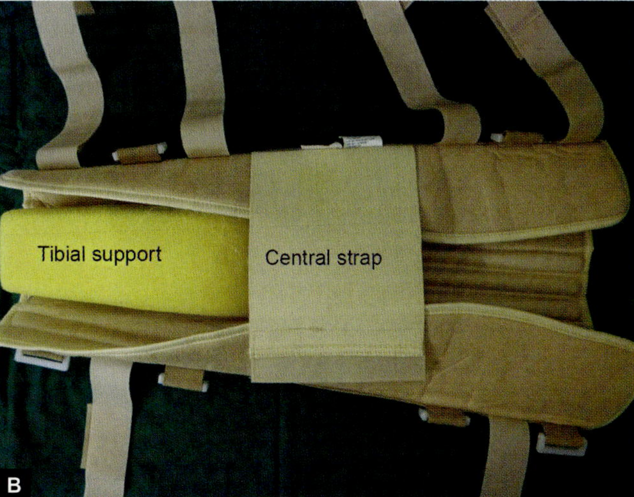

Figures 41.5A and B Image of a modified extension brace for posterior cruciate ligament (PCL) support. (A) Image shows a side view of a PCL support brace where 2-inch thick commercial sponge is glued over the distal aspect of brace where the tibia/leg rests. This acts as posterior support to the tibia preventing its subluxation. (B) Image shows the top view of brace. The central strap of brace is tied over the patella; the femoral straps are kept tight whereas tibial straps are kept loose

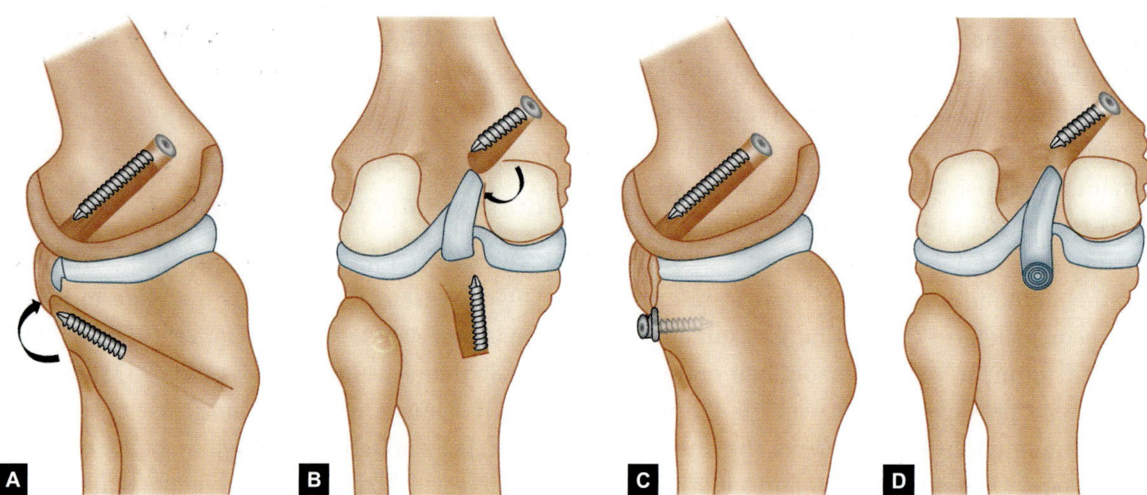

Figures 41.6A to D Diagrammatic representation of tunnel and inlay techniques. (A) Image shows lateral view of diagrammatic represents an acute 90° turn of graft behind the tibia to ascend upward toward femur (black arrow). (B) Image shows a posterior view of the posterior cruciate ligament (PCL) graft where it takes another 90° turn in the femoral tunnel (black arrow). (C) Image shows lateral view of the inlay technique showing the absence of acute turn of graft at the tibial end as graft is fixed in the PCL trough with a screw. (D) Image shows lateral view of the inlay technique

cross-sectional area and the soft tissue end can be split into two strands to be used as DB. Concern with B-PT-B and Quad-B is about anterior knee pain and weakening of synergist required in PCL deficient knee.

'Tibial Tunnel' or 'Inlay' Technique

The tunnel technique involves placement of graft through a transtibial tunnel. In the tunnel technique, the graft must make an acute 90° turn as it emerges out of the tibial tunnel at the back of the tibia to enter the knee joint. This acute 90° turn forms a killer turn as the graft is subjected to abrasive and elongation forces[46] (**Figures 41.6A and B**). Inlay technique involves open, anatomical placement of graft and fixation at tibia at PCL trough (**Figures 41.6C and D**). This technique avoids killer turn. Femoral placement remains essentially same in both techniques. Markolf et al. performed an *in vivo* experiment over 62 cadaveric knees in which 31 knees underwent PCL reconstruction by tibial inlay and other 31 by tibial tunnel technique using B-PT-B graft.[47] These knees were subjected to 2000 cyclical loading through 50–300 N force at an angle of 45°. All inlay grafts survived the test whereas 10 out of 31 of tunnel techniques failed the loading before 2000 cycles. The grafts fixed by inlay technique showed significantly less thinning (12.5% versus 40.6%) at acute angles and lengthening (5.9 mm versus 9.8 mm) as compared with the tunnel technique after cyclical loading. Bergfeld et al. also concluded in a cadaveric study on six paired knees that inlay technique results in better graft survival, lesser mechanical degradation and better placement of graft at the footprint as compared with the tunnel technique.[48]

Tunnel technique is all-arthroscopic, lesser morbidity and easy revision but higher chance of failure. Inlay technique involves open approach, more morbidity and difficult to revise with an implant at back of the knee. However, due to ease of graft preparation, lesser morbidity and surgeon's comfort, the tunnel technique seems to be more popular. The outcome of tunnel technique can be improved with thicker graft, appropriate tunnel placement, back-up/hybrid fixation and slower rehabilitation.

Single Bundle (SB) or Double Bundle (DB)

Single Tunnel AL Bundle (Technically Single Bundle)

This remains the most popular PCL reconstruction technique. Currently, the data comparing the two techniques is not enough to prove the superiority of one over other. SB scores over technical ease, less morbidity, cost effectiveness and easier revision.

Double-Bundle Technique

Wherein both ALB and PMB are reconstructed making two tunnels on the femoral footprint, seems to be more anatomical. But, it comes with a tag of technically demanding procedure, increased morbidity, difficult revision, and, of course, an increased cost of the procedure.

Various studies fail to prove the difference between the two. In a study on 42 patients of PCL reconstruction (tibial tunnel technique; 23 SB, 19DB) with a minimum follow-up of 2 years, Kim et al. concluded that there was no statistical difference between the two techniques when posterior and rotatory laxity, Lysholm, and IKDC scores were compared.[49] Kohen et al. did a systematic review on comparing two techniques of SB and DB PCL reconstruction and concluded that superiority of one procedure over other remains uncertain. The comparison between two remains complicated due to usage of different grafts, inlay or tunnel techniques and tensioning patterns.[13]

Fixation Option

The purpose of graft fixation is to provide mechanical support to the graft in the bone tunnel, while it heals with the bone during early postoperative phase. To achieve a strong fixation with optimal pull out strength and stiff construct, the knowledge of *in vivo* and *in vitro* forces over the PCL is necessary. Morrison et al. revealed that peak force in PCL varies in different position of the knee; 330 N in walking, 950 N during knee extension and 2500 during full squat and leg press.[50,51] So, fixation option for the PCL graft should be able to counteract such pullout forces and should be strong enough to let the graft heal in tunnel while the patient undergoes rehabilitation. Various options are described in the literature e.g., interference screw (metal/bioabsorbable), endobutton, staple, suture post and screw washer for PCL graft fixation. In various cadaveric studies, the pull out strength of these fixation options varies from 200–900 N in isolation. Hoher et al. concluded that alone metal interference screw on femoral side for 'hamstring graft' seems to have least pullout strength (242 ± 91 N) as compared with bioabsorbable screw (480 ± 133 N) and endobutton (520 ± 50 N). However, the pull out strength on tibia side between metal and bioabsorbable screw is nearly same for the hamstring graft (419 N versus 507 N). Screw and washer provide maximum pull out strength of 821 ± 219 N.[52] In conclusion, the pullout strength and stiffness of the construct can be increased by using backup fixation like staple, screw, and washer at the end of the graft especially on tibia side where the bone is softer due to its cancellous nature. If femoral side fixation is doubtful or bone seems to be soft, the back-up fixation on the femoral side too should be added up. The detailed biomechanical analysis of all the implants used in PCL graft fixation is out of scope this chapter.

Femoral End Graft Fixation

- *Anatomic fixation:* Inside-out/outside-in femoral tunnel: interference screw (metal/bioabsorbable).
- *Extra-anatomic fixation:* Endobutton, button on the cortex.
- *Over the cortex:* Staple, screw with washer.

Tibial End Graft Fixation

a. *Bone tunnel technique:*
   Anatomic—interference screw.
   Extra-anatomic—screw post, staple over graft tissue.
b. *Inlay technique*—lag screw with washer over the bone plug, staple.

SINGLE-BUNDLE TIBIAL TUNNEL TECHNIQUE PCL RECONSTRUCTION USING QUADRUPLED HAMSTRING GRAFT

Patient Position

After appropriate anesthesia, spinal or GA, pneumatic tourniquet is applied. Prophylactic antibiotic (1.5 gm intravenous cefuroxime) should be administered 30 minutes prior to inflation of tourniquet. Examination under anesthesia is performed to confirm the grade of posterior drawer and other associated injuries, if any. The medial and lateral tibiofemoral step-off of the injured and normal knee is palpated. This information is used during tensioning of the PCL reconstruction to confirm restoration of the injured knee to the 'neutral' position. It is particularly important to examine the medial and posterolateral ligamentous structures. Failure to treat associated ligamentous injuries is one of the most common causes of a failed PCL reconstruction as it increases stress on the reconstructed PCL by 30%.[27] A side-post on the side of thigh should be applied to support the thigh in flexed position while performing arthroscopy. Routine sterile preparation of the index limb should be done as per standard protocol. If autograft QHG harvest is planned from index knee, it may be prudent to keep the other limb also prepared as occasionally the graft diameter may be quite less (less than 8 mm) which is inappropriate for PCL reconstruction. We believe that PCL graft diameter should be at least 8 mm or preferably 9 mm in order to overcome the stress over the graft at the killer turn.

Standard Arthroscopy and Probing

After inflation of tourniquet, diagnostic arthroscopy is performed through a high AL portal that is close to patellar tendon (PT) and at the level of inferior pole of patella. Placing this portal at the height of the inferior pole of the patella places the arthroscope above the fat pad and allows a better view of the posteromedial (PM) aspect of the knee joint. Too far lateral and low AL portal will deflect the scope toward MFC making access toward PM recess difficult. The anteromedial (AM) portal is established under direct vision using an 18 gauge spinal needle to determine the optimal position. In general, this portal is as close as possible to the medial border of the PT and at the height of the inferior pole of the patella. It is important not to make this portal too low as this may cause difficulty when attempting to insert instrumentation through the AM portal into the PM compartment of the knee. After establishing the AL and AM portals, a standard arthroscopic examination of the knee joint is performed, and any meniscal and or chondral injuries are appropriately addressed. It is important not to mistake pseudolaxity of the ACL for a torn ACL. In chronic PCL tear, the PCL is replaced by fibrotic lax remnant tissue covered by synovium (unlike in chronic ACL tear where notch and lateral wall is empty) that remains lax after posterior drawer. In chronic PCL tear, 'lax ACL sign' is apparent (**Figure 41.7**). Because the tibia is subluxated posteriorly, the ACL remains lax and could be wrongly interpreted as chronic ACL tear. Taking down such an ACL could prove disastrous.

The PCL reconstruction is facilitated by the use of a PM portal. A PM portal is necessary to resect tissue at the PCL tibial attachment site. Viewing through a PM portal also provides the best view of the PCL tibial attachment site and eliminates the need to use a 70° arthroscope. The posteromedial portal is established during preparation of the PCL tibial attachment site and will be described later in the chapter.

Graft Harvest and Preparation

An inch long incision is made, 1 cm medial to tibial tuberosity. Pes anserinus fascia is incised and semitendinosus and gracilis tendon is harvested in standard fashion. The tendon is prepared in usual way and quadrupled. Minimum length of graft required for the tibial tunnel technique is 10 cm. Four centimeter is required for intra-articular portion of graft and 2.5 cm each for tibial and femoral tunnels. That makes it 9 cm. When tibia is pulled anteriorly while fixing the tibial side of graft, additional 1 cm is pulled inward making the length required to be 9 + 1 cm, i.e. 10 cm. Opposite side semitendinosus tendon should be harvested in order to increase the diameter of graft to a minimum of 8 mm if ipsilateral tendons fail to make it up to the minimum requirement.

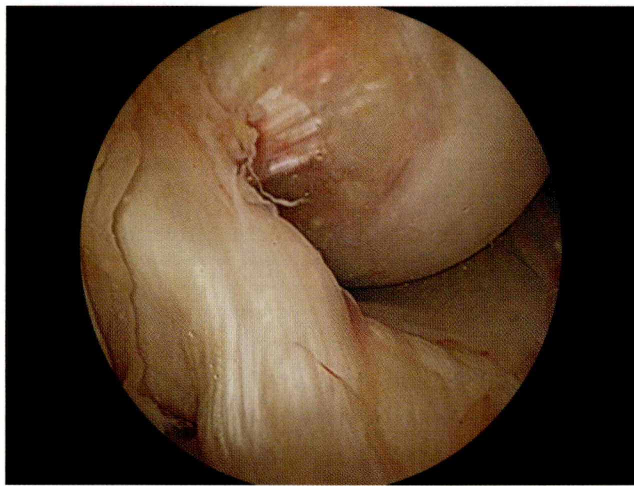

Figure 41.7 Arthroscopic view of the right knee with posterior cruciate ligament tear shows intact but lax anterior cruciate ligament

Fat Pad and Notch Debridement

The intercondylar area should be debrided of inferior plica and any synovitis. Retropatellar fad pad should be judiciously shaved off for easy visualization. The space between the PCL undersurface and MFC lateral wall should be cleared of synovium and loose fibers of PCL for easy access and visualization of PM recess.

Establish Posteromedial Portal

Once the scope is pushed into the PM recess, the posteromedial (PM) portal is established. 'PM portal is kept high and away from MFC.' The PM portal is created under direct vision. With the arthroscope in the AL portal, the arthroscope is first advanced past the medial border of the ACL and then between the medial border of the PCL and the MFC into the posteromedial compartment of the knee. This maneuver is often facilitated by hanging the leg over the side of the operating room table and applying a varus force to the foot. This will open up the space between the medial border of PCL and the MFC allowing the arthroscope to pass into the posteromedial compartment of the knee. With the arthroscope in the posteromedial compartment, the room lights can be turned down and the skin illuminated by the light from the arthroscope. This step will assist with locating the correct position for the skin puncture. It is important that the location of this portal not be too low. If the portal is placed too low, difficulty will be encountered reaching the distal part of the PCL tibial attachment site when the portal is used to introduce instrumentation into the back of the knee to prepare the PCL tibial attachment site. An 18 gauge spinal needle is used to locate the proper location for the portal. A #11 knife blade on a long handle is passed along the path of the spinal needle and is used to make a small incision in the posterior capsule. Care must be taken to avoid breaking or losing the knife blade in the knee joint or the posteromedial soft tissues. Failure to incise the posterior capsule will make it extremely difficult to pass a plastic cannula into the posteromedial compartment. Insertion of a 5.5/7 mm plastic cannula into the posteromedial compartment is facilitating by first inserting a switching stick into the knee joint and then screwing the cannula into place over the switching stick. Cannula insertion will prevent fluid leakage and repeated struggle to insert instrument or scope through the PM portal. Adequate distension of posterior compartment is the key of all arthroscopic technique of PCL reconstruction. Shift the scope into PM portal and visualize the PCL origin and also assess the extent of synovium, scar tissue and fat pad at the back of PCL remnant.

Preparation of PCL Tibial Attachment Site

While viewing the PM compartment with a 30° or 70° arthroscope in the AL portal, insert the 4.5 mm motorized shaver through the PM portal. Judicious debridement of scar tissue, synovium and fat pad should be done so that PCL tibial footprint should be adequately visualized. If the residual PCL stump has to be preserved, the footprint should not be disturbed. Otherwise, the whole mass of the defunct PCL should be taken down with help of PCL elevator (Smith and Nephew Endoscopy, Andover, MA), shaver, punches and occasionally radio frequency (RF) device. A PCL elevator is introduced through the anteromedial portal into the posteromedial compartment of the knee. The PCL elevator is carefully used to bluntly dissect the posterior capsule from the posterior aspect of the PCL and the back of the tibia. Blunt dissection with the PCL elevator is extended inferiorly along the back of the tibia until the tip of the elevator encounters a bony ridge, which represents the most inferior part of the PCL tibial attachment site. This point is usually reached when the PCL elevator is inserted to the 25 mm mark. This step frees the posterior capsule and allows the posterior capsule to displace with capsular distension from the back of the tibia and the PCL tibial attachment site, thus increasing the distance between the PCL and the posterior neurovascular structures. Under direct vision, a 4.5 mm curved motorized shaver blade is inserted through the PM portal cannula and the PCL remnant resected. It is important to resect the tissue until the shaver blade can be felt to be hitting the posterior cortex of the tibia. An RF probe can be used to further clear soft tissue at the PCL tibial attachment site. The area behind and around the PCL origin at the tibia should be debrided enough so that the tip of the PCL guide, guidewire and tibial drill coming off the tibial tunnel should be easily visualized. Nonvisualization of guidewire or tibial drill can endanger the safety of the neurovascular bundle in the popliteal fossa.

Tip—The face of shaver blade should be kept away from the posterior capsule. If the posterior capsule is opened, the fluid would leak into the posterior compartment of the leg and can cause compartment syndrome. Also, it can endanger the neurovascular bundle in the popliteal fossa.

Drilling of Tibial Tunnel

Whether to drill a femoral tunnel first or tibial is usually the surgeon's preference. We drill the tibial tunnel first and block the mouth of the tunnel with a plastic conical cap to prevent fluid loss. A 3 cm vertical skin incision is placed just medial to the tibial tuberosity. The PCL tibia aimer (Smith and Nephew Endoscopy, Andover, MA) is set at a 50°–55° angle and inserted through the AM portal onto the posterior cortex of the tibia. The aimer tip is positioned midway between the medial and lateral mammillary prominences that places the aimer in the middle of the PCL tibial attachment site in the medial-lateral direction. The 30° arthroscope and sheath are then inserted into the PM portal cannula. This approach gives an excellent view of the PCL tibial attachment site and eliminates the need to use a 70° arthroscope. While viewing through the PM portal, the tip of the PCL tibial aimer is advanced down the back of the tibia about 20 mm below the tibial articular surface to the posterior capsule attachment site (**Figure 41.8A**). Placing the tip of the tibial aimer in this location will result in the tip of the tibial guide pin lying 5 mm superior to site of the capsular attachment on the back on the tibia. The aimer bullet is inserted into the aimer handle and the aimer bullet advances through the anteromedial incision onto the anteromedial surface of the tibia. The PCL safety stop (Smith and Nephew Endoscopy, Andover, MA) is attached to the drill guide and a 2.4 mm PCL safety guide pin (Smith and Nephew Endoscopy, Andover, MA) drilled into the tibia until the laser mark on the guide pin contacts the PCL safety stop. These steps prevent the tibial guide pin from advancing beyond the tip of the PCL aimer. The PCL tibia aimer is backed away from the posterior cortex of the tibia and the tip of the guide pin tapped through the posterior tibial cortex with a small mallet (**Figure 41.8B**). The tibial guide pin position is confirmed with a lateral c-arm image (**Figure 41.8C**). It is important that the tibial guide pin not be positioned too proximal as this may result in insufficient bone proximal to the PCL tibia tunnel to prevent the PCL graft from migrating superiorly into the back of the knee joint when the PCL is loaded. All this time, a constant watch should be kept over the guide pin and should be protected with stylus over drill guide or a spoon from the PM portal. The PCL aimer should be removed and the PCL elevator is inserted through the anteromedial portal and the tip of the guide pin capped in the central recess of the elevator. The PCL tibial tunnel is drilled using a cannulated drill bit according to the size of graft. In order to ease the passage of the graft through the tibial tunnel,

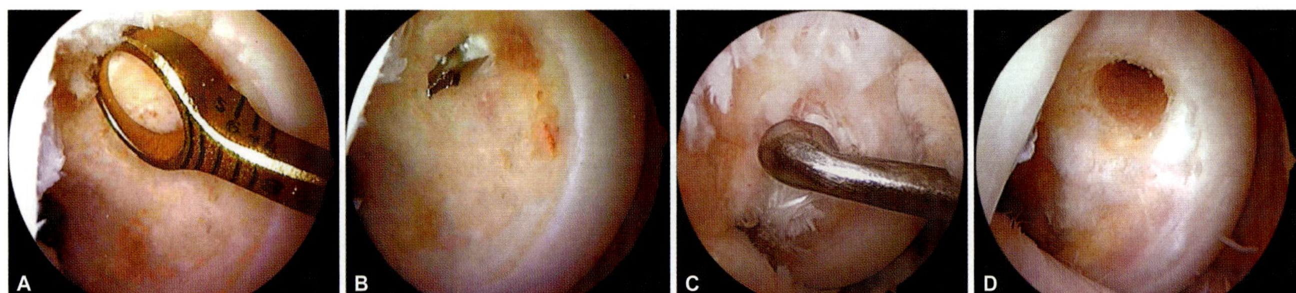

Figures 41.8A to D Arthroscopic image of right knee for preparing tibial tunnel; (A) Tibial jig in place 20 mm below the tibial plateau at the posterior cruciate ligament footprint; (B) Guidewire in place protected by tip of tibial jig; (C) Intraoperative X-ray lateral view of right knee shows correct placement of guidewire for the tibial tunnel; (D) Rasp at the mouth of the tibial tunnel exit at the back of tibia smoothening the tunnel to prevent abrasive damage to graft at killer angle

it is recommended that the PCL tibial tunnel be drilled 1 mm greater than the measured diameter of the PCL graft. The PCL tibial tunnel is reamed under power until the resistance of posterior tibial cortex is felt. The remainder of the posterior cortex is drilled by hand. The superior edge of the tibial tunnel is chamfered with a rasp to prevent abrasive damage to the graft (**Figure 41.8D**).

Once the tibial tunnel is drilled, tibial passing suture (No. 5 Ethibond, Ethicon, Johnson and Johnson, USA) should be placed with the help of an arthroscopic grasper at the posterior mouth. This loop end is further grasped by a long curved hemostat and pulled out from the AM portal. Suture passage at this point is much easier than later when fluid extravasation and posterior fossa swelling can make it difficult to visualize and triangulate. After the tibial tunnel is drilled, the tunnel mouth entry adjacent to tibial tuberosity should be plugged with commercially available conical plastic plugs to prevent saline leakage.

Drilling of Single Femoral Tunnel

Single bundle PLC reconstruction means reconstruction of the AL bundle of the PCL. The point selected over the MFC is high and shallow and about 8–10 mm behind the shallow cartilage margin. This marks the footprint of AL bundle (**Figure 41.9A**).

The femoral tunnel can be drilled inside-out or outside-in. The inside-out technique involves making of another accessory low AL portal that is used to mark and drill the femoral tunnel. After keeping the knee in 100°–110° flexion, the guide pin is placed at an appropriately marked point. Tunnel is drilled free hand, through and through so that the outer cortex can be kept intact depending upon which fixation method is planned. First, the tunnel can be drilled with 4.5 mm cannulated drill bit over the guide pin. Then over drilling is done with appropriate size femoral reamer. The advantage of inside-out is a precise placement of femoral tunnel and smaller incision on outer aspect of MFC. The disadvantage is the placement of a short tunnel and difficult visualization in the hyperflexed position.

The outside-in technique involves the usage of a femoral guide. The femoral guide is placed through the AM portal at the desired point. The angle of drill guide is kept between 55° to 60°. The incision is made over the skin of MFC along the axis of the knee and subcutaneous tissue dissected. Guide pin is drilled over guide sleeve. The exit of pin is observed with the scope in the AL portal. After the pin is placed in the desired position, the drill guide is removed (**Figure 41.9B**). The guide pin is over drilled with appropriate size femoral reamer, through and through. During this step, the tip of the guide pin is protected with a curette placed through the AM portal to prevent accidental over migration into the joint causing damage to the lateral femoral cartilage or over the scope lens (**Figure 41.9C**). Once the femoral tunnel is drilled, the lower part of the femoral tunnel inlet is rasped in order to blunt sharp edges. This prevents the graft from abrasive damage while insertion and further during rehabilitation. The average length of femoral tunnel is 35–40 mm. The final position of the single femoral tunnel in flexed position is described as shallow and high (**Figure 41.9D**).

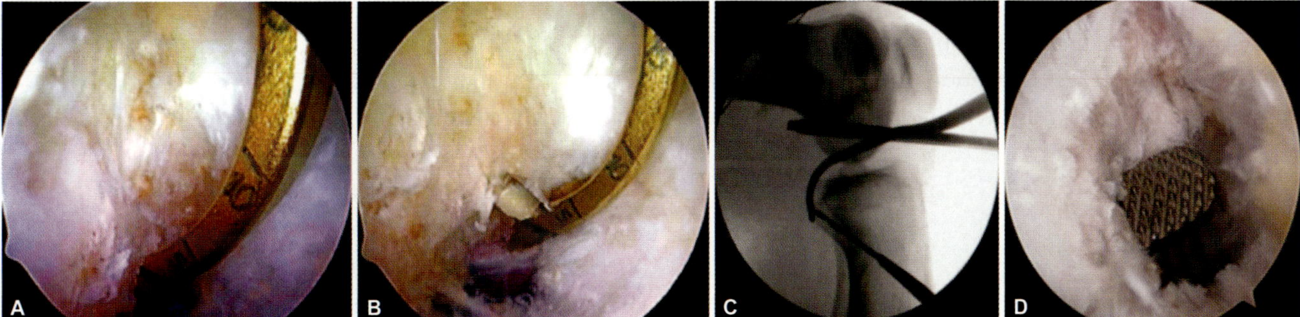

Figures 41.9A to D Arthroscopic image of right knee for making of femoral tunnel; (A) Femoral jig in place; (B) Guidewire in place with outside-in drilling; (C) Protecting the guidewire tip with curette through the AM portal; (D) Femoral tunnel for the anterolateral bundle single bundle posterior cruciate ligament reconstruction; note shallow and high positions of the femoral tunnel

Femoral Passing Suture

Now the tibial passing suture loop is pulled into the femoral tunnel using the grasper.

Passage of Graft in Tibial Tunnel

The prepared graft is loaded over the passing/leading suture that is placed in the tibial and femoral tunnel. The suture is pulled gradually and slowly. The scope is placed now in the PM portal. The leading suture is grasped with arthroscopic grasper that is placed through the AM portal and suture is pulled in increments. The other end of suture remains in the femoral tunnel and the assistant keeps pulling the increments gained each time. This maneuver places least stress on leading suture and prevents graft abrasion at the back of tibial tunnel while pulling the graft. Once graft negotiates the killer turn of tibia, pulling into the femoral tunnel is easy. Once the 2.5 cm mark on the graft crosses the femoral inlet, graft should not be pulled further.

Fixation of Graft in the Femoral Tunnel

The guidewire is placed in the tunnel anterior (shallow) to the graft. Appropriate size bioabsorbable/titanium interference screw is selected (usually one size smaller than tunnel size) and inserted over the guidewire. Graft is pulled from the tibial end to check the adequacy of fixation. In case the fixation strength is doubtful, supplementary fixation can be performed. Sutures at the femoral end of the graft can be tied over a button/suture disk or screw and post. The graft can also be fixed on the femoral tunnel using endobutton (Smith & Nephew, Andover, USA) or tightrope (Arthrex, USA). Fixation options are according to the surgeon's preference. There is no method that is superior over other.

Tibial Fixation

The tibial end of graft suture can be marked as single knotted (semitendinosus) and double knotted (gracilis). Keeping all the sutures in tension (single and doubly knotted), the knee is taken into 10–15 motion cycle to take away the slack in the graft. Cycling of the knee should be performed if femoral fixation is performed using suspensory fixation (endobutton/tightrope) that helps in settling the button over the cortex. Holding the graft in tension and keeping the knee in anterior drawer, the graft is fixed in the tibial tunnel at 70° flexion with the help of interference screw. This screw should be advanced up to the mouth of the tibial tunnel posteriorly. Supplementary fixation in form of button/staple/screw-washer post should be used to improve the pullout strength and prevent graft slippage. The tension in the graft is confirmed by probing. If PCL is adequately tensioned and posterior translation is restored to normal, the ACL tension is restored which initially appeared lax (**Figure 41.10**).

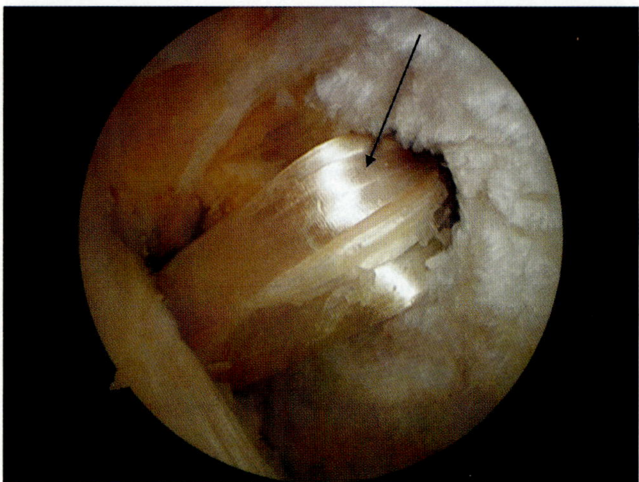

Figure 41.10 Arthroscopic image of right knee with the posterior cruciate ligament graft in place

Joint Irrigation and Wound Closure

Thorough irrigation of the joint is performed in order to remove the soft tissue and bony debris. The wound is closed in layers. Placing an intra-articular drain for 24 hours is debatable as no study has proven its efficacy. It remains the surgeon's or institutional preference. We believe that it should be used in combined ACL–PCL reconstruction where there are four tunnels opening into the joint and are potential for major hemarthrosis. Three layers of compression bandage should be applied which ensures minimal postoperative joint effusion.

Postoperative Care

The limb is placed in posterior tibial support splint after the surgery. Three-layer compression bandage is continued for 4 days. Drain is removed by 24–48 hours. IV antibiotic is continued till 24 hours. Appropriate analgesics should be continued for a week. Postoperative radiograph should be done to confirm the accurate placement of fixation device.

Rehabilitation

The PCL rehabilitation is way different than the ACL as the forces acting on the graft are completely different. There is active gravitational force and weight of the leg acting over the graft that can stretch and abrade the graft especially in the tunnel technique. So, the rehabilitation program is quite conservative till 12–16 weeks where the graft is allowed to heal in the tunnels and protected from stretching and abrasive forces. An aggressive rehabilitation can be lead to graft failure. Principles of PCL rehabilitation involve slow mobilization, activation and strengthening of quadriceps, avoiding activation of hamstring in early phase of rehabilitation and protection of graft from gravitational force. We follow slow rehabilitation protocol that is illustrated in **Table 41.1** and the outcome in last few years has been encouraging with conservative protocol. Fanelli too recommended a slow rehabilitation protocol for PCL.[53]

DOUBLE-BUNDLE PCL RECONSTRUCTION USING QUADRICEPS TENDON-BONE GRAFT

Introduction

Double-bundle PCL (DB PCL) reconstruction has been proposed as a possible surgical technique to improve the inconsistent results in restoring posterior stability historically reported for single-bundle PCL reconstructions that reconstruct only the ALB fibers. Although current clinical studies have not conclusively demonstrated a significant difference in restoring posterior stability between single- and DB PCL reconstructions, there are several theoretical advantages to performing a DB PCL reconstruction.[13] Similar to an ACL reconstruction, a DB PCL reconstruction will restore more of the native PCL femoral attachment site. The femoral attachment site of the PCL is very large making it difficult to restore with a single strand PCL graft.[54-56]

TABLE 41.1 Postoperative rehabilitation protocol

Weeks	*Movements*	*Weight bearing, brace*	*Strengthen*	*Avoid*
0–3	Knee brace in extension No movements allowed	Non weight bearing gait with axillary crutch, brace kept locked	Static isometric quadriceps, straight leg raising with brace	Knee flexion and weight bearing
4–6	Gradual passive knee flexion and active knee extension in lateral position	Partial weight bearing with axillary crutch and with brace kept locked in extension	Static isometric quadriceps, straight leg raising with brace	Sitting knee flexion or active knee flexion that activates hamstring
7–12	Aim to achieve full range of motion, mostly passive, in lateral position	Gradual full weight bearing. PCL brace if available	Quadriceps	Sitting knee flexion that activates hamstring
13–24	Full range of motion	PCL brace to continue	Quadriceps	Resisted hamstring
25–52	Progressive strength, agility, and proprioceptive training, return to sports when index knee is similar to normal knee in terms of strength, stability, range of motion, proprioception, and agility			

Abbreviation: PCL, posterior cruciate ligament.

Adding a second graft strand to the PCL replacement graft will restore a larger percentage of the native PCL attachment site by placing additional collagenous tissue within the PCL femoral attachment site.[56] The additional collagenous tissue will also increase the strength and cross-sectional area of the PCL graft. If the second PCL graft strand is placed in the appropriate location in the native PCL femoral attachment site, a load-sharing PCL graft construct can be created.[56,57] Having two graft strands share the tensile load will decrease the tensile force in each graft strand.[56,57] Decreasing the graft force in each PCL graft strand may decrease graft elongation and failure. Finally, biomechanical studies using human cadaveric knees have demonstrated that DB PCL reconstructions better restore posterior tibial translation and knee kinematics compared with single-bundle PCL reconstructions.[11,13] This is particularly true in combined PCL and PLC injuries.[13]

Indications for Double-Bundle (DB) PCL Reconstruction

- Young, active patients with isolated grade III PCL injury who desire, 'the best knee possible'
- Patients with grade III PCL with PLC injury.

Contraindications for DB PCL Reconstruction

1. *Knee dislocation:* Theoretical advantage of DB PCL reconstruction is offset by additional surgical time and complexity of procedure.
2. *Reconstruction for grade III PCL with combined MCL and posteromedial corner injury:* This requires drilling of tunnels in MFC for PCL femoral attachment, superficial MCL and posterior oblique ligament for reconstruction. This can increase risk of fracture of MFC. In this situation a single-bundle PCL reconstruction is performed.

Graft Selection

The optimal graft for DB PCL reconstruction should have a large cross-sectional area, be long enough to meet the longer length of the PCL, be able to be split into two graft strands, and should allow for secure fixation on both ends of the graft so that an early range of motion can be started in the immediate postoperative period. Of the autograft options available, the quadriceps tendon best meets these requirements.[56,58-60] The cross-sectional area of a 10 mm width, full-thickness quadriceps tendon graft is 1.8 times greater than a 10 mm width bone-PT-bone graft.[52,60] In most knees, a 10–12 mm width, full-thickness quadriceps tendon graft can be harvested with or without a patellar bone block. Harvesting a patellar bone block as part of the quadriceps tendon graft allows secure graft fixation to be achieved in the tibial tunnel with an absorbable interference screw and back-up suture screw/washer post fixation. The soft tissue end of the quadriceps tendon graft can be split into two graft strands that are passed into the two femoral tunnels. The donor site morbidity of the quadriceps tendon graft includes all of the issues seen with harvest of a bone-PT-bone graft. Similar to the bone-PT-bone grafts, donor site morbidity can be minimized by a meticulous surgical technique, harvesting a small 20–22 mm length patellar bone block and bone grafting of the patellar defect. A quadriceps tendon autograft is preferred in young patients with isolated grade III PCL injuries who require surgery and young patients with combined ACL/PCL and grade III PCL and MCL injuries.

In patients with combined grade III PCL and PLC injuries or knee dislocations, allograft tissue is preferred for the PCL, ACL and collateral ligaments. In these situations, allograft tissue has the advantages of eliminating donor site morbidity, unlimited size and length of the graft tissue and bone blocks, smaller incisions, less surgical dissection and decreased operative time. An Achilles tendon allograft with calcaneal bone block is the ideal allograft tissue for a DB PCL reconstruction. The calcaneal block allows for secure fixation of the PCL graft in the tibial tunnel with an absorbable interference screw and back-up suture screw/washer postfixation. The soft tissue end of the Achilles tendon allograft is long and wide and can be easily split into two strands. However, availability and high cost of allograft is an issue in most of the countries.

How to Harvest a Quadriceps Tendon Autograft?[61]

Graft Harvest

The quadriceps tendon graft should be harvested with the knee flexed to 90°. Flexing the knee to 90° creates tension in the extensor mechanism that facilitates graft harvesting. The graft is usually harvested with the tourniquet inflated. Prior to inflating the tourniquet, the suprapatellar pouch is injected with a mixture of 30 cc of local anesthesia and 30 cc of normal saline. The step inflates the suprapatellar pouch which helps identify the synovium during graft harvest. The quadriceps tendon is exposed through a vertical incision, centered slightly medial to the midline of the thigh (**Figure 41.11**). The incision starts at the superior pole of the patella and extends 5 cm in the superior direction. Sharp dissection is carried down through the skin and subcutaneous tissue until the investing fascia of the thigh and the prepatellar retinaculum are identified. The subcutaneous tissue is retracted with Army-Navy type retractors. The investing fascia of the thigh and prepatellar retinaculum is sharply incised exposing the quadriceps tendon and the superior pole of the patella. The prepatellar retinaculum is preserved for later closure. Incise and dissect the paratenon off the underlying quadriceps tendon. Using blunt and sharp dissection, identify the entire length of the quadriceps tendon up to the musculotendinous junction. Typically, a 70–80 mm soft tissue graft is required for single or DB PCL reconstruction. Additional tendon length can be obtained by using a Cobb periosteal elevator to dissect the superficial fibers of the vastus medialis and vastus lateralis off of the rectus femoris tendon. Identify and mark the center of the superior pole of the patella and the quadriceps tendon. A metal template of the appropriate width is useful to mark the quadriceps tendon. The template is centered at the superior pole of the patellar and at the center of the proximal portion of the quadriceps tendon. The template should be positioned parallel with the quadriceps tendon fibers. It is important to leave a 3–4 mm cuff of tendon medially. Failure to leave a medial cuff of quadriceps tendon intact will detach and weaken the VMO. In order to optimize the cross-sectional area of the PCL graft, it is necessary to harvest a full-thickness graft. For a DB PCL reconstruction, a full thickness, 10–12 mm width graft is harvested. This graft width will usually allow the soft tissue end of the graft to be split into two strands of equal width with each strand being approximately 7–8 mm in diameter after tubularization with a whipstitch. The medial edge of the tendon quadriceps tendon is incised with a #10 knife blade (**Figure 41.12A**). Typically, the cut can be made to the full depth of the scalpel blade. The tendon is incised down to the synovium, which is easily visible if the suprapatellar pouch was previously inflated with fluid. The lateral edge of the tendon graft is incised in a similar fashion. The superior border of the tendon is incised at the required graft length (**Figure 41.12B**). A large Allis clamp is used to grasp the proximal portion of the tendon and curved Metzenbaum scissors used to develop a tissue plane of the required depth down to the superior pole of the patella. Care should be taken not to enter the synovium. However, if the synovium is entered this is not a problem as a watertight closure can be obtained by suturing the synovium using a running, locked 2-0 absorbable suture. To harvest the patellar bone block, the knee is placed in extension and traction is applied to the quadriceps tendon using the Allis clamp. This will deliver the superior pole of the patella into the incision. A 10 or 11 mm width × 22 mm length bone block is marked on the superior surface of the

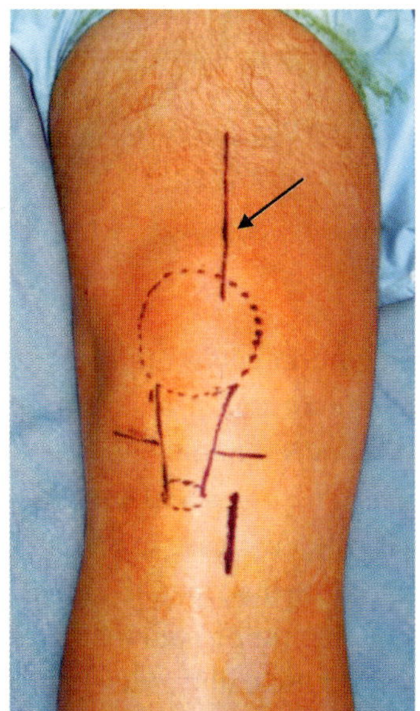

Figure 41.11 Black arrow pointing toward the incision for quadriceps tendon harvesting

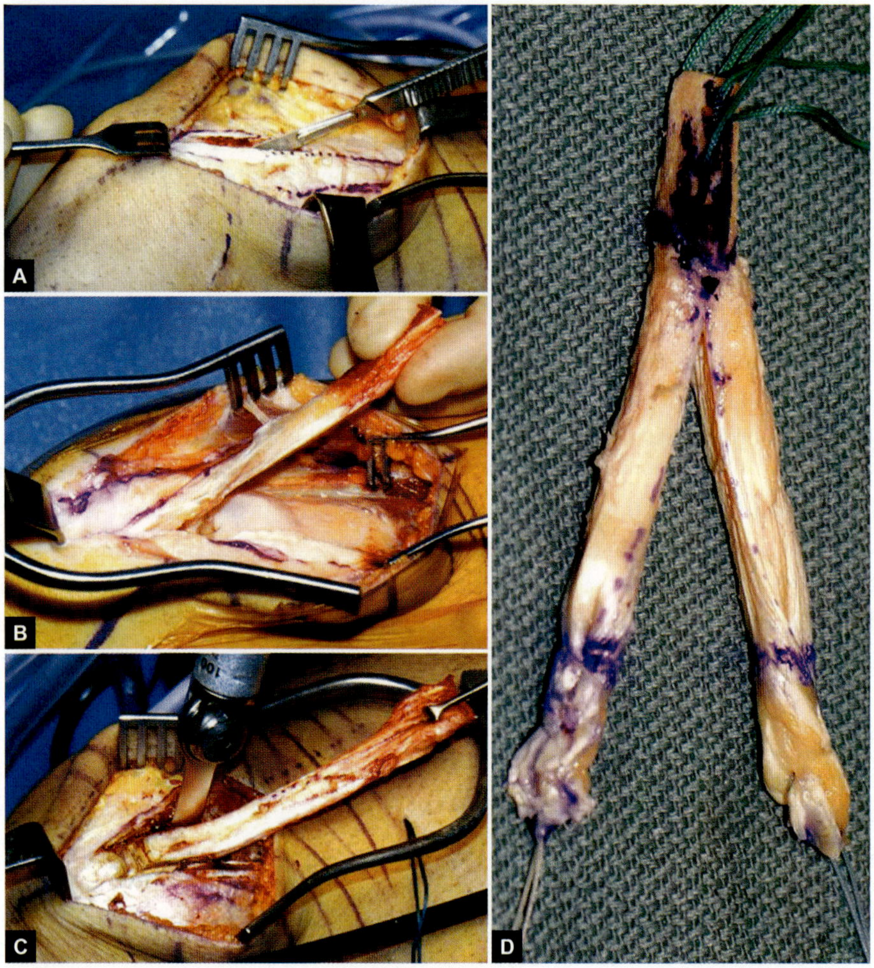

Figures 41.12A to D Technique of quadriceps graft harvest; (A) Incision of quadriceps graft with #10 blade; (B) Appropriate length of quadriceps graft excised; (C) Osteotomy of patella bone plug; (D) Prepared quadriceps graft

patella using an electrocautery pencil. A microsagittal saw with a blade width of 10 mm is used to harvest the patellar bone block (**Figure 41.12C**). The anterior cortex is cut at an angle of 70° from the plane of the anterior surface of the patella to depth of 8 mm creating a trapezoidal bone block. The proximal end of the quadriceps tendon is retracted inferiorly, and the saw is used to undercut the superior pole of the patella in the coronal plane. This step helps prevent propagation of cracks into the articular surface when removing the bone block and also ensures that the entire quadriceps tendon attachment on the superior pole of the patella is removed with the soft tissue part of the graft. A 1/4-inch curved Lambotte type osteotome is used to gently remove the bone block. If the synovium is inadvertently entered it is closed with running, locked 2-0 absorbable suture.

Closure

The quadriceps tendon edges are loosely approximated in layers with interrupted 0 absorbable sutures. It is important to avoid over tightening the tendon as this may result in quadriceps tightness and restricted postoperative knee flexion and or an increase in patellofemoral contact pressure that can cause postoperative patellofemoral pain. Bone harvested with a coring reamer from the tibial tunnel is used to bone graft the patellar defect at the completion of the procedure. In order to restore the normal tension band effect of the anterior soft tissues of the extensor mechanism, it is important to close the prepatellar retinaculum securely. A small sponge is packed into the incision and the thigh wrapped down to the superior pole of the patella with a 4-inch elastic bandage. This step will help minimize fluid extravasation from the quadriceps tendon harvest site. After the PCL reconstruction is completed, it is important to close the subcutaneous tissue in layers with 2-0 and 3-0 absorbable sutures to optimize the cosmetic appearance of the incision. The skin is closed with a running 3-0 nylon pullout subcuticular suture.

Postoperative Care

Avoid applying Steri-strips to the incision in the early postoperative period until the soft tissue swelling has subsided. The postoperative fluid extravasation and soft tissue swelling may cause skin blisters to form at the site of application of the Steri-strips. Apply Steri-strips and vitamin E oil to the incision for 3 months to minimize spreading of the incision. The patient is instructed to avoid direct sunlight on the incision for 1 year. Patellar mobilization, electrical muscle stimulation to the quadriceps muscles and isometric quadriceps contractions are important to minimize scarring in the suprapatellar pouch. Quadriceps stretching is started at 3 months to prevent quadriceps tightness.

Double-Bundle PCL Quadriceps Tendon Graft Preparation

The patellar bone block is trimmed with a bone rongeur to fit through an 11 mm sizing block or tube. Three, evenly spaced 2 mm drill holes are placed in the bone block followed by three #5 nonabsorbable polyester sutures. High-strength sutures such as FiberWire, OrthoCord, or UltraBraid should not be used as these sutures may cut through the bone block when they are tensioned and tied around a screw and washer for backup tibial fixation. The full thickness of the quadriceps tendon graft is split into two equal width strands. Each strand is sutured over a distance of 25 mm using #2 FiberWire running locked whipstitches (**Figure 41.12D**). Each graft strand is sized and circumferentially marked with a surgical marker 25 mm from the free end. Insure that both graft strands and the entire quadriceps tendon graft and attached patellar bone block pass easily through an 11 mm sizing block or tube. The quadriceps tendon graft is wrapped in a moist sponge and placed on a graft tensioning board and pretensioned to 10–15 lb until the graft is ready to be inserted into the knee.

Operating Room Setup, Examination Under Anesthesia

The setup and examination are similar to single bundle reconstruction.

Establishing the Arthroscopic Portals and Diagnostic Arthroscopy

This is similar to the single bundle PCL reconstruction technique.

PCL Femoral Tunnel Location

In order to properly place the two PCL femoral tunnels, it is important to understand the native anatomy of the PCL femoral attachment site and the influence that different femoral tunnel locations have on the length-tension of the PCL graft. The goal of DB PCL reconstruction is to create a load-sharing graft. By creating a load-sharing PCL graft, each graft strand will carry part of the load, thus decreasing the load on each strand. The native PCL femoral insertion site extends from high in the notch (12 o'clock) along the lateral aspect of the MFC to approximately the 5 o'clock (right knee), 7 o'clock (left knee).[55,56,62] The PCL femoral attachment site extends high in the roof of the notch and the anterior portion follows within 2–3 mm of the distal articular cartilage border, moving away until it is around 5 mm from the distal cartilage border at the posterior part of the attachment site.[55,56,62] The proximal edge of the PCL attachment site is straight or oval and tapers in width along its posterior portion.

The femoral location of a PCL graft strongly influences graft tension and the ability of the reconstruction to restore posterior stability.[56,57,62] The proximal-distal location of a PCL graft within the PCL femoral attachment site is the most important factor determining the length-tension of the graft.[3] PCL grafts placed in the proximal part of the PCL attachment site tighten in extension and loosen in flexion, while PCL grafts placed in the distal part of the PCL attachment site tighten in flexion and loosen in extension.[55] The anterior-posterior placement of the PCL graft in the PCL attachment site has little influence on the tension in the graft and the ability of the PCL reconstruction to control posterior stability.[55] According to the biomechanical study of Shearn et al., placing one strand of the PCL graft at the anterior-distal part of the PCL attachment site and the second strand at the middle-middle or middle-distal part of the PCL attachment site will create a load-sharing PCL graft construct which restores posterior stability from 0° to 120° of flexion.[57] Positioning the two graft strands of the PCL reconstruction at these locations resulted in lower peak graft tension in each strand compared with a reciprocal loading graft placement.

Drilling the PCL Femoral Tunnels

When performing a single-bundle PCL reconstruction, it is often possible and desirable to preserve intact remnants of the PCL and the MFLs. Due to the large size of the two PCL graft strands; this is not usually possible when performing a DB PCL reconstruction using a quadriceps tendon autograft or Achilles tendon allograft. The PCL is viewed with the 30° arthroscope in the AL portal. The PCL is resected, leaving 3–4 mm at the femoral attachment site to aid with identification. The borders of the PCL femoral attachment site are marked with an RF probe.

An outside-in technique is preferred for drilling the two femoral tunnels as this approach allows for good visualization of the PCL graft strands at the time of femoral fixation with interference screws and allows backup suture/post fixation to be used on femoral side. The Acufex PCL femoral aimer (Smith and Nephew Endoscopy, Andover, USA) is inserted into the intercondylar notch through the anteromedial portal. The PCL femoral aimer is tentatively placed at the PCL femoral attachment site at the 1 o'clock position (right knee) or 11 o'clock position (left knee) and the aimer bullet inserted until the tip contacts the skin on the medial aspect of the distal thigh. The bullet should lie at least 15 mm proximal to the articular cartilage border of the MFC. The bullet location is marked on the skin with a surgical marker and the bullet removed from the aimer. If a quadriceps tendon autograft was harvested, it is often possible to retract the medial edge of the incision and expose the location of the aimer bullet. If this can be done without excessive traction on the skin, then it is not necessary to make an additional medial incision. If an Achilles tendon allograft is used for the PCL graft, or if excessive skin retraction of the quadriceps tendon harvest incision is required, then it is necessary to make a separate medial incision. A 3–4 cm incision is made parallel to the femoral shaft at the previously marked spot. Dissection is carried down to the VMO fascia that is split. A subvastus elevation of the VMO is made and a z-type retractor is used to retract the VMO, exposing the femoral shaft. The PCL femoral aimer is placed at the PCL femoral attachment site at a 1 o'clock position (right knee) in the notch. This will place the first PCL tunnel in the anterior third of the PCL femoral attachment site. The center of the PCL femoral aimer is placed 6 mm proximal to the articular cartilage border, placing the first tunnel in the distal third of the PCL femoral attachment site (**Figure 41.13A**). The bullet is advanced to the femoral cortex and a 2.4 mm drill tipped guide pin drilled into the PCL attachment site (**Figure 41.13B**). The tip of the guide pin is grasped with a curved hemostat and the first femoral tunnel drilled using a cannulated drill bit which matches the diameter of the PCL graft strand (**Figure 41.13C**). The intra-articular edges of the tunnel are beveled with an ACL chamfer rasp to decrease graft abrasion. The first femoral tunnel is plugged with a plastic tunnel plug.

The second PCL femoral tunnel is drilled in similar fashion. For the second PCL tunnel, the PCL femoral aimer is centered at a 4 o'clock position (right knee) in the notch (**Figure 41.13D**). This will place the second tunnel in the middle-posterior region of the PCL femoral attachment site. It is important to leave a 2–3 mm bone bridge between the two femoral tunnels. The center of the PCL femoral aimer is placed 8 mm proximal to the articular cartilage border, placing the second tunnel in the middle-third of the PCL femoral attachment site. The bullet is advanced to the femoral cortex. There should be at least a 1.5 cm

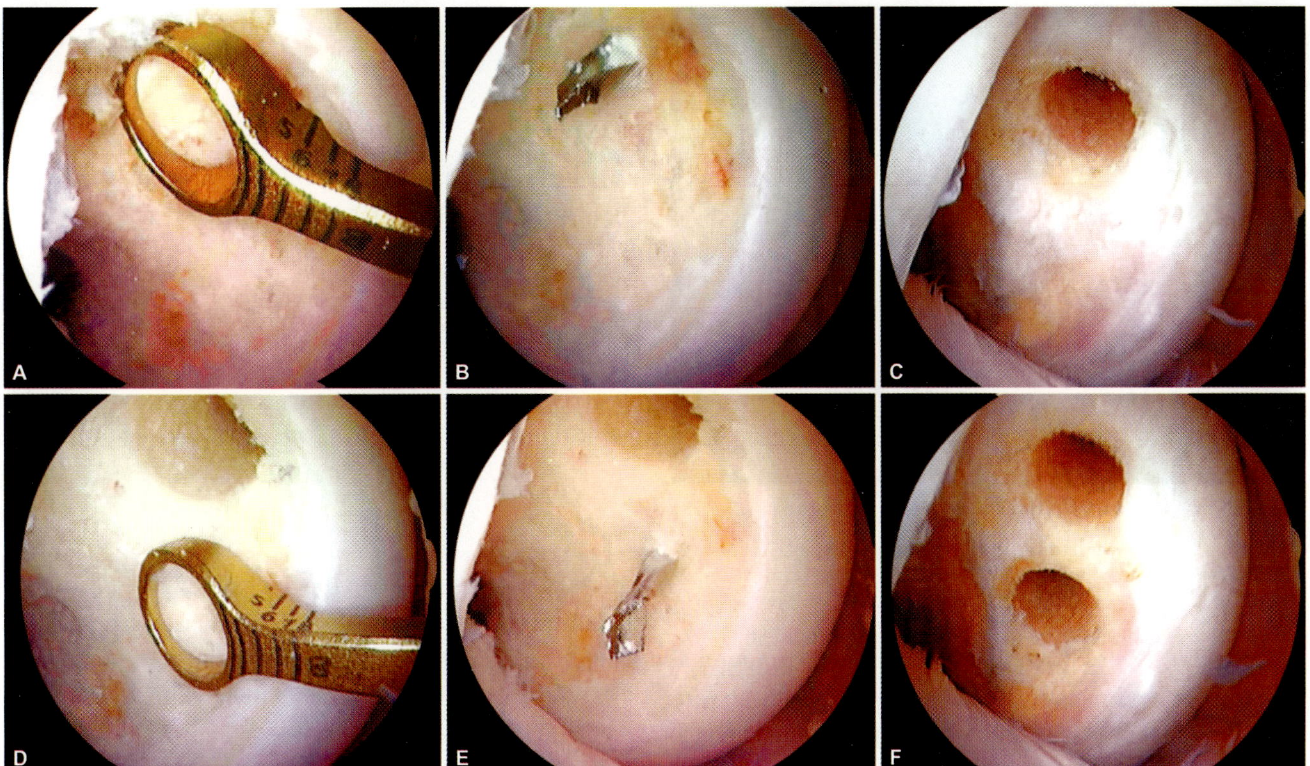

Figures 41.13A to F Arthroscopic image reveals placement of double femoral tunnels for double-bundle posterior cruciate ligament reconstruction; (A) Femoral jig in place; (B) Guidewire; (C) Tunnel for the anterolateral (AL) bundle; (D) Femoral jig in place for the posterolateral (PM) bundle; (E) Guidewire in place; (F) Final two tunnels for the AL and PM bundle

distance between the second guide pin and the first femoral tunnel (**Figure 41.13E**). The 2.4 mm drill tipped guide pin is drilled into the PCL attachment site and the second PCL femoral tunnel drilled as previously described (**Figure 41.13F**). After rasping the intra-articular edges of the second femoral tunnel, the tunnel is plugged with a plastic tunnel plug.

Establish Posteromedial Portal

Established as discussed in the SB technique section.

Preparation of the PCL Tibial Attachment Site

In order to ensure ease in passing the DB PCL graft, it is important to remove the entire native PCL remnant at the PCL tibial attachment site. Failure to remove this tissue can prevent the two graft strands from exiting the PCL tibial tunnel and passing into their femoral tunnels. Rest of the preparation is similar to single bundle technique section.

Drilling the PCL Tibial Tunnel

The PCL tibial tunnel is prepared in standard fashion as described in SB section. However, the PCL tibial tunnel is drilled using a cannulated drill bit if an Achilles tendon allograft is used or a coring reamer if a quadriceps tendon autograft has been harvested. The bone from the coring reamer is used to bone graft the defect in the superior pole of the patella. In order to ease passage of the two graft strands through the tibial tunnel, it is recommended that the PCL tibial tunnel be 1 mm greater than the measured diameter of the PCL graft.

PCL Graft Passage

While viewing through the AL portal, a looped 20-gauge wire is passed through the PCL tibial tunnel and retrieved with a grasper and advanced into the intercondylar notch up to the two femoral tunnels. A second grasper is passed down the first PCL femoral tunnel into the intercondylar

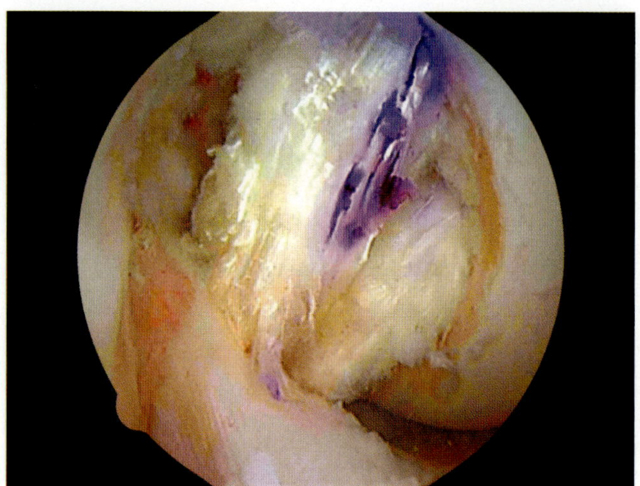

Figure 41.14 Arthroscopic image of double-bundle posterior cruciate ligament graft in the anterolateral and posterolateral tunnels of the right knee

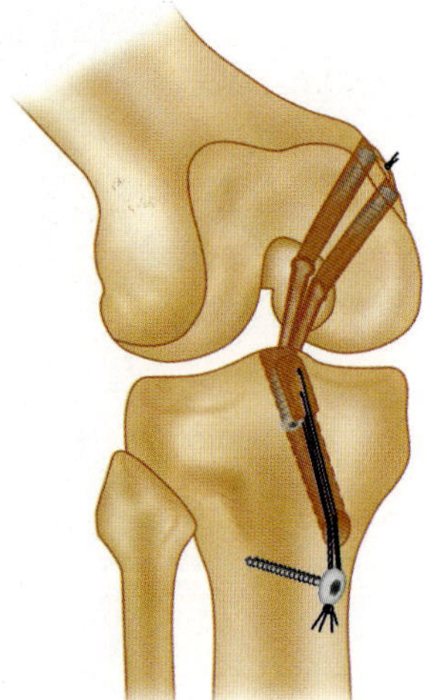

Figure 41.15

notch and the wire loop pulled out through the medial incision. A #5 polyester suture is passed through the wire loop and the looped end of the suture pulled out the PCL tibial tunnel. This step is repeated using a different colored suture for the second PCL femoral tunnel. The two looped #5 polyester sutures exiting the PCL tibia tunnel are used to pass the whipstitches on each graft strand of the PCL graft across the knee joint and out the medial incision. The junction of the PCL bone block and the PCL soft tissue graft is marked circumferentially with a surgical marker. This mark is used to determine the depth of insertion of the bone block in the PCL tibial tunnel. The two PCL graft strands are passed together through the PCL tibial tunnel by applying tension to the whipstitches exiting the medial incision. The two graft strands are passed into their respective femoral tunnels (**Figure 41.14**). The PCL graft strands are pulled into their femoral tunnels until the previously placed mark on the PCL bone block is positioned at the exit of the PCL tibial tunnel. This will position the bone block at the back edge of the tibial tunnel, decreasing graft abrasion at the so-called 'killer angle.'

Graft Fixation and Tensioning

The bone block of the PCL graft is fixed in the tibial tunnel using an absorbable interference screw inserted inferior to the bone block. Typically a 9 × 25 mm screw is used. The #5 polyester sutures in the bone block are tied around a 3.5 mm AO screw and washer, thus providing double fixation on the tibial side (**Figure 41.15**). The knee is cycled 30 times with tension applied to the whipstitches of the two graft strands. The knee is flexed to 90°, neutral tibial rotation and an anterior tibial force applied against the posterior aspect of the calf to reduce the tibia. The tibiofemoral step-off of the normal knee that was measured at the beginning of the procedure is recreated. While maintaining tension on the whipstitches, each graft strand is fixed with a 9 × 25 mm absorbable interference screw. It is important that the screws be inserted until flush with the femoral cortex. Leaving the screws prominent will irritate the VMO and cause pain. The knee is taken through 0°–130° of flexion and the tibiofemoral step-off palpated at 90° of flexion.

Postoperative Care and Rehabilitation

The neurovascular status of the operative leg is confirmed to be normal before leaving the operating room. A sterile compression dressing and cold pack or Cryocuff (DJO Global Orthopaedics, Vista, CA) followed by a hinged knee brace or extension knee brace with posterior support for the tibia locked at 0° is applied in the operating room. The knee is elevated with a pillow placed under the calf to prevent posterior sagging of the tibia. Quadriceps isometrics, straight leg raises and ankle pumps are started immediately with the brace on. Passive knee flexion from 0° to 90°, three times a day with the tibia supported by the physical therapist is performed for the first 2 weeks. After the passive range of motion is increased to 0-120 degrees at 3-4 weeks and 0-135 degrees, active knee extension is started from 90-0 degrees. No active flexion is allowed for the first 12 weeks. The weight bearing status is determined by whether associated medial or posterolateral procedures have been performed. If associated medial or posterolateral procedures have been performed, the patient is kept toe-touch weight bearing for the first 6–8 weeks. For isolated PCL reconstruction, 25% weight bearing is allowed at 2 weeks if the patient has regained quadriceps control. For a detailed postoperative rehabilitation protocol consult reference.[63]

Factors Responsible for Poor Results after PCL Reconstruction

a. Nonanatomic graft placement.
b. Inadequate graft fixation.
c. Too thin graft.
d. Failure to correct the malalignment of the limb.
e. Failure to recognize and treat associated ligament injuries.
f. Presence of medial compartment or patellofemoral arthritis.
g. Poor rehabilitation.

REFERENCES

1. Butler DL, Noyes FR, Grood ES. Ligamentous restraints to anterior-posterior drawer in the human knee. A biomechanical study. J Bone Joint Surg Am. 1980;62(2):259-70.
2. Kennedy JC, Hawkins RJ, Willis RB, Danylchuck KD. Tension studies of human knee ligaments. Yield point, ultimate failure, and disruption of the cruciate and tibial collateral ligaments. J Bone Joint Surg Am. 1976;58(3):350-5.
3. Marinozzi G, Pappalardo S, Steindler R. Human knee ligaments: mechanical tests and ultrastructural observations. Ital J Orthop Traumatol. 1983;9(2):231-40.
4. Girgis FG, Marshall JL, Monajem A. The cruciate ligaments of the knee joint. Anatomical, functional and experimental analysis. Clin Orthop Relat Res. 1975;106:216-31.
5. Harner CD, Livesay GA, Kashiwaguchi S, et al. Comparative study of the size and shape of human anterior and posterior cruciate ligaments. J Orthop Res. 1995;13(3):429-34.
6. Harner CD, Xerogeanes JW, Livesay GA, et al. The human posterior cruciate ligament complex: an interdisciplinary study. Ligament morphology and biomechanical evaluation. Am J Sports Med. 1995;23(6):736-45.
7. Makris CA, Georgoulis AD, Papageorgiou CD, Moebius UG, Soucacos PN. Posterior cruciate ligament architecture: evaluation under microsurgical dissection. Arthroscopy. 2000;16(6):627-32.
8. Hatsushika D, Nimura A, Mochizuki T, et al. Attachments of separate small bundles of human posterior cruciate ligament: an anatomic study. Knee Surg Sports Traumatol Arthrosc. 2013;21(5):998-1004.
9. Race A, Amis AA. PCL reconstruction. *In vitro* biomechanical comparison of 'isometric' versus single and double-bundled 'anatomic' grafts. J Bone Joint Surg Br. 1998;80(1):173-9.
10. Van Hoof T, Cromheecke M, Tampere T, et al. The posterior cruciate ligament: a study on its bony and soft tissue anatomy using novel 3D CT technology. Knee Surg Sports Traumatol Arthrosc. 2013;21(5):1005-10.
11. Harner CD, Janaushek MA, Kanamori A, et al. Biomechanical analysis of a double-bundle posterior cruciate ligament reconstruction. Am J Sports Med. 2000;28(2):144-51.
12. Mannor DA, Shearn JT, Grood ES, Noyes FR, Levy MS. Two-bundle posterior cruciate ligament reconstruction. An *in vitro* analysis of graft placement and tension. Am J Sports Med. 2000;28(6):833-45.
13. Kohen RB, Sekiya JK. Single-bundle versus double-bundle posterior cruciate ligament reconstruction. Arthroscopy. 2009;25(12):1470-7.
14. Kusayama T, Harner CD, Carlin GJ, Xerogeanes JW, Smith BA. Anatomical and biomechanical characteristics of human meniscofemoral ligaments. Knee Surg Sports Traumatol Arthrosc. 1994;2(4):234-7.
15. Gupte CM, Smith A, Jamieson N, et al. Meniscofemoral ligaments—structural and material properties. J Biomech. 2002;35(12):1623-9.
16. Gupte CM, Bull AM, Thomas RD, Amis AA. A review of the function and biomechanics of the meniscofemoral ligaments. Arthroscopy. 2003;19(2):161-71.

17. Covey DC, Sapega AA, Riffenburgh RH. The effects of sequential sectioning of defined posterior cruciate ligament fiber regions on translational knee motion. Am J Sports Med. 2008;36(3):480-6.
18. Grood ES, Stowers SF, Noyes FR. Limits of movement in the human knee. Effect of sectioning the posterior cruciate ligament and posterolateral structures. J Bone Joint Surg Am. 1988;70(1):88-97.
19. Shelbourne KD, Davis TJ, Patel DV. The natural history of acute, isolated, nonoperatively treated posterior cruciate ligament injuries. A prospective study. Am J Sports Med. 1999;27(3):276-83.
20. Fanelli GC, Edson CJ. Posterior cruciate ligament injuries in trauma patients: Part II. Arthroscopy. 1995;11(5):526-9.
21. Petrie RS, Harner CD. Evaluation and management of the posterior cruciate injured knee. Oper Tech Sports Med. 1999;7(3):93-103.
22. Kim JG, Lim HC, Kim HJ, et al. Delayed detection of clinically significant posterior cruciate ligament injury after peri-articular fracture around the knee of 448 patients. Arch Orthop Trauma Surg. 2012;132(12):1741-6.
23. Logan M, Williams A, Lavelle J, Gedroyc W, Freeman M. The effect of posterior cruciate ligament deficiency on knee kinematics. Am J Sports Med. 2004;32(8):1915-22.
24. Fontbote CA, Sell TC, Laudner KG, et al. Neuromuscular and biomechanical adaptations of patients with isolated deficiency of the posterior cruciate ligament. Am J Sports Med. 2005;33(7):982-9.
25. Skyhar MJ, Warren RF, Ortiz GJ, Schwartz E, Otis JC. The effects of sectioning of the posterior cruciate ligament and the posterolateral complex on the articular contact pressures within the knee. J Bone Joint Surg Am. 1993;75(5):694-9.
26. Strobel MJ, Weiler A, Schulz MS, Russe K, Eichhorn HJ. Arthroscopic evaluation of articular cartilage lesions in posterior-cruciate-ligament-deficient knees. Arthroscopy. 2003;19(3):262-8.
27. Harner CD, Vogrin TM, Hoher J, Ma CB, Woo SL. Biomechanical analysis of a posterior cruciate ligament reconstruction. Deficiency of the posterolateral structures as a cause of graft failure. Am J Sports Med. 2000;28(1):32-9.
28. Hoher J, Vogrin TM, Woo SL, et al. *In situ* forces in the human posterior cruciate ligament in response to muscle loads: a cadaveric study. J Orthop Res. 1999;17(5):763-8.
29. Esmaili Jah AA, Keyhani S, Zarei R, Moghaddam AK. Accuracy of MRI in comparison with clinical and arthroscopic findings in ligamentous and meniscal injuries of the knee. Acta Orthop Belg. 2005;71(2):189-96.
30. Rubinstein RA, Jr, Shelbourne KD, McCarroll JR, VanMeter CD, Rettig AC. The accuracy of the clinical examination in the setting of posterior cruciate ligament injuries. Am J Sports Med. 1994;22(4):550-7.
31. Fischer SP, Fox JM, Del Pizzo W, et al. Accuracy of diagnoses from magnetic resonance imaging of the knee. A multi-center analysis of one thousand and fourteen patients. J Bone Joint Surg Am. 1991;73(1):2-10.
32. Fowler PJ, Messieh SS. Isolated posterior cruciate ligament injuries in athletes. Am J Sports Med. 1987;15(6):553-7.
33. Geissler WB, Whipple TL. Intra-articular abnormalities in association with posterior cruciate ligament injuries. Am J Sports Med. 1993;21(6):846-9.
34. Hamada M, Shino K, Mitsuoka T, et al. Chondral injury associated with acute isolated posterior cruciate ligament injury. Arthroscopy. 2000;16(1):59-63.
35. Parolie JM, Bergfeld JA. Long-term results of nonoperative treatment of isolated posterior cruciate ligament injuries in the athlete. Am J Sports Med. 1986;14(1):35-8.
36. Torg JS, Barton TM, Pavlov H, Stine R. Natural history of the posterior cruciate ligament-deficient knee. Clin Orthop Relat Res. 1989;246:208-16.
37. Mariani PP, Margheritini F, Christel P, Bellelli A. Evaluation of posterior cruciate ligament healing: a study using magnetic resonance imaging and stress radiography. Arthroscopy. 2005;21(11):1354-61.
38. Jung YB, Jung HJ, Yang JJ, et al. Characterization of spontaneous healing of chronic posterior cruciate ligament injury: analysis of instability and magnetic resonance imaging. J Magn Reson Imaging. 2008;27(6):1336-40.
39. Shelbourne KD, Jennings RW, Vahey TN. Magnetic resonance imaging of posterior cruciate ligament injuries: assessment of healing. Am J Knee Surg. 1999;12(4):209-13.
40. Fanelli GC, Giannotti BF, Edson CJ. Arthroscopically assisted combined posterior cruciate ligament/posterior lateral complex reconstruction. Arthroscopy. 1996;12(5):521-30.
41. Jansson KS, Costello KE, O'Brien L, Wijdicks CA, Laprade RF. A historical perspective of PCL bracing. Knee Surg Sports Traumatol Arthrosc. 2013;21(5):1064-70.

42. Safran MR, Allen AA, Lephart SM, et al. Proprioception in the posterior cruciate ligament deficient knee. Knee Surg Sports Traumatol Arthrosc. 1999;7(5):310-7.
43. Ahn JH, Yang HS, Jeong WK, Koh KH. Arthroscopic transtibial posterior cruciate ligament reconstruction with preservation of posterior cruciate ligament fibers: clinical results of minimum 2-year follow-up. Am J Sports Med. 2006;34(2):194-204.
44. Kim SJ, Kim SH, Chun YM, et al. Clinical comparison of conventional and remnant-preserving transtibial single-bundle posterior cruciate ligament reconstruction combined with posterolateral corner reconstruction. Am J Sports Med. 2012;40(3):640-9.
45. Jung HJ, Kim JH, Lee HJ, et al. The isometry of two different paths for remnant-preserving posterior cruciate ligament reconstruction. Knee Surg Sports Traumatol Arthrosc. 2013;21(5):1029-35.
46. Cooper DE, Stewart D. Posterior cruciate ligament reconstruction using single-bundle patella tendon graft with tibial inlay fixation: 2- to 10-year follow-up. Am J Sports Med. 2004;32(2):346-60.
47. Markolf KL, Zemanovic JR, McAllister DR. Cyclic loading of posterior cruciate ligament replacements fixed with tibial tunnel and tibial inlay methods. J Bone Joint Surg Am. 2002;84-A(4):518-24.
48. Bergfeld JA, McAllister DR, Parker RD, Valdevit AD, Kambic HE. A biomechanical comparison of posterior cruciate ligament reconstruction techniques. Am J Sports Med. 2001;29(2):129-36.
49. Kim SJ, Jung M, Moon HK, Kim SG, Chun YM. Anterolateral transtibial posterior cruciate ligament reconstruction combined with anatomical reconstruction of posterolateral corner insufficiency: comparison of single-bundle versus double-bundle posterior cruciate ligament reconstruction over a 2- to 6-year follow-up. Am J Sports Med. 2011;39(3):481-9.
50. Morrison JB. The mechanics of the knee joint in relation to normal walking. J Biomech. 1970;3(1):51-61.
51. Zheng N, Fleisig GS, Escamilla RF, Barrentine SW. An analytical model of the knee for estimation of internal forces during exercise. J Biomech. 1998;31(10):963-7.
52. Hoher J, Scheffler S, Weiler A. Graft choice and graft fixation in PCL reconstruction. Knee Surg Sports Traumatol Arthrosc. 2003;11(5):297-306.
53. Fanelli GC. Posterior cruciate ligament rehabilitation: how slow should we go? Arthroscopy. 2008;24(2):234-5.
54. Harner CD, Baek GH, Vogrin TM, et al. Quantitative analysis of human cruciate ligament insertions. Arthroscopy. 1999;15(7):741-9.
55. Noyes FR. Function of the posterior cruciate ligament and posterolateral structures. Noyes' Knee Disorders Surgery, Rehabilitation, Clinical Outcomes, Chapter 20. Saunders; United States; 2010.
56. Noyes FR. Posterior cruciate ligament: diagnosis, operative techniques, and clinical outcomes. Noyes' Knee Disorders Surgery, Rehabilitation, Clinical Outcomes, Chapter 21. Saunders; United States; 2010.
57. Shearn JT, Grood ES, Noyes FR, Levy MS. Two-bundle posterior cruciate ligament reconstruction: how bundle tension depends on femoral placement. J Bone Joint Surg Am. 2004;86-A(6):1262-70.
58. Fulkerson JP, Langeland R. An alternative cruciate reconstruction graft: the central quadriceps tendon. Arthroscopy. 1995;11(2):252-4.
59. Staubli HU. The quadriceps tendon-bone construct for ACL reconstruction. Sports Med Arthroscopy Rev. 1997;5:59-67.
60. Staubli HU, Schatzmann L, Brunner P, Rincon L, Nolte LP. Quadriceps tendon and patellar ligament: cryosectional anatomy and structural properties in young adults. Knee Surg Sports Traumatol Arthrosc. 1996;4(2):100-10.
61. Morgan CD LE. Quadriceps tendon autograft harvesting. Tech Knee Surgery 2005;4:152-7.
62. Noyes FR. PCL Reconstruction with the Acufex Director Drill Guide. A Smith & Nephew Technique Plus Illustrated Guide; 2001.
63. Noyes FR. Rehabilitation of posterior cruciate ligament and posterolateral reconstructive procedures. Chapter 23, In Noyes' Knee Disorders Surgery, Rehabilitation, Clinical Outcomes: Saunders Elsevier Publishers; 2010.

Chapter 42

Posterolateral Complex Knee Injuries

Pranjal Kodkani

INTRODUCTION

The posterolateral complex of knee has been a 'dark side of the knee' for a long duration. Very little was understood of its complex anatomy. Different anatomists labeled various structures differently. There is a wide degree of variation in the anatomy of structures themselves to add to its complexity. Collaborating, comparing, documenting, and treating these injuries, therefore, could not be standardized till the recent past.

With a number of studies focusing on the anatomy and biomechanics of the posterolateral complex, there is some extent of light shed on this dark side of the knee. We now have some clarity on the nomenclature of structures of the posterolateral complex, their anatomy, and the important stabilizing structures.

Poor understanding of the anatomy, biomechanics, and modalities of management for injuries to these structures resulted in a neglect of these injuries. However, we have now come to realize the importance of the posterolateral complex in restoring normal kinematics of the knee. The awareness in identifying and addressing these injuries has therefore increased.

A better understanding has given rise to various surgical modalities of treating injuries to the posterolateral complex. A number of surgeons have advocated various procedures for managing injuries to the posterolateral complex; however, the last word on it is far from being said.

Management of these injuries cannot be overlooked or neglected. This can lead to nonresolution or recurrence of symptoms. In cases with multiligamentous involvements, it can lead to failure of other ligament reconstructions. It is, therefore, important to address these injuries especially in conditions where there is a multiligamentous involvement. A high rate of intra-articular ligament reconstruction failures (to the extent of up to 30%) have been associated with nonrecognition of the associated posterolateral complex injuries.

There is a high incidence of posterolateral complex involvement in a knee dislocation that is very often under reported. Under reporting is either the result of a tunnel vision on part of the surgeon with importance given to assess and address only the intra-articular cruciate ligaments or due to neglect despite a suspicion. There has been a wide variation in documentation of this injury in knee dislocations varying from 5% to as high as 28.5%.

The documentation of this injury on MRI in acute cases is higher than those clinically diagnosed. It is therefore necessary to look out for these injuries on radiography and correlate them clinically.

The acute injuries to posterolateral complex are most commonly associated with posterior cruciate ligament (PCL) injuries followed by its association with the anterior cruciate ligament (ACL) injury. However, they may occur in isolation as well. In Fanelli's series of knee dislocations, 62% of PCL injuries and 12% of ACL injuries were associated with posterolateral complex injuries.

Posterolateral complex laxity may also occur secondary to a chronic neglect of cruciate ligament injuries, especially in presence of a varus aligned knee. Chronic laxity can lead to early degeneration with irreversible chondral damage. These therefore need to be identified and treated early (**Flow chart 42.1**).

NORMAL ANATOMY AND FUNCTIONAL BIOMECHANICS

A number of anatomists have described structures of the posterolateral complex. However, there has been little consistency in the descriptions and nomenclature of the structures among the anatomists themselves. This therefore further complicates the understanding of an already poorly understood aspect of the knee.

Recent studies on the anatomy and biomechanics by LaPrade, Engebretsen et al. have, however, resolved most of the controversies. The layer concept as advocated by Marshall et al. may not be all that applicable on the lateral side as for the medial. A number of variations and inconsistencies in the structures of the middle layer on the posterolateral aspect may complicate its understanding.

The much addressed to 'arcuate complex' is a reinforcing structure of the posterolateral capsule. The structures comprising the 'arcuate complex', however, are highly inconsistent and play a secondary role in stability of the posterolateral corner. The arcuate ligament complex as proposed was debatably a combination of the posterior oblique ligament, the fabellofibular ligament, the popliteofibular ligament, and the capsular arm of short head of biceps. The presence of fabella in the knee is, however, highly inconsistent and therefore even that of the arcuate complex. The term 'arcuate ligament' henceforth is avoidable in the description of posterolateral complex.

The fibular collateral ligament (FCL), popliteus tendon, popliteofibular ligament (**Figure 42.1**), and biceps are the primary stabilizing structures of the posterolateral aspect of knee. The surgical anatomy of these structures therefore needs to be essentially understood in detail.

The FCL: This strong cord-like ligament extends from the lateral femoral condyle to the fibula. The attachment of the ligament on the femoral condyle is just posterior and

Flow chart 42.1 Chronic posterolateral complex laxity

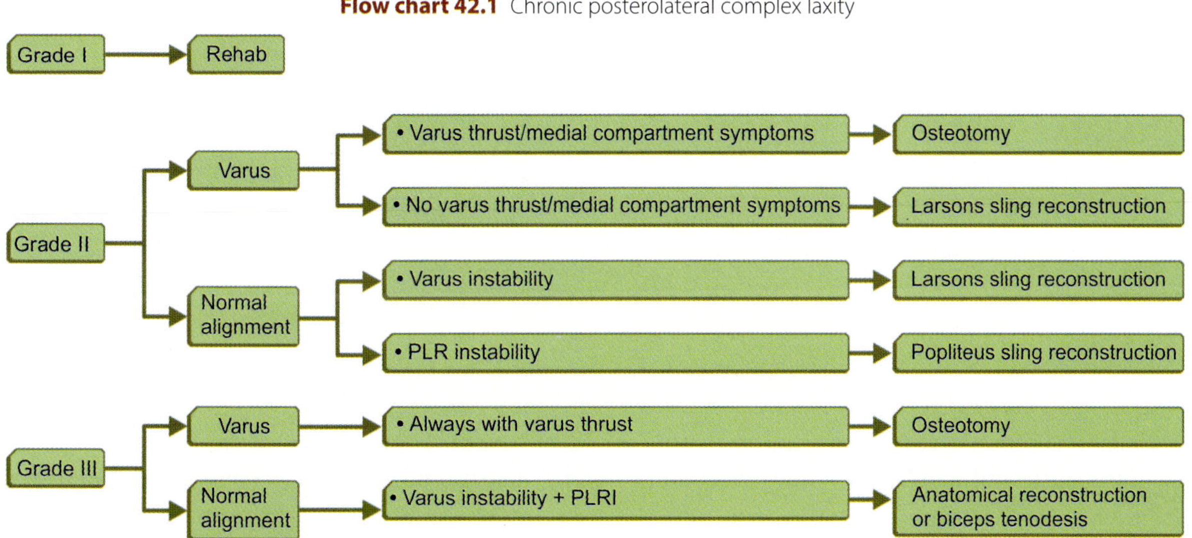

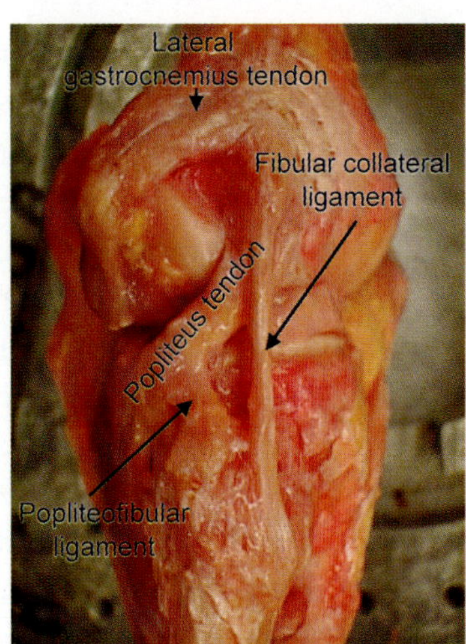

Figure 42.1 Important anatomic structures of the posterolateral corner—popliteus, popliteofibular ligament, fibular collateral ligament (Adapted from LaPrade; Posterolateral Knee Injuries)

proximal to the lateral epicondyle. On the fibular head it has a highly variable point of attachment, but more consistently, it is on the anterolateral surface of the fibular head.

The popliteus: The insertion of this tendon is intracapsular and flush with the chondro-osseous junction on the lateral femoral condyle. It is at an average of 18 mm distal and anterior to the attachment of the FCL on the femur. The tendon exits the joint through a popliteal hiatus to form the musculotendinous junction of the popliteus. Within the popliteal hiatus, it has attachments to the lateral meniscus through posterosuperior, posteroinferior, and anteroinferior popliteomeniscal ligaments.

The popliteofibular ligament: It is an extra-articular structure spanning from the posteromedial aspect of fibular head to the popliteus at its musculotendinous junction. It is a flat-broad ligament that becomes taut on flexion beyond 70° and in external rotation. Along with the popliteus tendon, it is an important stabilizer of the posterolateral corner.

Biceps femoris: It has two heads of origin—a long head and a short head. The long head biceps has six attachments on the posterolateral aspect of the knee. The direct arm attaching primarily onto the posterior and lateral aspect of the fibular head and the anterior arm attaching on the lateral aspect of fibular head forming the lateral wall of the biceps bursa. In addition to these two tendinous arms, it has four additional fascial attachments—the reflected arm, a lateral aponeurosis, an anterior aponeurosis, and the distal fascial expansions. Its other attachments are onto the iliotibial tract, the FCL, extension onto the anterior compartment fascia, and the lateral gastrocnemius and soleus muscle.

The short head of biceps has its primary attachment to the common biceps tendon, a capsular arm, a capsulo-osseous layer to the iliotibial band, a direct arm on the tip of fibula, an anterior arm deep to the FCL, and a lateral aponeurotic expansion to the posteromedial aspect of the FCL.

Cadaveric studies have been conducted to assess the contribution of individual structures of the posterolateral corner (PLC) toward stability of the knee. Each structure was sectioned selectively and its contribution to varus, rotational, and anteroposterior stability was examined.

The FCL and posterolateral capsule contribute primarily to the varus stability in all angles of flexion with a lesser role in resisting external rotation. The maximum varus instability following FCL sectioning is at 30°. The FCL sectioning in isolation does not cause posterior translation. However, in combination with the deep ligament complex causes posterior translation.

The popliteus tendon resists excessive external rotation of the tibia during knee flexion from 20° to 130°, and it resists excessive varus of the tibia during flexion from 0° to 90°. The popliteofibular ligament is a primary static restraint for external rotation. It is a secondary restraint for primary varus moment, posterior translation, and coupled external rotation. Sectioning of the posterolateral complex in isolation does not increase internal rotation of tibia. However, in association with sectioning of the ACL, it results in an increased internal rotation in 30° and 60° flexion. The biceps is a dynamic lateral restrain against varus forces. However, it does not play a role in the posterolateral rotatory stability.

PLC is found to be a secondary restraint to posterior translation (the PLC being the primary restraint). However, vice versa isolated PLC sectioning does not affect varus or external rotation stability significantly. A grade III posterior laxity always suggests an associated posterolateral complex involvement along with a PCL insufficiency. Sectioning of the PLC along with the PCL has also been found to increase the patellofemoral contact pressures significantly more than in isolated PCL sectioning. The posterolateral structures, therefore, play a primary role in maintaining varus and posterolateral rotatory stability of the knee.

INJURIES TO THE POSTERO-LATERAL COMPLEX

Mechanisms of Injuries

The posterolateral complex injury often occurs in association with other ligament disruptions as in cases of knee dislocation. This is commonly seen in sports injuries and motor vehicular accidents. However, it is evident even in low-velocity dislocations in overweight individuals, where a low-velocity injury is converted to a high-energy trauma resulting in a dislocation. It may therefore be found to occur even in cases of domestic falls and other injuries occurring in day-to-day activities like a fall while getting off a bus or train, a fall at home, from stairs, or even dancing.

Isolated injuries to the posterolateral complex are also known to occur. One needs to have a high degree of suspicion to identify and diagnose these cases. These otherwise go undetected, without a diagnosis and result in a neglect with an irreversible sequel.

A varus hyperextension type of injury leads to forces acting directly on the posterolateral complex leading to its disruption. Other mechanisms of injury include combined hyperextension and external rotation such as a direct hit from the front while standing. Contact and noncontact hyperextension injuries in sports such as football, rugby, and skiing can result in PLC injuries. A severe varus bending moment or a severe external rotation torque as in a wrestling tackle can lead to rotational dislocations with PLC injury. When a posteriorly directed force acts on the tibia that is externally rotated in a flexed knee position, the PLC is prone to injury. With further force even, even the PCL may be injured.

Types of PLC Injuries

The posterolateral complex has a multitude of structures. It may not be necessary for all structures to be injured at the time of trauma. The structures injured would depend on factors such as mode of injury, severity, direction, position of foot and knee along with strength of the ligaments and bone.

The extra-articular structures may be conceptualized as structures cocooning the intra-articular tissues. These have certain degree of resilience to injury. However, beyond a threshold, they would give way. An external injuring varus force when applied therefore gets transmitted primarily onto the PLC beyond that the forces get transmitted onto the cruciates.

A high degree of variability exists in the nature of injury to the posterolateral structures. There may be bony avulsions from the sites of insertion. Avulsions may be of the popliteus, FCL, the biceps with the fibular head, the popliteofibular ligament, or a Segond avulsion fracture. There may be intrasubstance tears or stretching of ligaments or at the musculotendinous junctions. There may be midsubstance tears of the ligaments; however, tears within the intracapsular substance of popliteus tendon itself are rarely noted. Most consistent finding is stretching or a tear in the posterolateral capsule.

In severe injuries with grade III laxities, there may be an associated injury to the common peroneal nerve. The nerve is prone to injury as it courses posteromedial to the biceps and is relatively fixed in its course around the neck of fibula. All acute PLC injuries therefore need to be examined for this commonly associated nerve involvement.

Depending on the structures involved and the extent of involvement, one can elicit either varus instability or posterolateral rotatory instability (**Figure 42.2**) or there may be a combination of the both. The degree of tears would determine the extent of laxity. The Fanelli classification would therefore indicate the structures involved and the Hughston classification would indicate the degree of involvement.

Fanelli Classification

- *Type A:* Increased external rotation only. Suggestive of injury to popliteofibular ligament and popliteus tendon complex only
- *Type B:* Increased external rotation with mild varus laxity of 5 mm difference at 30° flexion. Suggestive of popliteofibular ligament and popliteus tendon injury with attenuation of FCL

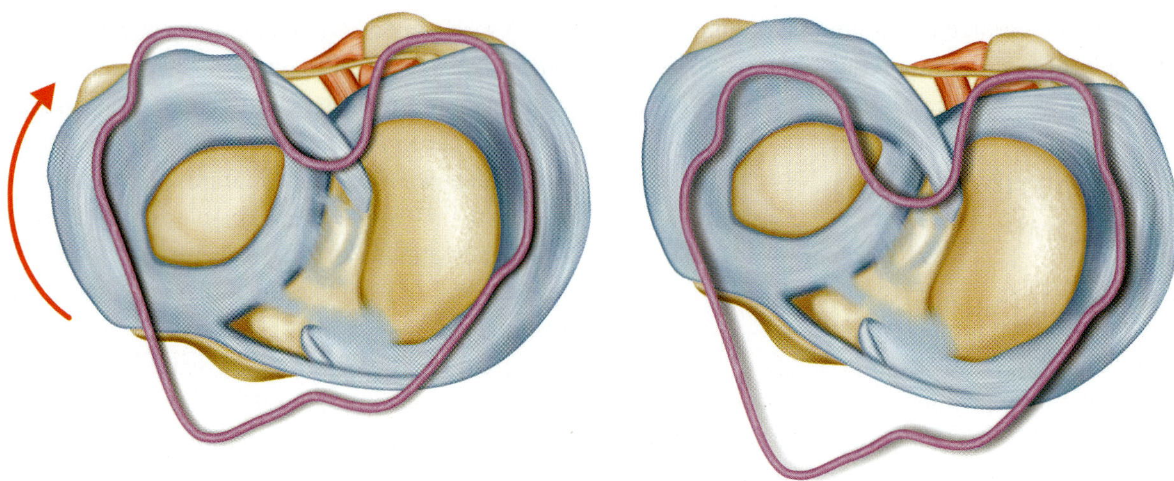

Figure 42.2 Posterolateral rotatory instability

- *Type C:* Increased external rotation with varus laxity of 10 mm or more at 30° knee flexion. Suggestive of injury to all structures of PLC including the capsule that may be associated with cruciate ligament injury.

Hughston and Baker Classification

- *Mild (grade I/1+):* 0–5 mm with a definite end point
- *Moderate (grade II/2+):* 6–10 mm with definite end point
- *Severe (grade III/3+):* >10 mm with soft or no appreciable end point.

A long-standing cruciate-deficient knee in presence of varus results in overloading of the normal posterolateral complex. The adductor momentum causing distraction forces onto the lateral aspect of the knee are normally shared by the cruciates and the PLC. In absence of the cruciate ligaments, the forces exclusively load the PLC. A cyclic loading of the PLC results in stretching of the posterolateral capsuloligamentous structures. This, in turn, further enhances the varus thrust causing overloading of the medial compartment and resulting in early degeneration. These are conditions where there is laxity of the posterolateral structures despite no anatomical disruption.

Sequel of PLC Injuries

A long-standing posterolateral complex laxity can lead to secondary changes. The sequel may be a result of the varus rotation instability, external rotation instability, or a combination of both. A prolonged neglect of an ACL-deficient knee can lead to secondary laxity of the PLC structures in a varus aligned knee. Vice versa a neglect of the PLC injury can lead to early failure of an ACL or PCL reconstruction.

Forces on the ACL graft increase with varus loading due to a PLC deficiency and further increase when varus loading is coupled with external rotation forces. The lateral joint opening as a result of the PLC deficiency causes cyclic overloading and stretching of the reconstructed ACL, resulting in early failure of the reconstruction.

The PCL graft is likewise overloaded in absence of the PLC structural stability due to the varus loading and absence of resistance otherwise offered to posterior translation and external rotation by the PLC structures. It is therefore essential to address the PLC laxity in presence of a cruciate reconstructed knee to avoid these long-term sequel and early failures.

Repeated varus overloading of the medial compartment occurs due to the adductor momentum and varus thrust during heel strike and stance phase of gait. This leads to early wearing off of the medial compartment. It may occur even in knees with a neutral alignment with a PLC laxity and therefore the importance in managing these early. Knees with grade III laxity may result in early arthrosis. However, with isolated grade II laxity, there are no definitive reports suggesting early development of osteoarthrosis in a neutral aligned knee.

The rotatory component of posterolateral instability may result in tears of the lateral meniscus and early lateral compartment degeneration. It also overloads the patellofemoral joint and may result in anterior knee pain and early patellofemoral arthrosis. Laxity of posterolateral structures is therefore a precursor to irreversible degenerative changes in all compartments and therefore should not be neglected.

Diagnosis of PLC Injuries

Posterolateral complex injuries often occur in association with other ligament injuries. One therefore needs to be thorough with ones clinical evaluation of the knee joint for all ligamentous injuries. Patient history, physical examination, radiology, and arthroscopic findings often need to be correlated to reach a diagnosis and plan the correct line of management.

In acute cases of knee dislocations, one may not be able to elicit all clinical tests for examination. One may therefore need to rely on radiology findings, examination under anesthesia, and arthroscopic findings before proceeding with a surgical line of treatment.

Patient History

Careful history taking is essential with attention paid to the details in mode of injury narrated by the patient. The patient may give history of pain, instability or at times may have neurologic symptoms related to the common peroneal nerve.

Acute posterolateral knee injuries may occur due to a varus overload injury such as a direct hit on the medial aspect of the knee. Hyperextension type of injury may occur as in kicking or due to a direct hit on the anterior aspect of the knee. Rotational injuries may occur in a twisting injury to the knee with a planted foot as stopping and throwing during fielding in cricket or in a tackle as in wrestling. Road traffic accidents very often result in knee dislocations and all should be examined for posterolateral complex involvement. Knee dislocations commonly reduce spontaneously at the time of injury and one should have a high degree of suspicion, depending on the mode of injury to avoid missing these.

Pain is either on the lateral, anterolateral, or posterolateral aspect or in chronic cases medial joint pain may develop. The instability symptoms include giving way into hyperextension during activities such as negotiating stairs, slopes, or on uneven surfaces. Some patients may give history of the knee having an outward thrust while walking. In sporting activities, one may experience instability with cutting, pivoting, and twisting maneuvers. These symptoms may present acutely or after a prolonged neglect of a mild posterolateral rotatory instability. Neurologic symptoms may be present related to peroneal nerve involvement.

Physical Examination

Acute presentation may be of a dislocated knee or a spontaneously reduced dislocation. Ecchymosis, edema, and induration are present on the posterolateral and lateral aspect of the knee. Tenderness is at the site of injured structures. Neurological examination should be done to rule out peroneal nerve injury.

Chronic cases may have a demonstrable varus thrust during heel strike and stance phase of the gait. One should carefully examine the limb alignment for presence of varus. Some patients may voluntarily keep the knee in flexion to avoid the hyperextension instability. Some may be able to demonstrate their rotatory instability actively.

PLC injuries may result in varus instability or posterolateral rotatory instability. These may be present either in isolation or may present as combined instability. While assessing posterolateral complex laxity, one should therefore assess both these components of the instability. All tests should be performed on both sides to compare the involved side with the contralateral normal knee.

Standard tests performed for PLC laxity:

- Varus stress test
- Varus recurvatum test
- Dial test (tibial external rotation)
- Posterolateral drawers test
- Reverse pivot shift test
- Standing apprehension test.

Varus stress test (Figure 42.3): The test is to be performed in extension and 30° flexion.

With the leg kept by the bedside, the examiner palpates the joint line with one hand and the other hand gives a varus force to the knee. One ensures opening of the lateral joint line and can assess the degree of opening as well. One should avoid mistaking a closing of the medial joint space for a lateral joint line opening.

Opening of the lateral joint line more than the opposite normal knee is suggestive of varus instability due to PLC laxity. If the laxity is only in 30° flexion, then it is suggestive of isolated FCL involvement. If laxity is even in extension, then it is suggestive of associated posterolateral structures involvement. A grade III laxity is always indicative of a combined injury.

Varus recurvatum external rotation test: The test was described by Hughston et al. Hanging both the legs by their great toes a comparison with the normal side shows increased recurvatum and external rotation. This is indicative of laxity in posterolateral structures. If associated with a varus, it is indicative of varus instability due to FCL laxity.

Dial test (Figure 42.4): The test is performed for diagnosing posterolateral rotatory instability.

It is to be performed in 30° and 90° of knee flexion in supine or prone position. In presence of PCL laxity, the test is to be performed in prone position to allow for reduction in posterior tibial subluxation. The examiner externally rotates the tibia holding the foot with ankle locked in dorsiflexion. A difference of 15° or more from the normal side indicates posterolateral rotatory laxity. One should differentiate posterolateral rotatory subluxation of tibia from anteromedial rotatory instability. It is best to observe the posterolateral rotation of the tuberosity and palpate the anteromedial and anterolateral joint line to differentiate it from anteromedial rotatory instability. It is important to hold the ankle in locked position to avoid a misdiagnosis due to rotations at the ankle. The test is very sensitive and therefore can diagnose even minor grades of rotatory instabilities.

Posterolateral drawers test: The test was described by Hughston and Norwood for diagnosis of posterolateral rotatory instability.

The knee is kept in 90° flexion with 15° external rotation. The test may be performed with the examiner being seated over the planted foot in external rotation. A posterolateral force on the upper end tibia results in rotatory subluxation of the tibia that can be reduced with an anteriorly directed rotatory force. Keeping the foot planted in internal rotation reduces this posterolateral laxity. Some patients may be able to demonstrate this rotatory instability actively by alternate contraction of the biceps and quadriceps.

Reverse pivot shift: The test was described by Jacob et al. for diagnosing posterolateral rotatory instability.

Unlike the pivot shift test, the reverse pivot shift test is carried out with leg in external rotation. The pivot shifts posteriorly beyond 70° flexion due to posterolateral rotatory subluxation of lateral tibial plateau and relocates

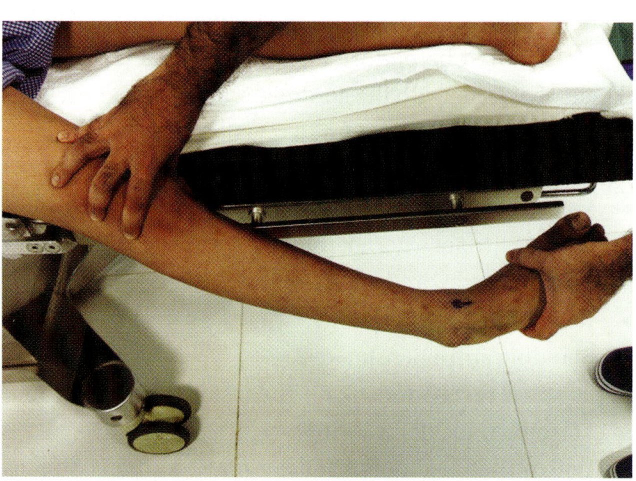

Figure 42.3 Varus stress test

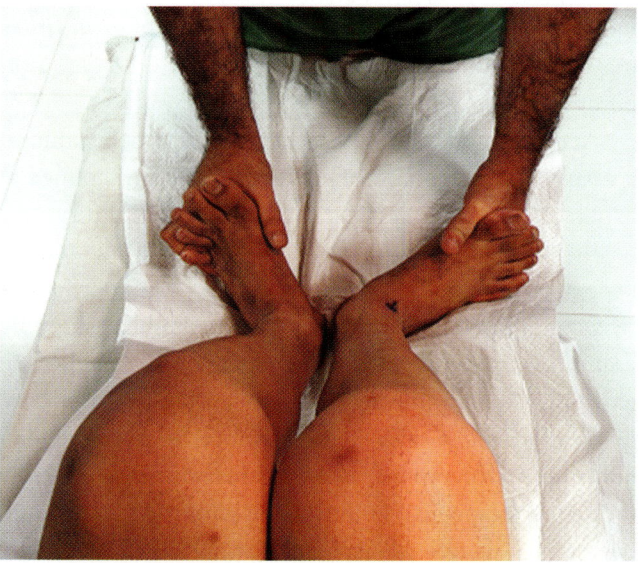

Figure 42.4 Dial test

to normal on extension at near 30°. As the knee is brought from flexion to extension with a valgus external rotation at the knee, it reduces back with a clunk. The test is most evident in grade III posterolateral complex injuries. The test may not be positive in cases with grade II posterolateral laxity.

Standing apprehension test: The test was described by Ferrari et al. for posterolateral rotatory instability.

A positive test results from tibiofemoral displacement that occurs while the patient stands on the affected knee slightly flexed and the examiner's thumb pushes on the anterolateral part of the lateral femoral condyle. Movement of the condyle relative to the tibial plateau can be palpated while the patient experiences a giving-way sensation reproducing his instability symptoms.

Radiography

Plain X-rays should be done in all cases including anteroposterior and lateral views. Weight-bearing films should be done with comparative films of the opposite normal side. In cases suspected with alignment abnormalities, a scannogram should be performed. A comparative varus/valgus stress view is helpful in documenting and assessing the degree and significance of laxity. These may, however, be avoided in acute cases to avoid additional injury. MRI is necessary for diagnosis of musculotendinous and ligamentous injuries especially in acute cases and for correlation with X-ray findings.

Plain X-rays may reveal a Segond fracture, avulsion of the Gerdy tubercle, an arcuate fracture of the fibular head, fibular head avulsion, popliteus avulsions (**Figure 42.5**), or lateral femoral epicondyle avulsion. PLC injuries may also be associated with medial tibial plateau fractures. In presence of a PLC injury, avulsion fractures of posterior tibial spine may be present. Chronic cases may show arthritic changes in medial, lateral, or patellofemoral compartments.

Varus stress X-rays of the knee at 30° flexion would show a difference in the lateral joint line opening compared with the opposite normal knee. A difference of up to 2.7 mm indicates an isolated FCL injury. Difference of more than 4 mm indicates a combined PLC injury along with the FCL.

MRI confirms the X-ray diagnosis. Bone contusions are seen in the medial femoral condyle and corresponding tibial plateau. Bone contusions may also be seen on anterolateral tibial plateau and posterior lateral femoral condyle in cases of rotatory dislocations. Bone contusions on anteromedial femoral condyle and tibial plateau may be seen in varus extension injuries. Seventy-degree oblique coronal cuts may be done to appreciate the PLC structures better. It is advisable to have high-density scans to avoid missing out on the posterolateral structures. Injuries to the FCL, popliteus, popliteofibular ligament, arcuate ligament complex, biceps, iliotibial tract, and lateral capsule can be appreciated on an MRI. A hyperintense signal of the popliteus should alert ones attention toward a PLC injury (**Figure 42.6**).

Figure 42.5 Popliteus avulsion

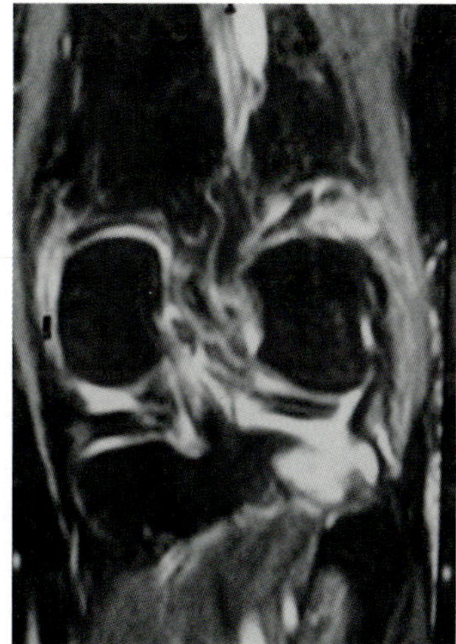

Figure 42.6 Popliteofibular complex injury

It is mandatory to know the normal anatomy and MRI appearance of the PLC structures before one is able to detect abnormalities. Coronal, oblique, and transverse cuts are most useful in reaching a diagnosis. The importance of an MRI diagnosis is crucial to correlate clinical findings for decision on management. This is especially true since many of these structures or their injuries cannot be identified arthroscopically.

The radiologist concerned plays a key role and should therefore be very well versed with these injuries and take appropriate high-density cuts to identify these. Routine cursory scans would miss out on diagnosing these injuries.

Normally, the PLC structures appear as low-intensity structures on T2-weighted fat subtraction fast spin echo images. When injured they appear as intermediate or high-intensity structures that may appear thickened or may show discontinuity.

Arthroscopic Evaluation

The lateral gutter examination may reveal it to be more capacious due to stretching of lateral capsule.

The popliteus tendon should be examined throughout its length. One may find popliteus avulsions with bone fragments in the lateral gutter or the popliteal hiatus. In acute presentations, one may find capsular tears with a floating lateral meniscus.

Quite consistently in these injuries, one finds the popliteomeniscal ligaments torn or absent with the popliteus tendon lax and lying more posteriorly in the hiatus than normal. If the popliteus has been avulsed subsynovial, one may find the normal insertion site of the popliteus on the femoral condyle devoid of the tendon on arthroscopic palpation. An avulsed popliteus often finds its attachment on the adjacent lateral capsule.

The 'Drive-through' sign: The lateral compartment normally does not open more than 5 mm on varus stress between 30° and 90° flexion. In presence of a posterolateral complex laxity, this opening is more than 5 mm and one is able to easily drive the scope across the middle of lateral compartment up to the posterior capsule without resistance (**Figure 42.7**). Grade III opening is found only in presence of FCL injury. In case of isolated popliteus or popliteofibular ligament injury, one may not find the 'Drive through' sign positive since it affects primarily rotatory stability. Also injuries at the musculotendinous junctions of the popliteus cannot be identified arthroscopically since they are extra-articular. One therefore needs to rely on clinical examination and radiological diagnosis for management.

TREATMENT OPTIONS

The treatment is tailored depending on the clinical presentation. This may be conservative or a surgical line of management. More often these injuries present as multiligament injuries, and the management therefore needs to be tailored accordingly.

Present reports do not advocate surgical treatment for isolated grade II varus laxity and these may be treated conservatively provided, they are asymptomatic. Symptomatic grade II laxities, however, necessitate management. In presence of a multiligament injury, it may be advisable to address these grade II laxities to prevent long-term failures of cruciate reconstructions. Surgical management is advisable for all grade III laxities.

The surgical treatment options are repairs, reconstructions, ligament advancement procedures, and in certain cases osteotomy may be necessary.

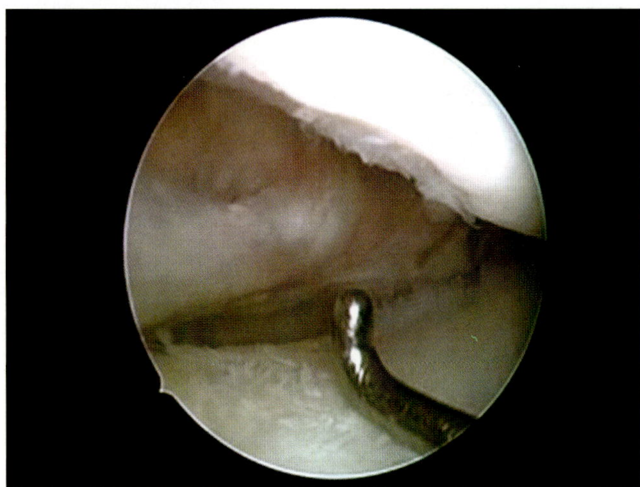

Figure 42.7 Grade III posterolateral corner injury with 'drive through sign'

In an Acute Presentation

- One may proceed with the management of ligament injuries once neurovascular injury is ruled out. In presence of a neurovascular injury, these would take precedence over management of the ligament injuries. However, the ligament injuries should not be neglected and the knee should be maintained in a reduced, neutral rotation position in 30° flexion. On recovery of the neurovascular status, one attends to the ligament instability. If a neurovascular repair is to be performed, the ligament repairs may be performed in the same sitting.
- A quick arthroscopic examination should be performed before an open repair, to assess intra-articular injuries and extent of PLC injury. Meniscus tears and impinging ligament tears should be cleared at this stage
- Repairs should be attempted in all grade III injuries
- Bony avulsions and capsular tears provide good stability following fixation and repair
- Midsubstance tears on repair may not give the desired result and stability. It is therefore advisable to augment these with a reconstruction. Attenuated ligaments and musculotendinous junction injuries of the popliteus require a reconstruction
- It is advisable to proceed with these surgeries 7–10 days following the injury, which is the golden period for repairs. Operating immediately following injury may not achieve good repairs and if performed too late one may not be able to identify individual structures to achieve anatomical repairs
- The approach used for repairs is a lateral 'hockey stick' incision (**Figure 42.8**)
- Bony avulsions are fixed by anchors, screws, or transosseous sutures
- Popliteus avulsions can be fixed by a 'recessing' procedure
- Repairs should be performed anatomically and in layers. One should start with repairs of the deepest layer and end with repairs of the most superficial layer. The popliteus is therefore repaired first. This is followed by repair of the posterolateral capsule, then the FCL. The biceps and the iliotibial tract are repaired last
- The cruciate ligament may be addressed to either in the same stage or at a second stage depending on age, preinjury activities, presence of arthrosis, bone bruises, associated injuries, graft availability, expected patient compliance with rehabilitation, and patient expectations.

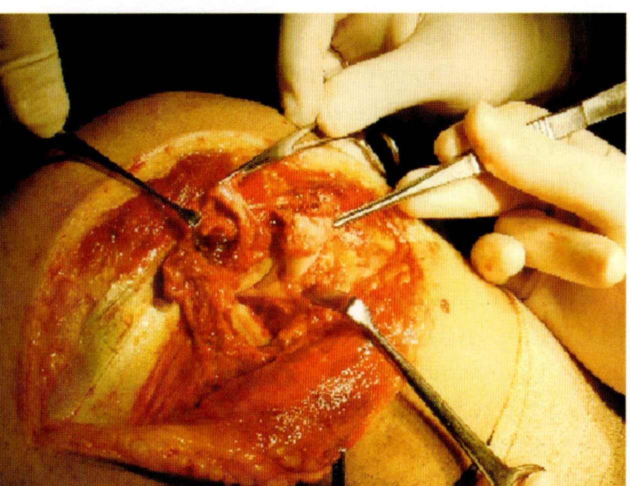

Figure 42.8 Lateral hockey stick incision for exposure of posterolateral corner injuries

In a Chronic Presentation

The PLC laxity may be the result of a neglected primary PLC injury or it may be secondary to a prolonged neglect of a cruciate injury. Varus knees may also present with a PLC laxity due to cyclic overloading of these structures without a history of any previous injury.

The factors determining the modality of treatment are as follows:

- Primary post-traumatic/secondary laxity
- Grade of laxity
- Presence of deformity
- Presence of secondary changes like arthrosis
- Planes of ligament instability—varus/rotational/combined
- Patients expectations and demands from treatment

- Graft availability
- Condition of bone/presence of osteoporosis.

The treatment modalities are as follows:

- Reconstruction/augmentation—anatomical or nonanatomical
- Ligament advancement procedures—acute or gradual
- Osteotomy.

In case of laxity as a result of primary post-traumatic PLC injury, it is not advisable to perform ligament advancement procedures as there may be a residual discontinuity in the structures and therefore may be ineffective following advancements.

Ligament advancements such as distal transport of fibular head or proximal advancement of FCL with popliteus (Hughston) from the femoral condyle may be effective in nontraumatic secondary PLC laxity.

All grade III laxities require a surgical line of treatment. However, depending on the age of patient, demand in activities, presence of secondary changes one needs to decide, if a joint salvage with ligament reconstructions may be advisable or a joint replacement needs to be considered.

In presence of a varus deformity or in knees with medial compartment arthrosis with even neutral alignment, it is advisable to perform a valgusization upper tibial osteotomy. One may perform a supratuberosity 'dome osteotomy' with a 'dome stabilizer' to permit early mobilization (**Figure 42.9**). However, any type of valgusization upper tibial osteotomy may be as effective. There is no comparative data to suggest superiority of one osteotomy over other for management of PLC laxity.

Various PLC sling reconstruction procedures have been advocated by different authors with a wide variation in the degree of success. The variation in results with no common consensus is due to variability in the type and extent of injury, type of grafts used and methods of reconstructions. However, the history of various ligament reconstructions in the past suggests anatomical reconstructions to give best results. It may therefore be advisable to perform anatomical reconstructions in post-traumatic cases. One may expect these to have the best potential for a long-term excellent result.

The anatomical reconstruction consists of reconstruction of the FCL that would primarily counter the varus rotations or reconstruction of a popliteus sling that counters primarily the posterolateral rotatory instability. Both are reconstructed in presence of a combined varus and posterolateral rotatory instability. This reconstruction may be performed by a standard open technique with a 'hockey stick' incision or may be performed through a mini open technique (**Figure 42.10**). A sling reconstruction as advocated by Larson is a good option for cases with chronic

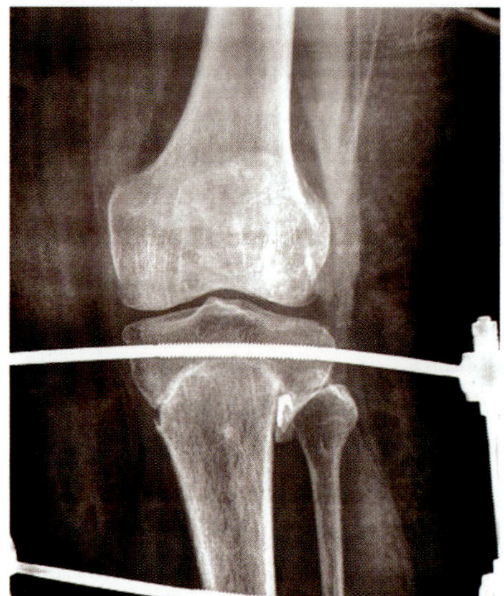

Figure 42.9 Dome osteotomy of upper tibia with 'dome stabilizer' for valgusization

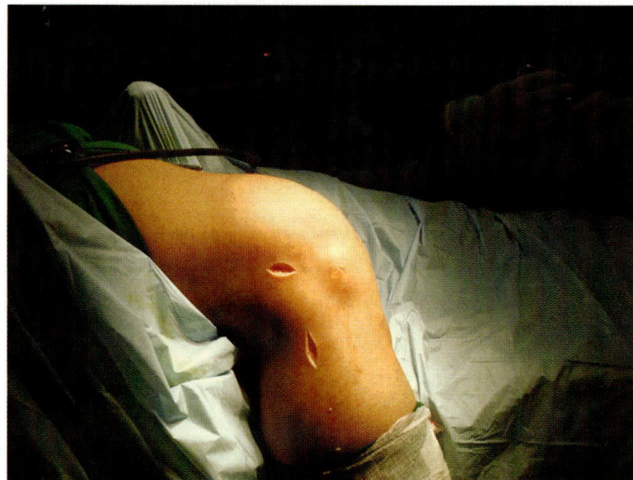

Figure 42.10 Mini-incision approach for posterolateral corner reconstruction

PLC insufficiency where one expects all the posterolateral structures to be attenuated along with the capsule.

In the Indian scenario, graft choices for PLC reconstructions are very limited especially in a multiligament injured knee. The preferred grafts are autologous semitendinosus or the gracilis from the ipsilateral knee. One may at times need to resort to grafts from the contralateral knee in case of multiligament reconstructions. In case of nonavailability of grafts, one may need to proceed with biceps tenodesis as advocated by Clancy. However, this procedure substitutes only for the FCL and is best reserved for revision surgery or to salvage a failed PLC reconstruction. Some authors do not advocate the Clancy biceps tenodesis since it obliterates the dynamic stabilization provided by the biceps. One may therefore perform a split biceps tenodesis to retain the dynamic stabilization by the biceps. This, however, forms a weaker construct as compared to the biceps tenodesis.

Presence of osteoporosis would determine the kind of fixation and the proportion of tunnel diameters for the ligament reconstructions. Various fixation devices may be used such as interference screws for direct fixation, suspensory devices, anchors, or transosseous sutures to avoid implants.

TECHNIQUE OF PLC RECONSTRUCTION

Numerous techniques of PLC reconstruction have been described in literature. The procedure described here is an adaptation from the technique developed by LaPrade et al. consequent to their anatomical studies of the posterolateral complex.

The technique advocated by Laprade et al. describes the anatomical reconstruction of the FCL with a popliteus sling reconstruction and the popliteofibular ligament. The construct, however, has the popliteofibular ligament construct passing from the posteromedial aspect of fibular head to the posterolateral part of the lateral tibial plateau where the popliteus sling tunnel exits. In my personal opinion, this part of the reconstruction conceptualizes more as a posterior tibiofibular ligament in the region rather than the popliteofibular ligament, since it has no attachment on the lateral femoral condyle. I therefore

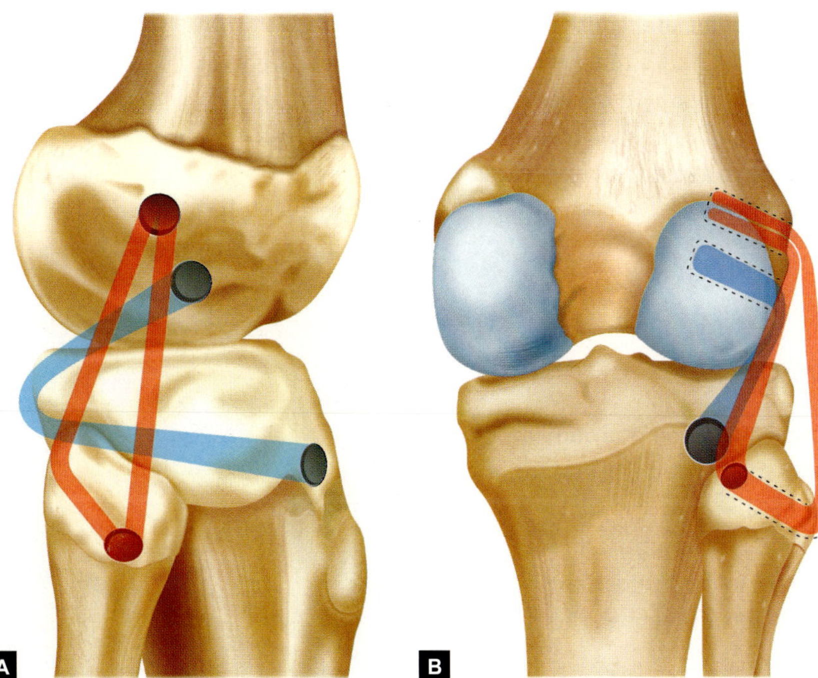

Figures 42.11A and B Posterolateral corner reconstruction (modified anatomical) (Adapted and modified from LaPrade, Posterolateral Knee Injuries)

prefer to follow the concept as advocated in the Larson procedure for reconstructing the popliteofibular ligament (**Figures 42.11A and B**).

The reconstructions may be performed as open procedures using the standard lateral hockey stick incision to identify all the PLC structures. Or one may perform these as mini-open procedures using more smaller cosmetic incisions. In cases of knee dislocation with associated common peroneal nerve involvement, it is best to utilize the open approach to identify, isolate and if necessary decompress the common peroneal nerve. In cases where the anatomy of common peroneal nerve may not be altered, one may perform the reconstructions with a mini-open approach. In the mini-open approach one incision is at the level of lateral femoral epicondyle and the second on the fibular head. Through the femoral incision the insertion of FCL and the insertion of popliteus can be accessed. Through the fibular incision the entry and exit points of the fibular tunnel and the exit point of the tibial tunnel can be accessed.

My graft preference for the popliteus sling is a double-stranded Gracilis autograft and for the Larson part of the reconstruction I prefer to use the semitendinosus autograft.

The popliteus sling reconstruction procedure can also be performed as an all arthroscopic procedure (Journal of techniques in knee surgery. Vol 10. March 2011, Pranjal Kodkani). In presence of multiligament reconstruction with associated PCL reconstructions, one may perform these by mini open technique to avoid fluid extravasation and risk of a compartment syndrome.

Technical Tips

Popliteus Sling Reconstruction

- Insertion of popliteus on lateral femoral condyle is just adjacent to the articular cartilage and 18 mm distal and anterior to insertion of FCL
- Reconstruction on femoral site is intra-articular
- Construct passes extra-articular through the popliteal hiatus and exits through the anteroposterior tunnel in tibia
- Tibial tunnel exits at the level of musculotendinous junction of the popliteus below the popliteus ridge
- Plicate posterolateral capsule
- Fixation of construct is in 70° knee flexion, valgus and keeping the foot in 15° internal rotation.

Larson Sling Reconstruction

- Fibular tunnel should not be too superficial nor too deep in the fibular head. It should be parallel to the proximal tibiofibular joint. It starts just distal and anterior to insertion of FCL and exits superomedially at the level of popliteofibular ligament attachment
- The construct is deep to the Biceps tendon and the iliotibial tract
- Femoral tunnel insertion is extracapsular. The most isometric point is at the femoral epicondyle.
- Passage of graft across tissue planes can be eased with the especially designed (Dr Kodkani's) tissue elevator-suture passer (**Figure 42.12**)
- Femoral fixation of construct is keeping the knee in 30° flexion, valgus and foot in 15° internal rotation.

The postoperative rehabilitation should delay full weight-bearing to 6 weeks and start of range of motion only after 1 month. Concentrate on quadriceps toning and strengthening exercises. Hamstring toning and strengthening should be delayed to 6 months postoperatively.

SUMMARY

The posterolateral structures form a complex unit providing varus and posterolateral rotatory stability to

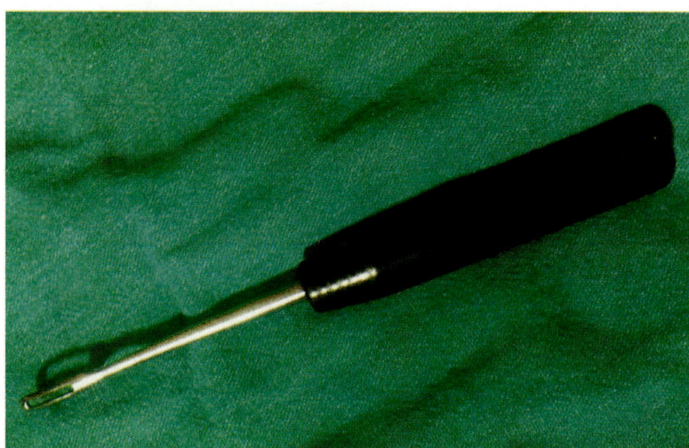

Figure 42.12 Kodkani's tissue elevator—suture passer

the knee. The three primarily important structures are the FCL, popliteus tendon, and the popliteofibular ligament. These may be injured in isolation or as a combination along with other ligament injuries. Often these injuries may be missed or overlooked and can lead to long-term sequel leading to failure in getting desired results. A high degree of suspicion to detect these injuries is therefore necessary. A careful examination is important to decide on the plan of management.

It is essential that all acute grade III injuries are treated by primary surgical repairs. Reconstructions and augmentations are often required in chronic ligament laxities. Option of osteotomy needs to be considered, wherever necessary. Numerous techniques of reconstructions are described in literature. However, none has been shown to be superior to others by randomized trials. It is best to therefore tailor ones management depending on the clinical presentation.

A mismanagement of posterolateral complex injuries can result in deleterious irreversible secondary changes and failure to achieve desired results. It is therefore important to address, these injuries appropriately to restore normal knee kinematics and these should not be overlooked or neglected.

Chapter 43

Revision Options in Failed ACL and PCL Reconstruction

Nishith Shah, Rohan K Vakta

INTRODUCTION

The significance of addressing and treating anterior cruciate ligament (ACL) and posterior cruciate ligament (PCL) revision is that with the increase in the number of primary ligament surgeries being performed, there are a larger number of revisions that need to be done. It is estimated that at this moment approximately 25,000 ACL reconstruction surgeries are being done in India every year (Source: Industrial data). All over the world, the failure of ligament reconstruction surgery is approximately 10–12%, so India is likely to have a big surge in the number of revision ligament surgery in coming years.

Treatment of the failed ACL and PCL reconstruction is complex and technically challenging. It is, therefore, important to follow a specific approach to evaluate, diagnose, and treat potential revision ACL and PCL cases. Revision surgery is done to achieve a stable, painless, and functional joint once again. Revision surgery is done not only due to complications of previous surgery but also after a perfect primary ligament reconstruction. After the 1st surgery, these patients tend to resume their two-wheeler driving and athletic activities very fast that results into ligament failure. Arthroscopically, the assisted revision ACL reconstruction is performed similar to the standard techniques for the primary reconstruction. But there are certain areas that need special attention. These include the removal of previous fixation devices, drilling tunnels, graft harvesting, and fixation. Revision surgery is not easy. There are many factors that can make this surgery very difficult and the success rate is low as compared with primary surgery. For a successful revision ligament reconstruction, we need to understand the philosophy of the primary ACL and PCL reconstruction.

FAILED ACL RECONSTRUCTION

When Revision ACL Reconstruction will be Needed?

- Motion limiting arthrofibrosis that is not relieved after adequate conservative management
- Retrauma resulting into instability
- Locking of the knee
- Pain repeated infusions and synovitis (sending swelling).

Postoperative Arthrofibrosis

Postoperative arthrofibrosis manifests as a postoperative restriction of motion in flexion as well as in extension. One needs to check generalized ligament laxity of the patient (Ehler–Danlos syndrome). Most of the patients will complain of tightness/stiffness in the anterior knee with difficulty in stair climbing and squatting. Patellofemoral crepitus is a late sequel.

Postoperative imitation of motion can be due to (**Figure 43.1**).

- Cyclops syndrome
- Intra-articular adhesions
- Ossifications
- Tunnel-related problems
- Posterior capsular fibrosis (especially in the case of associated PCL injury).

How to Diagnose?

Radiograph

A good quality anteroposterior (AP) and lateral X-ray in neutral rotation are a must. The lateral X-ray should be in maximum extension. It will show the main cause of limitation of movements many times. This view helps in evaluating the tibial tunnel placement in relation to the intercondylar roof, which appears as a linear density (Blumensaat's line). If the screw is not properly fixed in the femoral tunnel or if the screw becomes loose, it can produce a mechanical block in the extension.

MRI

This modality can show various causes of limited motion, especially 'cyclops lesion' as well as the tunnel placement.

Arthroscopy

Arthroscopy can show different types of scar formation in the intercondylar area, fat pad, and in the suprapatellar area. This modality cannot only diagnose but can also treat the pathology at the same time.

Management of Arthrofibrosis

After adequate physiotherapy and medical management, if there is no substantial increase in the ROM, arthroscopic adhesiolysis ± quadricepsplasty is the treatment of choice. Forcible manipulation under anesthesia for a stiff knee is not to be done because it can cause various grades of muscle injuries, from few fiber tears to a complete rupture of quadriceps femoris. Forcible extension is known to produce partial or complete tears of the posterior capsule. After such manipulation, blood collects in the popliteal fossa that can result into fibrosis or calcification in the posterior capsule. This can further limit the ROM.

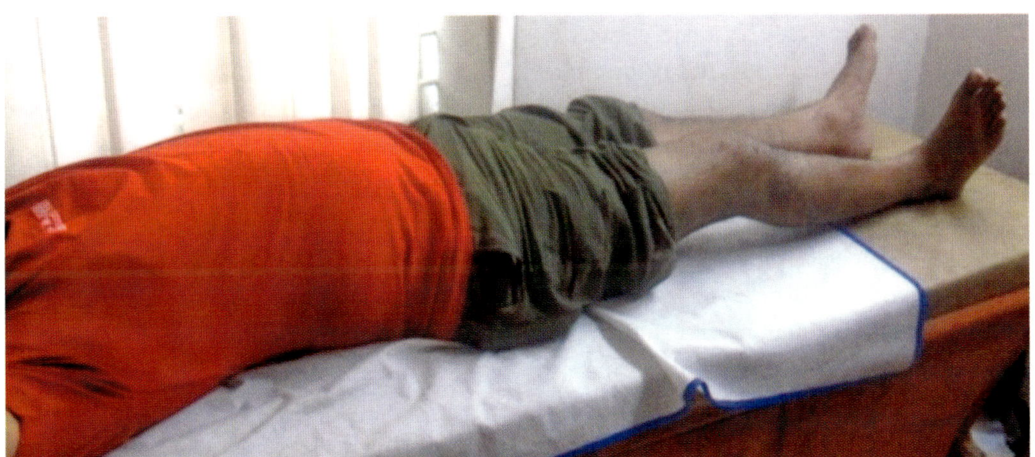

Figure 43.1 Postoperative imitation of motion

- For *cyclops lesion*, one can shave the scar tissue anterior to the reconstructed ACL with a radio-frequency (RF) device. A notchplasty might be needed if graft impingement is observed after the removal of the scar tissue.
- *Anteriorly placed tibial tunnel:* If notchplasty and thinning of the reconstructed ACL do not solve this problem, then the complete removal of the graft should be done.
- *Notch stenosis:* An extremely narrow notch can cause an extension deficit. A standing PA radiograph X-ray in 45° flexion (Rosenberg view) will show the narrowing of the intercondylar notch. Usually, more notch stenosis is seen on arthroscopy compared with radiography finding due to cartilaginous involvement in stenosis of the notch. Previously, the transtibial tunnel technique was used to reconstruct the ACL. In this, there were more chances of the anterior placement of the tunnel, resulting into high chances of graft impingement and failure. Adequate notchplasty with osteophytes resection should be done to gain full extension. Currently, the medial portal technique is being used to create a femoral tunnel, so chances of graft impingement and need of notchplasty are almost eliminated.
- *Meniscal tear:* If there is a bucket handle or flap tear that might produce the restriction of flexion, it should be tackled either by debridement or meniscus repair.
- *Problems with fixation hardware:* If hardware is visible in the notch or if it is already loose, it should be removed to prevent further damage to the graft and to increase the ROM (**Figure 43.2**).
- *Intercondylar area adhesions:* Adhesions can exist between the infrapatellar fat pad, patellar tendon and intercondylar area. Due to this, the quadriceps force is not totally transferred across the patella and patellar tendon. The passive knee extension is possible, but the active knee extension is not possible. Arthroscopic adhesiolysis with a shaver, RF device, and basket punches will solve the problem in more than 80% cases. In few long-standing cases, one might have to combine quadricepsplasty with adhesiolysis, to regain full flexion.

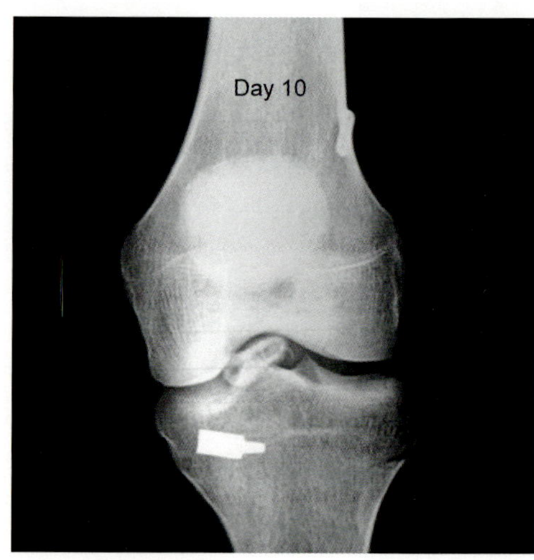

Figure 43.2 Loose fixation device

- *Loose bodies:* Though it is rare, a large corticocancellous bone fragment that remains in the joint after creating the bone tunnels may behave as an intra-articular loose body and can block movements. Therefore, it is always advisable to lavage the joint thoroughly before the placement of a new ligament.
- *Posterior capsular contracture:* If there is no mechanical obstruction, the intra-articular scar tissue or ligamentous calcification, posterior capsular fibrosis should be kept in mind for the post-ACL reconstruction limitation of the extension. This is more problematic if ligament reconstruction surgery is done within few days of injury. If the problem persists and if arthroscopic adhesiolysis with aggressive rehabilitation does not bring the desired result, posterior capsulotomy should be considered.
- *Flexion deficit:* Far anterior femoral tunnel placement, suprapatellar pouch adhesions, or the calcification of the medial collateral ligament can result into flexion deformity. MRI is helpful to see the femoral tunnel placement.

Graft Deficiency and Reinjury

Causes of Graft Failure

Graft failure can be due to technical, mechanical, and biological causes (**Table 43.1**). The time of graft failure

TABLE 43.1 Causes for graft failure

Preoperative	*Intraoperative*	*Postoperative*
Failure to diagnose injury to secondary restraints especially posterolateral corner	Inadequate notchplasty	Improper graft incorporation
	Improper tunnel placement	Trauma
	Improper tensioning	Improper rehabilitation
	Inadequate fixation	Infection
	Faulty selection/ harvest of graft	

occurrence after the first reconstruction may help us in determining the cause of failure. Failures within the first 6 months can be due to poor surgical technique, failure of graft healing, postoperative infection or too aggressive rehabilitation. Failures that occur after 1 year are usually due to another injury, the most common being varus injury in two wheeler's accidents. Interstitial failure is the most common, as opposed to failure at the tunnel interface. Gradual failure is more likely to occur than acute failure from a sudden overload. Other factors that can lead to an unsatisfactory outcome of ligament reconstruction are injuries to other knee structures or leg alignment.

If the patient does not give a history of trauma but describes the feeling of increasing laxity, one must keep in mind the about-mentioned causes. Usually, the patient complains of pain, instability, or both. More and more patients come with primary complains of pain and not laxity. A thorough examination will reveal single or multiple ligaments' laxity. Few of these patients may present with repeated effusion, degenerated joint or Morrant Baker cyst. Some patients may give the history of a bloody aspiration and a careful history is important. Diagnosis is done by the routine tests. The pivot shift test, valgus and varus stress tests, and external rotation in 30° and 90° flexion are cornerstone tests for the diagnosis of reappearance of laxity (**Figure 43.3**). The knee is also palpated for insertional tendinopathy like pes bursitis or popliteal tendonitis. In long standing cases, thigh muscle atrophy should be noted.

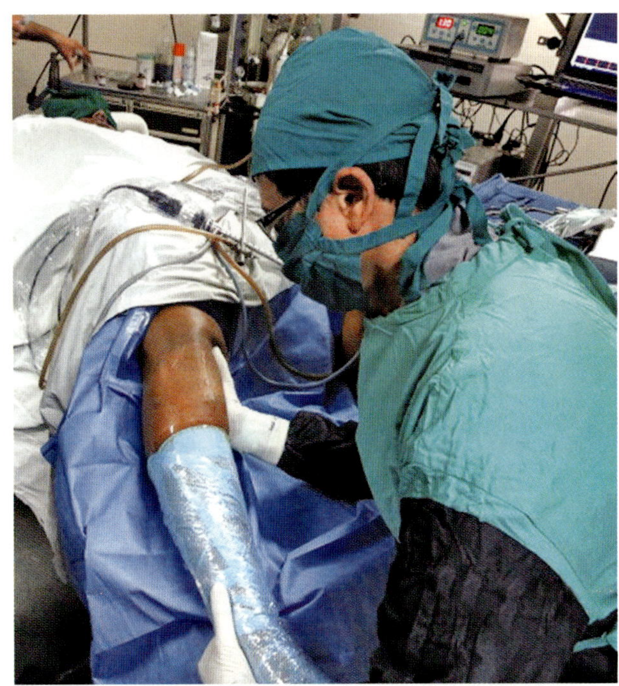

Figure 43.3 Examination under anesthesia is a must prior to surgery

Radiographs

Both knees AP (standing) in neutral rotation are mandatory. In the case of suspected medial compartment arthrosis, Rosenberg view is advised as it throws light on many areas of the knee, which are not seen on routine films. Stress radiographs in AP and lateral in different positions can show the MCL/LCL and ACL/PCL laxity (**Figures 43.4A and B**). More displacement in the lateral view will be seen as per the damage to peripheral ligament structures. Attention should also be paid to hardware, bone tunnels and tunnel enlargement (**Figure 43.5**).

CT Scan

This modality is important when a plain X-ray shows tunnel enlargement (**Figure 43.6**). Tunnel size cannot be accurately documented with MRI because of the metallic artifact (stainless steel implant or debris from reamer).

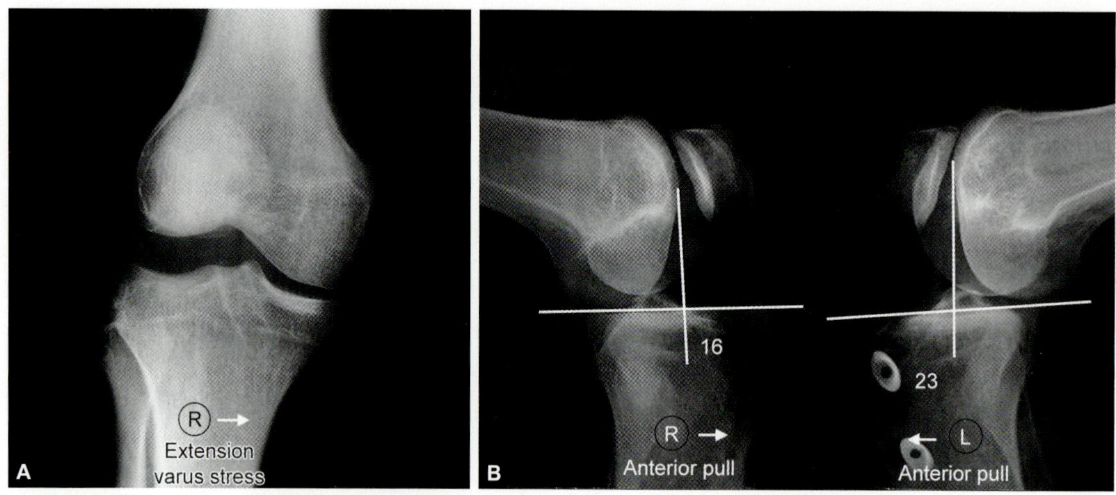

Figures 43.4A and B Stress radiographs (Anteroposterior and lateral)

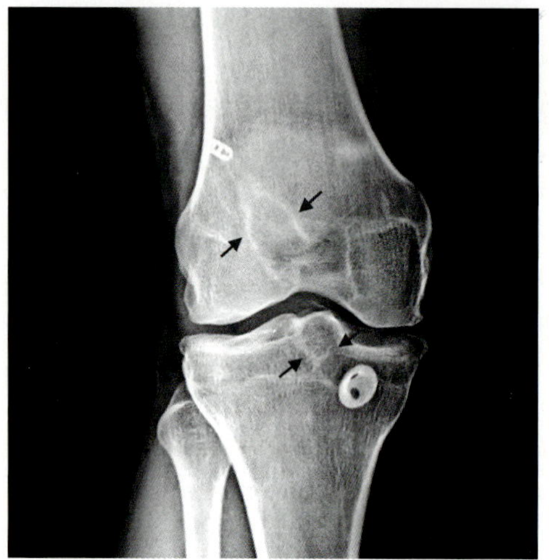

Figure 43.5 Plain X-ray showing tunnel enlargement

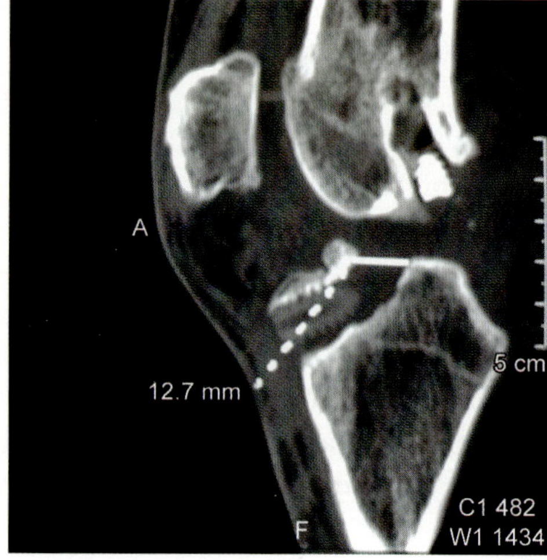

Figure 43.6 CT scan showing for tunnel enlargement and size

The 3D construction is always more helpful but is not a must.

MRI

It does not add to the diagnosis or management of the failed ligament. Revision surgery is based on clinical examination.

Management

In a ligament deficient knee, we may encounter multiple problems and its awareness is important. Full diagnostic arthroscopy of the knee joint is performed. If needed, articular cartilage as well as meniscus surgery are performed. The total removal of the failed graft is done with shaver and punches. The patellofemoral joint is evaluated along with the PCL and anterior horn of lateral meniscus.

It is difficult to define a standard therapeutic approach in any revision reconstruction surgery. To finish revision in a single stage, it is important to study the previous surgery in detail for many aspects.

Which graft was used for 1st reconstruction and from where?

Available grafts for revision surgery are as follows:

Autografts: The harvesting graft from the same limb has the disadvantage of adding further insult to the already injured knee, though it allows graft harvesting through the

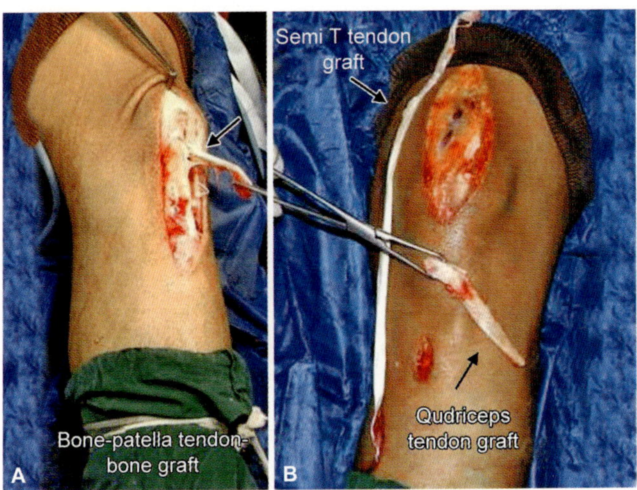

Figures 43.7A and B Graft options

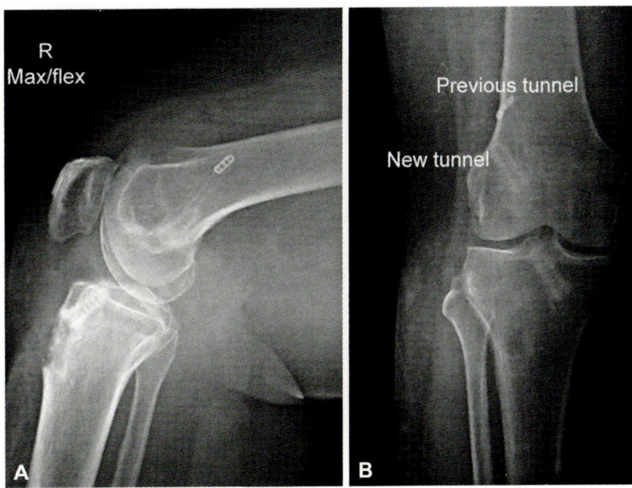

Figures 43.8A and B Previous small implants such as Endobutton need not be removed as it can be left *in situ*, if there was no infection

same or slightly longer incisions. It also spares contralateral extremity or the risks of using allograft.

Graft options include the bone-patellar tendon-bone (BPTB) graft, hamstring tendons, and quadriceps tendon (Q tendon) depending upon the previously used graft. Harvest of all three grafts from the ipsilateral extremity would increase the donor site morbidity (**Figures 43.7A and B**).

Graft/s from the contralateral knee can be obtained without further insulting the injured knee. The practice does result in morbidity to the normal knee and may decrease the postoperative patient's mobility but is the only option where allografts are not available. For any revision surgery, preoperative consent for the possible contralateral graft harvest from the opposite extremity must be obtained.

Observing surgical scars, palpation of graft areas and review of the previous operative chart, if available, will give good information about what was already used. One will have to plan revision surgery according to graft availability from the same as well as opposite limb. Various synthetic materials such as Ethibond and Mersilene tape along with the remaining ACL must be removed before placing the new ligament, so that recurrent synovitis does not occur. Previous small implants like Endobutton need not be removed as it can be left *in situ* if there was no infection (**Figures 43.8A and B**).

Allografts: A popular way to treat failed multiple ligament reconstruction in Western countries is with the use of allografts. The advantage of eliminating graft site morbidity is appealing. Allografts provide a readily available source of the tissue that can be prepared simultaneously before or during the surgical procedure. Efficient time management is important in revision surgeries where fluid extravasation and tourniquet time are concerns. Many types of allografts are available. The wide variety of allograft choices allows more anatomic reproduction of the injured ligament.

Disadvantages of allografts include the slight but definite risk of disease transmission. The risk should be explained to the patient during preoperative discussion. The incorporation of the allograft proceeds more slowly than that of the autograft, and rehabilitation protocols need to be modified.

Artificial graft: More than five varieties of artificial grafts are available. These are rarely used, as allografts have shown excellent results in revision surgery.

Tunnel Placement for New Ligament

If previous tunnels were correctly placed and were of less than 8 mm diameter, usually one will not face any difficulty in removing the hardware and do a revision surgery using the same tunnels in a single sitting. Whether it is a revision

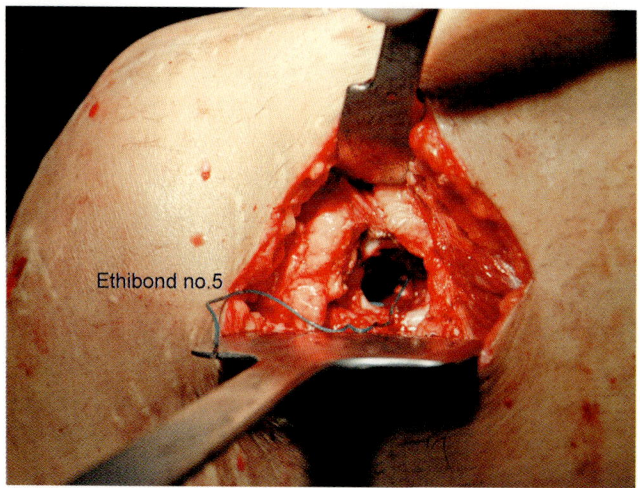

Figure 43.9 Previous tunnel being cleared of all old suture, implants and graft material

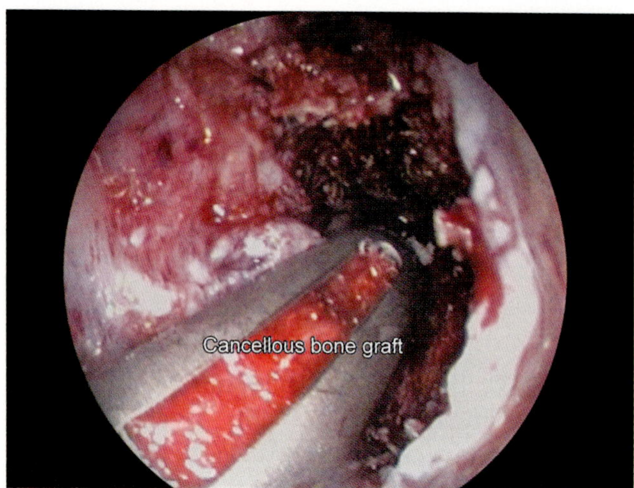

Figure 43.10 Older tunnels filled with cancellous bone graft

surgery or primary surgery, one has to check for graft impingement in the intercondylar notch when the knee is fully extended.

One must study whether original bone tunnels will come in the way of new tunnels or not. If there is a chance of mixing of old and new tunnels on either side, it will be better to do a two-stage surgery. In the first surgery, all allograft material is removed along with sutures and implants, tunnels are freshened, and cancellous bone harvested from iliac crest fills up the tunnels **(Figures 43.9 and 43.10)**. One should wait for at least 3 months before new tunnels are made.

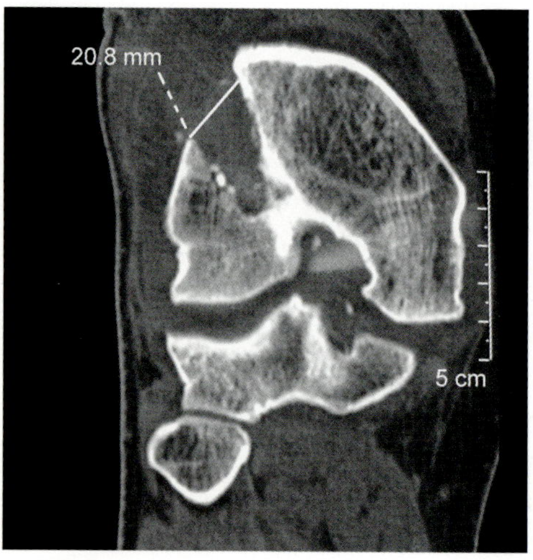

Figure 43.11 CT scan showing tunnel enlargement

Tunnel Enlargement

This well recognized problem is seen after ACL reconstruction with the hamstring graft. Femoral tunnel enlargement is common with fixation done away from the tunnel by using Endobutton or cross pin fixation. This is known as the 'windshield wiper effect' or 'bungee effect' due to the mobile hamstring graft. If the new ligament becomes lax and the patient is symptomatic due to tunnel enlargement, it becomes important. Due to chemical reaction with bioabsorbable screws, osteolysis or painful cyst formation can be seen in the X-ray or MRI.

One needs to know how much tunnel has enlarged before revision surgery. The best modality for this is CT scan (**Figure 43.11**). If the primary tunnels are anatomical but are of more than 20 mm diameter, cancellous or corticocancellous bone grafting should be done as a primary surgery for the revision ligament reconstruction.

Hardware Removal

A variety of hardware components are used in modern ligament reconstruction surgery. These hardware components might need removal for revision surgery. Hardware removal sometimes becomes the most difficult part of the procedure. Preoperative radiographs in the form of normal X-rays and CT scan with or without 3D reconstruction must be assessed thoroughly to decide direction, numbers and position of screws, buttons, staples, pins, and wires. If not needed, old hardware should not be touched unless until ligament failure is due to infection or comes in the way of revision surgery.

When femoral fixation is done with a metal interference (IF) screw and needs removal, few points need to be kept in mind. One may require multiple sizes of screwdrivers as well as coring reamers to remove the firmly embedded screw. SS cancellous screws if used for the BPTB graft may need appropriate screwdrivers for the removal of such screws. If the screw was inserted at a steep angle, an accessory low anterolateral portal needs to be created with a spinal needle. The tibial tunnel screw removal is not difficult as the tunnel is short.

If the screw is deep inside the tunnel, it will be difficult to locate the screw head. Image intensifier fluoroscopy might be required to locate the screw exactly. Small microfracture chisels and gouges can be helpful for removing any bone covering the screw. Also, one might need an RF device to take away the fibrous tissue between the tunnel and the head before screw removal. All the scar tissues surrounding the screw must be removed before removal is attempted. It would be better to place a K wire in the hole of the IF screw before screw removal is attempted with a cannulated screwdriver. This will lessen the chances of screw loss in the intercondylar area in presence of scar tissue.

Biodegradable screws need not be removed because either they were already absorbed or will be broken while making a new tunnel. Its debris must be removed. Staples can be removed most easily by using an elevator rather than an extractor or osteotome. On the femoral site, notch debridement might be needed before locating intra-articular staple. A sharp trocar is inserted between the bone and the staple to loosen it. Once it is loose, it is grasped firmly with forceps and removed under arthroscopic vision. The PCL injury or damage to the shaver tip can occur, so surgeon has to be very careful. One has to check the bony bridges between the staple and the tunnel. Sometimes removal of serrated staple requires great force and this might produce unstable bone areas that may be detrimental to revision surgery. In cases where removing hardware might result in excessive loss of bone, necessitating bone grafting or staging of the procedure, it is better to leave it in place and change the tunnel direction.

In case of an artificial ligament like carbon fiber or gore tax removal, one may encounter chronic synovitis with repeated effusions. In such scenario, many times bone grafting procedure will be needed before new graft is placed. If the ACL failure was secondary to postoperative infection, synovectomy, removal of hardware, lavage of the joint, and suitable antibiotics will be needed for a long time with repeated blood investigations before revision is attempted. It is always advisable to use good quality titanium or bioabsorbable implants during primary surgery so that revision surgeon will not face difficulties during revision surgery.

Removal of Interference Screw from the Popliteal Fossa (Posterolateral Capsule)

Very occasionally an IF screw breaks the posterior wall of femoral tunnel or comes out of graft and lodges itself into PL area. Not only this can result into ligament laxity but also retrieval can be a challenging task. If it cannot be removed arthroscopically, a small incision on the PL aspect and help of an arthroscope can make this difficult task of screw removal easy. Image intensifier (IITV) must be kept ready as an important stand-by tool (**Figures 43.12 and 43.13**).

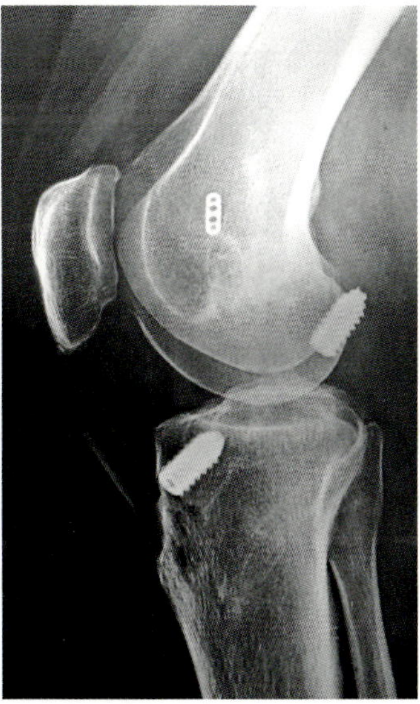

Figure 43.12 X-ray screw outside the femoral tunnel

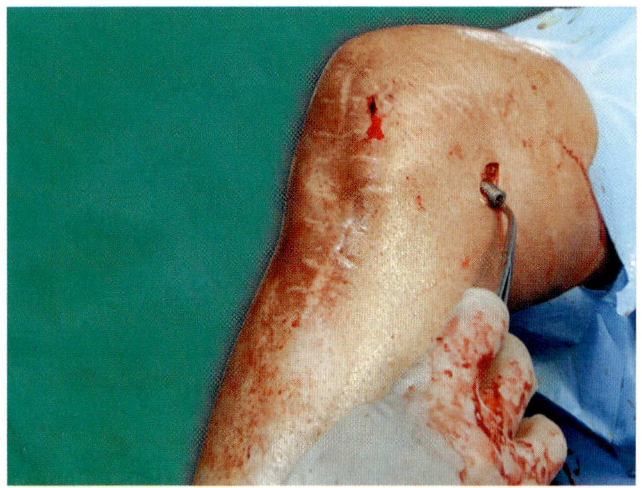

Figure 43.13 Screw removed through a small posterolateral incision

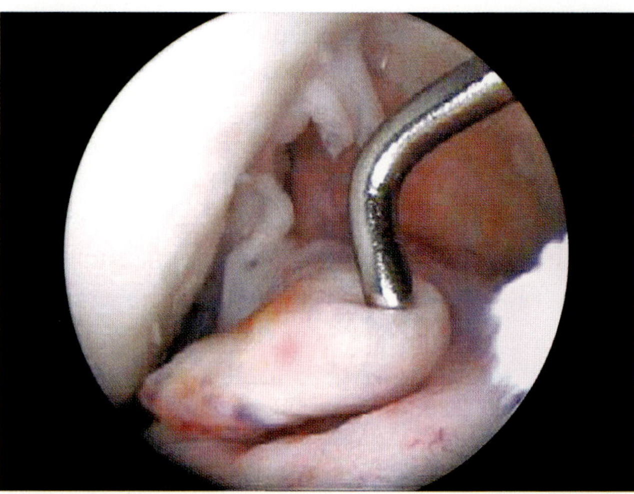

Figure 43.14 Cyclops

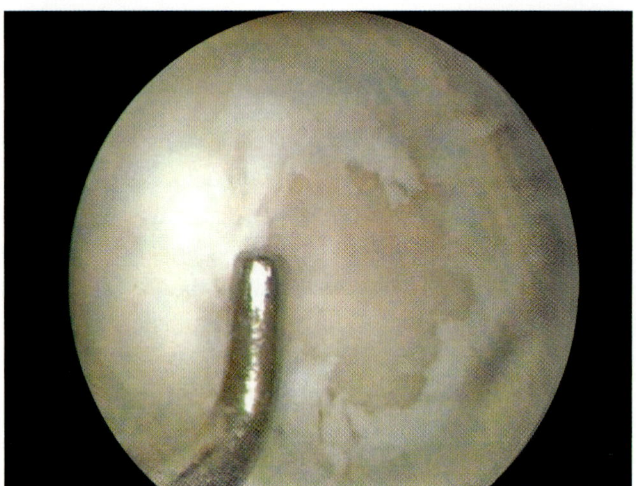

Figure 43.15 Osteochondral defect

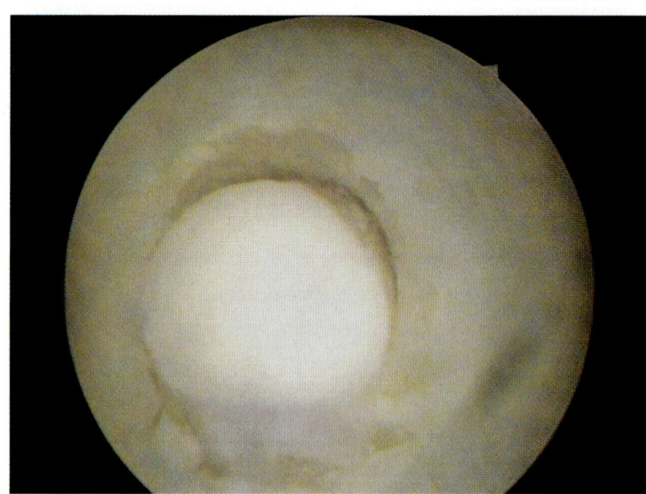

Figure 43.16 Mosaicplasty

Locking

Locking of knee is not very common after ACL reconstruction.

Causes: If it occurs, then it can be due to torn meniscus, chondral or osteochondral lesion, cyclops lesion, hardware problem, or due to loose screw/body in the joint (**Figure 43.14**).

Management

Whatever the cause of locking is, it should be tackled as soon as possible if conservative treatment fails. If there is a loose body or loose implant in the intercondylar notch, it is easy to remove after excising scar tissue in which the screw/loose body is embedded.

Meniscus can be debrided or repaired if there is a peripheral separation. Repair should be done especially in young knees to prevent further cartilage damage. Full thickness cartilage lesions can be treated with various modern modalities starting from microfracture to cartilage implantation depending on the area and depth of cartilage loss (**Figures 43.15 and 43.16**). The range of movements must be checked after removal of any pathology.

Pain

In many patients with ligament laxity, the presenting symptom is pain and not gross instability. Courses for pain can be many after primary ligament reconstruction procedure.

Causes:

- Synovitis
- Limited range of movements
- Meniscus lesion
- Anterior knee pain due to problems of the patella, tibial tuberosity, and fat pad
- Insertional tendinopathy
- Reflex sympathetic dystrophy
- Fibrous nodule at tibial tunnel due to bioscrew.

Careful history for pain must be elicited. When doing a knee examination, in patients with BPTB graft reconstruction, particular attention should be paid to the scar, apex of the patella, patellar tendon, fat pad, and tibial tuberosity. Also tightness of hamstring, quadriceps, IT band, and gastroc soleus muscle must be checked.

MRI: MRI can show cartilage lesions, loose bodies, meniscus tears, and protuberant bioabsorbable screw as possible causes.

Management

Arthrofibrosis, meniscus lesion, and chondral lesion should be treated arthroscopically as described before. If pain at the donor site of the BPTB graft is present, then it is treated as per the site of the pain. Anterior knee pain after the BPTB bone graft in Asian patients is not so frequent when compared with Western literature.

- *Patellofemoral joint:* Few patients complain of crepitations in the patellofemoral joint ± pain after the BPTB reconstruction. Stretching and strengthening of quadriceps and iliotibial tract is more beneficial than arthroscopic chondroplasty. If there is increased lateral pressure due to patella malposition, selective lateral release can be performed arthroscopically.
- *Patellar apex pain:* It is important to bone graft the donor site of the patellar bone plug at the time of ligament reconstruction surgery. Surgeon should also be careful in not leaving palpable sharp edges after harvesting the graft. Quadriceps shortening should be excluded and if it is present then stretching exercises should be started. Conservative management in form of hot and cold fomentation, medicines, and ultrasound should be tried before surgery. Local hydrocortisone injection should be avoided as it can produce patellar tendon rupture. Scar revision with surgery might help but it has not produced consistent result. If problem persists, patient should be advised not to sit on the ground and squat.
- *Tibial tuberosity:* If there are sharp edges at the graft harvest site, kneeling might be painful. Pain might be due to tibial fixation hardware like staples, screw, or washers. Removal might give benefit to the patient.
- *Insertional tendinopathies:* Tendinopathies on the lateral and posterolateral corner (PLC) of the knee due to involvement of the biceps femoris, IT band, and occasional popliteal tendon are common. This particularly seen after semitendinosus reconstruction. Besides medicines, ultrasound, deep friction massage, and physiotherapist should concentrate on stretching the shortened muscle. Taping might be beneficial. Serum magnesium level should be checked in the chronic patients.
- *Semitendinosus tendon donor site:* Patient complains of pain at the upper third or middle part of the medial side of the thigh immediately after surgery or after few days of physiotherapy. This might be due to spontaneous or late rupture of the muscle fibers. Hamstring tightness might be seen during examination. Treatment is in form of ultrasound with ionophoresis, gentle massage, and supervised stretching exercises.
- *Patellar tendon problems:* If the patient has pain, giving way symptoms, and a feeling of instability with a palpable defect in the patellar tendon after harvest suggestive of a patellar tendon rupture, external bracing should be done as a diagnostic modality. Occasionally, herniation of infrapatellar fat pad through the defect can cause pain. Patellar tendon rupture mandatory relieves pain, surgical reapproximation of patellar tendon with possibly hamstring augmentation.
- Patellar tendon pain after the BPTB graft is a very debilitating condition. The ACL reconstruction will relieve patient of his instability symptoms but pain can

be very debilitating. The treatment of the donor site morbidity does not have good success rate.

- Wherever possible primary ACL reconstruction should be done only with the hamstring graft so that sensitive extensor mechanism is spared.

Recurrent Swelling

An effusion for a few days after ACL reconstruction is not uncommon.

Causes: The most frequent cause is reactive synovitis, which might be due to a left meniscus fragment, loose body, or scar tissue mass arising from reconstructed ACL. Postoperative infection can also cause recurrent swelling, which should be ruled out by C-reactive protein.

The X-ray and MRI might reveal cartilage pathology, meniscus fragment, or a loose body.

Management

- *Acute effusion:* In the initial stages, effusion is aspirated and the joint is rested. If there is no instability or meniscal pathology, intra-articular hydrocortisone injection might relieve the symptoms. Physiotherapy should be restricted for 1–2 weeks. If effusion persists, rearthroscopy should be done.
- *Chronic effusion:* If effusion occurs after the reconstruction and is still present at 4–5 weeks, intra-articular cortisone injection is recommended, since the joint fluid contains cytokines that have a catabolic effect on the graft. Total graft absorption is seen in cases of chronic effusion treated only with rest and dressings (second look arthroscopy showed an empty intercondylar area with no ACL).
- If the effusion develops several months after the reconstruction, differential diagnosis should include a reinjury or progressive degenerative changes. Conservative measures should be started followed by an intra-articular cortisone injection. In resistant cases one might need to perform a repeat arthroscopy and partial or total synovectomy.
- *Limitation of motion:* Once an extension deficit is corrected, it is common for other intra-articular pathology to subside.

IMPORTANT STEPS TO BE CONSIDERED IN REVISION ACL RECONSTRUCTION

The new femoral tunnel should be placed at 9 or 9.30 positions for right knee or at 3 or 3.30 positions for the left. It is important to achieve a PL femoral tunnel by drilling through the anteromedial or accessory anteromedial portal in order to control rotation as well as anterior translation of the knee. One might be able to avoid old tunnel femoral tunnel, if it was at 12, 11, or 1 o'clock position. This new placement will not only be able to control anterior displacement but also rotational instability.

Radiographically, the tibial tunnel should be placed directly posterior to the intersection point of the Blumensaat's line and the tibial joint line (on lateral view in full knee extension). Placement of the tibial tunnel too anteriorly might lead to an extension deficit due to the graft impingement, which possibly can result into a graft failure. Also, an excessively anterior tibial tunnel can cause high-tension forces to the graft in knee flexion ('nutcracker knee'). In addition to the graft elongation and secondly failure, this may lead to a flexion deficit. In countries of Southeast Asia as well as in Muslim countries, when a person sits on the ground for daily activities, such forces might result in early and massive chondral defects, and eventually lead to painful knees, especially when the femoral tunnel is anteriorly placed.

- *ACL graft removal:* If the patient's clinical symptoms do not improve after 1–2 revision reconstruction surgeries by an expert, graft removal should be considered. Either this patient will have extension deficit, flexion deficit and/or pain. Clinical comparison of both knees should be done, and if operated graft is tight as compared with opposite side, this should be considered as pain generator. If any laxity testing machine is available, this can be quantified. The pain does not allow the patient to fully extend the knee. Here is a perplexing situation. The knee is stable but the graft removal has to be done for persistent clinical pain in spite of one or two revision surgeries. This should be done only as a last resort. One should never ever ignore a patient who complains of persistent pain with deformity after ligament reconstruction surgery because the cause is more likely to the mechanical and technical errors.

Notchplasty: Inadequate notchplasty may lead to graft impingement of the ACL reconstruction with attenuation and subsequent graft failure. Usually, the anterior margin of the intercondylar notch has reformed with fibrocartilage. Before planning a new tunnel, complete removal of this fibrocartilage and osteophytes should be performed. After the removal of this material superiorly and laterally, the bony notch is addressed. Now, the bony notch is enlarged superiorly and laterally creating a vault, to make visualization of the old tunnel as well as the site of the new tunnel easier. It is helpful to view from anteromedial portal, which gives a clear picture of the posterior notch. In extension, there should be 6 mm of clearance between the graft and the superior notch, while throughout flexion there should be no contact between the graft and the inner wall of the lateral femoral condyle.

Final adjustments to the notch must await insertion of the graft. If additional notchplasty is needed once the graft has been fixed to the femur, to protect the graft, either additional bone can be removed by small curved osteotomy and mallet (safe) or by a specialized type of a burr. This burr should be used with a blunt surface keeping towards the graft. Suction should not be used while using the motorized burr.

Arthroscopic confirmation of adequacy of notchplasty is performed as the knee is ranged from full flexion to extension, ensuring that the graft does not impinge against the PCL, the anterior roof, or the lateral wall of the notch.

Graft fixation: In choosing a fixation technique following points should be considered:

- Circumferential (360°) healing of graft against tunnel wall (IF screw cannot achieve this)
- Bioabsorbable material
- Strong initial fixation.

Although there are a variety of fixation methods available, the most popular is the Endobutton and/or IF screw on the femoral side and cortical screw or IF screw on the tibial side. If there is slightest doubt regarding intratunnel fixation, it will be nice to add cortical fixation on both side with simple screw and a washer or a suture disk (**Figures 43.17A and B**).

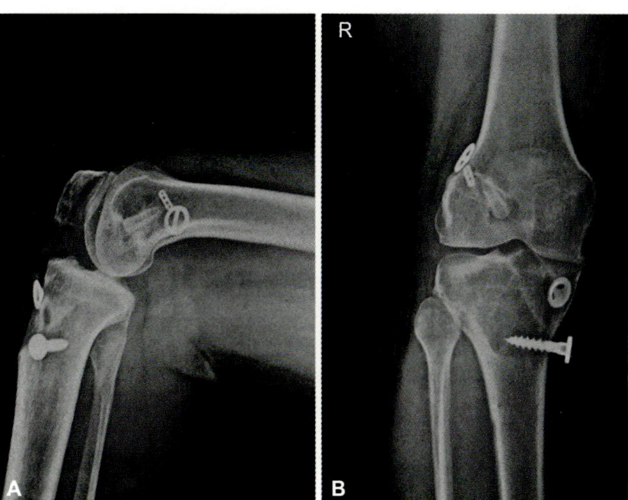

Figures 43.17A and B Additional fixation with cortical screw and suture disc

- *ACL with (PLC) or MCL laxity:* This combination of injuries is frequently not recognized until after failure of an ACL reconstruction, which may have been technically well performed. In PL laxity there is increased external tibial rotation at 30° of flexion, associated varus laxity and hyperextension of knee joint. This kind of laxity loads the newly constructed ACL especially when a patient gets up from sitting on the ground. Restoration of lateral collateral ligament (LCL), popliteus tendon, and PL capsule are critical to successful repair. This is normally done with SemiT harvested from opposite side (modified Larson's technique) but with more laxity, one should be ready to reconstruct popliteofibular complex as well as the LCL separately. Iliotibial and biceps tenodesis are additional salvage procedures that one needs to know while addressing PLC injury (**Figure 43.18**). In chronic case of ACL with MCL laxity grade 3, both the ACL and MCL need to be reconstructed.

REVISION POSTERIOR CRUCIATE LIGAMENT (PCL) RECONSTRUCTION

Our knowledge about the problems after the PCL deficient knee is definitely increasing, so is the PCL reconstruction surgery. The PCL is more difficult ligament to reconstruct and so the failure is also more. Most of the patients will find it very difficult to sit on the ground and to squat, if

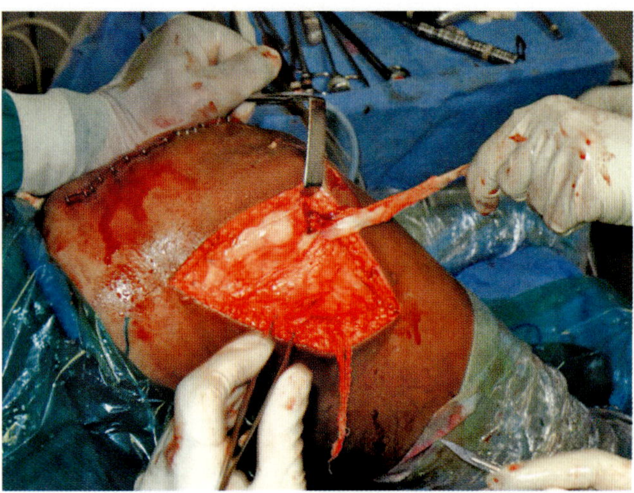

Figure 43.18 Addressing PLC injury

there is a PCL deficient knee. These problems will become more profound if there is an associated posteromedial or posterolateral corner (PLC) laxity. The failed PCL reconstruction can result in pain, instability, or stiffness, especially after sitting for a few minutes on a chair or a couch. There can be rapid secondary arthritic changes of the patellofemoral joint as well as medial compartment if this issue is not addressed in time. It is important to identify the causes for failure of the PCL reconstruction surgery. These can be divided into primary or secondary.

Primary failures can be due to poor tunnel placement, especially the tibial tunnel, failure to identify combined laxity, improper autograft tensioning or fixation, and postoperative infection. If meniscus or articular cartilage pathology was not addressed properly at the time of initial reconstruction surgery, it can also contribute to graft failure.

Secondly failures can be due to improper aggressive rehabilitation, inadequate graft healing, new trauma, or a noncompliant patient. In the countries where people have to sit on the ground, failure to address PLC laxity at the time of primary PCL reconstruction surgery is the single largest cause of failure of primary ligament reconstruction surgery.

Noyes et al. studied multiple causes of failure of PCL reconstruction surgery. They could identify 41% patients had untreated PLC injury and 39% of patients had poorly placed tunnels. The third most common cause was untreated varus malalignment. So it is important to have a hip knee ankle. X-ray (alignment X-ray) along with MRI when one plans a revision PCL reconstruction surgery.

How to Manage a Revision PCL Reconstruction?

Thorough preoperative history and a proper clinical examination of patient is very important; it should start with patient standing and taking weight on both knees. A patient should be made to walk to appreciate varus thrust or recurvatum if there is any. If there is varus deformity, there is an increased load on the PL structures that ultimately results into the failure of the ligament reconstruction. The preoperative range of movements as well as medial or lateral laxity must be recorded property. If the posterior displacement is more than 10 mm, it is important to check for PL laxity. The record of previous surgery should give an insight to which graft material will be available for revision. It is important to understand whether the presenting complaint is pain or instability. For most of the patients of PCL injury, instability is not the main problem. Simple examination from lateral side in approximately 70° knee flexion in a relaxed patient will show posterior sag of affected side. To elicit clinical picture of the PCL sag, one needs to be proficient in conducting tests for ligament laxity, especially posterior drawer, Lachman's test, step off test of Harner, and Godfrey's test (relaxed patient, hip, and knees flexed at 90°; posterior displacement of tibia is seen in the case of PCL deficiency). To rule out associated PLC injury, dial test should be done at 30° and 90° of knee flexion. If tibial external rotation increases at 30°, it is consistent with the isolated PLC injury while if external rotation increases in both 30° and 90°, then it is indicating of PCL\PLC injury. In this situation, a biplanar osteotomy is indicated for simultaneous correction of varus and to increase the tibial slope to make PCL tight by open wedge osteotomy (**Figures 43.19A and B**). Some patients may not require ligament reconstruction surgery after a good biplanar osteotomy. It is also very important to recognize fixed posterior capsular contracture in the long-standing PCL failure cases because this needs to be corrected before any other surgery is done. Proper evaluation of neurovascular status as well as examination of spine

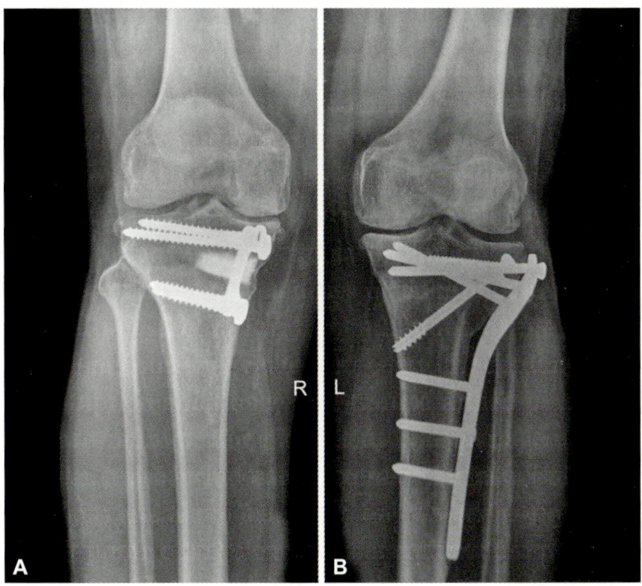

Figures 43.19A and B Open wedge osteotomy

cannot be over emphasized. Special attention should be given to any signs of pre-existing injury to popliteal vessels or peroneal nerve. If that is any doubt about was vascular insufficiency, Doppler study ± arteriogram should be done. Before surgical intervention for revision surgery, preoperative planning, and discussion is a must with the patient as well as the surgical team.

Following imaging modalities can help for better outcome of surgery:

- *X-ray—AP and lateral:* This will not only show patellar changes but also the tunnels as well as hardware.
- PA flexion weight-bearing in 45° flexion (for notch constriction and joint line narrowing) and Merchant's view of patella.
- HKA X-ray (full-standing view to have hip, knee, and ankle in a single cassette) to calculate varus of valgus deformity. This needs to be corrected first if it is not in acceptable range (**Figure 43.20**).
- Stress radiography should be done by an orthopedic surgeon himself or by a competent radiologist who understands the importance of such views. The radiographic analysis can be helpful to diagnose degree of fixed posterior tibial capsular contracture and to diagnose other injuries that may affect the treatment. Posterior capsular contracture is more common than

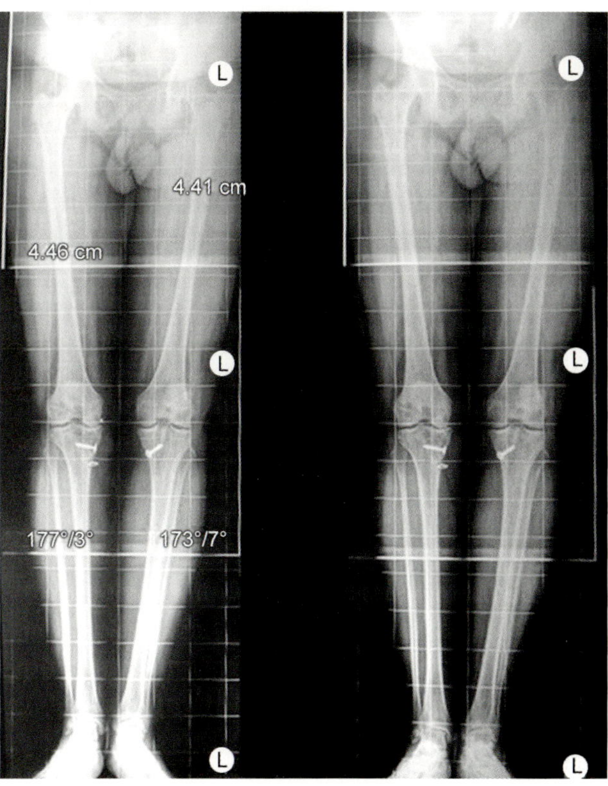

Figure 43.20 Hip, knee, ankle (HKA) standing X-rays

we think, and plain neutral rotation radiograph of both knees in 90° flexion will show the obvious deformity.

- *CT scan:* If there was postoperative infection or tunnel dilatation on the X-ray, CT scan is the most important modality before surgery. It helps to measure the tunnel diameter and will also detect other bony changes like osteophytes and loose bodies.
- *MRI:* It is very important to know about all the injuries, especially of articular cartilage before revision PCL surgery. For this purpose MRI has proved to be a very important imaging modality. Not only it does show meniscus or ligament injury but also can throw light on cartilage injuries as well as synovitis. CT scan has its role to measure tunnel enlargement especially in postoperative infection failure.

Graft Choice

If the primary reconstruction was done by Hamstring graft, either the Q tendon or BPTB autograft can be used from either limb. Q tendon graft with 20 mm bone plug or

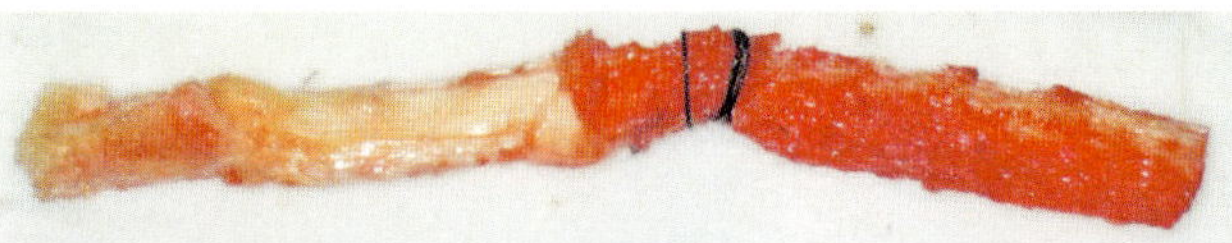

Figure 43.21 Bone patellar tendon bone (BPTB) graft

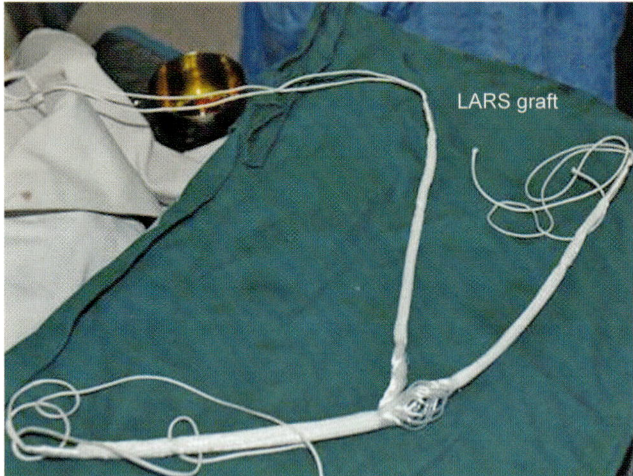

Figure 43.22 LARS artificial graft

BPTB graft with 50 mm or more long tibial plug with a total length of 100–110 mm should be used for revision surgery (**Figure 43.21**). Availability of allograft will definitely reduce morbidity but it has its own problems. Long-term results of the PCL revision surgery with artificial grafts like the LARS (**Figure 43.22**), neo-ligament, and carbon fiber are not encouraging. Carbon fiber is already discarded for routine ligament reconstruction surgery.

PCL RECONSTRUCTION: SURGICAL TECHNIQUE

After making an accurate diagnosis of the pathologies, it is important to do counseling of the patient because there is a gap between expectations and ultimate results as far as revision PCL reconstruction surgery is concerned. All scars of previous surgery are checked for their mobility as well as for surgical planning. Contraindications for surgery are arthrofibrosis and the restricted ROM, a fixed posterior drawer that cannot be reduced. In such cases double pin traction for few days is given to stretch posterior capsule first and bring it to neutral status.

Essential requirements in the operation theater are availability of 3 L normal saline bottles, injection epinephrine, all the implants and instrumentation and an efficient surgical team where each member knows his or her role. Fluid pressure pump, IITV, and radio-frequency device like arthrocare can facilitate the surgery but are not absolutely a must. It is always important to take prior permission from the patient to use graft material from the contralateral limb, especially in case of multiple ligaments reconstruction revision surgery. Also, the surgeon should be aware about IT band usage for ligament surgery as well as biceps tenodesis.

Transtibial Tunnel Technique

Under spinal anesthesia and tourniquet control, examination is done once again of both lower limbs before undertaking surgery. The range of movements is recorded. Diagnostic knee scopy is done with a 30° scope. Anatomy and pathology is assessed. A double bundle PCL reconstruction might be a preferred method in case of a revision PCL reconstruction but nonavailability of the allograft or artificial graft may limit one to use single bundle revision surgery. In rare situation split Q tendon graft can be used for two bundles reconstruction (**Figure 43.23**). If the primary surgery was by hamstring grafts, the graft choices now available are either Q tendon or BPTB graft. We believe that there is no role of a 7 or 8 mm. Hamstring graft for a revision surgery. The ideal width should be 10 mm or more and length of 100 mm (10 cm) or more. Once diagnostic arthroscopy is finished, the graft is harvested and prepared. Its diameter is carefully measured. Q tendon graft can be with or without the bone plug. The bone plug length when used for femoral tunnel should be of approximately 20 mm length. If it is longer than this, then it can be extremely difficult to negotiate it in the femoral tunnel if the intercondylar area is small.

Removal of Old PCL

With 30° scope from anterolateral portal, remnant of PCL is debrided if it was completely torn. In the case of a stretched PCL (usually AL bundle), we try to preserve the

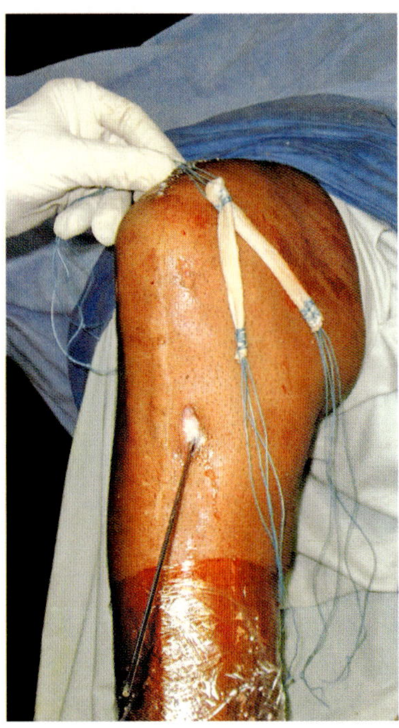

Figure 43.23 Q tendon graft

PM bundle and augment PCL. A space is created between the ACL and PCL to insert the scope in the popliteal region. A 70° scope can be of great help but it is not a must. A tissue elevator-cum-wire catcher (ACUFEX) from AM portal helps to elevate torn fibers as well as fibrous tissue from posterior tibia. One can measure the depth of cleaning up of the tissue by observing the depth markings on the tissue elevator. Clearing up to 20–25 mm is adequate for a successful revision surgery. Shaver is inserted in the popliteal region to clean the tissue as well as the stump. It is absolutely a must to keep the tip of the shaver blade under scope vision all the time. High flow of normal saline is required to keep the posterior capsule away. 3 L bottles of normal saline at approximately 4–6 feet above the top of the table are sufficient. Portals should be placed in such a manner that there will be minimal leakage. For good tissue clearance, Use of a curved shaver blade is useful. If multiple ligament reconstruction surgery is being considered with the revision PCL reconstruction, one ampoule of epinephrine should be added to first two bottles of normal saline to reduce blood oozing and this facilitates arthroscopic surgery. Fluid pressure pump can be used but one needs to constantly monitor fluid extravasation in the popliteal the region that can cause compartment syndrome after few hours.

Drilling a Tibial Tunnel (Figure 43.24)

Posteromedial portal is created and the 30° arthroscope is transferred to this portal. PCL tibial attachment is visualized. A PCL jig with tibial aimer is fixed at 60° to 65° angles. This reduces 'Killer angle turn' on the back of the tibia and facilitates passing of autograft or allograft. Tibial aimer is passed from AM portal to the popliteal area and its position is fixed under vision at an anatomical point on the posterior tibia. Drill tipped passing pin or a K wire is drilled from anterior or anteromedial tibia to posterior very gently. It is stopped as soon its tip is seen in the vision of the scope. Anterolateral bundle of PCL needs to be recreated so it is important to verify proper placement of the drill tipped pin. Image intensifier can be used for this but it is not essential. Once the position of the pin is confirmed, a flower head reamer of same or 1 mm less than the diameter of harvested/prepared graft is placed on the pin. From the anteromedial portal, tissue elevator-cum-wire catcher is passed in the popliteal region before drilling and tip of the drill is firmly secured with this instrument. This can also be done with the help of a curved scoop. The idea is that the pin should not migrate backwards while drilling and injure the neurovascular structures in the popliteal region. Tibial tunnel is created from the center or anteromedial side of

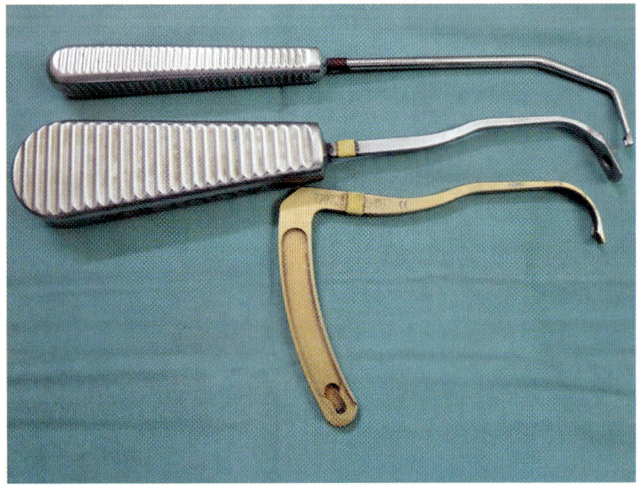

Figure 43.24 PCL jig and instruments to facilitate arthroscopic PCL reconstruction

the tibia to the center of the joint where the tip of the tibial aimer is placed for an anatomical revision; PCL surgery drilling is done all the time under vision. The tunnel is cleared of any remnants of old ligament, suture material or tissue. A dilator of same diameter of the graft dilates the tunnel by compressing the bone inside the tunnel. A 24-gauge long wire loop is passed from tibia to popliteal fossa. With the help of a Grabber or a Crochet hook, this wire is brought in the intercondylar notch and placed in the back part of the intercondylar notch.

Femoral Tunnel

Femoral tunnel can be done either by the outside-in technique with the help of a PCL femoral aimer or by the inside-out freehand technique. In both the techniques, one has to be careful that when a pin is placed at an anatomical place on medial femoral condyle, it should not pass very near the lateral femoral condyle. There should be enough gaps left to make femoral tunnel without injuring articular cartilage of medial femoral condyle, especially while using inside out technique. A 20 mm socket is created in the medial femoral condyle from inside and rest of the tunnel is drilled with a 4 mm drill to facilitate pulling of the graft. All the soft tissue around the femoral hole is also cleared.

Previously placed 24 gauge wire is pulled out of the femoral tunnel with the help of two Crochet hooks. This needs patience. Once the SS wire is passing through both the tunnels, the tunnel dilator is inserted in the tibial tunnel to confirm that no tissue is in the way on a new PCL graft.

Graft Passage

The BPTB or Q tendon graft prepared with Ethibond no. 5 is placed in the wire loop at tibial end. With the help of the probe and gentle constant pull, femoral bone plug is carefully pulled into the femoral tunnel of medial femoral condyle. The new ligament is checked for its lightness, placement as well as impingement by other structures or bony overgrowth. Femoral end is either fixed with a titanium screw or a bioscrew. It is important to have very sound fixation so that the early ROM exercises can be initiated. This can help in graft incorporation as well as

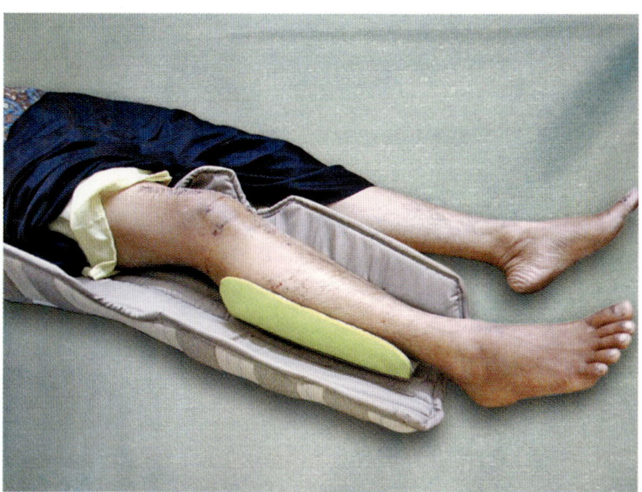

Figure 43.25 Posterior cruciate ligament (PCL) brace

maintaining healthy articular cartilage. On the tibial side, if the bone of the plug is sufficiently long, it can be fixed by the metal or IF screw. In the case of any doubt, a suture disk or a ligament screw can be used to work for fixing a new PCL on the tibial side. It is important to keep the knee in 70°–90° of flexion and translated anteriorly while tightening or inserting the tibial screw. The knee is finally checked for the elimination of laxity.

Surgeon and anesthetist should check the distal perfusion of the operated limb once tourniquet is released. A PCL brace that supports the upper-half of the posterior tibia is applied in the operation theater before shifting the patient to the room (**Figure 43.25**).

On the next day of surgery, patient is allowed full weight-bearing walker ambulation if fixation is sound and only isolated revision PCL reconstruction surgery is done. Patient is encouraged due to static quadriceps, straight leg raising (SLR), ankle pumps and passive patella mobilization exercises with in the limit of tolerance of pain. Distal pulsation is monitored for the next 24 hours at least. Before sending the patient home, patient is explained about potential hazard of deep vein thrombosis and the need for thromboprophylaxis.

If there is already substantial varus deformity with ligament laxity, it is important to do a varus correction with alteration of the tibial slope with medial open wedge osteotomy before attempting revision surgery for the ACL or PCL deficient knees. If there is still PL laxity is present, PL reconstruction must be done (**Figure 43.26**). In cases of

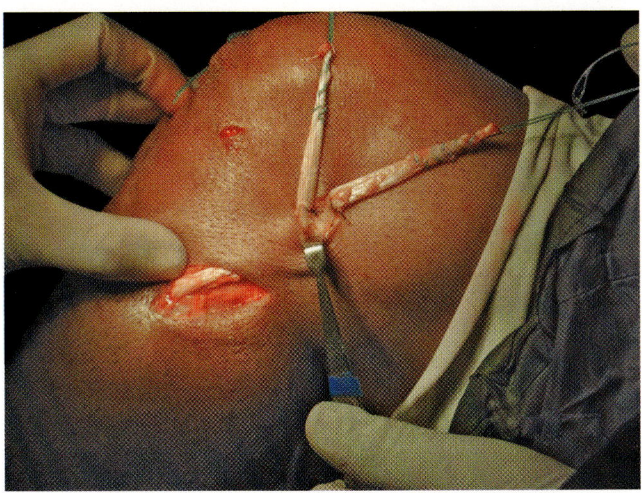

Figure 43.26 Posterolateral corner reconstruction

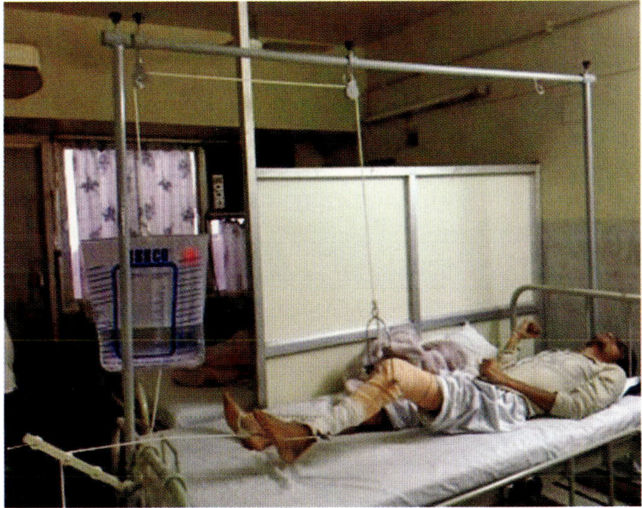

Figure 43.27 Double pin traction

the old primary PCL reconstruction that came with fixed posterior capsular contracture, we may need to consider applying a double pin traction to stretch posterior capsule (**Figure 43.27**) and bring tibia to normal position. Very rarely posterior capsulotomy might be required in resistive case. After full correction, the revision PCL reconstruction should be attempted.

Postoperative Rehabilitation

In revised ligament reconstruction surgery, one should not be very aggressive about using different kinds of modalities in the initial stages of rehabilitation. Before the revision surgery, it is very important for a surgeon to discuss with the patient regarding physiotherapy he/she will be required to do and for how long. It is useful to counsel the patient by teaching them SLR, static quadriceps exercises and ankle pumps. Postoperative brace and use of support like a walker, elbow crutch, or a stick will be required for almost 3 months. If additional ACL reconstruction is done with cartilage surgery like microfracture or mosaicplasty, it is advisable to use a CPM and delay weight-bearing.

For PCL rehabilitation, the dictum is to go slow. PCL being an anti-antigravity ligament, it is important to protect the revision reconstruct for long time against damaging forces. Usually a PCL brace is continued for three months at night. Patient usually is not allowed to sit in a chair in 90° flexion knee for 6 weeks. The knee bending is allowed in prone position as soon as possible after the surgery depending on the fixation of the graft and additional procedures done for revision surgery. This ensures cartilage nourishment as well as has the muscles around the knee. In case of multiple ligamentous reconstruction, a plaster application for 4–6 weeks will not have that detrimental effect as compared to the experience of laxity if immediate exercises are started. Sporting activities are not allowed for six months to one year. A sports person will require an additional rehabilitation under the care of a professional physiotherapist for proprioception, muscle strength, agility and strength training. Also, the surgeon should discuss about possibility returning to sports at a reduced level as compared to his/her primary ligament surgery level.

Guidelines for Revision Ligament Reconstruction Surgery

- *Perfect planning:* Clinical examination, radiography, availability of implants
- Efficient anesthetist (epidural anesthesia might be needed) and theater team
- *Good tourniquet and enough saline for arthroscopy:* Fluid at height or infusion pump
- *Prepare both the limbs for graft harvest:* Take prior consent

- Confirm your diagnosis, especially of PLC and MCL laxity under anesthesia
- Knee in 90° flexion for both revision surgeries
- Remove essential hardware only, along with all suture and other nonabsorbable material
- Harvest required grafts and ask assistant to prepare them
- *Make perfect tunnels:* The same as the diameter of the prepared graft
- *Pass the graft gently:* BPTB graft for PCL reconstruction difficult to pass
- *Fix the graft properly in both tunnels:* If needed use double fixation on both sides
- Confirm your reconstruction by doing re-arthroscopy
- *PCL brace to protect the graft from failure:* For 2–3 months
- Spend time with the patient after surgery for explaining rehabilitation
- *Do not hesitate to do two-stage revision or osteotomy:* Results are better
- Long-term follow-up is needed.

BIBLIOGRAPHY

1. Amendola AS, Giffin JR, Sanders DW. Osteotomy for knee stability: the effect of increasing tibial slope on anterior tibial translation. Paper presented at: American Association for Orthopaedic Sports Medicine, Specialty Day; San Francisco; 2001.
2. Clatworthy M, Amendola AS. The anterior cruciate ligament and arthritis. Clin Sports Med. 1999; 18:173-98.
3. Colville MR, Bowman RR. The significance of isometer measurements and graft position during anterior cruciate ligament reconstruction. Am J Sports Med. 1993;21:832-5.
4. Dejour H, Neyret P, Bonnin M. In: Fu F (Ed), Knee Surgery. Baltimore, MD: Williams & Wilkins; 1994. pp. 859-75.
5. Dejour H, Walch G, Chambat P, et al. Active subluxation in extension: a new concept of study of the ACL deficient knee. Am J Knee Surg. 1988; 1:204-11.
6. Fanelli GC, Edson CJ, Manish DR. Revision anterior cruciate ligament reconstruction. Associated patholaxity, tibiofemoral malalignment, rehabilitation, and results. Am J Knee Surg. 2001; 14(3):201-4.
7. Fanelli GC. Complications in PCL surgery. In: Fanelli GC (Ed.), Posterior Cruciate Ligament Injuries. A Practical Guide to Management. New York: Springer-Verlag; 2001. pp. 291-302.
8. Fanelli GC. The multiple ligament injured knee: a practical guide to management; New York: Springer; 2004. pp. 227-40.
9. Gillogly SD, Andrews JR, Schaeffer RA, et al. Pitfalls of intra-articular anterior cruciate ligament reconstruction. Orthop Trans. 1993;16:820.
10. Hegyes MS, Richardson MW, Miller MD. Knee dislocation: complications of nonoperative and operative management. Clin sports Med. 2000; 19:519-43.
11. Hughston JC, Jacobsen KE. Chronic posterolateral rotatory instability of the knee. J Bone Joint Surg Am. 1985; 67:351-9.
12. Kartus J, Stener S, Lindahl S, Erikkson BL, Karlsson J. Ipsi- or contralateral patellar tendon graft in anterior cruciate ligament revision surgery. A comparison of two methods. Am J Sports Med. 1998;26(4):499-504.
13. Kurosaka M, Yoshiya S, Andrish JT. A biomechanical comparison of different surgical techniques of graft fixation in anterior cruciate ligament reconstruction. Am J Sports Med. 1987;15:225-9.
14. Markoff KL, Bargar WL, Shoemaker SC, et al. The role of joint load in knee stability. J None Bone Joint Surg Am. 1981; 63(4): 570-85.
15. Matthews L, Lawrence S, Vahiro MA, et al. Fixation strengths of patellar tendon bone grafts. Arthroscopy. 1993;9:76-81.
16. Morgan CD, Kalmam VR, Grawl DM. Isometry testing for anterior cruciate ligament revisited. Arthroscopy. 1995;11:647-59.
17. Naudie D, Amendola A, Fowler P. Opening wedge high tibial osteotomy for chronic posteror instability. Proceedings of the meeting of the American Association for Orthopedic Sports Medicine; Keystone, CO; 2001.
18. Noyes FR, Barber-Westin SD, Hewett TE. High tibial osteotomy and ligament reconstruction for varus angulated anterior cruciate ligament-deficient knees. Am J Sports Med. 2000; 28(3):282-96.
19. Penner DA, Daniel DM, Wood P, et al. An in vitro study of anterior cruciate ligament graft placement and isometry. Am J Sports Med. 1988;16:238-43.

20. Prodromos CC, Joyes BT, Shi K, Keller BL, et al. A meta-analysis of stability after anterior cruciate ligament reconstruction as a function of hamstring versus patellar tendon graft and fixation type. Arthroscopy. 2005;21:1202.
21. Robertson DB, Daniel DM, Biden E. Soft tissue fixation to bone. Am J Sports Med. 1986;14:398-403.
22. Strobel MJ. Manual of Arthroscopic Surgery. New York: Springer-Verlag; 2001.
23. Strobel MJ. Posterior Cruciate Ligament. New York: Springer-Verlag.
24. Yaru NC, Daniel DM, Penner D. The effect of tibial attachment site on graft impingement in an anterior cruciate ligament reconstruction. Am J Sports Med. 1992; 20:217-20.
25. Zarins B, Marder R. Revision of failed arthroscopic and ligament surgery. Blackwell Science; New Jersey, USA; 1998.

Chapter 44

Dislocation of the Knee

Ashok Rajgopal, Vivek Dahiya, Vipin Tyagi

Dislocation of the knee is defined as a complete disruption of the tibiofemoral joint (**Figures 44.1A and B**). A subluxation is a partial disruption of the joint with some tibiofemoral contact remaining. Apart from the damage to the intra-articular and stabilizing structures, the neurovascular bundle too can be damaged resulting in a limb-threatening situation. The following structures can be damaged when a knee dislocates: cruciate ligaments, collateral ligaments, menisci, articular cartilage, medial and lateral capsular structures, popliteal artery, tibial, and peroneal nerves. These injuries require a timely and accurate diagnosis, stabilization, and treatment.

INCIDENCE

The yearly incidence of knee dislocation has been reported to range from 1/10,000 to 1/100,000.[1] However, accurate data are difficult to obtain on account of the fact that a number of dislocations reduce spontaneously, leading to a wrong diagnosis at presentation. In case a knee presents with a gross instability of two or more ligaments, it must be evaluated on the lines of a dislocated knee.

MECHANISM OF INJURY

Severe high-energy trauma to the knee (vehicular accidents) accounts for the majority of knee dislocations. These are more destructive to the soft-tissue envelope of the knee and have a higher incidence (32%) of associated vascular injury.[2] Sports-related low energy trauma also lead to knee dislocations with football (35%) and wrestling (15%) being the more common ones contributing to this.[3] The incidence of vascular complications is also low (4.6%).[4]

CLASSIFICATION

Kennedy in 1963 classified knee dislocations on the basis of the direction of displacement of the tibia in relation to the femur (**Table 44.1**).[5]

This classification was simple to follow and remember, but it did not portray the specific injury patterns and did not guide the treatment.

Schenk[6] in 1994 proposed a classification focusing on the pattern of ligament injury with the presence or absence of fractures. Yu[7] further modified it by the

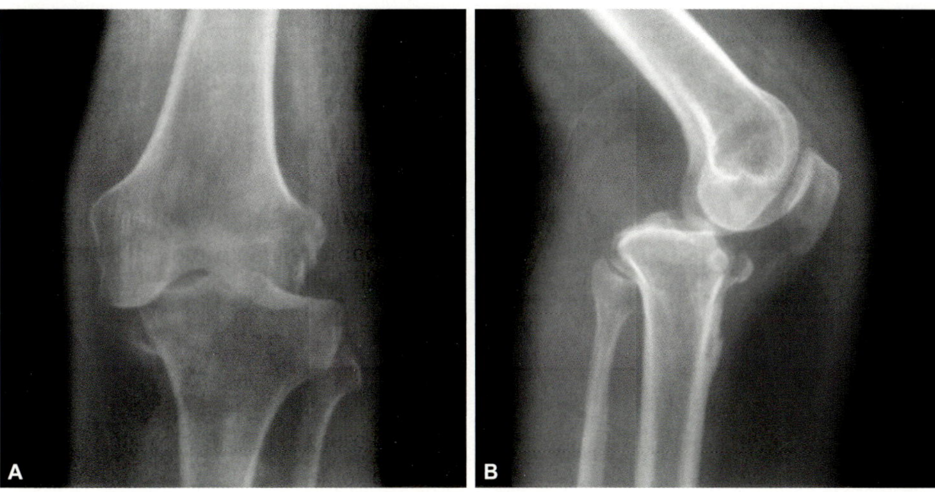

Figures 44.1A and B X-rays showing knee dislocation

TABLE 44.1 Kennedy classification of knee dislocations

Type of dislocation	Incidence[2,5]	Mechanism	Structures involved (in order of giving way)
Anterior	40%	Hyperextension High or low energy	Posterior capsule ACL PCL Popliteal artery (at 50° of hyperextension)
Posterior	33%	High energy dashboard injuries	PCL ACL MCL/LCL Popliteal artery
Medial	18%	High-energy varus trauma	MCL + LCL ACL/PCL Associated fractures
Lateral	4%	High-injury valgus trauma	MCL + LCL ACL/PCL Associated fractures
Rotatory	5%	Rotatory force	Both collaterals Both cruciates

Abbreviations: ACL, anterior cruciate ligament; PCL, posterior cruciate ligament; MCL, medial collateral ligament; LCL, lateral collateral ligament.

TABLE 44.2 Schenk classification of knee dislocations (modified by Yu)

Classification	Subclass	Associated ligament injury
KD-I		Single cruciate: ACL or PCL
KD-II		Bicruciate: ACL and PCL
KD-III		Bicruciate and posteromedial or posterolateral: ACL + PCL + MCL or ACL + PCL + LCL/PLC
KD-IV		Bicruciate and posteromedial and posterolateral: ACL + PCL + MCL + LCL/PLC
KD-V		Dislocation with associated fracture
	KD-V1	Single cruciate: ACL or PCL
	KD-V2	Bicruciate: ACL and PCL
	KD-V3M	Bicruciate and posteromedial: ACL + PCL + MCL
	KD-V3L	Bicruciate and posterolateral: ACL + PCL + LCL/PLC
	KD-V4	Bicruciate and posteromedial and posterolateral: ACL + PCL + MCL + LCL/PLC

Abbreviation: PLC, posterolateral corner.

addition of arterial or neural injury. Injuries are classified according to the number of ligaments injured from I to IV, and V denotes a fracture. This number is preceded by KD denoting knee dislocation. C and N are used to denote associated vascular and neurologic injury, respectively (**Table 44.2**).

More recently, a pathophysiological classification has been proposed by SOFCOT (The French Society of Orthopedic Surgery and Traumatology) that combines the direction of dislocation and the pattern of ligament injury (**Table 44.3**).[8]

VASCULAR INJURY

The incidence of vascular injury associated with a knee dislocation varies from 5% to 80% in the literature.[9] The

TABLE 44.3 The French Society of Orthopedic Surgery and Traumatology (SOFCOT) Classification

Type 1		Simple bicruciate lesion without dislocation
	Type 1a	Medial
	Type 1b	Lateral
	Type 1c	Posterior
Type 2		Pure dislocation without peripheral tear
	Type 2a	Anterior
	Type 2b	Posterior
Type 3		Dislocation with single cruciate lesion
	Type 3a	ACL
	Type 3b	PCL
Type 4		Combined lesions associating peripheral tear and dislocation
	Type 4a	Medial (lateral dislocation)
	Type 4b	Lateral (medial dislocation)
	Type 4c	Complex (rotational medial and lateral tear)

treatment of vascular injury takes precedence over the dislocation, and a vascular surgeon should be involved at the outset. Delay in vascularization of more than 8 hours from the time of injury increases the amputation rates from 13% to 86%.[2] The popliteal artery lies in the subcutaneous tissue of the popliteal fossa tethered proximally at the adductor hiatus and distally by a fibrous band covering the soleus. This immobility predisposes it to injury during a knee dislocation. Anterior dislocations more often result in traction injuries (> 50° of hyperextension) to the popliteal artery, whereas posterior dislocations result in a higher rate of arterial transection as the proximal tibia is thrust posteriorly into the vessel.[5]

NEUROLOGIC INJURY

Neurologic injury, after a dislocated knee, has an incidence of 16–50%.[1,10] Most commonly, the peroneal or posterior tibial nerve is injured in a posterolateral dislocation, though all types of dislocations can result in nerve injury. The peroneal nerve is at the greatest risk on account of its tethering around the fibular head. The mechanism of injury is most commonly a traction injury, resulting in various degrees of neuropraxia or axonotmesis. Only about 50% of patients regain function after a peroneal nerve injury.[11]

EVALUATION

The evaluation of a dislocated knee begins with a detailed history and an attempt to elicit the mechanism of injury. Particular attention must be paid to identify the potential-associated injuries. There should be a high index of suspicion to exclude the possibility of knee dislocation followed by spontaneous reduction. Beware of the patient who walks in with complaints of instability. There may be no effusion, and at times minimal pain but on clinical examination gross instability may be noted. The surgeon in the emergency focuses on the inspection of the limb, skin integrity, color, vascular assessment, and visual and tactile joint examination. A neurovascular examination must be done and documented prior to and after reducing a dislocated knee. Vascular surgery consultation must be sought after immediately if the pulses are absent or decreased and/or the postreduction ankle brachial index is >0.9. Sensation in the distribution of both superficial and deep peroneal nerves should be assessed and peroneal nerve motor function documented. Radiographs are obtained to determine the direction of dislocation and assess the presence of any fractures. After the reduction radiographs are obtained again to verify the reduction and if the joint is grossly unstable, some form of splintage or external fixation may be deemed essential. Ligamentous damage is then assessed using the standard tests, and instability patterns are documented. Once the patients are medically stabilized, an MRI scan of the knee is done to evaluate the integrity of the ligaments, menisci, and cartilage in the knee joint.

PRINCIPLES OF MANAGEMENT OF A KNEE DISLOCATION

The treatment of knee dislocation has evolved from conservative management to early surgical repair/reconstruction. Conservative management involved the closed reduction of the dislocation followed by 6–9 weeks of immobilization in a splint or cast. This led to the increased incidence of residual instability and poor ranges of motion.[5,12-14] There is enough evidence in the published literature that surgical treatment provides better results.[15]

However, a few questions need to be answered conclusively when managing the knee dislocations surgically. Timing of surgery, repair or reconstruct, sequence of ligament repair, and graft choices are the controversies currently not solved.

Urgent surgical intervention is required in the case of a vascular injury, open dislocations[16] or irreducible dislocations[17] (most commonly a posterolateral dislocation with button holing of the medial femoral condyle through the medial joint capsule with subsequent invagination of the capsule into the joint). Fractures associated with knee dislocations ought to be fixed urgently.

Early surgery (within 2–3 weeks) has shown to give better International Knee Documentation Committee (IKDC) scores, higher rates of return to work and return to sports.[5,12-14] In an acute setting, all bony avulsion injuries must be repaired, and the reconstruction of PCL and ACL must be done.[12,13] The repair of the cruciates has a higher rate of flexion loss, posterior sag, and inability to return to preinjury activity levels. Hence, the reconstruction of cruciate ligaments is the preferred option.

Delay in the treatment of collateral ligaments compromises the surgeon's ability to repair the tissues. Grade I and II MCL tears can be treated conservatively in a long hinged knee brace. Grade III MCL tears need repair/reconstruction or a posterior oblique ligament advancement. Avulsion injuries may be fixed and mid-substance tears can be augmented using autologous semitendinosus or gracilis grafts.

The treatment of lateral collateral ligament/posterolateral complex injuries follows the same principles. Reconstruction is advisable as the repair has shown a higher rate of failure.[18]

In the case of concomitant vascular injury, which was repaired, a delay of 10–14 days is recommended and the surgery is performed without a tourniquet.

Autografts are desirable, but in a dislocated knee gives rise to a few problems, namely limitation in number, trauma to an already injured knee, donor site morbidity, and increased surgery time. These disadvantages are circumvented by using allografts with the knowledge of increased cost, delayed incorporation of graft and minimal risk of disease transmission.[19] The bone-patellar tendon-bone allograft is preferred for the ACL. Achilles tendon allograft is used for the PCL with the calcaneal bone plug rigidly fixed in the femoral tunnel. LCL is reconstructed with the bone-patellar tendon-bone or the calcaneus tendon allograft.

REHABILITATION

Rehabilitation after knee dislocation is largely dependent on the nature of injury to the ligaments and vascular structures. The primary aim of rehabilitation is to protect the repair/reconstruction, maximize muscle strength, and regain the maximum range of motion and proprioception. In the first phase, after surgery, i.e. till the end of 6 weeks postoperative, the knee is immobilized in a straight knee brace and the focus is on maintaining quadriceps strength by means of isometric exercises. In this phase, the patient is non-weight bearing with the help of a walker or crutches. Thereafter, in the second phase, i.e. week 7–12, the brace is changed to a dial loc type that allows the patient to control knee flexion. Closed-chain knee-bending exercises are started with a progressively increasing range of motion. These may be in the form of heel slides in supine and sitting position. Cycling is another non-weight-bearing closed-chain exercise that is very good for regaining the knee range of motion and increasing strength and endurance. At this stage, the patient progresses to partial weight-bearing ambulation, gradually progressing to full weight-bearing by the end of this phase. In the third phase, from week 13 onward, the knee brace is changed to a functional knee support, and the patient is put on a combination of open- and closed-chain exercises with progressively increasing resistance along with knee proprioceptive exercises. As the strength improves, the patient is put on a progressive-resisted exercise program along with agility exercises and plyometrics, the target being to return to active sports by the end of 6 months from surgery.

CONCLUSION

Knee dislocation is a severe injury with a high potential of being missed and associated neurovascular injuries. It requires an early diagnosis and early appropriate surgical intervention to achieve a satisfactory result.

REFERENCES

1. Meyers MH, Moore TM, Harvey JP Jr. Traumatic dislocation of the knee joint. J Bone Joint Surg Am. 1975;57(3):430-3.
2. Green NE, Allen BL. Vascular injuries associated with dislocation of the knee. J Bone Joint Surg Am. 1977;59(2):236-9.
3. Shelbourne KD, Porter DA, Clingman JA, McCarroll JR, Rettig AC. Low velocity knee dislocation. Orthop Rev. 1991;20:995-1004.
4. Shelbourne KD, Klootwyk TE. Low velocity knee dislocation with sports injuries: Treatment principles. Clin Sports Med. 2000;19:443-56.
5. Dedmond BT, Almekinders LC. Operative versus nonoperative treatment of dislocations: a meta-analysis. Am J Knee Surg. 2001;14:33-8.
6. Schenk RC. Classification and treatment of knee dislocations. Orthop Spec Educ. 1998;4:35.
7. Yu JS, Goodwin D, Salonen D, et al. Complete dislocation of the knee : spectrum of associated soft tissue injuries depicted by MR imaging. AJR Am J Roentgenol. 1995;164(1):135-9.
8. Boisgard S, Versier G, Deschamps S, et al. French Society of Orthopaedic Surgery and Traumatology (SOFCOT): bicruciate ligament lesions and dislocation of the knee: mechanisms and classification. Orthop Traumatol Surg Res. 2009;95(8):627-31.
9. Hoover NW. Injuries of the popliteal artery associated with fractures and dislocations. Surg Clin North Am. 1961;41: 1099.
10. Wascher DC, Dvirnak PC, DeCoster DC. Knee dislocation: initial assessment and implications for treatment. J Orthop Trauma. 1997;11:525.
11. Wood MB. Peroneal nerve repair: surgical results. Clin Orthop Relat Res. 1991;267:206.
12. Harner CD, Waltrip RL, Bennett CH, et al. Surgical management of knee dislocations. J Bone Joint Surg Am. 2004;86:262.
13. Liow RY, McNicholas MJ, Keating JF, Nutton RW. Ligamant repair and reconstruction in traumatic dislocation of the knee. J Bone Joint Surg Br. 2003;85:845.
14. Richter M, Bosch U, Wippermann B, Hofmann A, Krettek C. Comparison of surgical repair or reconstruction of the cruciate ligaments versus nonsurgical treatment in patients with traumatic knee dislocations. Am J Sports Med. 2002;30:718-27.
15. Levy BA, Dajani KA, Whelan DB, et al. Decision making in the multiligament -injured knee—an evidence based systematic review. Arthroscopy. 2009;25(4):430-8.
16. Rihn JA, Cha PS, Groff YJ, Harner CD. The acutely dislocated knee: evaluation and management. J Am Acad Orthop Surg. 2004;12:334.
17. Urguden M, Bilbasar H, Ozenci AM, Akyildiz FF, Gür S. Irreducible posterolateral knee dislocation resulting from a low energy trauma. Arthroscopy. 2004;20(Suppl 1):50-3.
18. Montgomery JB. Dislocation of the knee. Orthop Clin North Am. 1987;18:149.
19. Harner CD, Olson E, Irrgang JJ, et al. Allograft versus autograft anterior cruciate ligament reconstruction: 3 to 5 years outcome. Clin Orthop. 1996:324:134.

Chapter 45

Illustration of Knee MRI

Jatinder Pal Singh

IMAGING PROTOCOL AND MRI ANATOMY

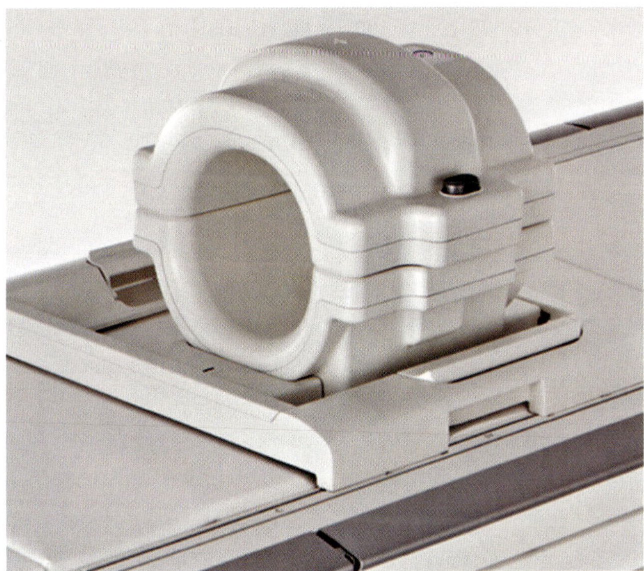

Figure 45.1 A 15-channel knee coil for obtaining dedicated knee MRI scans. Knee is positioned in full extension and 5° of internal rotation

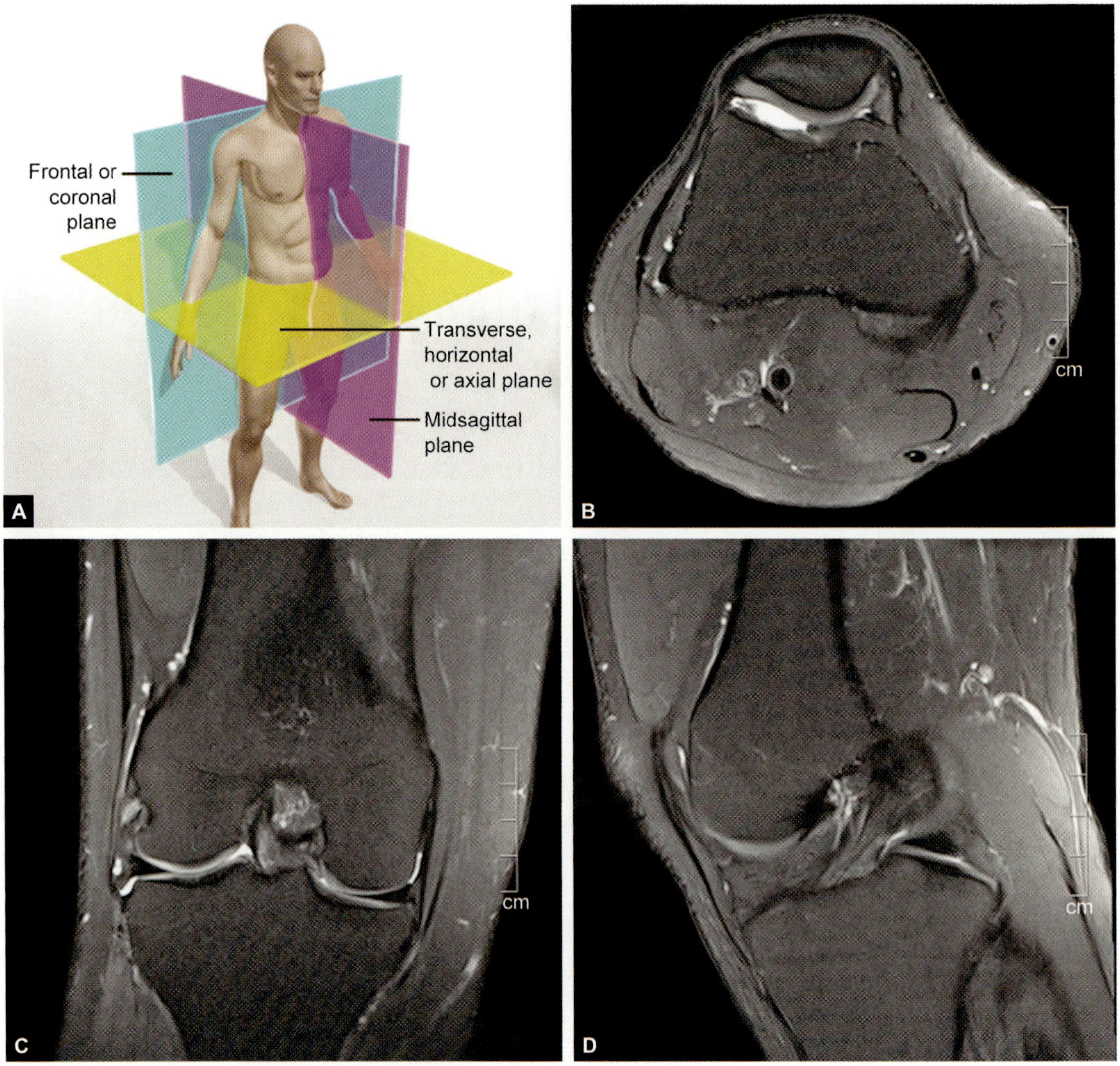

Figures 45.2A to D The knee MR acquisition planes. 3D representation (A) of three planes in which MR imaging is performed. These are axial (B), coronal (C) and sagittal oblique (D)

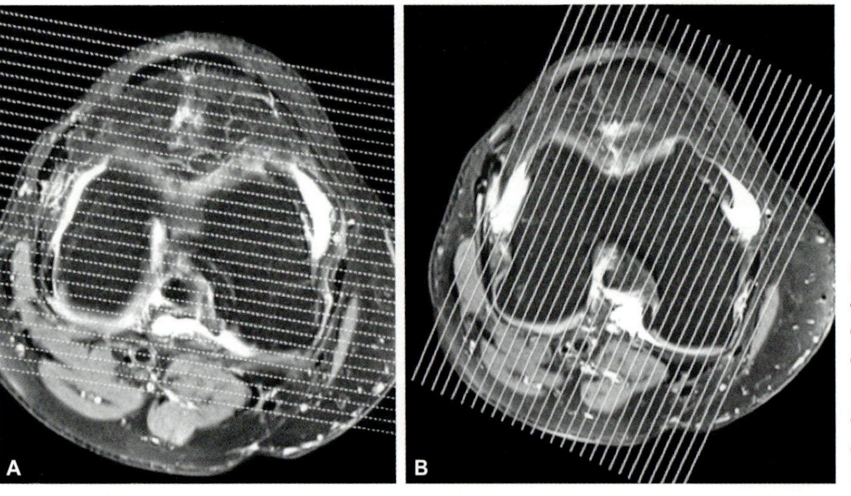

Figures 45.3A and B Knee MRI technique. The axial cuts are used to plan coronal (A) and sagittal oblique (B) sequences. The coronal images are oriented parallel to the posterior intercondylar line and sagittal oblique images are oriented in an anteromedial to posterolateral direction to allow better visualization of the anterior cruciate ligament

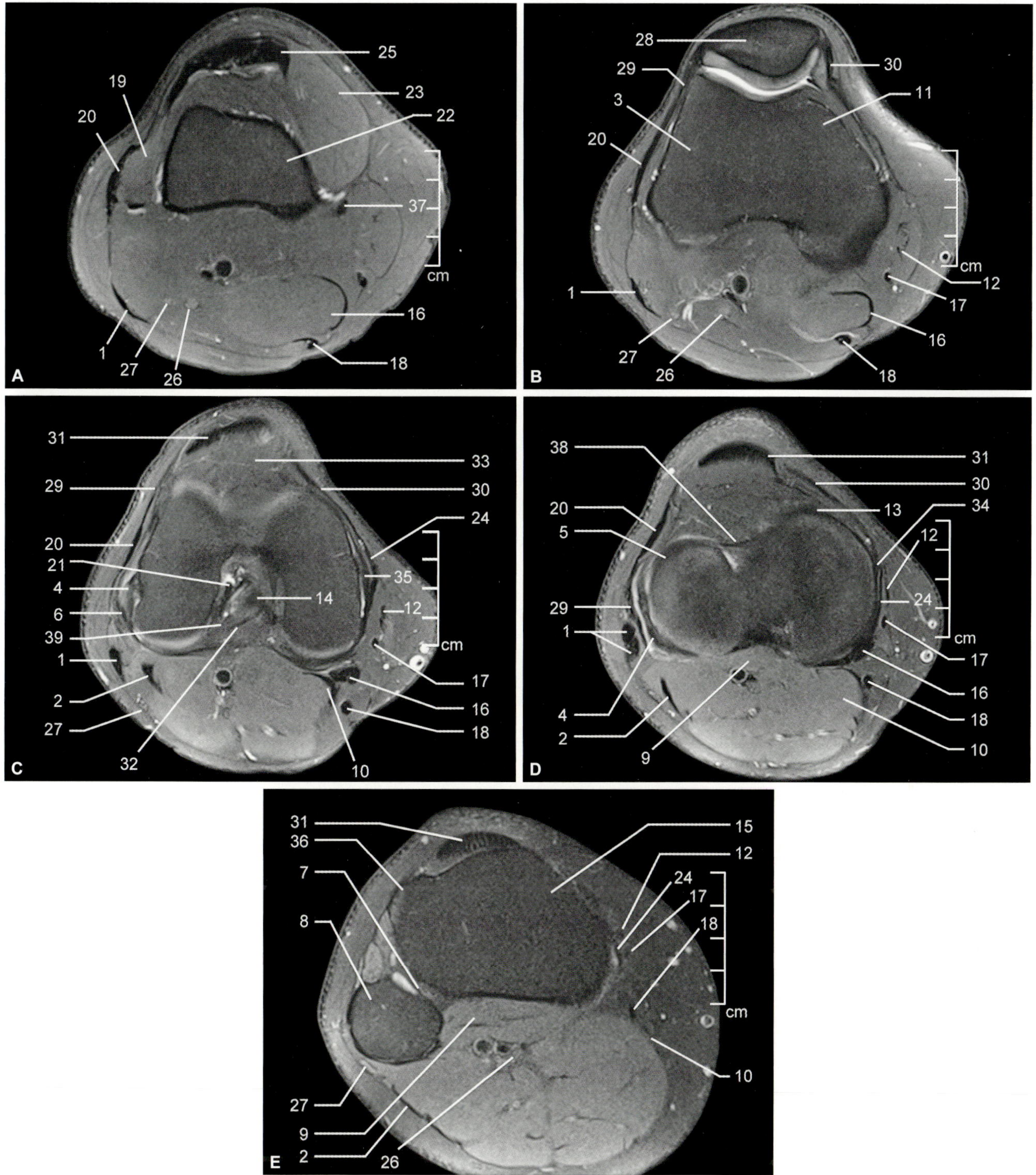

Figures 45.4A to E MR anatomy in axial plane. 1. Biceps femoris tendon. 2. Gastrocnemius muscle and tendon lateral head. 3. Lateral femoral condyle. 4. Popliteus tendon. 5. Lateral meniscus. 6. Fibular collateral ligament. 7. Superior tibiofibular joint (not seen). 8. Fibula (not seen). 9. Popliteus muscle. 10. Gastrocnemius muscle and tendon medial head. 11. Medial femoral condyle. 12. Sartorius. 13. Medial meniscus. 14. Posterior cruciate ligament. 15. Tibia. 16. Semimembranosus tendon. 17. Gracilis tendon. 18. Semitendinosus. 19. Vastus lateralis muscle. 20. Iliotibial tract. 21. Anterior cruciate ligament. 22. Femur. 23. Vastus medialis. 24. Tibial collateral ligament. 25. Quadriceps tendon. 26. Tibial nerve. 27. Common peroneal nerve. 28. Patella. 29. Lateral patellar retinaculum. 30. Medial patellar retinaculum. 31. Patellar tendon. 32. Posterior meniscofemoral ligament of Wrisberg. 33. Hoffa's fat. 34. Meniscotibial ligament. 35. Meniscofemoral ligament. 36. Gerdy's tubercle. 37. Adductor magnus tendon. 38. Transverse ligament. 39. Anterior ligament of Humphery.

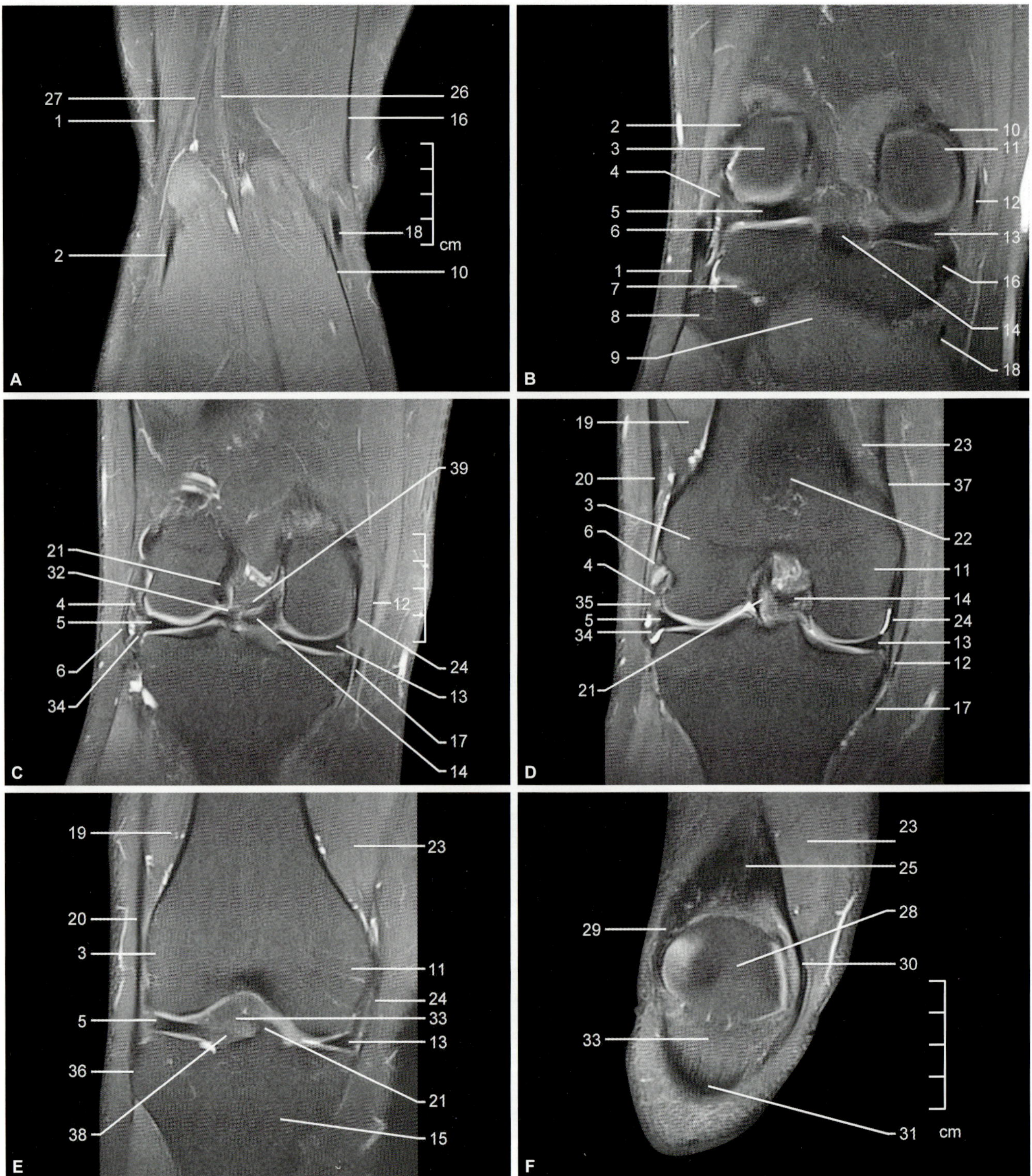

Figures 45.5A to F MR anatomy in coronal plane. 1. Biceps femoris tendon. 2. Gastrocnemius muscle and tendon lateral head. 3. Lateral femoral condyle. 4. Popliteus tendon. 5. Lateral meniscus. 6. Fibular collateral ligament. 7. Superior tibiofibular joint. 8. Fibula. 9. Popliteus muscle. 10. Gastrocnemius muscle and tendon medial head. 11. Medial femoral condyle. 12. Sartorius. 13. Medial meniscus. 14. Posterior cruciate ligament. 15. Tibia. 16. Semimembranosus tendon. 17. Gracilis tendon. 18. Semitendinosus. 19. Vastus lateralis muscle. 20. Iliotibial tract. 21. Anterior cruciate ligament. 22. Femur. 23. Vastus medialis. 24. Tibial collateral ligament. 25. Quadriceps tendon. 26. Tibial nerve. 27. Common peroneal nerve. 28. Patella. 29. Lateral patellar retinaculum. 30. Medial patellar retinaculum. 31. Patellar tendon. 32. Posterior meniscofemoral ligament of Wrisberg. 33. Hoffa's fat. 34. Meniscotibial ligament. 35. Meniscofemoral ligament. 36. Gerdy's tubercle. 37. Adductor magnus tendon. 38. Transverse ligament. 39. Anterior ligament of Humphery

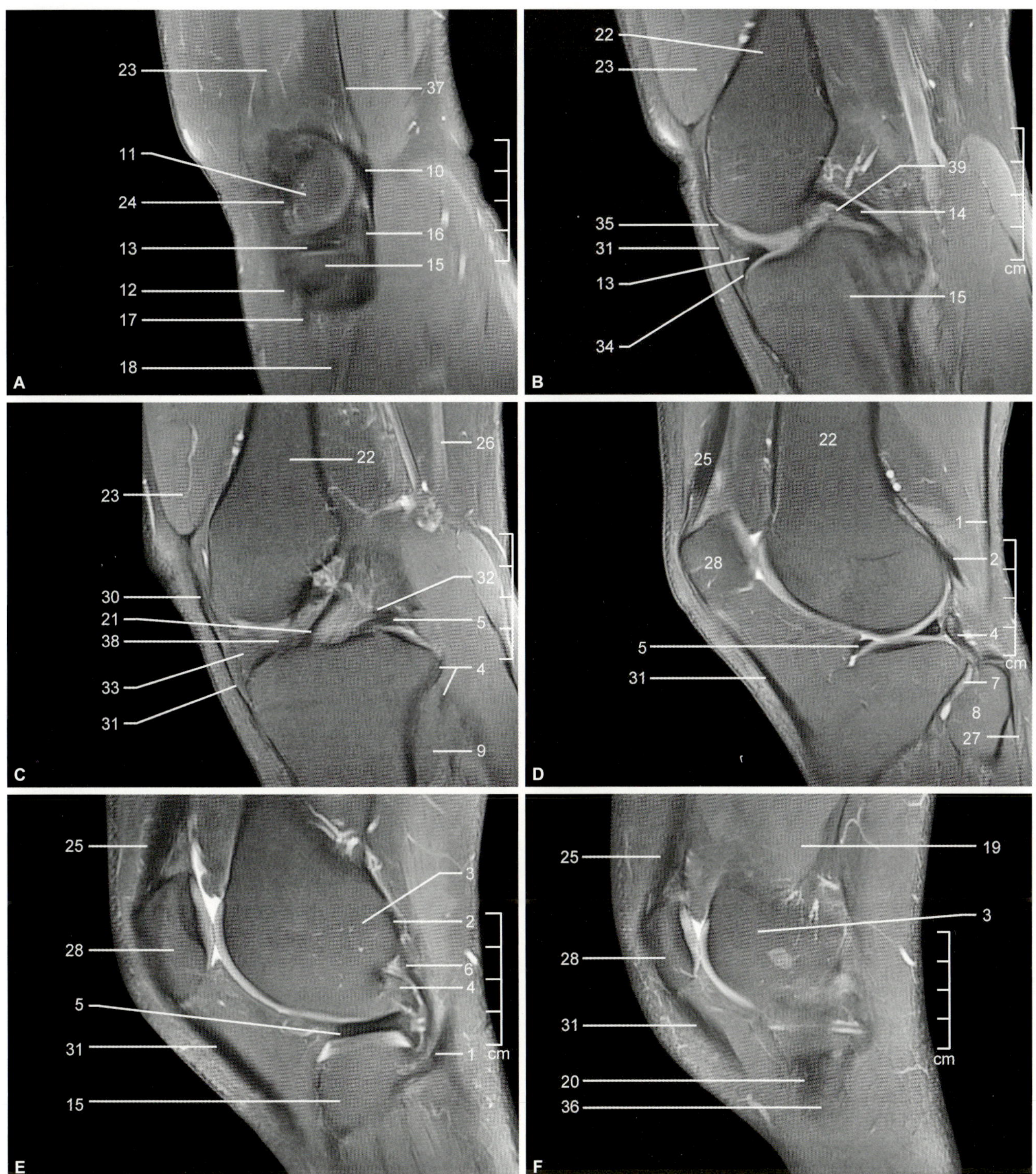

Figures 45.6A to F MR anatomy in sagittal plane. 1. Biceps femoris tendon. 2. Gastrocnemius muscle and tendon lateral head. 3. Lateral femoral condyle. 4. Popliteus tendon. 5. Lateral meniscus. 6. Fibular collateral ligament. 7. Superior tibiofibular joint. 8. Fibula. 9. Popliteus muscle. 10. Gastrocnemius muscle and tendon medial head. 11. Medial femoral condyle. 12. Sartorius. 13. Medial meniscus. 14. Posterior cruciate ligament. 15. Tibia. 16. Semimembranosus tendon. 17. Gracilis tendon. 18. Semitendinosus. 19. Vastus lateralis muscle. 20. Iliotibial tract. 21. Anterior cruciate ligament. 22. Femur. 23. Vastus medialis. 24. Tibial collateral ligament. 25. Quadriceps tendon. 26. Tibial nerve. 27. Common peroneal nerve. 28. Patella. 29. Lateral patellar retinaculum (not shown). 30. Medial patellar retinaculum. 31. Patellar tendon. 32. Posterior meniscofemoral ligament of Wrisberg. 33. Hoffa's fat. 34. Meniscotibial ligament. 35. Meniscofemoral ligament. 36. Gerdy's tubercle. 37. Adductor Magnus tendon. 38. Transverse ligament. 39. Anterior ligament of Humphery

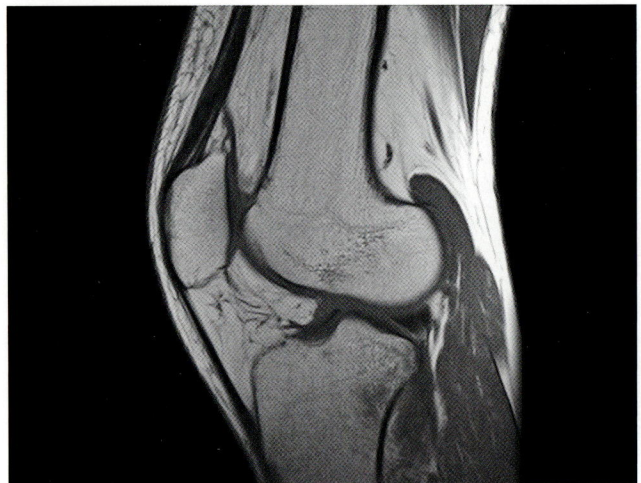

Figure 45.7 Identifying the MR sequence. Sagittal T1 weighted image shows fat in the subcutaneous tissues and within the bone marrow as high signal. The fluid within the joint is of low signal intensity, as is the signal from the cartilage and the muscles

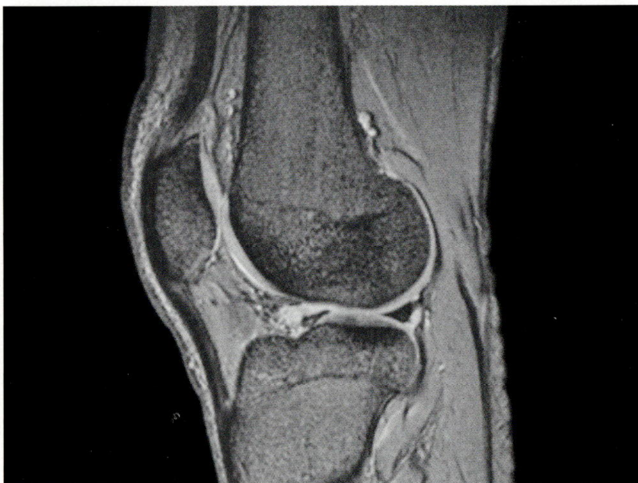

Figure 45.9 Identifying the MR sequence. Sagittal gradient sequence is a fluid sensitive sequence and shows increased signal intensity through the joint fluid and cartilage. The signal from the bone is reduced with coarse granular hypointensity. Note the borders of the muscles are clearly delineated and the signal from the muscle is lower than seen in PD fat sat images

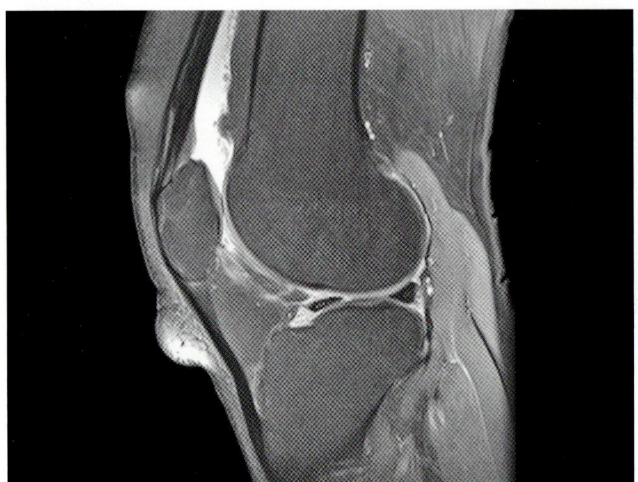

Figure 45.8 Identifying the MR sequence. Sagittal PD fat sat weighted image is a fluid sensitive sequence and shows increased signal intensity through the joint fluid and cartilage. Note the signal from the muscles is similar to articular cartilage. The signal from the subcutaneous and marrow fat is suppressed

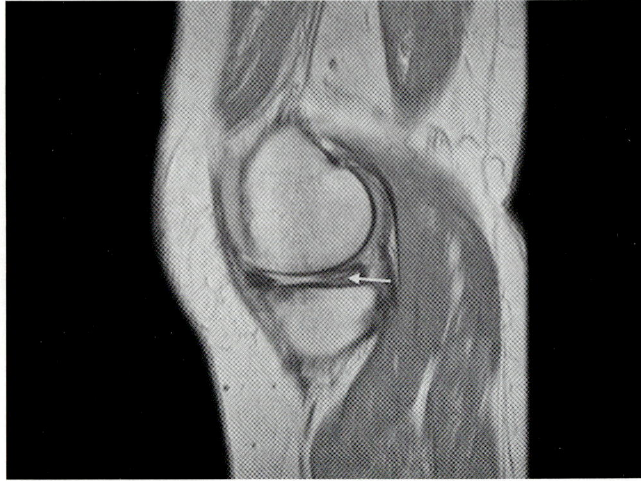

Figure 45.10 Identifying the MR sequence. Sagittal PD weighted image is a fluid sensitive sequence and shows increased signal intensity through the joint fluid and cartilage. The signal from the subcutaneous fat and bone marrow is similar to that seen in T1 weighted images. Note the signal from the muscles is more than seen in T1 weighted image. Also noted in this case is a complex medial meniscal tear (arrow)

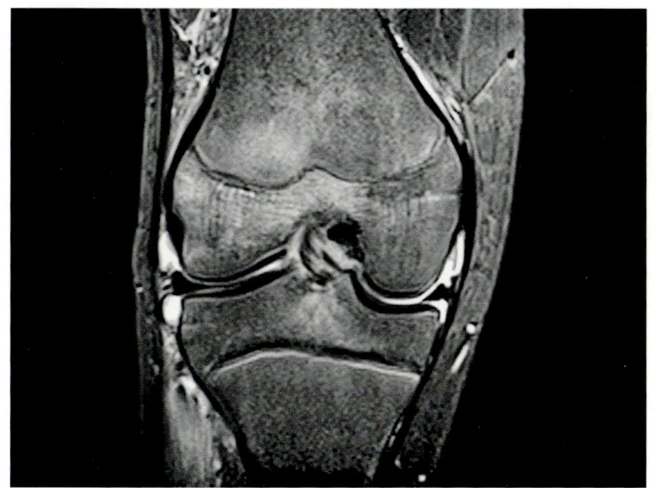

Figure 45.11 Identifying the MR sequence. Coronal STIR weighted image shows increased signal intensity through the joint fluid. Note the signal from the muscle and cartilage is low. The signal from the subcutaneous and marrow fat is suppressed

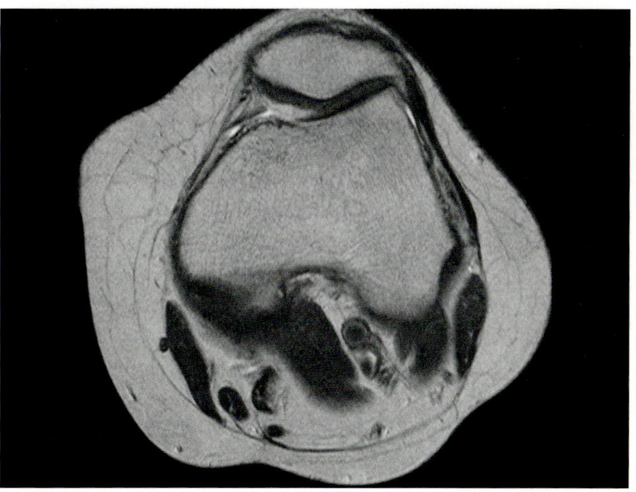

Figure 45.12 Identifying the MR sequence. Axial T2 weighed image shows increased signal intensity through the joint fluid. Note the signal from the subcutaneous fat and bone marrow is similar to that seen in T1 weighted images. The signal from the muscle and cartilage is low

CRUCIATE LIGAMENT PATHOLOGIES

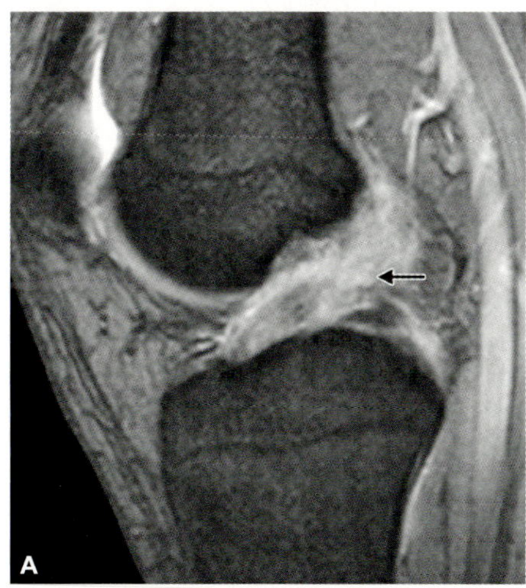

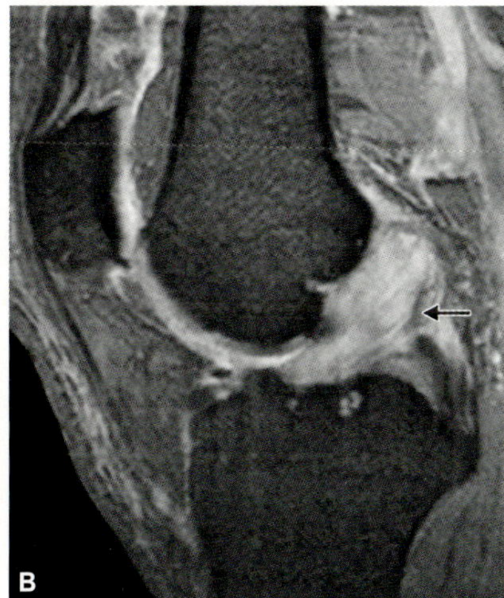

Figures 45.13A and B Anterior cruciate ligament (ACL) pathology. Sagittal gradient image shows: (A) Cloud like amorphous signal intensity (arrow) representing ACL tear and (B) intrasubstance high signal with linear striations (positive celery stick sign) secondary to ACL mucoid degeneration

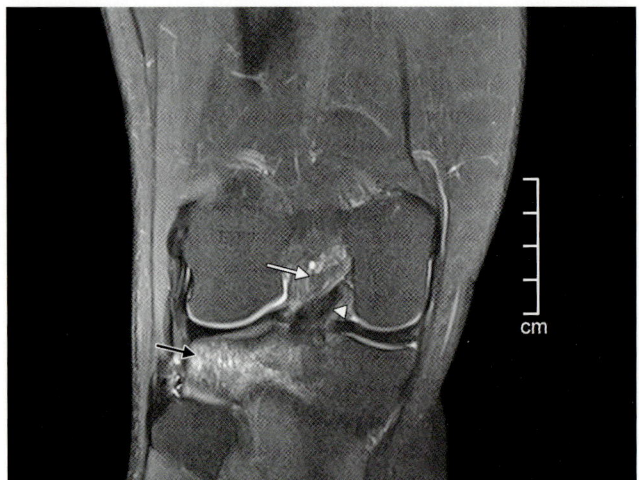

Figure 45.14 Coronal proton density (PD) fat saturated image shows ACL tear with an empty notch sign. Torn ACL leaves an empty space in the superolateral portion of the intercondylar notch (white arrow) above the intact PCL (arrowhead). Bone marrow edema (black arrow) seen as increased signal intensity in the posterior part of lateral tibial plateau is secondary to kissing bone contusion

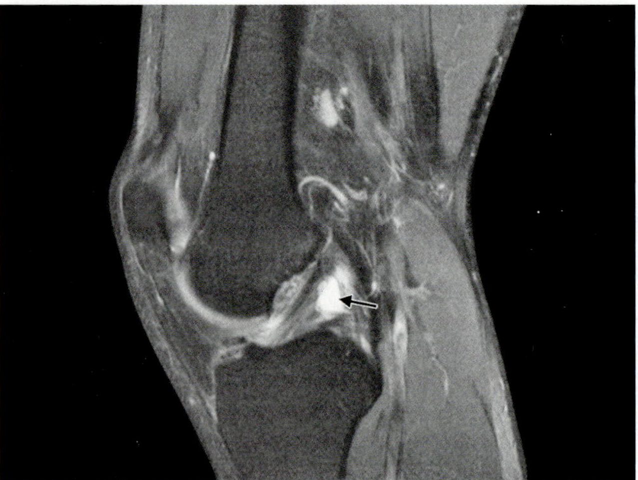

Figure 45.15 Sagittal PD fat sat weighted image shows a ganglion cyst (arrow) arising from the anterior cruciate ligament. The hypointense signal of the ACL is preserved suggestive of intact ligament

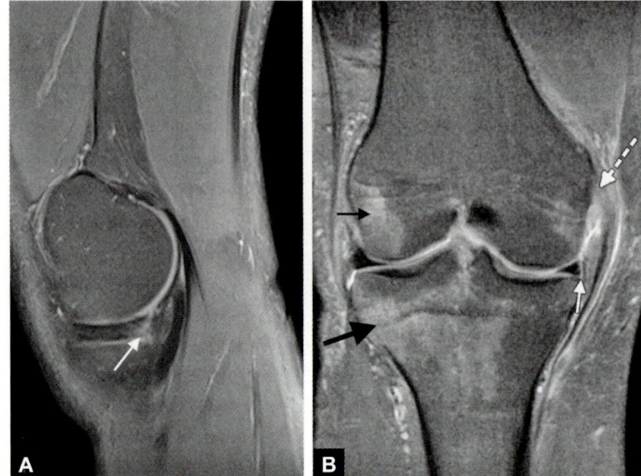

Figures 45.16A and B Abnormality of multiple supporting structures: O' Donoghue's triad. Sagittal PD fat sat weighted image (A) shows longitudinal vertical tear (arrow) on the medial meniscus. (B) Coronal PD fat sat weighted image shows torn anterior cruciate ligament, medial meniscal tear (broken white arrow), longitudinal vertical medial meniscal tear (white arrow) and classic bone bruising in the mid portion of lateral femoral condyle (thin black arrow) and medial tibial plateau (thick black arrow)

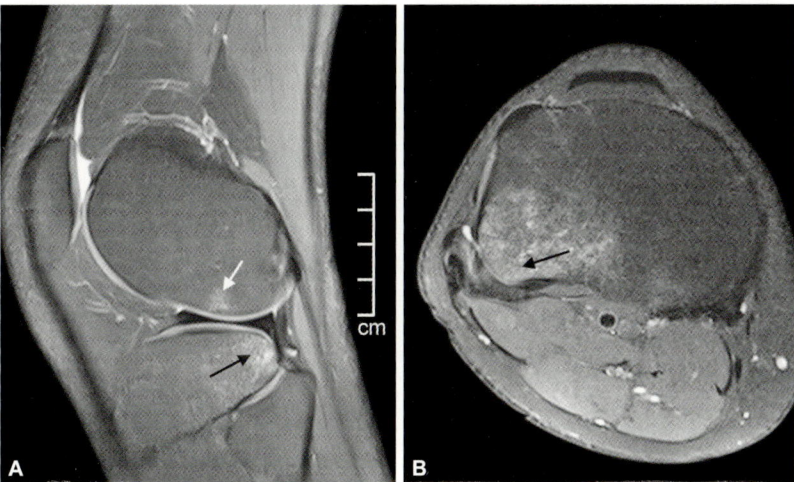

Figures 45.17A and B Anterior cruciate ligament injuries. Sagittal (A) and axial (B) PD fat sat image shows classic bone bruise in the mid portion of lateral femoral condyle (white arrow) and in the posterior aspect of lateral tibial plateau (black arrow). The lesions reflect contact of two bones during internal rotation of the tibia. This pattern, designated anterolateral rotatory instability, is a common cause of disruption of anterior cruciate ligament

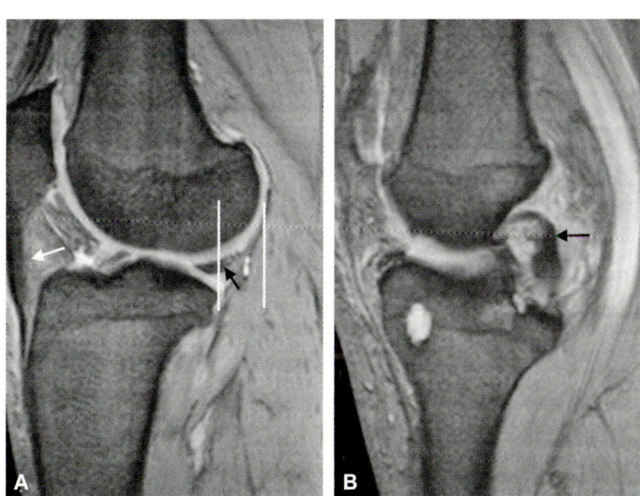

Figures 45.18A and B Anterior cruciate ligament injuries. Sagittal gradient sequences show acute complete anterior cruciate ligament tear with forward shift of the tibia with respect to femur. This can be measured by determining the distance between the two vertical grey lines in (A). Note the "wrinkled" patellar tendon (arrow), further evidence of forward movement of the tibia. Also note the uncovering of the posterior horn of lateral meniscus (short black arrow). In (B), note the buckling of the posterior cruciate ligament (arrow)

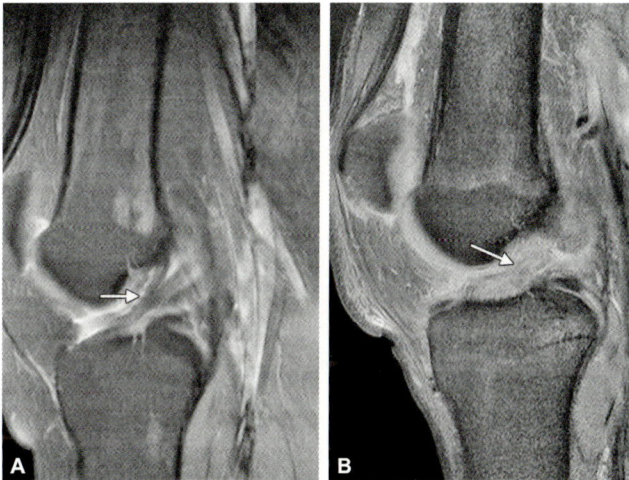

Figures 45.19A and B Anterior cruciate ligament injuries. Sagittal PD fat sat images show torn anterior cruciate ligament (arrow) with altered morphology and depression of its fiber (A) or a wavy contour (B) and lack of anterior band of hypointensity

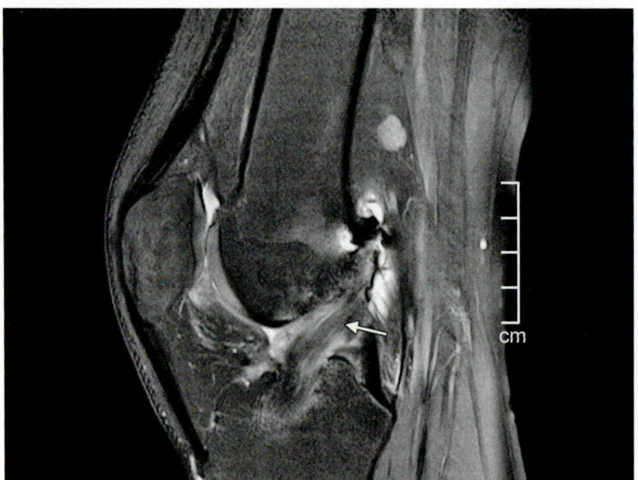

Figure 45.20 ACL reconstruction. Sagittal PD fat sat weighted image reveals an intact ACL graft (arrow)

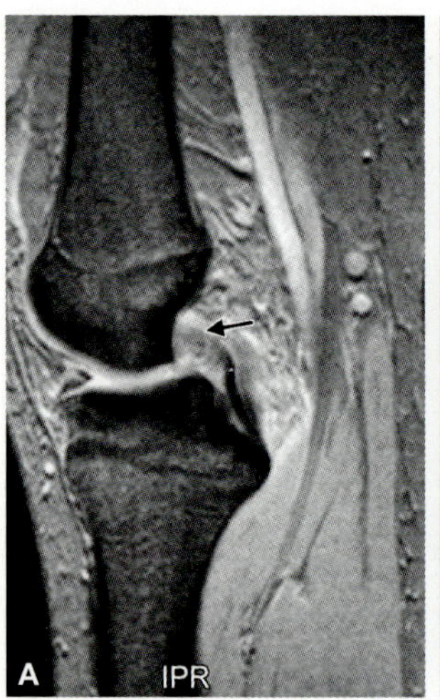

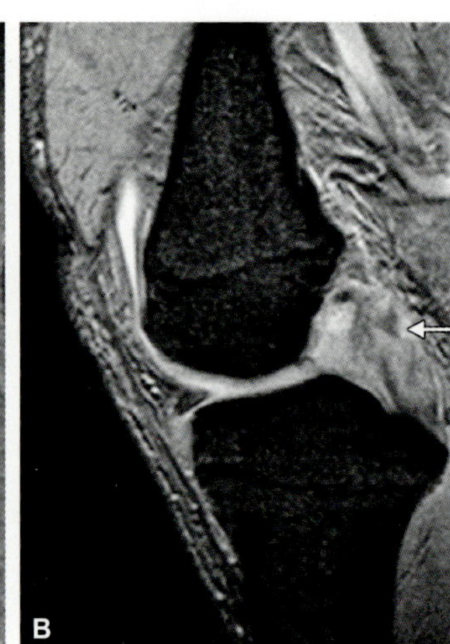

Figures 45.21A and B Posterior cruciate ligament (PCL) tear. (A) Sagittal gradient sequence with high signal within the proximal attachment (black arrow) and lack of normal hypointensity suggestive of a grade two tear of PCL. (B) Sagittal gradient sequence with high signal within whole of the PCL (white arrow) with wavy contour suggestive of grade 3 tear

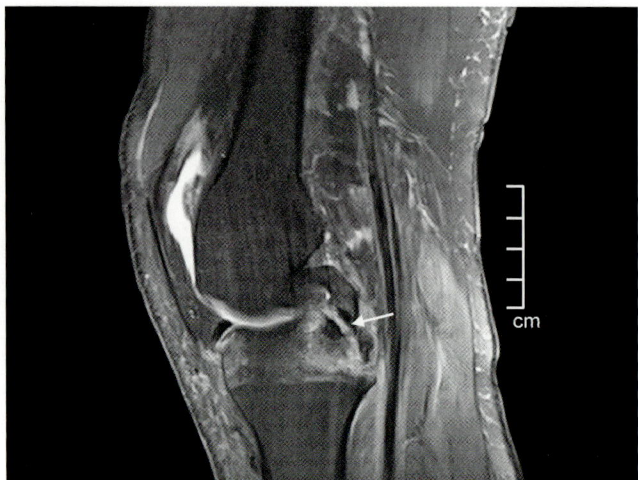

Figure 45.22 Acute avulsion fracture of posterior cruciate ligament. Sagittal PD fat sat image shows presence of an avulsion fracture and displacement of the bone fragment (arrow) attached to the posterior cruciate ligament

MENISCAL PATHOLOGIES

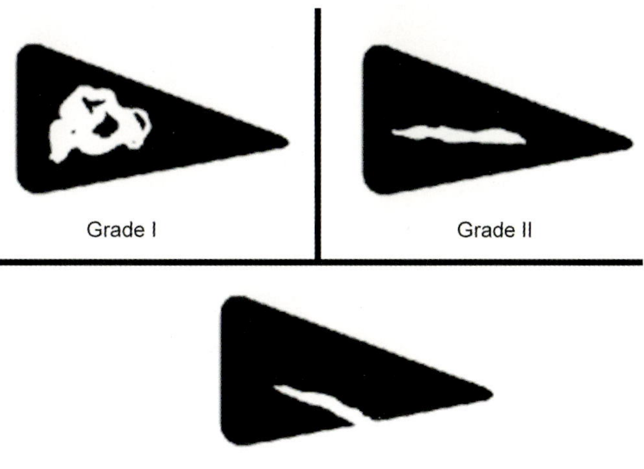

Figure 45.23 Grades of intrameniscal signal intensity. The meniscus may appear of uniform low signal intensity (grade 0); it may contain one or several circular foci of signal change (grade I); a linear signal intensity that does not extend to an articular surface (grade II); or a linear or irregular signal intensity that extends to the articular surface (grade III)

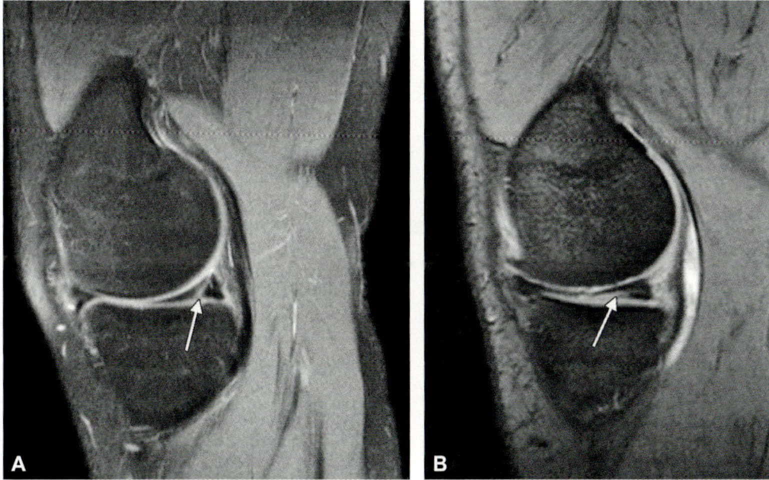

Figures 45.24A and B Meniscal tear: longitudinal tear. Sagittal PD fat sat image (A) shows a complete longitudinal oblique tear (arrow) in the posterior horn of medial meniscus and on the right a sagittal gradient image (B) shows a complete longitudinal horizontal tear (arrow) in the posterior half of body of medial meniscus

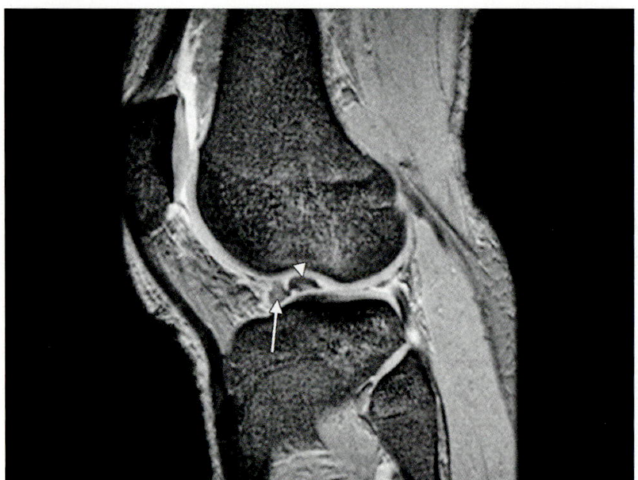

Figure 45.25 Meniscal detachment and flipped meniscus. Sagittal gradient image shows a detached posterior horn of the medial meniscus that is inverted (arrow) and located anterior to the anterior horn the medial meniscus (arrowhead)

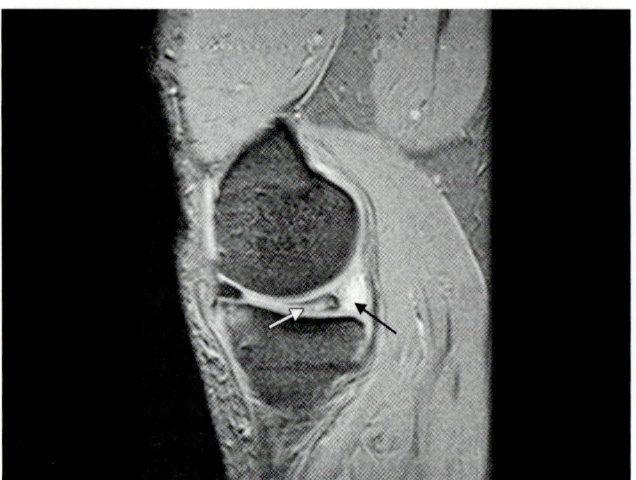

Figure 45.26 Meniscocapsular separation. Sagittal gradient image shows fluid signal between the posterior portion of medial meniscus and the joint capsule (black arrow). A longitudinal oblique tear is seen through the posterior horn (white arrow)

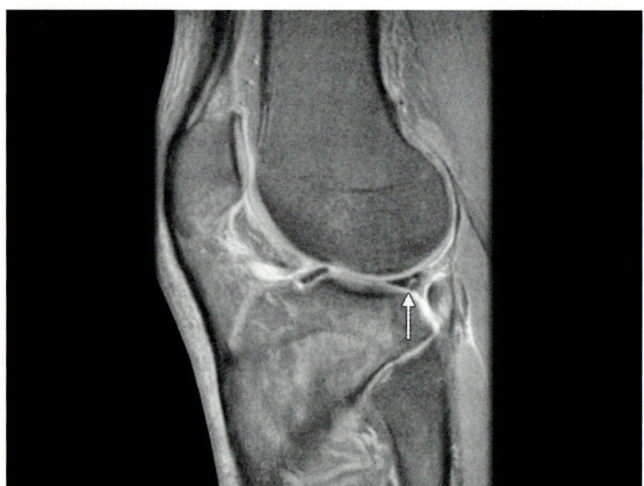

Figure 45.27 Peripheral vertical tear of lateral meniscus. Sagittal PD fat sat image shows a longitudinal vertical high signal (arrow) in the posterior horn of lateral meniscus

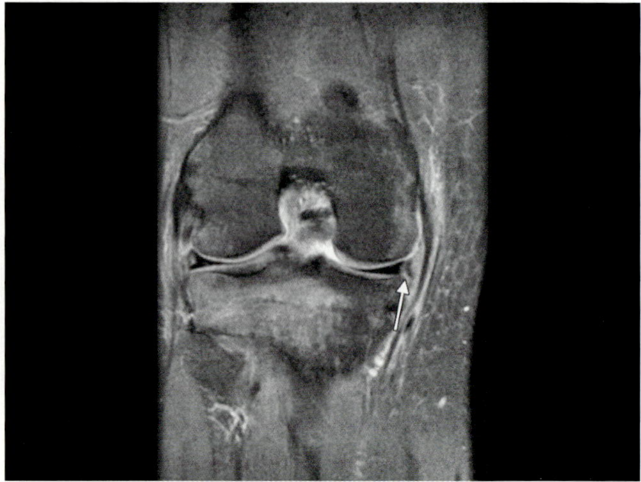

Figure 45.28 Peripheral vertical tear of medial meniscus. Coronal PD fat sat image shows a longitudinal vertical high signal (arrow) in the peripheral portion of body of medial meniscus

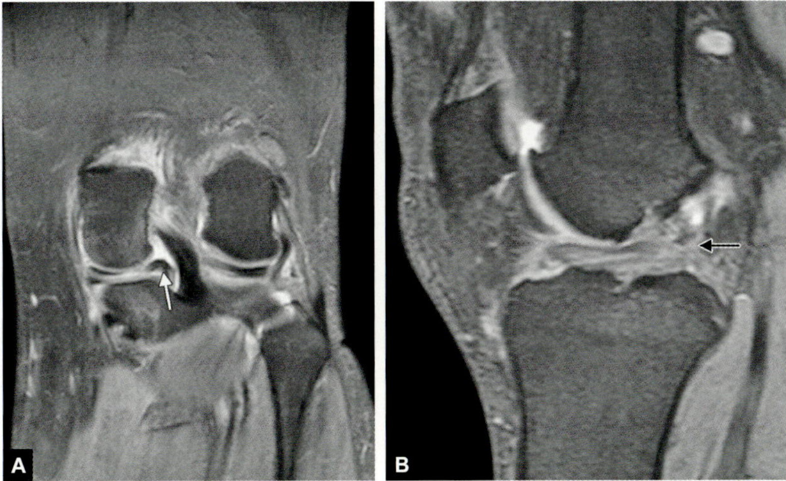

Figures 45.29A and B Bucket handle displaced meniscal tear. Coronal PD FS image (A) shows a torn displaced meniscal fragment (arrow) in the intercondylar notch and the sagittal PD fat sat image (B) shows the displaced bucket handle fragment of the meniscus adjacent to the posterior cruciate ligament and producing a double PCL sign

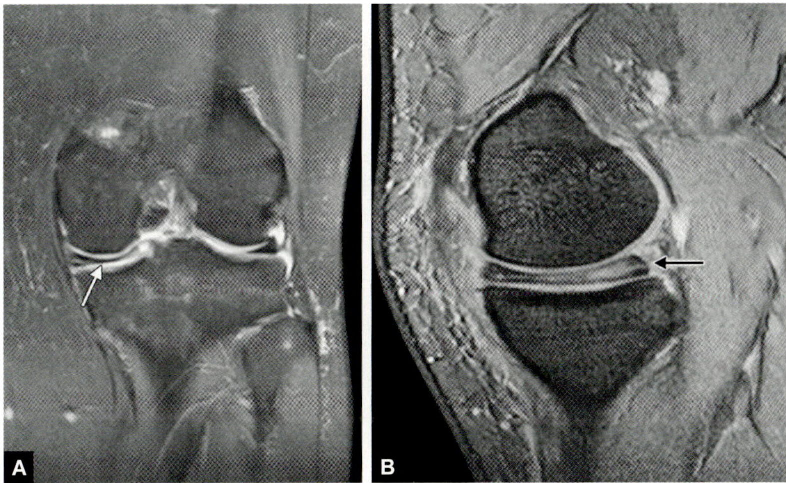

Figures 45.30A and B Discoid medial meniscus. Coronal PD fat sat image (A) and sagittal gradient image (B) shows an altered disk shaped medial meniscus (arrow) with abnormal diffuse increased signal intensity, generally indicative of a cavitatory type of longitudinal horizontal tear

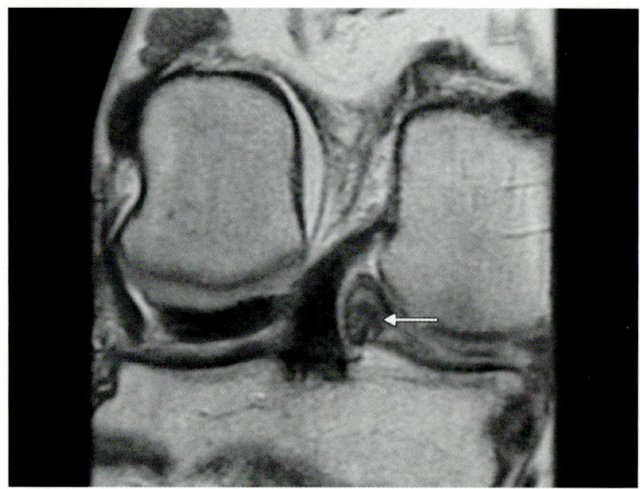

Figure 45.31 Folded meniscal tear. Coronal PD image shows a folded medial meniscus fragment displaced in the posterior intercondylar region (arrow)

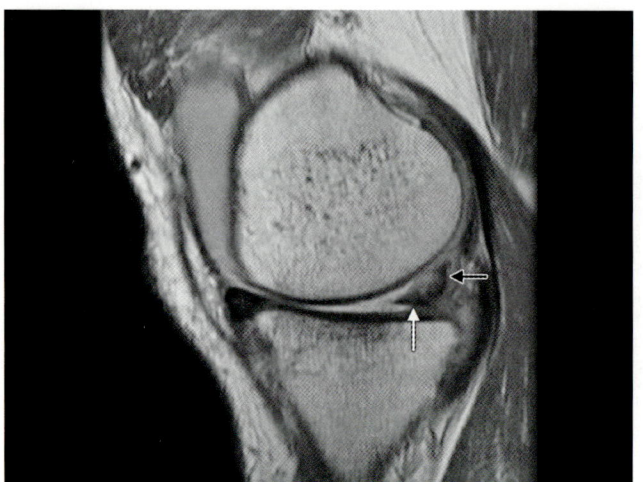

Figure 45.32 Detached meniscal fragment. Sagittal PD image displays a free meniscal fragment (black arrow) with signal intensity identical to that of the torn posterior horn of medial meniscus (white arrow)

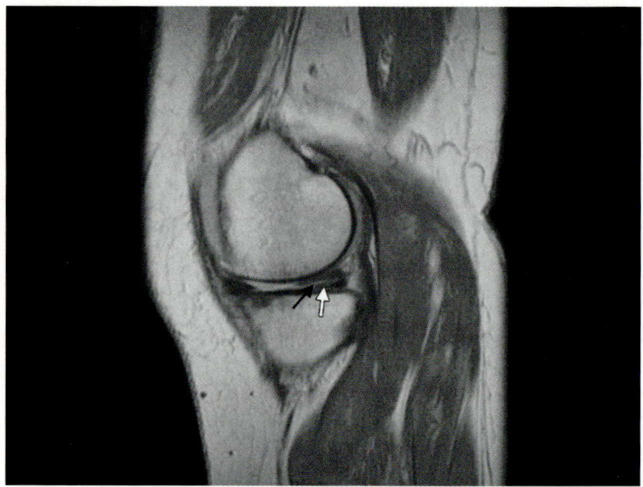

Figure 45.33 Complex medial meniscal tear. Sagittal PD image shows a longitudinal oblique (white arrow) and a horizontal (black arrow) area of increased signal (representing tear) in the posterior horn of medial meniscus

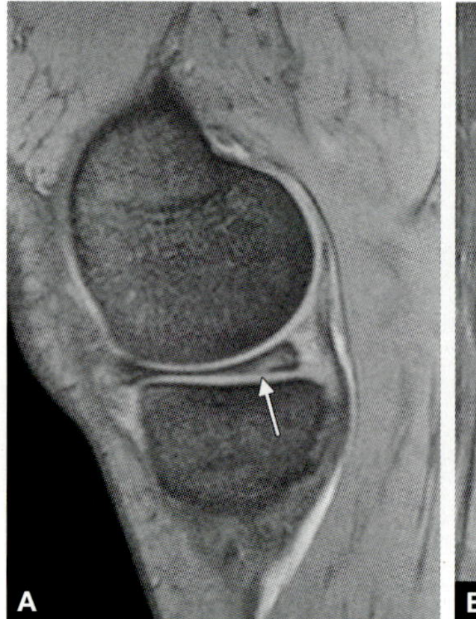

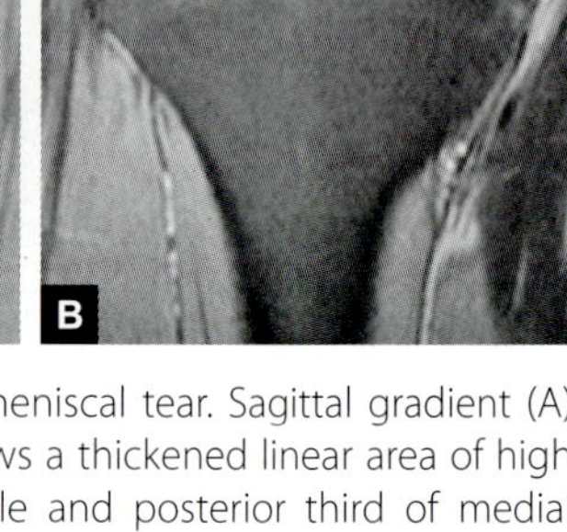

Figures 45.34A and B Healed meniscal tear. Sagittal gradient (A) and coronal PD fat sat (B) MR shows a thickened linear area of high signal near the junction of middle and posterior third of medial meniscus that is extending to the inferior surface and is covered by a thin hypointense line (arrow)

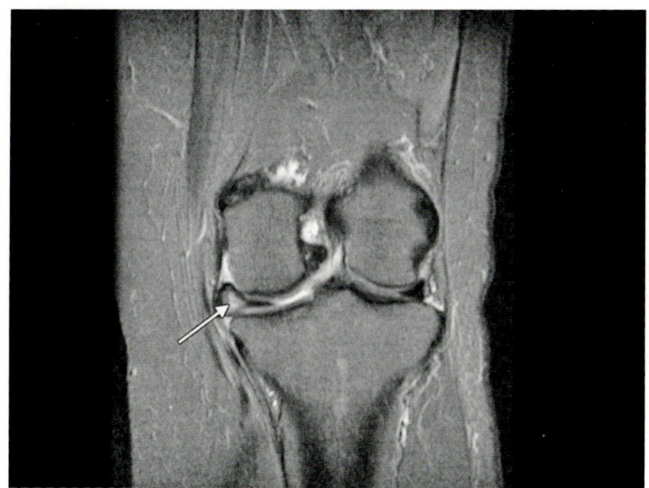

Figure 45.35 Meniscal cyst. Coronal PD fat sat MR image shows an intrameniscal cyst within the body of medial meniscus

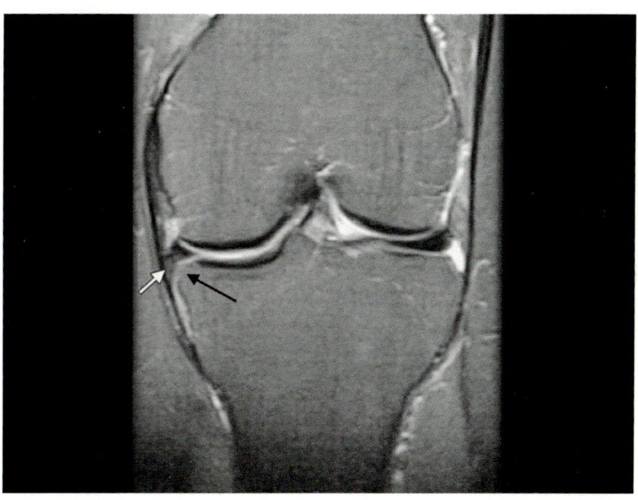

Figure 45.37 Displaced flap meniscal tears. Coronal PD fat sat image shows an inferiorly displaced torn meniscal fragment (arrow) in the medial gutter, between the medial collateral ligament and the medial tibial plateau. Note subjacent marrow edema in the tibial plateau (long black arrow)

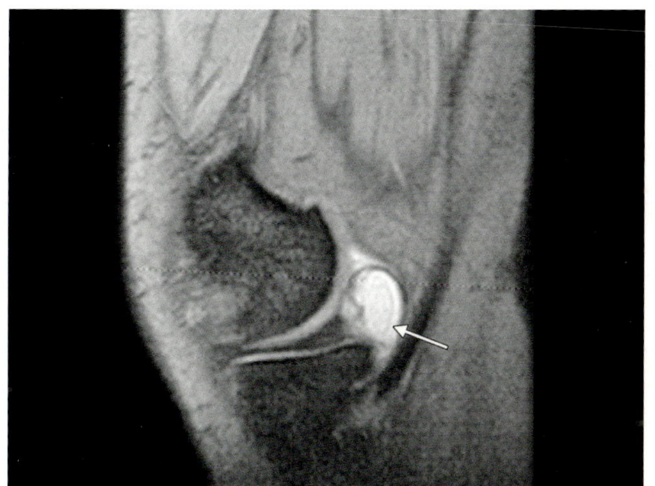

Figure 45.36 Meniscal cyst. Sagittal gradient image shows a perimeniscal cyst (arrow) behind the posterior horn of medial meniscus

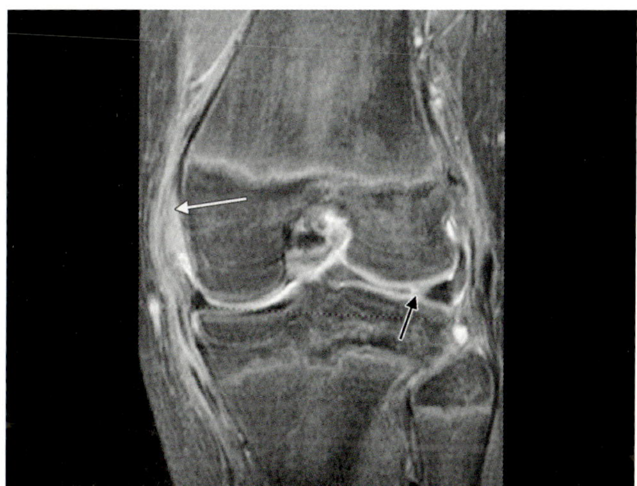

Figure 45.38 Radial tear of lateral meniscus. Coronal PD fat sat image shows a radial tear near the junction of middle and posterior third of lateral meniscus (black arrow). Note grade two tear of femoral attachment of medial collateral ligament (white arrow) seen as intra-substance high signal

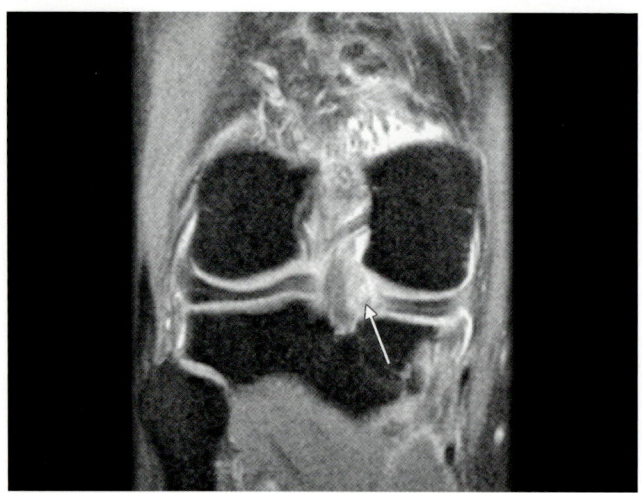

Figure 45.39 Medial meniscus radial tear (posterior root tear). Coronal PD fat sat image shows site of radial tear (white arrow) of posterior horn of medial meniscus. A gap at the site meniscal failure relates to medial displacement of the intact portion of the posterior horn. The posterior root ligament is not visualized and may be avulsed

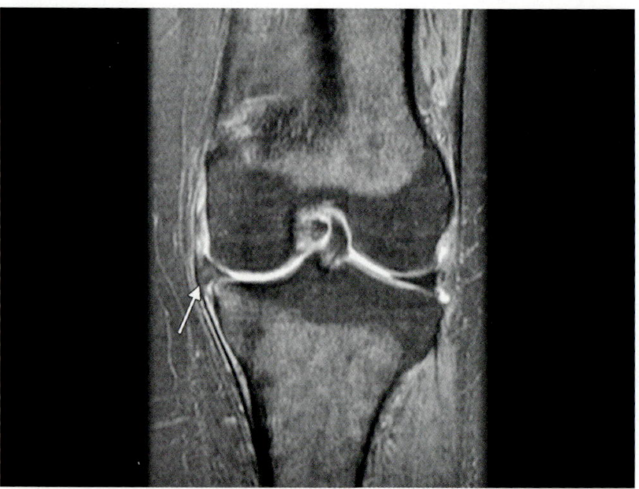

Figure 45.40 Medial meniscus radial tear (posterior root tear). Coronal PF fat image shows medial displacement of body of the medial meniscus (white arrow) beyond the articular margin secondary to a large radial tear of the posterior horn (Fig. 45.38)

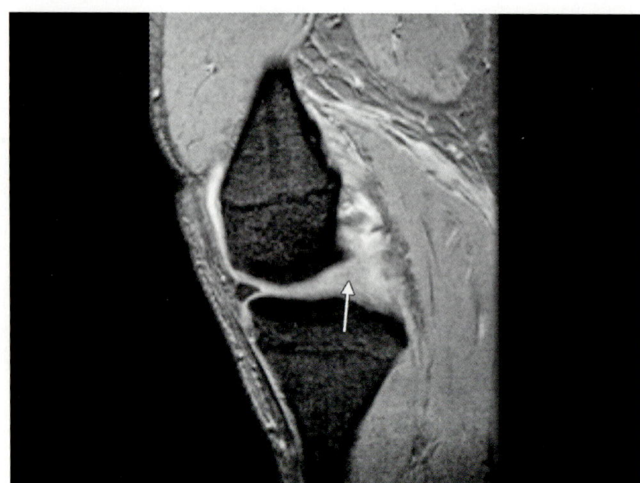

Figure 45.41 Medial meniscus radial tear (posterior root tear). Sagittal gradient weighted image with non-visualization of the posterior horn of the medial meniscus and a faint hypointensity (arrow) representing ghost meniscus

COLLATERAL LIGAMENT PATHOLOGIES

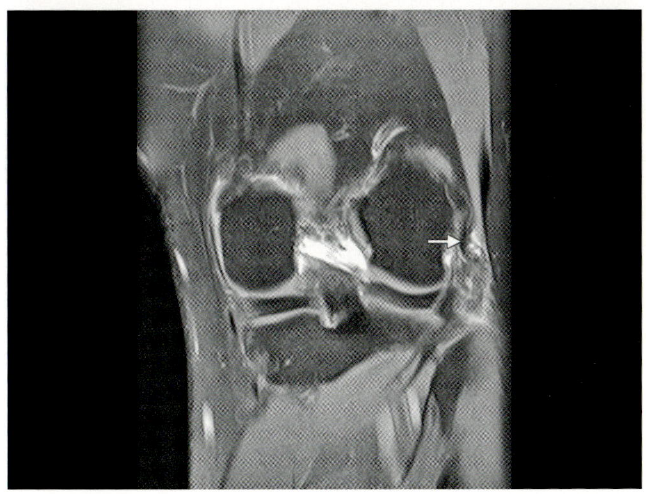

Figure 45.42 Lateral collateral ligament injury. Complete tear of the lateral collateral ligament from its fibular attachment in this left knee coronal PD fat sat weighted MR image. Note the wavy torn ligament (arrow) with adjacent soft tissue high signal

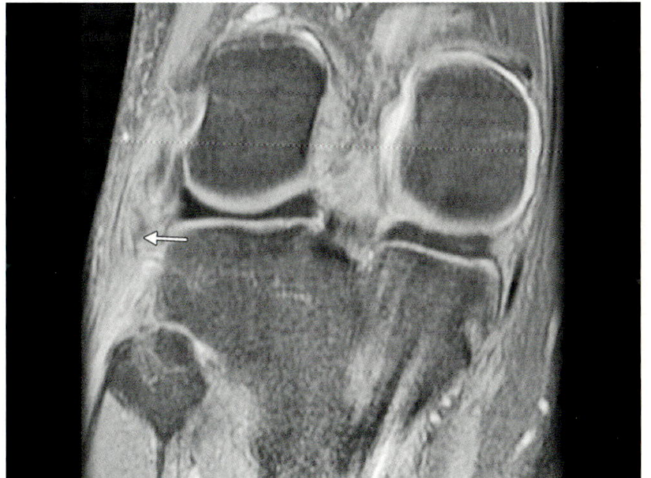

Figure 45.43 Lateral collateral ligament injury. Complete tear of the lateral collateral ligament from its fibular attachment in this right knee coronal PD fat sat weighted MRI image. Note the wavy torn ligament (arrow) with adjacent soft tissue high signal

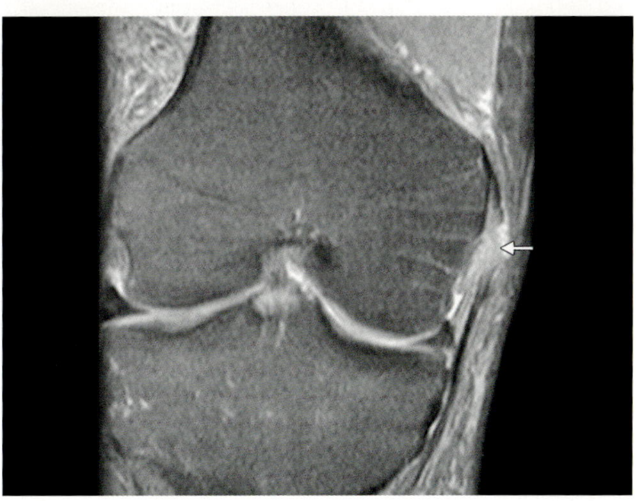

Figure 45.44 Medial collateral ligament injury. Complete disruption of the proximal portion of tibial collateral ligament (arrow) suggestive of a grade 3 tear

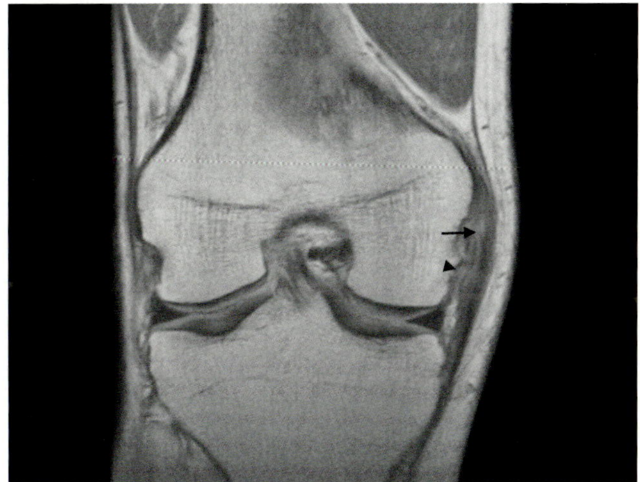

Figure 45.45 Medial collateral ligament injury (MCL). Coronal PD weighted MR image shows minimal high signal along the femoral attachment of tibial collateral ligament (arrow) with slight blurring of the ligament edges; suggestive of a grade I tear. Note disruption of the meniscofemoral ligament (arrowhead)

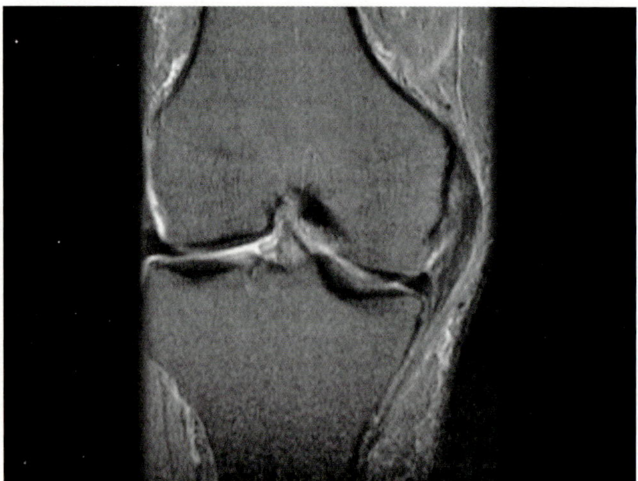

Figure 45.46 Medial collateral ligament injury. Coronal PD fat sat weighted MR image shows swelling and high signal with the proximal tibial collateral ligament; representing grade 2 tear. The meniscofemoral and meniscotibial ligaments were noted to be intact (not shown)

ANTERIOR STRUCTURES OF THE KNEE

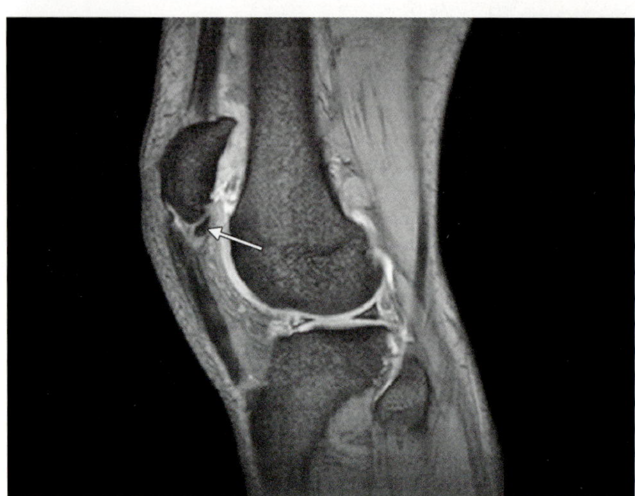

Figure 45.47 Sinding-Larsen-Johansson disease. A sagittal gradient MR image in a 12-year-old boy shows fragmentation (arrow) of the lower pole of patella with increased signal intensity in the adjacent portion of the patellar tendon. The remaining portion of the patellar tendon is thickened due patellar tendinopathy

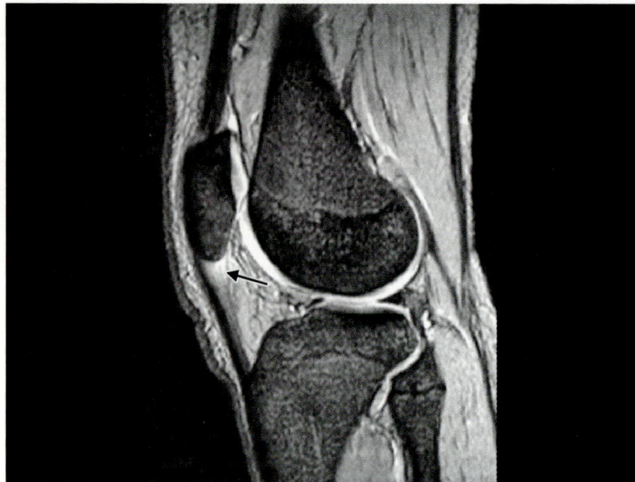

Figure 45.48 Proximal patellar tendon pathology. Sagittal gradient images show high signal in the posterior part of proximal patellar tendon in an adult patient suggestive of proximal patellar tendinopathy or jumper's knee

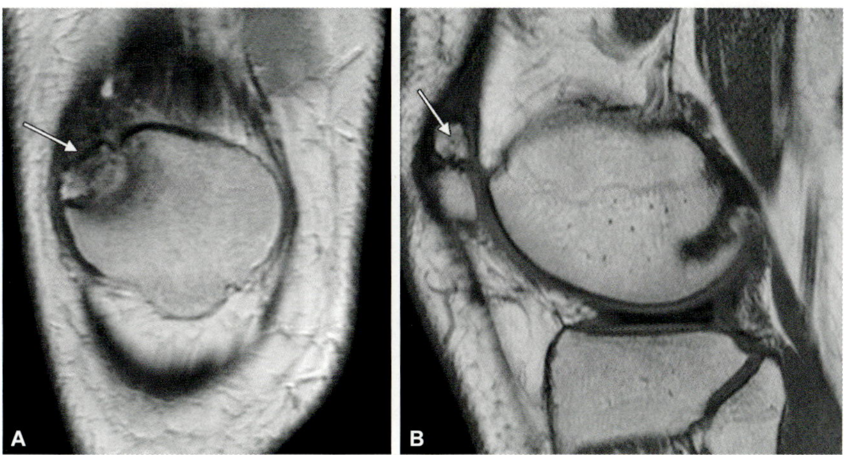

Figures 45.49A and B Bipartite patella. Coronal (A) and sagittal (B) PD image shows an accessory ossification center in the superolateral aspect of patella (arrows)

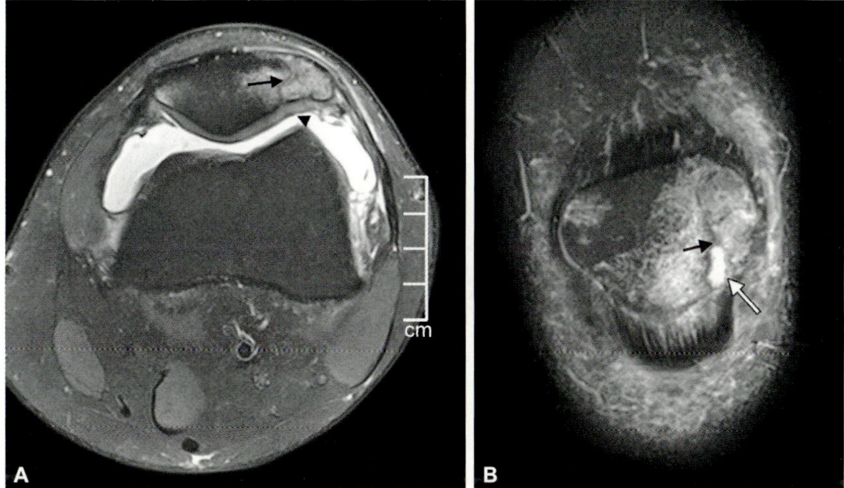

Figures 45.50A and B Fracture of patella. Axial (A) and coronal (B) PD fat sat images reveal fracture line through the lateral aspect of patella with surrounding bone marrow edema. The underlying articular cartilage (arrowhead) appears intact. Note the fluid cleft (white arrow in B) in the inferior portion of the fracture line

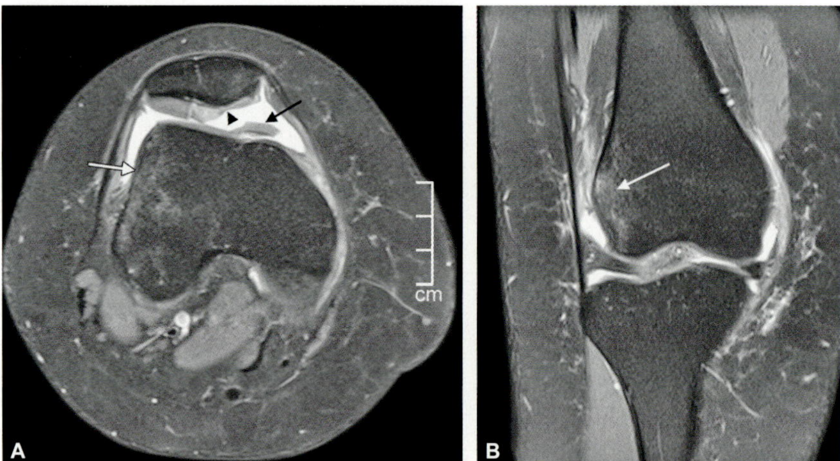

Figures 45.51A and B Lateral patellar dislocation—relocation injury. Axial PD fat sat image (A) shows a region of patella devoid of articular cartilage (arrowhead) with the detached articular cartilage fragment (black arrow) within the joint. Note the residual marrow edema in the lateral femoral condyle (white arrows) in both (A) and (B) indicative of a recent lateral patellar dislocation

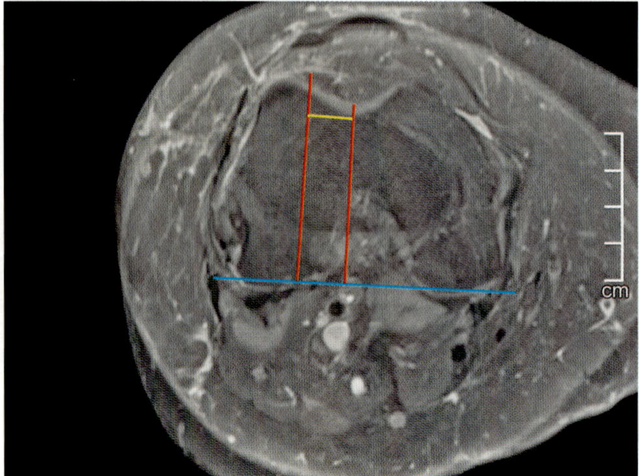

Figure 45.52 Patellar instability—Tibial Tubercle to Trochlear Groove Distance (TT-TG). To obtain the TT-TG, one draws a line through the trochlear groove (red line) that is perpendicular to a line drawn across the backs of the femoral condyles (blue line). At the level of the tibial tubercle, a second line is drawn though the tibial tubercle (red line) exactly parallel to the trochlear groove line. The distance between these two lines (yellow line) is the TT-TG distance; normally 10–15 mm drawing these lines is easiest if one is able to superimpose the two images on each other, as shown. The second method is by using axial MR images on Picture archiving and communication system (PACS) monitor and keeping the measurement cursor fixed in the middle of tibial tubercle and scrolling till we reach the image with trochlear groove and then drawing a measurement line up to the center point of the trochlear groove

IMPINGEMENT SYNDROMES

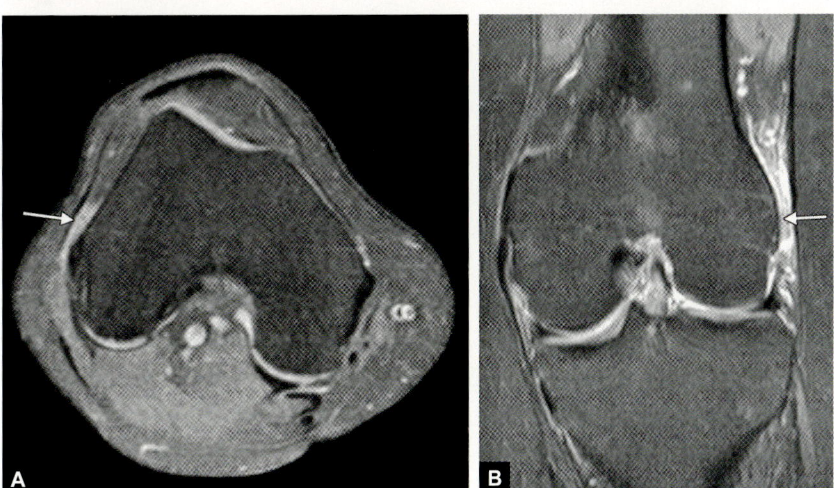

Figures 45.53A and B Iliotibial band friction syndrome. Axial (A) and coronal (B) PD fat sat images in different patients show high signal (white arrows) in the fat between the iliotibial band and lateral femoral condyle

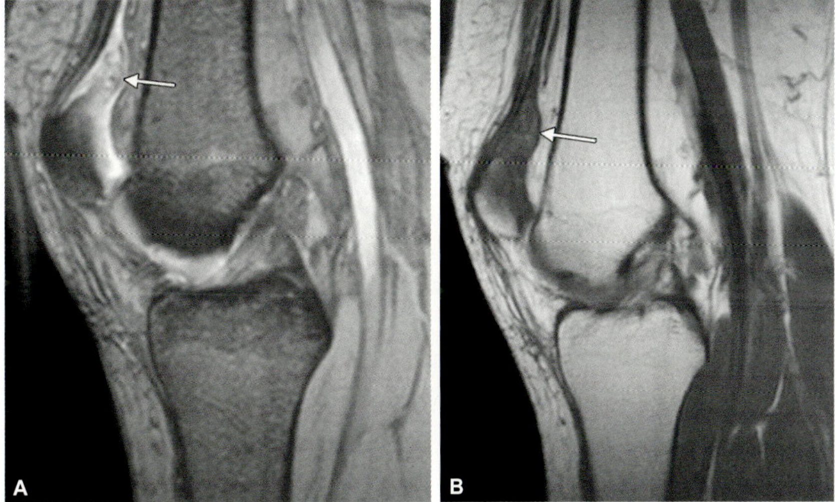

Figures 45.54A and B Suprapatellar fat pad impingement syndrome. Sagittal gradient (A) and sagittal T1 (B) weighted MR images show inflammatory changes in the suprapatellar, or quadriceps, fat pat seen as high signal on fluid sensitive sequence and low signal on T1 weighted sequence. Note the posterior contour bulge (arrows)

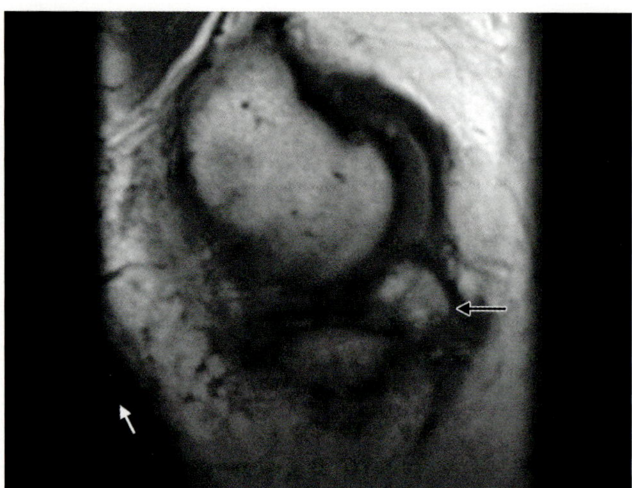

Figure 45.55 Knee locking due to fat impingement. Sagittal T1 weighted image shows a globular area of herniated fat (black arrow) entrapped between the posterior horn of medial meniscus and posterior joint capsule

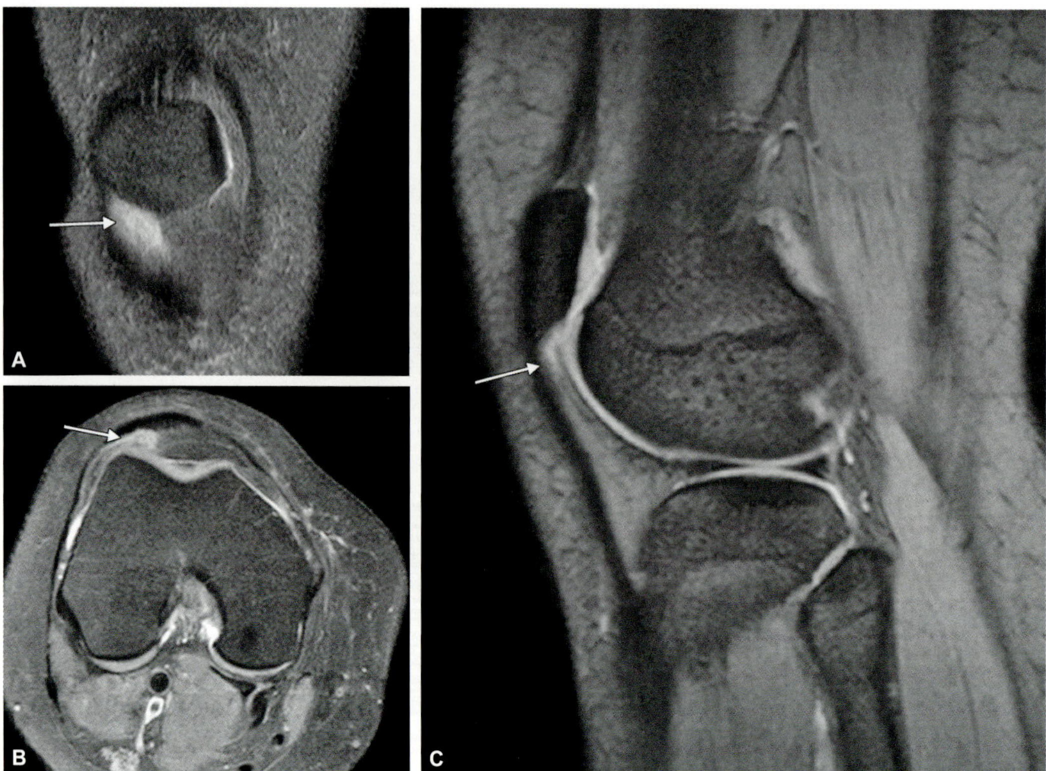

Figures 45.56A to C Patellar tendon-lateral femoral condyle impingement syndrome (fat pad impingement syndrome. Coronal (A), axial (B) and sagittal (C) PD fat sat images show inflammatory change in the superolateral aspect of Hoffa's fat pad (white arrows) seen as high signal between the patellar tendon and anterior part of lateral femoral condyle

SYNOVIAL PATHOLOGIES

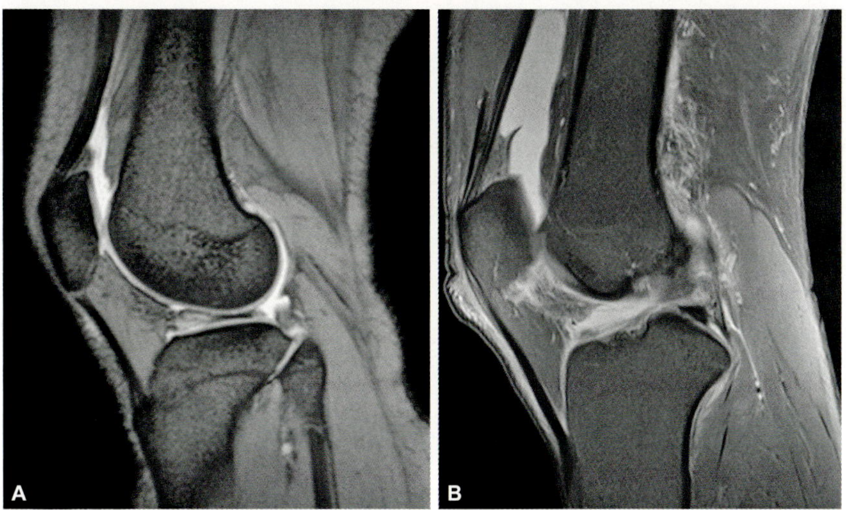

Figures 45.57A and B Suprapatellar knee joint effusion. Sagittal gradient (A) image shows mild effusion in the suprapatellar pouch and (B) sagittal PD fat sat image shows a large knee joint effusion

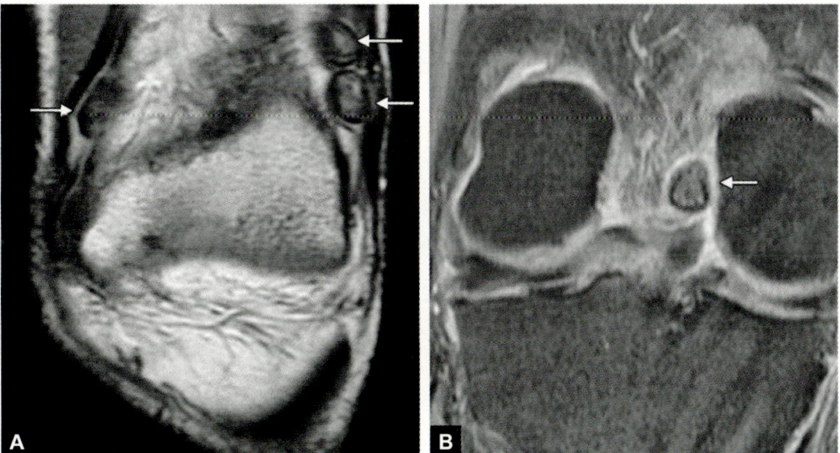

Figures 45.58A and B Synovial osteochondromatosis. Coronal PD (A) and PD fat sat (B) images show multiple rounded loose bodies (arrows) within the joint

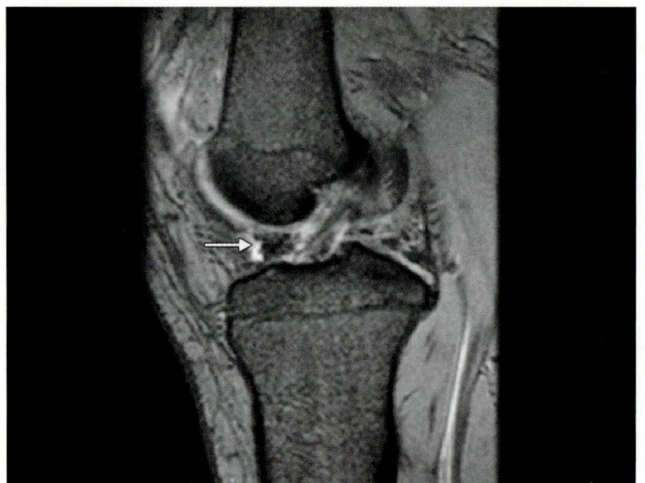

Figure 45.59 Pigmented villonodular synovitis (PVNS). Sagittal gradient sequence shows a nodular soft tissue area of reduced signal intensity due to hemosiderin deposition, located in the anterior joint recess (arrow)

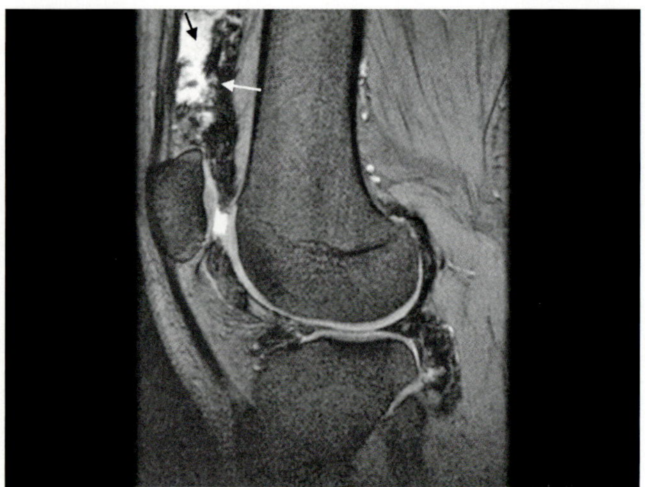

Figure 45.60 Pigmented villonodular synovitis (PVNS). Sagittal gradient sequence shows classic features of the disease. A joint effusion (black arrow) of high signal intensity in the suprapatellar region. Hemosiderin deposition accounts for the low signal intensity in the synovial nodules along the joint lining (white arrow)

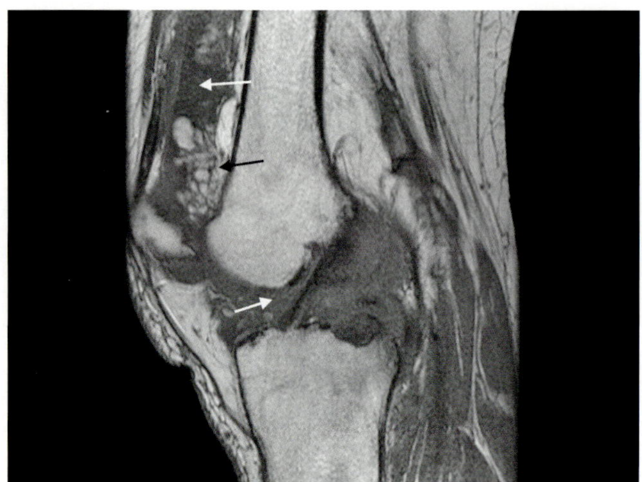

Figure 45.61 Lipoma arborescence. Sagittal T1 weighted image shows rounded frond like projection (black arrow) in the suprapatellar region that are of fat signal intensity. Note associated joint effusion (white arrows)

CARTILAGE PATHOLOGIES

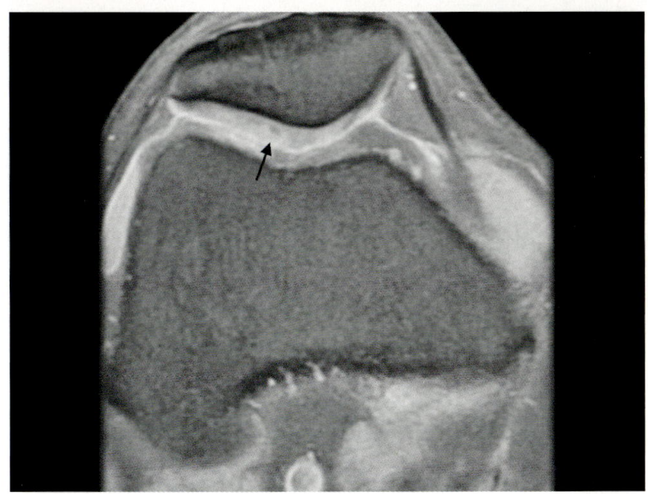

Figure 45.62 Chondromalacia patellae grade 1. Axial PD fat sat weighted image shows fibrillation of the articular cartilage behind the lateral facet of patella

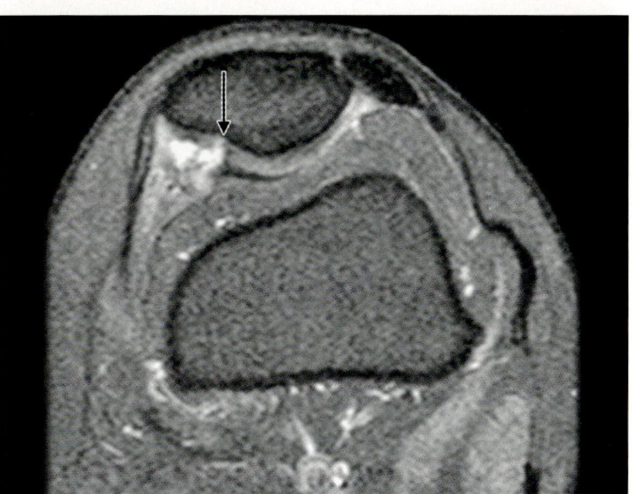

Figure 45.64 Chondromalacia patellae grade 3. Axial PD fat sat weighted image shows a full thickness articular cartilage defect behind the lateral facet of patella. Note no underlying bone marrow edema or subchondral cyst formation

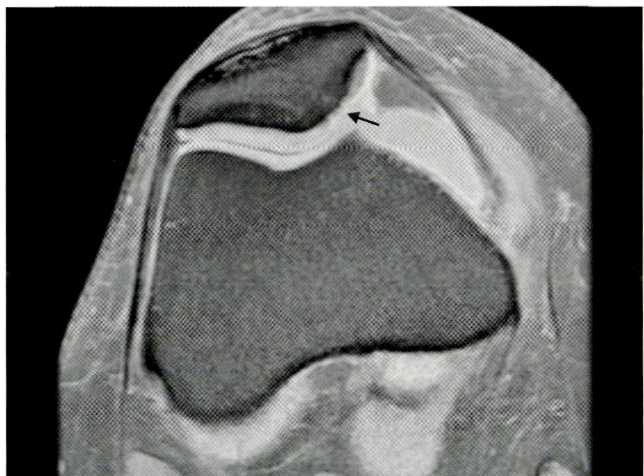

Figure 45.63 Chondromalacia patellae grade 2. Axial PD fat sat weighted image shows partial thickness articular cartilage defect (arrow) behind the medial facet of patella

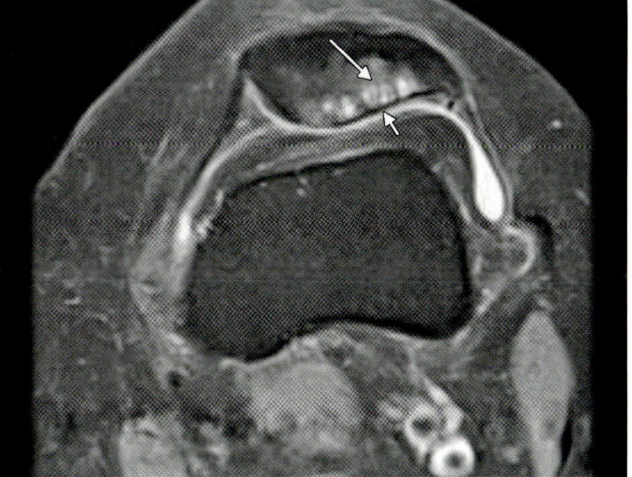

Figure 45.65 Chondromalacia patellae grade 4. Axial PD fat sat weighted image shows full thickness articular cartilage defect (short arrow) behind the lateral facet of patella with underlying subcortical cystic degeneration and marrow edema (long arrow)

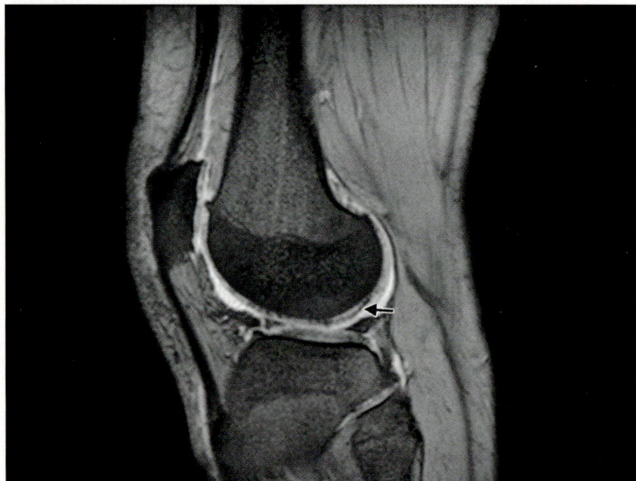

Figure 45.66 Chondrocalcinosis. Sagittal gradient image shows hypointensities within the articular cartilage over the lateral femoral condyle, lateral tibial plateau and behind the patella in this known case of calcium pyrophosphate dihydrate (CPPD) crystal deposition disease

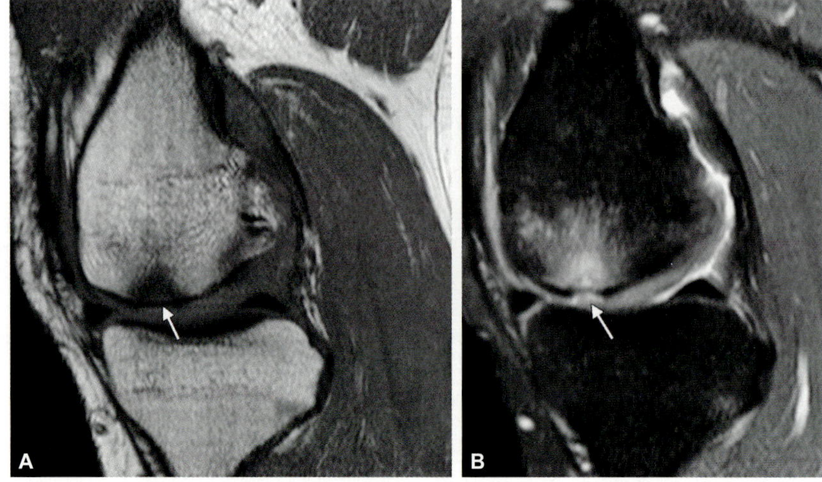

Figures 45.67A and B Acute chondral lesion. Sagittal T1 (A) and STIR (B) weighted images show a full thickness chondral lesion (arrow) with sharp margins and extensive subjacent marrow edema in the medial femoral condyle

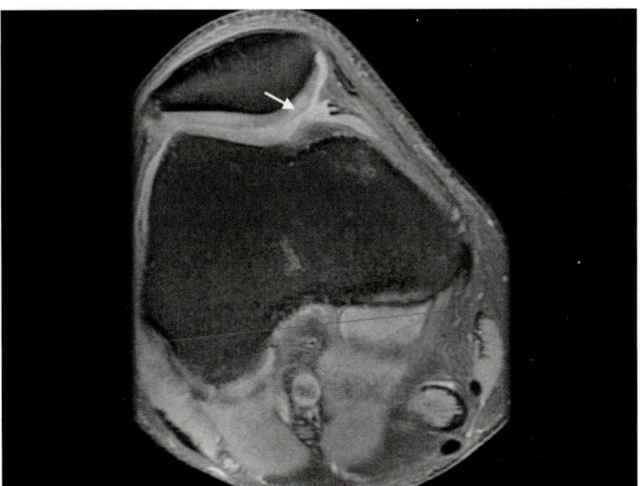

Figure 45.68 Delamination articular cartilage tear. Axial PD fat sat weighted image shows a bright fluid cleft (arrow) extending from articular cartilage over the apex of patella into the medial side representing delamination of the articular cartilage. Note absence of underlying bone marrow edema

MARROW PATHOLOGIES

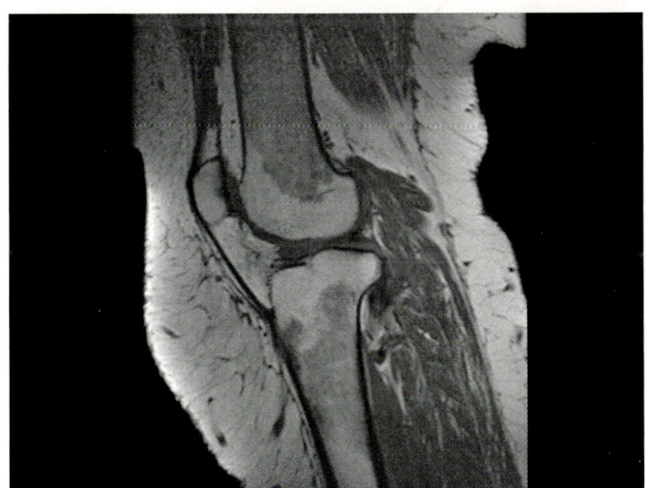

Figure 45.69 Hematopoietic hyperplasia. Sagittal T1-weighted image shows low-signal intensity hematopoietic marrow in metaphyses. Signal intensity of marrow is similar to that of muscle. High signal intensity in distal epiphyses represents normal fatty marrow. STIR image (not shown), reveals signal intensity of hematopoietic marrow in distal femurs to be slightly more than that of muscle

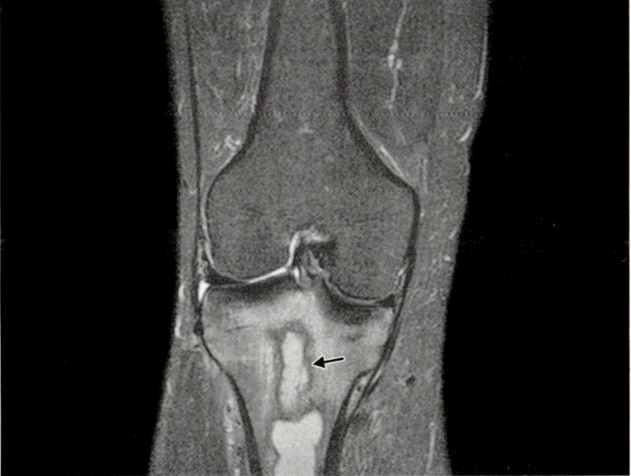

Figure 45.70 Brodies abscess. Coronal STIR weighted image shows localized osteomyelitis in the proximal tibial metadiaphyseal region seen as a well-circumscribed area of hyperintensity with a hypointense margin (arrow) and surrounding marrow edema

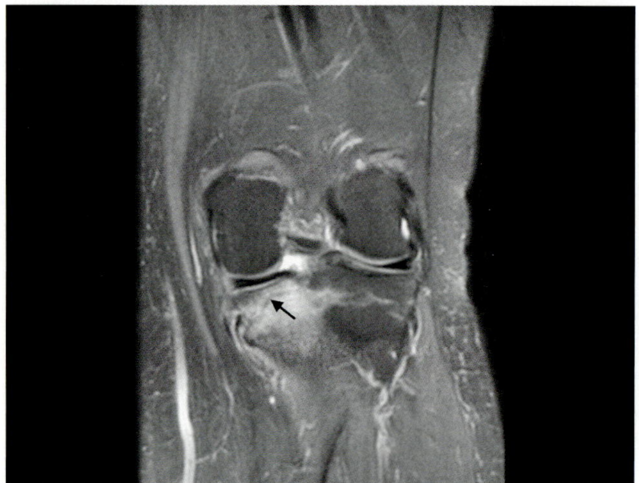

Figure 45.71 Medial tibial plateau fracture. Coronal PD fat sat weighted images reveal a horizontal fracture line (arrow) through the medial tibial plateau with surrounding bone marrow edema

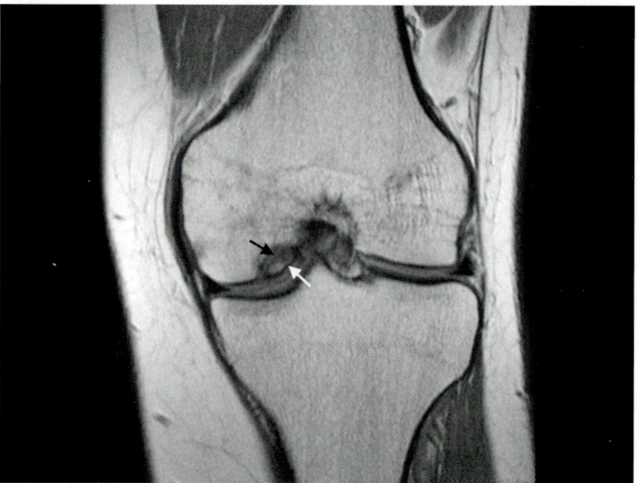

Figure 45.72 Osteochondritis dissecans. Coronal T1 weighted image shows an osteochondral fragment (arrow) with a low signal line (black arrow) surrounding the low signal necrotic fragment indicating instability. Note the fragment is located in the lateral aspect of medial femoral condyle, away from the weight bearing area

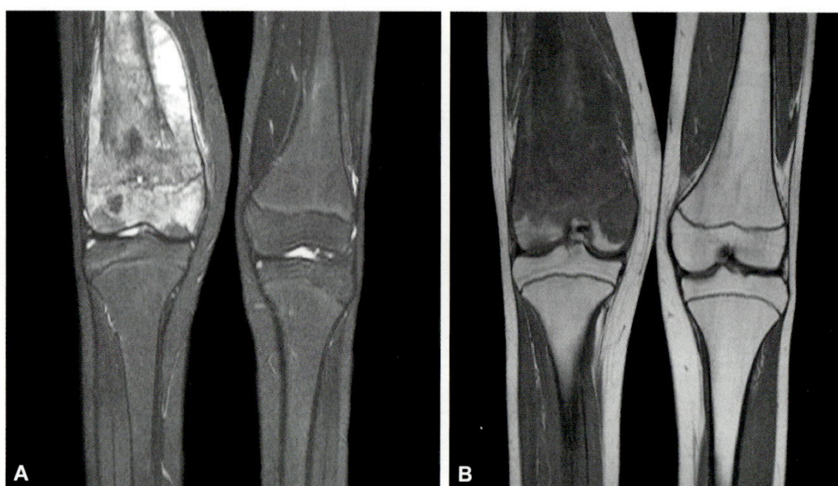

Figures 45.73A and B Osteogenic sarcoma of right distal femur. Coronal STIR (A) and T1 (B) weighted images show an irregular circumferential heterogeneous mass arising from the lower metadiaphyseal region of the right femur with cortical destruction, speculated periosteal reaction, medullary infiltration and new bone formation

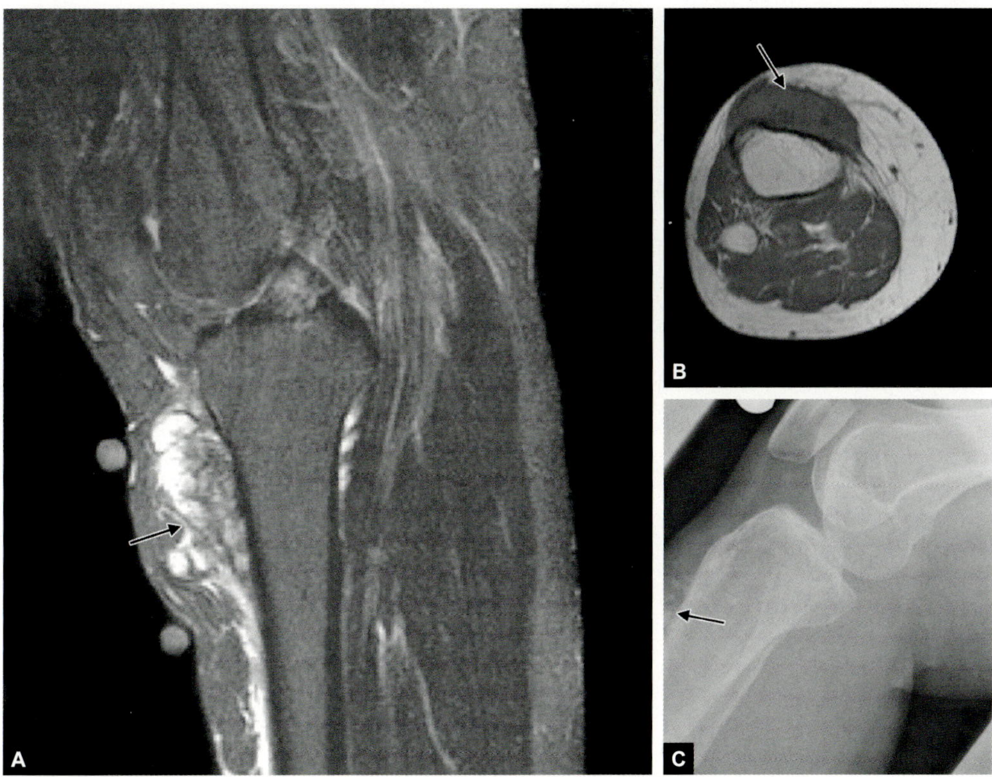

Figures 45.74A to C Paraosteal osteosarcoma of proximal tibia. Sagittal STIR image (A) shows a heterogeneous intensity mass (arrow) anterior to the proximal metadiaphyseal region of the tibia. This is hypointense on axial T1 weighted image (B) and the lateral knee radiograph (C) reveals perpendicular periosteal reaction (arrow) extending into broad-based soft-tissue mass without cortical thickening or erosion

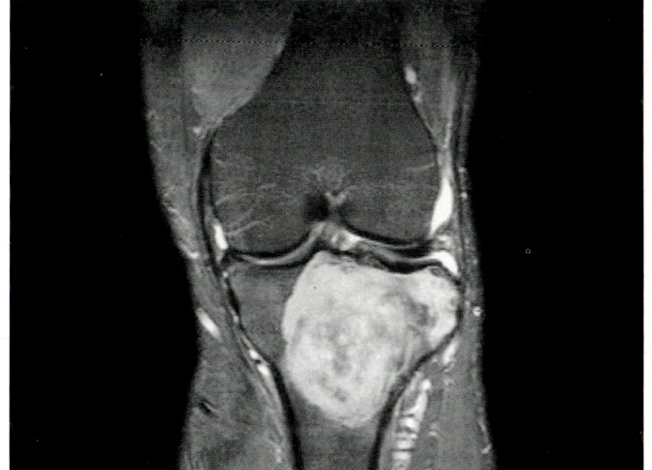

Figure 45.75 Giant cell tumor of proximal tibia. Coronal PD fat sat weighted image shows a large expansile metaepiphyseal lesion in the proximal tibia. Histopathological examination revealed a giant cell tumor

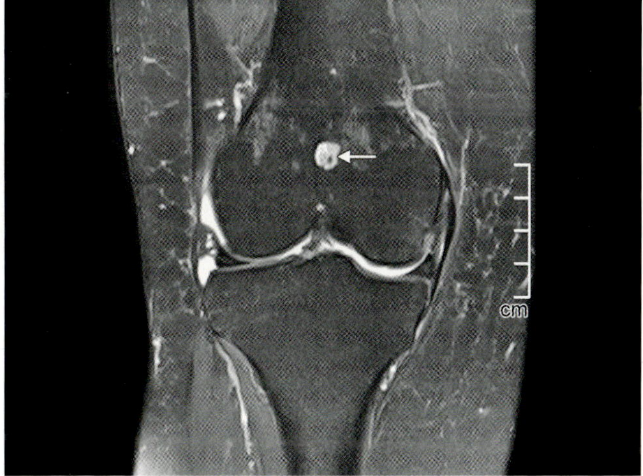

Figure 45.76 Enchondroma distal femur. Coronal PD fat sat-weighted MR image shows a small lobulated lesion (arrow) in the medullary cavity of the distal femur, a typical appearance of a benign enchondroma. Note tiny central hypointensities representing calcification. Patients with a small, painless, lobulated lesion such as this need not be referred to an orthopedic oncologist

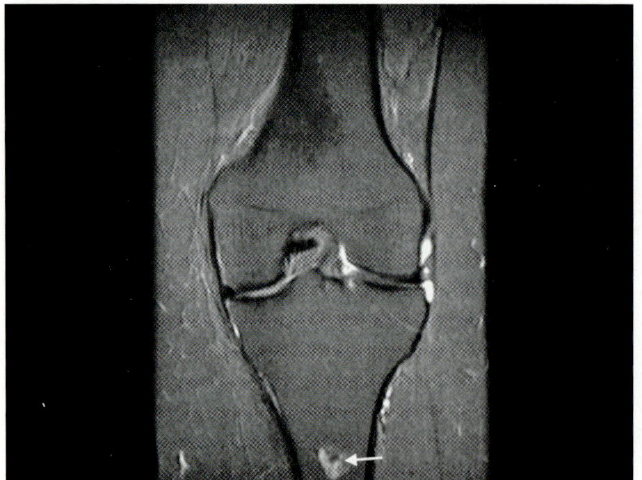

Figure 45.77 Enchondroma proximal tibia. Coronal PD fat sat-weighted MR image shows a small lobulated lesion (arrow) in the medullary cavity of the proximal tibia, a typical appearance of a benign enchondroma. Note tiny central hypointensity representing calcification

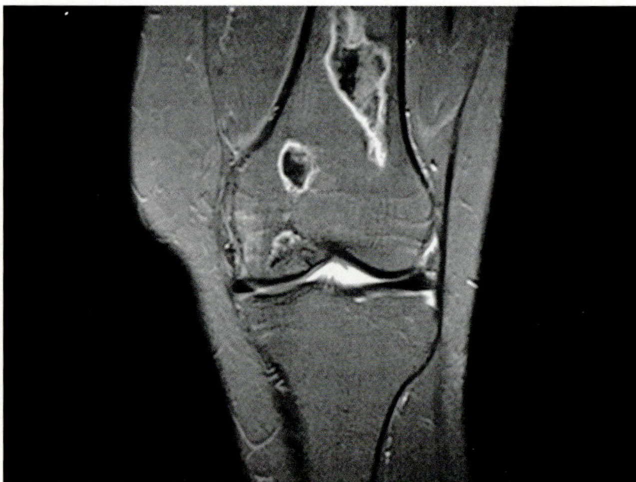

Figure 45.78 Osteonecrosis. Coronal PD fat sat image in a patient receiving corticosteroids therapy reveals classic morphological features of osteonecrosis involving the femur. Note the serpentine-like outline of the fat-containing lesions

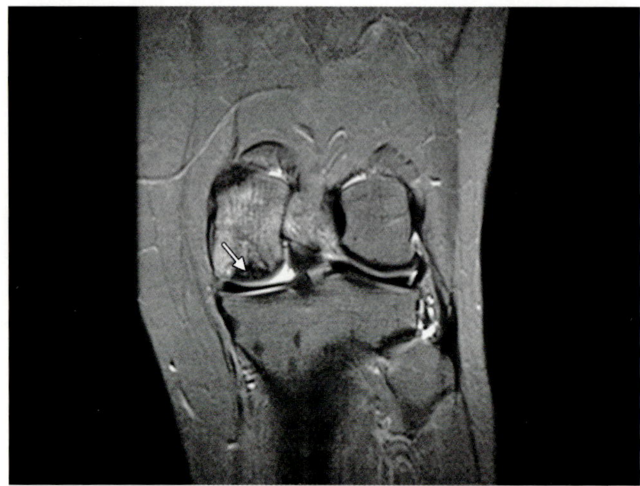

Figure 45.79 Spontaneous osteonecrosis of the knee (SONK). Coronal PD fat sat image shows a wide subchondral area of low signal intensity (arrow) with underlying bone marrow edema. Note no evidence of cortical flattening or any subcortical fracture related fluid cleft

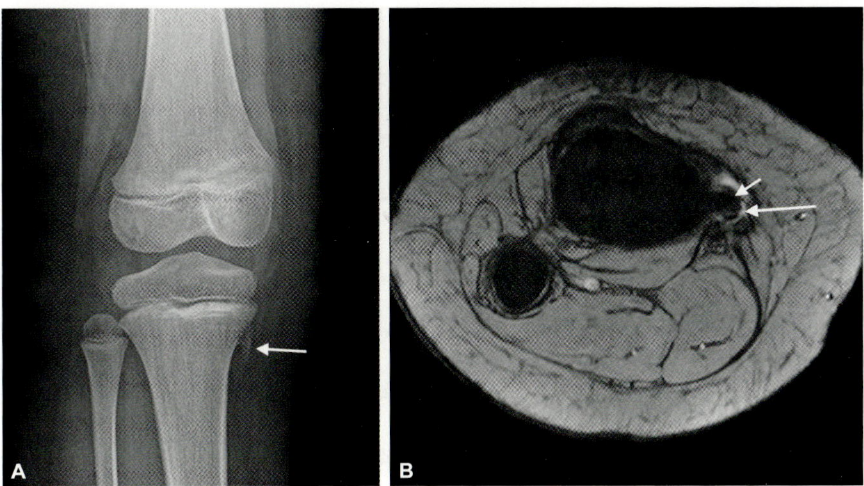

Figures 45.80A and B Solitary osteochondroma. AP knee radiograph (A) shows an exostosis as a bony outgrowth (arrow) from the medial aspect of the metadiaphyseal portion of tibia. Axial gradient image (B) reveals the osteochondroma (short arrow) with a thin hyperintense cartilaginous cap (long arrow). Note the indentation and displacement of the overlying conjoint pes anserine tendons

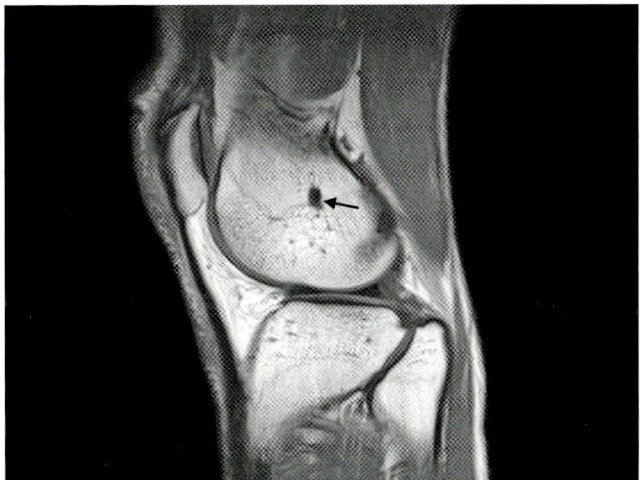

Figure 45.81 Bone island. Sagittal T1 weighted image shows a well define hypointense lesion within the lateral femoral condyle representing enostosis or bone island

CYSTS AND BURSAE

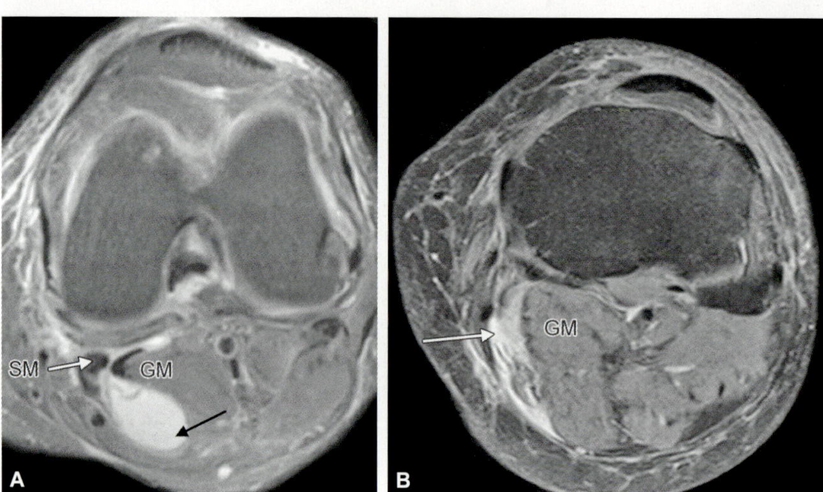

Figures 45.82A and B Synovial/Baker's cyst. Axial PD fat sat image (A) shows a synovial cyst located between the semimembranosus (SM) and medial head of gastrocnemius tendon (GM) and projecting posteriorly on the medial side of popliteal fossa. (B) shows fluid of high signal intensity (arrow) overlying the medial head of gastrocnemius tendon and muscle (GM) as a result of ruptures popliteal cyst

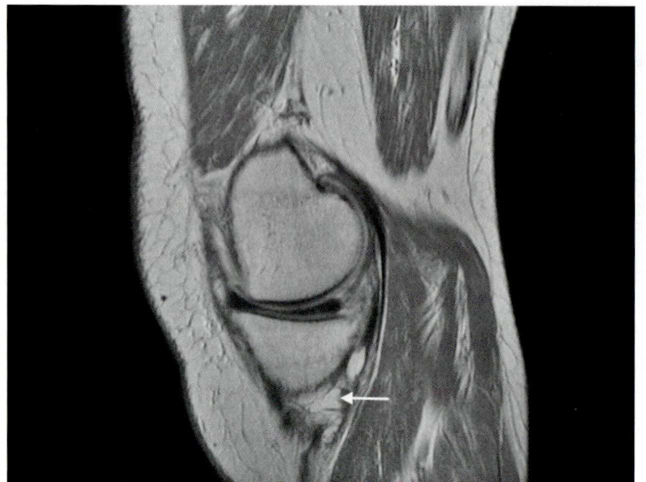

Figure 45.83 Pes Anserine bursitis. Sagittal PD image shows fluid signal intensity (arrow) in the medial aspect of tibia, along the conjoint tendons of Sartorius, gracilis and semitendonosus suggestive of inflammatory bursitis

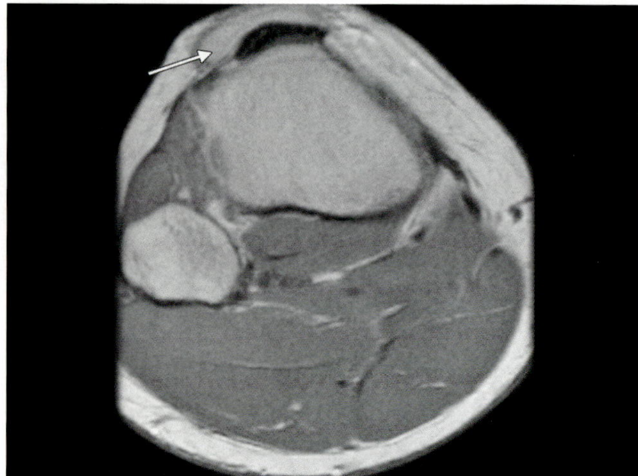

Figure 45.84 Prepatellar bursitis. Axial PD image shows a fluid collection (arrow) anterior to patellar tendon suggestive of prepatellar bursitis

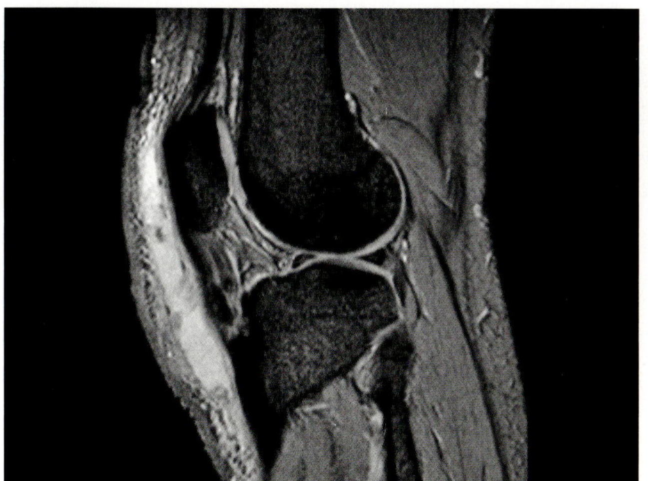

Figure 45.85 Prepatellar bursitis. Sagittal gradient image shows a fluid collection anterior to patella and patellar tendon suggestive of prepatellar bursitis

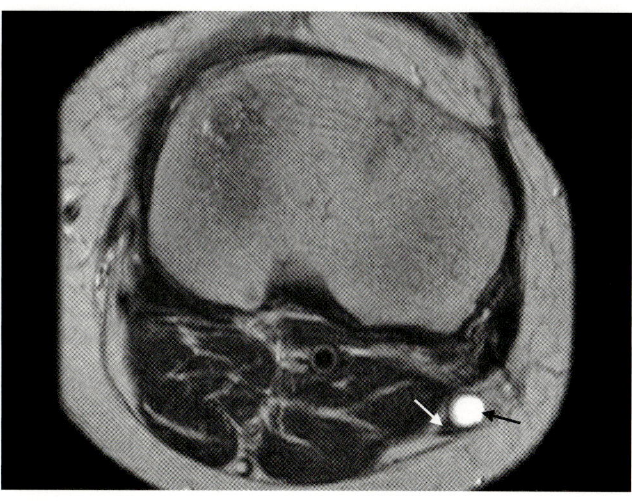

Figure 45.86 Peroneal nerve ganglion cyst. Axial PD weighted image shows a rounded cyst (black arrow) along the course of the common peroneal nerve (white arrow) in a patient presenting with foot drop

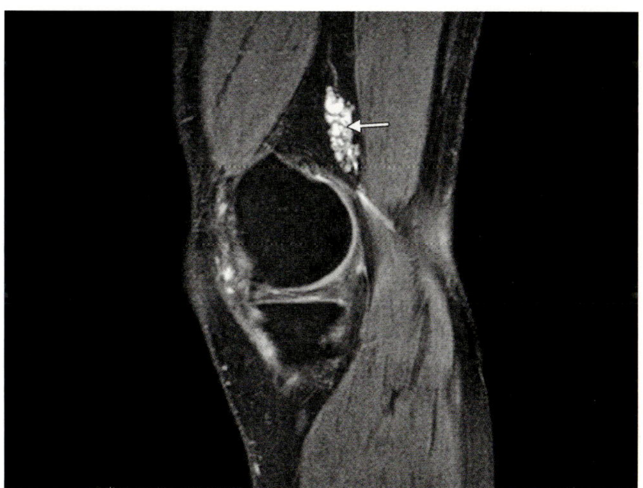

Figure 45.87 Slow flow vascular malformation. Sagittal PD fat sat weighted image shows a lobulated hyperintense cystic appearing soft tissue abnormality (arrow) in the intermuscular tissue plane suggestive of a slow flow vascular malformation

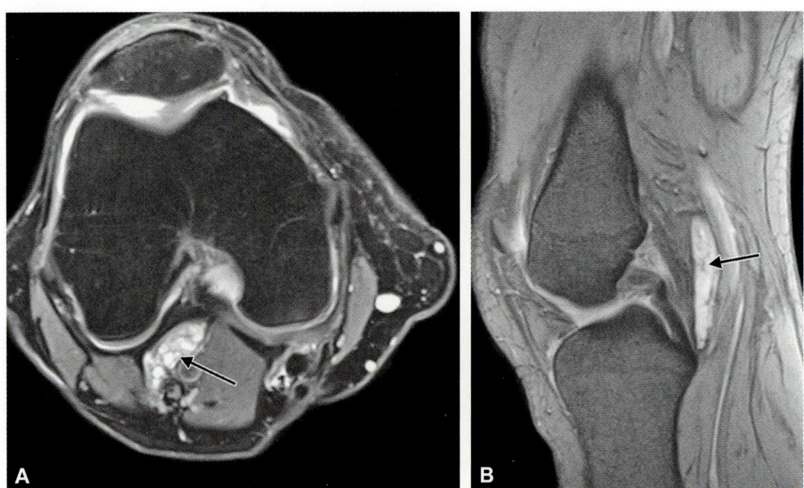

Figures 45.88A and B Capsular ganglion cyst. Axial (A) and sagittal (B) PD fat sat images show a lobulated fluid filled structure, along the posterior joint capsule suggestive of capsular ganglion cyst

Chapter 46

Atlas: Arthroscopy

Ashok Rajgopal, Attique Vasdev, Vivek Dahiya, Vipin Tyagi, Himanshu Gupta

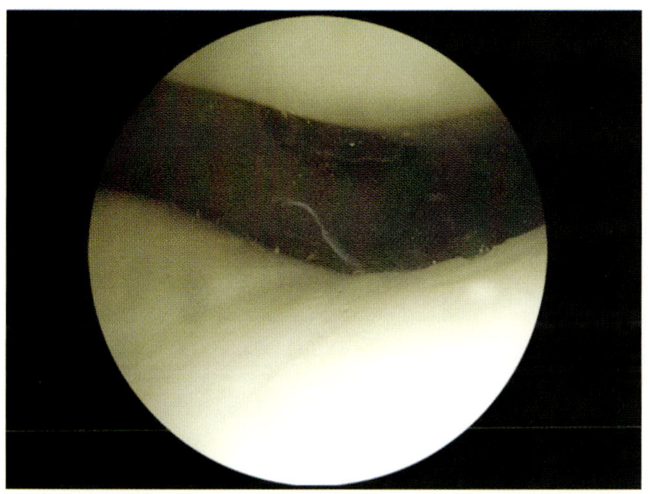

Figure 46.1 Normal patellofemoral cartilage

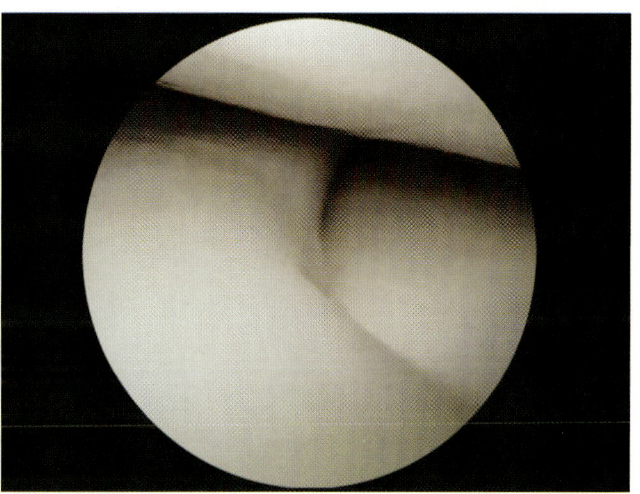

Figure 46.2 Normal medial meniscus

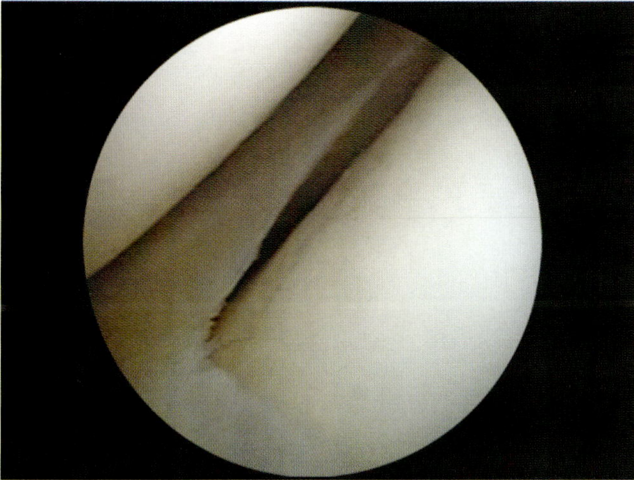

Figure 46.3 Normal lateral meniscus

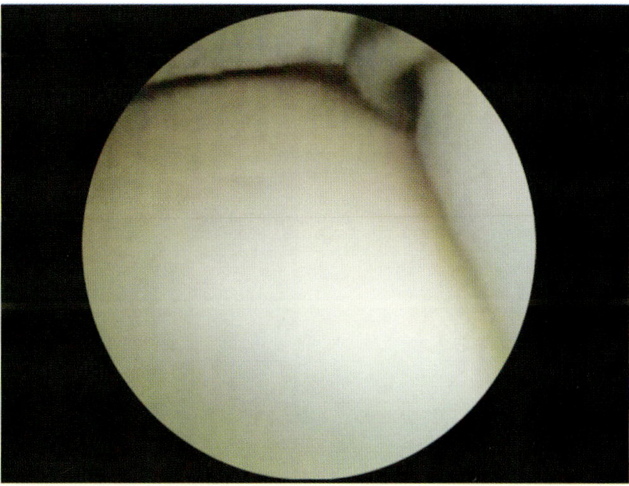

Figure 46.4 Probing of normal meniscus

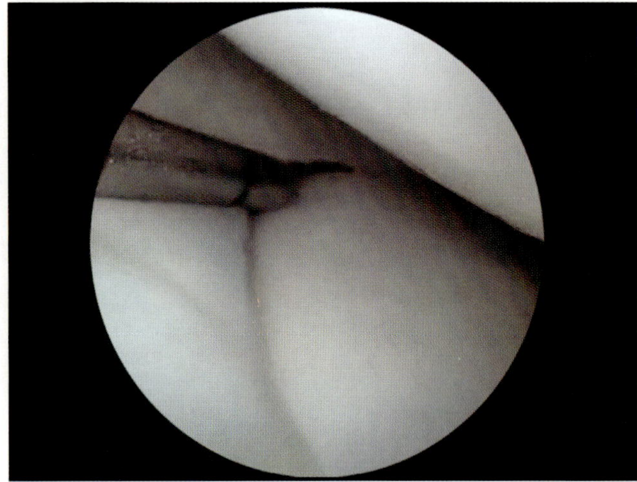

Figure 46.5 Normal medial meniscus probing

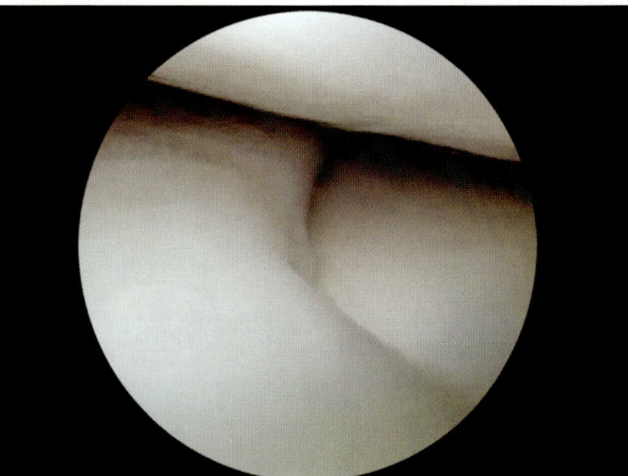

Figure 46.6 Normal medial meniscus top view

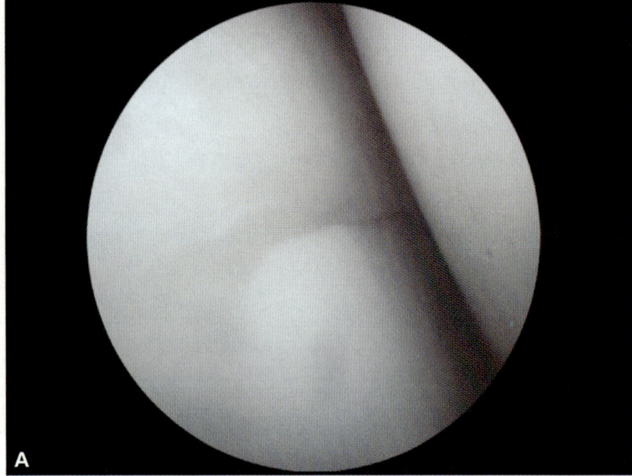

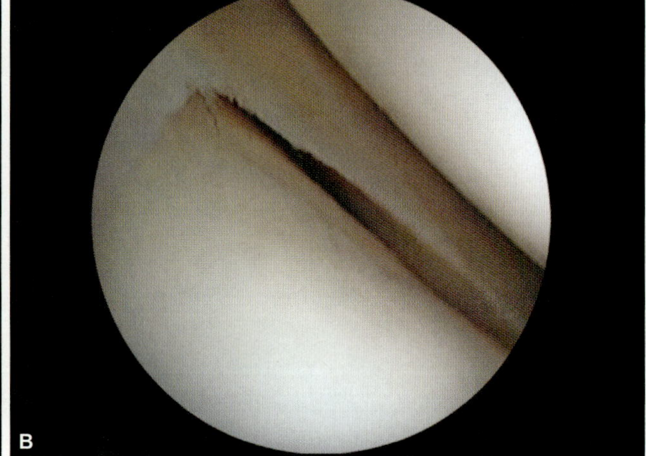

Figures 46.7A and B Normal meniscus

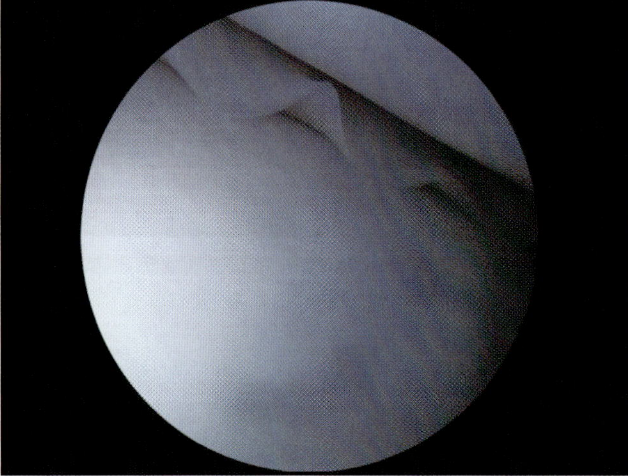

Figure 46.8 Normal variation of medial meniscus

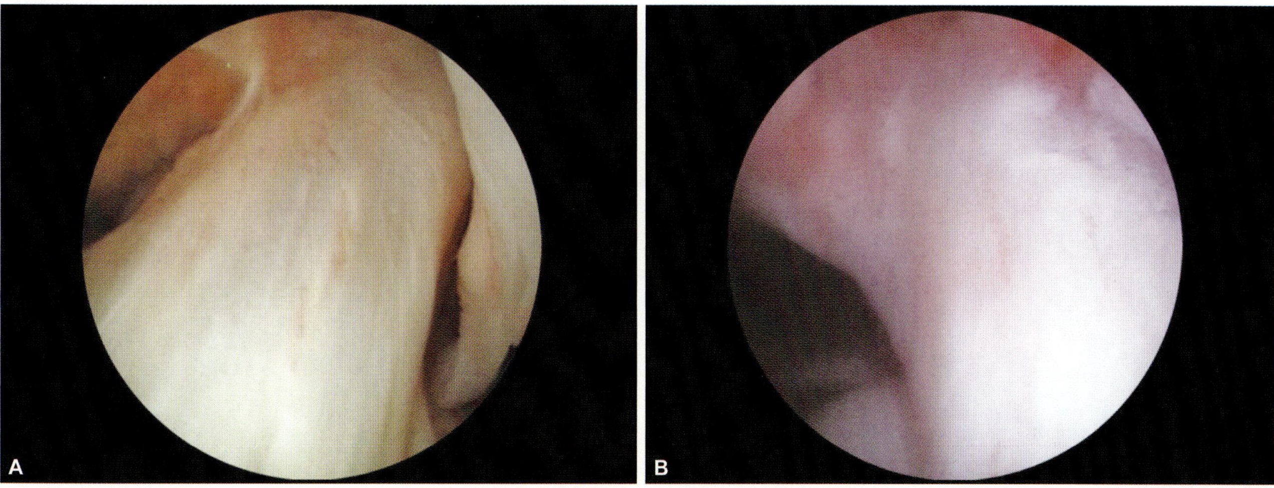

Figures 46.9A and B Normal ACL

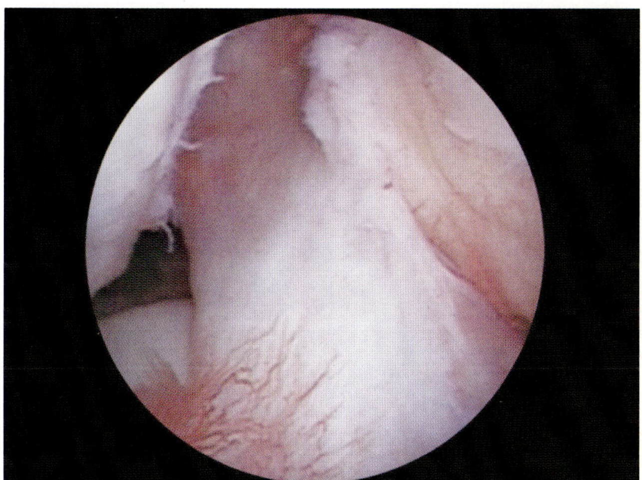

Figure 46.10 Normal ACL with excessive vascularization

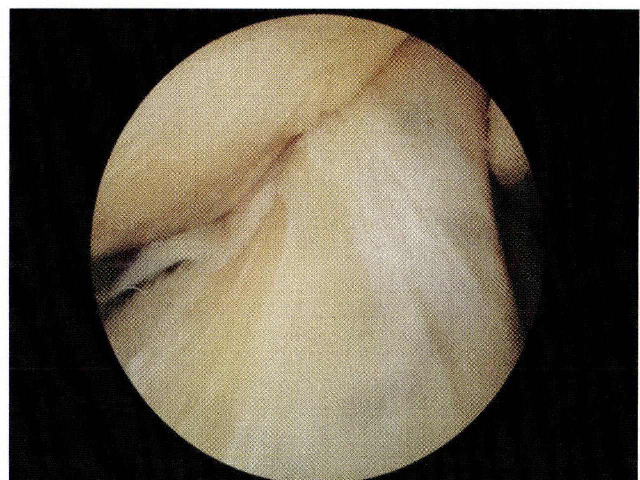

Figure 46.11 Normal ACL with spiral orientation of fibers of both bundles

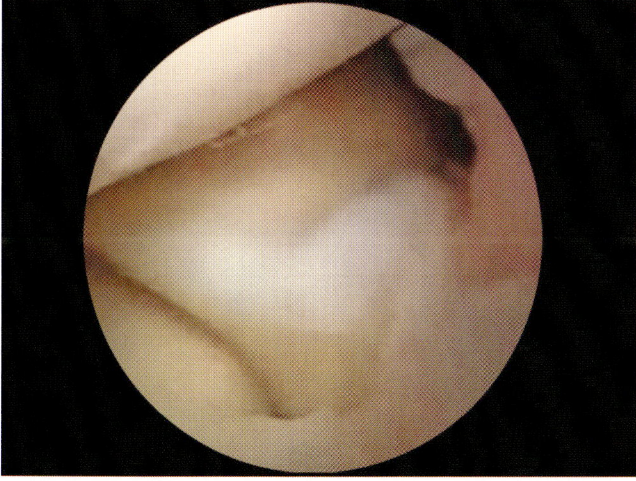

Figure 46.12 Normal posterior horn

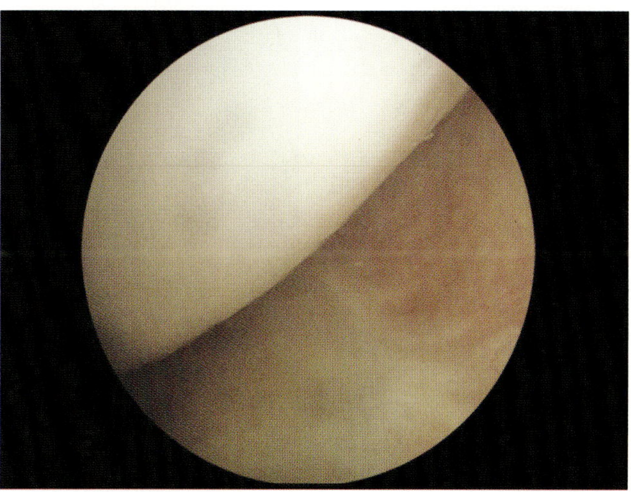

Figure 46.13 Normal meniscus capsule junction

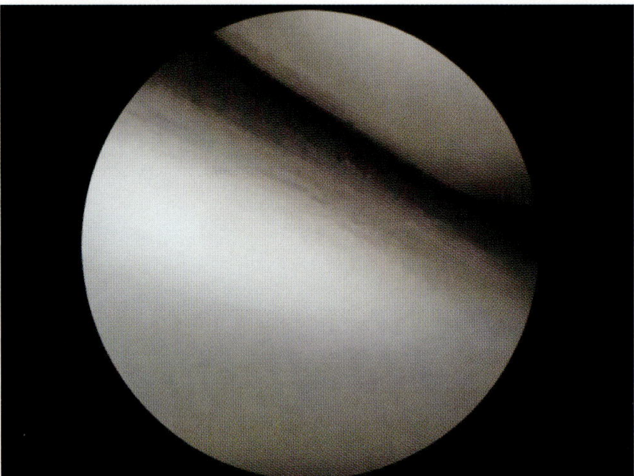

Figure 46.14 Normal cartilage

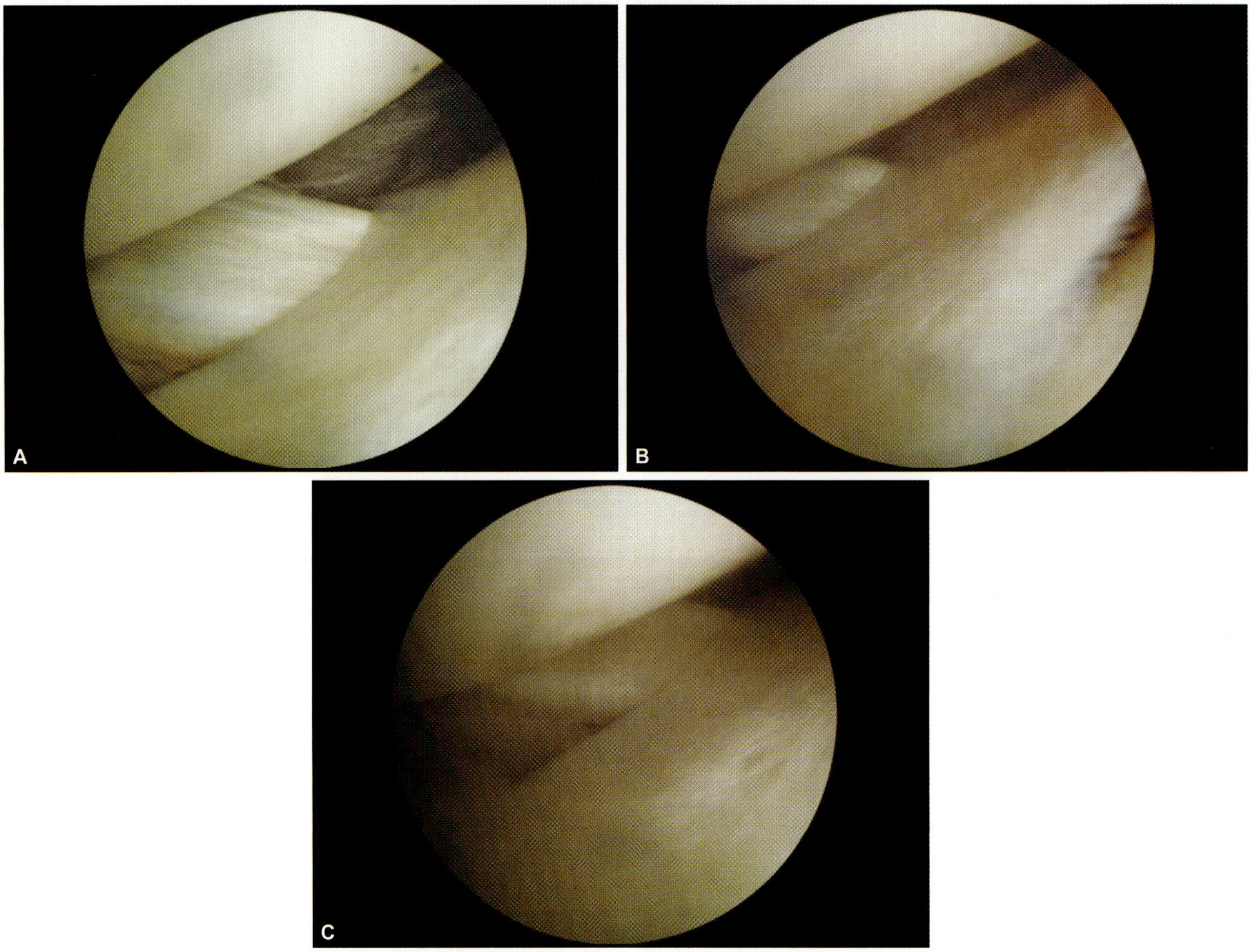

A B C

Figures 46.15A to C Normal popliteus

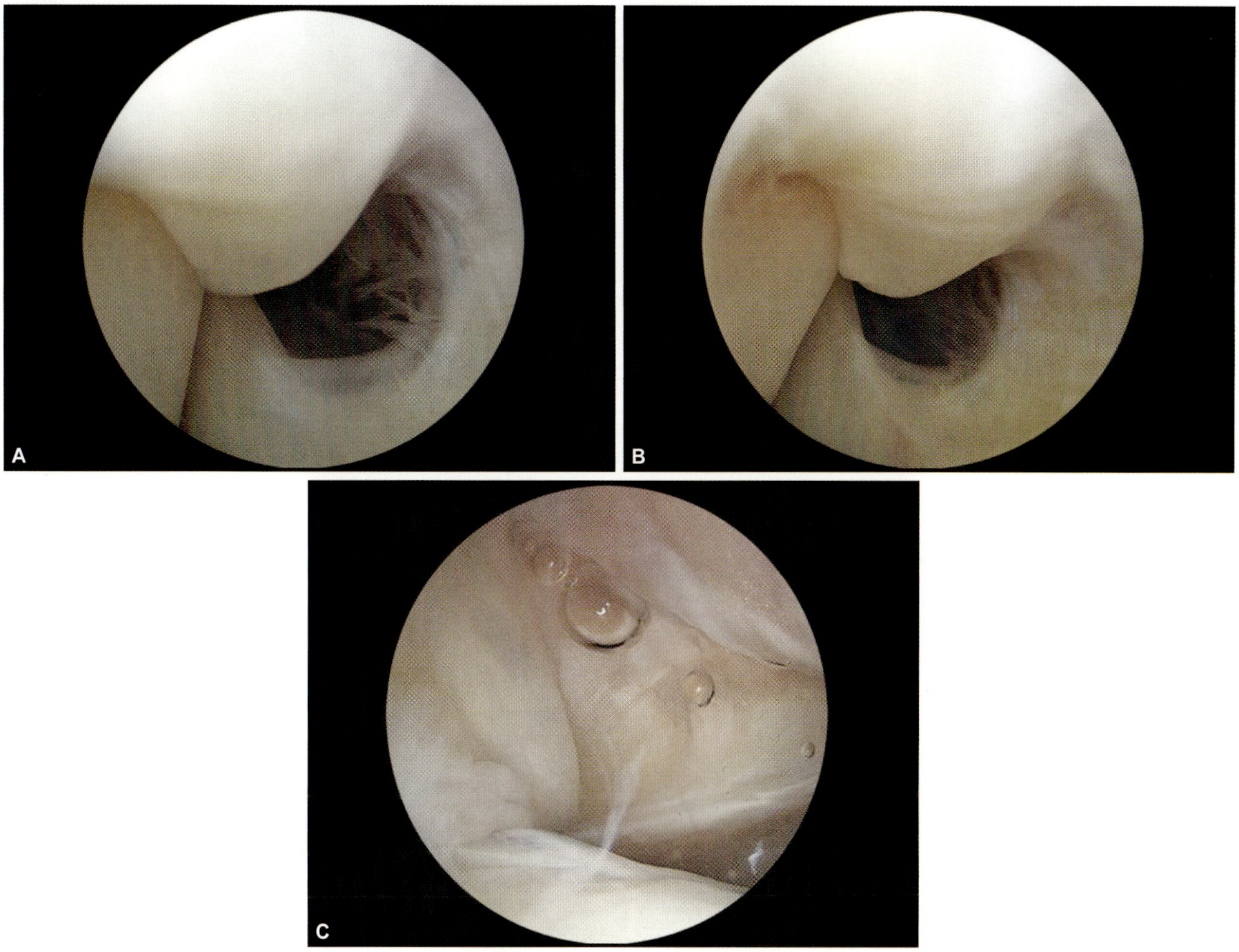

Figures 46.16A to C Popliteal hiatus

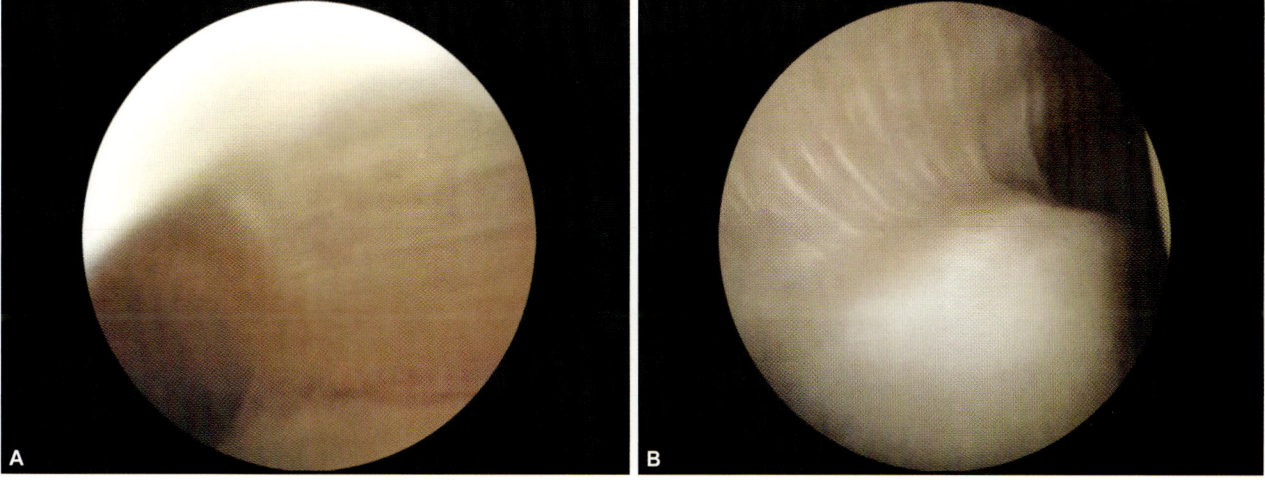

Figures 46.17A and B Lateral gutter

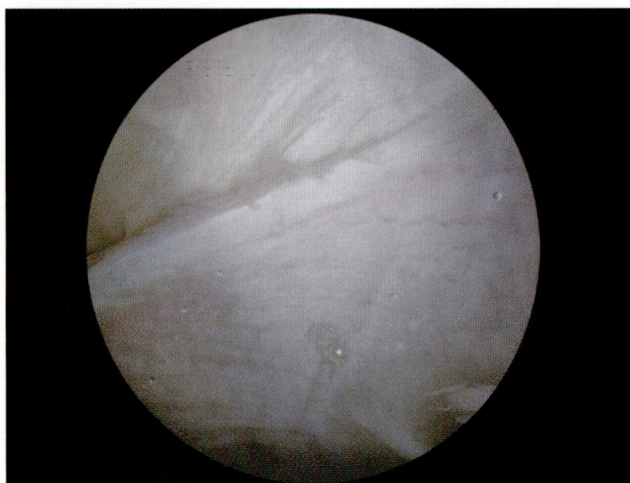

Figure 46.18 Medial gutter

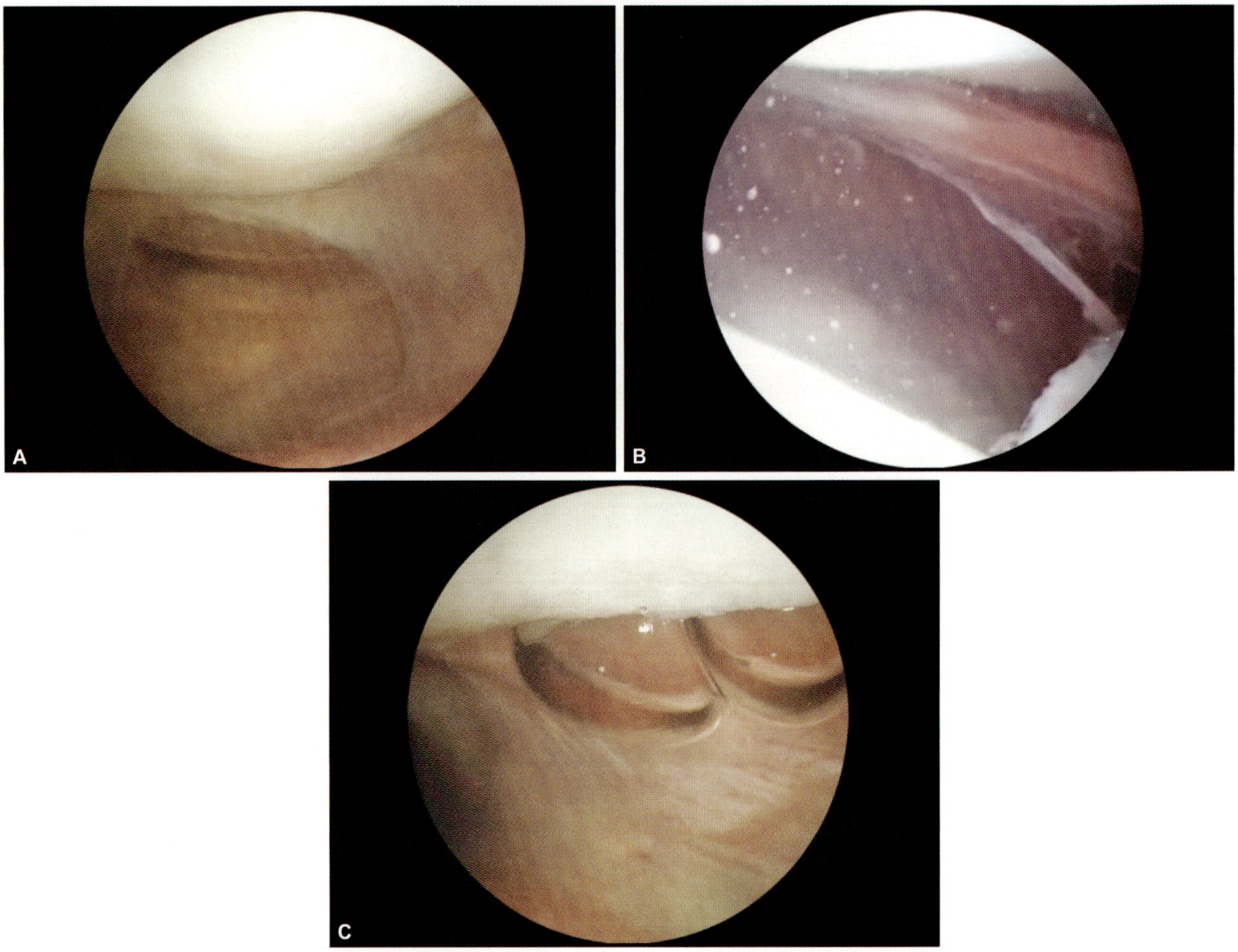

A B C

Figures 46.19A to C PLICA suprapatellar pouch

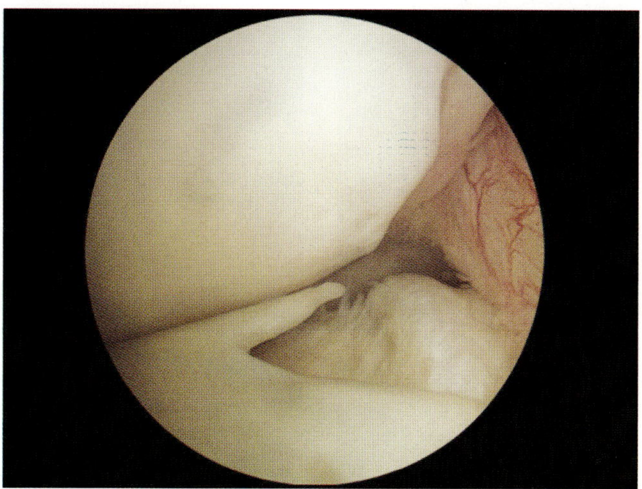

Figure 46.20 Lateral discoid meniscus—incomplete

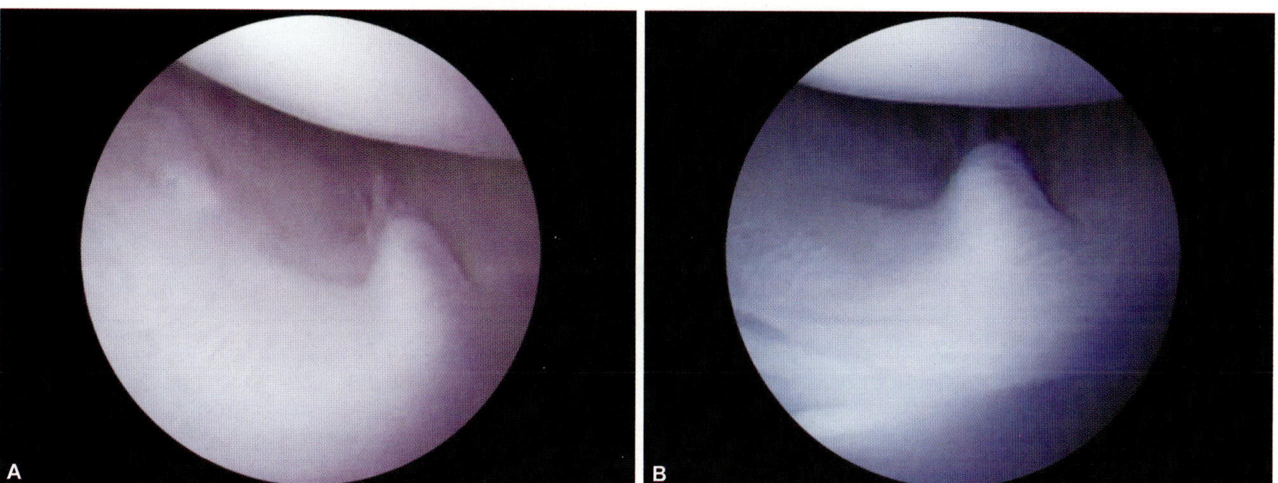

Figures 46.21A and B Discoid lateral meniscus complete type

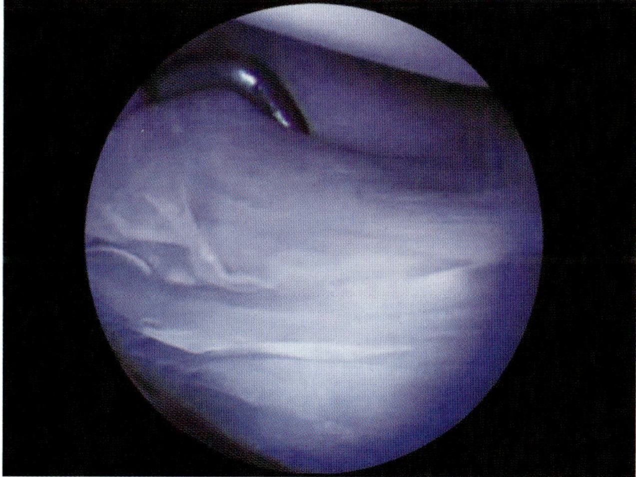

Figure 46.22 Probing discoid lateral meniscus

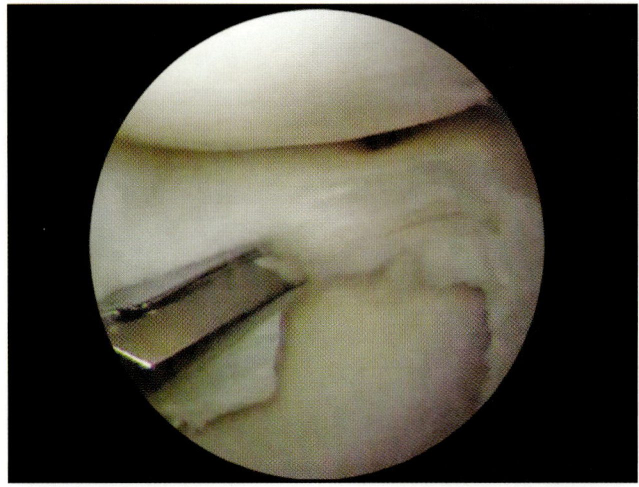

Figure 46.23 Meniscectomy lateral discoid meniscus

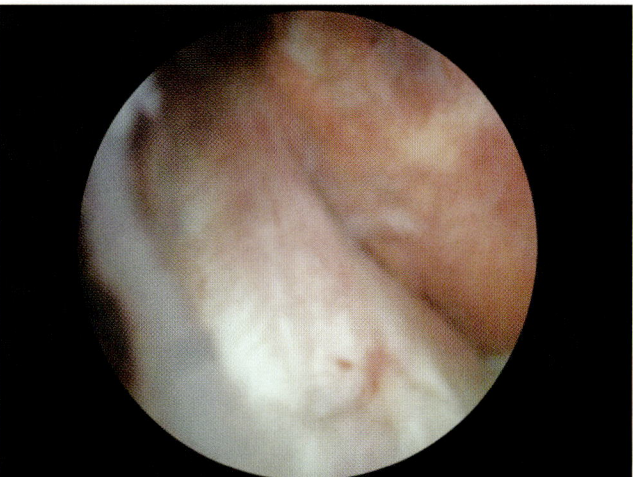

Figure 46.24 Inflammatory reaction around anterior cruciate ligament

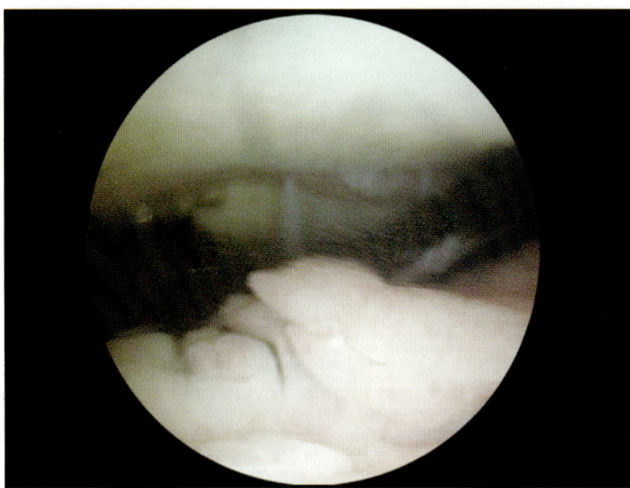

Figure 46.25 Synovial hypertrophy patellofemoral joint

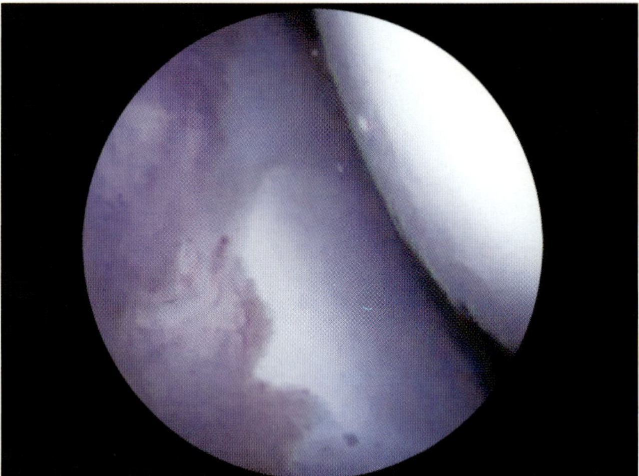

Figure 46.26 Anterior horn medial meniscus with synovial hypertrophy

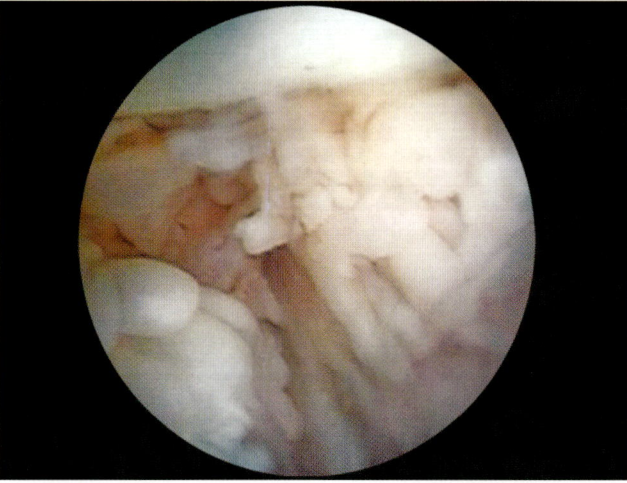

Figure 46.27 Synovitis

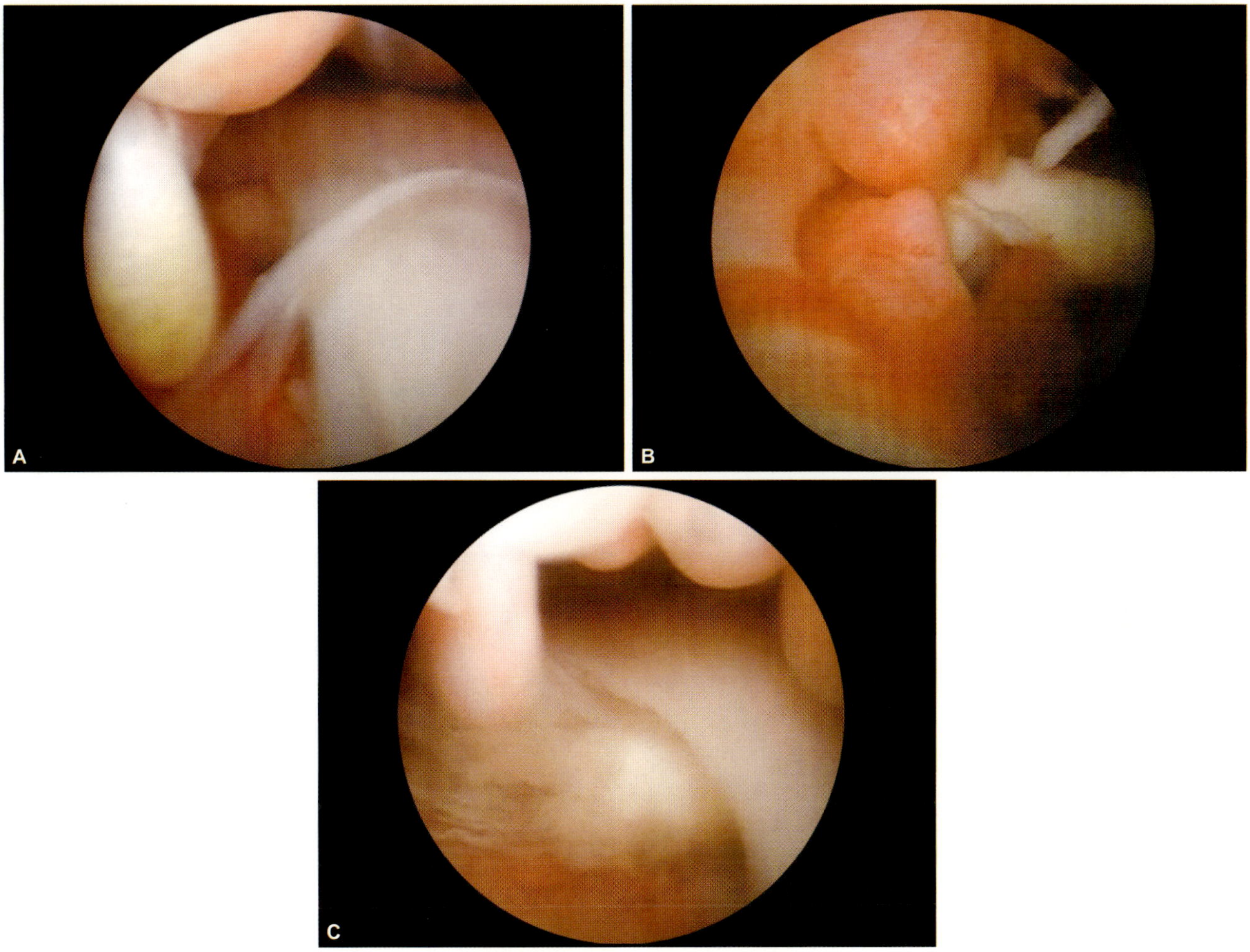

Figures 46.28A to C Inflammatory synovitis

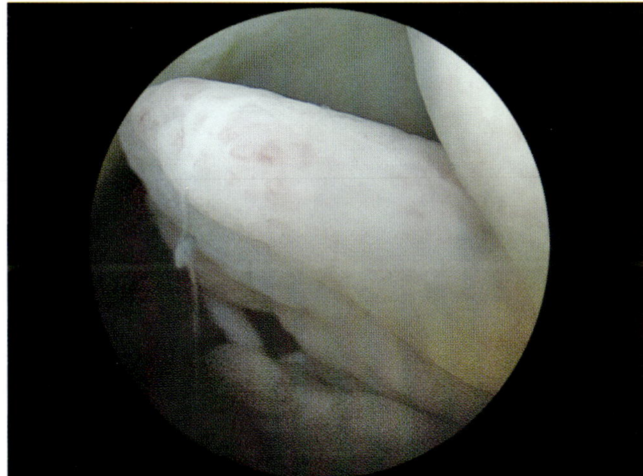

Figure 46.29 Synovial hypertrophy

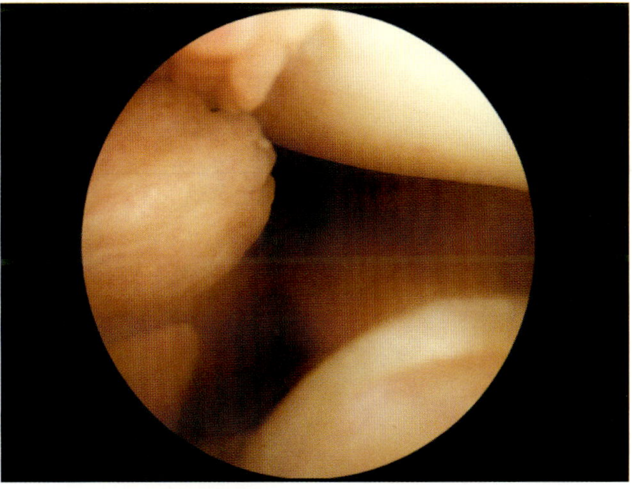

Figure 46.30 Inflammatory synovitis

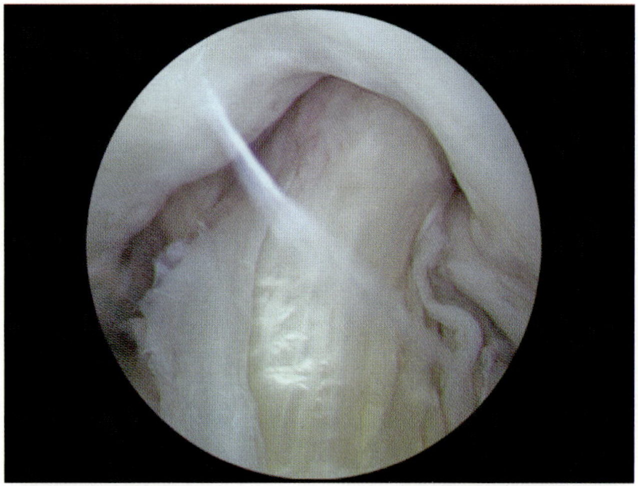

Figure 46.31 ACL with notch impingement

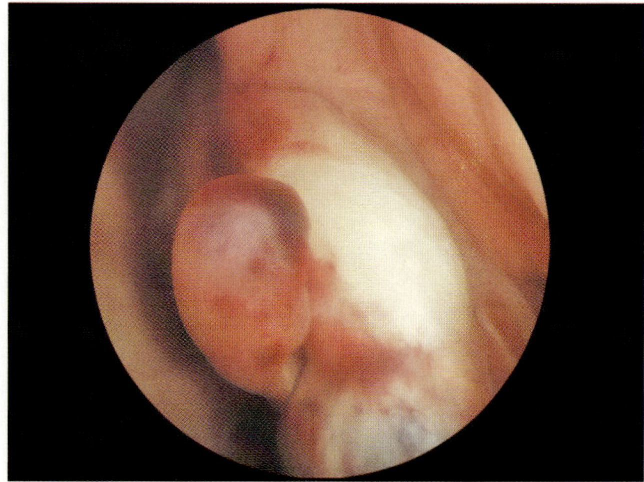

Figure 46.32 Inflammatory synovitis

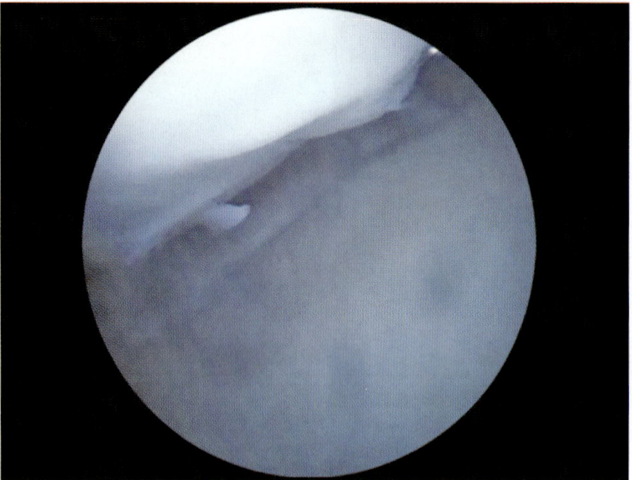

Figure 46.33 Grade 1 chondromalacia (softening) demonstration with probe

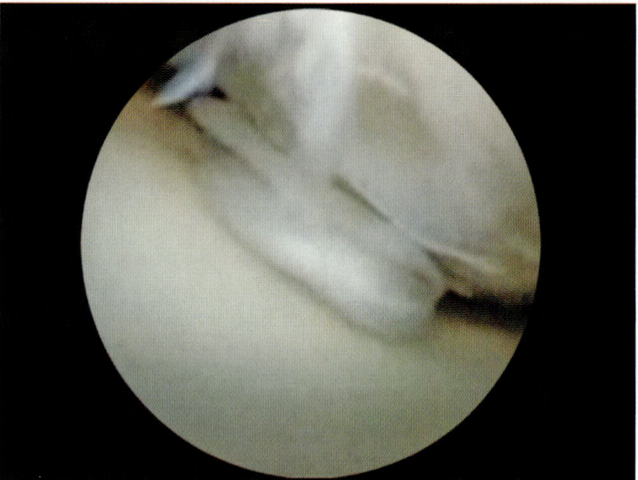

Figure 46.34 Loose femoral chondral fragment

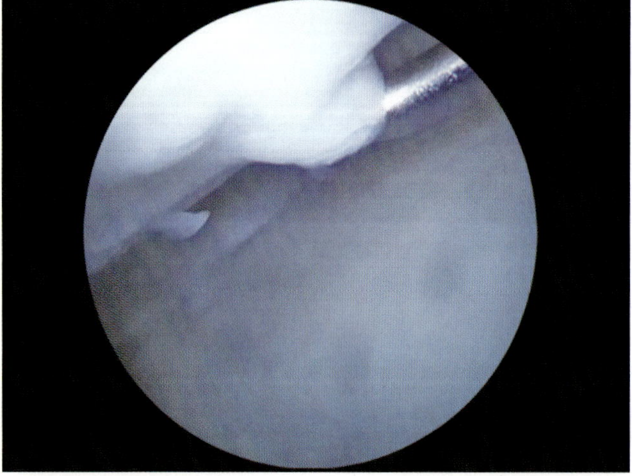

Figure 46.35 Femoral cartilage delamination demonstration with probe inside defect

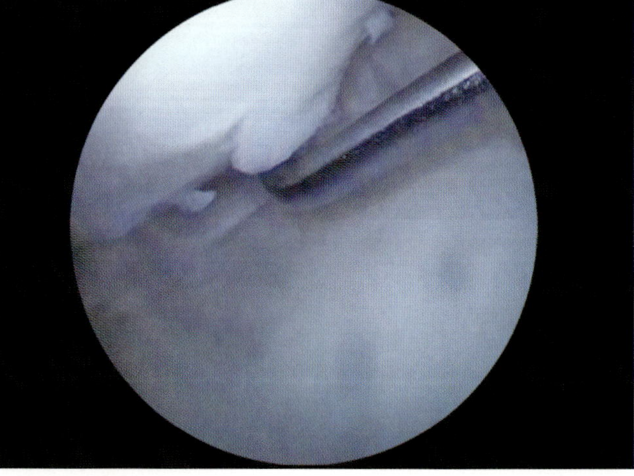

Figure 46.36 Femoral cartilage delamination demonstration with help of probe

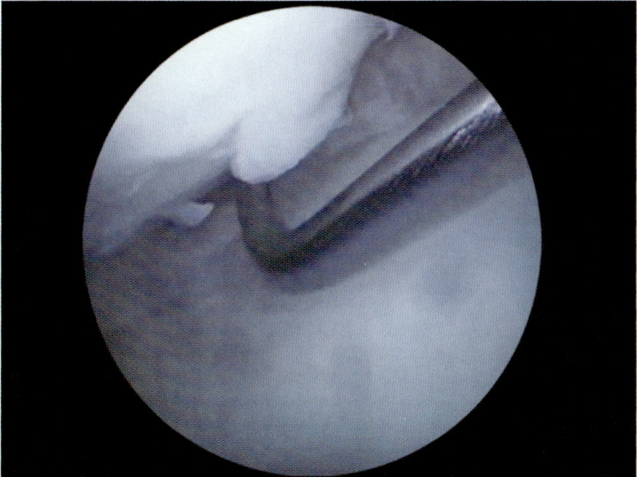

Figure 46.37 Attached chondral flap

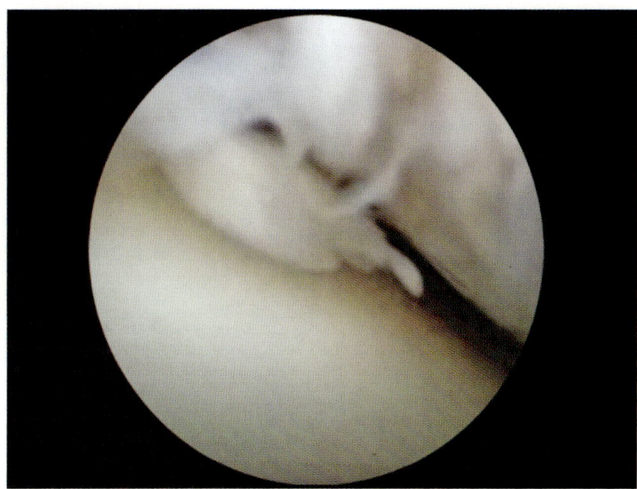

Figure 46.38 Chondromalacia femur with free chondral fragment

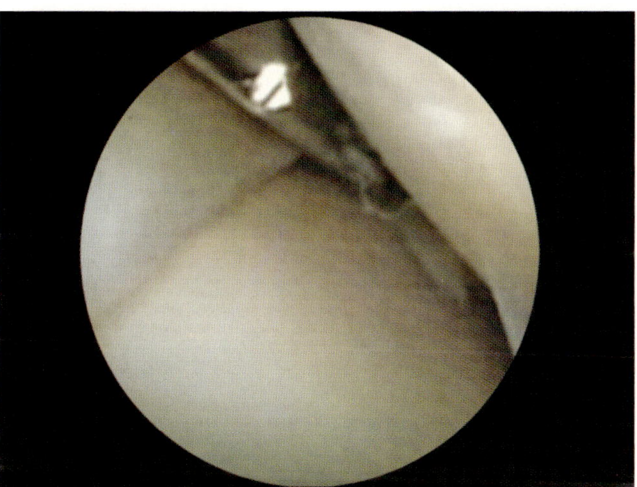

Figure 46.39 Grade 2 chondromalacia

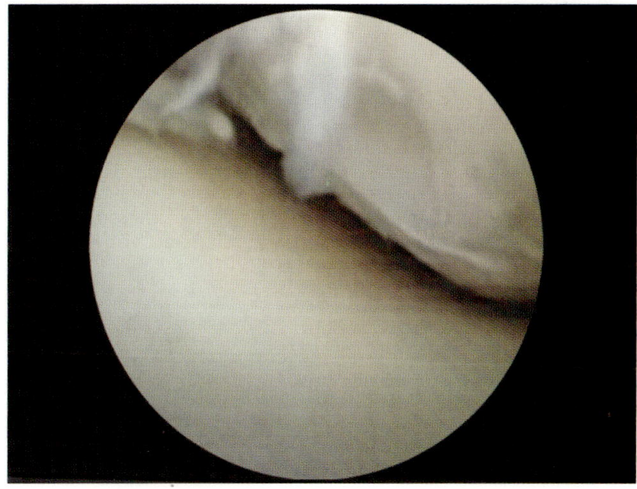

Figure 46.40 Grade 3 chondromalacia in femur

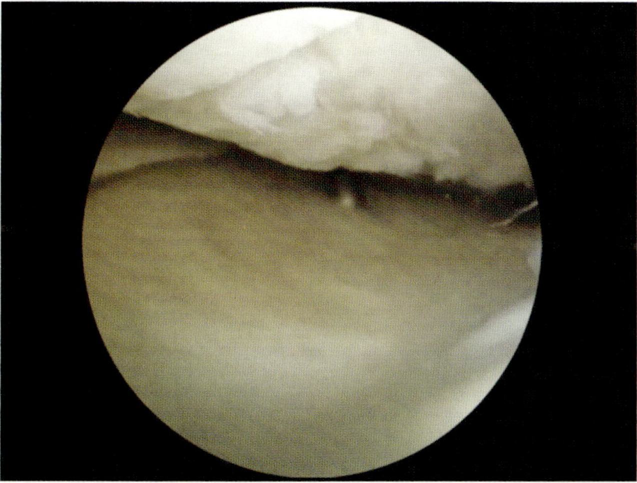

Figure 46.41 Grade 1 chondromalacia in tibia and grade 2 in femur

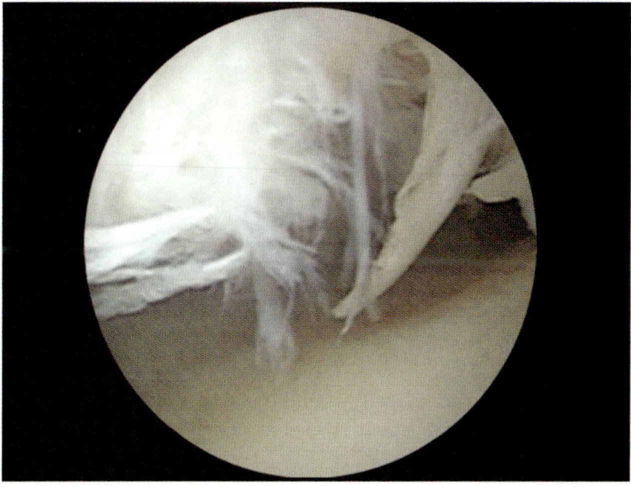

Figure 46.42 Grade 3 chondromalacia with fraying of cartilage

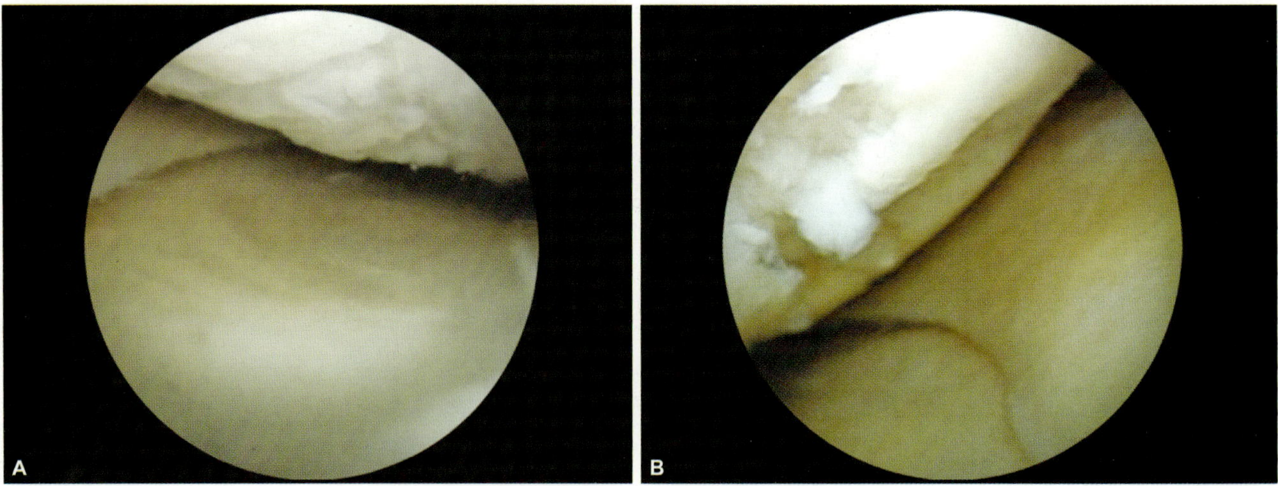

Figures 46.43A and B Grade 3 chondromalacia in femur

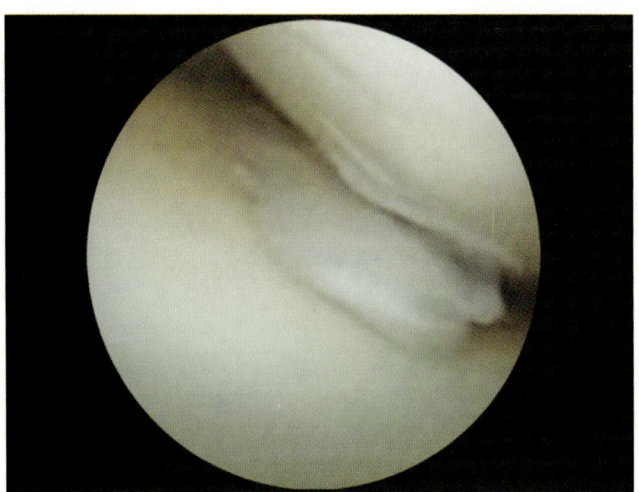

Figure 46.44 Loose body (chondral fragment)

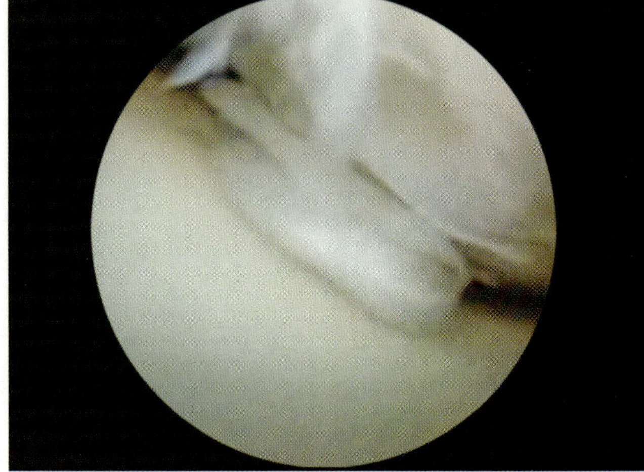

Figure 46.45 Grade 3 chondromalacia with free chondral fragment

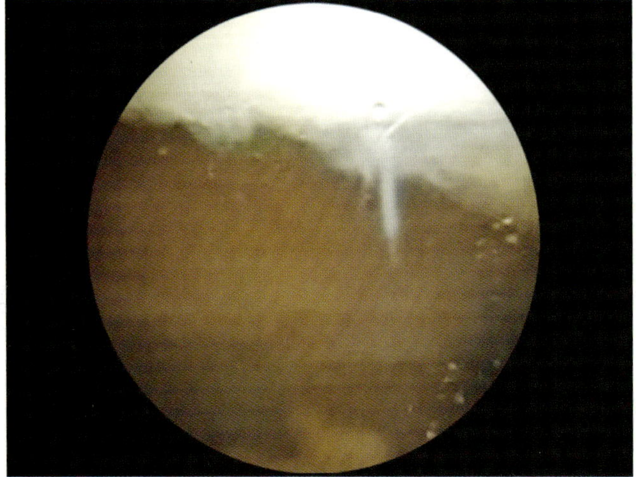

Figure 46.46 Grade 3 chondromalacia patella

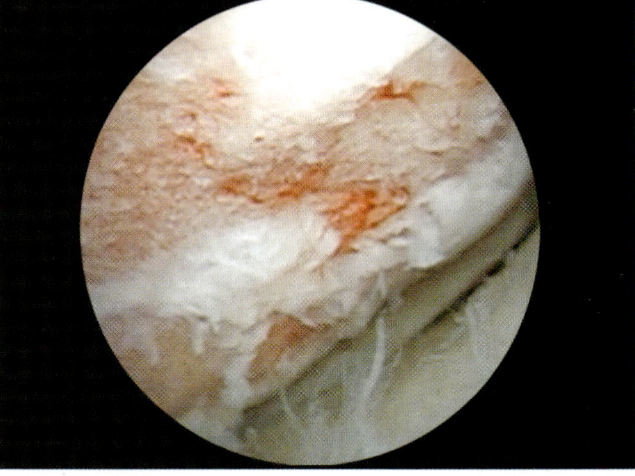

Figure 46.47 Osteochondral defect (chondromalacia grade 4)

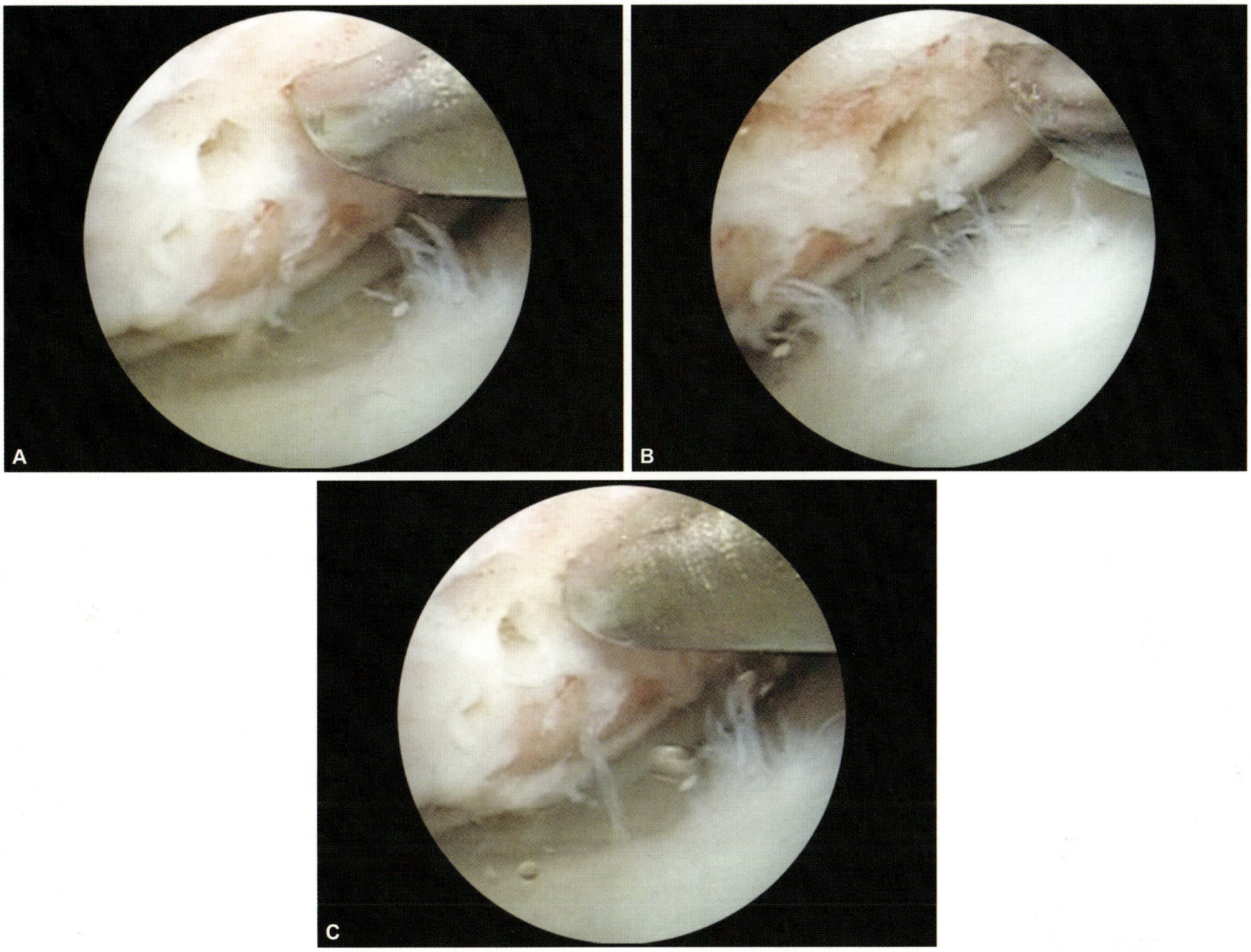

Figures 46.48A to C Microfracture in osteochondral defect

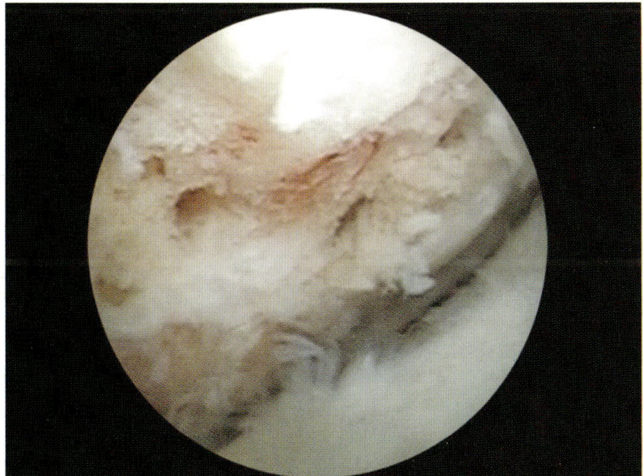

Figure 46.49 Femur osteochondral defect

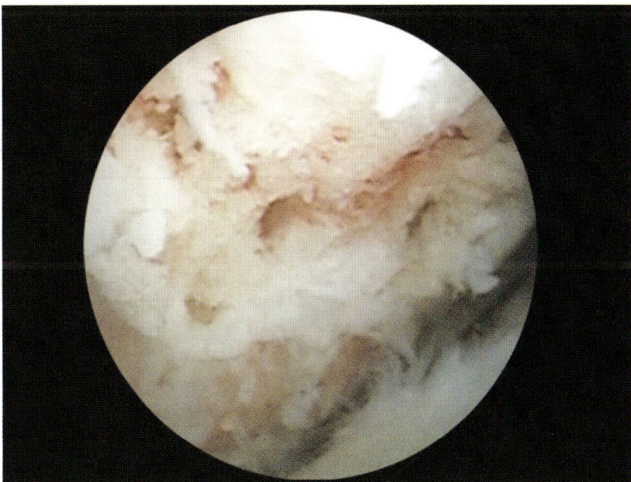

Figure 46.50 Microfracture (Osteochondral)

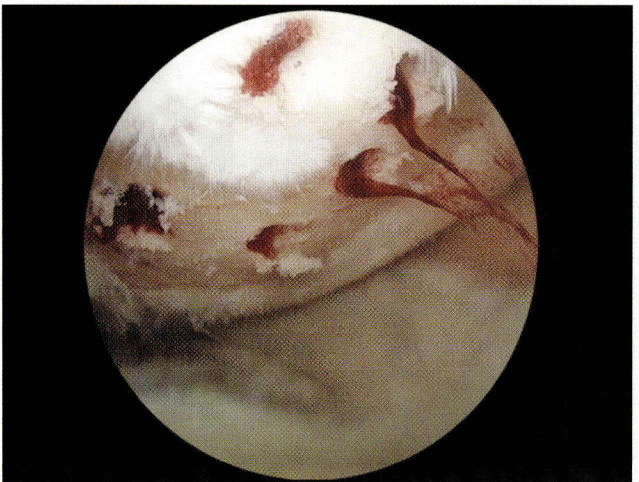

Figure 46.51 Hematoma formation in microfracture

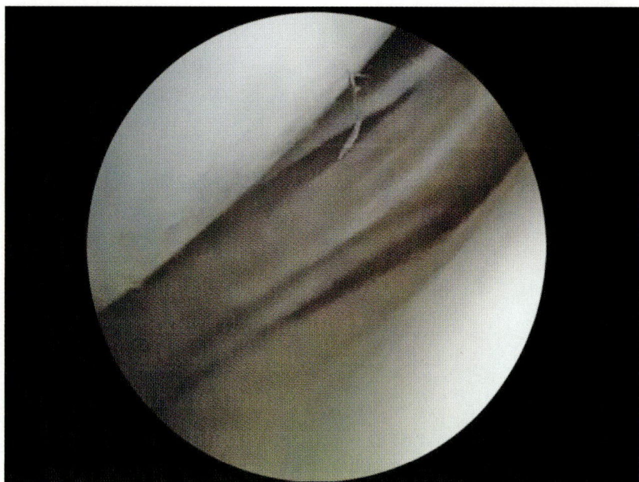

Figure 46.52 Lateral meniscus vertical tear

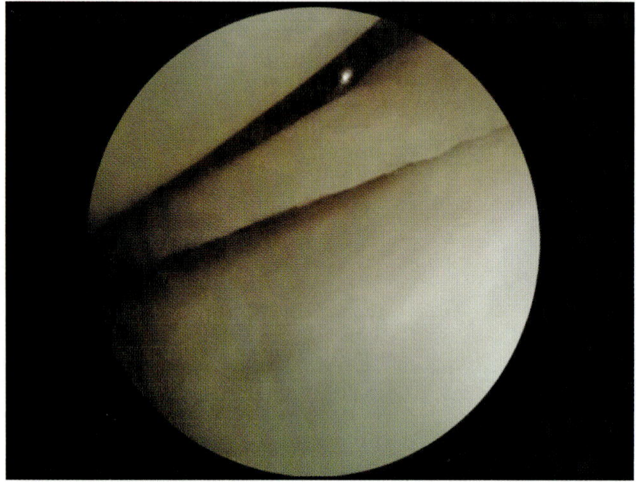

Figure 46.53 Vertical incomplete tear

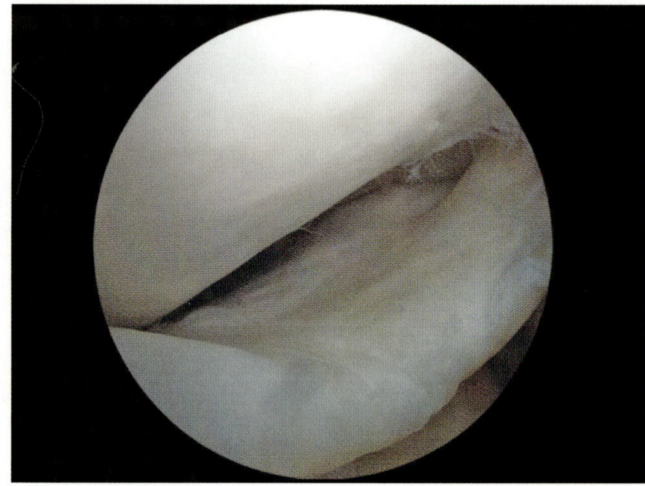

Figure 46.54 Medial meniscus bucket handle tear displaced in notch

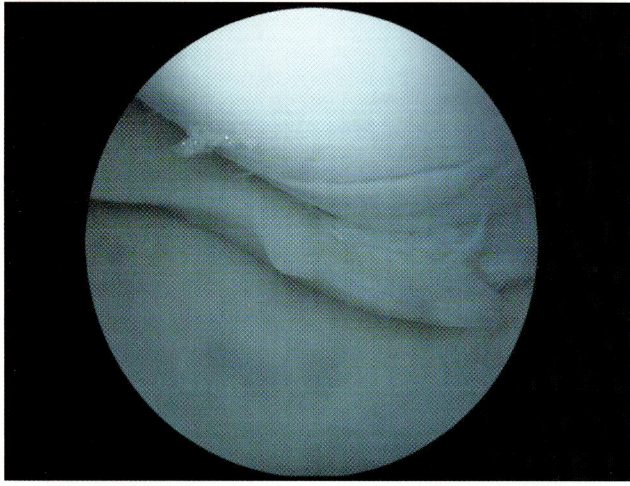

Figure 46.55 Bucket handle tear with femoral cartilage fissuring grade 2 chondromalacia

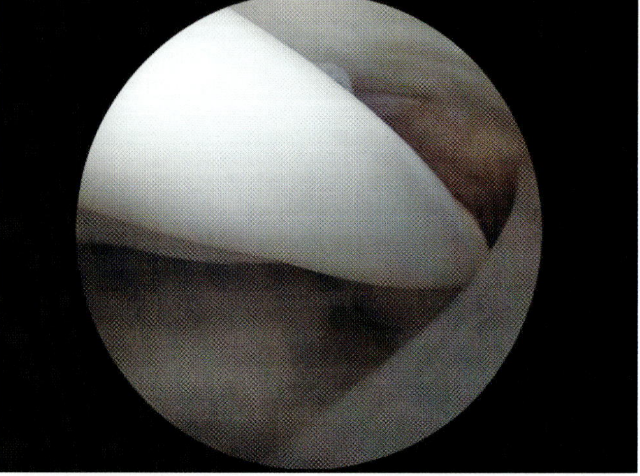

Figure 46.56 Bucket handle displaced in notch

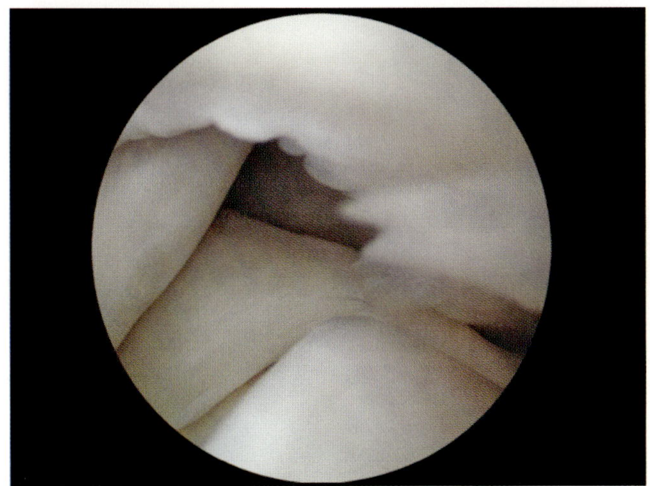

Figure 46.57 Bucket handle tear displaced

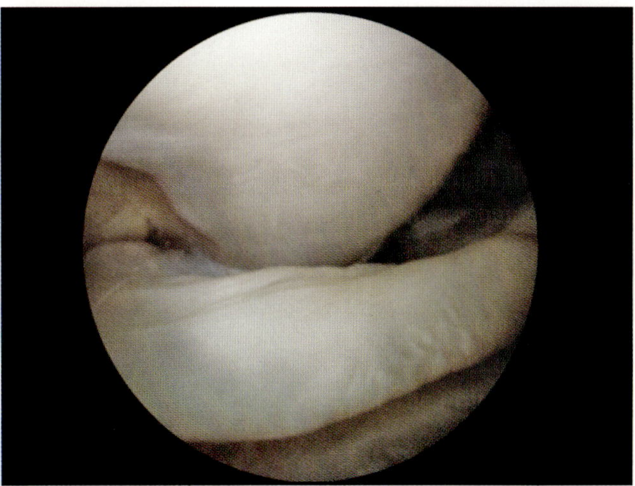

Figure 46.58 Displaced bucket handle tear

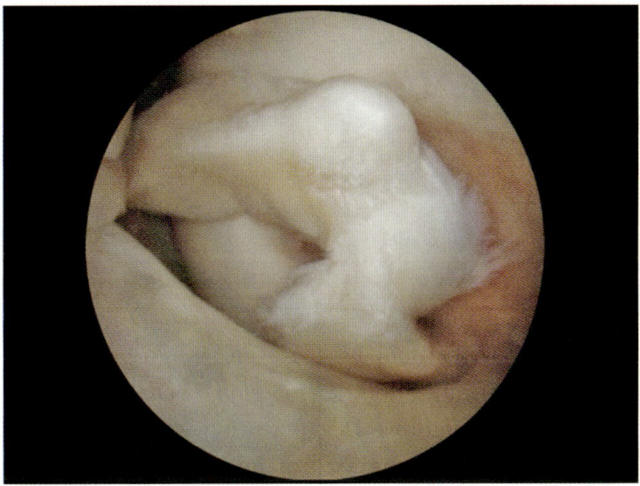

Figure 46.59 Bucket handle tear in notch

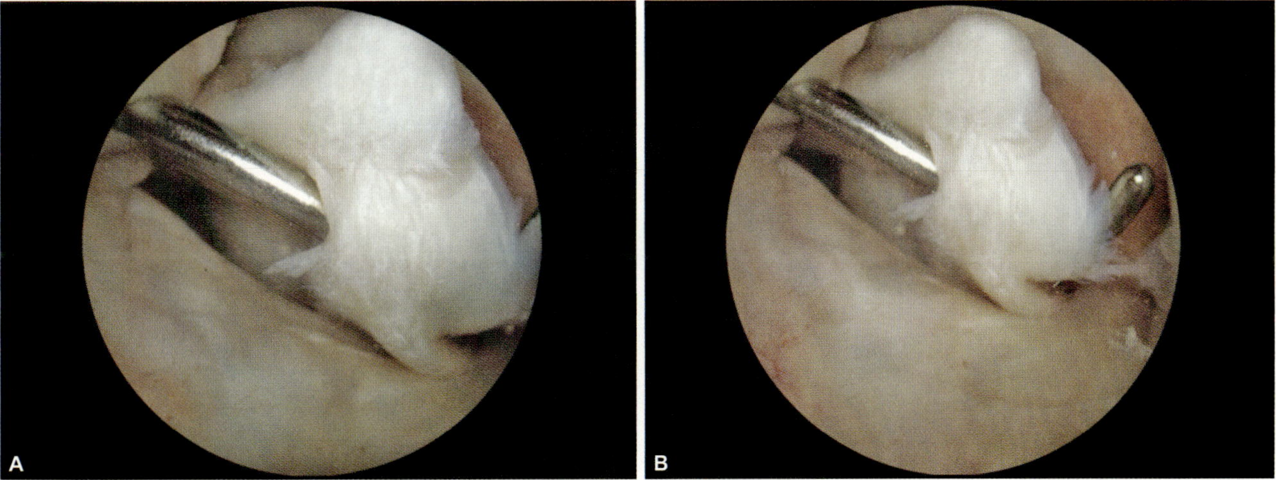

Figures 46.60A and B Probing bucket handle tear

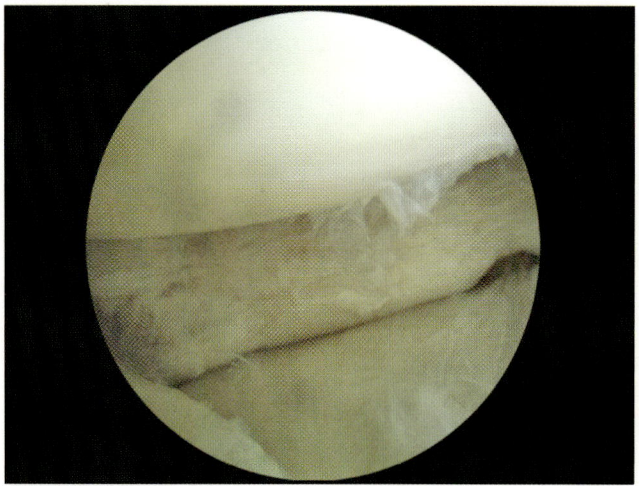

Figure 46.61 Partial meniscectomy of body and posterior horn

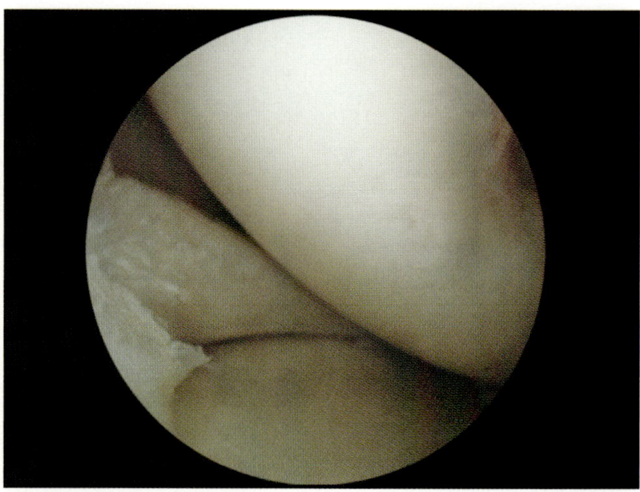

Figure 46.62 Bucket handle tear after partial medial meniscectomy

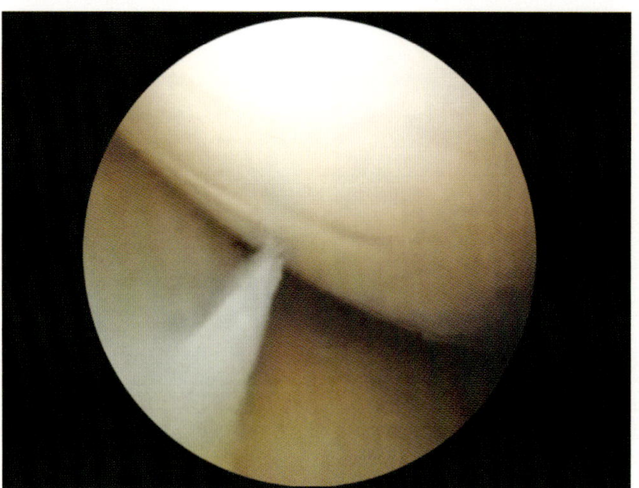

Figure 46.63 Peripheral tear

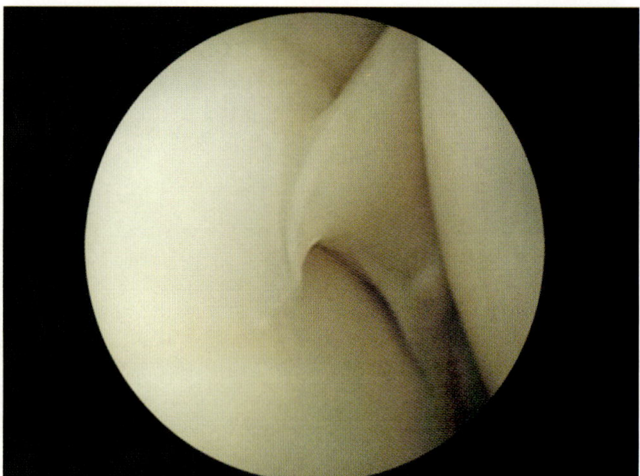

Figure 46.64 Oblique tear

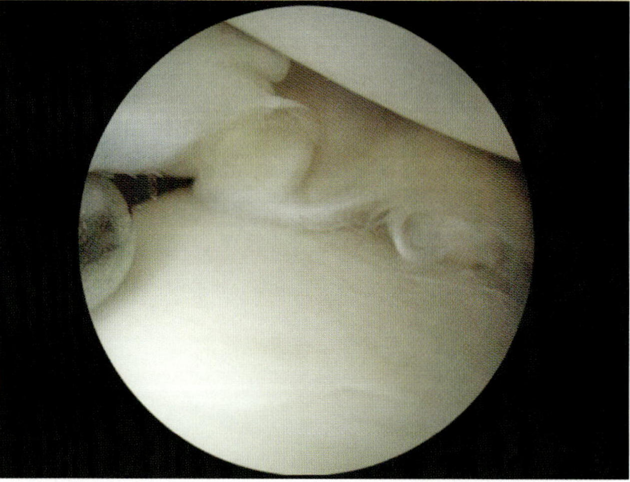

Figure 46.65 Complex tear

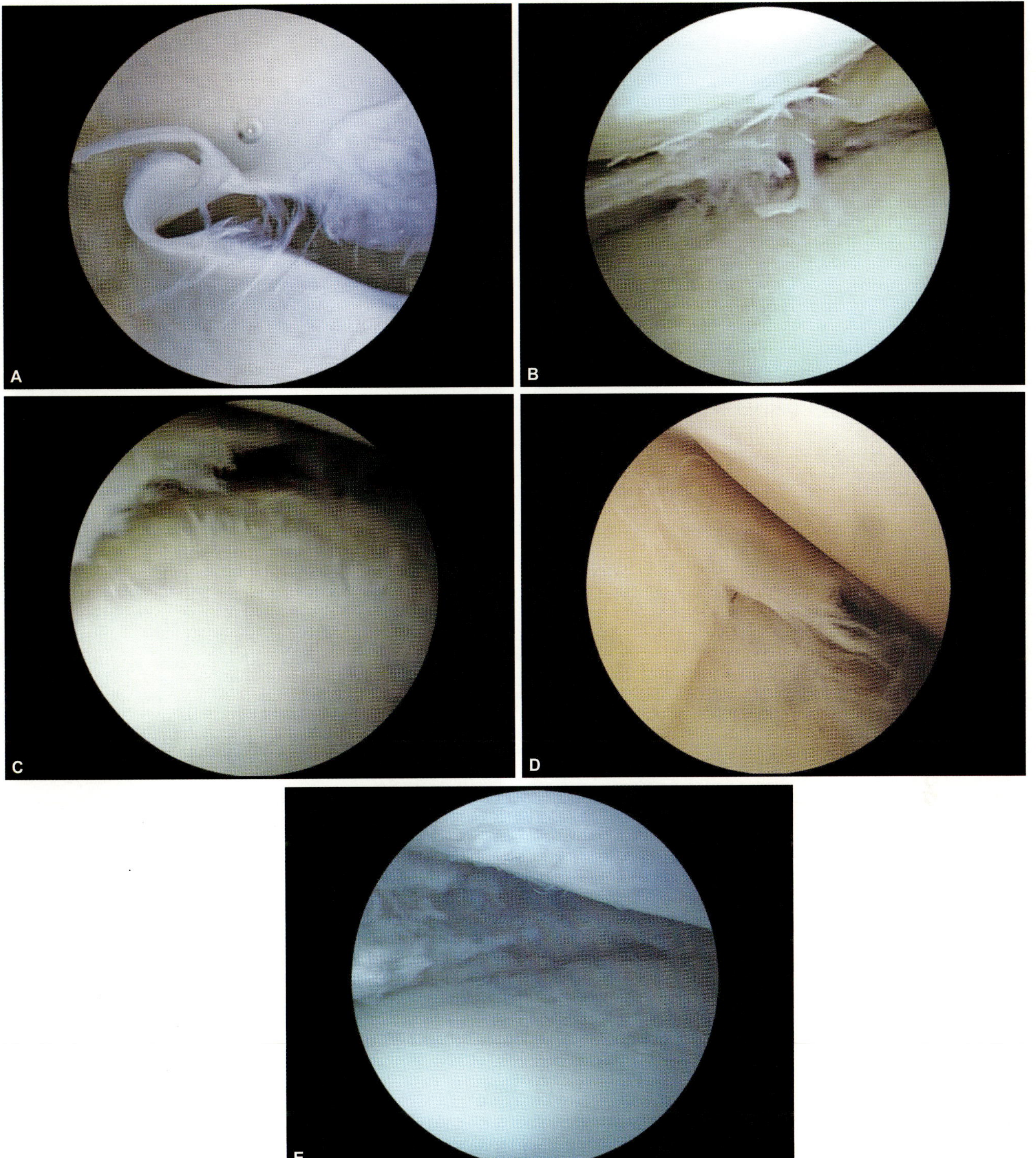

Figures 46.66A to E Degenerative tears of the meniscus

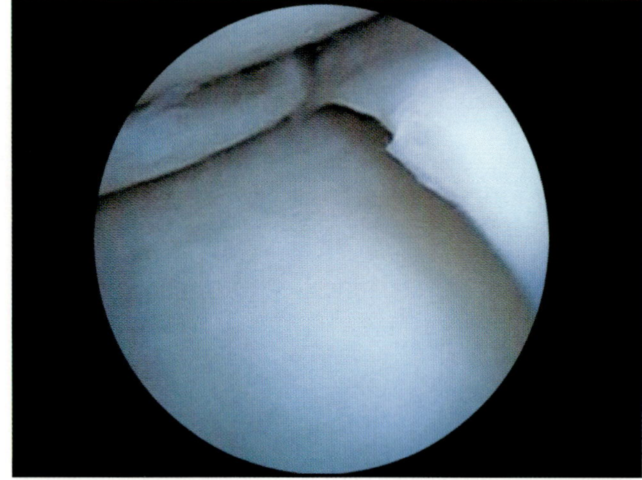

Figure 46.67 Flap tear or parrot beak tear

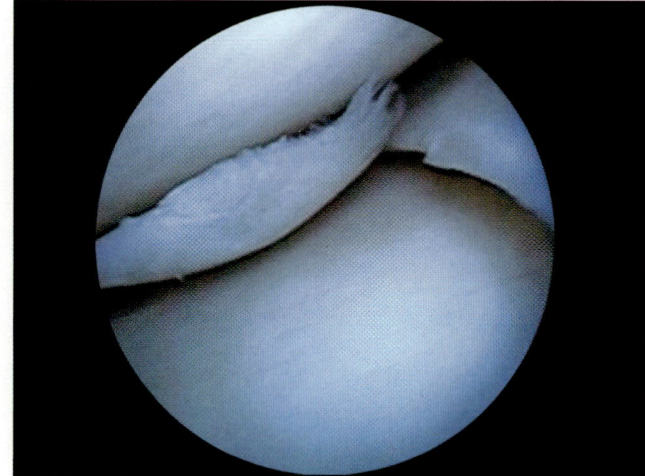

Figure 46.68 Parrot beak or Flap tear

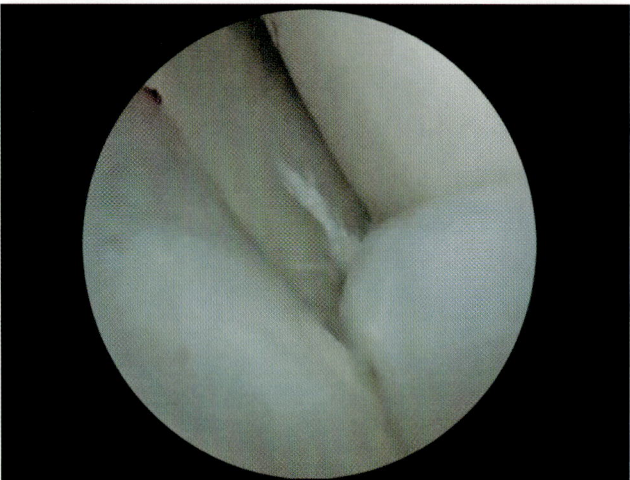

Figure 46.69 Parrot beak tear

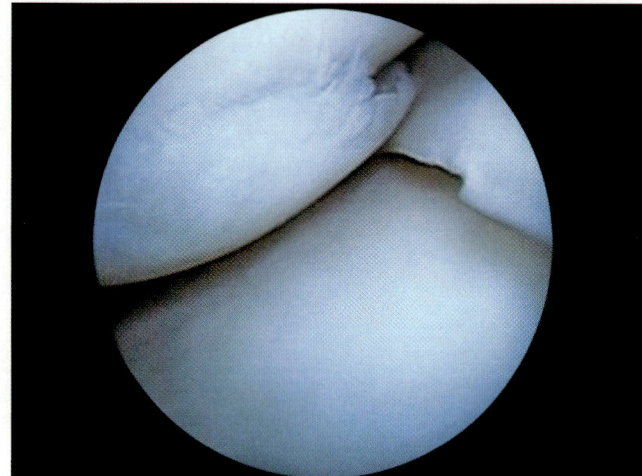

Figure 46.70 Parrot beak or Flap tear

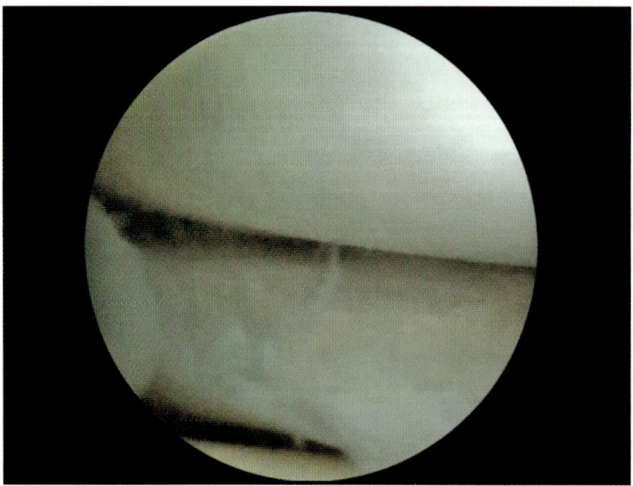

Figure 46.71 Parrot beak tear

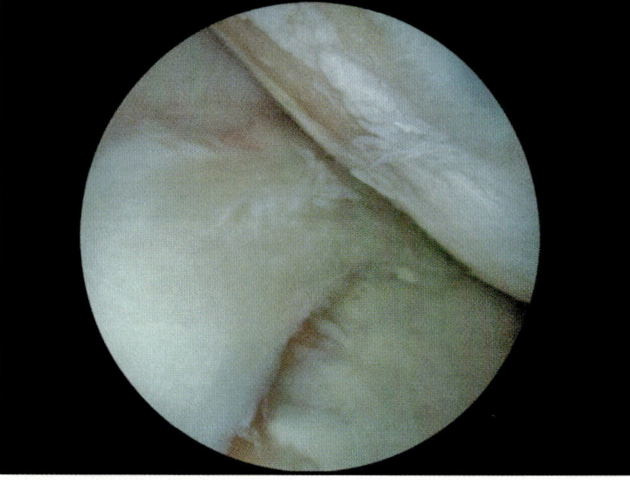

Figure 46.72 Degenerative joint disease

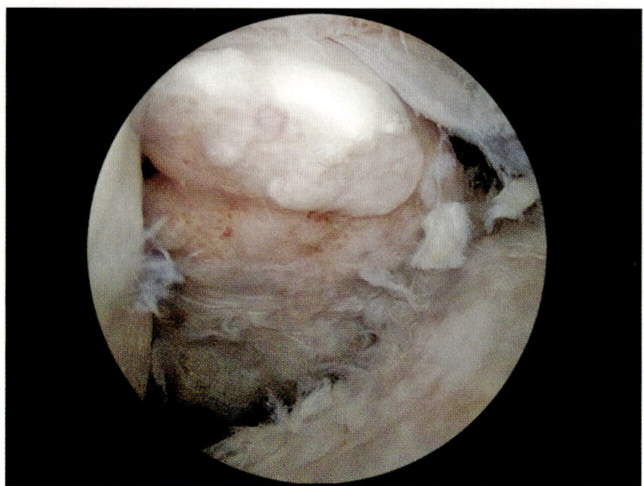

Figure 46.73 Degenerative joint disease with osteophyte in notch

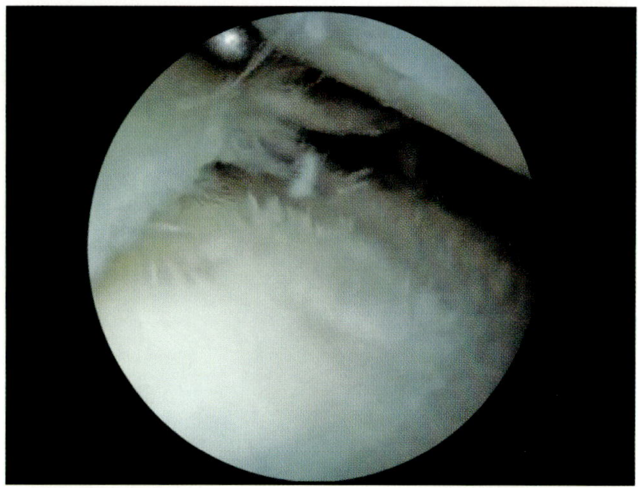

Figure 46.74 Degenerative joint disease

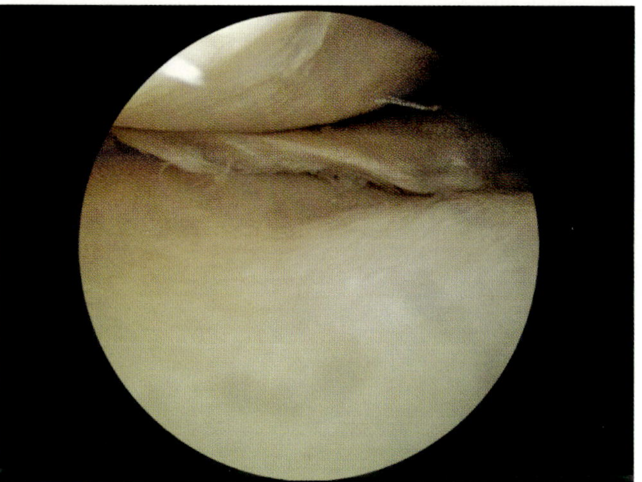

Figure 46.75 Grade 2 chondromalacia with degenerative meniscal tear

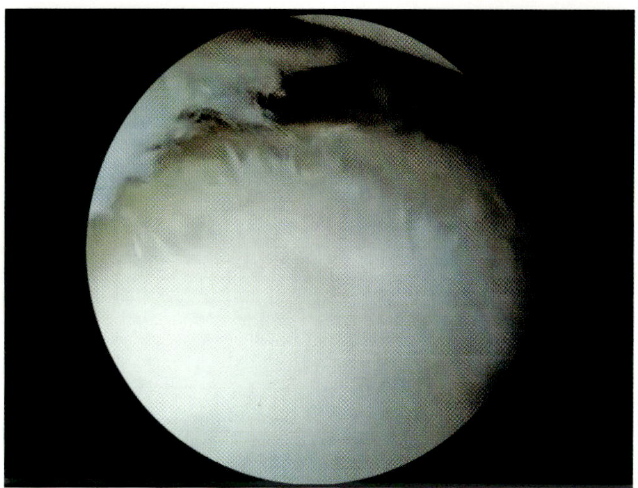

Figure 46.76 Degenerative changes in medial meniscus and tibial condyle

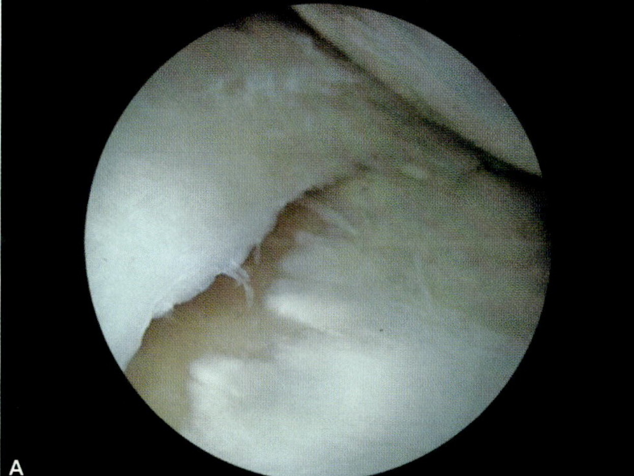

Figures 46.77A and B Degenerative joint disease

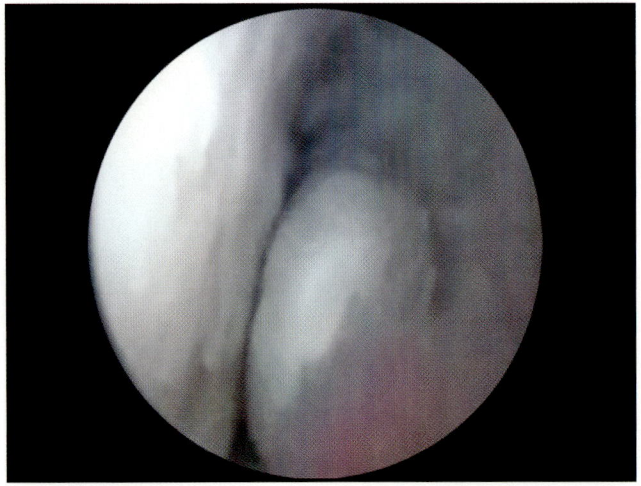

Figure 46.78 Loose body in intercondylar notch

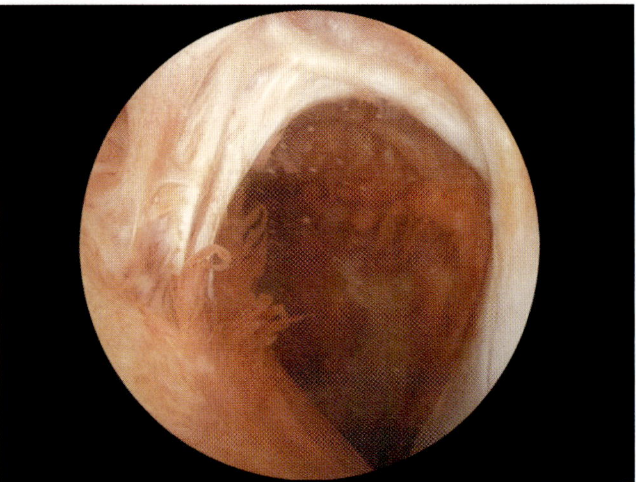

Figure 46.79 Empty wall sign in ACL deficient knee

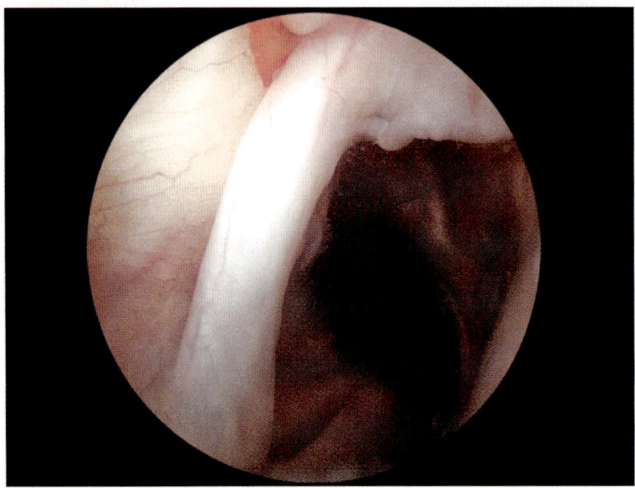

Figure 46.80 Empty wall sign in ACL deficiency

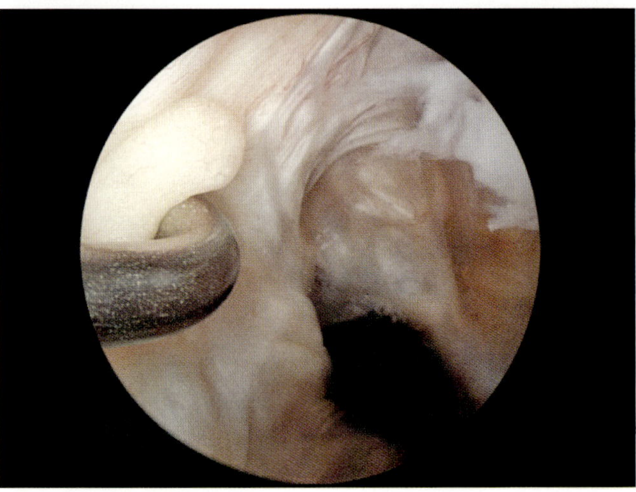

Figure 46.81 ACL deficient knee

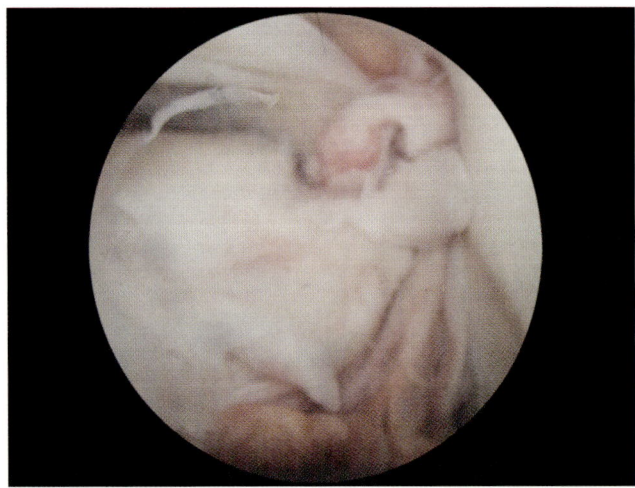

Figure 46.82 Torn ACL

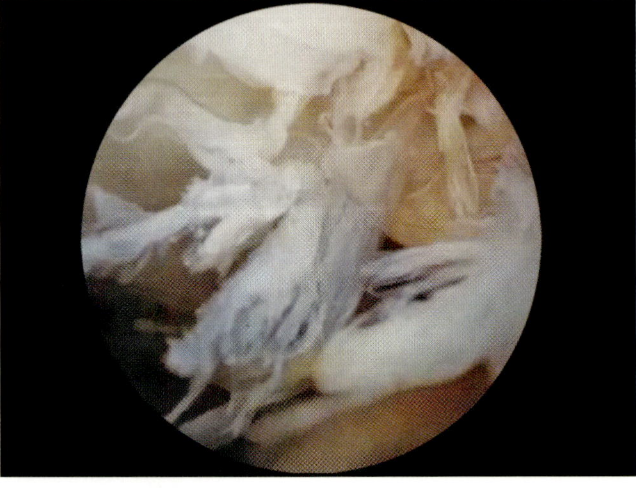

Figure 46.83 Torn femoral ACL stump

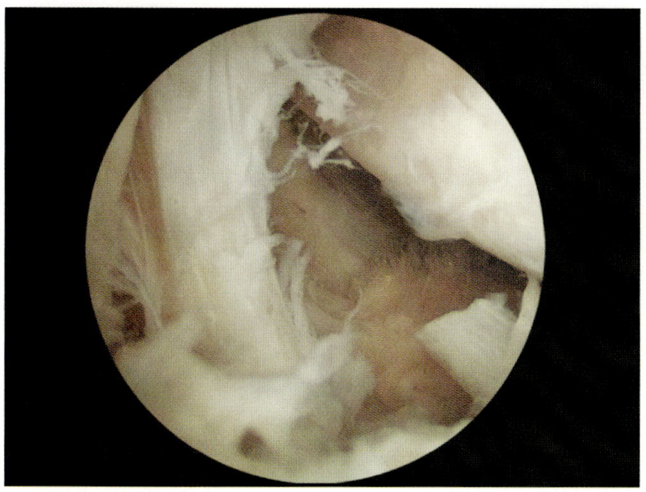

Figure 46.84 Chronic ACL with PCL tear

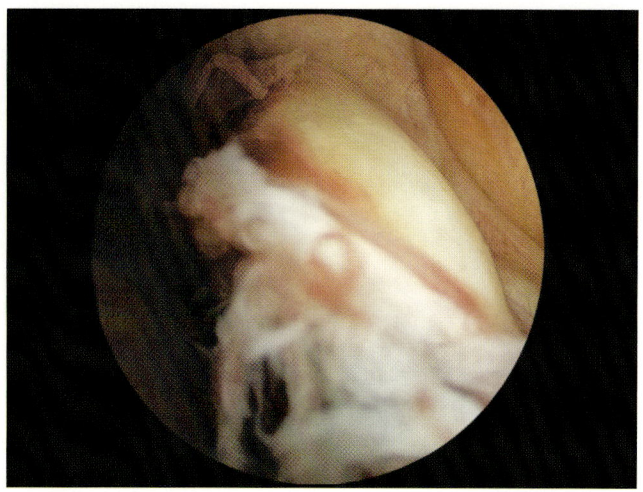

Figure 46.85 Partial ACL tear

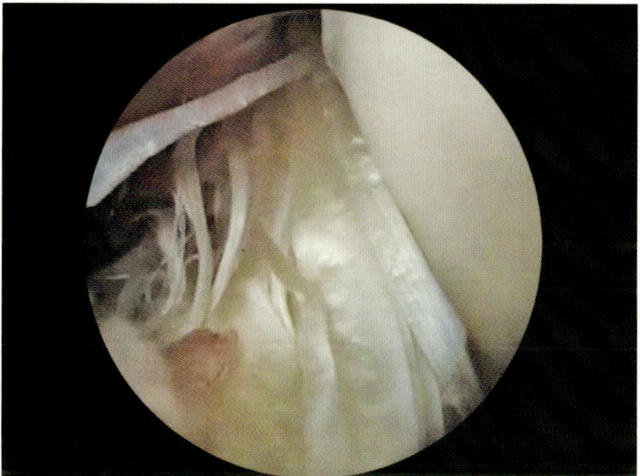

Figure 46.86 Torn reconstructed ACL

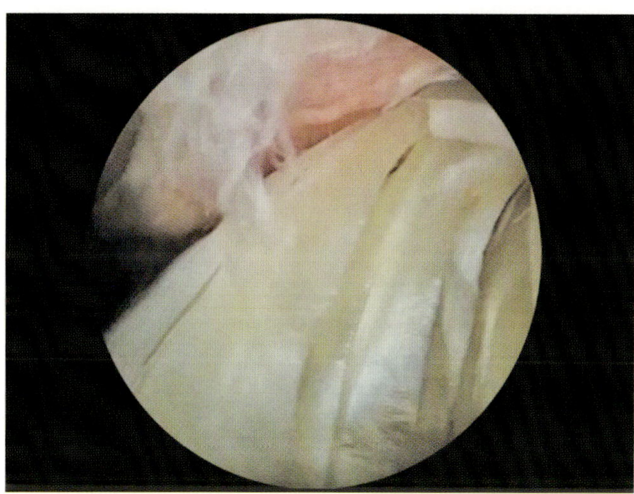

Figure 46.87 Torn reconstructed anterior cruciate ligament

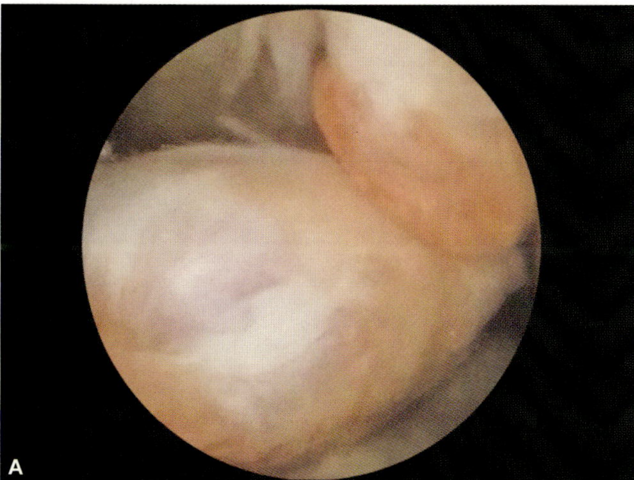

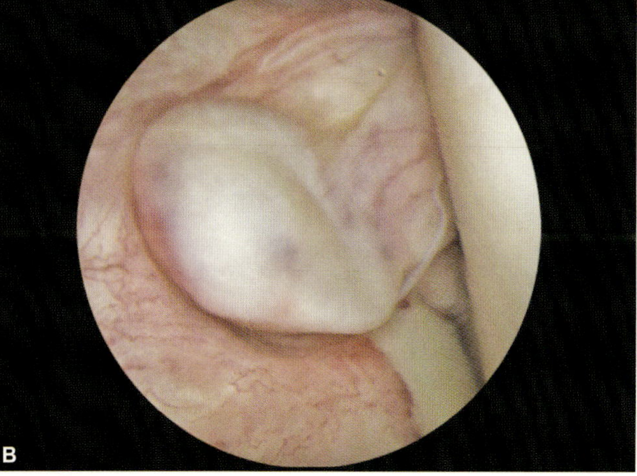

Figures 46.88 A and B

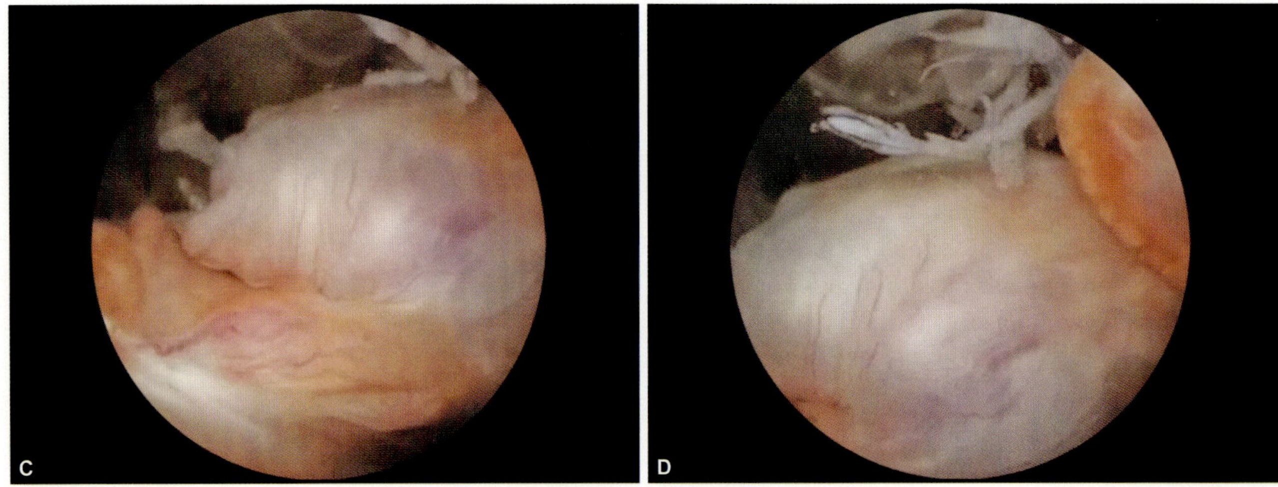

Figures 46.88 C and D

Figures 46.88 A to D Torn reconstructed ACL

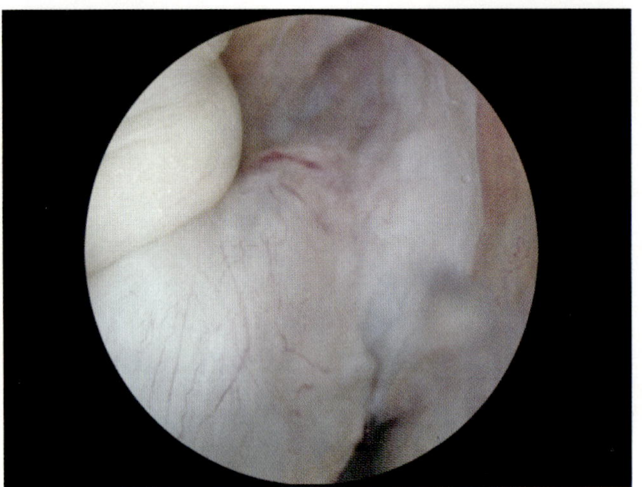

Figure 46.89 ACL attached to posterior structures lambda sign

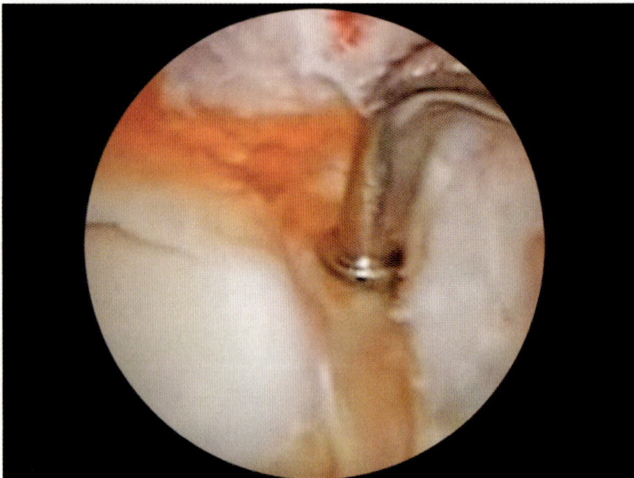

Figure 46.90 Positioning of ACL guide

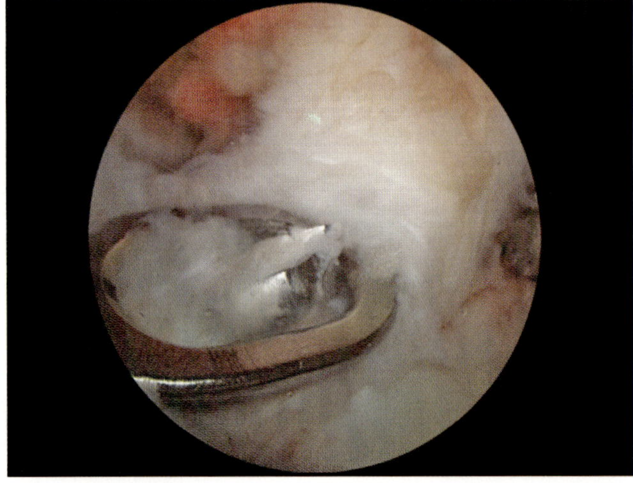

Figure 46.91 Tibial tunnel positioning in ACL stump

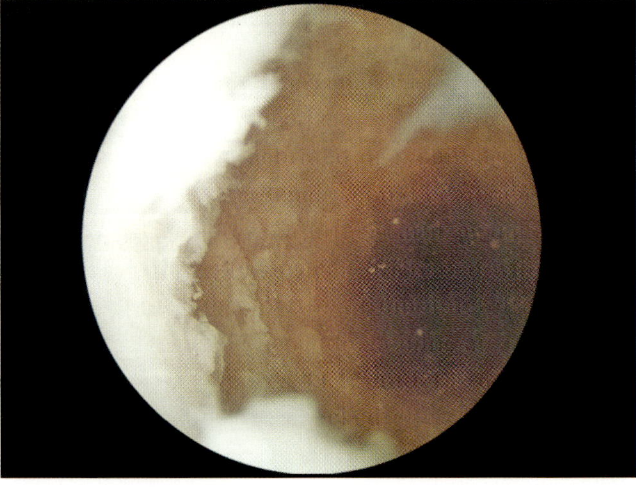

Figure 46.92 Tibial tunnel positioning

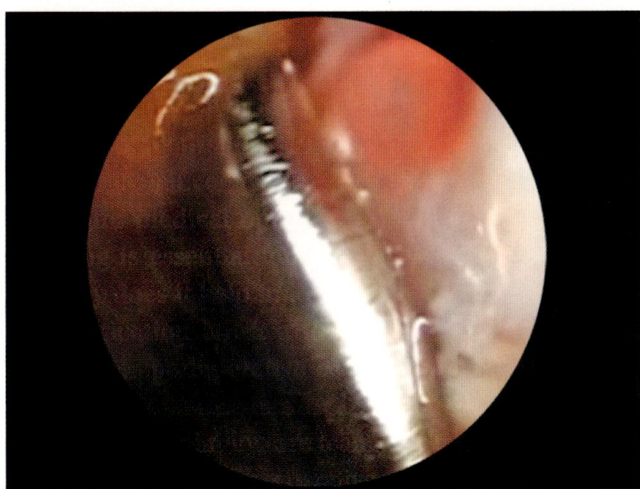

Figure 46.93 Transtibial positioning of femoral tunnel

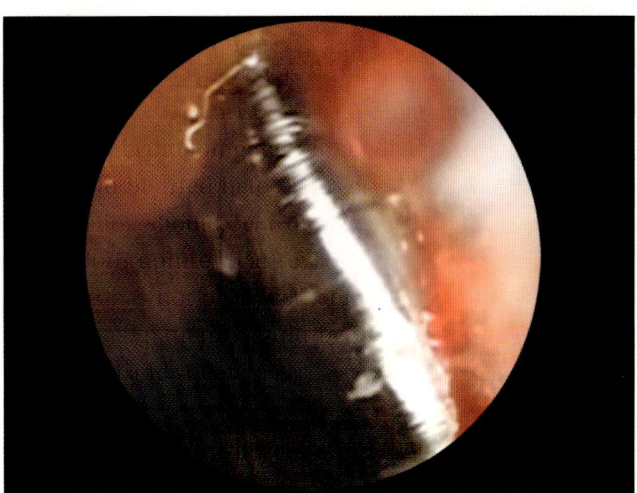

Figure 46.94 Femoral guidewire positioning in transtibial reconstruction

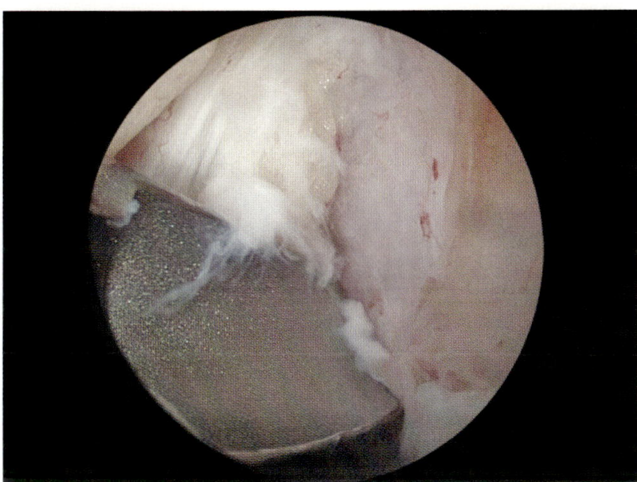

Figure 46.95 Femur zig positioning (anteromedial)

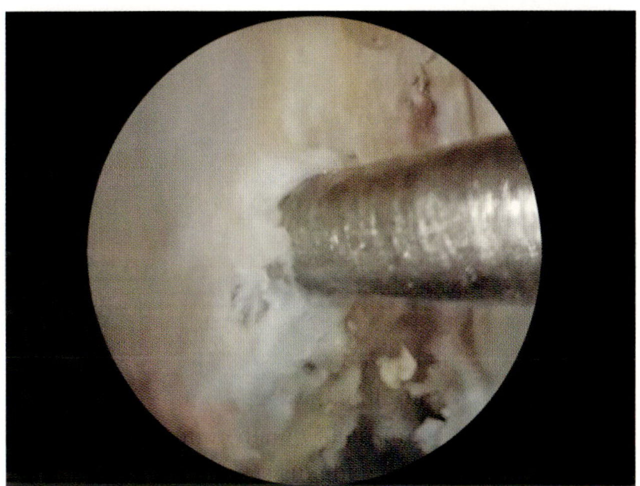

Figure 46.96 Guidewire placement for femoral tunnel

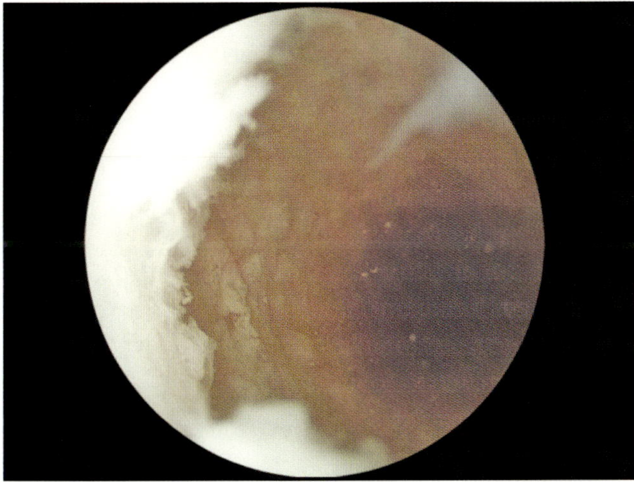

Figure 46.97 Femoral tunnel

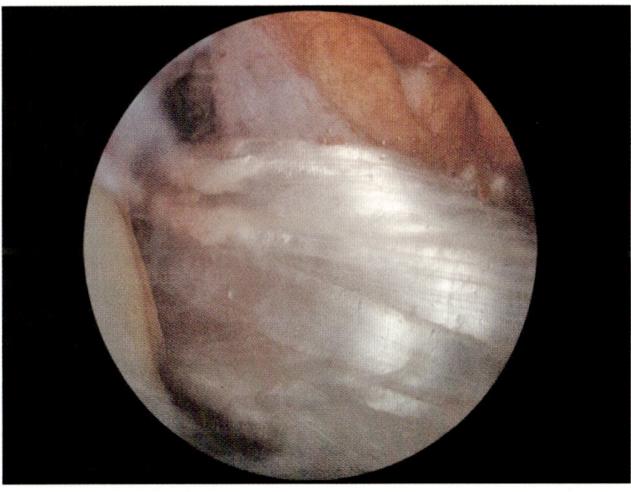

Figure 46.98 Reconstructed ACL hamstring graft

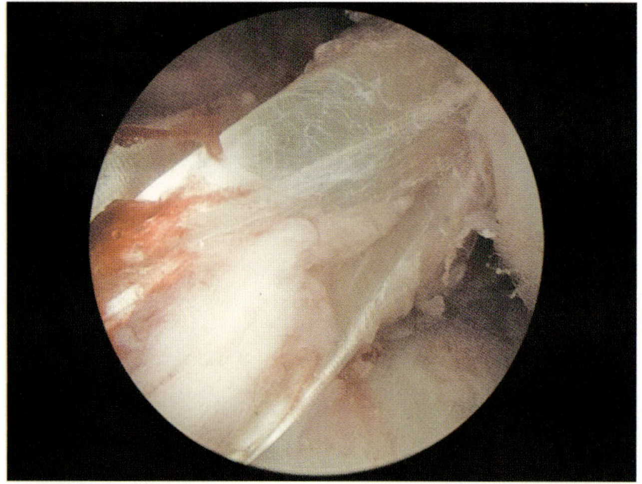

Figure 46.99 Reconstructed ACL (bone patella tendon graft)

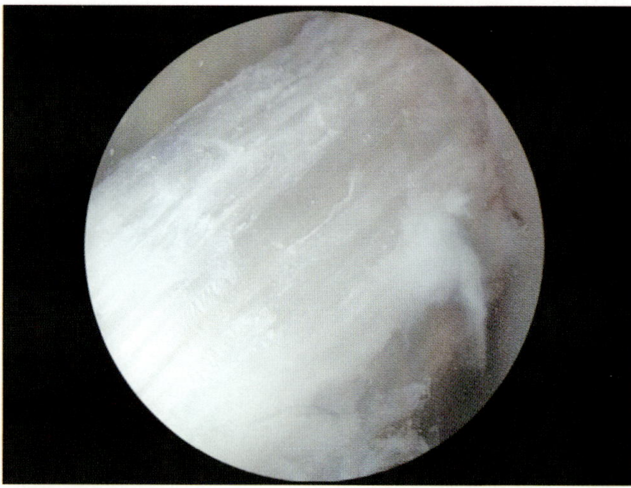

Figure 46.100 Reconstructed bone patella tendon graft as ACL

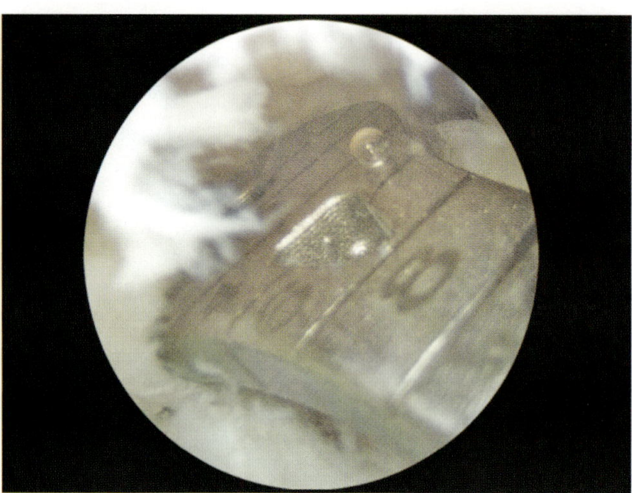

Figure 46.101 PCL positioning guide

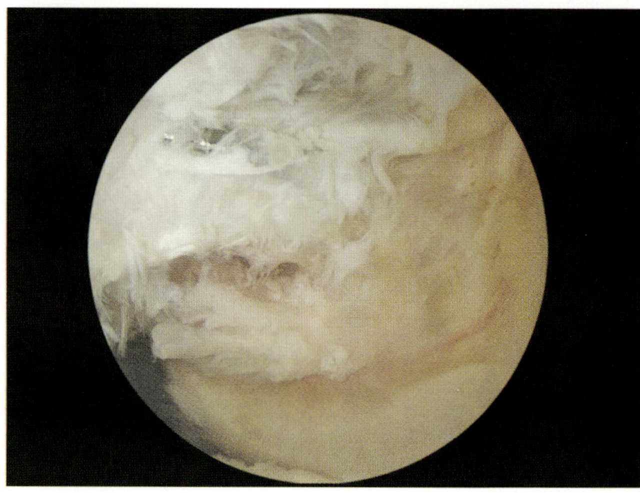

Figure 46.102 Femoral entry site for guidewire in PCL reconstruction

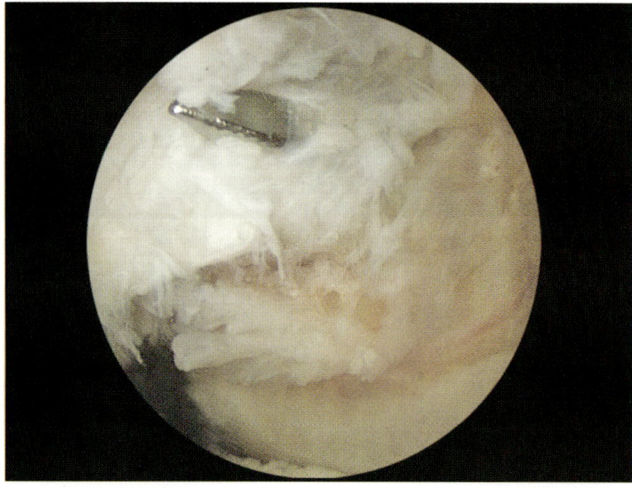

Figure 46.103 Femoral entry site for guidewire for PCL

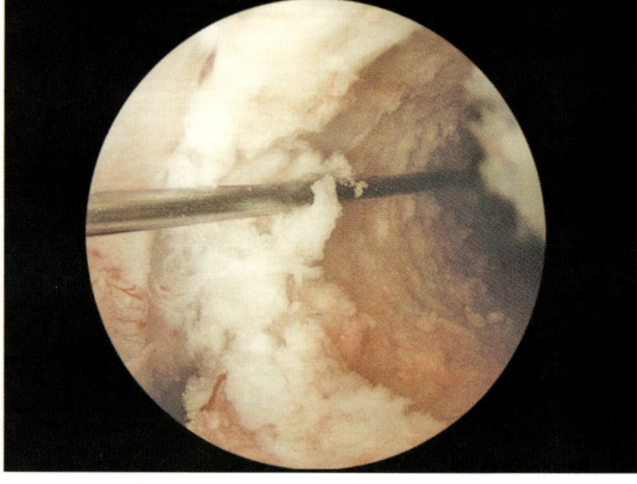

Figure 46.104 Femoral tunnel for PCL graft

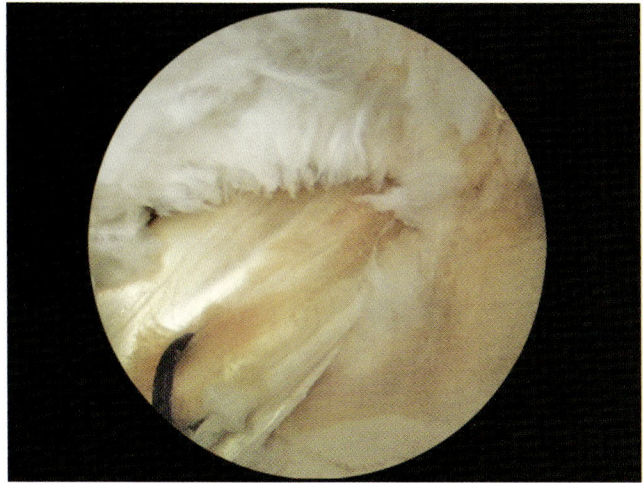

Figure 46.105 Reconstructed PCL using hamstring graft

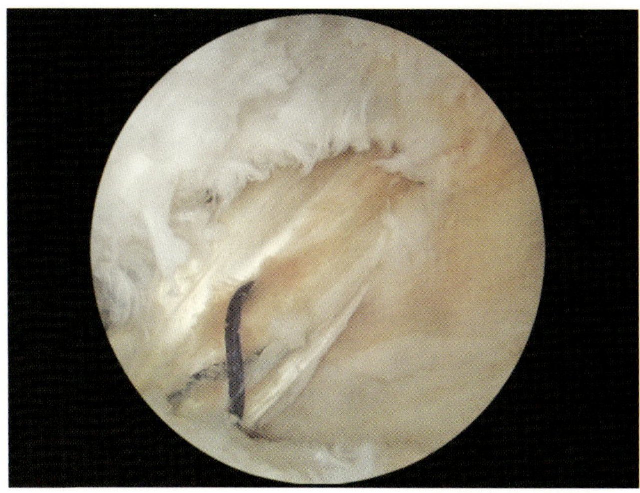

Figure 46.106 Reconstructed PCL

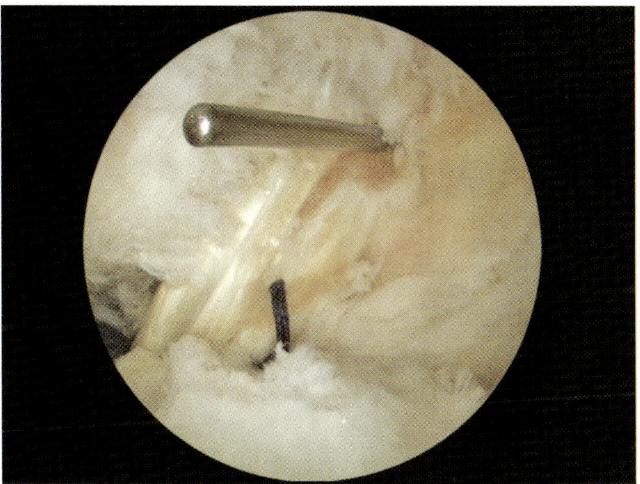

Figure 46.107 Guidewire position in PCL reconstruction for screw insertion

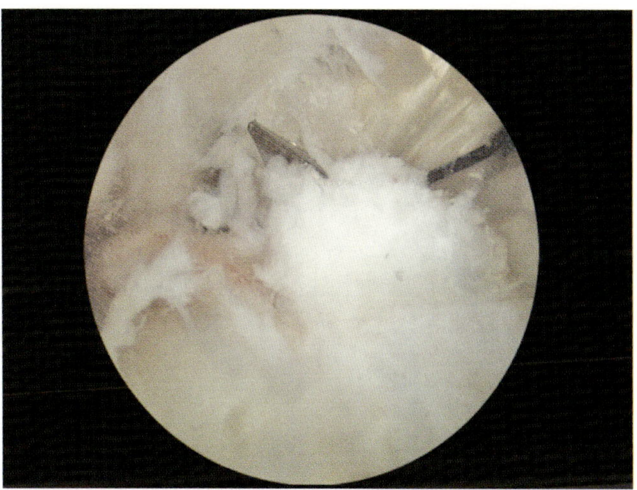

Figure 46.108 ACL guidewire position in front of reconstructed ACL

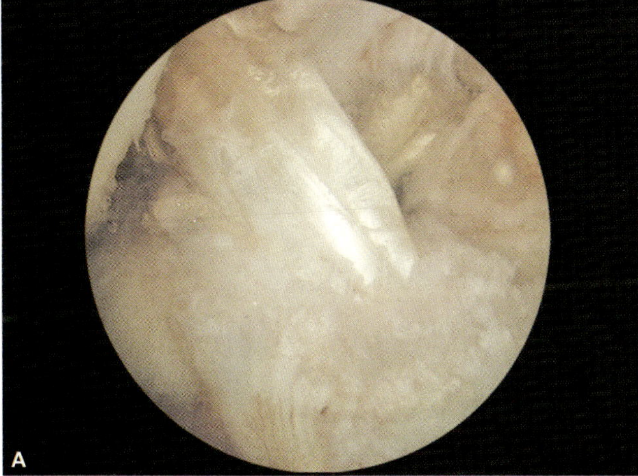

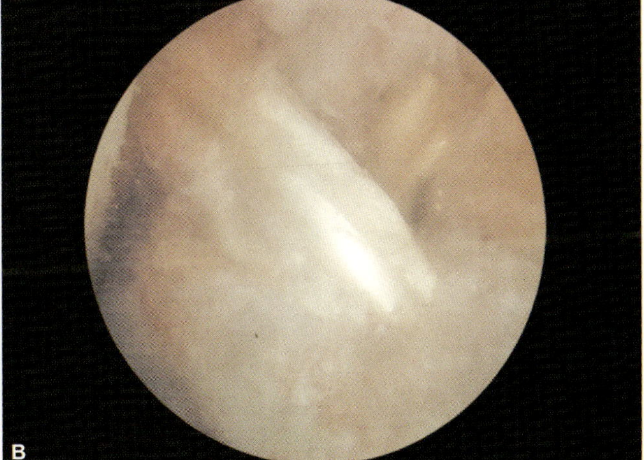

Figures 46.109A and B Reconstructed ACL and PCL

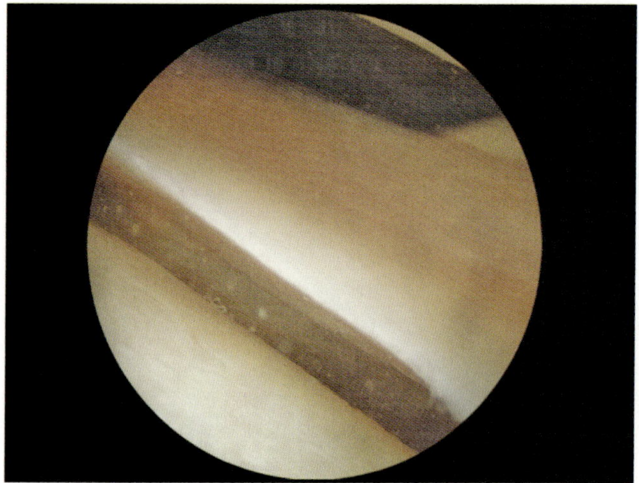

Figure 46.110 Drive through sign in posterolateral corner injuries

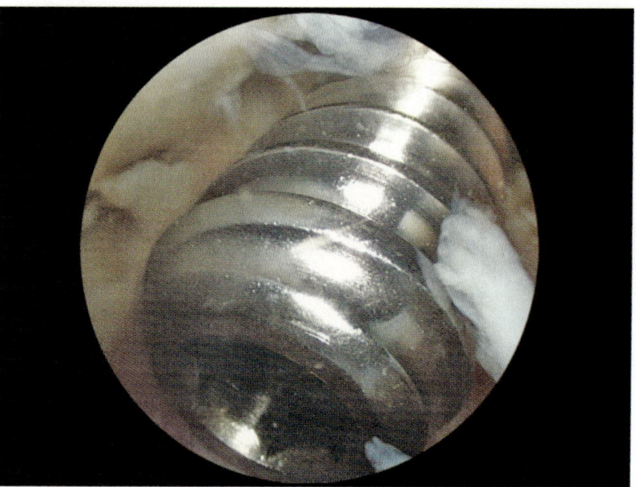

Figure 46.111 Interference screw migration into notch

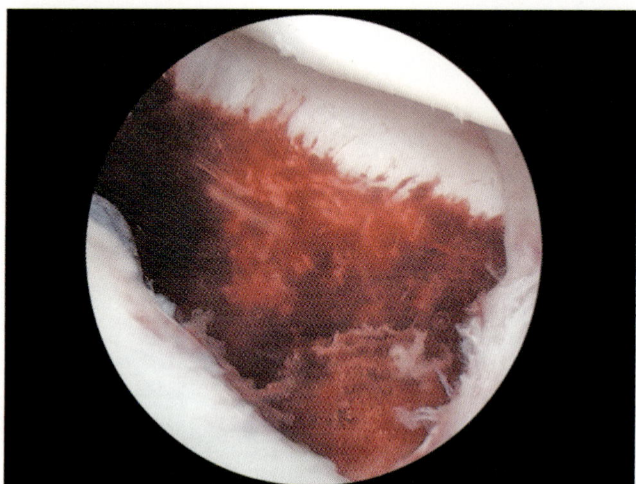

Figure 46.112 Osteochondral fracture

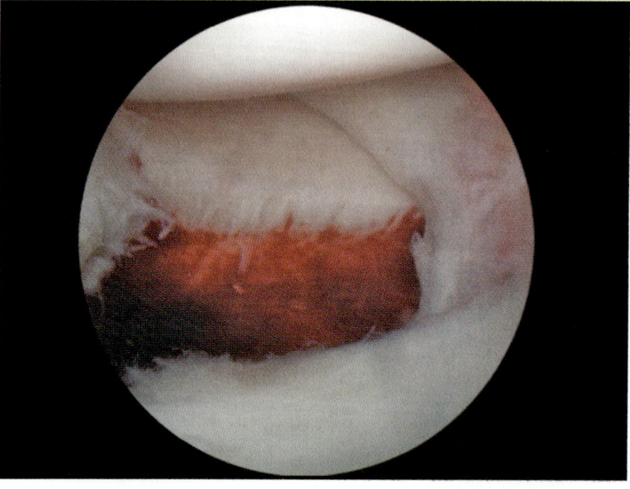

Figure 46.113 Fractured osteochondral fragment

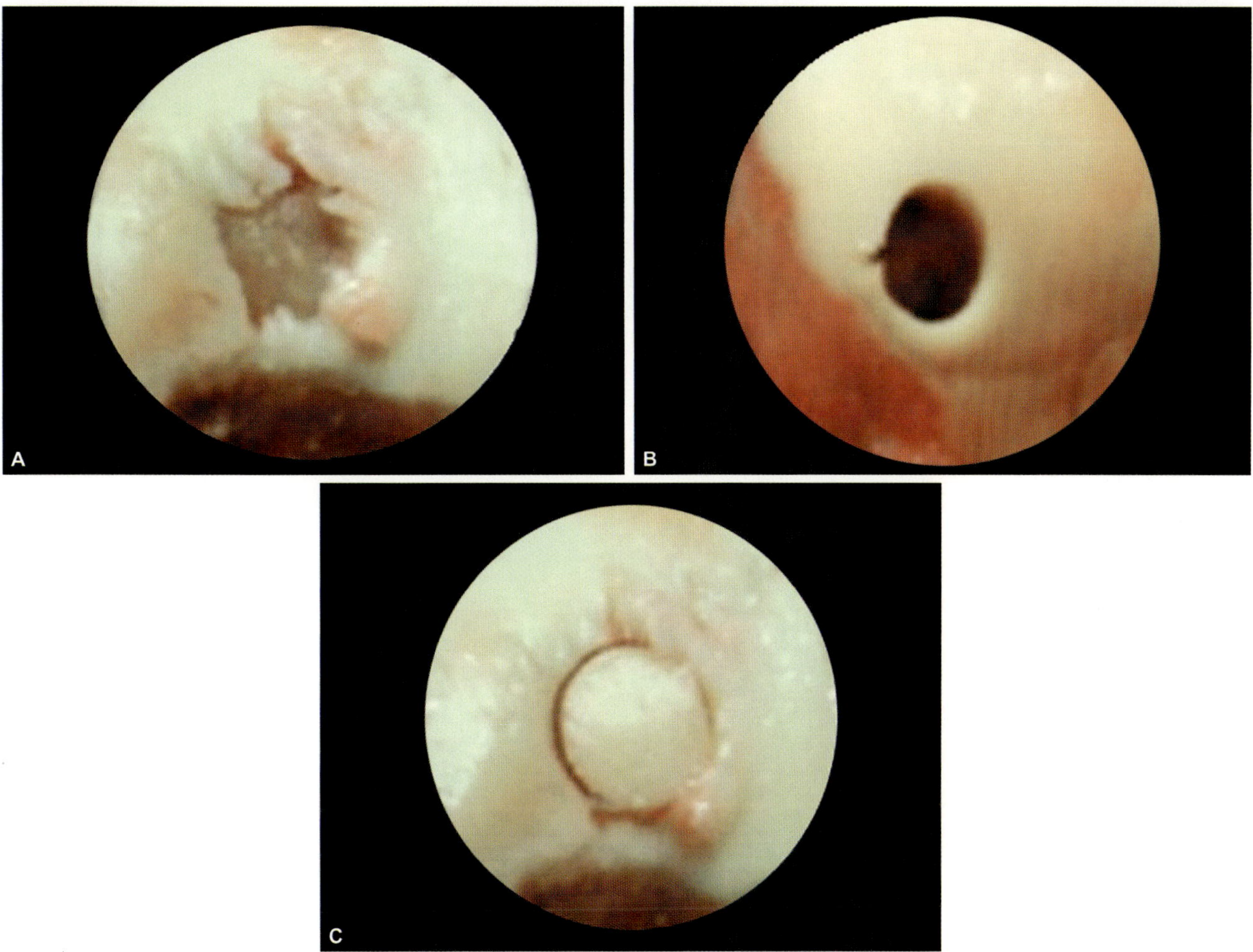

Figures 46.114A to C (A) Mosaicplasty–osteochondral defect; (B) Mosaicplasty–before graft placement; (C) Mosaicplasty–post-grafting

INDEX

Page numbers followed by *f* refer to figure and *t* refer to table

B

C

D

E

G

H

I

J

K

L

N

O

P

Q

R

S

U

V